Neinstein's

Adolescent and Young Adult Health Care

A Practical Guide

Neinstein's
Adolescent and Young Adult Health Care

A Practical Guide

Sixth Edition

EDITOR-IN-CHIEF

Lawrence S. Neinstein, MD, FACP

Professor of Pediatrics and Medicine
Executive Director
USC Engemann Student Health Center
Chief, Division of College Health
Department of Pediatrics
USC Keck School of Medicine
Assistant Provost of Student Health
and Wellness
University of Southern California
Los Angeles, California

SENIOR ASSOCIATE EDITOR

Debra K. Katzman, MD, FRCPC

Professor of Pediatrics, Division of
Adolescent Medicine, Department
of Pediatrics
The Hospital for Sick Children and
University of Toronto
Senior Associate Scientist, Research
Institute
Director, Health Science Research
Undergraduate Medical Education,
University of Toronto School of Medicine
Toronto, Ontario, Canada

ASSOCIATE EDITORS

S. Todd Callahan, MD
Catherine M. Gordon, MD, MSc
Alain Joffe, MD
Vaughn I. Rickert, PsyD

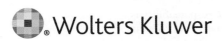
. Wolters Kluwer

Philadelphia • Baltimore • New York • London
Buenos Aires • Hong Kong • Sydney • Tokyo

Acquisitions Editor: Jamie M. Elfrank
Product Development Editor: Ashley Fischer
Editorial Assistant: Brian Convery
Marketing Manager: Stephanie Kindlick
Production Project Manager: Priscilla Crater
Design Coordinator: Teresa Mallon
Manufacturing Coordinator: Beth Welsh
Prepress Vendor: S4Carlisle Publishing Services

6th edition

Library of Congress Cataloging-in-Publication Data
Names: Neinstein, Lawrence S., editor. | Katzman, Debra, editor. | Callahan, Todd.
Title: Neinstein's adolescent and young adult health care: a practical guide / editor-in-chief, Lawrence S. Neinstein, MD, FACP; senior associate editor, Debra K. Katzman; associate editors, Todd Callahan [and three others].
 Other titles: Adolescent health care. | Adolescent and young adult health care
 Description: 6th edition. | Philadelphia, PA : Wolters Kluwer, [2016] | Includes bibliographical references.
 Identifiers: LCCN 2015034565 | ISBN 9781451190083
 Subjects: LCSH: Adolescent medicine.
 Classification: LCC RJ550 .N45 2016 | DDC 616.00835—dc23 LC record available at http://lccn.loc.gov/2015034565

Contributors

Matthew C. Aalsma, PhD
Associate Professor
Department of Pediatrics
Indiana University School of Medicine
Indianapolis, Indiana

William P. Adelman MD, FAAP
Associate Professor
Department of Pediatrics
F. Edward Hebert School of Medicine
Uniformed Services
University of the Health Sciences
Chair
Division of Adolescent Medicine
Walter Reed National Military Medical Center
Bethesda, Maryland

Mark E. Alexander, MD
Assistant Professor of Pediatrics
Department of Pediatrics
Harvard Medical School
Co-Director of Exercise Physiology and Arrhythmia Service
Department of Cardiology
Boston Children's Hospital
Boston, Massachusetts

Martin M. Anderson, MD, MPH
Director of Adolescent Medicine
Professor of Clinical Pediatrics
Mattel Children's Hospital
UCLA Department of Pediatrics
Los Angeles, California

Colette L. Auerswald, MD, MS, FSAHM
Associate Professor
Community Health and Human Development
Director, MS Program
University of California–University of California
    San Francisco Joint Medical Program
University of California
Berkeley, California

Gregory N. Barnes, MD, PhD
Spafford Ackerly Chair in Child and Adolescent Psychiatry
Director
University of Louisville Autism Center
Associate Professor of Neurology and Pediatrics
Department of Neurology University of Louisville
Kosair Children's Hospital
Louisville, Kentucky

Romina L. Barral, MD
Assistant Professor
Department of Pediatrics
University of Missouri - Kansas City
Faculty
Division of Adolescent Medicine
Children's Mercy Hospital and Clinics
Kansas City, Missouri

Michael A. Beasley, MD
Instructor of Orthopedics
Harvard Medical School
Staff Physician
Division of Sports Medicine
Boston Children's Hospital
Boston, Massachusetts

Madeline Beauregard, BA
Research Study Assistant II
Primary Care at Longwood
Division of General Pediatrics
Boston Children's Hospital
Boston, Massachusetts

Meera S. Beharry, MD, FAAP
Regional Vice-President (North America)
International Association for Adolescent Health
Assistant Professor
Department of Pediatrics
Texas A & M Health Science Center
Section Chief, Adolescent Medicine
Department of Pediatrics
McLane Children's Scott & White Health Hospital
Temple, Texas

Marvin E. Belzer, MD
Professor of Clinical Pediatrics
Department of Pediatrics
University of Southern California
Director
Division of Adolescent and Young Adult Medicine
Department of Pediatrics
Children's Hospital Los Angeles
Los Angeles, California

William R. Betts, PhD
Assistant Professor
Department of Pediatrics
University of Colorado School of Medicine
Denver, Colorado
Director for Behavioral Health
The Kempe Center-Children's Hospital Colorado
Aurora, Colorado

Candice Biernesser, LSW, MPH
Research Program Administrator
Department of Child and Adolescent Psychiatry
Western Psychiatric Institute and Clinic
Graduate Student Researcher
Department of Behavior and Community Health Sciences
University of Pittsburgh
Pittsburgh, Pennsylvania

Margaret J. Blythe, MD, FAAP, FSAHM
Professor Emeritus of Pediatrics
Department of Pediatrics
Indiana University School of Medicine
Indianapolis, Indiana

Joshua S. Borus, MD, MPH
Instructor in Pediatrics
Harvard Medical School
Co-Director of Medical Student and Resident Training
Division of Adolescent/Young Adult Medicine
Boston Children's Hospital
Boston, Massachusetts

Paul Boxer, PhD
Associate Professor
Department of Psychology
Senior Fellow
School of Criminal Justice
Rutgers University
Director
Center on Youth Violence and Juvenile Justice
Newark, New Jersey

Terrill D. Bravender, MD, MPH
Professor of Pediatrics and Psychiatry
Ohio State University College of Medicine
Adolescent Medicine Physician
Nationwide Children's Hospital
Columbus, Ohio

Paula K. Braverman, MD
Professor of Pediatrics
Department of Pediatrics
Division of Adolescent and Transition Medicine
Children's Hospital Medical Center
University of Cincinnati College of Medicine
Cincinnati, Ohio

David A. Brent, MD
Academic Chief
Child and Adolescent Psychiatry
Professor of Psychiatry, Epidemiology, and Pediatrics
Endowed Chair, Suicide Studies
Director
Services for Teens at Risk Western Psychiatric Institute and
   Clinic
Pittsburgh, Pennsylvania

Cora Collette Breuner, MD, MPH
Professor of Pediatrics and Adolescent Medicine
Department of Pediatrics
University of Washington
Professor of Pediatrics and Adolescent Medicine
Adjunct Professor of Orthopedics/Sports Medicine
Seattle Children's Hospital
Seattle, Washington

Gale R. Burstein, MD, MPH
Clinical Professor of Pediatrics
State University of New York at Buffalo School of Medicine and
   Biomedical Sciences
Commissioner
Erie County Department of Health
Buffalo, New York

S. Todd Callahan, MD, MPH
Associate Professor
Division of Adolescent and Young Adult Health
Department of Pediatrics
Monroe Carell Jr. Children's Hospital, Vanderbilt
Vanderbilt University Medical Center
Nashville, Tennessee

Jeremi M. Carswell, MD
Assistant in Medicine
Department of Pediatrics
Harvard Medical School
Instructor of Medicine
Department of Medicine
Boston Children's Hospital
Boston, Massachusetts

Mariam R. Chacko, MD
Professor
Department of Pediatrics
Section of Adolescent Medicine & Sports Medicine
Baylor College of Medicine
Texas Children's Hospital
Houston, Texas

J. Aimée Coulombe, PhD
Research Associate
Better Nights, Better Days Pediatric Sleep Team
Department of Psychology and Neuroscience
Dalhousie University
Halifax, Nova Scotia, Canada

Joanne E. Cox, MD
Associate Professor
Department of Pediatrics
Harvard Medical School
Associate Chief
Division of General Pediatrics
Boston Children's Hospital
Boston, Massachusetts

Nancy A. Crimmins, MD
Assistant Professor of Pediatrics
Department of Pediatrics
University of Cincinnati College of Medicine
Division of Endocrinology
Cincinnati Children's Hospital Medical Center
Cincinnati, Ohio

Lawrence J. D'Angelo, MD, MPH
Professor
Department of Pediatrics, Medicine, and Epidemiology
George Washington University
Chief
Division of Adolescent and Young Adult Medicine
Children's National Health System
Washington, District of Columbia

Anthony H. Dekker, DO
Director of Addiction Medicine
United States Department of Defense
Fort Belvoir, Virginia

Diana Deister, MD
Assistant in Medicine
Developmental Medicine Center
Boston Children's Hospital
Boston, Massachusetts

Amy D. Divasta, MD, MMSc
Assistant Professor
Department of Pediatrics
Harvard Medical School
Attending Physician
Division of Adolescent Medicine
Division of Pediatric Gynecology
Boston Children's Hospital
Boston, Massachusetts

Wendi G. Ehrman, MD
Associate Professor of Pediatrics
Department of Pediatrics
Medical College of Wisconsin
Milwaukee, Wisconsin
Consultant Staff
Department of Pediatrics
Children's Hospital of Wisconsin
Milwaukee, Wisconsin

Abigail English, JD
Director
Center for Adolescent Health and the Law
Chapel Hill, North Carolina

Dillon J. Etter
Section of Adolescent Medicine Indiana
    University School of Medicine
Indianapolis, Indiana

Amy Fleischman, MD, MMSc
Assistant Professor
Division of Endocrinology
Boston Children's Hospital
Boston, Massachusetts

Joseph T. Flynn, MD, MS
Dr. Robert O. Hickman Endowed Chair in Pediatric Nephrology
Professor of Pediatrics
University of Washington School of Medicine
Chief
Division of Nephrology
Seattle Children's Hospital
Seattle, Washington

Michelle Forcier, MD, MPH
Associate Professor of Pediatrics
Clinical Department of Pediatrics
Division of Adolescent Medicine
The Warren Alpert School of Medicine
Brown University
Providence, Rhode Island

J. Dennis Fortenberry, MD, MS
Professor of Pediatrics and Medicine
Section of Adolescent Medicine
Department of Pediatrics
Indiana University School of Medicine
Indianapolis, Indiana

Lynette A. Gillis, MD
Assistant Professor
Department of Pediatrics
Vanderbilt University
Nashville, Tennessee

Melanie A. Gold, DO, DABMA, MQT
Professor
Department of Pediatrics
Division of Child and Adolescent Health
Section of Adolescent Medicine
Columbia University Medical Center
Heilbrunn
Department of Population & Family Health
Columbia University Mailman School of Public Health
Medical Director
School Based Health Centers
New York Presbyterian Hospital
New York, New York

Neville H. Golden, MD
The Marron and Mary Elizabeth Kendrick Professor of Pediatrics
Department of Pediatrics
Stanford University School of Medicine
Chief
Division of Adolescent Medicine
Lucile Packard Children's Hospital
Stanford, California

Rachel Gonzales-Castaneda, PhD, MPH
Associate Professor
Department of Psychology
Azusa Pacific University
Azusa, California
Associate Research Psychologist
Semel Institute/Geffen School of Medicine
University of California, Los Angeles, Integrated
    Substance Abuse Programs
Los Angeles, California

Holly C. Gooding, MD, MSc
Instructor
Department of Pediatrics
Harvard Medical School
Division of Adolescent/Young Adult Medicine
Boston Children's Hospital
Boston, Massachusetts

Catherine M. Gordon, MD, MSc
Professor
Department of Pediatrics
University of Cincinnati College of Medicine
Director
Division of Adolescent and Transition Medicine
Cincinnati Children's Hospital Medical Center
Cincinnati, Ohio

Kevin M. Gray, MD
Associate Professor
Department of Psychiatry and Behavioral Sciences
Medical University of South Carolina
Charleston, South Carolina

Rebecca Gudeman, JD, MPA
Senior Attorney
National Center for Youth Law
Oakland, California

Tamara S. Hannon, MD, MS
Associate Professor
Department of Pediatrics
Indiana University School of Medicine
Director
Riley Diabetes Program
Riley Hospital for Children at Indiana University Health
Indianapolis, Indiana

Dougal S. Hargreaves, MBBS, MSc
Honarary Research Associate
University College London (UCL) Institute of Child Health
London, United Kingdom

Scott B. Harpin, PhD, MPH, RN
Assistant Professor
University of Colorado, College of Nursing
Aurora, Colorado

Erin N. Harrop, MSW
School of Social Work
University of Washington
Social Worker
Adolescent Medicine Clinic
Seattle Children's Hospital
Seattle, Washington

Kimber L. Hendrix, ABD
Doctoral Candidate
Purdue University
West Lafayette, Indiana

Devon J. Hensel, PhD, MS
Assistant Research Professor
Department of Pediatrics
Section of Adolescent Medicine
Indiana University School of Medicine
Assistant Professor
Department of Sociology
Indiana University—Purdue University Indianapolis
Assistant Professor
Department of Epidemiology
Fairbanks School of Public Health
Indianapolis, Indiana

Todd I. Herrenkohl, PhD
Co-Director
3DL Partnership
Professor
School of Social Work
University of Washington
Seattle, Washington

Paula J. Adams Hillard, MD
Professor
Department of Obstetrics and Gynecology
Stanford University School of Medicine
Director of Pediatric and Adolescent Gynecology
Lucile Packard Stanford Children's Hospital
Stanford, California

Nicole Hubner, MD, FRCSC
Fellow
Section of Pediatric and Adolescent Gynaecology
Department of Endocrinology
The Hospital for Sick Children
Toronto, Ontario, Canada

Jeffrey W. Hutchinson, MD
Assistant Professor
Department of Pediatrics
Associate Dean of Clinical Affairs and Chief Diversity Officer
F. Edward Hébert Uniformed Services University (USU) of the Health Sciences School of Medicine
Bethesda, Maryland

James R. Jacobs, MD, PhD
Medical Director
USC Engemann Student Health Center
Los Angeles, California

Marc S. Jacobson, MD
Professor
Department of Pediatrics
Nassau University Medical Center
East Meadow, New York

Raysenia L. James, DO, MPH
Family and Community Medicine
University of Arizona
Tucson, Arizona

Mary Anne Jamieson, MD, FRCSC
Associate Professor
Departments of Obstetrics & Gynecology, and Pediatrics
Queen's University
Kingston, Ontario, Canada

Carolyn B. Jasik
Assistant Professor
Department of Pediatrics
University of California
San Francisco, California

M. Susan Jay, MD
Professor of Pediatrics
Medical College of Wisconsin
Milwaukee, Wisconsin

Walter M. Jay, MD
Professor of Ophthalmology
Loyola University Medical Center
Maywood, Illinois

Alain Joffe, MD, MPH
Associate Professor
Department of Population, Family and Reproductive Health
John Hopkins Bloomberg School of Public Health
Director
The Johns Hopkins University Student Health and Wellness Center
Baltimore, Maryland

Jessica A. Kahn, MD, MPH
Professor
Division of Adolescent Medicine
Department of Pediatrics
Cincinnati Children's Hospital Medical Center
University of Cincinnati College of Medicine
Cincinnati, Ohio

Debra K. Katzman, MD, FRCPC
Professor of Pediatrics, Division of Adolescent Medicine, Department of Pediatrics
The Hospital for Sick Children and University of Toronto
Senior Associate Scientist, Research Institute
Director, Health Science Research
Undergraduate Medical Education, University of Toronto School of Medicine
Toronto, Ontario, Canada

Laura M. Kester, MD, MPH
Assistant Professor of Clinical Pediatrics
Department of Pediatrics, Section of Adolescent Medicine
Indiana University
Indianapolis, Indiana

Sari L. Kives, MD
Associate Professor
Department of Obstetrics and Gynecology
University of Toronto
The Hospital for Sick Children
Toronto, Ontario, Canada

Michael R. Kohn, MD, FRACP
Senior Staff Specialist
Department of Adolescent Medicine
Sydney Children's Hospital Network
Westmead, New South Wales, Australia

Daphne J. Korczak MD, MSc
Assistant Professor
Department of Psychiatry
University of Toronto
Director
Paediatric PostgraduateTeaching in Psychiatry
Department of Psychiatry
The Hospital for Sick Children
Toronto, Ontario, Canada

Daniel P. Krowchuk, MD
Professor of Pediatrics and Dermatology
Department of Pediatrics
Chief
Department of General Pediatrics and Adolescent Medicine
Wake Forest School of Medicine
Winston-Salem, North Carolina

Cecilia A. Larson, MD
Instructor
Department of Medicine
Harvard Medical School
Boston, Massachusetts
The Joslin Diabetes and Endocrine Clinic
Needham, Massachusetts

Katherine S. L. Lau, PhD
Postdoctoral Fellow
Department of Pediatrics
Indiana University School of Medicine
Indianapolis, Indiana

Sharon Levy, MD, MPH
Assistant Professor of Pediatrics
Harvard Medical School
Director, Adolescent Substance Abuse Program
Division of Developmental Pediatrics
Boston Children's Hospital
Boston, Massachusetts

Carol Lewis, MD
Director
Refugee Health Program
Primary Care Associate
Hasbro Children's Hospital
Professor of Pediatrics
Clinical Alpert Medical School of Brown University
Providence, Rhode Island

Keith J. Loud, MD, CM, MSc
Associate Professor of Pediatrics and Orthopaedic Surgery
Geisel School of Medicine at Dartmouth
Children's Hospital at Dartmouth-Hitchcock
Lebanon, New Hampshire

Lilia C. Lovera, MD
Neurology Chief Resident
Department of Neurology
Stritch School of Medicine
Loyola University Chicago
Maywood, Illinois

M. Joan Mansfield, MD
Assistant Professor of Pediatrics
Harvard Medical School
Associate in Medicine
Departments of Adolescent/Young Adult Medicine and
    Endocrinology
Boston Children's Hospital
Boston, Massachusetts

Bethany A. Marston, MD
Assistant Professor
Departments of Pediatrics and Medicine
University of Rochester
Rochester, New York

Anne McGlynn-Wright, MA
Pre-Doctoral Candidate
Department of Sociology
University of Washington
Seattle, Washington

William P. Meehan III, MD
Assistant Professor of Pediatrics and Orthopedics
Harvard Medical School
Director of The Micheli Center for Sports Injury Prevention
Division of Sports Medicine
Boston Children's Hospital
Boston, Massachusetts

Eric T. Meininger, MD, MPH
Gillette Children's Specialty Healthcare
St. Paul, Minnesota

Lora Melnicoe, MD, MPH
Advanced Instructor
Department of Pediatrics
University of Colorado
Denver Health Medical Center
Denver, Colorado

Melissa Mirosh, MD, FRCSC
Assistant Professor
Department of Obstetrics, Gynecology, and Reproductive Sciences
University of Saskatchewan College of Medicine
Attending Staff
Department of Obstetrics and Gynecology
Royal University Hospital
Saskatoon, Saskatchewan, Canada

Laurie A. P. Mitan, MD
Associate Professor of Pediatrics
Division of Adolescent & Transition Medicine
Cincinnati Children's Hospital Medical Center
Department of Pediatrics
The University of Cincinnati College of Medicine
Cincinnati, Ohio

Suneeta Monga, MD, FRCPC
Assistant Professor
Department of Psychiatry
University of Toronto
Director of Scholarship and Professional Development
Department of Psychiatry
The Hospital for Sick Children
Toronto, Ontario, Canada

Megan A. Moreno, MD, MSED, MPH
Associate Professor of Pediatrics
Adjunct Associate Professor of Health Services
University of Washington
Principal Investigator
Social Media and Adolescent Health Research Team
Seattle Children's Research Institute
Seattle, Washington

Anna-Barbara Moscicki, MD
Professor
Department of Pediatrics
University of California, San Francisco
Pediatric Vice-Chair
Clinical Translational Research
San Francisco, California

Shelly T. Ben Harush Negari, MD
Clinician
Division of Adolescent and Transition Medicine
Cincinnati Children's Hospital Medical Center
Cincinnati, Ohio

Anita L. Nelson, MD
Professor
Department of Obstetrics and Gynecology
David Geffen School of Medicine at UCLA
Los Angeles, California

Blaise A. Nemeth, MD, MS
Associate Professor (CHS)
Department of Orthopedics and Rehabilitation
Department of Pediatrics
American Family Children's Hospital
University of Wisconsin School of Medicine and Public Health
Madison, Wisconsin

Dennis K. Norman, EdD, ABPP
Associate Professor of Psychology
Department of Psychiatry
Harvard Medical School
Faculty
John F. Kennedy School of Government
Chair
Harvard University Native American Program
Cambridge, Massachusetts

Johanna Olson, MD
Assistant Professor of Pediatrics
Division of Adolescent and Young Adult Medicine
Children's Hospital Los Angeles
USC Keck School of Medicine
Los Angeles, California

Donald P. Orr, MD
Professor
Department of Pediatrics, Adolescent Medicine
Indiana University School of Medicine
Health Information & Translational Sciences
Director
Pediatric Adolescent Medicine
Indiana University School of Medicine
Indianapolis, Indiana

Elizabeth M. Ozer, PhD
Professor
Division of Adolescent & Young Adult Medicine
Department of Pediatrics
UCSF Benioff Children's Hospital
Director of Research
Office of Diversity & Outreach
University of California
San Francisco, California

Sherine Patterson-Rose, MD, MPH
Assistant Professor of Pediatrics
Division of Adolescent and Transition Medicine
Cincinnati Children's Hospital Medical Center
Cincinnati, Ohio

Sarah Pitts, MD
Assistant Professor of Pediatrics
Department of Adolescent/Young Adult Medicine
Boston Children's Hospital
Harvard Medical School
Boston, Massachusetts

Judith J. Prochaska, PhD, MPH
Associate Professor of Medicine
Stanford Prevention Research Center
Department of Medicine
Stanford University
Stanford, California

Mari Radzik, PhD
Assistant Professor of Clinical Pediatrics
USC Keck School of Medicine
Children's Hospital Los Angeles
Los Angeles, California

Vaughn I. Rickert, PsyD
Donald P. Orr Professor of Adolescent Medicine
Director
Section of Adolescent Medicine
Department of Pediatrics
Indiana University School of Medicine
Indianapolis, Indiana

Cynthia L. Robbins MD, MS
Assistant Professor of Clinical Pediatrics
Indiana University School of Medicine
Indianapolis, Indiana

Mary E. Romano, MD MPH
Assistant Professor
Division of Adolescent and Young Adult Health
Department of Pediatrics
Monroe Carell Jr. Children's Hospital at Vanderbilt
Nashville, Tennessee

Amanda P. Roper, MD
Resident Physician
Department of Psychiatry and Behavioral Sciences
Medical University of South Carolina
Charleston, South Carolina

Peter C. Rowe, MD
Professor of Pediatrics
Division of General Pediatrics and Adolescent Medicine
School of Medicine
The Johns Hopkins University School of Medicine
Baltimore, Maryland

Mark L. Rubinstein, MD
Associate Professor
Division of Adolescent & Young Adult Medicine
UCSF Benioff Children's Hospital
University of California, San Francisco
San Francisco, California

Gretchen J. Russo, RN, BSN, JD

Mandakini Sadhir, MD
Fellow
Department of Pediatrics
Medical College of Wisconsin
Clinical Instructor
Department of Adolescent Medicine/Pediatrics
Children's Hospital of Wisconsin
Milwaukee, Wisconsin

John Santelli, MD, MPH
Harriet and Robert H. Heilbrunn Professor
Chair, Population and Family Health
Department of Population and Family Health
Columbia University Mailman School of Public Health
New York, New York

Susan M. Sawyer, MBBS, MD, FRACP, FSAHM
Geoff and Helen Handbury Chair of Adolescent Health
Department of Paediatrics
The University of Melbourne
Director
Centre for Adolescent Health
Royal Children's Hospital
Melbourne, Victoria, Australia

Beth I. Schwartz, MD
Clinical Instructor
Division of Gynecology
Cincinnati Children's Hospital Medical Center
Department of Obstetrics & Gynecology
University of Cincinnati College of Medicine
Cincinnati, Ohio

Katherine Schwartz, JD, MPA
Research Associate
Department of Pediatrics
Section of Adolescent Medicine
Indiana University School of Medicine
Indianapolis, Indiana

Sara Sherer, PhD
Assistant Professor of Clinical Pediatrics
Department of Pediatrics
USC Keck School of Medicine
Director of Behavioral Services
Division of Adolescent and Young Adult Medicine
Children's Hospital Los Angeles
Psychology Training Director
USC UCEDD Mental Health
Division of General Pediatrics
Children's Hospital Los Angeles
Los Angeles, California

Lydia A. Shrier, MD, MPH
Associate Professor
Department of Pediatrics
Harvard Medical School
Senior Associate in Medicine
Division of Adolescent and Young Adult Medicine
Boston Children's Hospital
Boston, Massachusetts

David M. Siegel, MD, MPH
Professor
Department of Pediatrics
School of Medicine and Dentistry
University of Rochester
Chief
Division of Pediatric Rheumatology
Golisano Children's Hospital
Rochester, New York

Lisa K. Simons, MD
Instructor of Pediatrics
Department of Pediatrics
Northwestern University Feinberg School of Medicine
Division of Adolescent Medicine
Ann & Robert H. Lurie Children's Hospital of Chicago
Chicago, Illinois

Earl J. Soileau Jr, MD, FSAHM
Assistant Professor
Department of Family Medicine
Louisiana State University Health Sciences Center
School of Medicine, New Orleans
Lake Charles, Louisiana

Diane E. J. Stafford, MD
Assistant Professor
Department of Pediatrics
Harvard Medical School
Attending Physician
Training Program Director
Department of Medicine
Boston Children's Hospital
Boston, Massachusetts

Cynthia J. Stein, MD, MPH
Instructor in Orthopedic Surgery
Harvard Medical School
Division of Sports Medicine
Boston Children's Hospital
Boston, Massachusetts

Jonathan M. Swartz, MD
Instructor in Pediatrics
Division of Endocrinology
Harvard Medical School
Boston Children's Hospital
Boston, Massachusetts

Diane Tanaka, MD
Assistant Professor of Clinical Pediatrics
Division of Adolescent Medicine
Medical Director
Teenage and Young Adult Health Center
Children's Hospital of Los Angeles
Los Angeles, California

Heather Taussig, PhD
Professor and Associate Dean for Research
Graduate School of Social Work
University of Denver
Adjoint Professor
Kempe Center for the Prevention and Treatment of Child Abuse and Neglect
Department of Pediatrics
University of Colorado School of Medicine
Denver, Colorado

Shamir Tuchman, MD
Pediatric Nephrologist
Children's National Health System
Washington, District of Columbia

Sarah A. Van Orman, MD, MMM
Executive Director
University Health Services
University of Wisconsin–Madison
Madison, Wisconsin

Russell M. Viner, MBBS, PhD
Professor of Adolescent Health
University College London (UCL) Institute of Child Health
London, United Kingdom

Leslie R. Walker, MD
Professor of Pediatrics
Chief
Division of Adolescent Medicine
University of Washington
Seattle Children's Hospital
Seattle, Washington

Roger Dale Walker, MD
Professor
Departments of Psychiatry and Public Health and Preventive
  Medicine
Director
Center for American Indian Health, Education and Research
Director
One Sky Center: National Native Health Resource Center
Oregon Health and Science University
Portland, Oregon

Curren Warf, MD, MSEd, FAAP, FCPS, FSAHM
Clinical Professor of Paediatrics
Department of Paediatrics Head
Division of Adolescent Health and Medicine
British Columbia Children's Hospital/University of British
  Columbia
Vancouver, British Columbia, Canada

Shelly K. Weiss, MD, FRCPC
Professor
Division of Neurology
Department of Pediatrics
The Hospital for Sick Children
University of Toronto
Toronto, Ontario, Canada

Merill Weitzel, MD
Clinical Instructor of Obstetrics and Gynecology
Harvard Medical School
Attending Physician
Department of Medicine
Boston Children's Hospital
Boston, Massachusetts

Elissa R. Weitzman, ScD, MSc
Assistant Professor
Department of Pediatrics
Harvard Medical School
Assistant Professor
Division of Adolescent Medicine
Boston Children's Hospital
Boston, Massachusetts

Elizabeth R. Woods, MD, MPH
Professor
Department of Pediatrics
Harvard Medical School
Associate Chief
Division of Adolescent and Young Adult Medicine
Boston Children's Hospital
Boston, Massachusetts

Alan D. Woolf, MD, MPH
Professor
Department of Pediatrics
Harvard Medical School
Chief
Pediatric Environmental Health Center
Boston Children's Hospital
Boston, Massachusetts

Kimberly A. Workowski, MD
Professor of Medicine
Division of Infectious Diseases
Emory University
Atlanta, Georgia

Kristin Wunder, MPH
Department of Population and Family Health
Columbia University Mailman School of Public Health
New York, New York

Stavra A. Xanthakos, MD, MS
Associate Professor of Pediatrics
Department of Pediatrics
University of Cincinnati College of Medicine
Associate Professor of Pediatrics
Division of Gastroenterology, Hepatology and Nutrition
Cincinnati Children's Hospital Medical Center
Cincinnati, Ohio

Foreword

Written by Catherine DeAngelis, Roberta G. Williams, and Pierre-André Michaud

I am delighted and honored to write a foreword to the sixth edition of *Neinstein's Adolescent and Young Adult Health Care: A Practical Guide*. In this text, Larry Neinstein and his associate editors provide a practical, data-enriched, and easy-to-read resource for anyone who deals with adolescents, including not only those in the health care fields. While physicians, nurse practitioners, nurses, physician assistants, psychologists, social workers, health educators, nutritionists, and pharmacists comprise the main intended audience, I believe there is much valuable information herein for teachers and parents too.

While the first edition was designed for daily office use, subsequent editions, including the sixth, expand on that design and incorporate all areas where adolescents and young adults (AYAs) are cared for. This edition builds on the firm foundations of the previous editions and adds greater emphasis in several areas. One area includes more information on young adults, with the title adding *Young Adult Health Care*, to exemplify the emphasis. Other areas of greater emphasis are special populations, including the juvenile justice system, military service, immigrants, and Native Americans. There is also greater emphasis on global issues of AYA care.

Adolescent medicine has come a long way from the small training program for physicians interested in school health that began in Boston in the early 1950s. Currently, adolescent medicine is required in all pediatric training programs, it is a board-certified subspecialty, and there are a number of journals dedicated to the specialty.

We can only guess what the future might hold as epigenetics, neuroimaging, information technology, and social media (or is it really antisocial media?)—and who knows what else—might contribute to understanding the complex pathophysiology of the physical, emotional, and behavioral aspects of AYAs. Whatever they might be, Larry Neinstein, his associate editors, and those whom they train will be well prepared to continue publishing the defining text for the field.

Catherine DeAngelis, MD, MPH
University Distinguished Service Professor, Emerita
Professor of Pediatrics, Emerita
The Johns Hopkins University School of Medicine
Professor of Health Policy and Management
School of Public Health
Editor-in-Chief Emerita, JAMA
Baltimore, Maryland

It is an honor to write a foreword to the sixth edition of *Neinstein's Adolescent and Young Adult Health Care: A Practical Guide*. This comprehensive compendium of wisdom about health promotion and disease recognition and management has long been a reliable source of information. Previous editions have been a trusted and easily navigated reference guide for all health professionals caring for adolescents. The scope of this body of work not only encompasses the developmentally specific issues of the healthy AYAs, but also provides expansive information on commonly encountered complaints and disorders. Not only is this guide relevant to the healthy AYAs, but it is also very useful for the management of those with chronic disease. It is often unrecognized that even patients with *severe* disability face many of the social, sexual, and substance use issues encountered by their healthy counterparts. Health management requires a clear understanding of the psychosocial behaviors and motivations that are characteristic of this age-group and consideration of the specific emerging morbidities, such as mental health problems, that occur during this transformative period.

The world as experienced by AYAs will continue to change—emerging diseases and treatments, new technologies, impermanent social and economic structures, and modes of health care delivery are in flux. Dissemination of health information is rapidly evolving along with the roles of provider and patient. Nowhere is this more prescient than in the period of adolescence through emerging adulthood. The very concept of youth, its beginning and end, is being challenged with the delay of perceived and actual independence compared with previous generations. For both healthy AYAs and those with chronic disease, these changes will have massive social and legal implications for the future. Certainly, today's AYAs face a challenging world, with need for preparation for different skills, self-advocacy, communication style, and virtual presence.

What remains unchanged is the impact of AYA health on social capital and disease burden in future years. Anticipatory care during this developmental stage will yield great dividends, yet this is the very time when both healthy AYAs and those with chronic disease drop out of health care. Maintaining a partnership with them requires an understanding of their aspirations, needs, and specific health issues. That is why this broad-based, specifically targeted, and conveniently organized text has such a dedicated following.

Roberta G. Williams, MD
Professor and Past Chair of Pediatrics
USC Keck School of Medicine
Children's Hospital Los Angeles
Los Angeles, California

For many years, Neinstein's textbook has been a major reference for interdisciplinary professionals involved in the care of AYAs, who live not only in the United States but also in other regions of the world. The newest edition of this textbook adds to the previous publications not only in providing a comprehensive review of all the major conditions affecting the health of AYAs, but also in depicting the state of the health of this population around the world. While the United States represents the cradle of adolescent medicine, more and more countries from different regions of the world are sensitized to the specific needs of the AYA population. Since the 1980s, there have been many significant global developments that support professionals in the health care of AYAs. For instance, the World Health Organization has worked on the health of adolescents with a focus on sexual and reproductive health,[1] and more recently, they have created a framework to support health professionals in the improvement of health services in school settings[2] and in the training of school health professionals in developing specific curricula in adolescent health.[3] Around the same time, the International Association for Adolescent Health[4] was established and launched its quadrennial international scientific congress, where professionals gathered from all over the planet. The Journal of Adolescent Health, the official publication of the Society of Adolescent Health and Medicine, publishes cutting edge research from AYA researchers around the world. Another indication of the growing interest in AYA health was the creation of the European Training in Effective Adolescent Care and Health (Euteach).[5] In fact, Dr. Larry Neinstein was a collaborator with other European colleagues on the Euteach training package, which provides training modules and tools in the field of adolescent health.

Indeed, there are no miraculous or sophisticated technologies to address the health problems of AYAs. The solution quite often lies in training health professionals to adequately communicate with their young people and to improve their knowledge and skills, involving young people in decisions or preventive strategies, and providing a safe and effective environment such as the one developed under the concept of "Youth Friendly Health Service."[6] A textbook such as the Neinstein's sixth edition provides the essential ingredients for the training of all health professionals who care for AYAs. The sixth edition of *Neinstein's Adolescent and Young Adult Health Care: A Practical Guide* constitutes an invaluable resource to improve and update the competencies of adolescent health professionals worldwide.

Prof. Pierre-André Michaud, MD
Honorary Professor
Faculty of Biology and Medicine
University of Lausanne
Independent Consultant in School, Adolescent
Health and Medical Education
Euteach Coordinator
Lausanne, Switzerland

[1]Venkatraman Chandra-Mouli, Joar Svanemyr, Avni Amin, et al. Twenty Years After International Conference on Population and Development: Where Are We With Adolescent Sexual and Reproductive Health and Rights? 2015;(1): Supplement, S1–S6
[2]http://www.euro.who.int/__data/assets/pdf_file/0003/246981/European-framework-for-quality-standards-in-school-health-services-and-competences-for-school-health-professionals.pdf
[3]http://apps.who.int/iris/bitstream/10665/148354/1/9789241508315_eng.pdf?ua=1
[4]http://iaah.org/
[5]www.euteach.com
[6]http://www.who.int/maternal_child_adolescent/documents/fch_cah_02_14/en.

Preface

It has been extremely exciting and enlightening to cast our memories back more than 30 years, to the first edition of Adolescent Health Care, and reflect on the many changes in the field of adolescent and young adult (AYA) health. During this period, the field has grown and changed significantly. For us, some of the most significant changes include expansion of the field of adolescent health care to include systems of care as diverse as school-based health clinics and transitional health clinics; mandatory inclusion of adolescent health in pediatric education; new discoveries in neuroscience on the continuing development of the brain into young adulthood; the importance of the emerging young adult population; the continued growth and need for quality AYA health care both within the United States and globally; and the significant impact of mental health and substance abuse morbidities and mortalities in this population. These are but a few of the many changes documented throughout the textbook. Naturally, with these continued changes, the book continues to evolve. It is these exciting developments, coupled with our passion for caring for our patients and their families, that have inspired us to improve the sixth edition.

The book contains many new additions, continuing to make it the most comprehensive text in AYA health and the most utilized over the past 30 years. For the first time ever, we have included young adults into the scope of this book. The sixth edition is organized into 16 sections, including 80 chapters. All chapters include new information, the latest research findings, and up-to-date clinical recommendations. New chapters have been added such as the health of AYAs globally, the use of technology, transgender AYAs, youth in the military, youth in foster placement, immigrant youth, and American Indians and Alaskan Native youth. Each chapter contains excellent illustrations, figures, and tables to help the reader better understand and remember important points. There are new full-color designs and more clinical photos that provide visual appeal and clarity. Web sites, appropriate for teenagers, parents, and professionals, are in both the text and in the reference section, and are expanded to access up-to-date information where relevant. Many readers have asked for an e-edition, and this has been accomplished with the sixth edition. The sixth edition has both a print and a companion e-edition. The sixth edition is for a wide variety of health professionals including pediatricians, family practitioners, gynecologists, internists, psychiatrists, psychologists, nurses, nurse practitioners, physician assistants, medical students, residents, and fellows. It is also ideal for a multitude of sites including school-based clinics, college health centers, juvenile detention centers, pediatric emergency rooms, and other facilities that serve AYAs.

The intent of the book has always been to provide practical, easy-to-read information and resources to assist health-care providers in the care of AYAs and ultimately improve the health and well-being of this population. We continue to try and meet these standards in the sixth edition. It is our goal that this book is the best place to find all of the authoritative, state-of-the-art clinical answers on AYA health that students and health professionals need.

We have been so grateful to have the expertise of our associate editors, Dr. Todd Callahan, Dr. Catherine Gordon, Dr. Alain Joffe, and Dr. Vaughn Rickert. It is with deep sadness that toward the end of this edition's work, Dr. Vaughn Rickert died suddenly. We have a memorial tribute to our friend and colleague on page xix. Our associate editors are among the most recognized and respected authorities in the field of adolescent health care. They provide a wide range of expertise ranging from gynecology, endocrinology, mental health issues, and preventive health issues to substance abuse and sexually transmitted infections. They have been invaluable in continuing to raise the standards of this textbook. In addition to these four associate editors, we have brought together the field's most influential authors in AYA health care to write these chapters and share their expertise.

This edition also includes a special acknowledgment to our dear friend and treasured colleague David Scott Rosen, MD, who passed away on February 11, 2013, from cancer. David was a wonderful adolescent medicine physician, educator, and mentor, and an associate editor of Neinstein's fifth edition. David dedicated his professional life in medicine to caring for AYAs, to training students and residents to care for AYAs, and to finding better ways to prevent and treat diseases that are serious problems for teenagers and young adults. In many ways, this book exemplifies everything David stood for. In addition to being a wonderful physician, David was an incredibly accomplished photographer. David's work primarily consisted of portraits of children and teenagers. To honor David's memory, we have put together a collection of his photographs (see page xx–xxi) that we believe capture the teen spirit and energy.

Writing a book that accurately reflects the excitement, controversies, and uncertainties in AYA health was a formidable and humbling experience. We hope that this book will educate interdisciplinary health-care professionals about this exciting and growing field, teach the next generation of clinicians about AYA health, and ultimately impact and improve the care we provide to young people and their families. There is no greater honor.

Finally, we dedicate this book to young people and to their health-care providers. AYAs continue to inspire us to write this book and sustain our desire to make sure that we provide them with the best possible health. We hope that the sixth edition will provide a wealth of information for those who care for AYAs.

Debra K. Katzman, MD, FRCPC

Lawrence S. Neinstein, MD

I would also like to thank with all my heart the first senior associate editor this book has had for her incredible contributions. Debra Katzman has been an amazing colleague and so important in achieving this sixth edition.

Lawrence S. Neinstein, MD

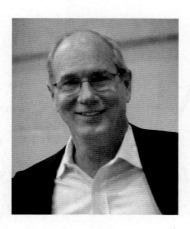

Vaughn I. Rickert, Jr, PsyD, HSPP
March 16, 1953–June 17, 2015

On June 17, 2015, our dear friend, colleague, scholar, advocate, husband, father, son, and associate editor for *Neinstein's* sixth edition, Vaughn I. Rickert, Jr, unexpectedly passed away.

Vaughn's dedication to and passion for helping professionals improve the health and health care of adolescents, young adults, and their families as the Director of Adolescent Medicine, and the Donald P. Orr Professor of Adolescent Medicine at Indiana University School of Medicine in Indianapolis, Indiana, will be truly missed. He had a gift for bringing professionals and communities together for the betterment of young people, and was particularly skilled at fostering a culture of connection and belonging. Vaughn's contributions to *Neinstein's* sixth edition and to adolescent health in general were outstanding in scope and impact.

Vaughn will be sorely missed by many, but never will he be forgotten by those who were fortunate enough to have known him well. We will miss his wry sense of humor, his beautiful smile, his boundless energy, his infectious enthusiasm, and his never-ending warmth. He is survived by his loving wife, Cynthia, and his three adored sons, Jeffrey, Ryan, and Mason.

...In
Memory

of our dear friend and colleague,
David Scott Rosen, MD
1959–2013

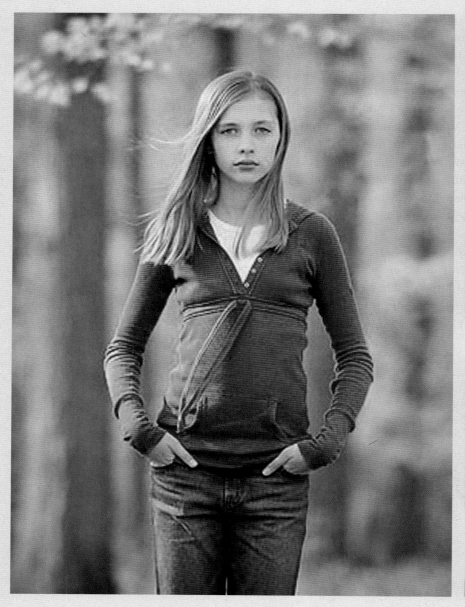

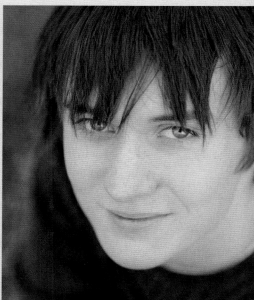

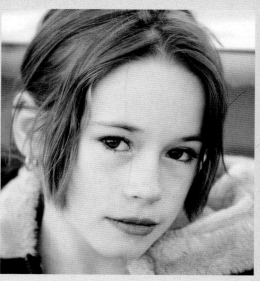

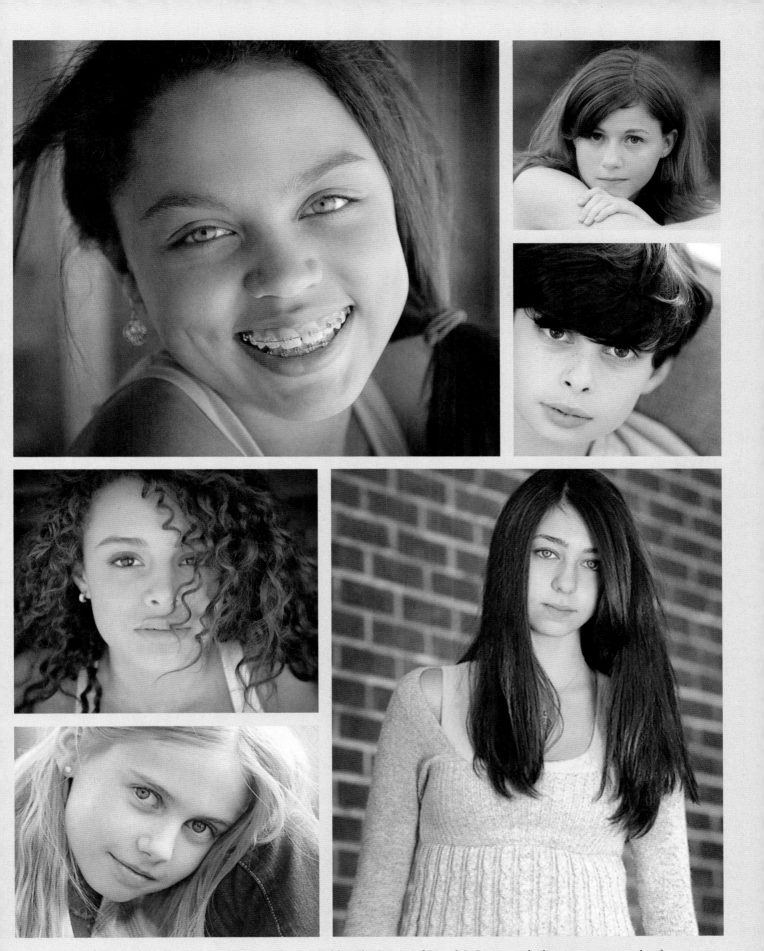

Photographs by David Scott Rosen and provided by The Estate of David S. Rosen with the sincere gratitude of *Neinstein's Adolescent and Young Adult Health Care* editorial team.

Table of Contents

General Considerations in Adolescent and Young Adult Health Care

CHAPTER 1

Health of the World's Adolescents and Young Adults

Dougal S. Hargreaves
Kristin Wunder
Russell M. Viner
John Santelli

KEY WORDS

- Demography
- Global health
- Health disparities
- Health status
- Morbidity and mortality
- Social determinants of health

The world now has the largest generation of adolescents and young adults (AYAs) in history: 1.2 billion aged 10 to 19 years (17.3% of the world population) and 1.8 billion aged 10 to 24 years (26.3% of the world population).[1] This "youth bulge," seen particularly in rapidly developing low- and middle-income countries (LMICs), has the potential to deliver a substantial economic and productivity dividend for countries as this better educated generation of youth enter the workforce.[2]

Adolescence and young adulthood have been considered the healthiest times of life, and therefore have received little attention in terms of global health policy and perspectives. However, recently there has been greater focus on AYA health, highlighting emerging patterns of global mortality, high rates of health-risk behaviors, and morbidity, and recognizing that health patterns among AYAs have lifelong consequences. Recent decades have seen rapid reductions in global mortality among young children, but much smaller reductions in mortality among AYAs. Indeed, AYA mortality from motor vehicle crashes (MVCs) and other transport injuries, suicide, and homicide is rising in many countries.[3] As a result, AYAs now have higher mortality rates than children 1 to 4 years old in high-, middle-, and some low-income countries.[3] Economic development and the conquering of infectious diseases have resulted in improved child survival and created the "youth bulge" seen globally and in many LMIC. Yet, the same rapid social and economic change appears to be inimical to the health of AYAs.[3]

Globally, there are large numbers of avoidable deaths among AYAs from a range of causes, including intentional and unintentional injuries, maternal mortality, and human immunodeficiency virus (HIV) infection. Behaviors and attitudes acquired during adolescence and young adulthood are also critical determinants of future health. Five of the ten major risk factors for poor lifelong health identified in the Global Burden of Disease study largely originate during adolescence and young adulthood[4]: smoking, excess alcohol intake, obesity/overweight, poor diet, and physical inactivity.

Within the US, AYA health trends are similarly concerning. From 2000 to 2012, little progress has been made in improving most AYA outcomes, including those related to overall health (violence, mental health, health care access, substance use, obesity). Some indicators were significantly improved during this period, including unintentional injuries, assaults, cigarette smoking, and condom use. However, significant increases were reported in

chlamydia/HIV infections, hearing loss, and 'screen time' for AYAs and for obesity rates among young adults.

Health concerns of young adults increasingly resemble those of adolescents (aged 10 to 19 years), given intersecting social trends toward longer engagement in formal education and delays in marriage and childbearing, leading to extended social transitions from adolescence into the adult years. As a result, the time span from puberty to adult social and financial independence in developed countries has increased from 6 years in the 1950s to over 15 years today. This is a global phenomenon, with similar trends in high-income countries and LMICs. Young adults have a spectrum of health behaviors that are similar to adolescents, and frequently higher prevalence of risky behaviors and worse outcomes.

The first part of this chapter provides an integrated conceptual framework or perspective on social determinants, developmental influences, and life-course perspectives on the health of AYAs (Fig. 1.1).[6] The second part of the chapter includes the US and global data to characterize variations in AYA health and health determinants. The third part of the chapter highlights a series of recommendations for health care providers and policy makers responsible for AYA health. Finally, the last part of this chapter includes supplementary information devoted to the morbidity and mortality of AYAs in the US.

SOCIAL DETERMINANTS

The World Health Organization (WHO) defines social determinants of health as 'the conditions in which people are born, grow, live, work, and age'.[7] Health services often focus on individual-level risks and behaviors (see Chapters 4 and 5), while the social determinants approach recognizes the health impact of social factors at family, peer group, school, community, national, and even global levels. As illustrated in the model shown in Figure 1.2, social determinants may have positive effects on resilience and health-enhancing behaviors as well as on the development or exposure to risky or harmful behaviors and situations.

The WHO Commission on the Social Determinants of Health[7] differentiates fundamental structural factors (e.g., political, economic, education, and welfare systems) and more proximal factors that influence the "circumstances of daily life." Proximal factors include social institutions (e.g., families, peers, and schools), food, housing, recreation, access to education and employment, and social and financial independence. The importance of various structural and proximal influences on AYA health is discussed below.

Structural Determinants of Health

Structural determinants of health include social policies and programs, economic policies, and politics that may create poor and

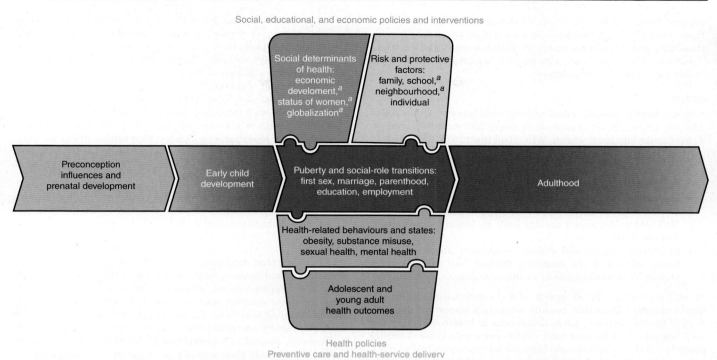

FIGURE 1.1 Conceptual framework for adolescent health. (From Sawyer SM, Afifi RA, Bearinger LH, et al. Adolescence: a foundation for future health. *Lancet* 2012;379(9826):1630–1640. Available at http://www.thelancet.com/journals/lancet/article/PIIS0140-6736(12)60072-5/fulltext)

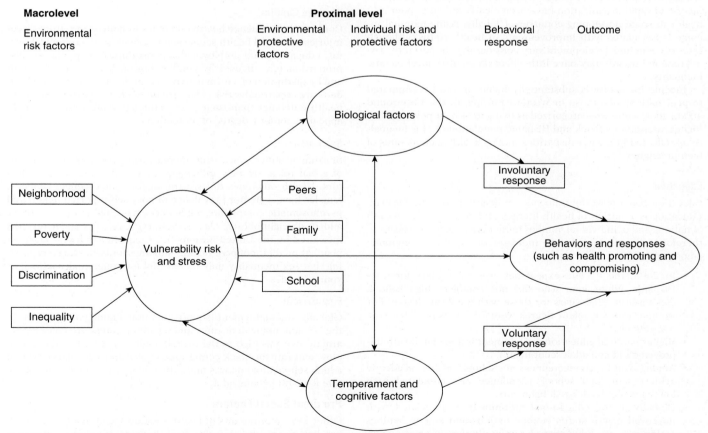

FIGURE 1.2 A model of resilience in adolescence. (Adapted from The Johns Hopkins University and Blum RW. Resilience in adolescence, section C: factors that buffer and exacerbate stress. 2011. Available at http://a1.phobos.apple.com/us/r30/CobaltPublic/v4/93/fd/f3/93fdf355-4462-4ec7-cbe4-55ff7e5dd182/210-9012651533345481912-AHDLecture9.pdf)

unequal living conditions, which affect the health of populations. These structural determinants operate within countries, but increasingly operate between countries as the effects of globalization. Structural determinants are significantly responsible for the poor health experienced by populations.

Income

National wealth and disparities in household income within countries are important determinants of many AYA health outcomes. With regard to national wealth, WHO data from 2011 show that:

- Mortality rates for 15- to 19-year-olds varied from over 200/100,000 in some middle-income countries to under 50/100,000 in Japan, Singapore, and some European countries.[8]
- Pregnancy rates for 15- to 19-year-old females are as high as 200/1,000 in the poorest nations, compared to less than 10/1,000 in developed nations such as Japan, Norway, Italy, and the Netherlands.
- In contrast, injury and violence rates were unrelated to national income in the countries studied, and smoking rates among AYAs were higher in wealthier countries.[8]

In addition to the overall wealth of a country, inequality in per capita income within that country is also an important determinant of health outcome. Large differences in health outcomes are seen among countries that have similar per capita gross domestic product—both among low- and high-income countries (e-Fig. 1.1). Income inequality within a country appears to be of approximately equal importance to per capita national income with regards to rates of bullying, pregnancy, and mortality.[8] In contrast, rates of smoking, violence, and injuries do not seem to be significantly related to country-level income inequality. High youth unemployment and rapid urbanization have been clearly linked to poor AYA health in some developing countries. Globally, rising national income is associated with improvements in health status, although rates of economic development vary considerably. Importantly, rising national wealth may have little effect on country-level income inequality.

Income inequality is substantially higher in the US compared to peer nations like those in Western Europe. In the US, around 40% of adolescents are categorized as living in or near poverty, with higher rates among Black and Hispanic populations.[6] This inequality is reflected in greater disparities in AYA health such as rates of teen pregnancy.[9]

Education

Education has a powerful influence on health across the lifespan. Education is a marker of health literacy and practices. The wealth of nations and of individual families influences access to education; therefore, education is also an indicator of social and economic empowerment.

- In 2008, the US life expectancy was 67.5 years for non-Hispanic White men who did not complete high school, compared to 80.4 years for those with a college degree. For women, the equivalent figures were 73.5 versus 83.9 years, respectively.[10]
- Higher parental educational attainment is associated with improved child and adolescent health.
- Among youth, connectedness to school, higher academic achievement, and school attendance are associated with lower rates of health-risk behaviors.
- Globally, rising educational attainment is associated with improved health status, among nations and among families within nations. Education is commonly perceived as a gateway to social advancement by families and political leaders. Financial insecurity and family instability may reduce the ability of youth to continue education.

- Between 2000 and 2010, the number of children attending elementary or primary school increased by 50 million worldwide. However, there were smaller increases in enrollment in secondary schools. Globally, there are still an estimated 71 million children of lower secondary age (11 to 14 years) who are out of school.[11]
- In the least developed countries, one-quarter of AYA males (15- to 24-year-olds) and one-third of females are illiterate.[11]
- Higher rates of attendance in secondary education are associated with lower rates of injuries, teen births, HIV prevalence, and overall mortality. The health effects are particularly marked among females, who are less likely to attend secondary school in some countries.

Educational and parenting support for young mothers significantly improves health outcomes of their children in adolescence (see Life-Course Perspective section below)[11,12] (e-Fig. 1.2).

Migration

Another structural determinant of health is migration. Internal migration is found in movement from rural to urban areas, particularly in developing nations, which have sizeable rural populations. Many of these internal migrants are AYAs seeking employment. International AYAs is relatively uncommon before age 18, but then increases rapidly and peaks among young adults (e-Fig. 1.3).

Globally, around 175 million people (2.9% of the world's population) live outside their country of origin. While immigrants are healthier on average than the general population in high-income countries (sometimes referred to as the "healthy immigrant effect"), migration may have adverse health consequences, particularly in regards to mental health.

War and Conflict

Conflict may influence health outcomes in many ways, from direct injuries to mental health sequelae and effects on food supply, housing, education, and employment opportunities. AYAs may be disproportionately affected by conflict—through direct involvement and by disruption of a formative period in the life course. Child soldiers are at particular risk. They are more likely to experience poor health outcomes than their peers, although education and family appear to confer a degree of protection.

Sex Inequality

Starting at puberty, sex is an increasingly important determinant of social roles, strongly influenced by cultural and religious factors. Health outcomes diverge throughout adolescence. Globally, females have a greater prevalence of poor self-reported health and psychosomatic complaints, while males have higher rates of injury and overweight/obesity. At the country level, sex inequality (as measured by the United Nations Sex Inequality Index) is an independent predictor of poor health outcomes for both sexes,[8] suggesting that sex inequality may be harmful for young males as well as young females.

Employment

Globally, unemployment is more common among young adults. In the US, unemployment rates among young adults are consistently around twice as high as the overall adult rate. In 2013, the unemployment rate for Black young adults (aged 19 to 24 years) without a high school diploma was more than 50%, nearly twice that of the rate for White young adults.[6]

Proximal Social Factors

Other key determinants of health include social institutions (e.g., families, peers, and schools), food, housing, recreation, access to education and employment, and health behaviors that directly influence AYAs. These social factors have been shown to influence a wide variety of AYA health outcomes (Fig. 1.3).

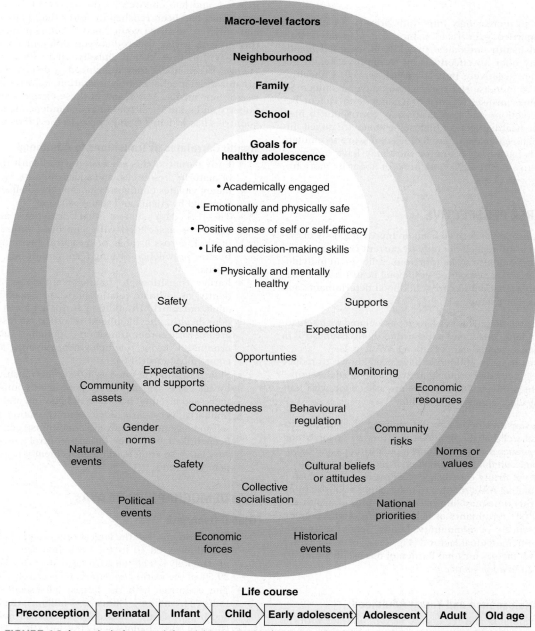

FIGURE 1.3 An ecologic framework for adolescent health. (From Blum RW, Bastos F, Kabiru C, et al. Adolescent health in the 21st century. *Lancet* 2012;379(9826):1567–1568. Available at http://www.thelancet.com/journals/lancet/article/PIIS0140-6736(12)60407-3/fulltext)

Neighborhood

Living in a poor area is associated with a range of adverse adolescent outcomes, including lower educational attainment, poorer mental health, and higher rates of teenage pregnancy and youth violence. In addition to the structural effects of poverty described above, area-level deprivation is partly mediated through reduced social capital, which reduces resilience and opportunities available to AYAs.

School

Enjoyment and engagement with school (often described as school-connectedness) is associated with reduced substance use, better mental health, and a range of other health outcomes.[12] Schools can also play an important role in improving health, both through public health interventions (e.g., alcohol programs) or through on-site health services, which have been shown to improve the quality of services young people receive and increase use of appropriate contraception.[13]

Families

While family influences are less dominant in adolescence and young adulthood than in early childhood, family connectedness and parental involvement remain important protective factors. Conversely, parental behaviors such as smoking, alcohol, and violence are all associated with higher rates of these behaviors among their children.

Peers

Peer approval is an increasingly important priority for most adolescents.[12] Supportive peer relationships are associated with improved mental health outcomes. In addition, peer-led health interventions may offer an effective way to improve health behaviors. Peers can negatively impact health as well. Unhealthy behaviors by peers increase the risk of many adverse outcomes, including substance misuse, teenage pregnancy, and violent behavior. Peer interactions and popularity may contribute to high self-esteem.[12] The health effects of high self-esteem are mixed. Individuals with high self-esteem may feel less pressure to emulate negative health behaviors of peers, or they may have increased exposure to negative health behaviors brought about by more frequent socializing with peers.

LIFE-COURSE PERSPECTIVE

A life-course perspective is derived from an increasing body of evidence that health is influenced not only by current risk factors and social determinants, but also by factors from earlier in an individual's life. Adolescence is a key period in lifelong health trajectories, with links both to prenatal and early childhood determinants and lifelong outcomes. For example:

- Micronutrient deficiencies in utero are associated with schizophrenia in adolescence, and exposure to diethylstilbestrol in utero can cause vaginal cancer among AYA females.[9]
- Interventions in early childhood have been shown to reduce teenage pregnancy and criminal activity among adolescents.
- Teen smoking and sexual behaviors are associated with lung and genitourinary cancers in later life.[9]

Adolescence is a sensitive period for determining lifelong trajectories in health and well-being.[8] While exploratory behavior is normal during adolescence and young adulthood, attitudes and habits acquired at this age can determine lifelong health risks. Patterns of behavior are not yet firmly established, leading to greater clustering of behaviors among AYAs relative to older adults. Holistic interventions during this time may improve a wide range of health and other outcomes.[12] Determinants of behaviors are often complex, with interacting effects of community, family, school, area, and peers, in addition to individual factors[8] (Fig. 1.4). As noted earlier, 5 of the top 10 risk factors for total burden of disease in adults are initiated or shaped in adolescence.[12]

Transitions in Adolescence and Young Adulthood

Both social determinants and life-course factors interact with the intrinsic biologic, psychological, and social transitions that take place during adolescence. Biologic transitions are influenced by nutritional and environmental factors, with the age of puberty falling in rich countries during the 19th and early 20th century. Subsequently, the timing has been fairly stable in rich countries since the 1960s.

The World Bank describes several key aspects of the social transition from childhood to adulthood.[2]

- Dependent child to autonomous adult
- Primary (elementary) to secondary/later education into the workforce
- Transition into responsible and productive citizenship (growing up global)
  - Developmental markers such as age at first sex, marriage, and childbearing
  - Age at leaving education and entering workforce
- Recipient of health care to responsibility for own health care

In the US during the 1960s, 77% of women and 67% of men completed their education, left home, achieved financial independence, married, and had children by the age of 30. By 2000, these five milestones had been reached by fewer than half of young women and only one in three young men.[14] Young adults' experience of this process varies widely between different countries and cultures. Within the US and globally, there have also been rapid changes in recent decades, influenced by diverse factors, including urbanization, mechanization, migration, industrialization, and the rise of new media. As a result of these changes, the gap between puberty and adult social and financial independence in developed countries has widened from 6 years in the 1950s to 15+ today.

Health Correlates of Transitions to Adulthood

- Early parenthood is associated with health risks, due to lack of maturity, resources, and social support. Where early pregnancy violates community norms, these effects may be compounded by stigma and social isolation.
- The US data suggest that delaying parenthood until age 34 is associated with improved future health of the mother, across a range of measures including self-reported health, prevalence of long-term conditions, and functional status.[15]
- Earlier transitions to financial autonomy, living independently, or intimate relationships are associated with poorer adult outcomes. In addition to higher rates of anxiety and poor health, the likelihood of other adverse outcomes increase with earlier transitions, including substance misuse, criminal behavior, unemployment, divorce, and lower socioeconomic status (SES).
- Slow transition (defined as little or no transition to adult roles by age 24) is also associated poor health outcomes, including increased criminal behavior and poor mental health.
- Similarly, very early adolescent transition to independent self-management of chronic conditions such as diabetes has been linked to poorer disease control outcomes; however, very late transition to self-management is also associated with poor outcomes.

DEMOGRAPHICS OF AYAs

Global Overview

- The world now has the largest generation of AYAs in history— 1.2 billion aged 10 to 19, 1.8 billion aged 10 to 24, and approximately 2.0 billion AYAs aged 10 to 26 (17.3%, 26.3%, and 29.5% of the world population, respectively)[1] (Fig. 1.5).
- The countries with the largest adolescent populations are India (243 million), China (207 million), the US (44 million), and Indonesia and Pakistan (both with 41 million each).
- Globally, 88% of adolescents live in LMICs. The proportion of the world's adolescents living in urban areas was estimated at 50% in 2009, and is projected to increase to 70% by 2050, due to the increasing urbanization of developing nations.
- In the last two decades, rapid improvements in childhood survival have produced so-called "youth bulges" (i.e., increases in youth as a percentage of the total population) in many countries, particularly rapidly developing countries. This can exacerbate youth unemployment, with too many workers for too few jobs.
- The region with highest growth in its AYA population is sub-Saharan Africa, where numbers of adolescents are projected to overtake South Asia and East Asia and Pacific Regions by 2050 (e-Figs. 1.4 to 1.7).

Population Structure and Composition

- Low replacement fertility and low rates of childhood mortality have produced a situation where some world regions currently have a greater number of AYAs than younger children. For every 10 children in the first decade of life in Europe,

Risk Factors	Substance Abuse	Delinquency	Teen Pregnancy	School Dropout	Violence	Depression & Anxiety
Community						
Availability of drugs	✓				✓	
Availability of firearms		✓			✓	
Community laws and norms favorable towards drug use, firearms, and crime	✓	✓			✓	
Media portrayals of violence					✓	
Transitions and mobility	✓	✓		✓		✓
Low community attachment and disorganization	✓	✓			✓	
Extreme economic deprivation	✓	✓	✓	✓	✓	
Family						
Family history of the problem behavior	✓	✓	✓	✓	✓	✓
Family management problems	✓	✓	✓	✓	✓	
Family conflict	✓	✓	✓	✓	✓	✓
Favorable parental attitudes and involvement in the problem behavior	✓	✓			✓	
School						
Academic failure beginning in late elementary school	✓	✓	✓	✓	✓	✓
Lack of commitment to school	✓	✓	✓	✓	✓	
Individual/Peer						
Early and persistent antisocial behavior	✓	✓	✓	✓	✓	✓
Alienation and rebelliousness	✓	✓		✓		
Friends who engage in the problem behavior	✓	✓	✓	✓	✓	
Favorable attitude towards the problem behavior	✓	✓	✓	✓		
Early initiation of the problem behavior	✓	✓	✓	✓	✓	
Constitutional factors	✓	✓			✓	✓

FIGURE 1.4 Risk factors for adolescent problem behaviors. (From Institute of Medicine, National Research Council. *The science of adolescent risk-taking: workshop report. Committee on the science of adolescence*. Washington, DC: The National Academies Press, 2011:Table 6-1. Available at http://www.ncbi.nlm.nih.gov/books/NBK53411/)

there are 10.6 young people in the second decade of life and 13.6 in the third decade. This imbalance is even greater in some countries, such as Russia (16.4 in third decade for every 10 in first decade) and Japan (29.4 in third decade for every 10 in first decade).

- Conversely, data from sub-Saharan Africa show continued high fertility and child mortality. For every 10 children in the first decade of life, there are 7.6 young people in the second decade and 6.0 in the third decade.
- 2012 US Census data show that there were 42.0 million adolescents aged 10 to 19 (13.4% of population) and 73.2 million AYAs aged 10 to 26 (23.3%).[6,16] Compared to many other countries, the US has a more equal balance between first, second, and third decades. For every 10 children aged 0 to 9 years, there are 10.5 young people in the second decade and 10.6 in the third decade of life.[1]

- The racial and ethnic composition of the AYA population in the US is changing rapidly. In 1980, 80% of AYAs aged 15 to 24 were White. In 2010, that figure was closer to 60%, and by 2040 it is projected to be under 50%.[12] Non-White populations are now spread much more widely throughout the US rather than living in concentrated areas, which was common in the past.[6]

MORTALITY OF AYAs

Global Mortality

- Globally, an estimated 2.1 million deaths occurred among AYAs (10 to 24 years) in 2010.[17]
- In a study of 50 low-, middle-, and high-income countries, the mortality rate decreased more rapidly among young children than AYAs from 1955 to 2004. Compared to a decrease

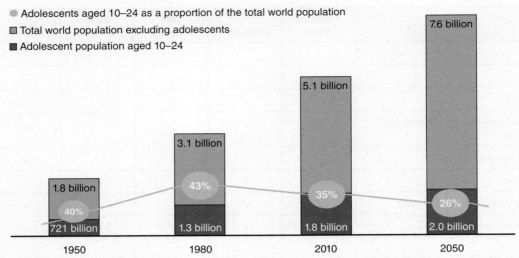

● Adolescents aged 10–24 as a proportion of the total world population

▨ Total world population excluding adolescents

■ Adolescent population aged 10–24

FIGURE 1.5 Population of adolescents 10 to 24 years old as a proportion of the total population, 1950 to 2050. 2050 estimates are based off of medium fertility rates. Fertility rates are grossly grouped into three categories: high, medium, and low; and fertility is more likely to have sizable impacts on future population size, growth and age structure than changes in mortality. Thus, population estimates for 2050 were selected using medium fertility rate data. Medium fertility rate is defined as a crude birth rate of 20–30/1000. (From United Nations, Department of Economic and Social Affairs, Population Division. *World population prospects: the 2012 revision*, DVD edition. 2013.)

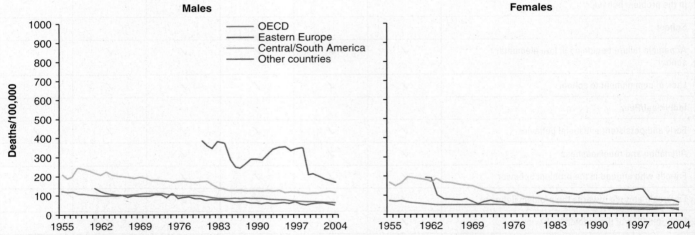

FIGURE 1.6 Trends in mortality rates 1955 to 2004, ages 10 to 24 years old, by country group. (From Viner RM, Coffey C, Mathers C, et al. 50-year mortality trends in children and young people: a study of 50 low-income, middle-income, and high-income countries. *Lancet* 2011;377(9772):1162–1174. Available at http://www.thelancet.com/journals/lancet/article/PIIS0140-6736(11)60106-2/fulltext)

in mortality of 1.6% to 2.0% per year among children aged 1 to 9 years,[17] mortality decreased by 1.4% to 2.0% per year among early adolescents (10 to 14 years), 1.2% to 1.7% per year in AYA females (15 to 24 years), and by 0.8% to 0.9% per year among AYA males (15 to 24 years) (Fig. 1.6). This is likely due to the health transition from infections to injuries and non-communicable diseases, which acts to shift disease burden from childhood to adolescence (e-Fig. 1.7).

• Mortality from communicable diseases among AYAs decreased by 20 to 50 times over the last 50 years (i.e., to 2% to 5% of the baseline level). Communicable diseases are now relatively uncommon causes of death, even in low-income countries. Similarly, there are low overall rates of mortality from nutritional disorders in this age-group, although nutrition is still a significant concern in certain populations and in some countries.

• Over the last 50 years, rates of maternal mortality (mortality related to pregnancies ending in birth, miscarriage, and abortion) decreased 12-fold in 21 high-income countries

belonging to the Organization for Economic Cooperation and Development (OECD)*. Mortality decreased seven-fold in Central and South American countries and 40-fold in other countries. From 2000 to 2004, maternal mortality accounted for 6% of mortality among young women in Central and South American countries, but only 1% of deaths in other regions.

• Despite declines in maternal mortality, adolescents are at higher risk of maternal death than older women; Latin American data show that death rates are 3 to 4 times higher among girls under 16 years old than women in their 20s.[18]

• In addition, an estimated 1 to 4 million unsafe abortions are performed on adolescent girls in developing world.[19] Unsafe abortion is estimated to be responsible for 13% of maternal deaths.

---

*OECD members included here are Australia, Austria, Canada, Denmark, Finland, France, Greece, Iceland, Ireland, Italy, Japan, Luxembourg, Netherlands, New Zealand, Norway, Portugal, Spain, Sweden, Switzerland, United Kingdom, and the US.

- Mortality due to AYA injuries (10 to 24 years old) increased between the 1950s and the late 1970s for both sexes in OECD, Central and South American countries. Since 1978 to 1982, injuries have been the leading cause of death in AYA males in all regions, causing 70% to 75% of overall mortality. Injuries have been the leading cause of mortality for AYA females in OECD and eastern European countries (53% to 55%). Relative to other causes, injuries are an important but less common cause of mortality among women in Central and South America (35%).

- MVCs and other transport injuries caused the greatest proportion of injury-related deaths in AYAs (10 to 24 years old) across most of the study period in all regions, with the exception of young men in Central and South American countries, where more injuries were due to violence.

- Violence-related mortality increased in males and females aged 10 to 24 years across all regions during the study period, both in absolute rate and as a proportion of overall mortality. By 2000 to 2004, violence accounted for one-third of deaths in males within this age-group in Central and South American countries and two-fifths of deaths in eastern European countries. For females, and for males in other regions, violence accounted for 8% to 15% of mortality (e-Figs. 1.8 to 1.10ab).

- There are an estimated 71,000 adolescent suicides every year, and the number who attempt suicide may be 40 times greater—almost 3 million. By 2000 to 2004, suicide accounted for 14% to 16% of deaths in young men in all regions except Central and South American countries (7%). Suicide was responsible for 11% of deaths in young women in OECD countries, 6% in Central and South American countries, 8% in eastern European countries, and 13% in other countries.

- It is unknown how many injury deaths are due to domestic or sexual violence. However, these deaths are prevalent to varying degrees in all countries. Accurate figures are difficult to obtain, but domestic or sexual violence was reported by 65% of adolescent females aged 15 to 19 in Uganda.

- The US data show that 4% of adolescent males and 11% of females reported that they had been forced to have sex[20] (e-Fig. 1.11).

The US Mortality

- The US data mirror global data in showing much smaller declines in age-specific mortality among AYAs than younger children. Between 1970 and 2010, young adult males have had the smallest declines of any age-group except for the very elderly[21] (e-Fig. 1.12).

- The US AYAs also have high rates of mortality compared to AYAs in comparable countries. In early adolescence (10 to 14 years), there is no difference in all-cause mortality between the US and comparable OECD countries. However, the US mortality among older AYAs (15 to 24 years) is significantly greater than peer countries, a finding that has been observed for many decades.[9]

- The causes of high AYA mortality in the US compared to other rich countries are not well understood. However, high levels of mortality are associated with poor ranking across a wide range of health outcomes and risk factors.[9]

- Cancer is the fourth highest cause of death among AYAs in the US, with the most common forms being lymphoma, leukemia, malignant melanoma, and central nervous system (CNS) cancers[6] (e-Fig. 1.13).

The US Mortality Related to Injuries

- Deaths in AYAs are dominated by unintentional injuries (particularly MVCs), homicide, and suicide. Together, these causes make up 47% of deaths among 10-year-olds, 81% among 18-year-olds, and equally high rates among young adults.

- Although high-quality health care services can save the lives of individuals suffering injuries, effective strategies to reduce injury-related deaths require public health interventions. For example, death rates from MVCs fell by 38% between 1988 and 1992. The decline in MVCs has been attributed to implementation of the 1984 Uniform Drinking Age Act, which required states to raise the legal age for drinking alcohol to 21.[12]

- The US is an outlier among developed countries on youth violence, with 3.4 million adolescents becoming victims of youth violence every year. The difference is particularly striking for firearms injuries. Among 26 high-income countries with populations exceeding 1 million, the US has more deaths among children and young people than the other 25 countries combined; rates of firearm-related death were nearly 12 times higher in the US than the other 25 countries.[22]

- Suicide is the third most common cause of death among AYAs in the US, and 17% of young people report having considered suicide. There is evidence that suicide is influenced by different factors among AYAs than older groups. Relative to older groups, suicide among young veterans was more likely to be associated with relationship problems or misuse of alcohol and other substances. In contrast, suicide among older veterans was more strongly related to financial and medical concerns.

- Similarly, suicide in younger groups is more commonly associated with impulsive and aggressive behaviors. The important role of impulsive behavior in AYA suicide reinforces the potential benefit of limiting access to firearms—around one in three firearms deaths among young people are self-inflicted.[6]

Disparities in the US Mortality

- The US mortality among all races increases throughout adolescence and young adulthood, and large racial disparities persist in all age-groups. Black AYAs have the highest mortality rates (122.4 deaths/100,000 20 to 24 year olds; 19.1/100,000 10 to 14 year olds). AYAs of Asian/Pacific Islander descent have the lowest rates (36.9 and 7.8 deaths/100 000, respectively).[6]

- Causes of mortality differ by racial groups and by sex in the US.
  - Among Black young adult males (aged 20 to 24 years), homicide is by far the most common cause of death (93.0/100,000/year—more than twice the rate of accidental deaths (37.8) and 6 times the rate of suicide (15.9).
  - In contrast, among White young adult females (age 20 to 24 years), accidents are the dominant cause of death (20.0/100,000), followed by suicide (5.0) and malignant neoplasms (3.4). Homicides are the 4th leading cause (2.6/100,000).
  - There were 2.7 homicides and 1.3 suicides/100,000 among Black males aged 10 to 14 years in the US. For White males in this age-group, the figures were 0.7 and 1.8/100,000, respectively.
  - See e-Table 1.1.

● MORBIDITY

Overview of Global and the US Morbidity

Years Lived with Disability (YLDs) and Disability Adjusted Life Years (DALYs) are measures of disease burden due to nonfatal health outcomes, or morbidity, and allow comparison of the relative disease burden associated with different risk factors and disease categories. As with mortality, adolescence and young adulthood is a time of transition from childhood patterns of morbidity—dominated at a global level by nutritional deficiencies and infections (diarrhea, pneumonia)—to adult patterns with high levels of mental health and musculoskeletal disorders[4,23] (e-Fig. 1.14).

More than 10% of American young adults (aged 18 to 24 years) report disability due to a physical, mental, or emotional condition.[6] Prevalence of many chronic conditions increases throughout adolescence and young adulthood. Some cause symptoms and influence quality of life in both the short and long term. For example, diabetes is diagnosed in about 1% of 18- to 25-year-olds and 2% of 26- to 34-year-olds (although others have diabetes which is undiagnosed). In contrast, rates of other conditions, such as hypertension, increase during adolescence and young adulthood; however, the effects may not be noticed until later in life.[6] Figure 1.7 illustrates the relative contribution of leading risk factors to overall morbidity (expressed as DALYs) in the US population, broken down by the causes of increased morbidity in each case.

Mental Health

- Approximately 20% of the world's adolescents are affected by mental health or behavioral problems.
- The prevalence of psychiatric disorders increases through adolescence in both males and females, peaking in late adolescence for males and the late 20s for females.
- Seventy-five percent of lifetime cases of mental health disorders (excluding dementia) present by 24 years.

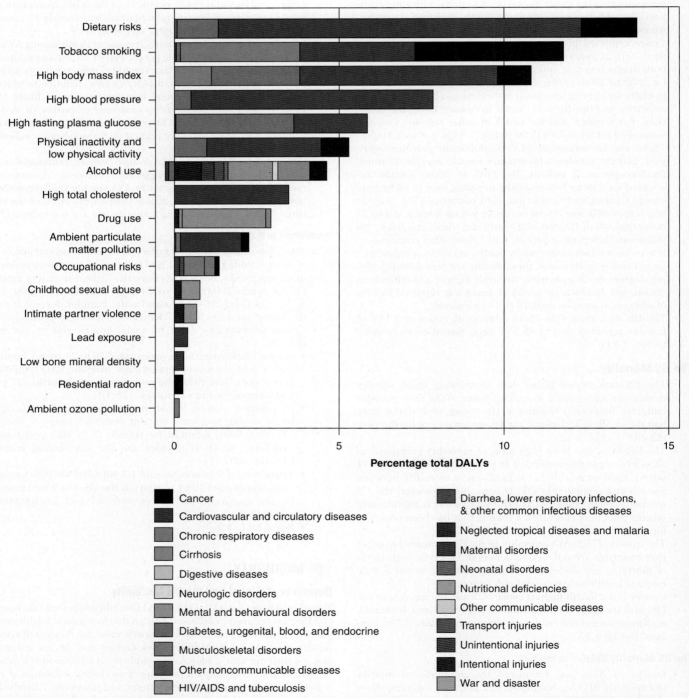

FIGURE 1.7 Percentage of DALYs attributable to the 17 leading risk factors, both sexes, all ages, US, 2010. (From Institute for Health Metrics and Evaluation. *The State of US Health: innovations, insights, and recommendations from the Global Burden of Disease Study*. Seattle, WA: IHME, 2013. Available at http://www .healthequity.umd.edu/documents/IHME_GBD_US_FINAL_PRINTED%20070513.pdf)

- Among AYAs, mental and behavioral disorders account for an estimated 184 million DALYs lost worldwide.[24] This measure combines years of life lost (YLLs) due to premature mortality and YLDs.
- A nationally representative longitudinal survey tracked youth in the US from early adolescence until their 30s. Overall, they found that around 20% met criteria for a psychiatric disorder within any 3-month period. Over half of these (11% of the total) met the criteria for two or more disorders.[25] By age 25, more than 60% had experienced a defined psychiatric disorder and an additional 20% reported psychiatric symptoms or impairment but did not meet formal diagnostic criteria[25] (e-Fig. 1.15).

Sexual and Reproductive Health

AYAs are an important age-group for prevention and treatment of sexually transmitted infections (STIs).

- Globally, 41% of behaviorally acquired HIV infections occurred in 15- to 24-year-olds.[26]
- The proportion of young women reporting that they had sex before the age of 15 is highest in Latin America and Caribbean (22% of women) and lowest in Asia.
- In the US, around half of all STI diagnoses each year occur in 15- to 24-year-olds.
- The US is an outlier among developed countries in teenage pregnancy, with rates 4 to 10 times higher than most Western European countries. Among 15- to 19-year-old girls, 8.4% become pregnant each year and 4% give birth (over 2,000 pregnancies and 1,100 deliveries/day).[6]
- Forty-seven percent of high school students report having had sexual intercourse, increasing from 12% of 7th graders to more than 60% of 12th graders. Fifteen percent of high school students reported having more than 3 partners. Teen birth rates in the US have fallen by approximately 50% between 1991 and 2012. Much of the decline in the US teen pregnancy since 1991 is the result of improved contraceptive use—with some contribution from youth who choose to remain abstinent.[27]
- Contraceptive methods are less likely to be effective among adolescents: 62% reported using a condom at last intercourse, of whom only two-thirds reported successful use.[6]
- Unmarried women in their 20s account for more than 2,700 unplanned pregnancies/day. About 1,600 abortions/day are performed on women in their 20s (around half of all abortions).
- About 20 million new STIs occur in the US/year, with about half among AYAs. Incidence of STIs is approximately equal in males and females.[6]
- Each year, young adults account for 4.6 million cases of human papillomavirus, 1.9 million cases of trichomoniasis, and 1.5 million cases of chlamydia.
- One in ten young adults in their 20s has genital herpes infection. The prevalence is estimated to be about one in three among Black, non-Hispanic young adults.
- Around 50,000 people in the US are diagnosed with HIV every year. The highest incidence is among young adults aged 20 to 29 years.[6]

Health Behaviors

The 2010 Global Burden of Disease study identified the 10 risk factors which were responsible for the highest burden of disability and premature death. Of these, two (smoking and drinking alcohol) are largely initiated during adolescence, while others such as diet, overweight/obesity, and physical inactivity are strongly determined by behaviors and attitudes acquired during this period.[28]

Morbidity in the US is broadly similar, although smoking and alcohol are responsible for less death and disability than in many other high-income countries, while obesity and dietary factors are more important.

- Prevalence of recommended physical activity for 15-year-olds is presented in Figure 1.8 for 43 high-income countries. e-Figures 1.16 to 1.18 present weekly smoking, weekly alcohol intake, and overweight/obesity among the same group.
- The US has the highest overall rates of physical activity, with 33% of males and 17% of females reporting at least one hour of moderate/vigorous physical activity daily (see Fig. 1.8).
- The US also has lower levels of smoking and alcohol use than many comparable countries (ranked fourth and fifth, respectively).
- However, the US has the highest rates of overweight/obesity (34% of males, 27% of females). Cross-country comparisons of the proportion of 15- to 19-year-old girls who are overweight and underweight are presented in Figures 1.9 and 1.10.

Smoking

- Approximately 80% of lifetime smokers initiate the habit as adolescents. Earlier age of initiation is linked to higher consumption in adulthood and greater mortality from smoking-related conditions.
- The US data show that 22% of 8th graders report smoking, increasing to 46.2% of 12th graders.
- Cigarette smoking in the US adolescents had declined steadily since the late 1990s, while the proportion using marijuana has plateaued during this time (e-Fig. 1.19).

Alcohol

- AYAs drink on fewer occasions per month, but are more likely to binge drink than older adults (e-Fig. 1.20).

Obesity/Overweight

- AYA obesity rates across OECD countries are high and have increased in recent decades.
- Among young people in the US, obesity rates tripled between 1991 and 1999. Subsequently, the trajectory has slowed; currently, 31.9% of children and youth are ≥85th percentile for body mass index.[6]
- 80% of the US adolescents who are obese at the age of 18 will remain obese throughout their lives.[6]
- In developed countries, dietary campaigns have focused on increasing consumption of fruit and vegetables. On average, young adults aged 18 to 25 years in the US eat about two portions of fruit or vegetables per day, compared with the recommended five.[6]
- Compared to other high-income countries, AYAs in the US have relatively high levels of physical activity.[29] Around 60% meet the recommended national guidelines.[6]
- Some developing countries are now seeing a "double nutrition" burden, where obesity is increasing alongside undernutrition. More than 20% of females aged 15 to 19 years are overweight in several developing countries.[19]
- In nine countries, more than half of all females aged 15 to 19 are anemic (India and eight countries in West/Central Africa). Underweight, anemia, and other nutritional deficiencies increase the risk of pregnancy and childbirth for both mother and baby[19] (e-Fig. 1.21).

The US Trends in Risk Factors among AYAs

Worsening trends[30]:

- Binge drinking
- Marijuana use among 12- to 17-year-olds
- Obesity rates
- Higher rates of chlamydia, attendance at family planning clinics and STI clinics.

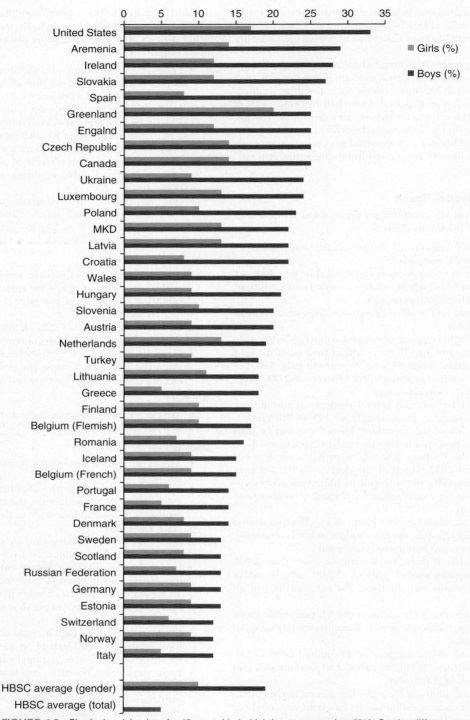

FIGURE 1.8 Physical activity data for 15-year-olds in high-income countries, 2010. Gender differences significant (at p < 0.05) for all countries except Greenland. (From Currie C, Zanotti C, Morgan A, et al., eds. *Social determinants of health and well-being among young people. Health Behaviour in School-aged Children (HBSC) study: international report from the 2009/2010 survey.* Copenhagen, WHO Regional Office for Europe (Health Policy for Children and Adolescents, No. 6). 2012:131. Available at http://www.euro.who.int/__data/assets/pdf_file/0003/163857/Social-determinants-of-health-and-well-being-among-young-people.pdf?ua=1)

Improving trends:

- Adolescents pregnancy (15- to 17-year-olds)
- More adolescents have never had sex
- Higher condom use among sexually active adolescents
- Smoking

No change in rates:

- Physical activity

HEALTH CARE UTILIZATION

Global Overview

- There is a lack of reliable data regarding health care utilization among AYAs—either at a regional or country level. Many countries report health care statistics in very broad age ranges (e.g., 15- to 44-year-olds or 15- to 64-year-olds). In a recent overview of adolescent health indicators, health service use

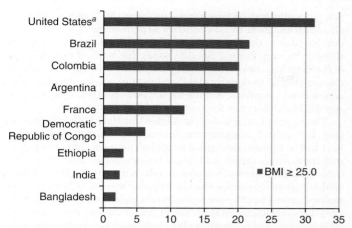

FIGURE 1.9 Percentage of adolescent girls 15 to 19 years old are overweight, by selected countries. Countries selected by top 40 in population and available data for specified age range. Data ranges from 2000 to 2007. [a]Age range for the US is 10 to 17 years old; BMI is calculated as at or above the 85th percentile of the CDC growth charts for age and gender. Age range for France is 15 to 24 years old. (Adapted from US Data: Child and Adolescent Health Measurement Initiative. 2011 National Survey of Children's Health, Data Resource Center for Child and Adolescent Health website. Available at http://www.childhealthdata.org/home. Accessed August 2014. All Other Data: World Health Organizations. *Nutrition Landscape Information Systems: Integrated WHO Nutrition Global Databases, User-defined customized data function: Body Mass Index.* Available at http://apps.who.int/nutrition/landscape/search.aspx?dm=53&countries=704&year=all&sf1=nb.dc.0710&sex=2)

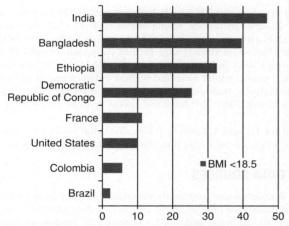

FIGURE 1.10 Percentage of adolescent girls 15 to 19 years old who are underweight, by selected countries. Countries selected by top 40 in population and available data for specified age range. Data ranges from 2000 to 2007. Age range for the US is 16 to 19 years old; Age range for France is 15 to 24 years old. (From World Health Organizations. *Nutrition Landscape Information Systems: Integrated WHO Nutrition Global Databases, User-defined customized data function: Body Mass Index.* Available at http://apps.who.int/nutrition/landscape/search.aspx?dm=53&countries=704&year=all&sf1=nb.dc.0710&sex=2)

was the only indicator for which no comparable country-level data were available.

- The WHO has advocated for universal access to health care among all age-groups and in all countries. In addition to financial barriers, many of the world's AYAs do not receive adequate health care for a variety of reasons, including lack of awareness/engagement with their health, concerns about the confidentiality or quality of the service offered, and practical and transport problems.
- Unmet health care needs in adolescence is associated with a range of poor health outcomes, including higher prevalence of physical and mental health symptoms, and higher rates of risk behaviors.
- In rich countries with universal access to health care, adolescence is a time of increasing health care utilization. This is especially true for females whose health service use is greater among adolescents than children aged 1 to 9 years.[31]

The US Overview

- In the US, average health care expenditures for both adolescents (12 to 17 years) and young adults (18- to 25-year-olds) are around $2,000/year. Among young adults, 17% of health care expenditure was out of pocket; a similar proportion of expenditure was out of pocket among adolescents (12 to 17 years) and older adults (≥26 years).[6]
- In 2010, AYAs (15- to 24-year-olds) accounted for 8.1% of all office visits, an average of 1.9 visits/person.
- In 2007, AYAs (15- to 24-year-olds) accounted for 16.3% of all emergency department (ED) visits, an average of 0.46 visits/person.
- Among the US adolescents aged 10 to 14 years, the most common reasons for attending an ED were superficial injuries, sprains/strains, upper respiratory infections, asthma, and abdominal pain. Among those who were admitted from the ED, the most common categories were asthma, appendicitis, mood disorder, attention deficit hyperactivity disorder and behavioral disorders, and fluid/electrolyte disorders.
- For those aged 15 to 17 years, the reasons were similar, although there were fewer visits/admissions for asthma, and higher rates of mood disorders and injuries.
- See e-Figs. 1.22 and 1.23.

Insurance Coverage and Access to Health Care

- The US is unique among developed countries in having significant numbers of AYAs with no or inadequate health care insurance.[16]
- AYA health care usage is influenced by insurance coverage. For example, young adults (18 to 24 years) are less likely to have health insurance and are more likely to access care at an ED, compared to adolescents (12 to 17 years).[32]
- The US survey data show a gradual reduction in the number of youth under 18 years old with no usual source of health care, from 7.7% in 1993 to 1994 to 4.7% in 2010 to 2011. However, the proportion is much higher among some subgroups (e.g., 7.9% of Hispanics, 12.8% who have been uninsured for up to 12 months, and 36.2% of those who have been uninsured for over 12 months).[33]
- The number of uninsured young adults decreased following passage of the Affordable Care Act (ACA), 2010. Under these reforms, young adults are entitled to be covered by their parents' insurance until age 26 years. Young adults are an important target group for the health insurance exchanges. Despite the ACA, young adults remain the most likely population to be uninsured in the US with over 20% of 19- to 26-year-olds lacking coverage. Among insured young adults, many have catastrophic health insurance coverage, which may not provide adequate access to care (e-Fig. 1.24).
- Prior to these health care reforms, young adults reported the lowest rates of insurance coverage of any age-group. This was due in part to the trend away from employer-provided insurance, which covered 31% of college graduates aged 21 to 24 in 2011, compared to 60% in 1989. Similar trends are seen among high school graduates aged 17 to 20, whose coverage dropped from 24% to 7% during this period.[6]
- Disparities in health care utilization reflect both differential access and health care need. Consistent with the high mortality rates from violence among young Black males, 2011 hospital data recorded 150,000 violent injuries among Black AYA males (aged 15 to 34), representing about 1 of every 41 males in this demographic.[6]

**Mental Health Services Utilization
by AYAs in the US**

- Only 1 in 4 young adults with a psychiatric disorder are receiving mental health services.[6]
- Poor communication and coordination between pediatric and adult mental health systems hinder continuity and care quality.[6]
- When attending mental health services, AYAs (aged 16 to 30 years) are more likely to drop out of treatment than older adults.[6]

Defining and Improving the Quality of AYA Health and Health Promotion Services.

Health Services

- Adolescence and young adulthood are often perceived as healthy times of life. Services for AYAs are often a low priority and do not meet the specific needs of this population.
- Most countries have few dedicated AYA services, although such services have been shown to improve quality of care.
- There is an increasing recognition and evidence base regarding the distinct health care needs and priorities of AYAs.[16] In many cases, these needs are similar for AYAs across the world.[34] For example, confidentiality and communications skills of health care providers are important in both the US and low-income countries, although distinct cultural factors are present for each country.
- Targeted age-appropriate health services can improve health outcomes in chronic conditions.[35]
- For many conditions, outcomes worsen in early adulthood as independent management coincides with transition to adult services and geographic movement for study/work.[36] Self-efficacy intervention improves quality of life among adolescents with chronic conditions.
- Since the publication of the 2002 WHO Agenda for Change, there have been policy efforts toward age-appropriate, adolescent friendly health care in every WHO region.[19]
- Several quality frameworks and tools have been published to support professionals in improving the quality of service for AYAs. They include an Australian framework for AYA inpatient care,[37] European primary care and inpatient tools, which have been endorsed by the WHO, and the US models like those for AYA mental health services and cancer care and follow-up.[6]

Health Promotion

- The US data show that provision of school-based health centers is associated with better experience of adolescent care and more healthy behaviors (e.g., use of appropriate contraception).
- Integrating the literature on social determinants of health, life-course perspectives, and evolving transition processes may inform more effective, evidence-based public health interventions in the future. For example, peer-led smoking interventions may be more likely to engage young people than awareness campaigns or interventions delivered purely by professionals.
- Similarly, programs that foster a positive and healthy self-identity may be more effective at reducing risk behaviors among AYAs than traditional interventions. Evaluation of programs that use fear to reduce risk behaviors (e.g., the anticrime Scared Straight program) or intensive professional/group support (Cambridge-Somerville Youth Study) has shown that outcomes among participants were sometimes worse than among controls.[38]

● SUMMARY: HEALTH OF THE WORLD'S AYAs

The current generation of AYAs represents the global workforce of the next 40 years; so maintaining and improving the health, happiness, and productivity of this population should be a priority.

Yet economic and social changes threaten the health of AYAs in all countries, from those countries experiencing rapid economic development to the "post-industrial" countries such as the US and those in Western Europe. Specific issues that warrant the attention of professionals, researchers, and policy makers include the shift in disease burden from early childhood to adolescence, youth bulges across many countries, and the impact and economic evaluation of specific health services for young people

The Lancet Commission on Adolescent Health and Wellbeing, launched in 2014, examines the diverse determinants of adolescent health. The Commission called for global, national, and local policy makers to work across traditional boundaries to improve health outcomes. This approach is equally relevant to the health of young adults: Potential gains for most health outcomes in AYAs will not be realized unless health care professionals engage more broadly with the issues highlighted in this chapter, including education systems, labor markets and economic policy, legislation governing substance use and driving licensing, access to clean water and healthy food, community and cultural influences on behavior, and opportunities for participation and volunteering.

The US has a very different pattern of AYA mortality and morbidity compared to other wealthy democratic countries. Aside from infancy, it is among AYA groups that the discrepancy is highest, with morbidity and mortality from violence central to this discrepancy. Resolving this discrepancy will require a focus on the social determinants of health related to inequalities, deprivation, and ethnicity.

● SUPPLEMENTAL DATA ON MORBIDITY AND MORTALITY OF AYAS IN THE US

While AYAs in the US face behavioral and nonbehavioral health risks, in most instances, young adults aged 18 to 25 face greater risks than either adolescents aged 12 to 17 or adults aged 26 to 34. In addition, some studies suggest that young adults aged 18 to 25 have the lowest perception of risk and the lowest access to care. Overall, young adults have the highest rates of motor vehicle injury and death, homicide, mental health problems, STIs, and substance abuse. They also have the lowest rates of health insurance coverage.[1]

Tables 1.1 and 1.2 review the health behavioral risks in adolescents versus young adults plus the trends in these behaviors.

● DATA SOURCES

AYA demographics, morbidity, mortality, and health behaviors change from year to year. The most current data are typically available on the Internet and can be accessed by readers seeking the most up-to-date information. Two excellent sources of data on AYAs are available at:

1. www.usc.edu/thenewadolescents. This comprehensive monograph compares morbidity and mortality across AYAs aged 12 to 17, 18 to 25, and 26 to 34 years.
2. http://www.jahonline.org/article/S1054-139X(14)00166-9/abstract?cc=y. Parks et al. provide a comprehensive review of the trends and risks in both the AYA population in the US (this is the source for **Tables 1.1, 1.2, and 1.3** in this chapter) (**Table 1.3**).[1]

In addition, the following resources provide important data about AYA health.

General

1. *Health US, 2014* (http://www.cdc.gov/nchs/data/hus/hus14.pdf): Health, US, 2013 is an annual report on trends in health statistics. The report consists of two main sections—a chartbook containing text and figures that illustrate major trends in the health of Americans and a trend tables section.

TABLE 1.1

Summary of Trends in Adolescent and Young Adult Health in the US, 2000 to 2012

Outcome	Ages	Year[a]	Time 1	Time 2	Change	Ages	Year	Time 1	Time 2	Change
Overall health, function, and mortality										
Health is excellent, very good, or good[b]	10–17	2000–2012	98.1%	97.3%	→	18–25	2000–2012	96.5%	95.4%	→
Limitation of activity[b]	10–17	2000–2012	8.5%	10.7%	→	18–25	2000–2012	4.3%	5.8%	→
Mortality (rate per 100,000)	15–19	2000–2010	66.8	51.2	↓	20–24	2000–2010	93.1	90.9	→
Injury										
MVC mortality (rate per 100,000)	15–19	2000–2010	25.3	13.6	↓	20–24	2000–2010	27.3	19.7	↓
Percent alcohol impaired among drivers involved in fatal crashes (BAC ≥ 0.08)	16–20	2002–2012	18%	18%	→	21–24	2002–2012	33%	32%	→
Drove under the influence of alcohol (past year)	12–17	2002–2012	10.6%	6.3%	↓	18–25	2002–2012	33.2%	22.5%	↓
Rode with drinking driver (past month)	9–12 grade	2001–2011	30.7%	24.1%	↓	ND				
Sometimes, most of the time, or always wore a seat belt[c]	9–12 grade	2001–2011	85.9%	92.3%	↑	18–24	2006–2010	94.3%	95.5%	→
Violence										
Homicide deaths (rate per 100,000)	15–19	2000–2010	9.4	8.3	→	20–24	2000–2010	15.8	13.2	→
Simple assault[d] (rate per 1,000)	15–17	2002–2012	44.6	28.0	↓	18–20	2002–2012	46.2	26.4	↓
Aggravated assault[e] (rate per 1,000)	15–17	2002–2012	12	3.5	↓	18–20	2002–2012	15	9.8	↓
Physical fighting (past year)	9–12 grade	2001–2011	33.2%	32.8%	→	ND				
Weapon carrying (past month)	9–12 grade	2001–2011	17.4%	16.6%	→	ND				
Mental health										
Suicide deaths (rate per 100,000)	15–19	2000–2010	8.0	7.5	→	20–24	2000–2010	12.5	13.6	→
Major depressive episode (past year)	12–17	2005–2012	8.6%	9.3%	→	18–25	2005–2012	8.7%	9.0%	→
Suicide attempt (past year)	9–12 grade	2001–2011	8.8%	7.8%	→	ND				
Used diet pills, powders and liquids, vomiting, or laxatives to lose weight (past month)	9–12 grade	2001–2011	9.2%	5.1%	↓	ND				
ADHD	10–17	(2001–2003)–(2010–2012)	8.8%	11.8%	→	ND				
Substance abuse										
Cigarette use (past month)	12–17	2002–2012	13.0%	6.7%	↓	18–25	2002–2012	40.8%	31.9%	↓
Alcohol use (past month)	12–17	2002–2012	17.6%	12.9%	↓	18–25	2002–2012	60.5%	60.2%	→
Binge alcohol use (past month)	12–17	2002–2012	10.8%	7.1%	→	18–25	2002–2012	41.0%	39.5%	→

(Continued)

TABLE 1.1

Summary of Trends in Adolescent and Young Adult Health in the US, 2000 to 2012 (*Continued*)

Outcome	Adolescents					Young Adults				
	Ages	Year[a]	Time 1	Time 2	Change	Ages	Year	Time 1	Time 2	Change
Substance abuse (*continued*)										
Heavy drinking: five or more binge episodes (past month)	12–17	2002–2012	2.6%	1.3%	→	18–25	2002–2012	15.0%	12.9%	→
Marijuana use (past month)	12–17	2002–2012	8.2%	7.3%	→	18–25	2002–2012	17.3%	18.5%	→
Sexual and reproductive health										
Never had vaginal intercourse: females[f]	15–19	2002–(2007–2010)	47.0%	52.6%	↑	20–24	2002–(2007–2010)	12.7%	12.9%	→
Never had vaginal intercourse: males[f]	15–19	2002–(2007–2010)	51.1%	56.3%	↑	20–24	2002–(2007–2010)	12.5%	15.5%	→
Never had same-sex sexual contact: females[f]	15–19	2002–(2006–2008)	89.4%	89.0%	→	20–24	2002–(2006–2008)	85.8%	84.2%	→
Never had same-sex sexual contact: males[f]	15–19	2002–(2006–2008)	95.5%	97.5%	→	20–24	2002–(2006–2008)	94.5%	94.4%	→
Contraceptive use by women at risk of unintended pregnancy[g]	15–19	2002–(2006–2010)	82.0%	82.0%	→	20–24	2002–(2006–2010)	87.9%	87.0%	→
Condom use at last intercourse	9–12 grade	2001–2011	57.9%	60.2%	→	ND				
Pregnancy[f] (rate per 1,000)	15–19	2001–2009	80.8	65.6	↓	20–24	2001–2009	173.7	153.8	↓
Births[f] (rate per 1,000)	15–19	2000–2012	47.7	29.4	↓	20–24	2000–2012	109.7	83.1	↓
Unintended births	15–19	2002–(2006–2010)	78.4%	77.2%	→	20–24	2002–(2006–2010)	44.0%	50.1%	↑
Chlamydia (rate per 100,000)	15–19	2001–2011	1408.0	2076.1	↑	20–24	2001–2011	1434.5	2,508.5	↑
Gonorrhea (rate per 100,000)	15–19	2001–2011	494.3	398.6	↓	20–24	2001–2011	584.6	516.0	↓
HIV diagnoses (rate per 100,000)	15–19	2008–2011	10.4	10.4	→	20–24	2008–2011	31.4	36.4	↑
Chronic conditions and related behaviors										
Special health care needs prevalence	12–17	(2005–2006)–(2009–2010)	16.8%	18.4%	→	ND				
Hearing loss (≥15 dB)	16–17	(1988–1994)–(2005–2006)	14.9%	21.5%	↑	18–19	(1988–1994)–(2005–2006)	15.2%	20.1%	↑
Current asthma prevalence	10–17	(2003–2005)–(2009–2011)	9.9%	11.1%	→	18–24	(2003–2005)–(2009–2011)	7.5%	8.7%	→
Lifetime asthma diagnosis prevalence	10–17	(2003–2005)–(2009–2011)	14.9%	17.5%	→	18–24	(2003–2005)–(2009–2011)	12.7%	16.5%	→
Obese	12–19	(2001–2002)–(2009–2010)	16.7%	18.4%	→	20–24	(2001–2002)–(2007–2008)	24.1%	28.7%	↑
Chronic conditions and related behaviors–Physical activity										
Adolescents: exercised for at least 60 min on ≥5 d	9–12 grade	2005–2011	35.8%	49.5%	↑	ND				
Young adults: met guidelines for physical activity (150 min/wk)	ND					18–24	(2001–2003)–(2010–2012)	53.1%	59.3%	↑
Television viewing (≥3 h/d)	9–12 grade	2001–2011	38.3%	32.4%	↓	ND				
Games/Internet (≥3 h/d)	9–12 grade	2003–2011	22.1%	31.1%	↑	ND				

(Continued)

TABLE 1.1

Summary of Trends in Adolescent and Young Adult Health in the US, 2000 to 2012 (*Continued*)

Summary of Trends in Health care Access and Utilization

Outcome	Adolescents (10–17)			Young Adults (18–25)		
	2000 (%)	2012 (%)	Change	2000 (%)	2012 (%)	Change
Full-year insured	84.8	88.9	↑	63.9	69.3	↑
Full-year uninsured	7.7	5.2	→	18.7	17.7	→
Partial-year uninsured	7.5	6.0	→	17.4	13.0	↓
Usual place when sick	91.6	94.8	→	74.8	73.1	→
Had doctor visit besides hospital, ER, and surgery (past year)	83.3	88.1	↑	73.3	70.7	→
Had well checkup (past year)	62.7	73.8	↑	ND	ND	
Had one or more ER visit (past year)	18.0	14.5	→	25.8	22.5	→
Dentist visit (past year)	81.4	87.2	↑	52.3	61.0	↑
Delay in care (past year)	7.2	8.7	→	9.3	10.5	→
Unmet need for dental care (past year)	7.3	7.1	→	11.7	13.4	→
Unmet need for prescriptions (past year)	2.4	2.6	→	7.6	7.3	→
Youth with special health care needs who received transition care	(2005–2006) 41.2	(2009–2010) 40.0	→	ND	ND	

↑ = Up; ↓ = Down; → = little or no change; Green = healthy change; Red = unhealthy change.
ADHD = attention deficit hyperactivity disorder; BAC = blood alcohol content; ER = emergency room; ND = no data.
[a]Although we aimed for data points spanning about 10 y, sources with at least 6 y are included. Two exceptions are for HIV incidence and young adult seat belt use, for which only 3 and 4 y of data, respectively, could be located. Trend data for HIV incidence are limited because of a change in data collection methodology in 2008. Another exception is the 17- span for the trend in hearing loss, a Healthy People 2020 core indicator.
[b]The measures "health is excellent, very good, or good" and "limitation of activity" are measures obtained from the National Health Interview Survey. Adolescent data were collected via parent report, whereas the data for young adults were self-reported.
[c]The adolescent and young adult seat belt data were collected from different sources, and the wording differs slightly. The adolescent measure, retrieved from Youth Risk Behavior Surveillance System, shows the percentage who "Sometimes, Most of the Time, or Always Wore a Seatbelt," and the question specifically asks the respondent to report on instances in which they are in the car while someone else is driving. The young adult measure, retrieved from Behavior Risk Factor Surveillance System, shows the percentage that "Sometimes, Nearly Always, or Always Wore Seatbelts."
[d]An attack or attempted attack without a weapon that results in no injury, minor injury (e.g., bruises, black eyes, cuts, scratches, or swelling), or an undetermined injury requiring <2 d of hospitalization.
[e]An attack or attempted attack with a weapon, regardless of whether the victim is injured, or an attack without a weapon when serious injury results.
[f]This review does not assess whether young adult trends in sexual experience, pregnancy, and childbirth are healthy or unhealthy; therefore, arrows are not color coded as healthy or unhealthy.
[g]"Women at risk of unintended pregnancy" refer to women who have a chance of becoming pregnant at the date of interview but do not want to become pregnant now: They are either (1) using a contraceptive method or (2) they are not using contraception, but they have had intercourse in the 3 mo before the interview and are not pregnant or trying to become pregnant.
From Park MJ, Scott JT, Adams SH, et al. Adolescent and young adult health in the US in the past decade: little improvement and young adults remain worse off. *J Adolesc Health* 2014;55:3–16.

2. *Abstract of the United States, 2012* (http://www.census.gov/library/publications/2011/compendia/statab/131ed.html): Each year the Census Bureau publishes data related to US demographics, health, education, and a wide range of other areas.

3. *Healthy People 2020* (http://www.healthypeople.gov/): This document outlines national health promotion and disease prevention objectives that are monitored and updated over time. New in this version is a section of AYA health ranging in age from 10 to 19 and 20 to 24.

4. *Add Health* (http://www.cpc.unc.edu/projects/addhealth): Add Health is a nationally representative study that explores the causes of health-related behaviors of adolescents in grades 7 through 12 and their outcomes in young adulthood. Add Health examines how social contexts (families, friends, peers, schools, neighborhoods, and communities) influence adolescents' health and risk behaviors. Wave 1, initiated in 1994, is the largest, most comprehensive survey of adolescents ever undertaken. Data at the individual, family, school, and community levels were collected in two waves between 1994 and 1996. In 2001 and 2002, Add Health respondents, 18 to 26 years old, were reinterviewed in a third wave to investigate

the influence that adolescence has on young adulthood. Numerous public and restricted release datasets are available. Longitudinal data are collected on such attributes as height, weight, pubertal development, mental health status (focusing on depression, the most common mental health problem among adolescents), and chronic and disabling conditions. Data are gathered from adolescents themselves, their parents, and school administrators. Already existing databases provide information about neighborhoods and communities

5. Childstats.gov (http://www.childstats.gov): This Web site offers easy access to federal and state statistics and reports on children and their families, including population and family characteristics, economic security, health, behavior and social environment, and education. Reports of the Federal Interagency Forum on Child and Family Statistics include *America's Children: Key National Indicators of Well-Being*, the annual federal monitoring report on the status of the nation's children, and *Nurturing Fatherhood*. In 2014, the Federal Interagency Forum on Child and Family Statistics published *America's Young Adults: Special Issue, 2014*, a one-time report on young adults in the US, aged 18 to 24.

TABLE 1.2

Current Health Status of AYAs in the US

Measure	Year	Adolescents[a]	Young Adults	Healthier
Overall health, function, and mortality				
Health is excellent, very good, or good[b]	2012	97.3%	95.4%	≈[c]
Limitation of activity[b]	2012	10.7%	5.8%	YA
Mortality (rate per 100,000)	2010	51.2	90.9	Adol
Injury				
Motor vehicle crash mortality (rate per 100,000)	2010	13.6	19.7	Adol
Percent alcohol impaired among drivers involved in fatal crashes (BAC ≥ 0.08)	2012	18%	32%	Adol
Drove under the influence of alcohol (past year)	2012	6.3%	22.5%	Adol
Sometimes, most of the time, or always wore a seat belt[d]	2011	92.3%	95.5% (2010)[e]	≈
Violence				
Homicide deaths (rate per 100,000)	2010	8.3	13.2	≈
Simple assault[f] (rate per 1,000)	2012	28.0	26.4	≈
Aggravated assault[f] (rate per 1,000)	2012	3.5	9.8	Adol
Mental health				
Suicide deaths (rate per 100,000)	2010	7.5	13.6	Adol
Major depressive episode (past year)	2012	9.3%	9.0%	≈
Substance use				
Cigarette use (past month)	2012	6.7%	31.9%	Adol
Alcohol use (past month)	2012	12.9%	60.2%	Adol
Binge alcohol use (past month)	2012	7.1%	39.5%	Adol
Heavy drinking: five or more binge episodes (past month)	2012	1.3%	12.9%	Adol
Marijuana use (past month)	2012	7.3%	18.5%	Adol
Sexual and reproductive health				
Never had vaginal intercourse: females	2007–2010	52.6%	12.9%	g
Never had vaginal intercourse: males	2007–2010	56.3%	15.5%	g
Never had same-sex sexual contact: females	2006–2008	89.0%	84.2%	g
Never had same-sex sexual contact: males	2006–2008	97.5%	94.4%	g
More than five opposite-sex sexual partners (past year): females[h]	2006–2010	3.5%	3.2%	≈
More than five opposite-sex sexual partners (past year): males	2006–2010	3.6%	6.8%	≈
Contraceptive use by women at risk of unintended pregnancy[i]	2006–2010	82.0%	87.0%	Adol
Pregnancy (rate per 1,000)	2009	65.6	153.8	g
Births (rate per 1,000)	2012	29.4	83.1	g
Unintended births	2006–2010	77.2%	50.1%	YA
Chlamydia (rate per 100,000)	2011	2076.1	2508.5	Adol

(*Continued*)

TABLE 1.2

Current Health Status of AYAs in the US (*Continued*)

Measure	Year	Adolescents[a]	Young Adults	Healthier
Sexual and reproductive health (*continued*)				
Gonorrhea (rate per 100,000)	2011	398.6	516.0	Adol
HIV diagnoses (rate per 100,000)	2011	10.4	36.4	Adol
Chronic conditions and related behaviors				
Dental decay present[j]	2007–2008	15.3%	27.9%	Adol
Hearing loss (≥15 dB)	2005–2006	21.5%	20.1%	≈
Current asthma prevalence	2009–2011	11.1%	8.7%	≈
Lifetime asthma diagnosis prevalence	2009–2011	17.5%	16.5%	≈
Obese	2009–2010	18.4%	28.7% (2007–2008)[e]	Adol
Health care access and utilization (past year)				
Full-year insured	2012	88.9%	69.3%	Adol
Full-year uninsured	2012	5.2%	17.7%	Adol
Partial-year uninsured	2012	6.0%	13.0%	Adol
Usual place when sick	2012	94.8%	73.1%	Adol
Had doctor visit besides hospital, ER, and surgery (past year)	2012	88.1%	70.7%	Adol
Had one or more ER visit (past year)	2012	14.5%	22.5%	Adol
Dentist visit (past year)	2012	87.2%	61.0%	Adol
Delay in care (past year)	2012	8.7%	10.5%	≈
Unmet need for dental care (past year)	2012	7.1%	13.4%	Adol
Unmet need for prescriptions (past year)	2012	2.6%	7.3%	Adol

[a]Specific age ranges vary. Age ranges for most indicators are presented in Table 1.2. For Table 1.3 indicators not in Table 1.2, age ranges are presented in the notes below.
[b]The measures "health is excellent, very good, or good" and "limitation of activity" are measures obtained from the National Health Interview Survey. Adolescent data were collected via parent report, whereas the data for young adults were self-reported.
[c]The symbol (≈) denotes that rates are similar.
[d]The adolescent and young adult seat belt data were collected from different sources, and the wording differs slightly. The adolescent measure, retrieved from Youth Risk Behavior Surveillance System, shows the percentage who "Sometimes, Most of the Time, or Always Wore a Seatbelt," and the question specifically asks the respondent to report on instances in which they are in the car while someone else is driving. The young adult measure, retrieved from Behavior Risk Factor Surveillance System, shows the percentage that "Sometimes, Nearly Always, or Always Wore Seatbelts."
[e]Indicates young adult assessment year different than year of adolescent assessment.
[f]Simple assault: An attack or attempted attack without a weapon that results in no injury, minor injury (e.g., bruises, black eyes, cuts, scratches, or swelling), or an undetermined injury requiring <2 d of hospitalization. Aggravated assault: An attack or attempted attack with a weapon, regardless of whether the victim is injured, or an attack without a weapon when serious injury results.
[g]This review does not assess whether young adult trends in sexual experience, pregnancy, and childbirth are healthy or unhealthy; therefore, they cannot be compared with adolescents.
[h]For the multiple partners indicator, adolescents are 15–19 y and young adults are 20–24 y for both males and females.
[i]"Women at risk of unintended pregnancy" refer to women who have a chance of becoming pregnant at the date of interview but do not want to become pregnant now: They are either (1) using a contraceptive method or (2) they are not using contraception, but they have had intercourse in the 3 mo before the interview and are not pregnant or trying to become pregnant.
[j]For the dental decay indicator, adolescents are 12–17 y and young adults are 18–25 y.
Adol, adolescents; BAC, blood alcohol content; ER, emergency room; YA, young adults.
From Park MJ, Scott JT, Adams SH, et al. Adolescent and young adult health in the US in the past decade: little improvement and young adults remain worse off. *J Adolesc Health* 2014;55:3–16.

Another source of national data is the Fed Stat gateway at (http://fedstats.sites.usa.gov/): This site has links to more than 70 federal agencies that collect national data on a wide range of areas.

Special Areas or Population

1. Healthy Campus 2020 (http://www.acha.org/healthycampus/): Healthy Campus 2020 provides a framework for improving the overall health status on campuses nationwide.

2. *National College Health Assessment (NCHA)* (http://www .acha-ncha.org/pubs_rpts.html): The American College Health Association (ACHA)-NCHA is a national research effort organized by ACHA to assist health care providers, health educators, counselors, and administrators in collecting data about college students' habits, behaviors, and perceptions on the most prevalent health topics. Topics include alcohol, tobacco, and other drug use; sexual health; weight, nutrition,

TABLE 1.3

National Data Sources for Monitoring AYA Health by Health Area in the US

Name and Web site	Source and/or Method	Periodicity
Overall health, function, and mortality		
WONDER http://wonder.cdc.gov/ucd-icd10.html	Death certificates	Data released every 1–2 y on online database, timing varies; detailed mortality data 2010 current; since 1999
National Health Interview Survey (NHIS) http://www.cdc.gov/nchs/nhis.htm	Household interview survey	Annual data and reports; usually out in September; 2006 current (out September 2007); current survey model since 1995
Injury		
Youth Risk Behavior Surveillance System (YRBSS) http://www.cdc.gov/healthyyouth/yrbs/index.htm	Surveys in high schools	Data and reports released in June every 2 y; 2007 current (out June 2008); since 1991
National Highway Traffic Safety Administration/FARS/NCSA http://www.nhtsa.dot.gov/	Police reports, fatal crash records	Annual traffic safety facts reports released in Fall every year; 2007 current (out November 2008); since 1993
WISQARS http://www.cdc.gov/injury/wisqars/	Death certificates	Data released every 1–2 y on online database, timing varies; 2005 current (out January 2008); since 1981
National Survey on Drug Use and Health (NSDUH) http://oas.samhsa.gov/nsduh.htm	Household interview survey	Annual reports and tables released in November or December; 2007 current (out November 2008); since 1994
BRFSS http://www.cdc.gov/brfss/	Telephone survey, national	Data released every year in online database; timing varies; 2007 current; since 1990
Violence		
Bureau of Justice Statistics–National Crime Victimization Survey: http://www.ojp.usdoj.gov/bjs/	FBI crime reports	Annual reports released in November or December every 2–3 y; 2005 current (out December 2006); since 1996
YRBSS http://www.cdc.gov/healthyyouth/yrbs/index.htm	Surveys in high schools	Data and reports released in June every 2 y; 2007 current (out June 2008); since 1991
WISQARS http://www.cdc.gov/injury/wisqars/	Death certificates	Data released every 1–2 y on online database, timing varies; 2005 current (out January 2008); since 1981
Mental health		
WONDER http://wonder.cdc.gov/ucd-icd10.html	Death certificates	Data released every 1–2 y on online database, timing varies; detailed mortality data 2010 current; since 1999
YRBSS http://www.cdc.gov/healthyyouth/yrbs/index.htm	Surveys in high schools	Data and reports released in June every 2 y; 2007 current (out June 2008); since 1991
NHIS http://www.cdc.gov/nchs/nhis.htm	Household interview survey	Annual data and reports; usually out in September; 2006 current (out September 2007); current survey model since 1995
Monitoring the Future http://monitoringthefuture.org/	Surveys in schools	Annual reports; usually out in June; 2007 current (out September 2008); since 1975
WISQARS http://www.cdc.gov/injury/wisqars/	Death certificates	Data released every 1–2 y on online database, timing varies; 2005 current (out January 2008); since 1981
NSDUH http://oas.samhsa.gov/nsduh.htm	Household interview survey	Annual reports and tables released in November or December; 2007 current (out November 2008); since 1994
Substance use		
NSDUH http://oas.samhsa.gov/nsduh.htm	Household interview survey	Annual reports and tables released in November or December; 2007 current (out November 2008); since 1994
Monitoring the Future http://monitoringthefuture.org/	Surveys in schools	Annual reports; usually out in June; 2007 current (out September 2008); since 1975
YRBSS http://www.cdc.gov/healthyyouth/yrbs/index.htm	Surveys in high schools	Data and reports released in June every 2 y; 2007 current (out June 2008); since 1991

(Continued)

TABLE 1.3

National Data Sources for Monitoring AYA Health by Health Area in the US (*Continued*)

Name and Web site	Source and/or Method	Periodicity
Sexual and reproductive health		
Birth data–NVSS http://www.cdc.gov/nchs/births.htm	Birth certificates	Annual reports released in November or December every year (online database now available); 2006 current (out January 2009); since 1968
Pregnancy data–National Vital Statistics http://www.cdc.gov/nchs/births.htm and Guttmacher Institute http://www.guttmacher.org/sections/pregnancy.php	Vital statistics calculations	Vital Statistics: Data released every 2 y; timing varies; 2004 current (out April 2008); since 1976 Guttmacher: Data and/or reports released every 2–3 y; timing varies; 2002 current (out September 2006); since 1986
National Survey of Family Growth http://www.cdc.gov/nchs/nsfg.htm	Interviews	Data and/or reports from 2002 (out July 2005); conducting 2007 survey now; since 1973
HIV/AIDS and STDs Surveillance Statistics http://www.cdc.gov/hiv/topics/surveillance/basic.htm http://www.cdc.gov/nchstp/dstd/Stats_Trends/Stats_and_Trends.htm	Cases from states and/or areas; confidential reporting system	Annual reports released in November and/or December every 1–2 y; 2007 current (out November 2008); since 1981 (STDs) and 1982 (HIV/AIDS)
YRBSS http://www.cdc.gov/healthyyouth/yrbs/index|.htm	Surveys in high schools	Data and reports released in June every 2 y; 2007 current (out June 2008); since 1991
Chronic conditions and related behaviors National Health and Nutrition Examination Survey (NHANES) http://www.cdc.gov/nchs/nhanes.htm	Interviews, physical examinations, clinical measurements, or tests	Data and reports released in April every 2 y; 2003–2006 current (out February 2009); since 1976
BRFSS http://www.cdc.gov/brfss/	Telephone survey, national	Data released every year in online database; timing varies; 2007 current; since 1990
YRBSS http://www.cdc.gov/healthyyouth/yrbs/index.htm	Surveys in high schools	Data and reports released in June every 2 y; 2007 current (out June 2008); since 1991
NHIS http://www.cdc.gov/nchs/nhis.htm	Household interview survey	Annual data and reports; usually out in September 2006 current (out September 2007); current survey model since 1995
Health care access and utilization		
National Survey of Children's Health http://www.nschdata.org/	Interviews	Online database; timing varies; 2003 current (out September 2005); since 2003
National Survey of Children with Special Health Care Needs; http://www.cdc.gov/nchs/slaits/cshcn.htm	Interviews	Online database; timing varies; 2005 or 2006 current (out October 2007); since 2001
National Hospital Ambulatory Medical Care Survey: http://www.cdc.gov/nchs/about/major/ahcd/ahcd1.htm	Patient records	Reports; timing varies; 2005 current (out June 2007); since 1992
NHIS http://www.cdc.gov/nchs/nhis.htm	Household interview survey	Annual data and reports; usually out in September; 2006 current (out September 2007); current survey model since 1995
Medical Expenditure Panel Survey http://meps.ahrq.gov/mepsweb/	Household interviews	Reports and/or tables released every year; timing varies; 2005 current; since 1996
Population and education		
US Census Bureau–Population, Poverty http://www.census.gov/	Surveys	Data and reports released in summer every year; 2006 current (out September 2007); since 1970
National Center for Education Statistics http://www.nces.ed.gov/	Surveys	Annual Digest of Education Statistics released in summer every year; 2006 current (out June 2008); since 1995
Online data analysis		
University of Michigan Inter-university Consortium for Political and Social Research http://www.icpsr.umich.edu/icpsrweb/landing.jsp	Surveys, interviews, and so forth	Online Data Analysis tool providing access to different data series, including NSDUH, NHANES, NHIS, and more. All years or the most recent data may not be available.
Health Data Interactive http://www.cdc.gov/nchs/hdi.htm		Online Data Analysis tool providing access to different data series, including NHIS, NHANES, NVSS, and more. All years or the most recent data may not be available.

BRFSS, Behavior Risk Factor Surveillance System; FARS, Fatality and Analysis Reporting System; NCSA, National Center for Statistics and Analysis; NVSS, National Vital Statistics System; STD, sexually transmitted diseases; WISQARS, Web-based Injury Statistics Query and Reporting System; WONDER, Wide-Ranging Online Data for Epidemiologic Research. From Park MJ, Scott JT, Adams SH, et al. Adolescent and young adult health in the US in the past decade: little improvement and young adults remain worse off. *J Adolesc Health* 2014;55:3–16.

and exercise; mental health; and injury prevention, personal safety, and violence.

3. *National Center for Injury Prevention and Control (NCIPC)* (http://www.cdc.gov/injury/): The NCIPC has a vast array of data and information on injuries and injury prevention in all age-groups. Also at this site is the interactive data tool WISQARS.

4. *National Survey of Children with Special Health Care Needs* (http://www.cdc.gov/nchs/slaits/cshcn.htm): This survey assesses the prevalence and impact of special health care needs among children in all 50 states and the District of Columbia.

5. Cancer data: *National Cancer Institute, Surveillance Epidemiology and End Results (SEER)* (http://seer.cancer.gov/index.html): The SEER Public-Use Data include SEER incidence and population data associated by age, sex, race, year of diagnosis, and geographic areas (including SEER registry and county).

6. Chronic Disease: (http://www.cdc.gov/nccdphp/). Statistics and information on chronic diseases from National Center for Chronic Disease Prevention and Health Promotion. In addition, Centers for Disease Control and Prevention published a special report on the "Indicators for Chronic Disease Surveillance—US, 2013 in *Morbidity and Mortality Weekly Report (MMWR)* vol. 64 RR-1 http://www.cdc.gov/mmwr/preview/mmwrhtml/rr6401a1.htm?s_cid=rr6401a1_e

7. Infectious diseases: The *Summary of Notifiable Diseases* is available each year in *MMWR* (www.cdc.gov/mmwr).

8. Sports injury data: The National Center for Catastrophic Sport Injury Research (http://nccsir.unc.edu/) collects and disseminates death and permanent disability sports injury data that involve brain and/or spinal cord injuries. Three annual reports are compiled each spring: (a) Annual Survey of Football Fatalities, (b) Annual Survey of Catastrophic Football Injuries, and (c) Annual Report of All Sports Catastrophic Injuries.

DEMOGRAPHICS

General

In 2012, the proportion of AYAs in the US was:
- Adolescents (10 to 19 years): 42 million or 13.5% of the US population.
- Young adults:
  - (aged 20 to 24 years): 21.8 million or 7.1% of the US population.

- (aged 25 to 29 years): 20.9 million or 6.8% of the US population.

In the US, males slightly outnumber females among 18- to 25-year-olds. Whites are the largest racial/ethnic group in the US, accounting for approximately 60% of the population in each age-group. However, there is significant variation in ethnic/racial in certain states. For example, in California, Hispanics/Latinos are the largest racial/ethnic group among AYAs, accounting for 48% of adolescents, 43% of 20- to 24-year-olds, and 42% of 25- to 29-year-olds.

Figure 1.11 demonstrates population projection trends by age-group in the US from 2010 to 2030. Figure 1.12 demonstrates population projection adjusted by number of years per age-group.

MORTALITY

Quick Facts Regarding Mortality Risks for Adolescents in the US

- Rates of fatal unintentional injuries are much higher among AYAs than for younger children. According to the National Safety Council, rates in 2010 were[39]:

Age 11	4.0/100,000
Age 15	9.3/100,000
Age 16	14.9/100,000
Age 19	31.3/100,000
Ages 20 to 24	35.8/100,000
Ages 25 to 29	34.9/100,000

- Gunfire kills a child every 3 hours, 7 children every day, and 51 children a week.[39]
- Every 5 hours, a child or adolescent commits suicide.[40]

Leading Causes of Death

The top five causes are the same in AYAs, but rates are triple or more among young adults (Table 1.4).

Unintentional Injuries

Unintentional injuries are the leading cause of mortality among AYAs aged 12 to 34. MVCs account for the largest percentage of unintentional injuries, with the highest rates among 18- to 25-year-olds. Among AYAs, 47% of deaths are due to unintended injuries, and half of these involve MVC. In 2010, MVC-related hospitalization and ED

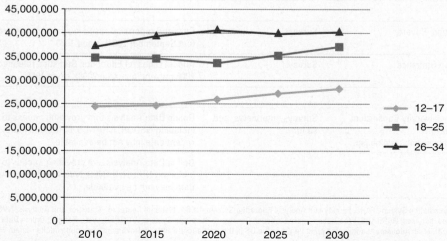

FIGURE 1.11 Population projection trends by age-group, in the US, 2010 to 2030 (Courtesy of Lawrence S. Neinstein, with permission. Available at www.usc.edu/thenewadolescents [figure 1.2a]).

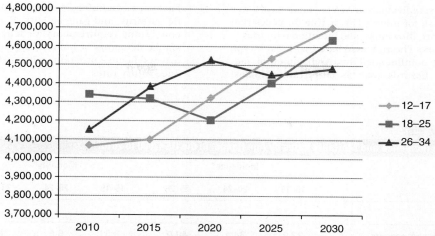

FIGURE 1.12 Population projection trends 2010 to 2030 by age-group/year, in the US, adjusted by number of years/age-group. (Courtesy of Lawrence S. Neinstein, with permission. Available at www .usc.edu/thenewadolescents [figure 1.2b]).

treatment of young adults cost the US health care system $9 billion. Among youth aged 1 to 19 years, unintentional injuries are responsible for more deaths than homicide, suicide, congenital anomalies, cancer, heart disease, respiratory illness, and HIV combined.[41]

Leading Causes of Injuries

Four types of injury—being struck by or against an object or person, falls, motor vehicle traffic-related injuries, and being cut by a sharp object—account for approximately 60% of all injury-related visits to EDs by adolescents. Of these four causes, only motor vehicle traffic-related injuries are a significant source of mortality. Sports injuries make up >40% of injuries classified as "being struck by or against an object or person."

Factors Contributing to AYA Injuries

- Age: AYAs are at highest risk for MVC.
- Gender: For nearly all injuries, the male death rate exceeds the rate in females. Males are more likely than females to engage in risky driving behaviors, drive after drinking alcohol, and are less likely to wear seat belts.[42]
- Race and ethnicity: Injury death rates vary substantially by race and ethnicity. The highest injury fatality rates are among Black and Native American adolescents, and the lowest rates are among Asian youth.
- Driving hours: In 2012, 41% of MVC deaths among adolescents occurred between 9 p.m. and 6 a.m., and 53% of adolescent MVC occurred on Friday, Saturday, or Sunday.[43]
- Alcohol: Alcohol involvement in crashes is highest among men aged 21 to 30 years. Alcohol-related crashes peak at night and are higher on weekends than on weekdays. Among passenger vehicle drivers who were fatally injured between 9 p.m. and 6 a.m. in 2012, 58% had blood alcohol concentrations (BACs) $\geq$ 0.08% compared with 19% during other hours. In 2012, 46% of all fatally injured passenger vehicle drivers on weekends (from 6 p.m. Friday to 6 a.m. Monday) had BACs $\geq$ 0.08%. At other times, the proportion was 24%.[44]

TABLE 1.4

Leading Causes of Death, Rates (per 100,000) by Age-Group, in the US (2008)

	Age					
Rank	12–17 y Cause of Death	Annual deaths per 100,000	18–25 y Cause of Death	Annual deaths per 100,000	26–34 y Cause of Death	Annual deaths per 100,000
1	Unintentional injury	11.9	Unintentional injury	39.1	Unintentional injury	27.1
2	Homicide	4.0	Homicide	14.5	Suicide	12.9
3	Suicide	3.8	Suicide	12	Homicide	11
4	Malignant neoplasms	2.7	Malignant neoplasms	4.4	Malignant neoplasms	9
5	Heart disease	1.1	Heart disease	3.2	Heart disease	8.3
6	Congenital anomalies	0.9	Congenital anomalies	1.1	HIV	2.5
7	Cerebrovascular	0.3	Diabetes mellitus	0.6	Diabetes mellitus	1.5
8	Chronic lower Respiratory disease	0.3	HIV	0.6	Cerebrovascular	1.4
9	Influenza & pneumonia	0.3	Influenza & pneumonia	0.6	Liver disease	1.1
10	Benign neoplasms	0.2	Cerebrovascular	0.5	Congenital anomalies	0.9

Source: Center for Disease Control and Prevention, National Center for Health Statistics. Underlying Cause of Death 1999–2008 on CDC WONDER Online Database.

- Socioeconomic factors: Individuals in AYA populations of lower SES are at greatest risk for injury. This is true for pedestrian injuries, fires and burns, drownings, and intentional injuries.
- Environmental factors: The risk associated with each type of AYA injury is also influenced by environmental factors. These include hazards such as all-terrain vehicles, backyard swimming pools, firearms, kerosene heaters, traffic patterns, and gang activity. Policies such as regulations concerning requirements for fences around private pools, smoke detectors in homes, bicycle helmets, and graduated drivers' license programs with night restrictions also influence injury rates.

TABLE 1.5

Cancer Incidence and Mortality Rates by Age Range, in the US (2006 to 2010)

Age (y)	Incidence[a]			Mortality[a]		
	15–19	20–24	25–29	15–19	20–24	25–29
Males						
All malignant cancers	**22.2**	**34.4**	**48.0**	**3.5**	**5.6**	**7.2**
Leukemia	3.6	3.3	3.1	1.0	1.3	1.3
Lymphoma	5.3	7.8	8.1	0.3	0.7	0.9
Hodgkin lymphoma	3.1	4.7	4.2	0.1	0.2	0.3
Non-Hodgkin lymphoma	2.1	3.2	3.9	0.3	0.5	0.6
Brain and nervous system	2.3	2.6	3.2	0.5	0.6	1.0
Bones and joints	1.8	1.2	0.7	0.6	0.7	0.4
Soft tissue	1.1	1.3	1.6	0.3	0.4	0.5
Skin[b]	1.0	3.0	4.8	0.0	0.2	0.4
Respiratory system	0.4	0.8	1.2	0.1	0.1	0.3
Male genital system	3.7	12.8	14.0	0.1	0.4	0.5
Digestive system	0.7	1.7	3.7	0.2	0.4	0.1
Females						
All malignant cancers	**20.0**	**37.2**	**64.8**	**2.5**	**3.6**	**6.2**
Leukemia	2.6	2.3	2.2	0.7	0.8	0.8
Lymphoma	4.5	6.5	7.1	0.2	0.4	0.6
Hodgkin lymphoma	3.2	4.6	4.2	0.1	0.2	0.2
Non-Hodgkin lymphoma	1.3	1.9	2.8	0.1	0.2	0.3
Brain and nervous system	1.8	2.2	2.3	0.4	0.4	0.6
Bones and joints	0.9	0.7	0.5	0.4	0.3	0.2
Soft tissue	1.2	1.2	1.2	0.3	0.3	0.3
Skin[b]	1.6	5.9	10.1	0.0	0.1	0.3
Respiratory system	0.2	0.4	0.8	0.0	0.1	0.2
Breast	0.2	1.6	8.6	—	0.1	0.7
Female genitourinary	1.7	3.9	9.7	0.1	0.3	1.0
Digestive system	0.6	1.6	3.4	0.1	0.4	0.9

[a]Rates are per 100,000.
[b]Excluding basal and squamous cancers.
Statistics could not be calculated based on limited number of cases for the time interval.
Adapted from SEER Cancer Statistics Review 1975-2010 Section 32. Adolescent and Young Adult Cancer by Site (Tables 32.12-14).
Available at http://seer.cancer.gov/archive/csr/1975_2010/results_merged/sect_32_aya.pdf

- Developmental factors: The developing AYA brain may be a factor contributing to risk-taking behaviors and unintentional injuries.

Intentional Injuries
Homicides
Homicides and suicides are the second and third leading causes of death, respectively, in AYAs aged 12 to 34. Homicide remains the number two cause of death in both AYAs, accounting for 16% of deaths. Homicide continues to be a major public health problem in the US, particularly for young Black males. It is the number one cause of death among Black AYA males aged 15 to 24 years.

Suicides
Suicides have changed from a problem of predominantly older persons to one that affects primarily AYAs. Adolescent suicide rates remained stable between 1900 and 1955 and then began to rise dramatically. Currently, suicide is the third leading cause of death for AYAs, accounting for 12% of deaths in this population.

Cancer
Excluding intentional and unintentional injuries, cancer is the leading cause of death in adolescents and is the leading cause of death by disease. It is the second cause of death among younger adolescents 10- to 14-years old and ranks fourth among AYAs aged 15 to 24-years.[45] Cancer has a higher incidence rate in AYAs aged 15 to 39 years than in younger children, but much lower than in older adults. According to NCI's Surveillance, Epidemiology, and End Results program, about 70,000 AYAs aged 15 to 39 years are diagnosed with cancer in the US each year (Table 1.5).[46] AYAs frequently have different types of cancer than either younger children or older adults. For example, more common AYA cancers are Hodgkin lymphoma, melanoma, testicular cancer, thyroid cancer, and sarcoma. The 5-year overall survival rate among adolescents ages 15 to 19 years with cancer exceeds 80%, similar to that among younger children. Young adults aged 20 to 35 have the lowest improvements in cancer survival rates in many malignancies during the past 25 to 35 years, potentially related to differences in involvement in treatment protocols, treatment centers, and access to health care.[47]

PREVENTION OF INJURIES
Many unintentional injury deaths of children and AYAs can be prevented. The three key approaches to injury prevention are education, environment and product changes, and legislation or regulation. Education can serve to promote changes in individual behaviors that increase the risk of injury and/or death. Environment and product modifications can make the adolescent's physical surroundings, toys, equipment, and clothes less likely to facilitate an injury. Legislation and regulation are among the most powerful tools to reduce adolescent injury, but they also require the most energy and concentrated efforts on the part of individuals and groups.

Motor Vehicle Injuries
1. Adopt graduated licensing laws and policies that keep adolescent drivers off the streets during late night and early morning hours.
2. Have parents impose restrictions and limitations of driving privileges on their teenage children.
3. Adopt laws restricting the number and age of passengers carried by teenage drivers.
4. Promote administrative license revocation that authorizes police to confiscate the licenses of drivers who either fail or refuse to take a chemical test for alcohol.
5. Promote primary safety belt laws that allow police to stop vehicles if the occupants are not using safety belts.
6. Strictly enforce zero-tolerance laws for blood alcohol in drivers younger than 21 years.
7. Evaluate strategies to limit access to alcohol and promote safety belt use among AYAs.
8. Continue to evaluate the separate components of graduated licensing systems to determine which ones are most effective.

MORBIDITY
Mortality rates for adolescents are low compared with those for adults; nonetheless, there is significant morbidity among AYAs. Table 1.6 lists the morbidity rates for selected diseases among AYAs during 2012. As with AYA deaths, many of the diseases that are contracted by AYAs are a result of health-related behaviors and lifestyle choices. For example, STIs are more prevalent among AYAs than any other population group (Table 1.6).[48]

Mental Health
AYAs have high rates of depression and anxiety. Serious mental illness often emerges during young adulthood. Compared to adults aged 26 to 34, young adults have higher rates of serious psychological distress and suicidal thoughts, plans, and attempts.

TABLE 1.6

Reported Cases of Selected Notifiable Diseases among Children, Adolescents, and Young Adults, in the US (2012)

Disease	5–14 y	15–24 y	25–39 y	Total (All Ages)
HIV diagnoses	119	7,500	13,957	35,361
Chlamydia	NA	987,412	365,410	1,422,976
Gonorrhea	NA	196,772	106,054	334,826
Hepatitis A (acute)	82	262	360	1,562
Hepatitis B (acute)	3	129	1,146	2,895
Hepatitis C (acute)	1	448	786	1,782
Lyme disease (confirmed and probable)	4,297	3,063	3,452	30,831
Measles	19	2	12	55
Meningococcal disease	28	95	81	551
Mumps	54	23	37	229
Pertussis	21,852	5,636	3,377	48,277
Syphilis (primary and secondary)	NA	4,160	6,683	15,667
Toxic shock syndrome	16	33	7	65
Tuberculosis	226	1,020	2,421	9,945

NA, data not available.
Adapted from Centers for Disease Control and Prevention. Summary of notifiable diseases—US, 2012. *MMWR* 2014;61(53):1–121.

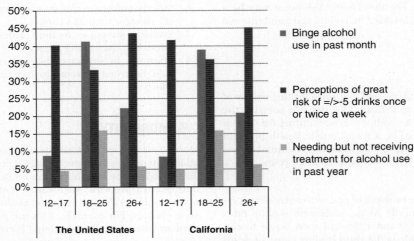

FIGURE 1.13 Binge drinking, perceptions of risk, and access to care by age-group, in the US and California, 2008 to 2009. (Courtesy of Lawrence S. Neinstein, 2013).

Substance Abuse

Young adults are a population with the "perfect storm" of alcohol risk: that is, the highest rate of past-month binge drinking but the lowest perception of risk and the greatest need for services but lowest access to services (Fig. 1.13). In addition, in the US, young adults have the highest rates of past-month tobacco and cigarette use, as well as higher rates of marijuana, cocaine, and other illicit drug use.

Reproductive Health

Birth rates peak in young adults aged 25 to 29. Trends reflect a decrease in birth rates since 1980 in AYAs until age 29. However, there has been a continuing rise in the percentage of pregnancies, resulting in a live birth in this age-group.

Sexually Transmitted Infections

The highest incidence rates of chlamydia and gonorrhea are in young adult males aged 20 to 24 and in older AYA females aged 15 to 24. New HIV cases are most frequent in young adults aged 20 to 24. Human papillomavirus infections are the most frequent STIs in the young sexually active US population, with 74% of the 6.2 million new infections each year occurring in AYAs age 15 to 24.

Chronic Diseases

In the US, there are over 16.3 million cases of the top seven common chronic diseases—cancer, diabetes, heart disease, hypertension, stroke, mental disorders, and pulmonary conditions. Three—cancer, heart disease, and mental disorders (suicide)—are among the top five causes of mortality in young adults. Many of the most frequent chronic diseases either start or continue in the AYA years. Others (e.g., heart disease, stroke, and diabetes) can be prevented with interventions during adolescence and young adulthood.

UTILIZATION AND ACCESSIBILITY OF SERVICES

Young adults have:

- The highest uninsured rates in both the US with males more likely to be uninsured than females.
- The lowest number of outpatient health care visits per person per year but the highest number of emergency room visits.
- The highest prevalence of $0 spending per person per year (26%).

REFERENCES

1. Population Division, United National Department of Economic and Social Affairs. *World population prospects: the 2012 revision* [Internet]. United Nations. Available at http://esa.un.org/unpd/wpp/Excel-Data/population.htm
2. The International Bank for Reconstruction and Development. *World development report 2007: development and the next generation.* Washington, DC: The World Bank, 2006.
3. Viner RM, Coffey C, Mathers C, et al. 50-year mortality trends in children and young people: a study of 50 low-income, middle-income, and high-income countries. *Lancet* 2011;377(9772):1162–1174.
4. Lim SS, Vos T, Flaxman AD, et al. A comparative risk assessment of burden of disease and injury attributable to 67 risk factors and risk factor clusters in 21 regions, 1990–2010: a systematic analysis for the Global Burden of Disease Study 2010. *Lancet* 2012;380(9859):2224–2260.
5. Park MJ, Scott JT, Adams SH, et al. Adolescent and young adult health in the United States in the past decade: little improvement and young adults remain worse off than adolescents. *J Adolesc Health* [Internet]. Available at http://www.sciencedirect.com/science/article/pii/S1054139X14001669
6. Stroud C, Mainero T, Olson S, et al. *Improving the health, safety, and well-being of young adults: workshop summary.* Washington, DC: The National Academies Press, 2013.
7. Commission on Social Determinants of Health; World Health Organization. *Commission on social determinants of health—final report* [Internet]. Geneva: World Health Organization. [cited 2014 Mar 6]. Available at http://www.who.int/social_determinants/thecommission/finalreport/en/
8. Viner RM, Ozer EM, Denny S, et al. Adolescence and the social determinants of health. *Lancet* 2012;379(9826):1641–52.
9. Woolf SH, Aron L, eds.; Panel on Understanding, Cross-National Health Differences Among High-Income Countries; Committee on Population; Division of Behavioral and Social Sciences and, Education; et al. *U.S. health in international perspective: shorter lives, poorer health.* Washington, DC: The National Academies Press, 2013.
10. Olshansky SJ, Antonucci T, Berkman L, et al. Differences in life expectancy due to race and educational differences are widening, and many may not catch up. *Health Aff (Millwood).* 2012;31(8):1803–1813.
11. UNICEF; UNESCO. *Envisioning education in the post-2015 development agenda* [Internet]. 2013. Available at http://www.unicef.org/education/files/Post-2015_EN_web.pdf
12. Committee on the Science of Adolescence; Board on Children, Youth, and, Families; Institute of Medicine and National Research Council. *The science of adolescent risk-taking: workshop report* [Internet]. The National Academies Press, 2011 [cited 2013 Oct 11]. Available at http://www.nap.edu/catalog.php?record_id=12961
13. Gibson EJ, Santelli JS, Minguez M, et al. Measuring school health center impact on access to and quality of primary care. *J Adolesc Health* 2013;53(6):699–705.
14. Henig RM. What is it about 20-somethings? *The New York Times* [Internet]. 2010 Aug 18 [cited 2014 Feb 23]. Available at http://www.nytimes.com/2010/08/22/magazine/22Adulthood-t.html
15. Mirowsky J. Age at first birth, health, and mortality. *J Health Soc Behav* 2005;46(1):32–50.
16. National Research Council; Committee on Adolescent Health Care Services and Models of Care for Treatment Prevention and Healthy Development, Institute of Medicine; Lawrence RS, Appleton-Gootman J, Sim LJ. *Adolescent health services: missing opportunities.* Washington, DC: The National Academies Press, 2009.
17. Wang H, Dwyer-Lindgren L, Lofgren KT, et al. Age-specific and sex-specific mortality in 187 countries, 1970–2010: a systematic analysis for the Global Burden of Disease Study 2010. *Lancet* 2012;380(9859):2071–2094.
18. Conde-Agudelo A, Belizán JM, Lammers C. Maternal-perinatal morbidity and mortality associated with adolescent pregnancy in Latin America: cross-sectional study. *Am J Obstet Gynecol* 2005;192(2):342–349.
19. UNICEF. *UNICEF state of the world's children 2011—adolescence: an age of opportunity.* 2011.

20. Center for Disease Control and Prevention. Youth risk behavior surveillance—United States, 2005. *MMWR Surveillance Summ* 2006;55(5). Available at http://www.cdc.gov/mmwr/PDF/SS/ss5505.pdf

21. Institute for Health Metrics and Evaluation. *The State of US Health: innovations, insights and recommendations from the global burden of disease study.* [Internet]. Seattle, WA: Institute for Health Metrics and Evaluation, 2013. Available at http://www.healthmetricsandevaluation.org/sites/default/files/policy_report/2013/IHME_GBD_US_FINAL_PRINTED%20070513.pdf

22. Center for Disease Control and Prevention. Rates of homicide, suicide, and firearm-related death among children—26 industrialized countries. *MMWR* 1997;46(05):101–105.

23. Murray CJL, Vos T, Lozano R, et al. Disability-adjusted life years (DALYs) for 291 diseases and injuries in 21 regions, 1990–2010: a systematic analysis for the Global Burden of Disease Study 2010. *Lancet* 2012;380(9859):2197–223.

24. Whiteford HA, Degenhardt L, Rehm J, et al. Global burden of disease attributable to mental and substance use disorders: findings from the Global Burden of Disease Study 2010. *Lancet* 2013;382(9904):1575–1586. Available at http://www.thelancet.com/journals/lancet/article/PIIS0140-6736(13)61611-6/abstract

25. Copeland W, Shanahan L, Costello EJ, et al. Cumulative prevalence of psychiatric disorders by young adulthood: a prospective cohort analysis from the Great Smoky Mountains Study. *J Am Acad Child Adolesc Psychiatry* 2011;50(3):252–261.

26. UNICEF. *Opportunity in crisis: preventing HIV from early adolescence to young adulthood [Internet].* UNICEF; 2011. Available at http://www.unicef.org/media/files/Opportunity_in_Crisis_LoRes_EN_05182011.pdf

27. Santelli JS, Melnikas AJ. Teen fertility in transition: recent and historic trends in the United States. *Annu Rev Public Health* 2010;31:371–383.

28. Murray CJL, Ezzati M, Flaxman AD, et al. GBD 2010: design, definitions, and metrics. *Lancet* 2012;380(9859):2063–2066.

29. Currie C, Zanotti C, Morgan A, et al., eds. *Social determinants of health and well-being among young people. Health Behaviour in School-aged Children (HBSC) study: international report from the 2009/2010 survey. [Internet].* WHO Regional Office for Europe, 2012. Available at http://www.hbsc.org/publications/international/

30. Jiang N, Kolbe LJ, Seo D-C, et al. Health of adolescents and young adults: trends in achieving the 21 Critical National Health Objectives by 2010. *J Adolesc Health Off Publ Soc Adolesc Med* 2011;49(2):124–132.

31. Hargreaves DS, Viner RM. Adolescent inpatient activity 1999–2010: analysis of English Hospital Episode Statistics data. *Arch Dis Child* 2014;99(9):830–833.

32. Callahan ST, Cooper WO. Changes in ambulatory health care use during the transition to young adulthood. *J Adolesc Health* 2010;46(5):407–413.

33. Centers for Disease Control and Prevention. *National health interview survey.* Available from: http://www.cdc.gov/nchs/nhis.htm

34. Viner RM. Adolescents' health needs: the same the world over. *Arch Dis Child* 2013;98(1):2.

35. Harden PN, Walsh G, Bandler N, et al. Bridging the gap: an integrated paediatric to adult clinical service for young adults with kidney failure. *BMJ* 2012;344:e3718.

36. Crowley R, Wolfe I, Lock K, et al. Improving the transition between paediatric and adult healthcare: a systematic review. *Arch Dis Child* 2011;96(6):548–553.

37. Sawyer SM, Ambresin A-E, Bennett KE, et al. A measurement framework for quality health care for adolescents in hospital. *J Adolesc Health* 2014;55(4):484–490.

38. Wilson TD. Redirect: the surprising new science of psychological change. *J Posit Psychol* 2012;7(6):530–532.

39. National Safety Council. *Injury Facts: 2014 edition.* Itasca, IL. National Safety Council, 2014. Children's Defense Fund. *Protect children not guns.* Washington, DC: Children's Defense Fund, 2013. Available at http://www.childrensdefense.org/child-research-data-publications/data/protect-children-not-guns-2013.html. Accessed October 3, 2014.

40. Children's Defense Fund. *The state of America's children 2014.* Washington, DC: Children's Defense Fund, 2014. Available at http://www.childrensdefense.org/child-research-data-publications/data/2014-soac.pdf?utm_source=2014-SOAC-PDF&utm_medium=link&utm_campaign=2014-SOAC. Accessed October 2, 2014.

41. Deal L, Gomby D, Zippiroli L, et al. *The future of children: unintentional injuries in childhood.* Vol. 10. Los Altos, CA: David and Lucile Packard Foundation, 2000.

42. Kann L, Kinchen S, Shanklin SL, et al. Youth risk behavior surveillance—United States, 2013. *MMWR CDC Surveill Summ* 2014;63 (suppl 4):1–168.

43. Insurance Institute for Highway Safety. *Fatality facts: teenagers.* Arlington (VA): Insurance Institute for Highway Safety, 2012. Available at http://www.iihs.org/iihs/topics/t/teenagers/fatalityfacts/teenagers. Accessed October 3, 2014.

44. Insurance Institute for Highway Safety. *Fatality facts: alcohol. 2012.* Available at http://www.iihs.org/iihs/topics/t/alcohol-impaired-driving/fatalityfacts/alcohol-impaired-driving/2012. Accessed October 3, 2014.

45. Heron M. Deaths: leading causes for 2010. *Natl Vital Stat Rep* 2013;62:1–96.

46. National Cancer Institute (U.S.). Cancer Statistics Branch. *SEER cancer statistics review 1975–2011.* Bethesda, MD: National Cancer Institute, 2014. Available at http://purl.access.gpo.gov/GPO/LPS3349. Accessed October 3, 2014.

47. Neinstein L. *The new adolescents: an analysis of health conditions, behaviors, risks, and access to services in the United States compared to California, among adolescents (12–17), emerging young adults (18–25) and young adults (26–34).* 2013. Available at www.usc.edu/thenewadolescents. Accessed October 3, 2014.

48. Adams DA, Jajosky RA, Ajani U, et al. Summary of notifiable diseases—United States, 2012. *MMWR* 2014;61:1–121.

📶 **ADDITIONAL RESOURCES AND WEBSITES ONLINE**

CHAPTER 2

Normal Physical Growth and Development

Jeremi M. Carswell
Diane E. J. Stafford

Accelerated growth, maturation of sexual characteristics, and the attainment of adult height and body proportions are the physical hallmarks of adolescence. Underlying these changes are the complicated activation and interplay of several hormonal axes that have been previously quiescent. This chapter provides an overview of the normal pubertal process and highlights the wide variation in the onset and duration of puberty in healthy adolescents and between male and female adolescents. Understanding these variations will provide the health care provider a framework for differentiating normal variations from abnormal pubertal development. The focus of Chapter 11 is abnormalities in growth and pubertal development.

⬤ MAJOR ENDOCRINE AXES AFFECTING GROWTH AND PUBERTAL MATURATION

Although there is activity and change in most hormonal systems during adolescence, the three that are primarily responsible for many of the physical changes are the hypothalamic–pituitary–gonadal (HPG) axis, the hypothalamic–pituitary–adrenal (HPA) axis, and the growth hormone (GH) axis.

HPG Axis

This axis is ultimately responsible for the release of estradiol and testosterone from the ovaries and testes, respectively, via the pituitary hormones, luteinizing hormone (LH), and follicle-stimulating hormone (FSH). This process originates with the release of gonadotropin-releasing hormone (GnRH) from the hypothalamic pulse generator that then signals release of LH and FSH from the anterior pituitary. The mechanisms by which this system is activated are not completely understood, although it appears that it is released/inhibited by the central nervous system, which in turn enables a positive feedback loop that results in pubertal maturation (Fig. 2.1).

HPA Axis

The products of HPA maturation in the context of puberty are the adrenal androgens, primarily dehydroepiandrosterone (DHEA) and its sulfate ester, dehydroepiandrosterone-sulfate (DHEA-S). These hormones exert their effects primarily by acting as precursors for

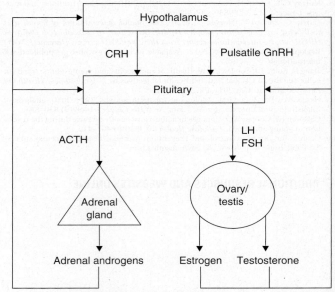

FIGURE 2.1 The hypothalamic–pituitary–gonadal and the hypothalamic–pituitary–adrenal axes. CRH, corticotropin-releasing hormone; GnRH, gonadotropin-releasing hormone; ACTH, adrenocorticotropic hormone; LH, luteinizing hormone; FSH, follicle-stimulating hormone.

the more potent androgens testosterone and dihydrotestosterone. It is important to recognize that production of these androgens is independent of the changes occurring in the HPG axis and that maturation may occur at different times.

GH Axis

Pituitary secretion of GH is positively regulated by GH-releasing hormone (GHRH) and negatively by somatostatin. GH is released in a pulsatile manner, with maximum secretion at the onset of slow-wave sleep.

The effects of GH are primarily modulated through proteins called insulin-like growth factors (IGFs) and their binding proteins (BPs). The major mechanism for growth appears to be through stimulation of IGF-1 by GH, which affects bone growth. Measurement of IGF-1 and IGFBP-3 levels serves as a surrogate measure of GH production because of significant diurnal variation in GH levels. Serum IGF-1 levels increase with age and pubertal development (Fig. 2.2).

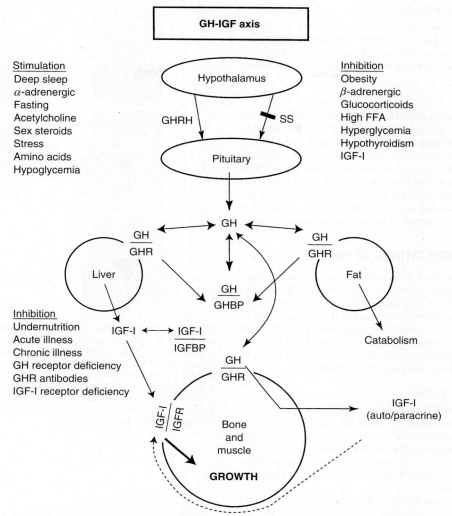

FIGURE 2.2 Simplified diagram of GH–IGF-1 axis involving hypophysiotropic hormones controlling pituitary GH release, circulating GHBP and its GH receptor source, IGF-1 and its largely GH-dependent BPs, and cellular responsiveness to GH and IGF-1 interacting with their specific receptors. FFA, free fatty acids; GHRH, growth hormone–releasing hormone. (From Rosenbloom AL, Guevara-Aguirre J, Rosenfield RG, et al. *Trends in endocrinology and metabolism;* vol 5. *Growth in growth hormone insensitivity.* New York, NY: Elsevier Science, 1994:296, with permission.)

MATURATION OF THE HPG AXIS

Gonadal Steroids

Estrogen

Estradiol (E2) from the ovary accounts for most of the *circulating* estrogens, although there is a small amount of extraovarian conversion from androstenedione (to estrone) and testosterone (to estradiol). In addition to stimulating breast growth and maturation of the vaginal mucosa, estrogen has profound effects on the skeleton, being the primary hormone responsible for epiphysial closure. At higher doses, estrogen causes epiphyseal fusion and, therefore, termination of linear growth. The mechanism by which this occurs is thought to involve estrogen's stimulation of chondrogenesis on the epiphyseal growth plate.[1]

Testosterone

Although the testes represent the primary source of this hormone, a small amount is generated from the extratesticular conversion of the adrenal hormone androstenedione in both males and females. Testosterone is the primary hormone responsible for the voice change in males and attainment of male body habitus, but it is

dihydrotestosterone, the product of conversion of testosterone by 5α-reductase, that causes phallic and prostate growth.

GnRH Pulse Generator and Its Regulators

GnRH Pulse Generator

The exact triggers for the pulsatile hypothalamic release of GnRH that occurs around the time of puberty are incompletely understood, although three distinct changes are observed.

1. Nocturnal sleep-related augmentation of pulsatile LH secretion begins as a result of the increase in the pulsatile release of GnRH.[2] When measuring LH levels to assess for the onset of hormonal activation, levels will initially only be detectable in the early morning, with inherent implications for testing the activity of the HPG axis in early puberty.
2. The sensitivity of the hypothalamus and the pituitary to estradiol (E2) and testosterone (T) decreases such that the gonadotropins LH and FSH begin to increase.
3. A positive feedback system develops in females so that rising levels of estrogen trigger GnRH release, stimulating LH to initiate ovulation.

Kisspeptins and the KISS1/GPR54 System

Kisspeptins refer to a class of peptides encoded by the *KISS1/Kiss1* gene that act through the receptor, *GPR54*. These compounds appear to stimulate LH through GnRH at the hypothalamic level and are implicated as necessary for pubertal onset, as well as normal reproductive function.[3]

Leptin

This product of the *ob* gene produced by fat cells was initially thought to have a gateway role in pubertal development. It was discovered to play a key role in the regulation of appetite, food intake, and energy expenditure, providing a signal to the central nervous system regarding satiety and the amount of energy stored in adipose tissue.[4] With further investigation, its role has been identified as more modest; it appears that leptin is permissive for pubertal advancement at the hypothalamic level by modulation of the GnRH system, although it has also been shown to have effects at other levels of the HPG axis.[5]

PHYSICAL MANIFESTATIONS OF PUBERTY

What are commonly thought of as pubertal secondary sexual characteristics should be separated into gonadarche and adrenarche, arising from activation of the HPG axis and HPA axis, respectively. In girls, gonadarche is represented by thelarche, or the onset of breast budding, and in boys by testicular enlargement to 4 mL and above, or 2.5 cm in the longest axis. Pubarche, or the growth of terminal sexual hair in girls, is mainly the result of adrenarche. In boys, both testicular and adrenal androgens contribute.

Sexual Maturity Rating Scales

Sexual maturity rating (SMR) scales (also called *Tanner staging)* as developed by Marshall and Tanner[6,7] allow for accurate classification of physical pubertal maturation. For both boys and girls, there are five stages categorizing secondary sexual characteristics (pubic hair and breast development in females, pubic hair and genitalia in males). These stages are described as follows and are shown in drawings in Figures 2.3 to 2.5.

Males (testicular volumes as measured by a Prader Orchidometer)

1. Genital stage 1 (G1): Prepubertal
   a. Testes: Volume, <4 mL, or long axis, <2.5 cm
   b. Phallus: Childlike
2. Genital stage 2 (G2)
   a. Testes: Volume, 4 to 8 mL, or long axis, 2.6 to 3.3 cm
   b. Scrotum: Reddened, thinner, and larger
   c. Phallus: No change
3. Genital stage 3 (G3)
   a. Testes: Volume, 10 to 15 mL, or long axis, 3.4 to 4.0 cm
   b. Scrotum: Greater enlargement
   c. Phallus: Increased length
4. Genital stage 4 (G4)
   a. Testes: Volume, 15 to 20 mL, or long axis, 4.1 to 4.5 cm
   b. Scrotum: Further enlargement and darkening
   c. Phallus: Increased length and circumference
5. Genital stage 5 (G5)
   a. Testes: Volume, >25 mL, or long axis, >4.5 cm
   b. Scrotum and phallus: Adult

Females

1. Breast stage 1 (B1)
   a. Breast: Prepubertal; no glandular tissue
   b. Areola and papilla: Areola conforms to general chest line
2. Breast stage 2 (B2)
   a. Breast: Breast bud; small amount of glandular tissue
   b. Areola: Areola widens
3. Breast stage 3 (B3)
   a. Breast: Larger and more elevation; extends beyond areolar parameter

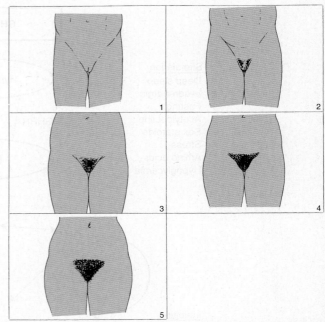

FIGURE 2.3 Female pubic hair development. SMR 1*:* Prepubertal; no pubic hair. SMR 2: Straight hair is extending along the labia and, between ratings 2 and 3, begins on the pubis. SMR 3: Pubic hair has increased in quantity, is darker, and is present in the typical female triangle but in smaller quantity. SMR 4: Pubic hair has increased in quantity, is darker, and is more dense, curled, and adult in distribution but less abundant. SMR 5: Abundant, adult-type pattern; hair may extend onto the medial aspect of the thighs. (From Daniel WA, Palshock BZ. A physician's guide to sexual maturity rating. *Patient Care* 1979;30:122, with permission. Illustration by Paul Singh-Roy.)

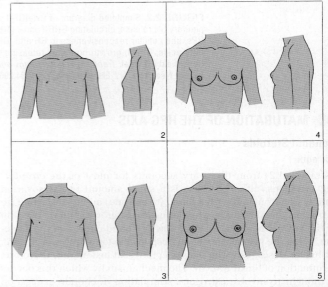

FIGURE 2.4 Female breast development. SMR 1, not shown: Prepubertal; elevations of papilla only. SMR 2: Breast buds appear; areola is slightly widened and projects as small mound. SMR 3: Enlargement of the entire breast with protrusion of the papilla or of the nipple. SMR 4: Enlargement of the breast and projection of areola and papilla as a secondary mound. SMR 5: Adult configuration of the breast with protrusion of the nipple; areola no longer projects separately from remainder of breast. (From Daniel WA, Paulshock BZ. A physician's guide to sexual maturity rating. *Patient Care* 1979;30:122, with permission. Illustration by Paul Singh-Roy.)

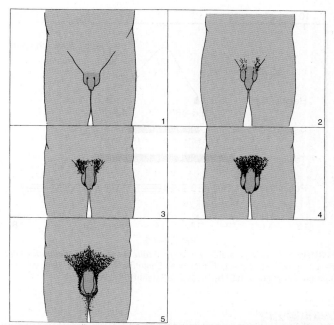

FIGURE 2.5 Male genital and pubic hair development. Ratings for pubic hair and for genital development can differ in a typical boy at any given time, because pubic hair and genitalia do not necessarily develop at the same rate. SMR 1: Prepubertal; no pubic hair. Genitalia unchanged from early childhood. SMR 2: Light, downy hair develops laterally and later becomes dark. Penis and testes may be slightly larger; scrotum becomes more textured. SMR 3: Pubic hair has extended across the pubis. Testes and scrotum are further enlarged; penis is larger, especially in length. SMR 4: More abundant pubic hair with curling. Genitalia resemble those of an adult; glans has become larger and broader, and scrotum is darker. SMR 5: Adult quantity and pattern of pubic hair, with hair present along the inner borders of the thighs. The testes and the scrotum are adult in size. (From Daniel WA, Paulshock BZ. A physician's guide to sexual maturity rating. *Patient Care* 1979;30:122, with permission. Illustration by Paul Singh-Roy.)

   b. Areola and papilla: Areola continues to enlarge but remains in contour with the breast
4. Breast stage 4 (B4)
   a. Breast: Larger and more elevation
   b. Areola and papilla: Areola and papilla form a mound projecting from the breast contour
5. Breast stage 5 (B5)
   a. Breast: Adult (size variable)
   b. Areola and papilla: Areola and breast in same plane, with papilla projecting above areola

Male and Female: Pubic hair

1. Pubic hair stage 1 (PH1)
   a. None
2. Public hair stage 2 (PH2)
   a. Small amount of long, slightly pigmented, downy hair along the base of the scrotum and phallus in the male or the labia majora in female; vellus hair versus sexual type hair (PH3)
3. Pubic hair stage 3 (PH3)
   a. Moderate amount of more curly, pigmented, and coarser hair, extending more laterally
4. Pubic hair stage 4 (PH4)
   a. Hair that resembles adult hair in coarseness and curliness but does not extend to medial surface of thighs
5. Pubic hair stage 5 (PH5)
   a. Adult type and quantity, extending to medial surface of thighs

Female Pubertal Changes
Events of Puberty
During puberty, the breasts develop and the ovaries, uterus, vagina, labia, and clitoris increase in size, with the uterus and ovaries increasing in size by approximately five-fold to seven-fold. Body composition changes, as girls accumulate fat mass at an average annual rate of 1.14 kg/year.[8]

Sequence
Often, the earliest physical sign of puberty in girls is thelarche, although few girls have pubic hair development as the first sign. On average, breast development starts at the age of 10 years for White girls and at 8.9 years for Black girls, according to a frequently cited large cross-sectional study.[9] The Breast Cancer and the Environment Research Program (BCERP) examined >1,200 girls longitudinally over 7 years in three urban areas and reported age at thelarche by both visual inspection as well as palpation (in contrast to the Pediatric Research in Office Settings (PROS) study which employed only inspection); median age of thelarche (SMR B2) was 8.8 for Black girls, 9.3 years for Hispanic, and 9.7 years for Caucasian and Asian participants. Notably, higher body mass index (BMI) was associated with earlier attainment of SMR 2.[10] These physical findings, however, may be preceded by the growth spurt by approximately 1 year. As a result, the growth curve is an essential tool in the evaluation of precocious or delayed puberty. The average length of time for completion of puberty is 4 years, but can range from 1.5 to 8 years.

Menarche
Menarche usually occurs during SMR B3 or B4, and approximately 3.3 years after the growth spurt, or roughly 2 years after breast budding. The normal range for menarche varies from 9 to 15 years and is dependent on such factors as race, socioeconomic status, heredity, nutrition, and culture. It occurs later at higher altitudes, in rural areas, and in larger families. Body composition also influences age at menarche, although controversy exists whether there is a necessary amount of adipose mass needed at the time of menarche.

Earlier menarche is usually correlated with shorter adult height, although this depends on the degree of estrogen stimulation before menses. Girls with higher or prolonged estrogen levels tend to grow less after menarche. On an average, girls grow 4 to 6 cm after menarche. The sequence of pubertal events in females is found in Figure 2.6. The age at menarche has gradually decreased during the last century. However, this trend has slowed significantly in the past few decades.

Several investigators have examined data from the Third National Health and Nutrition Examination Survey (NHANES III) conducted from 1988 to 1994.[11–13] One study[12] compared data from an earlier US survey 25 years previous to the NHANES III data and found that the average age at menarche had declined only minimally (i.e., by approximately 2.5 months, from 12.8 to 12.5 years). Another study cited up to a 4-month decrease in age at menarche.[12] Review of all available data in 2008 suggested a trend toward earlier menarche in the United States between 1940 and 1994, but with a magnitude of change of 2.5 to 4 months, revealing questionable clinical significance.[14] All studies that have examined race have demonstrated that Black girls reach menarche the earliest, followed by Mexican American and White girls.

Age at Puberty
Although there are slight differences in the ages of onset, the trend is for earlier pubertal onset, but almost no change in the age at menarche. On an average, girls of Black descent appear to enter puberty earlier than their Hispanic and White counterparts. The large study from the PROS group sampled >17,000 White and Black girls from around the United States with the SMR method and found that the earliest signs of puberty are occurring earlier than previously described.[8] In that study, the mean ages at onset of breast development were 8.9 years for Black girls and 10 years for White girls. Pubic hair development started at 8.8 years for Black girls and at 10.5 years for White girls. Similarly, Black girls experienced menarche at 12.2 years, and White girls at 12.9 years.

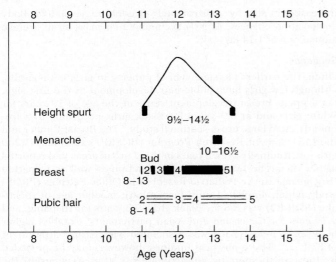

FIGURE 2.6 Biologic maturity in girls. (From Tanner JM. *Growth at Adolescence.* 2nd ed. Springfield, IL: Blackwell Scientific Publications, 1962, with permission. Copyright © 1962 by Blackwell Scientific Publications.)

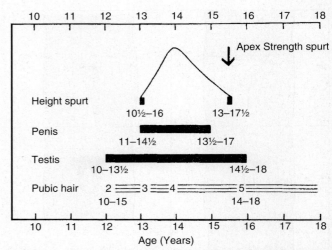

FIGURE 2.7 Biologic maturity in boys. (From Tanner JM. *Growth at Adolescence.* 2nd ed. Springfield, IL: Blackwell Scientific Publications, 1962, with permission. Copyright © 1962 by Blackwell Scientific Publications.)

Male Pubertal Changes

Events of Puberty

By the end of male puberty, the potential for reproduction is achieved. Internal and external genital organs increase in size, and body proportions change so that percentage of body fat actually declines[8] as opposed to the increase in females. Gynecomastia is a common issue in midpubertal boys that may cause significant concern (see Chapter 55). True gynecomastia is glandular development of at least 0.5 cm that is palpable. This may not be easily differentiated from pseudogynecomastia, which is an accumulation of fatty tissue.

Sequence

The earliest sign of physical pubertal development in approximately 98% of males is an increase in testicular volume to 4 mL or 2.5 cm in the long axis, although the first most noticeable event of male puberty is the growth of pubic hair. The growth spurt for boys is during mid- to late puberty, the time of rapidly rising testosterone levels. This is in contrast to an early growth spurt in girls. This is also the time when the voice changes, axillary hair develops, and acne may appear. Ejaculation occurs usually at SMR G3, as does the first evidence of spermarche, but fertility is not usually attained until SMR G4. Facial hair growth typically starts approximately 3 years after pubic hair growth. The hair on the face, chest, back, and abdomen may continue throughout and beyond puberty into adulthood, the amount and distribution being quite variable and dependent on ethnicity and family patterns. The average length of time for completion of puberty is 3 years, but it can range from 2 to 5 years. The sequence of events for an average male is shown in the following text in Figure 2.7. Table 2.1 lists testicular volume by SMR.

Age at Puberty

NHANES III data for boys demonstrate a similar trend regarding the initiation of puberty, but no change from earlier studies with regard to the attainment of SMR 5.[14] Also, as with girls, there were noticeable differences noted among racial groups, with Black boys entering puberty the earliest, followed by White boys, then Mexican American boys. A more recent review of data from the PROS study found the mean ages for onset of genital development to be 10.14 years for non-Hispanic White boys, 9.14 years for Black boys, and 10.04 years for Hispanic boys,[15] generally consistent with NHANES data and earlier (age-wise) than previously reported.[6] However, as with girls, the age at completion of genital development is not significantly different from previous studies,[16–18] with White boys completing puberty at 15.9 years, Black boys at 15.7 years, and Mexican

TABLE 2.1
Testicular Volume by SMR

| | Volume (cm³) | | | |
| | Left Testis | | Right Testis | |
SMR[a]	Mean	SD	Mean	SD
1	4.8	2.8	5.2	3.9
2	6.4	3.2	7.1	3.9
3	14.6	6.5	14.8	6.1
4	19.8	6.2	20.4	6.8
5	28.3	8.5	30.2	9.6

[a]Mean of genital and pubic hair ratings.
Adapted from Daniel WA Jr, Feinstein RA, Howard-Peebles P, et al. Testicular volumes of adolescents. *J Pediatr* 1982;101:1010.

American boys at 14.9 years. The overall trend, therefore, is earlier entry with prolonged progression. The potential causes of this trend are not entirely known. It is clear, however, that precocious puberty in boys should always prompt further evaluation as this condition is associated with pathology more often than in girls. Further evaluation should be undertaken if there is evidence of signs and symptoms of pubertal development before the age of 9 years or out of context of family history.

In both sexes, consequences of earlier maturation with regard to teen behavior, sexual activity, and pregnancy need to be addressed with age-appropriate interventions during middle childhood and the preteen years. In addition, the lifetime health consequences of early sexual maturation merit further study.

● ADRENARCHE

The increased secretion of androgens from the adrenals, called adrenarche, in the prepubertal and pubertal periods is independent of HPG changes. The two events are temporally related, with the increase in adrenal hormones preceding that of the gonadal sex steroids,[19] although the effects are evident later. It is important to note, however, that adrenal androgens are not necessary for pubertal development or the adolescent growth spurt. It is widely believed that adrenarche begins in mid-childhood, at around the age of 6 years, and adrenal androgen levels continue to rise until the age of 20 to 30 years. Evidence, however, suggests that the rise of DHEA-S is a more gradual process and occurs as early as the preschool years.[20,21]

Physical Manifestations

Local conversion of DHEA-S to testosterone then to dihydrotestosterone is responsible for hair growth in the androgen-dependent areas (face, chest, pubic area, axilla). Axillary and pubic areas are most sensitive to the effects of androgens, which is why these areas are the first to develop sexual hair. In addition, local conversion of DHEA-S within the apocrine glands of the axillae causes body odor, and conversion within sebaceous glands is responsible for the development of acne.

PHYSICAL GROWTH DURING PUBERTY

One of the most striking changes in adolescence is rapid growth velocity. This height spurt is dependent primarily on GH and the IGFs, but many other hormones may influence growth as well, especially the sex steroids. This is best illustrated by the example of the adolescent with isolated GH deficiency who grows throughout puberty but lacks a definitive growth spurt. Estrogens, and to a lesser extent, androgens, have a biphasic effect on the growth plate, stimulating bone formation early and inducing epiphyseal fusion late in puberty.[22] Premature or delayed puberty without prompt recognition and treatment may have marked effects on height.

GH during Puberty

Most linear growth is dependent on GH and its feedback loop. GH secretion is increased by GHRH, and decreased by hypothalamic somatostatin (Fig. 2.2). GH concentrations have been shown to double during the pubertal growth spurt. As with many hormones, GH is secreted in a pulsatile manner, with maximum rates at the onset of slow-wave sleep. It has been shown that the increased available GH is due to higher pulse amplitude and amount per pulse, as opposed to increased frequency or decreased clearance.[23,24] It is this pulsatile secretion which renders random GH testing unhelpful. GH exerts its effects through IGFs, mainly IGF-1 (or somatomedin-C) and IGF-2. Serum IGF-1 levels increase slowly and steadily during the prepubertal years, rise more steeply during puberty,[25] and remain elevated 1 to 2 years past the pubertal growth spurt. IGF levels among males and females must be interpreted with regard to pubertal stage and age.

Height Velocity

Height velocity during the pubertal growth spurt is at its highest levels outside of infancy. It should be noted that when calculating height velocity, it is important to use an interval of 6 to 12 months, as height growth is greatest during the spring and summer months. Although males and females are roughly the same height upon entry into puberty, males emerge taller by 13 cm on average. This is primarily due to the boys' 2-year lag behind girls in attainment of their peak height velocity, but a small amount of height may be accounted for by the higher peak velocity (Figs. 2.7 and 2.8). Girls gain their peak height velocity of 8.3 cm/year at an average age of 11.5 years and at SMR B2 to B3, whereas boys do not have their peak height velocity of 9.5 cm/year until the age of 13.5 years at SMR G3 to G4. Although there is great interindividual variation for height, one trend is for the peak height velocity to be higher, but not more sustained, in those who mature early. Therefore, there may not be a difference in final height. There are also curves available for early and late maturers (Figs. 2.8 and 2.9).

Prediction of Final Height

Predicting final height is a difficult task, and it should be emphasized that the methods available provide a general estimate.

Midparental Target Height

One method of predicting a general range for adult height is by the average of parental heights, accounting for the height difference of 13 cm (or 5 inches) between men and women. This is referred to as the midparental target height. One standard deviation from midparental height is 2 inches. As a result, 4 inches around the midparental height is within two standard deviations of the mean. For girls:

$$\frac{(\text{father's height} - 13 \text{ cm or } 5 \text{ inches}) + \text{mother's height}}{2}$$

For boys:

$$\frac{(\text{mother's height} + 13 \text{ cm or } 5 \text{ inches}) + \text{father's height}}{2}$$

Prediction Based on Bone Age

Skeletal maturation can be determined by comparing a radiograph of the adolescent's hand and wrist to standards of maturation in the normal population. Bone age is an index of physiologic maturation, providing an idea of the proportion of the total growth that has occurred. For example, if an adolescent is 15 years old and has a bone age of 12 years, there will be more potential growth than if the same adolescent's bone age were 15 years. The Bayley–Pinneau method uses the bone age to predict final height. This is based on obtaining a bone age (x-ray of the left hand and wrist) that is then matched to standards. Because sex steroids are known to cause bony maturations and epiphyseal fusion, this method is based on the percentage of final height as assessed by bone maturation. Various computer models have used these data to predict adult height. With these programs, basic information (e.g., height, weight, skeletal age) is entered and adult height is calculated using several methodologies, including that of Bayley and Pinneau. One such program can be found at http://www.bonexpert.com/adult-height-predictor. The use of skeletal age is discussed further in Chapter 11.

Weight Growth

1. Weight velocity increases and peaks during the adolescent growth spurt.
2. Pubertal weight gain accounts for approximately 50% of an individual's ideal body weight.
3. The onset of accelerated weight gain and the peak weight velocity (PWV) attained are highly variable. For example, normal weight gain during the year of PWV can vary from 4.6 to 10.6 kg in girls and from 5.8 to 13.2 kg in boys. Normal weight-for-age percentile curves are available through the Centers for Disease Control and Prevention (CDC) Web site www.cdc.gov/growthcharts/.

Pubertal Changes in Body Composition and Skeletal Mass

During childhood, boys and girls have relatively equal proportions of lean body mass, skeletal mass, and body fat. By the end of puberty, however, men have 1.5 times more lean body mass and skeletal mass than women and women have double the fat mass. Table 2.2 shows the effects of GH and the sex steroids on different aspects of body composition. The skeleton also undergoes epiphyseal maturation under the influence of estradiol (E2) and testosterone (T).

Lean Body Mass

1. Females: Lean body mass decreases from approximately 80% of body weight in early puberty to approximately 75% at maturity. The lean body mass increases in total amount, but decreases in percentage because adipose mass increases at a greater rate.
2. Males: Lean body mass increases from 80% to 85% to approximately 90% at maturity. This primarily reflects increased muscle mass from circulating androgens.

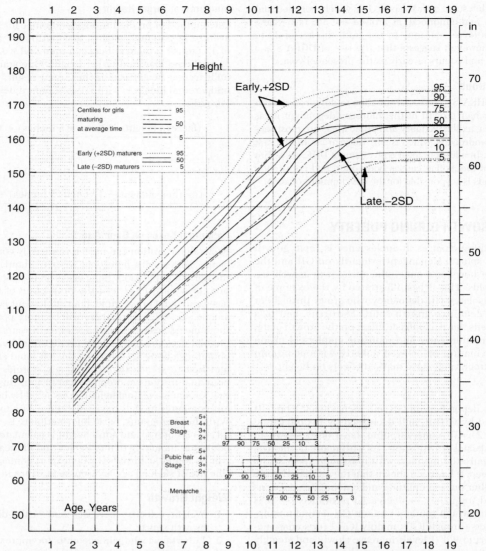

FIGURE 2.8 Height attained for American girls. (From Tanner JM, Davies PW. Clinical longitudinal standards for height and height velocity for North American children. *J Pediatr* 1985;107:317, with permission.)

Skeletal Mass

Changes in bone mass, or bone mineral density (BMD), parallel the alterations in lean body mass, body size, and muscle strength. Major determinants of BMD are physical activity level, heredity, nutrition, endocrine function, and other lifestyle factors. The accretion of skeletal bone mass during puberty is critical. Peak bone mass is acquired by early adulthood, serving as the "bone bank" for the remainder of life.[26] Bone mass is affected by the following:

1. Age at menarche: There is an inverse relation between the age at menarche and the risk of osteoporosis later in life, as demonstrated by epidemiological studies.[27]
2. Nutrition: Much has been studied about the effects of calcium and vitamin D, with mixed results. Currently, there are no studies that have been able to separate the effects of vitamin D from the effects of calcium on skeletal accrual, although there is a consensus that adequate consumption of both of these nutrients is important for optimal bone mineral accrual.
3. Exercise: Weight-bearing physical activity during pre- and early puberty has been shown to improve bone strength, but results have been less promising regarding the effects of exercise on postmenarcheal girls.[28]

Body Mass Index

BMI increases with puberty, although it should be pointed out that BMI does not quantitate body composition. BMI varies with age, gender, and ethnicity. In children and adolescents, BMI must be compared using age-stratified standardized percentiles. Charts and tables for BMI, which should be tracked in all children and teenagers, can be obtained from the National Center for Chronic Disease Prevention and Health Promotion of the CDC. (Web site addresses were listed previously in the section on Weight Growth.) There is a strong correlation between the timing of puberty and BMI: children with higher mean BMI mature earlier. BMI is determined by the following formula:

$$BMI = \text{Weight in kilograms} / (\text{height in meters})^2$$

or

$$BMI = (\text{Weight in kilograms} / \text{height in centimeters} / \text{height in centimeters}) \times 10,000$$

The BMI declines from birth and reaches a minimum between 4 and 6 years of age, before gradually increasing through adolescence and adulthood. The upward trend after the lowest point is referred

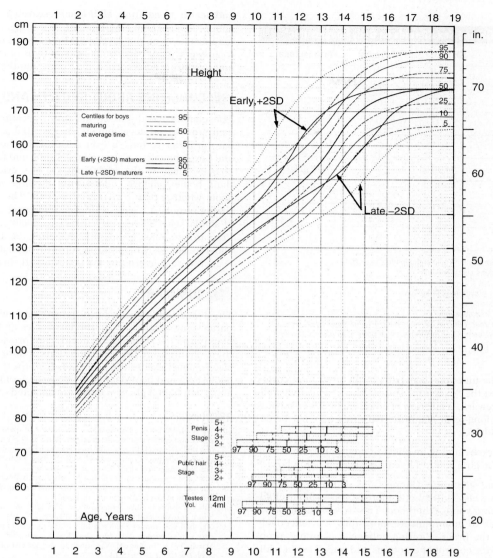

FIGURE 2.9 Height attained for American boys. (From Tanner JM, Davies PW. Clinical longitudinal standards for height and height velocity for North American children. *J Pediatr* 1985;107:317, with permission.)

to as the "adiposity rebound." Children with an earlier rebound are more likely to have an increased BMI.

Brain Maturation during Adolescence

Significant research in understanding brain development in adolescents and young adults (AYAs) is ongoing. This research has utilized new technologies (such as functional magnetic resonance imaging) that allow tracking of the growth of different regions of the brain, as well as investigating the connections within the brain. Some researchers are exploring the interactions between brain function, development, and behavior, while others have been investigating the sensitivity of the developing brain to effects of alcohol and other drugs. This research has resulted in some important new findings, including the discovery of significant changes in brain development even into the young adult years.

An understanding of brain development can assist in understanding the risk-taking behavior of AYAs. Brain development can play a significant role in these behaviors in conjunction with genetic makeup, childhood experiences, and environmental surroundings. Studies now indicate that the brain continues to develop in different ways and at different times into adolescence and young adulthood.

Developmental Stage

Early and Mid-adolescence: The brain undergoes significant growth and pruning. In general, this process moves from the back to front areas of the cerebral cortex.

Young Adulthood: Brain development that reflects sophisticated thinking and emotional regulation continues, but is not fully developed until mid-20s or sometimes later.[29] Of note, the brain is not fully mature at age 16, when many adolescents begin to drive, nor at age 18, the legal voting age, or at age 21, the legal drinking age. Rather, full maturity occurs at approximately age 25 in most individuals.

Area of the Brain

Prefrontal Cortex: Perhaps, the most widely studied areas for changes in young adulthood are in this brain region. The prefrontal cortex is associated with planning and problem-solving. Two aspects affecting the efficiency of this functioning are as follows:

1. Myelination: Enhanced myelination of nerve fibers contributes to signals being transmitted more efficiently.
2. Synaptic pruning: The wild patches of connections resulting from nerve growth are pruned back. This again allows for signals to be transmitted more efficiently.

TABLE 2.2

Primary Actions of GH and Sex Steroids on Body Composition[a]

	GH	Estradiol	Testosterone
Visceral fat[a,b]	↓↓	[c,d]	↓
Subcutaneous fat[a,e]	↓	↑	↓
Bone mineral[a,f]	↑	↑↑	↑↑
Muscle mass[a,e]	↑	[c]	↑↑
Extracellular water	↑ (acutely)	[c]	↑ (acutely)
Linear bone growth[a,e,f]	↑	↑↑	↑↑
Epiphyseal fusion[d,f]	[c]	↑↑	↑↑
Energy expenditure	↑	[c]	↑↑

[a]Possible synergy between somatotropic and gonadotropic signals.
[b]Nonaromatizable androgens also effectual.
[c]Limited or inconsistent data.
[d]Only in combination with a (synthetic) progestin.
[e]May differ in children and adults.
[f]Maximal effects require aromatization.
Adapted with permission from: Veldhuis JD, Roemmich JN, Richmond EJ, et al. Endocrine control of body composition in infancy, childhood and puberty. *Endocrine Reviews* 2005;26:114.

Executive Suite: The functions centering in the prefrontal cortex are sometimes called the "executive suite." This can include calibration of risk and reward, regulation of emotion, problem-solving, self-evaluation, and long-term planning. This area may not be developed until the mid-20s.

Cerebellum: This cerebellum is involved in emotional processing; it is at adult volume in girls before 11 years of age, but not in boys.[30]

Connections among Regions: Connections between different parts of the brain are also critical and increase throughout childhood, adolescence, and young adulthood. This development allows the prefrontal cortex to communicate more fully and effectively with other parts of the brain, allowing enhanced planning, problem-solving, and better control of emotions and impulses. In addition, these enhanced connections play an important role in growth of intellectual capacity and memory.

Brain Tissue

White Matter: The volume of white matter increases throughout childhood and adolescence.[29]

Gray Matter: This area of brain has an inverted U-shaped developmental curve overall.[31]

Rate of Development

It is clear that different parts of the brain mature at different rates. Overall, functional scans suggest that the parts of the brain that control basic functions, such as those controlling movement, mature first, while parts of the brain responsible for controlling impulses and planning ahead are mature the last.

While the brain of an adolescent or young adult may have a very high intellectual capacity and be "online," the areas of emotional and impulse control seem to reach maturity later. There is also the suggestion that the brain circuits involved in emotional responses are heightened in AYAs. These changes may relate to the risk-seeking behaviors and a tendency to act on impulse and without a regard for risk. In addition, some of these brain-based changes may even be involved in regulation of sleep and contribute to teens' preference for staying up late.

There continues to be much to learn and investigate into the development of the human brain and relationships with behaviors

and health. In addition, additional research is needed to better examine the effects of environment, parenting, and alcohol and others substances on the developing brain. Some of this work may lead to answers about why so many symptoms of mental disorders first emerge during adolescence and young adulthood.

CONCERNS ABOUT GROWTH AND DEVELOPMENT

This chapter has discussed most of the features of normal adolescent growth and development. As essential as it is for the healthcare provider to have a firm grasp of the facts of normal growth and development, a clear understanding and feeling for what these changes mean to the adolescent are also critically important. As their bodies change, adolescents develop tremendous concern about whether their bodies are "normal." The great variation in the timing of puberty, with resultant differences in physical maturity of similar-aged adolescents, serves to heighten teenagers' worries. Practitioners must be adept at detecting the adolescent's concerns about height, weight, pubic hair growth, or phallus size, for example, even if these concerns are not stated overtly in the initial complaint.

SUMMARY

The changes that occur during growth and puberty are a marvel of nature and a testimony to the intricacies and wonders of the human hormonal system. The health care provider must understand these changes and the wide variations of normalcy. He or she must also be able to sense the profound effect these changes have on the adolescent and be prepared to be a source of information, reassurance, and help if abnormalities are detected.

REFERENCES

1. Weise M, De-Levi S, Barnes KM, et al. Effects of estrogen on growth plate senescence and epiphyseal fusion. *Proc Natl Acad Sci USA* 2001;98:6871.
2. Marshall JC, Kelch RP. Gonadotropin-releasing hormone: role of pulsatile secretion in the regulation of reproduction. *N Engl J Med* 1986;315:1459.
3. Pinilla L, Aguilar E, Dieguez C, et al. Kisspeptins and reproduction: physiological roles and regulatory mechanisms. *Physiol Rev* 2012;92:1235–1316.
4. Zhang Y, Proenca R, Maffei M, et al. Positional cloning of the mouse ob gene and its human homologue. *Nature* 1994;372–425.
5. Sanchez-Garrido MA, Tena-Sempere, M. Metabolic control of puberty: roles of leptin and kisspeptins. *Horm Behav* 2013;64:187–194.
6. Marshall WA, Tanner JM. Variations in the pattern of pubertal changes associated with adolescence in girls. *Arch Dis Child* 1969;44:291.
7. Marshall WA, Tanner JM. Variations in the pattern of pubertal changes in boys. *Arch Dis Child* 1970;45:13.
8. Roche AF, Heysfield SB, Lohman TG, eds. *Human body composition. Total body composition: birth to old age*. Champaign, IL: Human Kinetics Publishers, 2001:230.
9. Herman-Giddens ME, Slora EJ, Wasserman RC, et al. Secondary sexual characteristics and menses in young girls seen in office practice: a study from the pediatric research in office settings network. *Pediatrics* 1997;99:505.
10. Biro FM, Greenspan LC, Galvez MP, et al. Onset of breast development in a longitudinal cohort. *Pediatrics* 2013;132:1019–1027.
11. Sun SS, Shumei S, Schubert CM, et al. National estimates of the timing of sexual maturation and racial differences among US children. *Pediatrics* 2003;111:815.
12. Chumlea WC, Schubert CM, Roche AF, et al. Age at menarche and racial comparisons in US girls. *Pediatrics* 2003;111:110.
13. Anderson SE, Dallal GE, Must A. Relative weight and race influence average age at menarche: results from two nationally representative surveys of US girls studied 25 years apart. *Pediatrics* 2003;111:815.
14. Euling SY, Herman-Giddens ME, Lee PA. Examination of US puberty-timing data from 1940 to 1994 for secular trends: panel findings. *Pediatrics* 2008;121:S172.
15. Herman-Giddens ME, Steffes J, Harris D, et al. Secondary sexual characteristics in boys: data from the pediatric research in office settings network. *Pediatrics* 2012;130:e1058.
16. Harlan WR, Grillo GP, Cornoni-Huntley J, et al. Secondary sex characteristics of boys 12-17 years of age: the US Health Examination Survey. *J Pediatr* 1979;95:293.
17. Lee PA. Normal ages of pubertal events among American males and females. *J Adolesc Health Care* 1980;1:26.
18. Villareal SF, Martorell R, Mendoza F. Sexual maturation of Mexican-American adolescents. *Am J Hum Biol* 1989;1:87.
19. Ducharme JR, Forest MG, De Peretti E, et al. Plasma adrenal and gonadal sex steroid in human pubertal development. *J Clin Endocrinol Metab* 1976;42:468.
20. Palmert MR, Hayden DL, Mansfield MJ, et al. The longitudinal study of adrenal maturation during gonadal suppression: evidence that adrenarche is a gradual process. *J Clin Endocrinol Metab* 2001;86:4536.
21. Remer T, Boye KR, Hartmann MF, et al. Urinary markers of adrenarche: reference values in healthy subjects, aged 3–18 years. *J Clin Endocrinol Metab* 2005;90:2015.
22. Vanderschueren D, Vandenput L, Boonen S, et al. Androgens and bone. *Endocr Rev* 2004;25(3):389.

23. Martha PMJ, Gorman KM, Blizzard RM, et al. Endogenous growth hormone secretion and clearance rates in normal boys as determined by deconvolution analysis; relationship to age, pubertal status, and body mass. *J Clin Endocrinol Metab* 1992;74:336.
24. Martha PM Jr, Rogol AD, Veldhuis JD. Alterations in the pulsatile properties of circulating growth hormone concentrations during puberty in boys. *J Clin Endocrinol Metab* 1989;69:563.
25. Juul A, Bang P, Hertel NT, et al. Serum insulin-like growth factor-I in 1030 healthy children, adolescents, and adults: relation to age, stage of puberty, testicular size, and body mass index. *J Clin Endocrinol Metab* 1994;78:744.
26. Bachrach LK. Making an impact on pediatric bone health. *J Pediatr* 2000; 136:137.
27. Seselj M, Nahhas RW Sherwood RJ, et al. The influence of age at menarche on cross-sectional geometry of bone in young adulthood. *Bone* 2012;51(1):38.
28. MacKelvie KJ, Khan KM, McKay HA. Is there a critical period for bone response to weight-bearing exercise in children and adolescents? A systematic review. *Br J Sports Med* 2002;36:250.
29. Lenoot RK, Nitlin G, Greenstein DK, et al. Sexual dimorphism of brain developmental trajectories during childhood and adolescence. *Neuroimage* 2007;36(4):1065–1073.
30. Caviness VSJ Jr, Kennedy DN, Richelme C, et al. The human brain age 7–11 years: a volumetric analysis based on magnetic resonance images. *Cere Cortex* 1996;6;726–736.
31. Giedd, JN, Rapoport JL. Structural MRI for pediatric brain development: what have we learned and where are we going? *Neuron* 2010;67:728–734.

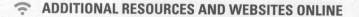 **ADDITIONAL RESOURCES AND WEBSITES ONLINE**

Psychosocial Development in Normal Adolescents and Young Adults

Sara Sherer
Mari Radzik

This chapter provides a framework of the psychosocial developmental process and discusses ways to enhance interactions between health care providers and adolescents and young adults (AYAs). General considerations are reviewed, including a review of the normal developmental phases and tasks of early adolescence (approximate ages 10 to 13), middle adolescence (approximate ages 14 to 17), late adolescence (approximate ages 17 to 21), and young adulthood (approximate ages 18 to 25). A review of the primary tasks for each of these phases includes a discussion of cognitive development, independence, body image, peer group, and identity development.

As modern Western societies lengthen the course of a lifetime, the end of adolescence and the initiation of adulthood has extended and become more fluid. The phase of life between adolescence and adulthood is now referred to as "emerging adulthood."[1,2] Today's emerging adults are known for their late entrance into formal adulthood and slow exit out of their parents' homes.[3] They are more educated than previous generations and enjoy connectedness to all forms of digital apparatus, resulting in far-reaching global influences impacting their identities.[4]

In terms of physical development, adolescence can be described as the period of life beginning with the appearance of secondary sexual characteristics and terminating with the cessation of somatic growth. In modern Western culture, the behavioral aspects of this developmental period have become equally important. Adolescence is, in fact, a biopsychosocial process that may start before the onset of puberty and last well beyond the termination of growth. Adolescence involves physical, psychological, emotional, and social growth and development, and each of these domains occurs at different rates. As such, adolescence is a period of increased vulnerability characterized by an ongoing process of transition and adjustment.[5] The events and challenges that arise during this period are often perplexing to parents, health care providers, and AYAs.

Over the past decade, advances in neuroimaging techniques have led to a greater understanding of the structural and functional development of the AYA brain, and the cognitive processes during this period of life. Studies have demonstrated that changes in brain structure continue beyond adolescence, with the most dramatic growth occurs in the development of executive functioning, organization, decision making and planning, and response inhibition.[6–8] Understanding biologic changes in brain structure and function during adolescence and young adulthood has important implications for understanding behaviors (see Chapter 2).

Health care professionals who are knowledgeable about normal adolescent psychosocial development are in a good position to identify the range of mental health problems, as well as the various emotional and behavioral issues that can affect the health and well-being of AYAs.[9]

THE PROCESS OF ADOLESCENCE

First, it is important to keep in mind that no outline of psychosocial development can adequately describe every AYA. Globally, 10- to 24-year-olds are now the largest generational group in history.[10] These AYAs are not members of a homogeneous group, but a diverse group that display wide variability in biologic, psychological, social, and emotional growth. Each AYA must meet his or her individual life demands and respond to the opportunities and challenges he or she faces in a unique and personal manner.[9,11]

Second, the transition from childhood to adulthood is not a continuous, uniform, or synchronous process. In fact, biologic, social, emotional, and intellectual growth may be totally asynchronous.[5] In addition, psychosocial growth may be accented by frequent periods of regression. It must be remembered that all of life, from birth to death, is a constant process of change and that adolescence and young adulthood is not the only challenging period.

Third, whereas adolescence has historically been described as a period of extreme instability, most adolescents do not experience difficulties during this time, and most are unperturbed by the developmental process.[12] This ability to cope with this developmental period reflects a resiliency that is often overlooked, as the behaviors of adolescents are often the primary focus of attention.[13] Recent studies that focus attention on parenting AYAs find that difficulties are far less prevalent than previously thought.[13] Only one in five families report difficult parent–child relationships. Overall, there is no evidence that intractable and major conflict between parents and their adolescent children is a "normal" part of adolescence,[14–16] and in fact most AYAs and their parents enjoy healthy relationships as adults.

Phases and Tasks of Adolescence

Adolescence and young adulthood can be conceptualized by dividing the process into four psychosocial developmental phases:

1. Early adolescence: approximate ages 10 to 13 years, or middle school years

2. Middle adolescence: approximate ages 14 to 17 years, or high school years
3. Late adolescence: approximate ages 17 to 21 years, or college or employment
4. Young or "emerging" adults: approximate ages 18 to 25 years

Regardless, by the end of adolescence, emerging adults strive to become emancipated from their parents and other adults. Some have attained a psychosexual maturity along with the necessary skills and resources from family, education, and community to begin to support themselves in an emotionally, socially, and financially satisfying way.[3] Others may still be supported as they attain the necessary skills and resources necessary to transition to adult independence.

Several tasks characterize the development of AYAs and are discussed in the following sections in conjunction with the various developmental phases. These tasks include the following:

1. Expanding cognitive development that allows young people to think in new, more complex ways
2. Achieving independence from parents
3. Accepting one's body image
4. Adopting peer codes and lifestyles
5. Establishing self, sexual, vocational, and moral identities

EARLY ADOLESCENCE (APPROXIMATE AGES 10 TO 13)

Early adolescent psychosocial development is heralded by rapid physical changes with the onset of puberty. These physical changes engender self-absorption and initiate the adolescent's struggle for independence. The onset of puberty occurs 1 to 2 years earlier for girls than for boys (see Chapter 2). Concomitantly, the psychosocial and emotional changes also occur 1 to 2 years earlier in girls.[17] Recent studies have provided evidence that the earlier age at onset of pubertal development in girls, the more challenging this developmentally period tends to be.[17]

Cognitive Development

Early adolescent development is characterized by cognitive abilities dominated by concrete thinking, egocentrism, and impulsive behavior. Young adolescents may start showing improvements in reasoning, information processing, and expertise.[5] The adolescent is at an early developmental stage in his or her abilities to long-range plan, see another's point of view and consider others' feelings.[18]

Movement Toward Independence

Early adolescence is characterized by the beginning of the shift from dependence on parents/caregivers to independent behavior. Common events at this time include the following:

1. Less interest in parental activities and more reluctance to accept parental advice or criticism; occasional rudeness; more realization that the parent is not perfect
2. An emotional void created by separation from parents, without the presence of a consistent alternative support group, which can create behavioral problems (e.g., a decrease in school performance)
3. Emotional lability (wide mood and behavior swings)
4. Increased ability to express oneself through speech
5. Search for new people to love in addition to parents

Body Image

Rapid physical changes lead the adolescent to be increasingly preoccupied with body image and the question of, "Am I normal?" Body image is a concept that changes with physical and psychosocial growth and development throughout adolescence and young adulthood. Male and female youth show increased dissatisfaction with their body image from middle school and can

persist into young adulthood. Weight dissatisfaction is especially pervasive among teenage girls and can lead to concerning health-compromising behaviors such as caloric restriction, dieting, binging, and purging (including excessive exercise, diuretics, diet pills, and laxatives). Girls who are precociously developed or less developed than their peers are prone to body dissatisfaction and low self-esteem. Dissatisfaction with body image may lead to dieting and eating disorders.[19]

The early adolescent's concern with body image is characterized by the following four factors:

1. Preoccupation with self
2. Uncertainty and concerns about appearance and attractiveness
3. Frequent comparison of own body with those of other adolescents
4. Increased interest in sexual anatomy and physiology, including anxieties and questions regarding menstruation or nocturnal emissions, masturbation, and breast or penis size.

Peer Group

With the beginning of separation from the family, the adolescent becomes more dependent on friends as a source of comfort.[18,20] The adolescent's peer group is characterized by the following:

1. Increasing focus on peers. Solitary friendships with a member of the same sex. These idealized friendships may become intense; boys, for example, may become "comrades-in-arms" with sworn pacts and allegiances, and young teenage girls may develop deep crushes on men as well as women.
2. Strongly emotional, tender feelings toward peers. The peer group usually consists of nonromantic friendships, which may lead to opposite-, same-, or both-sex attractions, exploration, fears, and/or relationships later on.
3. Peer contact primarily with the same sex, with some contact of the opposite sex made in groups of friends.

Identity Development

Associated with a steady increase in the complexity of the adolescent's cognitive abilities is the initiation of identity development, which is the complex process by which AYAs come to know themselves as unique individuals. According to Piaget's[21] cognitive theory, this corresponds to the cognitive evolution from concrete thinking (concrete operational thoughts) to abstract thinking (formal operational thoughts). During this early stage, the adolescent is expected to achieve academically and to prepare for the future. This period of identity development is characterized by the following:

1. Young adolescents apply their developing cognitive skills to the process of self-exploration, leading to increased self-interest and fantasy. For example, the young adolescent may feel himself or herself constantly "onstage."
2. Frequent daydreaming, which is not only normal but also an important component in identity development because it allows adolescents an avenue to explore, enact, problem solve, and recreate important aspects of their lives.
3. Setting unrealistic or idealistic (depending on the individual) vocational goals (e.g., musician, airplane pilot, or truck driver).
4. Testing authority is a common behavior in adolescents as they attempt to better define who they are, and is often a cause of tension between the adolescent and adults in authority such as parents or teachers.
5. A need for greater privacy often realized by adolescents' attempts to have more private physical spaces (closing doors to room), journal or diary writing, or Internet communications becoming more important.
6. Emergence of sexual feelings often relieved through masturbation or the telling of dirty jokes. Experimental curiosity, information seeking, and a lack of someone to discuss sexuality often drives adolescents to explore the Internet.[2]

7. Development of the adolescent's own value system, potentially leading to additional challenges to family and others.
8. Lack of impulse control and need for immediate gratification, which may result in dangerous risk-taking behavior.
9. Tendency to magnify one's personal situation (although adolescents often feel that they are continually onstage, conversely, they may also be convinced that they are alone and that their problems are unique).

MIDDLE ADOLESCENCE (APPROXIMATE AGES 14 TO 16)

Middle adolescence is characterized by an increased scope and intensity of feelings and by the rise in importance of peer group values.

Cognitive Development

During middle adolescence, the capacity to think and plan more abstractly develops with higher order abilities to plan for the future. Challenged by increasingly more complex academic and social challenges, adolescents become more efficient with abstract, multidimensional, planned, and hypothetical thinking.[5] However, if confronted with highly stressful events, adolescents may regress to more concrete thinking typical of early adolescence.[18]

Moving Toward Independence

Conflicts with parents and caretakers become more prevalent as the adolescent exhibits less interest in spending time with parents and devote more of his or her time to peers.

Body Image

Although the majority of the adolescents have experienced most of their pubertal changes, they continue to be preoccupied with their body image. Both girls and boys spend a lot of time focused on their physical appearance in order to "fit in" with their peer group. They spend a lot of time in grooming and trying to develop their own unique style. This is done in an effort to develop to achieve a satisfying and realistic body image. There appears to be an increased risk for eating disorders during this developmental phase.[19] In fact, anorexia nervosa has its peak onset in the mid- to late teenagers (15 to 19 years),[22] with a great prevalence of this disorder among girls (see Chapter 33).

Peer Group

The powerful role of peer groups is most apparent during middle adolescence.[18] Characteristics of this involvement include the following:

1. Intense involvement in the peer subculture
2. Conformity with peer values, codes, and dress, in an attempt to further separate from family
3. Peer groups expand to include romantic relationship, manifested by dating, sexual experimentation, and sexual activity.
4. Involvement with clubs, team sports, gangs, and other groups of interest

Evidence suggests that during middle adolescence, friends are the primary source of influence on youths' behavior, but estimates of peer pressure are often overstated especially if an authoritative parenting style is employed.[14]

Adolescents' reactions to peer pressure are extremely varied. Some are diverted from achieving educational and family goals, but many adolescents are propelled by peer pressure to excel in school, sports, and other positive activities.

Identity Development

As the young person's ability to abstract and to reason continues to increase in middle adolescence, they are better able to view themselves as unique individuals with a new sense of individuality. The middle adolescent's identity development is characterized by the following:

1. Increased scope and openness of feelings, with a new ability to emphasize and examine the feelings of others
2. Increased intellectual ability and creativity
3. More realistic vocational aspirations (adolescents with average and below-average intellectual abilities often realize their limitations at this time and may consequently experience lowered self-esteem and depression)
4. A feeling of omnipotence and immortality, leading to risk-taking behaviors, which is certainly a factor in the high rate of accidents, suicidal behaviors, drug use, risky sexual behaviors, resulting in pregnancies, and sexually transmitted diseases that become prevalent at this stage. At this developmental stage, these behaviors are enhanced in the presence of peers. Despite the fact that middle and late adolescents are often able to understand the risks involved in certain activities, in the presence of peers, and when emotionally aroused, they are more rewarded by the social stimuli associated with the peer group than by logical thinking.[23]

LATE ADOLESCENCE (APPROXIMATE AGES 17 TO 21)

Late adolescence is characterized by the development of personal identity and separation. If all has proceeded well in early and middle adolescence, especially the presence of a supportive family and peer group, the adolescent will be well on his or her way to handling the tasks and responsibilities of adulthood.[16] If the previously mentioned tasks have not been achieved, then problems such as depression, suicidal tendencies, substance use, or emotional disorders may worsen with the increasing independence and responsibilities of young adulthood.[24]

Cognitive Development

During late adolescence, the ability to think more abstractly and to plan for the future (i.e., career decisions) is more developed. Complex thinking processes are used to focus less on self-centered concepts and more on personal decision making. At this point, adolescents are able to make independent decisions about their life choices while weighing the costs and benefits more thoroughly.[18] In addition, late adolescents begin to focus on their emerging role in adult society. It is important to bear in mind that the maturational brain processes are still developing (and will continue into emerging adulthood) and are often lagging behind the challenges reflected by arousal and emotional motivation brought on by pubertal maturation.[23]

Moving Toward Independence

For most, late adolescence is a time of reduced restlessness and increased integration. The adolescent has become a separate entity from his or her family and may better appreciate the importance of his or her parents' values. Such an understanding may make it possible for the adolescent to seek and accept parental advice and guidance. However, it is not uncommon for some adolescents to be hesitant to accept the responsibilities of adulthood and to remain dependent on family and peers. Late adolescents often display the following:

1. A stronger personal identity
2. A greater ability to delay gratification
3. A better ability to solve problems and express ideas in words
4. A greater ability to make independent decisions and to compromise
5. A greater commitment to more stable interests

Body Image

The late adolescent has completed pubertal growth and development. However, body image issues may still be significant given the emphasis among peers and in the media. The emergence of disordered eating behaviors and eating disorders remain a significant problem.

Peer Group

As the late adolescent becomes more comfortable with his or her own identity and values, peer group values become less important. More time is spent in a relationship with one individual. Such relationships involve less experimentation and more sharing. The selection of a partner is based more on mutual understanding and enjoyment than on peer acceptance.

Identity Development

Identity development during late adolescence is characterized by the following:

1. The development of a rational and realistic conscience
2. The development of a sense of perspective, with the ability to delay gratification, compromise, and set limits
3. The development of practical vocational goals and the beginning of financial independence
4. The development of clear sexual identity
5. Further refinement of moral, religious, and sexual values

YOUNG OR "EMERGING" ADULTS (APPROXIMATE AGES 18 TO 25)

Although there is no specific definition of "young adulthood," it is thought to be a phase of the life that spans between late adolescence and early adulthood. It is felt to be a developmental period of exploration of possible life directions,[25] optimism, refined cognitive skills, and transition into adult roles.[3] Generally, young or "emerging" adulthood is the period between 18 and 25 years. A study of young people aged 18 to 29 years[3] describes young adults as optimistic and encourages a more positive view of this developmental phase. The study also describes emerging adults as fairly well educated across all the demographic groups and ready for adult responsibilities.[3] However, research also demonstrates that this generational period is often the time when mental disorders that commonly arise during mid- to late adolescence evolve more fully and follow the young adult into later adulthood.[26–28] In addition, there appears to be a progressively increasing delay in attaining "traditional" life milestones, including completing school, leaving home, becoming financially independent, marrying, and having a child. In 1960, 77% women and 65% of men at age 30 reached these five life "milestones." Among 30-year-olds in 2000, <50% of women and one-third of men had done so.[29,30]

Cognitive Development

During the emerging adulthood, brain development becomes more complex.[31] Brain imaging techniques reveal an extended period of maturation, especially in the frontal and parietal cortices, allowing for an increase in capacity for executive functioning (control and coordination of thought and behavior), the development of social cognition (what is perceived as important in the social world around the emerging adult), and perspective taking (taking on the viewpoint of another person)[6] (see Chapter 2). Emerging adults are therefore more successful in managing increased risk and the increased complexity of the adult world.[32] Toward the end of this stage, it is believed that the adolescent brain has fully matured.[31] Hence, by this period, a more complex cognitive facility is evident as emerging adults manage to cope with the nuances of the social and emotional constructs impacting their lives.

Moving Toward Independence

Moving away from home has a complex impact on the successful transition into adulthood. One study shows that an optimal and reasonable period of living with parents contributes to later psychological health.[15] Delayed transition to adulthood may help balance emotional health, while actual failure to fully transition to independent adulthood can become detrimental to the individual. This study recognized that failure to leave was often mitigated by social and financial difficulties, but emphasized that emerging adults fair better as adults following a timely transition.[15] The paths emerging adults take toward independence are unique and nonlinear; some emerging adults move forward and backward on the path to adulthood. Further, while on the course toward adulthood, emerging adults utilize varied timeframes to go through the different developmental tasks. Emerging adulthood may involve refining plans, moving back into a parents' home, quitting a job, or returning to school.[33] Indeed, in a large study of parents of emerging adults, it was found that parents and their emerging adult children had positive relationships and most emerging adults stayed at their parents homes while involved in attaining higher education.[15,33] Assessing the nature of the relationship between parents and emerging adults would help to understand if any stressors are present. In fact, it was found that after the adult child leaves the parental home, it is the parents who miss their children and struggle with adjusting to a childless home.[33]

Body Image

As the adolescent moves into adulthood, earlier body image issues such as eating disorders or obesity may follow. Studies have shown that body image issues, disordered eating, and obesity established in adolescence may persist into the emerging adult years.[19,34,35] This raises the urgency for the health care provider to assess and monitor body image, body mass index, and eating behaviors during the earlier phases of adolescence to mitigate lasting issues.

Peer Group and Identity Development

Most AYAs use this stage to complete the tasks associated with peer group and identity issues discussed earlier. As emerging adults become more independent of peer groups, and more able to apply the advanced cognitive skills now available to them, they become more involved in mature intimate relationships, and may delve further into identity exploration to refine their personal identities. Emerging adults may seem unfocused as they try out various life possibilities. They explore love and different levels of intimacy, seek work experiences that match possible occupational aspirations, try out different educational possibilities that may lead to different occupational futures, and consider a variety of world views reexamining earlier belief systems to develop their own set of values.[25] Consequently, as they move toward early adulthood, emerging adults are focused on refining their future goals and completing the pursuit of vocational goals, while taking greater responsibilities for their finances.[36]

CONCLUSION

Most AYAs will follow the psychosocial developmental trajectories outlined in this chapter. An understanding of this general pattern puts health care providers in a unique position to evaluate an adolescent or young adult's psychosocial development; so they can provide the support needed to attain a positive outcome.

REFERENCES

1. Tanner JL, Arnett JJ. Presenting "emerging adulthood": what makes it developmentally distinctive. In: Arnett JJ, Kloep M, Hendry LB, Tanner JL, eds. *Debating emerging adulthood: stage or process?* New York, NY: Oxford University Press, 2011:13–30.
2. Mitchell KJ, Ybarra ML, Korchmaros JD, et al. Accessing sexual health information online: use, motivations and consequences for youth with different sexual orientations. *Health Educ Res* 2014;29(1):147–157.
3. Arnett J, Schwab J. *The Clark University poll of young adults: striving, struggling, hopeful.* Worcester, MA: Clark University, 2012.
4. Jensen LA, Arnett JJ. Going global: new pathways for adolescents and emerging adults in a changing world. *J Soc Issues* 2012;68(3):473–492.
5. Steinberg L. Cognitive and affective development in adolescence. *Trends Cogn Sci* 2005;9(2):69–74.

6. Blakemore SJ, Choudhury S. Development of the adolescent brain: implications for executive function and social cognition. *J Child Psychol Psychiatry* 2006;47(3/4):296–312.
7. Casey B, Giedd JN, Thomas KM. Structural and functional brain development and its relation to cognitive development. *Biol Psychol* 2000;54(1):241–257.
8. Yurgelun-Todd D. Emotional and cognitive changes during adolescence. *Curr Opin Neurobiol* 2007;17(2):251–257.
9. Centers for Disease Control and Prevention. Youth risk behavior surveillance—United States, 2011. *MMWR* 2012;61(4):1–162.
10. World Health Organization. *Global health risks: mortality and burden of disease attributable to selected major risks*. Geneva, Switzerland: World Health Organization, 2009.
11. Gutgesell ME, Payne N. Issues of adolescent psychological development in the 21st century. *Pediatr Rev* 2004;25(3):79–85.
12. Freud A. Adolescence. *Psychoanal Study Child* 1958;13:255–278.
13. Sukarieh M, Tannock S. The positivity imperative: a critical look at the 'new' youth development movement. *J Youth Stud* 2011;14(6):675–691.
14. Steinberg L, Mounts NS, Lamborn SD, et al. Authoritative parenting and adolescent adjustment across varied ecological niches. *Adolescents and their Families: Structure, Function, and Parent–Youth Relations*. 2013;2(1):129.
15. Sacker A, Cable N. Transitions to adulthood and psychological distress in young adults born 12 years apart: constraints on and resources for development. *Psychol Med* 2010;12(2):301.
16. Johnson MD, Galambos NL. Paths to intimate relationship quality from parent–adolescent relations and mental health. *J Marriage Fam* 2014;76(1):145–160.
17. Mendle J, Turkheimer E, Emery RE. Detrimental psychological outcomes associated with early pubertal timing in adolescent girls. *Dev Rev* 2007;27(2):151–171.
18. Hornberger LL. Adolescent psychosocial growth and development. *J Pediatr Adolesc Gynecol* 2006;19(3):243–246.
19. Bucchianeri MM, Arikian AJ, Hannan PJ, et al. Body dissatisfaction from adolescence to young adulthood: findings from a 10-year longitudinal study. *Body Image* 2013;10(1):1–7.
20. Perry DG, Pauletti RE. Gender and adolescent development. *J Res Adolesc* 2011;21(1):61–74.
21. Piaget J, Inhelder, B, Weaver, H. *The psychology of the child*. New York, NY: Basic Books, 1969.
22. Hoek HW. Incidence, prevalence and mortality of anorexia nervosa and other eating disorders. *Curr Opin Psychiatry* 2006;19(4):389–394.
23. Steinberg L. Risk taking in adolescence new perspectives from brain and behavioral science. *Curr Dir Psychol Sci* 2007;16(2):55–59.
24. Adams SH, Knopf DK, Park MJ. Prevalence and treatment of mental health and substance use problems in the early emerging adult years in the United States: findings from the 2010 National Survey on drug use and health. *Emerg Adulthood* 2014;2(3):163–172.
25. Arnett JJ. Emerging adulthood: a theory of development from the late teens through the twenties. *Am Psychol* 2000;55(5):469.
26. Jones PB. Adult mental health disorders and their age at onset. *Br J Psychiatry Suppl* 2013; 54:s5–s10.
27. Neinstein L, Lu Y, Perez L, et al. *The new adolescents: an analysis of health conditions, behaviors, risks and access to services among emerging young adults*. Los Angeles, CA: University of Southern California, 2013.
28. Neinstein LS. Young adults remain worse off than adolescents. *J Adolesc Health* 2013;53(5):559–561.
29. Adams PE, Martinez ME, Vickerie JL, et al. *Summary health statistics for the US population: National Health Interview Survey, 2010*. Vital and health statistics. Series 10. Data from the National Health Survey. Hyattsville, MD: U.S. Department of Health and Human Services, 2011(251):1–117.
30. Henig RM. What is it about 20-somethings. *N Y Times Mag* August 22, 2010;18.
31. Giedd JN. Structural magnetic resonance imaging of the adolescent brain. *Ann N Y Acad Sci* 2004;1021(1):77–85.
32. Pharo H, Sim C, Graham M, et al. Risky business: executive function, personality, and reckless behavior during adolescence and emerging adulthood. *Behav Neurosci* 2011;125(6):970.
33. Arnett JJ, Schwab J. *The clark poll of parents of emerging adults*. Worcester, MA: Clark University, 2013.
34. Neumark-Sztainer D, Wall M, Guo J, et al. Obesity, disordered eating, and eating disorders in a longitudinal study of adolescents: how do dieters fare 5 years later? *J Am Diet Assoc* 2006;106(4):559–568.
35. Neumark-Sztainer D, Wall M, Larson NI, et al. Dieting and disordered eating behaviors from adolescence to young adulthood: findings from a 10-year longitudinal study. *J Am Diet Assoc* 2011;111(7):1004–1011.
36. Arnett JJ, Kloep M, Hendry LB, et al. *Debating emerging adulthood: stage or process?* New York, NY: Oxford University Press, 2010.

🛜 ADDITIONAL RESOURCES AND WEBSITES ONLINE

4

Office Visit, Interview Techniques, and Recommendations to Parents

Joshua S. Borus
Elizabeth R. Woods

KEY WORDS

- Communication
- Confidentiality
- HEEADSSS
- Interview techniques
- Office Visit
- Parental Advice
- Provider Advice
- Rapport

The skillful care of adolescent and young adult (AYA) patients requires competence that cannot be learned from a text alone. While we review some principles and goals of management in this chapter, the art of relating to AYAs is improved only with practice and reflection. Both process and content of an interview are important and one impacts the other. AYAs are much more likely to share concerns and information with a provider if the provider establishes rapport and trust. It is extremely difficult to care for an adolescent or young adult patient who is not open with his or her concerns; so time and energy invested in building rapport are essential.

 GENERAL GUIDELINES FOR THE OFFICE VISIT

Comfort with Adolescents and Young Adults

While it may seem self-evident, effective care of the adolescent or young adult requires the health care provider to feel comfortable with and enjoy working with this population. Providers who are uncomfortable with critical issues related to the care of AYAs (i.e., contraception, sexual health, substance use, independence) should refer their patients to providers who are comfortable working with this population.

There is significant overlap in the approach to AYAs, and as such these two populations are often grouped together in this chapter. However, there are some notable differences in the approach to the adolescent compared to the young adult based on chronologic and developmental age, especially with respect to consent, confidentiality, and privacy (see Chapter 9). We describe three approaches to the adolescent visit. Although these approaches translate well to the young adult population, we also review issues specific to young adults in more depth.

Meeting the Adolescent and Family: Initial Visit

The overarching goal of the AYA health visit is to improve outcomes for AYAs and help them establish good health practices as they move into adulthood. An important objective of the first visit is to build rapport with the patient and the family. Establishing the ground rules of the relationship, building trust, and focusing the visit on the adolescent's concerns can achieve this. Confidentiality and its limits (see below) must be discussed,[1–3] as well as giving practice and

provider contact information to both the adolescent and parent. This helps establish the adolescent as the principal participant in the visit while also recognizing the importance of the parent's role. Typically, one of three approaches is used to start the interview.

Start with Adolescent and Parent Together

Some providers prefer to start the interview with adolescent and parent(s) together. How the adolescent and parent(s) interact with one another (Does the parent speak for the adolescent instead of letting the patient answer? Are the parent and teen interacting with their phones and texting or using the time to talk and share?) can provide insight into the family interactions and inform the provider's strategy for addressing issues uncovered during the visit. Additionally, meeting together reinforces the importance of direct adolescent and parent communication. After introductions are delivered, a verbal outline or "roadmap" of the visit should be provided to the patient and the parent(s). This is often a time to discuss medical history, family history, and potentially nonsensitive social topics. Upon conclusion of this segment, the provider then asks the parent(s) to leave the room while the remainder of the history is completed with the adolescent alone.

Start with Parent Alone

Some providers like to include separate time at the initial visit with parent(s) and then conduct the confidential interview with the adolescent. This option offers an opportunity for the parent(s) to express concerns about the adolescent in private. After greeting everyone, the clinician explains the order of the visit and establishes confidentiality so that there is no confusion about the process or logistics of the visit. The clinician then meets with the parent(s) first, enabling them to express sensitive concerns at the beginning of the visit so that there is adequate time to address them. The clinician then meets with the adolescent alone to discuss the patient's concerns, obtain additional history, and conduct the physical examination. The visit concludes with the clinician summarizing with everyone. This approach ensures that the teen sees that the provider is not divulging confidential information to the family. Follow-up visits can start with a brief meeting with the parents alone if major issues persist, but should switch over to one of the other types of visits described.

Start with Adolescent Alone

An alternative approach is to meet first with the adolescent patient. This approach allows the provider to establish trust and focus attention on the adolescent. After meeting with the adolescent privately, the adolescent and parent(s) meet with the clinician together to complete the visit. It is important for the adolescent to understand that his or her parent(s) will likely be asked about the patient's past medical history as well as any parental concerns. Thus, confidentiality may need to be reviewed twice, once with adolescent alone so they feel comfortable and again when the parent is present so everyone understands the rules of the clinic.

Summarizing

The assessment usually concludes with a summary of the clinician's evaluation and management plan, including anticipatory guidance. Most of the discussion themes (e.g., concrete goals for eating healthier, resolution to get help from a math teacher, details about using a medication) can be done with the adolescent and family together, but sensitive concerns (e.g., smarter decision-making around sexual practices) should be discussed with the teen on his or her own. The parent's role in this process diminishes as the teen matures into young adulthood.

The Young Adult Visit

Typically, young adults come to medical visits alone, making these interactions more straightforward. However, when a parent(s) presents with the young adult, it is essential (particularly when a chronic disease is being addressed) that there is a clear understanding that the young adult is in charge of his or her health care. Legal age requirements governing the definition of adulthood vary across the globe (see Chapter 9) relative to who has control of and rights to medical information. It is important for the provider to understand these legal definitions. In most geographic locations, the provider will need verbal as well as written permission from the young adult to speak with a family member to help the patient with a treatment regimen or gain additional history. Regardless, young adults should be given an opportunity to consent to having their parent(s) involved in the summary of nonconfidential issues or participate in a discussion about how the parents can support the young adults in their health care.

Office Setup

Space

AYAs prefer their own waiting room (or separate area) that is relaxed, welcoming, and developmentally appropriate.[4] Some practices have separate blocks of time devoted to the AYAs in an effort to create this type of environment. If possible, clinic space should include an area that can accommodate larger groups for family or treatment team meetings. The examination room should include an examination table that has a curtain to promote a sense of privacy.

Clinic Staff

All clinic staff should have training on the developmental and health needs of AYAs. The clinic staff should adopt an AYA-friendly and nonjudgmental approach. Staff and receptionists should be familiar with issues such as confidentiality, crisis calls, and billing procedures. The staff should have flexible appointment booking procedures, including times to accept walk-in patients or a patient and his or her family who are in crisis. Every possible effort should be made to reduce wait times for young people.

Availability of Educational Materials

Age-appropriate magazines, hotline numbers, posters, and health education brochures both welcome the patient and signal that the provider is ready to talk about all topics, especially among youth who may be more reticent to discuss sensitive issues. Some practices place these materials in private places such as exam rooms and bathrooms to make them easier to obtain anonymously.

Appointments

Ideally (though perhaps not possible in some office settings), initial comprehensive visits should be given an hour in the schedule. Provision of after-school/early evening hours is critical for the patient to avoid missing school or employment. Discussion of who is needed at follow-up appointments (patient alone versus family and/or partner versus both patient and family and/or partner) should be identified at the end of the first visit. Finally, consult with the

adolescent or young adult alone on the best way to make contact for follow-up test results to protect his or her confidentiality.

Billing for Sensitive Services in the United States

In the United States, billing for services that the adolescent or young adult wishes to keep confidential is highly dependent on the patient's insurance. The legal age of majority (18 years in most US states) allows the young person to control his or her medical record. Insurance coverage now allows the parents to continue to maintain the adolescent or young adult on his or her health care plan through age 26 years. Thus, when confidential services are billed to the insurance, the patient's services will likely result in an explanation of benefits to the primary holder of the insurance plan (e.g., parent(s)) about the nature of the visit. Many issues can be disguised by billing under general symptom codes (e.g., "dysuria" or "cervicitis" instead of "chlamydia," if appropriate).

When a practice has general screening rules, it is much easier to explain certain tests. For example, "Mrs. Jones, our clinic policy is to run a pregnancy test on all females with abdominal pain." Some practices elect to bill the adolescent or young adult directly or absorb the costs of certain diagnoses or tests to protect the patient, but this is not always possible. Other options include directing the adolescent or young adult to obtain Medicaid funds for conditions such as pregnancy, family planning, or substance abuse or refer him or her to a health care setting that can provide low cost or free confidential services.

Note Taking/Electronic Communication

Patients should be aware that confidential aspects of care might be included in notes, letters, or electronic communication with other providers when appropriate. While there are benefits to electronic health records (EHRs), they also add layers of complexity around documenting sensitive diagnoses, patient information, and lab results (see Chapters 9 and 10). As more clinicians embrace EHRs, the ease with which accessing patient data increases, as does the ease with which confidentiality can be broken. For example, an emergency department provider sharing lab results with a patient and family may inadvertently reveal a positive screen for sexually transmitted infections or mistakenly disclose the adolescent's use of birth control when showing them a computer screen. To protect the AYAs' confidentiality when EHRs do not allow for sensitive information to remain confidential,[5] it may be necessary to establish mechanisms or protocols by which sensitive diagnoses or topics are not disclosed to parents. Patient portals, which allow patients access to their medical record or lab results remotely, also need to be considered carefully. The adolescent patient may be under pressure from a parent to allow unrestricted access to his or her record. Some strategies include creation of confidential diagnoses, fields, and/or medication sections that can only be accessed by in-system providers (see Chapters 9 and 10).

Interview Structure

It is not imperative to follow a rigidly proscribed format, but three central tasks must be addressed:

1. Introduction in which the adolescent or young adult is put at ease, a roadmap of the visit is presented, and confidentiality is discussed;
2. Definition of the patient's concerns/feelings and other information gathering; and
3. Summary in which the patient is informed about results of the examination, concerns are addressed, questions answered, nonconfidential issues summarized with the parents when appropriate and follow-up interval established.

Previsit Questionnaires

More providers are using written questionnaires completed by the patient either at home or in the waiting room to gather information. These questionnaires may help prompt the adolescent or young adult to consider important topics that he or she might want to address during the encounter. However, answers to sensitive questions may not be accurate if the surveys are completed in public spaces. Some providers use written screening tools to increase delivery of preventive services and screen for social determinants of health.[6,7] For mental health issues, the Patient Health Questionnaire (PHQ-9)[8] is a validated depression screen for teens and young adults (see Chapter 70), and the Self-Report for Childhood Anxiety Related Disorders (SCARED) has been validated as a screen for common anxiety disorders in adolescents.[9] The American Academy of Pediatrics has developed questionnaires for early, middle, and late adolescents/young adults to screen for a variety of issues at each visit through the Bright Futures project.[10]

Electronic Screening

With increased use of social media, many AYAs find the computer a nonthreatening way to disclose personal information that can be addressed in the clinical session.[11–13] Electronic screening allows collection of data before entry into the clinician's office, saving time in the encounter for discussing results rather than obtaining information.

Establish Rapport

Creating rapport is of paramount importance in the AYA patient–provider relationship, and it may require more than one visit to establish.[14,15] However, if rapport and trust are not built, subsequent visits will likely be ineffective. Helpful ways to engage AYAs include the following:

1. Begin by introducing yourself to the adolescent or young adult and parent(s), if present. Address/shake hands with the patient first.
2. Invest a few minutes chatting informally about nonsensitive topics such as friends, school, or hobbies. This decreases tension and may provide insights into the patient's personality, mood, and how she or he conceptualizes and articulates thoughts and feelings.
3. Let the adolescent or young adult talk for a while on topics of interest to him or her.
4. Treat all patients' comments seriously.
5. Start with nonthreatening health questions such as a review of systems if the patient is highly tense or suspicious.
6. Explore issues that concern the adolescent or young adult. These issues may differ dramatically from concerns expressed by the parents (see **Table 4.1**).

TABLE 4.1
Interviewing Suggestions for AYAs

1. Shake hands with the adolescent first.
2. Ask questions in context.
3. Focus initial history taking on the patient's complaints or problems.
4. Identify who has the problem (i.e., Is this problem the teen's concern or the parent's?).
5. Talk in terms that the adolescent will understand.
6. Highlight the positive.
7. Avoid lecturing and admonishing.
8. Take a neutral stance.
9. Usually, the less the interviewer says the better.
10. Avoid writing during the interview, especially during sensitive questioning.
11. Criticize the activity, not the adolescent, and explain why you have concern.
12. Assess your own ability to listen. A provider's difficulty in listening may be related to his or her own resentments or opinions of the adolescent's behavior.
13. When asking direct questions:
    a. use less personal questions before more personal questions,
    b. use open-ended questions, and
    c. avoid assumptions about gender and sexual preferences.

Ensure Confidentiality

Clinicians who care for AYAs must understand the concept of confidential care and the limits on confidentiality. Providers need to be cognizant that limits of confidentiality vary across geographic areas, and therefore, they must be familiar with their local standards and laws governing this core component of AYA care.[16,17]

It is the clinician's responsibility to explain this concept to the patient and parent(s). It is important that all parties involved with the patient be aware of the boundaries and exceptions to confidentiality. The patient should be made aware that if he or she is a danger to himself or herself or a danger to others, the provider will break confidentiality and report this information to the necessary parties. If the adolescent or young adult is accompanied by a parent to a clinic visit, the concept of confidentiality is best approached with the adolescent or young adult and his or her parent jointly.[18] This explanation may help the parents feel more comfortable about allowing the adolescent or young adult to meet with the clinician on his or her own. Discussing these complex concepts may also help dispel any conflicting beliefs the parent has about confidentiality.[19] For example, "Brian and Mrs. Jones, let me take a minute to review our clinic's confidentiality policy. We'll typically start our visits together so that everyone has a chance to put forward topics of discussion. Then there will be a time where I speak with Brian alone. Brian, this is an opportunity to talk about anything you want or to ask questions and I'll have some questions for you as well. You should know that what we talk about in that setting stays between you (Brian) and the health care team *unless* I am concerned about you hurting yourself or someone else. Your parents trust me to help care for you, and they need to know that if you tell me that you are in danger, are a danger to someone else, or are a danger to yourself, we would let them know together. This is all about keeping you safe. Do you have any questions?" Ensuring confidential health care will foster a more open discussion about sensitive topics between the adolescents or young adults and their provider.[17]

The clinician should make a reasonable effort to encourage the adolescent (and young adult, if appropriate) to involve parents in health care decisions. Some AYAs may be more willing to discuss sensitive topics with their parents in an environment where they feel safe and supported. For some AYAs, this may be the clinician's office. The clinician should be willing to help the adolescent or young adult communicate with his or her family. Often, AYAs are willing to disclose sensitive information to their parents, but may need help in framing the disclosure. It is often helpful when the provider offers to facilitate a discussion that includes difficult topics.

Structure of the Social History

To structure the psychosocial history, many clinicians use the HEEADSSS (home, education/employment, eating, activities, drugs, sexuality, suicide/depression, safety) screening framework (see Chapter 5).[20] This approach moves from less personal to more personal questions for each topic as the patient becomes more comfortable and rapport is developed. While some patients may be uncomfortable with some of the social history questions at their initial visit, this approach allows each adolescent or young adult to understand and appreciate what is acceptable to discuss at future encounters. This framework also allows the provider to praise strengths or good decision-making as well as comment on behaviors that may need modification or elimination in order to promote health and wellness. Below are some sample questions for each category that apply to all teens and young adults. Many are open ended to facilitate greater communication between the patient and the provider.

Home: Where do you live? What's it like in your neighborhood? Who lives with you? How does everyone at home get along? Have there been recent changes?

Education/Employment: Are you in school? What is the school like? Do you get extra support in any classes? What subjects do you do well in? Are there any favorite teachers/adults you can turn to for support? What do you want to do after finishing school? If out of school, Do you work? What is the job like and how long do you plan to stay with it? What's next?

Eating: What do you think about your weight? Do you follow a diet or are you aware of what you eat? Do you have meals with family, friends, or by yourself? Do you snack in front of a screen? How much fast food do you consume? How many sugar-sweetened drinks, calcium-containing foods, or fruits and vegetables do you have in a day? Have you ever thrown up, restricted your intake, or taken diet pills or laxatives to control your weight? Do you take any nutritional supplements or vitamins?

Activities: What do you do in your free time? What are you good at? What do you like to do for fun? Do you have a core set of friends? How do you get physical activity in your lives? How much screen time do you engage in? Are you involved in groups or clubs?

Drugs: Are there students at school who drink, smoke, or use other substances? Is there anybody at home who smokes, drinks, or uses other substances? Have you ever tried any of these things? How often do you use these now? How do you pay for substances? In addition to these questions, there are a variety of brief screening tools with good sensitivity for substance use.[21]

Sexuality: Are you in a relationship with anyone? Are you attracted to guys/men, girls/women, both, or neither? Have you had sex (clarify what sex is) or are you choosing to "hold off?" Do you have vaginal sex, meaning, and penis-in-vagina sex? Do you have anal sex, meaning, and penis-in-rectum/anus sex? How old were you when you first had sex? Have you had any problems with sex—is it what you thought it would be like? How many partners have you had? What are you using for protection? Do you know about plan B and how to get it? Most AYAs masturbate—do you have any questions about masturbating? Have you been pregnant or had an abortion?

Suicide/Depression: How is your mood? Do you think you get frustrated or upset more than your friends? How is your sleep? How is your level of interest in regular activities? Do you feel guilty or anxious about things? What is your energy level like? Do you find it hard to concentrate? Have your eating habits changed? Have you ever thought about hurting yourself or killing yourself? Should I be worried about you?

Safety: Do you feel safe at home, school, and in your neighborhood? Is there any bullying at school? Have you ever been hit, kicked, punched, or touched in an inappropriate way or against your will? How often do you wear a seatbelt while in a car?

Table 4.2 outlines some effective interviewing techniques that can be used in the assessment of an adolescent or young adult patient.

Physical Examination

Typically, AYAs are examined alone, though some younger or developmentally delayed teens may wish to have a parent present. The patient should be asked as to whether he or she would like a chaperone during the physical examination. Male providers are strongly advised to use a chaperone during genital or breast examination of all female patients, and this seems to be standard practice. While the converse should hold true, in practice, it is not atypical for female providers to examine male patients without a chaperone if the patient agrees.

While completing the physical examination, the clinician has an excellent opportunity to reassure the patient about his or her growth and physical development. The physical examination provides an opportunity to educate the adolescent or young adult about his or her changing body, especially for the younger adolescent. Pointing out normal findings may provide great relief of an unspoken concern, especially as it relates to the genital examination.

Closure

At the close of any visit, the health care provider should:

1. Summarize the diagnosis and treatment for the adolescent or young adult. Parents who accompany the patient may be

TABLE 4.2

Interviewing Techniques for AYAs

Open-ended questions often facilitate communication	What does your pain prevent you from doing?" or "Tell me more about the arguments with your mother" may uncover a richer response then "Does your pain stop you from playing sports?" or "Does it make you feel bad to argue with your mom?"
Restatement and summarization	This often clarifies a problem or encourages additional communication: "So what I'm hearing is you like Jim, but don't want to have sex with him. However, you're worried if you say no, he'll move onto someone else. Have I got it right or am I missing something?"
Clarification	The provider should not be afraid to ask the patient for help decoding slang. It demonstrates interest, that they are willing to ask for help, and allows the patient to be an authority.
Insight questions	Some questioning should focus on gaining a global understanding of the AYAs. "What do you see yourself doing in a year?" or "How would your friends describe you?"
Reassuring questions	Providing context and normalizing sensitive subjects through reassuring statements may facilitate discussion. For example, "Most of my patients your age masturbate—it is completely normal. Do you masturbate?"
Support and empathy	Acknowledging the patient's feelings is crucial to all clinical encounters regardless of age. "I'm sorry you've had to deal with this—is there a way I can be helpful?" demonstrates the clinician's empathy and support.
Reflection responses	The reflection response mirrors the adolescent's feelings. Consider the following example: MD: How do you like school? Teen: I hate it. MD: You hate it? Teen: Yeah, my teachers always…

included in the discussions of nonconfidential issues to provide support and assistance.
2. Discuss other resources available to the patient.
3. Allow time to address questions and concerns from the adolescent or young adult and parent.
4. Schedule a follow-up appointment.
5. The provider should inform the adolescent or young adult about the provider's office hours and availability should health concerns arise. The provider should encourage the patient to contact the office for all his or her health care needs.

PRINCIPLES TO APPROACHING THE ADOLESCENT OR YOUNG ADULT PATIENT

Avoid a Surrogate Parent Role

Rather than being a surrogate parent, the health-care provider should function as a concerned adult who is nonjudgmental when listening, advising, and providing guidance.

Avoid a Peer Role

Most AYAs want a provider who can be a sensitive and mature resource, rather than a friend. A lack of formality and a sense of humor may be inviting, but dressing and talking like a peer are not.

Sidestep Power Struggles

It is difficult to force adolescents and especially young adults into action. Avoiding power struggles, focusing on facts in a judgment-free way, and helping young people arrive at their own decision to make change in the clinical encounter are difficult, but much more effective in bringing about change. Motivational interviewing techniques, in which the provider helps the adolescent or young adult develop his or her own reasons to change behavior, facilitate change by emphasizing differences between desired goals and current behavior.[22,23]

Act as an Advocate

Providers should emphasize the patient's positive traits[24] and recognize that supporting the adolescent or young adult does not mean supporting inappropriate behavior.

Active Listening

It is important to emphasize the role of active listening and acknowledging the concerns of the patient. Focusing on what the adolescent or young adult communicates, understanding the patient's perspective, and refraining from giving advice without first getting permission will help open doors and provide the clinician with opportunities in conversation to discuss his or her priorities.

Instill Responsibility

Acknowledging the limits of the provider and promoting the patient's personal responsibility for his or her health and health care can lead to improved outcomes. The provider can be a willing coach but cannot make decisions for the adolescent or young adult. Ultimately, the patient (often with the assistance of his or her family or support system) needs to commit to staying healthy.[25]

Nonverbal Cues

It is important for the clinician to be aware of the patient's nonverbal interaction. Nonverbal communication such as facial expressions, gestures, eye contact, or posture provides important information and can help the provider connect with his or her patient.

Avoid Stereotyping

The clinician must avoid stereotyping AYAs. The clinician should be sensitive to cultural issues and the particular needs of his or her patients, particularly as it applies to his or her health care.

Behavioral Context

Recognizing there may be multiple reasons that lead to an action and exploring the thinking and context behind a decision may alter the provider's perception of a patient's behavior. For example, a clinician might think differently of a patient with poorly controlled ADHD skipping class because of excessive frustration than a patient skipping class because of wanting to see friends who are also skipping class. In addition, younger adolescents are often concrete thinkers who may alter behavior if given help considering alternative responses to a situation.

Hidden Agenda

AYAs may obscure the real reason for a visit due to concerns about confidentiality, embarrassment, or denial. The clinicians should clearly express they are open to all concerns and interested in assisting the patient. This can minimize, but may not eliminate, the patient's hesitancy to disclose his or her central reason for seeing the provider. For example, a female adolescent may complain about vague abdominal pain instead of verbalizing that she is really worried she may be pregnant or a male adolescent with chest pain may actually be concerned about gynecomastia. Reassurance about variations of normal clinical findings found on physical examination (i.e., "It looks like you have a small amount of tissue development around your chest—I see this in a number of young

men going through puberty. While this is completely normal, they are sometimes worried about it. Do you have any concerns?") and use of appropriate testing (i.e., "Sometimes many patients with abdominal pain are worried they might be pregnant. Is this something that you have a thought about? You know, we could do a simple test to help answer this question.") can bring these concerns to the surface.

Developmental Orientation

Providers must be sensitive to the developmental and behavioral trajectories of AYAs. The cognitive processes, emotional maturity, and developmental tasks of a 13-year-old are different than those of a 17-year-old, and both of these are different from a 22-year-old.[26] Being aware of the differences in developmental trajectories and modifying the interview approach around sensitive issues (i.e., body image, substance use, peer relationships, mental health, independence, sexual and reproductive health) to their unique context can result in a more complete understanding of the adolescent or young adult patient.

Special Interview Challenges

1. Garrulous patient: Overtalkative AYAs can often be directed by asking "I can see you like talking about this. Why?" or responding and then reframing the question with discrete answers "It sounds like you've got some strong opinions about gym class. Tell me, do you exercise almost every day, a few times a week, or not at all?"
2. Quiet patient: Try to activate the adolescents or young adults by talking about anything—their T-shirt, their phone, a current event, or sports to help break the silence.
3. Anxious patient: Reassurance and normalization are often useful—"Sometimes it's difficult to talk about---"
4. Angry patient: Clarify how you can help the patient. "It sounds like talking about these issues with your parents could be difficult—can I help with that?"

Family Considerations and Societal Determinants of Health

Family relationships are an important contributor to the adolescent or young adult's development. For the provider to effect change in an AYA, he or she must understand the strengths, weaknesses, interactions within, and stresses of the family and be willing to work with the entire family unit. Understanding the ability of the family to support and nurture the young person's development is critical to providing effective care. Change in the adolescent or young adult may be dependent on first initiating change within the family. Thus, conversations between the provider and the family can become an opportunity to effect change in the family as an initial step to improving the health and well-being of the patient. In addition, consulting with parents or other family members (with the consent of the young person) may help elucidate past medical family history, create support for the patient in complex treatment regimens,[27] and promote follow-up and referral care. Finally, the definition of family has evolved considerably over time, and asking the patient whom he or she considers his or her family is an important component of the history.

In addition to family considerations, providers should be attuned to the role of societal factors and constraints that impact AYAs.[28] Twenty percent of US adolescents live under the poverty line,[29] and economically disadvantaged AYAs rate their health status lower than those who are economically advantaged.[30]

Internal Considerations

Many practitioners recall their own experience as an adolescent or young adult to generate understanding and empathy for their patients. The provider may wish to disclose some personal experience with the adolescent or young adult about his or her own youth to reduce the distance between the clinician and the patient. However, there is a risk of making the patient feel uncomfortable; provider self-disclosure should be carefully considered before being used.

Optimize AYA–Provider Communication

The patient's perception of his or her provider's behavior contributes to his or her willingness to make a return visit as well as adhere to a treatment plan.[31] Providers who demonstrate honesty, listen attentively, answer questions, affirm confidentiality, show respect, exchange information, and enhance satisfaction will increase the probability that the adolescent or young adult will return for follow-up.[32]

RECOMMENDATIONS TO PARENTS OF ADOLESCENTS

Authoritative Parenting Style

Steinberg and colleagues[33] have conducted extensive research that has examined the impact of parenting styles on a variety of adolescent outcomes. These researchers have drawn from an economically and racially diverse group of adolescents and families from across the globe. A consistent finding in these studies is that the most positive adolescent outcomes appear to be found in families with parents who are identified as authoritative. Authoritative parents:

1. are warm and loving;
2. develop firm and consistent but not rigid family guidelines;
3. and foster a child's independence according to developmental stage. Independence helps a child develop a sense of self-direction. Not fostering independence and decision-making is associated with increasing levels of anxiety among adolescents.

Adolescents who have at least one parent with this parenting style demonstrated:

1. better academic performance,
2. fewer mental health problems,
3. fewer antisocial behaviors and diminished delinquency, and
4. higher self-esteem and self-reliance.

General Suggestions

Other suggestions for parents about navigating the challenges of adolescence and young adulthood include the following:

1. Listen and show interest in the adolescent or young adult's activities.
2. Avoid power struggles if possible and solve conflicts together using a collaborative approach.
3. Remain flexible.
4. Spend time together and create opportunities to have fun one-on-one.
5. Demonstrate trust.
6. Take opportunities to stress the positive when they arise.
7. Make resources available.
8. Ensure that standards and expectations are clear, but have some flexibility in how these are accomplished—for example, the time the trash is taken out does not matter as long as it is taken out in time for pick up.
9. Avoid minimizing problems while still giving perspective; conversely, do not overreact based on limited information.

Challenges of Adolescence

Parents should be aware of the developmental tasks (see Chapter 3) associated with adolescence as well as the impact of peers and technology (see Chapter 10) on the adolescent's social milieu. This translates into understanding what behaviors, feelings, and actions are normal and healthy during the adolescent years. Recognition and appreciation of normative teen behaviors can minimize difficulties between parents and their teen.

1. Peers play an increasingly important role in a teen's life as he or she seeks independence.
2. Parents must not overreact to rejection by the teen for a period of time. Parents should appreciate that most young people do not reject their parent's values and beliefs even as they may strive to be independent.
3. Adolescents need firm, fair, and explicit limits. Involvement of the adolescent in the limit-setting process is beneficial.
4. Parents need to be proactive about their adolescent's health and well-being. Proactive parents are defined as parents who anticipate potential conflicts and prepare their child to deal with these conflicts by discussion, modeling, and reason. While substance use experimentation by teens is predictable, data suggest that proactive parents had teens who were less likely to initiate early alcohol use and marijuana.[34,35] In addition, these parents were more likely to have their teens receive an annual visit, report more frequent discussions about health, and place a high value on physician discussions about health.[36]
5. Adolescents' sense of invulnerability adds to willingness to expose themselves to risks.
6. The societal pressures of the 21st century present challenges as most families have less support than before and are stretched thinner. Single parenting is more prevalent, extended families are less involved in care, and more families have no stay-at-home adult.
7. The lives of adolescents are increasingly saturated with media. Parents need to be available to decode messages engineered to exploit the vulnerabilities of this age group and promote unhealthy or unrealistic images to make a profit from the teen. In addition, ensuring that teens understand that the Internet and social media platforms can be used to ridicule and bully (see Chapter 10), leave a permanent digital footprint that may embarrass them in the future, and may convey inaccurate information is important.

Challenges of Young Adult Years

1. Young adults continue to work toward separation and individual identification. Parents should remember that the vast majority of young adults accept their parents' basic values.
2. Young adults typically seek to have a more equal relationship with parents even if they are not ready to be independent in all phases of their lives. This change in relationship will not occur instantaneously when attaining the age of majority but gradually over time.
3. Transitioning to adult health care, even when delayed into the mid-20s, may be difficult for the young adult.[37]

Establishing House Rules

House rules with AYAs should be clear, consistently enforced, and applied to all those living in the house. Uniformity and consistent application improves everyone's happiness. These can be discussed as a family and should involve the adolescent or young adult in the decision-making process. Keeping the rules to a manageable number (5–10) and writing them down, especially for young adolescents, is also advised.[38]

ACKNOWLEDGMENTS

Supported in part by the Leadership Education in Adolescent Health Training grant #T71MC00009 from Maternal and Children Health Bureau, Health Resources and Services Administration. We would also like to thank Griselda Potka, BA, for her administrative assistance with this chapter.

REFERENCES

1. *An overview of Minor's Consent Laws*; 2013. Available at http://www.guttmacher.org/statecenter/spibs/spib_OMCL.pdf. Accessed on April 24, 2014.
2. Gynecologists American College of Obstetricians and Gynecologists. *Guidelines for adolescent health care*. Washington, DC: American College of Obstetricians and Gynecologists, 2011.
3. Ford C, English A, Sigman G. Confidential health care for adolescents: position paper for the society for adolescent medicine. *J Adolesc Health* 2004;35:160–167.
4. Tivorsak TL, Britto MT, Klostermann BK, et al. Are pediatric practice settings adolescent friendly? An exploration of attitudes and preferences. *Clin Pediatr (Phila)* 2004;43:55–61.
5. Bourgeois FC, Taylor PL, Emans SJ, et al. Whose personal control? Creating private, personally controlled health records for pediatric and adolescent patients. *J Am Med Inf Assoc* 2008;15:737–743.
6. Ozer EM, Adams SH, Lustig JL, et al. Increasing the screening and counseling of adolescents for risky health behaviors: a primary care intervention. *Pediatrics* 2005;115:960–968.
7. Kenyon C, Sandel M, Silverstein M, et al. Revisiting the social history for child health. *Pediatrics* 2007;120:e734–e738.
8. Richardson LP, McCauley E, Grossman DC, et al. Evaluation of the Patient Health Questionnaire-9 Item for detecting major depression among adolescents. *Pediatrics* 2010;126:1117–1123.
9. Birmaher B, Khetarpal S, Brent D, et al. The Screen for Child Anxiety Related Emotional Disorders (SCARED): scale construction and psychometric characteristics. *J Am Acad Child Adolesc Psychiatry* 1997;36:545–553.
10. *Bright futures adolescent visit forms*. 2014. Available at http://brightfutures.aap.org/tool_and_resource_kit.html. Accessed on April 17, 2015.
11. Stevens J, Kelleher KJ, Gardner W, et al. Trial of computerized screening for adolescent behavioral concerns. *Pediatrics* 2008;121:1099–1105.
12. Olson AL, Gaffney CA, Hedberg VA, et al. Use of inexpensive technology to enhance adolescent health screening and counseling. *Arch Pediatr Adolesc Med* 2009;163:172–177.
13. Wylie SA, Hassan A, Krull EG, et al. Assessing and referring adolescents' health-related social problems: qualitative evaluation of a novel web-based approach. *J Telemed Telecare* 2008;18:392–398.
14. Hoffman ND, Freeman K, Swann S. Healthcare preferences of lesbian, gay, bisexual, transgender and questioning youth. *J Adolesc Health* 2009;45:222–229.
15. van Staa A, Jedeloo S, van der Stege H; On Your Own Feet Research Group. "What we want": chronically ill adolescents' preferences and priorities for improving health care. *Patient Prefer Adherence* 2011;5:291–305.
16. *State minor consent laws: a summary*, 3rd ed. 2009. Available at http://www.cahl.org/state-minor-consent-laws-a-summary-third-edition/. Accessed on April 24, 2014.
17. Ford CA, Millstein SG, Halpern-Felsher BL, et al. Influence of physician confidentiality assurances on adolescents' willingness to disclose information and seek future health care. A randomized controlled trial. *JAMA* 1997;278:1029–1034.
18. Duncan RE, Vandeleur M, Derks A, et al. Confidentiality with adolescents in the medical setting: what do parents think? *J Adolesc Health* 2011;49:428–430.
19. Hutchinson JW, Stafford EM. Changing parental opinions about teen privacy through education. *Pediatrics* 2005;116:966–971.
20. Klein DA, Goldenring JM, Adelman WP. HEADSSS 3.0 The psychosocial interview for adolescents updated for a new century fueled by media. *Contemp Pediatr* 2014:16–28.
21. Knight JR, Sherritt L, Harris SK, et al. Validity of brief alcohol screening tests among adolescents: a comparison of the AUDIT, POSIT, CAGE, and CRAFFT. *Alcohol Clin Exp Res* 2003;27:67–73.
22. Gold MA, Kokotailo PK. Motivational interviewing strategies to facilitate adolescent behavior change. *Adolesc Health Update* 2007;20:1–10.
23. Suarez N-K, Mariann S. *Motivational interviewing with adolescents and young adults*. New York, NY: Guilford Press, 2011.
24. Chung RJ, Burke PJ, Goodman E. Firm foundations: strength-based approaches to adolescent chronic disease. *Curr Opin Pediatr* 2010;22:389–397.
25. Duncan PM, Garcia AC, Frankowski BL, et al. Inspiring healthy adolescent choices: a rationale for and guide to strength promotion in primary care. *J Adolesc Health* 2007;41:525–535.
26. Johnson SB, Blum RW, Giedd JN. Adolescent maturity and the brain: the promise and pitfalls of neuroscience research in adolescent health policy. *J Adolesc Health* 2009;45:216–221.
27. Ellis D, Naar-King S, Templin T, et al. Multisystemic therapy for adolescents with poorly controlled type 1 diabetes: reduced diabetic ketoacidosis admissions and related costs over 24 months. *Diabetes Care* 2008;31:1746–1747.
28. Viner RM, Ozer EM, Denny S, et al. Adolescence and the social determinants of health. *Lancet* 2012;379:1641–52.
29. Baer TE, Gottlieb L, Sandel M. Addressing social determinants of health in the adolescent medical home. *Curr Opin Pediatr* 2013;25:447–453.
30. Johnson SB, Wang C. Why do adolescents say they are less healthy than their parents think they are? The importance of mental health varies by social class in a nationally representative sample. *Pediatrics* 2008;121:e307–e313.
31. Ginsburg KR, Slap GB, Cnaan A, et al. Adolescents' perceptions of factors affecting their decisions to seek health care. *JAMA* 1995;273:1913–1918.
32. Woods ER, Klein JD, Wingood GM, et al. Development of a new Adolescent Patient-Provider Interaction Scale (APPIS) for youth at risk for STDs/HIV. *J Adolesc Health* 2006;38:753. e1–e7.
33. Steinberg L. Gallagher lecture. The family at adolescence: transition and transformation. *J Adolesc Health* 2000; 27(3):170–178.
34. Hawkins JD, Graham JW, Maguin E, et al. Exploring the effects of age on alcohol use initiation and psychosocial risk factors on subsequent alcohol misuse. *J Stud Alcohol Drugs* 1997;58:280–290.
35. Kosterman R, Hawkins JD, Guo J, et al. The dynamics of alcohol and marjiana initiation: patterns and predictors of first use in adolescence. *Am J Public Health* 2000;90:360–366.
36. Gilbert AL, Aalsma MC. Proactive parents: an asset to the health and well-being of teens. *J Pediatr* 2014;164:1390–1395.
37. Lemly DC, Weitzman ER, O'Hare K. Advancing healthcare transitions in the medical home: tools for providers, families and adolescents with special healthcare needs. *Curr Opin Pediatr* 2013;25:439–46.
38. Patterson GR, Forgatch MS. *Parents and adolescents living together, Part 2: family problem solving*, 2nd ed. Champaign, IL: Research Press, 2005.

ADDITIONAL RESOURCES AND WEBSITES ONLINE

CHAPTER 5

Preventive Health Care for Adolescents and Young Adults

Carolyn B. Jasik
Elizabeth M. Ozer

KEY WORDS

- Electronic health records
- Preventive care
- Preventive counseling
- Preventive health guidelines
- Risk behavior
- Screening and counseling

Since the majority of adolescent and young adult (AYA) morbidity and mortality can be attributed to known preventable risk factors, preventive health care is the cornerstone of AYA Medicine. Behaviors initiated during adolescence, such as substance use and abuse, early sexual behavior, and risky driving, are responsible for the majority of deaths and disabling conditions in adolescence.[1] Motor vehicle deaths and homicide rates are highest during young adulthood as are rates of substance use, sexually transmitted infections (STIs), and mental health problems.[2] Unintentional injuries account for the most deaths during adolescence and young adulthood. Suicide and homicide are the 2nd and 3rd leading causes of death for adolescents and are tied for the 2nd leading cause of death among young adults.[3]

As discussed in other chapters in this book, the psychosocial and developmental milieu of adolescence and young adulthood fosters a risk-taking environment. The annual visit to a health care provider offers an opportunity to improve the health of AYAs through preventive screening and counseling. Visits to a health care provider should reinforce positive health behaviors, such as exercise and nutritious eating, and discourage health-risk behaviors such as those associated with unsafe sexual behaviors, unsafe driving, and use of tobacco or other drugs. Although the incidence of serious medical problems during adolescence and young adulthood is low, lifelong health habits are established during this time. It is therefore an ideal period for health professionals to invest time in health promotion and preventive services.

In this chapter, we review current best practices for preventive services for AYAs and highlight key aspects of preventive care, including preventive health guidelines, the health care delivery setting, the content of the visit, and emerging areas of efficiency such as electronic health records (EHRs).

PREVENTIVE SERVICES FOR AYAs

Clinical Guidelines for Preventive Services

Most AYAs visit primary care settings at least once a year; so primary care has been highlighted as an important setting for detection and early intervention for risk-taking behaviors and mental health issues in youth. Since many health problems during adolescence and young adulthood are preventable, primary care visits represent a key opportunity for preventive screening and intervention, with

evidence supporting the efficacy of certain clinical preventive services.[4] Interventions during adolescence and young adulthood may have long-term implications because unhealthy behaviors tend to continue into middle and late adulthood, and are linked to preventable chronic conditions and premature deaths.[2]

A broad consensus has emerged for comprehensive clinical preventive services for adolescents with the adoption of guidelines such as the American Medical Association's *Guidelines for Adolescent Preventive Services (GAPS): Recommendations and Rationale* and *Bright Futures: Guidelines for Health Supervision of Infants, Children, and Adolescents*. The third and most recent edition of Bright Futures, a professional consensus document created jointly by Health Resources and Services Administration's (HRSA's) Maternal and Child Health Bureau and the American Academy of Pediatrics (AAP), provides recommendations for the care of AYAs up to age 21 years.[5]

Adolescents

In general, preventive health guidelines recommend that all adolescents have an annual, confidential visit. During this visit, clinicians should provide screening, education, and counseling in a number of biomedical and sociobehavioral areas.[4] Adolescents should be screened for risky health behaviors, and strengths and competencies should be identified. The updated Bright Futures guidelines specifically encourage the promotion of positive youth development and recommend that clinicians focus on the strengths of the adolescent and his or her family in the annual visits.[5]

Health guidance should also be provided to parents to help them respond appropriately to the health needs of their adolescent child. This includes providing information about normative adolescent development, the signs and symptoms of disease and emotional distress, parenting behaviors that promote healthy adolescent adjustment, and methods to help adolescents avoid potentially harmful behaviors.

Young Adults

There are currently no specific guidelines developed for young adults regardless of the definition of age range for young adulthood.[4] The most comprehensive set of guidelines that intersect with the age group of 18 to 26 years are AAP's Bright Futures. Still, several other professional organizations have guidelines that are relevant to the care of young adults. The American College of Obstetricians and Gynecologists (ACOG) has created guidelines for both female adolescents and adults (aged 19 to 39 years). The American Academy of Family Physicians (AAFP) and the American College of Physicians (ACP) have developed guidelines that mirror the United States Preventive Services Task Force (USPSTF) recommendations.[6] **Table 5.1** compares guidelines for AYA preventive care, recommendations for screening, and recommended components of the physical examination from our review article in 2012.[4]

TABLE 5.1

Guidelines for AYA Preventive Health Care[a]

	USPSTF[8]		Bright Futures[14] Adolescent, Aged 11–21 y	ACOG[23,24]	
	Adolescent, Aged <18 y	Adult, Aged ≥18 y		Adolescent, Aged 13–21 y	Adult, Aged 19–39 y
Substance use					
Alcohol (screening and counseling)	NR	✓ All adults	✓	✓	✓
Tobacco (screening and counseling)	NR	✓ Adults, including pregnant women smokers >18	✓	✓	✓
Other illicit drugs (screening and counseling)	NR	NR	✓	✓	✓
Reproductive health					
STI screening (counseling)	✓ All sexually active adolescents and adults at increased risk for STI	✓ All sexually active adolescents and adults at increased risk for STI	✓ If sexually active	✓ If sexually active	✓
HIV	✓ All adolescents and adults aged 15 to 65	✓ All adolescents and adults aged 15 to 65	✓ If sexually active	✓ If sexually active	✓
Chlamydia (female)	✓ Sexually active at ≤24 y	Recommend against screening at >25 y, unless at risk	✓ If sexually active	✓ If sexually active	✓ Sexually active at <25 y
Chlamydia (male)	NR	NR	✓ If sexually active	✓ If sexually active	...
Syphilis	✓ All persons at increased risk for syphilis infection	✓ All persons at increased risk for syphilis infection	✓ If sexually active	✓ If sexually active and risk factors	✓
Gonorrhea	✓ All sexually active women if at increased risk for infection	✓ All sexually active women if at increased risk for infection	✓ If sexually active	✓ If sexually active	✓
Birth control methods	...	...	✓ If sexually active	✓ If sexually active	✓
Pregnancy	...	...	✓ Sexually active females without contraception, late menses, or amenorrhea	...	...
Mental health/depression					
Suicide screening	NR	NR	✓	✓	...
Depression	✓ 12–18 y when systems are in place to ensure accurate diagnosis, psychotherapy (cognitive-behavioral or interpersonal), and FU	✓ Adults, when staff-assisted depression care supports are in place to ensure accurate diagnosis, effective treatment, and FU	✓	✓	✓
Nutrition/exercise/obesity					
Cholesterol level	NR	✓ 20–35 y, screening for lipid disorders if at increased risk	✓ >20 y	✓	✓
Healthy diet	NR	✓ Adults with risk factors			
Hypertension/blood pressure	NR	✓ >18 y	✓	✓	✓
Obesity/BMI	✓ >6 y	✓ All adults	✓	✓	
Physical activity counseling	NR	NR	✓	...	...
Infectious disease/immunization (CDC)					
Td/Tdap	✓ >11 y, every 10 y, based on CDC	✓ >11 y, every 10 y based on CDC	CDC	...	CDC
Human papillomavirus	✓ 11–26 y, based on CDC	✓ 19–26 y, based on CDC	CDC	...	CDC
Varicella	✓ Based on CDC	Based on CDC	CDC	...	CDC
Measles, mumps, rubella	✓ Based on CDC	✓ Based on CDC	CDC	...	CDC
Influenza	✓ If risk factors, based on CDC	✓ Based on CDC	CDC	...	CDC
Pneumococcal (polysaccharide)	✓ If risk factors, based on CDC	✓ If risk factors, based on CDC	CDC	...	CDC

TABLE 5.1

Guidelines for AYA Preventive Health Care (*Continued*)

| | USPSTF[8] | | Bright Futures[14] | ACOG[23,24] | |
	Adolescent, Aged <18 y	Adult, Aged ≥18 y	Adolescent, Aged 11–21 y	Adolescent, Aged 13–21 y	Adult, Aged 19–39 y
Hepatitis A	✓ If risk factors, based on CDC	✓ If risk factors, based on CDC	CDC	...	CDC
Hepatitis B	✓7–18 y, based on CDC	✓ If risk factors, based on CDC	CDC	...	CDC
Meningococcal	✓11–18 y, based on CDC	✓ If risk factors, based on CDC	CDC	...	CDC
Polio	✓7–18 y, based on CDC	...	CDC	...	...
Safety/violence					
Family/partner violence	✓ Screening for all women of childbearing age, refer those at risk to relevant services	✓ Screening for all women of childbearing age, refer those at risk to relevant services	✓	✓	✓
Fighting	...	...	✓	...	✓
Helmets	...	...	✓	...	✓ Defined as recreational hazards
Seat belts	NR	NR	✓	...	✓
Alcohol while driving	NR	NR	✓	✓	...
Guns	...	...	✓	...	✓
Bullying	...	...	✓	...	...
Screening					
Cervical cancer screening	Recommend against	✓ age ≥21 (every 3 years)	✓ If sexually active	✓ ≥21 y[b]	✓ >21 y[b]
Testicular cancer screening	Recommend against	Recommend against		...	...
Vision	...	...	After risk assessment	...	...
Hearing	...	...	After risk assessment	...	✓
Anemia	...	...	After risk assessment	...	
Tuberculosis	...	...	After risk assessment	...	✓
Physical examination (as defined by *Bright Futures*)	...	...	Complete physical examination is included as part of every health supervision visit.	Physical examination should be included ≥1 time during early, middle, and late adolescence.	...
Measure blood pressure	...	✓	✓	...	✓
Calculate and plot BMI	✓	✓	✓	...	✓
Skin	...	...	✓	...	✓
Spine	...	...	✓	...	✓
Breast	...	...	✓	...	✓
Genitalia	..	...	✓	...	✓
BSE	Recommend against	Recommend against	...	...	✓ Despite a lack of definite data for or against BSE, BSE has the potential to defect palpable breast cancer and can be recommended

[a]"✓"Indicates a recommendation; NR, insufficient evidence to recommend for or against; "recommend against," recommend against or routinely providing the service based on the evidence.
[b]Updated November 20, 2009.
ACOG, American Congress of Obstetricians and Gynecologists; BMI, body mass index; BSE, breast self-examination; CDC, Centers for Disease Control and Prevention; ellipses, no mention; FU, follow-up; HIV, human immunodeficiency virus; NR, no recommendation; STI, sexually transmitted infection; Td/Tdap, tetanus, diphtheria/tetanus, diphtheria, pertussis; USPSTF, US Preventive Services Task Force.
Ozer EM, Urquhart JT, Brindis CD, et al. Young adult preventive health care guidelines: there but can't be found. *Arch Pediatr Adolesc Med* 2012;166(3):240–247.

TABLE 5.2

Consistency of Preventive Health Care Recommendations for Young Adults[a]

	USPSTF[8]		Bright Futures[14] Adolescent, Aged 11–21 y	ACOG[23,24] Young Adult, Aged 18–26 y	AAFP[25] Young Adult, Aged 18–26 y	ACP[26] Young Adult, Aged 18–26 y
	Adolescent, Aged 11–17 y	Young Adult, Aged 18–26 y				
Substance use						
Alcohol (screening and counseling)		✓	✓	✓	✓	✓
Tobacco (screening and counseling)		✓	✓	✓	✓	✓
Other illicit drugs (screening and counseling)				✓		
Reproductive health						
STI screening and counseling	+	+	+	✓	+	+
HIV	✓	✓	+	✓	+	+
Chlamydia (female)	+		+	+		
Chlamydia (male)			+			
Syphilis	+	+	+	✓		
Gonorrhea	+	+	+	✓	+	+
Birth control methods			+			
Pregnancy			+			
Mental health/depression						
Suicide screening			✓	✓		
Depression	✓	✓	✓		✓	✓
Nutrition/exercise/obesity						
Cholesterol level		+	✓	✓	+	+
Healthy diet		+	✓	✓	+	+
Hypertension/blood pressure		+	✓	✓	+	+
Obesity/BMI	✓	✓	✓	✓	✓	✓
Physical activity counseling			✓	✓		
Infectious disease/immunization (CDC)						
Td/Tdap	✓	✓	✓	✓	✓	✓
Human papillomavirus	✓	✓	✓	✓	✓	✓
Varicella	✓	✓	✓	✓	✓	✓
Measles, mumps, rubella	✓	✓	✓	✓	✓	✓
Influenza	+	✓	✓	✓	✓	✓
Pneumococcal (polysaccharide)	+	+	✓	✓	+	+
Hepatitis A	+	+	✓	✓	✓	+
Hepatitis B	✓	+	✓	✓	+	+
Meningococcal	✓	+	✓		+	+
Polio	✓		✓			
Safety/violence						
Family/partner violence	✓	✓				
Fighting			✓	✓		
Helmets			✓	✓		
Seat belts			✓	✓		
Alcohol while driving			✓			
Guns			✓	✓		
Bullying			✓			

[a]"✓" Indicates a recommendation; "+", if at risk.
AAFP, American Academy of Family Physicians; ACOG, American Congress of Obstetricians and Gynecologists; ACP, American College of Physicians; BMI, body mass index; CDC, Centers for Disease Control and Prevention; HIV, human immunodeficiency virus; STI, sexually transmitted infection; Td/Tdap, tetanus, diphtheria/tetanus, diphtheria, pertussis; USPSTF, US Preventive Services Task Force.
Ozer EM, Urquhart JT, Brindis CD, et al. Young adult preventive health care guidelines: there but can't be found. *Arch Pediatr Adolesc Med* 2012;166(3):240–247.

Table 5.2 provides a comparison of the evidence-based recommendations of the USPSTF and the guidelines issued by the four major professional organizations, reviewed above, whose members provide the majority of primary care to adolescents and adults.[4] These recommendations include screening for many of the major risks for morbidity and mortality among AYAs, including alcohol use, mental health, STIs, nutrition, exercise, and body mass index (BMI) screening.

Preventive Services and Insurance Coverage in the United States

As shown in **Table 5.2**, many of the recommendations included in the Bright Futures guidelines for adolescents are supported by sufficient evidence to be recommended by the USPSTF for older AYAs over the age of 18 years, such as screening and counseling for tobacco and alcohol use. However, there are areas in which Bright

Futures recommends screening or counseling, but the USPSTF does not. These include the following:

—Screening and counseling for illicit drug use
—Screening for suicide
—Counseling for physical activity
—Counseling for specific risks under the category of safety/violence

All USPSTF recommendations are also recommended by ACOG; however, ACOG recommends that women perform breast self-examinations despite the USPSTF recommendation against it.

Further, ACOG includes recommendations extending beyond those of the USPSTF, overlapping with the recommendations of Bright Futures.

Although the recommendations of Bright Futures target AYAs aged 11 to 21 years, the evidence for screening is stronger in several areas for adults (≥18 years), including tobacco and alcohol use, depression, cholesterol, and diet. Thus, for young adults, there is greater consistency between the USPSTF guidelines and the Bright Futures guidelines.[4] Table 5.3 displays a one-page clinician tool recently developed by The University of California, San Francisco's National Adolescent and Young Adult Health Information

---

TABLE 5.3

Summary of Recommended Guidelines for Clinical Preventive Services for Young Adults ages 18–26. UCSF Division of Adolescent and Young Adult Medicine

NAHIC

Guidelines as of 10/2014, subject to change.

	Preventive Services	All (√)	At Risk	Screening Test/Procedure and Other Notes
	Nutrition/exercise/obesity			
☐	**Hypertension/Blood pressure**[a]	√		**Screening every 2 y with BP <120/80**
☐	**Obesity/BMI**	√		**[Weight (lb.)/Height (in)] × 703**
☐	**Cholesterol level**		+	**Ages 20+; Test: Total cholesterol, HDL-C samples**
☐	**Healthy diet**		+	**Intensive behavioral dietary counseling**
	Substance Use			
☐	**Alcohol (screening and counseling)**	√		**NIAAA screening, AUDIT**
☐	**Tobacco (screening and counseling)**	√		**5-A framework (Ask, Advise, Assess, Assist, Arrange)**
☐	Illicit drugs (screening and counseling)	√		√ Bright Futures[b] and ACOG[c]
	Mental Health/Depression			
☐	**Depression (screening and treatment)**	√		**Screening questions; staff-assisted depression care supports should be in place**
☐	Suicide screening	√		√ Bright Futures and ACOG
	Safety/Violence			
☐	**Family/partner violence**	√		
☐	Fighting	√		√ Bright Futures and ACOG
☐	Helmets	√		√ Bright Futures and ACOG
☐	Seat belts	√		√ Bright Futures and ACOG
☐	Alcohol while driving	√		√ Bright Futures only
☐	Guns	√		√ Bright Futures and ACOG
☐	Bullying	√		√ Bright Futures only
	Reproductive Health			
☐	**HIV**	√		**HIV screening**
☐	**STI (screening and counseling)**		+	**High-intensity counseling interventions**
☐	**Syphilis**		+	**VDRL**
☐	**Gonorrhea (females)**		+	**NAATs; vaginal culture (Self swab preferred); test if ≤24 and sexually active or if ≥25 and at increased risk**

(Continued)

TABLE 5.3

Summary of Recommended Guidelines for Clinical Preventive Services for Young Adults ages 18–26. UCSF Division of Adolescent and Young Adult Medicine (Continued)

	Preventive Services	All (√)	At Risk	Screening Test/Procedure and Other Notes
☐	**Chlamydia (female)**		+	**NAATs; test if ≤24 and sexually active or if ≥25 and at increased risk**
☐	**Hepatitis C**		+	**Injection drug use, hemodialysis, incarceration and more**
☐	Chlamydia and Gonorrhea (male)		+	√ Bright Futures only
☐	Birth control methods	√	+	√ ACOG, + Bright Futures
☐	Pregnancy		+	+ Bright Futures; sexually active without contraception, late or absent menses, or heavy irregular bleeding
	Cancer Screening			
☐	**Cervical cancer**		+	**Females ages 21+: cytology (pap smear) every 3 y**
☐	**Testicular cancer**	√	–	**– USPSTF;** √ Bright Futures for all males 18–21
☐	**BRCA-related cancer**		+	**Family Hx of breast, ovarian, tubal, or perionteal cancer**
	Infectious Disease/Immunizations (CDC Recommendations) as of 02/2013			
☐	**Td/Tdap**	√		**Booster every 10 y**
☐	**Human papillomavirus**	√		**HPV 4 vaccine for males and females, 3 lifetime doses**
☐	**Varicella (Live Vaccine)**	√[d]		**2 lifetime doses (4–8 wk apart)[d] See below**
☐	**Measles, mumps, rubella**	√		**1 or 2 lifetime doses**
☐	**Influenza**	√		**1 dose annually**
☐	**Pneumococcal**		+	**PCV13: 1 lifetime dose	PPSV23: 1–2 lifetime doses**
☐	**Hepatitis A**	√		**2 lifetime doses**
☐	**Hepatitis B**	√		**3 lifetime doses**
☐	**Meningococcal**		+	**1 or more lifetime doses**

[a]At the time of publication, recommendation was being reviewed and updated.
[b]Bright Futures: recommendations are for annual visits, up to age 21.
[c]American Congress of Obstetricians and Gynecologists (ACOG) recommendations, up to age 26.
[d]The varicella vaccine should *not* be given to patients with these contraindications.
Bold, US Preventive Services Task Force (USPSTF) A or B Recommendation or CDC recommendations for immunizations; √, All young adults; +, Young adults at risk; –, Recommended against.
For more information, please view the appendix, and visit the official Web site.
National Adolescent and Young Adult Health Information Center. (2014). *Summary of recommended guidelines for clinical preventive services for young adults ages 18–26.* San Francisco, CA: National Adolescent and Young Adult Health Information Center, 2014. Available at http://nahic.ucsf.edu/cps/YAguidelines

Center (NAHIC) to facilitate the delivery of preventive care to young adults. This summary highlights the USPSTF evidence-based recommendations for young adult care and indicates additional preventive services guidelines that extend beyond the evidence base of the USPSTF (e.g., Bright Futures and ACOG).

In the United States, the enactment of the Patient Protection and Affordable Care Act of 2010 (ACA) has the potential to improve AYA health by increasing health insurance coverage and by requiring that preventive health care be provided to AYAs. The ACA allows young adults to remain on their parent's health insurance plan until age 26. Before the ACA was implemented, only 65% of young adults aged 19 to 25 were insured; by the end of 2011, this number of insured young adults had increased to 75%.[7]

The ACA also includes provisions to improve the content of care and increase access to and use of preventive services. New private health plans or policies in the United States must cover annual well visits until age 21, and private health insurance plans are required to cover a specified set of preventive services without cost sharing (copayments, deductibles, or coinsurance). As part of its preventive services mandate, the ACA requires that providers use professional guidelines, including (1) evidence-based services recommended by the USPSTF, (2) Advisory Committee for Immunization Practices (ACIP) recommended immunizations, (3) services outlined in Bright Futures, and (4) women's preventive services required by the HRSA. **Table 5.4** lists preventive services covered under ACA for AYAs without cost sharing by private insurers.

In addition to the ACA, other factors influence the delivery of preventive health services for AYAs in the United States. For example, insurance companies often monitor and audit provider performance on key aspects of preventive health care, including immunization rates and receipt of a periodic health examination. In some cases, receipt of individual preventive health services is

TABLE 5.4

Preventive Health Care Services for AYAs (aged 18–26) Covered under the 2010 Patient Protection and Affordable Care Act

Services for Adolescents and All Young Adults Covered by ACA (Aged 11–26)[a]
Alcohol misuse screening and counseling
Tobacco use screening
Blood pressure screening
Diabetes (type 2) screening for adults with high blood pressure[b]
Diet counseling[b]
Obesity screening and counseling
Cholesterol screening[b]
Depression screening
HIV screening
STI prevention counseling[b]
Syphilis screening (young adults only)[b]
Immunization vaccines
    Hepatitis A
    Hepatitis B
    HPV
    Influenza
    Measles, mumps, rubella
    Meningococcal
    Pneumococcal
    Tetanus, diphtheria, pertussis
    Varicella

Additional Services for Children Covered by ACA (Aged 11–17)
Behavioral assessments (not sure what this entails—could be the
    same as BF screening below)
Fluoride supplements[b]
Height, weight, and BMI measurements
Hematocrit/hemoglobin screening
Haemophilus influenza type b
Polio vaccine
Rotavirus vaccine
Lead screening[b]
Medical history
Oral Health-Risk assessment
Vision screening

Additional Services Covered for AYAs Aged 11–21 (Bright Futures Recommendations Only)
Annual wellness visit
Illicit drugs screening and counseling
Suicide screening
Safety/violence screening
    Family/partner violence (male and female)
    Fighting
    Helmets
    Seat belts
    Alcohol while driving
    Guns
    Bullying
Polio immunization

Additional Women's Services covered by ACA (Aged 18–26)
Well-woman visits
Contraception
Folic acid
Domestic and interpersonal violence screening and counseling
    (women of all ages)
Cervical cancer screening (if sexually active)
Chlamydia infection screening
Gonorrhea screening[b]
Breast Cancer Genetic Test Counseling (BRCA)[b]
Breast cancer chemoprevention counseling[b]
Hepatitis B screening for pregnant women
Rh incompatibility screening for pregnant women
Anemia screening for pregnant women
Gestational diabetes screening
Urinary tract or other infection screening for pregnant women
Breast-feeding comprehensive support and counseling

[a]These are overall guidelines with variability in interpretation by individual contracts and vendors.
[b]If at higher risk.

also monitored. The Healthcare Effectiveness Data and Information Set (HEDIS) is a tool used by more than 90% of US health plans to monitor provider performance. HEDIS includes 75 measures across 8 domains of care. Because many plans collect HEDIS data, and the measures are specifically defined, HEDIS makes it possible to compare the performance of health plans and providers. The HEDIS measures relevant to AYA health care are summarized in **Table 5.5**.

Important safety net services also cover preventive services for AYAs who otherwise might not have access. The Department of Health and Human Services' Title X provides funds for comprehensive family planning services and other preventive health care. The Early Periodic Screening, Diagnosis, and Treatment Program (EPSDT) is funded by Title V and administered by HRSA and the Maternal and Child Health Bureau. EPSDT provides preventive (and other) services to children who are enrolled in Medicaid or who are uninsured. Some states have added additional programming to address the preventive services family planning needs of uninsured AYAs, especially those seeking confidential care. In California, the Family Planning, Access, Care, and Treatment program provides preventive counseling for family planning and STIs.

Barriers to Providing Preventive Services

Health insurance coverage and clinical guidelines are important, but widespread implementation of preventive services for AYAs

TABLE 5.5

HEDIS Quality Measures for Preventive Services for AYAs

Adolescent well-care visit
Child and adolescents' access to primary care practitioners
Chlamydia screening in women
Childhood immunization status
Follow-up after hospitalization for mental illness
HPV vaccine for female adolescents
Immunization status for adolescents
Percentage of eligibles that received preventive dental services
Weight assessment and counseling for nutrition and physical activity for
    children/adolescents: BMI assessment for children/adolescents
Frequency and timeliness of ongoing prenatal care
Behavioral health-risk assessment for pregnant women
Cervical cancer screening
Cholesterol management for patients with cardiovascular conditions
Controlling high blood pressure
Comprehensive diabetes care
Antidepressant medication management

requires attention to many other factors. Current rates of screening and counseling for AYAs are lower than recommended, and there is inconsistency in screening across various risk areas.[8–12] Barriers to delivering preventive services within busy clinical practices have been well documented, including clinician factors (attitudes, lack of training, skills, and/or confidence to deliver services) and external factors (time constraints, lack of appropriate screening tools, and lack of reimbursement for services).[4,13,14] Access to preventive health care may also be limited by other issues such as concerns over confidentiality and transportation.

Improving Preventive Services Delivery

Offering alternate (and more convenient) locations for preventive services, policy changes that facilitate confidential care, using emerging technology for screening, and creating efficiencies for providers are all promising approaches to improving preventive service delivery for AYAs.[4,15]

Clinical Settings

To better serve AYAs, preventive services need to be available in a *wide range of health care settings* beyond clinicians' offices. AYAs feel "healthy" and may be reluctant health care consumers because they may not appreciate a direct benefit from preventive services. This is particularly true for male AYAs, who utilize fewer well-care preventive visits, receiving most of their care through acute care visits.[10,11,16] For this reason, acute care visits are an underutilized opportunity for the provision of preventive health screening and intervention.[10,17]

School-based and school-linked health resources are an increasingly important health services resource for adolescents (see http://www.gwu.edu/~mtg and http://www.nasbhc.org). Adolescents who use school-based health services are highly satisfied with the care they receive. Moreover, school-based and school-linked services often play a unique and complementary role in meeting the health needs of adolescents. For example, studies suggest that some teens may be more willing to access school-based health services than traditional health resources to address concerns about mental health, substance use, and reproductive health.[18] Similarly, community-based family planning and public health clinics also serve as an important safety net for AYAs.

Training and Screening Tools

Clinicians often cite inadequate training or insufficient confidence as a barrier to the provision of health services for AYAs. Clinician training to increase self-efficacy and clinical decision-making supports, such as screening and charting tools, have been shown to be effective in overcoming these barriers and thus increasing the delivery of preventive services to adolescents. These "training and tools" interventions have been evaluated across studies, usually in the context of a generalized approach (attempting to address multiple health behavior areas) but also in interventions that have targeted specific risk areas (e.g., substance use, tobacco use, and sexual health).[19] Examples include psychosocial screening assessments, and prompts and cues for providers. These tools have been integrated into patient charts, screening and charting forms, and office systems. A growing body of research is focused on the integration of technology to facilitate preventive service delivery using handheld devices, computerized behavioral screening, Internet-based approaches, and tablet-based screening modules.[19]

THE EHR AND PREVENTIVE SERVICES

Because of their widespread adoption, EHRs are increasingly important tools to facilitate and track preventive service delivery for individual patients and for entire patient populations. As of 2008, about half of children's hospitals had implemented an EHR.[20] Because of the Meaningful Use Program, which provides funds for institutions meeting core EHR technology requirements, most EHRs in the United States include a suite of features that can aid in the provision of preventive services for AYAs.

Challenges Related to Confidential Care

The provision of confidential care for adolescents seeking treatment for reproductive and mental health services is a well-established best practice.[21] However, most EHRs are not designed to provide granular control of access to and release of information that facilitates the provision of confidential care for adolescents.[22,23] Institutions are left with a dilemma—make do with existing tools, or invest institutional resources in modifications of existing technology. To minimize the risk of unintended release of information, some institutions turn off key functionality of the EHR for adolescent patients such as the patient portal, social histories, after-visit summaries, and problem lists. Unfortunately, this strategy excludes adolescents from many of the benefits of the EHR and also compromises institutional participation in federal programs, such as the Meaningful Use Program.

Key EHR Features for AYA Preventive Services

We summarize here the various features of the EHR as they relate to AYAs, paying particular attention to confidential care challenges and opportunities where the EHR can be leveraged to improve care.

Previsit Questionnaires

Automated screening offers several advantages to AYAs who may find it easier to disclose sensitive information electronically than to a provider. Automated screening also saves time, and the information can be directly placed into the electronic record. Automated screeners may be available separately from existing EHRs. They can also be developed within an EHR either using provided tools or custom formats. **Figure 5.1** shows a screen shot of the "Health e-Check" screening module that automates preventive health screening and allows for integration of adolescent responses into the EHR.[24]

Health Maintenance

Most EHR systems offer both provider and patient reminders when key health maintenance elements are due. For example, annual flu vaccine alerts can be set to remind providers to order the vaccine. Institutions use these alerts for vaccine reminders, but they can also be used for other AYA preventive services, such as pap and chlamydia screening. This is especially helpful when the guidelines are complex and differ by age, gender, or prior health conditions. EHRs also offer the ability to create standard order sets for periodic health examinations.

Population Health Management

EHRs may be used to determine rates of provision of preventive services on current patients in an individual practice. This type of population health management not only boosts receipt of preventive services, but also facilitates external reporting of HEDIS measures and internal quality control efforts.

Provider Documentation

Structured provider templates for preventive services visits that contain the key visit components can increase provider efficiency and assure that required elements for billing and compliance are documented. Documentation in an EHR may be more efficient, because information can automatically populate using data from other areas of the health record. However, these same features can pose challenges for the protection of confidential health information. For example, a prescription for birth control pills will appear on a shared medication list that will automatically appear in the notes of other providers. Thus, a visit to another health care professional could lead to a breach in confidential care by inadvertently listing confidential information from a primary care visit.

Patient Portal

The patient portal allows patients and/or parents to access personal health information online and to communicate with health care providers. AYAs are uniquely suited to benefit from the patient portal. In recent years, thousands of vendor-based patient portals have been implemented in response to Federal Meaningful Use criteria.

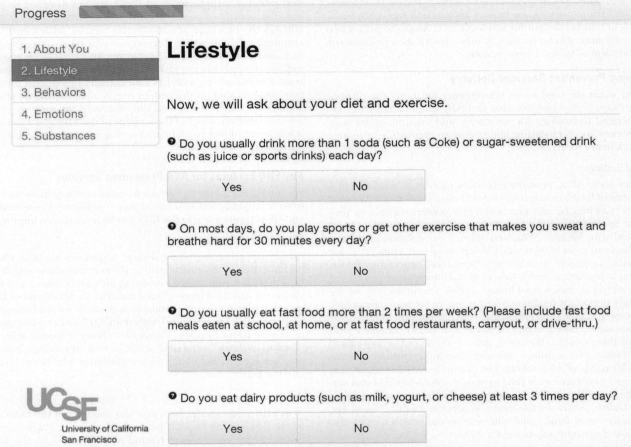

Progress

1. About You
2. Lifestyle
3. Behaviors
4. Emotions
5. Substances

Lifestyle

Now, we will ask about your diet and exercise.

❶ Do you usually drink more than 1 soda (such as Coke) or sugar-sweetened drink (such as juice or sports drinks) each day?

| Yes | No |

❷ On most days, do you play sports or get other exercise that makes you sweat and breathe hard for 30 minutes every day?

| Yes | No |

❸ Do you usually eat fast food more than 2 times per week? (Please include fast food meals eaten at school, at home, or at fast food restaurants, carryout, or drive-thru.)

| Yes | No |

❹ Do you eat dairy products (such as milk, yogurt, or cheese) at least 3 times per day?

| Yes | No |

UCSF
University of California
San Francisco

FIGURE 5.1 "Health e-Check" previsit screening module. (Ozer EM, Martin M, Jasik C, et al. The development of a clinic-based interactive behavioral health screening module for adolescents. Paper presented at the 2013 International Congress on Adolescent Health. Istanbul; 2013.)

Despite their widespread adoption, descriptive studies suggest that institutions often exclude adolescents or only allow access to parents because most EHRs do not yet have the flexibility to allow differential access to adolescents and parents.[22]

THE PREVENTIVE SERVICES VISIT

Caring for AYAs requires a different approach, format, and style than caring for children or adults; so it is not surprising that many health care providers report barriers to, or lack of confidence in, caring for these youth. The AYA preventive visit may potentially involve greater planning, sensitivity, expertise, and time than a visit with a younger child or adult. Most of the visit is spent taking a history or screening for health risks; so comfortable space is needed in which to conduct the interview. A plan for including the parent and/or guardian in the visit is also needed.

Setting the Stage for Preventive Care

To provide effective preventive services, the office visit must be organized and structured in an appropriate way for AYAs. This includes the physical space, services available, staff training, and provider training. The confidential psychosocial interview will be most successful if the environment is welcoming and the patient feels comfortable. Table 5.6 summarizes the key components for creating a friendly atmosphere for AYAs.[25]

Questionnaires and Screening Tools

To improve the efficiency of preventive care visits, screening questionnaires may be completed by the patient and/or parent prior to the visit. The standard previsit questionnaire for an adolescent or

young adult preventive services visit may assess health behaviors related to nutrition, physical activity, home life, education, substance use, mental health, sexual health, and exposure to violence. GAPS created a comprehensive screening questionnaire for use in primary care; and Bright Futures currently provides a sample previsit questionnaire.[5,26] Many clinics, programs, and practices elect to create their own questionnaires based on their knowledge of youth in their individual practices. In addition, several previsit questionnaires for AYA risk behavior screening have been developed using both written and electronic formats.[19]

Providers may also want to conduct screening in a particular risk area, either across all patients or specifically for those who demonstrate risk on prior general screens. Depression is one area in which there are several options for standardized screening. The Beck Depression Inventory is a well-validated and easily administered tool to screen for depression. There is also a shorter version (Beck Depression Inventory [BDI-PC]) that is developed for use in busy primary care settings. The TeenScreen Program also offers a shortened version of the Patient Health Questionnaire for Adolescents (PHQ-A).[27] Substance use is another area with valid screening tools. For example, the CRAFFT was developed for use in primary care settings to assess adolescent substance use.[28] Bright Futures and the NAHIC have toolkits with specific references and/or tools for dedicated screening in specific topics.[29]

History

As with any patient preventive visit history, essential domains include past medical history, family history, psychosocial history, and an age-appropriate review of systems. Any current health concerns should also be sought. When preventive services are

TABLE 5.6

Questions to Consider When Creating a Youth Friendly Environment

(?) Does your office/health center have...
- [ ] An atmosphere that is appealing to adolescents (pictures, posters, wallpaper)?
- [ ] Magazines that would interest adolescents and reflect their cultures and literacy levels?
- [ ] Appropriate-sized tables and chairs in your waiting and examination rooms (i.e., not for small children)?
- [ ] Private areas to complete forms and discuss reasons for visits?
- [ ] Facilities that comply with the Americans with Disabilities Act?
- [ ] Decorations that reflect the genders, sexual orientations, cultures, and ethnicities of your clients?

(?) Do you provide...
- [ ] Health education materials written for or by teens at the appropriate litency level and in their first languages?
- [ ] Translation services appropriate for your patient population?
- [ ] A clearly posted office policy about confidentiality?
- [ ] After-school hours?
- [ ] Opportunities for parents and adolescents to speak separately with a health care provider?
- [ ] Alternatives to written communications (i.e., phone calls, meetings, videos, audiotapes)?
- [ ] Health education materials in various locations, such as the waiting room, examination room, and bathroom, where teens would feel comfortable reading and taking them?
- [ ] Condoms?

(?) Does your staff...
- [ ] Greet adolescents in a courteous and friendly manner?
- [ ] Explain procedures and directions in an easy and understandable manner?
- [ ] Enjoy working with adolescents and their families?
- [ ] Have up-to-date knowledge about consent and confidentiality laws?
- [ ] Incorporate principles and practices that promote cultural and linguistic competence?
- [ ] Consider privacy concerns when adolescents check-in?
- [ ] Provide resource and referral information when there is a delay in scheduling a teen's appointment?

(?) When you speak to adolescents do you...
- [ ] Use nonjudgmental, jargon free, and gender-neutral language?
- [ ] Allow time to address their concerns and questions?
- [ ] Restate your name and explain your role and what you are doing?
- [ ] Ask gentle but direct questions?
- [ ] Offer options for another setting or provider?
- [ ] Explain the purpose and costs for tests, procedures, and referrals?
- [ ] Keep in mind that their communication skills may not reflect their cognitive or problem-solving abilities?
- [ ] Ask for clarification and explanations?
- [ ] Listen?
- [ ] Congratulate them when they are making healthy choices and decisions?

(?) Are you aware...
- [ ] That your values may conflict with or be inconsistent with those of other cultural or religious groups?
- [ ] That age and gender soles may vary among different cultures?
- [ ] Of health care beliefs and acceptable behaviors, customs, and expectations of different geographic, religions, and ethnic groups?
- [ ] Of the socioeconomic and environmental risk factors that contribute to the major health problems among the diverse groups you serve?
- [ ] Of community resources for youth and families?

AHWG

© Adolescent Health Working Group, 2003

delivered during a visit made for another reason or health concern (e.g., sports physical, acute medical problem), it is important to make sure that the patient's concerns are fully addressed.

Past Medical History

Past medical history is best obtained from both the adolescent or young adult and the parents and should include the following:

1. Childhood infections and illnesses
2. Prior hospitalizations and surgery
3. Significant injuries
4. Disabilities
5. Medications, including prescription medications, over-the-counter medications, complementary or alternative medications, vitamins, and nutritional supplements
6. Allergies
7. Immunization history
8. Developmental history, including prenatal, perinatal, and infancy history; peer relations; and school functioning
9. Mental health history, including a history of hospitalization, outpatient counseling, medications, school interventions, or other treatment

Family History

Often, information about family history is most accurately obtained from the parents. The family history should include the following:

1. Age and health status of family members
2. History of significant medical illnesses in the family, such as diabetes, cancer, heart disease, tuberculosis (TB), hypertension, or stroke
3. History of mental illness in the family, such as mood disorders, anxiety disorders, schizophrenia, or substance abuse

Psychosocial History

Given that the majority of morbidity and mortality among AYAs is related to behavioral risk factors, the "heart and soul" of the preventive visit for these populations is the psychosocial/behavioral history. Typically, this history is completed in person, but it can be facilitated by structured questionnaires and electronic screening as mentioned above. Collateral information from parents and family members is helpful and should be obtained whenever possible. One strategy is to complete the nonconfidential component with the parent present and the confidential sections after excusing the parent or guardian.

The key to a successful psychosocial interview is building rapport with the patient and providing a comfortable and safe space (see Table 5.6). Adolescents are more likely to seek care for family planning, mental health, and substance abuse counseling if they know the care is confidential.[21] Reassuring the adolescent that certain aspects of the interview can be kept confidential, as well as reviewing the circumstances under which information cannot be kept confidential, is helpful for establishing rapport. Clinicians within a practice should know the current local laws regarding confidential care and have a consistent approach. Chapter 4 summarizes the HEEADSSS assessment and psychosocial interview. The key components of a complete psychosocial history are summarized in Table 5.7.

Developmental Assessment

A comprehensive developmental assessment is a core part of the evaluation of the AYAs and is necessary to help the provider tailor preventive health screening and counseling. Chapter 2 has a detailed review of adolescent growth and development. Table 5.8 offers a description of adolescent psychological and social development with tips for developmentally appropriate counseling.[5] While age-based guidelines are useful, chronological age does not always match developmental age. For example, a 15-year-old female

TABLE 5.7

The Adolescent/Young Adult Psychosocial History: A Summary

Home	Who lives at home? Does the teen split time between households?
Education/ Employment	What grade are you in? Do you work? What are your plans for your future?
Eating	What did you eat yesterday? What did you drink yesterday? Is this typical? Do you skip meals? *Asses for disordered eating.* Are you happy with your current weight?
Activity	Do you have close friends? What do you do after school? Do you play sports?
Drugs	Have you ever smoked, drank alcohol, or done drugs? *Ask specifically about marijuana.* Do your friends use drugs? Do you ever drive, or ride with someone who has been drinking or using drugs? Do any of your family members use drugs or drink alcohol to excess?
Sexuality	Are you interested in guys, girls, or both? Have you ever been sexually active? *If yes,* how many partners have you had in your life? In the past 3 months? Do you use condoms? *For girls,* what do you use to prevent pregnancy?
Suicide (mental health)	Do you ever feel sad, down, or hopeless? Do you feel lonely or bored? Have you ever felt so sad or down that you didn't think life was worth living? Have you ever cut yourself? Do you feel anxious?
Safety	Do you wear a helmet when riding a bike or a skateboard? Do you wear a seat belt when riding in a car? Do you have guns in your home? Do you carry a gun? Do you feel safe in your home, school, and community? Have you ever not felt safe? Do you have a history of sexual or physical abuse?

patient who has the developmental progress of an early adolescent will require a different approach to preventive health counseling than a same-age peer in middle or late adolescence.

Review of Systems

The review of systems covers the following areas:

1. Vision: Trouble reading or watching television; vision correction
2. Hearing: Infections, trouble hearing, earaches
3. Dental: Prior care, pain, concerns (e.g., braces)
4. Head: Headaches, dizziness
5. Nose and throat: Frequent colds or sore throats, chronic rhinorrhea from allergies
6. Skin: Acne, moles, rashes, warts
7. Cardiovascular: Exercise intolerance, shortness of breath, chest pain, palpitations, syncope, and source of regular physical activity
8. Respiratory: Asthma, cough, sneezing, smoking, exposure to TB
9. Gastrointestinal: Abdominal pain, reflux, diarrhea, vomiting, bleeding, constipation
10. Genitourinary: Dysuria, bed-wetting, frequency, bleeding
11. Musculoskeletal: Limb pain, joint pain, or swelling
12. Central nervous system (CNS): Seizures, syncope
13. Menstrual: Menarche, frequency of menses, duration, menorrhagia or metrorrhagia, dysmenorrhea
14. Sexual: Sexual activity, contraception, pregnancy, abortions, STIs or STI symptoms

Measurements

Several key pieces of objective information are usually obtained and calculated by staff before the health provider evaluates the AYAs.

Height, Weight, and BMI Calculation

Yearly assessment of height, weight, and BMI calculation is essential to monitor adolescent growth and for early detection of overweight and obesity. All values should be plotted on the growth chart, or referenced in the EHR, and interpreted in the context of prior trends (see Chapters 32 and 33 for the evaluation and management of overweight/obesity and eating disorders, respectively.)

Blood Pressure

Blood pressure should be measured with an appropriate cuff and if abnormal, remeasured manually after allowing the patient to sit for 5 minutes. A diagnosis of hypertension is considered when the repeat blood pressure values on three separate visits (usually 2 weeks apart) are greater than the 95th percentile for age, gender, and height percentile using National High Blood Pressure Education Program Working Group (NHBPEP) tables. See Chapter 17 for additional information about the evaluation and management of hypertension in AYAs.

Other Vital Signs

Heart rate and temperature are also routinely measured. A high temperature could be a sign of current infection. A high heart rate could signal that the patient is in pain and/or, correlated with the history and physical, could be sign of a chronic health problem (i.e., hyperthyroidism, anemia). A heart rate below 50 or a temperature below 96° F could be a sign of an eating disorder and should be correlated with the history and growth chart.[30]

Vision Screening

Among 12- to 17-year-old adolescents, approximately 25% have visual acuity of 20/40 or less. This condition often develops during early adolescence. Adolescents should have a vision screening at the time of their initial evaluation and every 2 to 3 years thereafter. This can be done with a standard Snellen chart or a similar test. To "pass" a line on the Snellen chart, the adolescent should view the chart with one eye covered and be able to read at least one-half of the letters on that line correctly. Referral should be made for vision <20/30 in either or both eyes.

Hearing Screening

There is increasing concern about threats to hearing due to earphone/headphone use. Every patient should have at least one hearing screen performed during the adolescent years. It is important that this test be performed in a quiet room to allow for detection of subtle defects. Screening examinations are usually conducted at frequencies of 1,000, 2,000, and 4,000 Hz at 20 dB. Referral for more comprehensive hearing testing is indicated if there is a failure to hear 1,000 or 2,000 Hz at 20 dB or 4,000 Hz at 25 dB. The more comprehensive threshold test evaluates for the lowest intensity of sound heard at frequencies of 250, 1,000, 2,000, and 4,000 Hz. Evaluation is indicated with a threshold of 25 dB at two or more frequencies or at 35 dB for any frequency.

Physical Examination

The physical examination allows the clinician to assess growth and pubertal development and instruct the adolescent in methods of self-examination. The main elements of the physical examination are summarized below:

Sexual Maturity Rating

The sexual maturity rating (SMR), discussed in Chapter 2, is the method by which pubertal development is evaluated and described. Because many "normal values" in adolescence depend

TABLE 5.8

Adolescent Growth and Development

Characteristics	Early Adolescence	Middle Adolescence	Late Adolescence
Age range (These stages are variable and fluid.)	• Females: 9–13 y • Males: 11–15 y	• Females: 13–16 y • Males: 15–17 y	• Females: 16–21 y • Males: 17–21 y • The upper end varies and depends on cultural, economic, and educational factors.
Growth	• Secondary sexual characteristics appear. • Voice changes and body odor increases. • Growth rapidly accelerating; reaches peak velocity.	• Secondary sexual characteristics well advanced. • Menstruation begins in females. • Growth decelerating; stature reaches 95% of adult height.	• Physically mature; statural and reproductive growth virtually complete.
Cognition	• Concrete thought dominant. • Existential orientation. • Cannot perceive long-range implications of current decisions and acts.	• Rapidly gaining competence in abstract thought. • Capable of perceiving future implications of current acts and decisions but variably applied. • Reverts to concrete operations under stress.	• Established abstract thought processes. • Future oriented. • Capable of perceiving and acting on long-range options.
Psychological self and self-perception	• Preoccupation with rapid body change. • Former body image disrupted. • Concerned with privacy. • Frequent mood swings. • Very self-focused.	• Reestablishes body image as growth decelerates and stabilizes. • Extremely concerned with appearance and body. • Preoccupation with fantasy and idealism in exploring expanded cognition and future options. • Often risk takers. • Development of a sense of omnipotence and invincibility.	• Emancipation completed. • Intellectual and functional identity established. • May experience "crisis of 21" when facing societal demands for autonomy. • Body image and gender role definition nearly secured.
Family	• Defining independence—dependence boundaries. • Conflicts may occur but relate to minor issues.	• Frequency of conflicts may decrease, but their intensity increases. • Struggle for emancipation.	• Transposition of child-parent dependency relationship to the adult-adult model.
Peer group	• Seeks peer affiliation to counter instability generated by rapid change. • Compares own normality and acceptance with same-sex/age mates. • Same-sex friends and group activities.	• Strong need for identification to affirm self-image. • Looks to peer group to define behavioral code during emancipation process. • Cross-gender friendships more common.	• Group recedes in importance in favor of individual friendships and intimate relationships.
Sexuality	• Self-exploration and evaluation. • Limited dating. • Sexual fantasies are common and may serve as a source of guilt. • Masturbation begins during this period and may be accompanied by guilt. • Sexual activities are usually nonphysical. Early adolescents are often highly content with nonsexual interactions such as telephone calls to peers.	• Multiple plural relationships. • Heightened sexual activity. • Testing ability to attract boy/girl-friends and parameters of masculinity or femininity. • Preoccupation with romantic fantasy. • Experimentation with relationships and sexual behaviors. • More emphasis on physical contact. • Establishing sexual identity; fears/questions about homosexuality. • Dating and making out (petting) are common, and casual relationships with both noncoital and coital contacts are prevalent. • Denial of consequences of sexual behavior is typical.	• Forms stable relationships. • Capable of mutuality and reciprocity in caring for another rather than former narcissistic orientation. • Plans for future in thinking of marriage and/or family. • Intimacy involves commitment rather than exploration and romanticism. • Sexual orientation nearly secured.
Tips	• Effective communication tools must be very specific. • Use materials with pictures rather than tables and graphs. • Focus on issues that most concern these teens (weight gain, acne. physical changes, peer acceptance). • Early and late maturation can lead to difficulties. • Parents will welcome guidance on discipline, rules, and communication.	• Health care providers perceived as "friends" rather than authority figures help to develop trust with teens. • Teens must identify with the health care message to ensure follow-through and success. • Peer counseling, if carefully selected, can be effective with this age group. • Focus on supportive adult connections, health promotion, and harm reduction is key during this stage.	• More abstract reasoning allows for more traditional counseling approaches that rely on knowing consequences of behaviors. • Pediatric practices need to assist in transition to adult health care providers. • Provide the option to include close friends and/or partners for office visits.

Adapted from Greydanus D. Characteristics of early, middle, and late adolescence. *Delivering culturally effective health care to adolescents.* American Medical Association, 2002. Permission from Dr. Greydanus, December, 2002.

more on SMR than on age, evaluation of SMR is important not only in describing pubertal milestones but also in adequately assessing many physical parameters (e.g., BMI) and laboratory values (e.g., hemoglobin).

Skin

Check for evidence of acne, warts, fungal infections, and other lesions. Carefully inspect moles, especially in patients who are at particular risk for melanoma.

Teeth and Gums

Check for evidence of dental caries or gum infection. Look for signs of smokeless tobacco use. Enamel erosions are sometimes the first clue to the self-induced vomiting associated with some eating disorders.

Neck

Check for thyromegaly or adenopathy.

Cardiopulmonary

Check for heart murmurs or clicks.

Abdomen

Check for evidence of hepatosplenomegaly, tenderness, or masses.

Musculoskeletal

The musculoskeletal examination is especially important in adolescent athletes, in whom instabilities or other evidence of previous injury is the best predictor of future injury. Check for signs of overuse syndromes or osteochondroses. Check for scoliosis, particularly in premenarchal females.

Breasts

Examine for symmetry and developmental variations; in girls, assess SMR. Examine for masses or discharge; in boys, identify gynecomastia (present in approximately one-third of pubertal males). See Chapter 55.

Neurological

Test strength, reflexes, and coordination.

Genitalia (Male)

Examine the penis and testicles. Assess SMR. Look for signs of STIs. Retract the foreskin in uncircumcised patients. Check for hernia.

Pelvic Examination (Female)

A pelvic examination is indicated only for females who have an active complaint such as pelvic pain or vaginal discharge. Cervical cancer (Pap) screening is now only recommended starting at age 21 except in adolescent females with human immunodeficiency virus (HIV) or other immune deficiency.

Screening Tests

All screening tests in AYAs are completed based on an initial risk assessment, and there are no tests that are recommended for all AYAs.

Testing for TB Infection

The most accessible screening test for TB is a purified protein derivative (PPD) tuberculin skin test. A PPD should be considered based on an assessment of individual risk factors and recommendations of the local health department or school requirements. A PPD should be placed for patients with a known exposure to TB, immune deficiency or HIV, active symptoms, a country of origin that has high TB prevalence, at-risk housing or employment, or drug use. TB blood antibody tests, called interferon-gamma release assays or IGRAs, are also available, and two tests are currently approved in the United States: QuantiFERON and T-SPOT.

A positive test suggests that the patient has been infected with TB and further testing is needed to determine if the infection is latent or active. A negative test indicates that the patient does not have latent or active TB. Positivity is determined by risk factors for TB infection:

- 5 mm induration: Positive if the patient has a recent exposure to TB, HIV infection, or a chest x-ray consistent with TB.
- 10 mm induration: Positive if the patient has a high risk for disseminated TB such as lymphoma, diabetes, renal failure, malnutrition, or high risk for exposure to TB such as living in a high prevalence area, homelessness, incarceration, or illicit drug use.
- All other patients are considered positive at 15 mm of induration.

The Centers for Disease Control and Prevention (CDC) states that IGRAs are preferred over skin testing for patients who have received the bacille Calmette–Guérin (BCG) vaccine or those who have had a difficult time returning for their PPD reading (http://www.cdc.gov/tb/topic/testing/default.htm).

Hemoglobin or Hematocrit

A screening hemoglobin is only recommended if the nutrition screen is concerning for inadequate iron intake. AYAs with a vegetarian, vegan, or restrictive diet should be screened for anemia.

Metabolic Testing

Metabolic testing includes a lipid profile, diabetes screen, and liver enzymes. Dyslipidemia is determined by the measurement of a fasting lipid panel—total cholesterol (TC), low-density lipoprotein (LDL), triglycerides, and high-density lipoprotein (HDL). A diabetes screen includes a fasting glucose and hemoglobin A1C.

The National Heart, Lung, and Blood Institute and the AAP recommend screening based on patient and family risk factors. The primary reason to obtain these studies is if the patient is overweight or obese. Although the guidelines recommend fasting tests, many patients cannot present for fasting labs, and random testing may be necessary in those cases. Testing for dyslipidemia, diabetes, and nonalcoholic fatty liver is covered in other chapters in this text. Briefly, providers should consider screening tests for obese and overweight AYAs in the following cases:

1. Family history: Cardiovascular disease, hyperlipidemia, hypertension, stroke, obesity, or diabetes
2. Past medical history: Hypertension, diabetes/impaired fasting glucose, hyperlipidemia
3. BMI ≥85th percentile (if other risk factors are present), ≥95th percentile (all cases)

Labs should be repeated yearly for all youth with a BMI ≥ 95th percentile. Repeat testing depends on the level of abnormality, progression of the obesity, and degree of engagement in lifestyle change.

Gonorrhea and Chlamydia Screening

All sexually active AYAs should be screened yearly for chlamydia per guidelines. Gonorrhea screening is based on risk factors and local prevalence. Patients with high-risk sexual activity (multiple partners, prostitution, or men who have sex with men) or drug use should be tested yearly for gonorrhea. A combination test can be sent as a vaginal/cervical culture or urine/cervical polymerase chain reaction or PCR test.

Screening for Other STIs

Screening for HIV should be offered to all sexually active AYAs and should be encouraged for patients with any history of STI. Routine screening is not recommended for other STIs. But when a patient is diagnosed with one STI, he or she should be screened for others. Syphilis serology should be considered in high-risk populations, or where syphilis is prevalent. Men who have sex with men should receive annual screening for syphilis and HIV, in addition to chlamydia and gonorrhea. Hepatitis B status should also be confirmed for men who have sex with men.

IMMUNIZATIONS

The timely provision of immunizations is a key component of AYA health care. Changing immunization schedules and increasing vaccine refusal by patients and parents have complicated this process. With the advent of new requirements and vaccines, adolescents previously considered to be fully vaccinated suddenly find themselves "behind." In addition, AYAs frequently change providers and may have inadequate documentation of prior vaccines.

Recommended Vaccines

See Figures 5.2 and 5.3 for the CDC immunization schedule for AYAs. Immunization recommendations are updated annually by the CDC and can be found at http://www.immunize.org/cdc/child-schedule.pdf. Though prior immunization schedule versions had separate schedules for children and adolescents, there is now a single schedule. During adolescence, the vaccines that are typically given are those for meningococcus, human papillomavirus (HPV), and influenza. Many adolescents may need catch-up vaccines for hepatitis A and varicella, and a tetanus and pertussis booster depending on prior vaccination status.

Meningococcal Vaccine

Meningococcal disease usually presents as one of three syndromes: meningitis, bacteremia, or bacteremic pneumonia. *Neisseria meningitidis* serogroup B, C, and Y are the major causes of meningococcal disease in the United States. Each serogroup accounts for about one-third of disease; however, the proportion of diseases caused by each serogroup varies by age. About three-quarters of cases of disease among adolescents aged 11 or older are caused by serogroups C, W, or Y. *N. meningitidis* colonizes the nasopharyngeal mucosa and is transmitted by contact with respiratory tract secretions from those with disease or from asymptomatic carriers. Asymptomatic carriage rates are highest in the AYA population. Disease occurs infrequently as a result of nasopharyngeal colonization.

Currently, four meningococcal vaccines (MenACWY) have been licensed in the United States for the prevention of invasive disease caused by serogroups A, C, W, and Y. Two vaccines targeting serogroup B have been approved by the Food and Drug Administration. In 2015, the ACIP recommended that the vaccine series be administered to certain groups of AYAs (age > 10 years) at increased risk for meningococcal disease: persons with complement deficiencies, persons with anatomic or functional asplenia, microbiologists routinely exposed to isolates of the bacteria, and persons identified as being at increased risk because of a serogroup B meningococcal disease outbreak. Subsequently, the ACIP issued a permissive recommendation stating that the vaccine series may be administered to AYAs age 16-23 years (preferred age 16-18) to provide short term protection against serogroup B meningococcal disease.

Routine vaccination against meningococcal disease has been recommended by the ACIP since 2005 for adolescents. The ACIP recommends routine immunization of all adolescents aged 11 through 18 years with MenACWY. A single dose should be given at aged 11 or 12 years, with a booster dose administered at age 16 years. If the adolescent does not receive his or her first dose until age 13 through 15, the booster dose should be administered at age 16 through 18 years. If the first dose is given after the 16th birthday, a booster dose is not needed unless the adolescent is at increased risk for meningococcal disease (anatomical or functional asplenia, complement component deficiency). The ACIP does not recommend routine administration of MenACWY to young adults aged 19 through 21; however, the vaccine may be administered up to age 21 as catch-up for individuals who did not receive a dose after their 16th birthday. ACIP recommends that military recruits and first-year college students up to age 21 living in residence halls receive at least 1 dose of MenACWY prior to college entry. Ideally, the timing of the most recent dose should occur on or after the 16th birthday. If the young adult has had only one dose of vaccine before the 16th birthday, a booster dose is recommended before college enrollment. ACIP also recommends

two doses of MenACWY at least 2 months apart to adults with anatomical or functional asplenia, or persistent complement deficiencies. HIV infection is not an indication for routine vaccination.

Limited data suggest that the four MenACWY vaccine products can be used interchangeably; therefore, clinicians should administer the booster dose when indicated, regardless of the vaccine brand that was administered previously. Vaccination with MenACWY is contraindicated in those who have severe allergic reactions to any of its components (which include diphtheria and tetanus toxoid). No data are available on vaccination with MenACWY during pregnancy.

Human Papillomavirus

Three vaccines for prophylaxis against HPV have been recommended for AYAs, a bivalent vaccine (HPV2) (Cervarix, GlaxoSmithKline Inc.), a quadrivalent vaccine (HPV4) (Gardasil, Merck & Co.), and a 9-valent vaccines (HPV9) (Gardasil 9, Merck & Co.) (see Chapter 61). Each of the vaccines target HPV types 16 and 18 (the most common HPV types implicated in cervical cancer). HPV4 and HPV9 also target HPV types 6 and 11 (the most common HPV types associated with genital warts). HPV9 also targets HPV types 31, 33, 45, 52, and 58. The vaccines have been shown to be safe, highly immunogenic, and to prevent infections with HPV types 16 and/or 18 in randomized, double-blind, placebo-controlled trials. Approximately 66% of cervical cancer is related to HPV types 16 and 18 and an additional 15% is caused by HPV types 31, 33, 45, 52, and 58. About 90% of genital warts are related to types 6 and 11.

Currently, ACIP recommends routine vaccination of all adolescent females at age 11 or 12 years with 3 doses of either HPV2, HPV4, or HPV9. The series can be started as early as age 9 at the discretion of the health care provider. Vaccination is also recommended for AYA females aged 13 to 26 years who have not been vaccinated previously or who have not completed the series. For all males, ACIP recommends routine vaccination with HPV4 or HPV9 at age 11 or 12 years, but as early as age 9. Males, aged 13 through 21 years, who have not been vaccinated or who have not completed the three dose series should also be vaccinated. Young adult males aged 22 through 26 years may also be vaccinated. Ideally, vaccination should occur before the onset of sexual activity as the vaccine will not be effective against HPV subtypes that may have been already acquired.

Influenza

Two types of influenza vaccine are available, an inactivated vaccine and a live attenuated vaccine. Currently, both vaccine types are available as either trivalent (targeting three virus strains: two type A and one type B) or quadrivalent (targeting four virus strains: two type A and two type B), representing the strains most commonly found worldwide and predicted to be most likely to cause infections in the coming year. Vaccines are updated annually. Influenza in AYAs is discussed in Chapter 29.

Annual influenza vaccine is recommended for all individuals older than 6 months of age who do not have contraindications to receipt of the vaccine. Influenza vaccine should be received as soon as the vaccine becomes available each year. When vaccine supply is limited, priority should be given to AYAs with higher risk for influenza-related complications, including those with the following:

- Chronic pulmonary conditions (including asthma)
- Cardiovascular disease (with the exception of hypertension)
- Chronic renal, hepatic, neurologic, hematologic, or metabolic disorders
- Adolescents or young adults with immunosuppression (including those on immunosuppressing medication or who have HIV infection)
- Individuals who will be pregnant during influenza season
- Individuals on long-term aspirin therapy
- Residents of long-term care facilities
- American Indian/Alaskan natives
- Persons with morbid obesity (BMI ≥ 40)

Inactivated influenza vaccine is administered intramuscularly in the deltoid muscle. Only one dose is required for those older than

Recommended immunization schedule for persons aged 0 through 18 years – United States, 2015.

These recommendations must be read with the footnotes that follow. For those who fall behind or start late, provide catch-up vaccination at the earliest opportunity as indicated by the green bars in Figure 5.2. To determine minimum intervals between doses, see the catch-up schedule (Figure 5.4). School entry and adolescent vaccine age groups are shaded.

Vaccine	Birth	1 mo	2 mos	4 mos	6 mos	9 mos	12 mos	15 mos	18 mos	19–23 mos	2–3 yrs	4–6 yrs	7–10 yrs	11–12 yrs	13–15 yrs	16–18 yrs
Hepatitis B[1] (HepB)	1st dose	←――― 2nd dose ―――→			←――――――――――― 3rd dose ――――――――――――→											
Rotavirus[2] (RV) RV1 (2-dose series); RV5 (3-dose series)			1st dose	2nd dose	See footnote 2											
Diphtheria, tetanus, & acellular pertussis[3] (DTaP: <7 yrs)			1st dose	2nd dose	3rd dose		←―――― 4th dose ――――→					5th dose				
Tetanus, diphtheria, & acellular pertussis[4] (Tdap: ≥7 yrs)														(Tdap)		
Haemophilus influenzae type b[5] (Hib)			1st dose	2nd dose	See footnote 5		←― 3rd or 4th dose, See footnote 5 ―→									
Pneumococcal conjugate[6] (PCV13)			1st dose	2nd dose	3rd dose		←――― 4th dose ―――→									
Pneumococcal polysaccharide[6] (PPSV23)																
Inactivated poliovirus[7] (IPV: <18 yrs)			1st dose	2nd dose	←――――――――――― 3rd dose ――――――――――――→							4th dose				
Influenza[8] (IIV; LAIV) 2 doses for some: See footnote 8						Annual vaccination (IIV only) 1 or 2 doses					Annual vaccination (LAIV or IIV) 1 or 2 doses			Annual vaccination (LAIV or IIV) 1 dose only		
Measles, mumps, rubella[9] (MMR)					See footnote 9		←―――― 1st dose ――――→					2nd dose				
Varicella[10] (VAR)							←―――― 1st dose ――――→					2nd dose				
Hepatitis A[11] (HepA)							←――――― 2-dose series, See footnote 11 ―――――→									
Human papillomavirus[12] (HPV2: females only; HPV4: males and females)							See footnote 13							(3-dose series)		
Meningococcal[13] (Hib-MenCY ≥6 weeks; MenACWY-D ≥9 mos; MenACWY-CRM ≥2 mos)														1st dose		Booster

Legend:
- Range of recommended ages for all children
- Range of recommended ages for catch-up immunization
- Range of recommended ages for certain high-risk groups
- Range of recommended ages during which catch-up is encouraged and for certain high-risk groups
- Not routinely recommended

This schedule includes recommendations in effect as of January 1, 2015. Any dose not administered at the recommended age should be administered at a subsequent visit, when indicated and feasible. The use of a combination vaccine generally is preferred over separate injections of its equivalent component vaccines. Vaccination providers should consult the relevant Advisory Committee on Immunization Practices (ACIP) statement for detailed recommendations, available online at http://www.cdc.gov/vaccines/hcp/acip-recs/index.html. Clinically significant adverse events that follow vaccination should be reported to the Vaccine Adverse Event Reporting System (VAERS) online (http://www.vaers.hhs.gov) or by telephone (800-822-7967). Suspected cases of vaccine-preventable diseases should be reported to the state or local health department. Additional information, including precautions and contraindications for vaccination, is available from CDC online (http://www.cdc.gov/vaccines/recs/vac-admin/contraindications.htm) or by telephone (800-CDC-INFO [800-232-4636]).

This schedule is approved by the Advisory Committee on Immunization Practices (http://www.cdc.gov/vaccines/acip), the American Academy of Pediatrics (http://www.aap.org), the American Academy of Family Physicians (http://www.aafp.org), and the American College of Obstetricians and Gynecologists (http://www.acog.org).

FIGURE 5.2 CDC recommended immunization schedule for children and adolescents (see http://www.cdc.gov/vaccines/schedules/downloads/child/0-18yrs-schedule.pdf for schedule and footnotes).

Recommended Adult Immunization Schedule—United States - 2015

Note: These recommendations must be read with the footnotes that follow containing number of doses, intervals between doses, and other important information.

Recommended adult immunization schedule, by vaccine and age group[1]

VACCINE ▼ AGE GROUP ►	19-21 years	22-26 years	27-49 years	50-59 years	60-64 years	≥ 65 years
Influenza[*,2]	1 dose annually					
Tetanus, diphtheria, pertussis (Td/Tdap)[*,3]	Substitute 1-time dose of Tdap for Td booster; then boost with Td every 10 yrs					
Varicella[*,4]	2 doses					
Human papillomavirus (HPV) Female[*,5]	3 doses					
Human papillomavirus (HPV) Male[*,5]	3 doses					
Zoster[6]					1 dose	
Measles, mumps, rubella (MMR)[*,7]	1 or 2 doses					
Pneumococcal 13-valent conjugate (PCV13)[*,8]						1-time dose
Pneumococcal polysaccharide (PPSV23)[8]	1 or 2 doses					1 dose
Meningococcal[*,9]	1 or more doses					
Hepatitis A[*,10]	2 doses					
Hepatitis B[*,11]	3 doses					
Haemophilus influenzae type b (Hib)[*,12]	1 or 3 doses					

*Covered by the Vaccine Injury Compensation Program

(light gray)	For all persons in this category who meet the age requirements and who lack documentation of vaccination or have no evidence of previous infection; zoster vaccine recommended regardless of prior episode of zoster
(dark gray)	Recommended if some other risk factor is present (e.g., on the basis of medical, occupational, lifestyle, or other indication)
(white)	No recommendation

Report all clinically significant postvaccination reactions to the Vaccine Adverse Event Reporting System (VAERS). Reporting forms and instructions on filing a VAERS report are available at www.vaers.hhs.gov or by telephone, 800-822-7967.

Information on how to file a Vaccine Injury Compensation Program claim is available at www.hrsa.gov/vaccinecompensation or by telephone, 800-338-2382. To file a claim for vaccine injury, contact the U.S. Court of Federal Claims, 717 Madison Place, N.W., Washington, D.C. 20005; telephone, 202-357-6400.

Additional information about the vaccines in this schedule, extent of available data, and contraindications for vaccination is also available at www.cdc.gov/vaccines or from the CDC-INFO Contact Center at 800-CDC-INFO (800-232-4636) in English and Spanish, 8:00 a.m. - 8:00 p.m. Eastern Time, Monday - Friday, excluding holidays.

Use of trade names and commercial sources is for identification only and does not imply endorsement by the U.S. Department of Health and Human Services.

The recommendations in this schedule were approved by the Centers for Disease Control and Prevention's (CDC) Advisory Committee on Immunization Practices (ACIP), the American Academy of Family Physicians (AAFP), the America College of Physicians (ACP), American College of Obstetricians and Gynecologists (ACOG) and American College of Nurse-Midwives (ACNM).

Vaccines that might be indicated for adults based on medical and other indications[1]

VACCINE ▼ INDICATION ►	Pregnancy	Immuno-compromising conditions (excluding human immunodeficiency virus [HIV])[4,6,7,8,13]	HIV infection CD4+ T lymphocyte count[4,6,7,8,13] < 200 cells/µL	HIV infection CD4+ T lymphocyte count[4,6,7,8,13] ≥ 200 cells/µL	Men who have sex with men (MSM)	Kidney failure, end-stage renal disease, receipt of hemodialysis	Heart disease, chronic lung disease, chronic alcoholism	Asplenia (including elective splenectomy and persistent complement component deficiencies)[8,12]	Chronic liver disease	Diabetes	Healthcare personnel
Influenza[*,2]	1 dose IIV annually				1 dose IIV or LAIV annually	1 dose IIV annually					1 dose IIV or LAIV annually
Tetanus, diphtheria, pertussis (Td/Tdap)[*,3]	1 dose Tdap each pregnancy	Substitute 1-time dose of Tdap for Td booster; then boost with Td every 10 yrs									
Varicella[*,4]	Contraindicated				2 doses						
Human papillomavirus (HPV) Female[*,5]	3 doses through age 26 yrs				3 doses through age 26 yrs						
Human papillomavirus (HPV) Male[*,5]	3 doses through age 26 yrs				3 doses through age 21 yrs						
Zoster[6]	Contraindicated				1 dose						
Measles, mumps, rubella (MMR)[*,7]	Contraindicated				1 or 2 doses						
Pneumococcal 13-valent conjugate (PCV13)[*,8]	1 dose										
Pneumococcal polysaccharide (PPSV23)[8]	1 or 2 doses										
Meningococcal[*,9]	1 or more doses										
Hepatitis A[*,10]	2 doses										
Hepatitis B[*,11]	3 doses										
Haemophilus influenzae type b (Hib)[*,12]	post-HSCT recipients only	1 or 3 doses									

*Covered by the Vaccine Injury Compensation Program

(light gray)	For all persons in this category who meet the age requirements and who lack documentation of vaccination or have no evidence of previous infection; zoster vaccine recommended regardless of prior episode of zoster
(dark gray)	Recommended if some other risk factor is present (e.g., on the basis of medical, occupational, lifestyle, or other indications)
(white)	No recommendation

CDC U.S. Department of Health and Human Services Centers for Disease Control and Prevention

These schedules indicate the recommended age groups and medical indications for which administration of currently licensed vaccines is commonly recommended for adults ages 19 years and older, as of February 1, 2015. For all vaccines being recommended on the Adult Immunization Schedule: a vaccine series does not need to be restarted, regardless of the time that has elapsed between doses. Licensed combination vaccines may be used whenever any components of the combination are indicated and when the vaccine's other components are not contraindicated. For detailed recommendations on all vaccines, including those used primarily for travelers or that are issued during the year, consult the manufacturers' package inserts and the complete statements from the Advisory Committee on Immunization Practices (www.cdc.gov/vaccines/hcp/acip-recs/index.html). Use of trade names and commercial sources is for identification only and does not imply endorsement by the U.S. Department of Health and Human Services.

FIGURE 5.3 Adult immunization schedule. (see Centers for Disease Control and Prevention. Available at http://www.cdc.gov/vaccines/schedules/downloads/adult/adult-schedule.pdf for schedule and footnotes.)

9 years. It is contraindicated in persons with anaphylactic reactions to eggs and should be delayed in those with significant febrile illnesses (but not in those with minor upper respiratory infections). A recombinant influenza vaccine has been approved for adults aged 18 years and older that contains no egg protein and can therefore be administered to adults with egg allergies.

Live, attenuated influenza vaccine (LAIV) is marketed in the United States as FluMist. It is administered intranasally and is indicated for healthy persons aged 5 to 49 years, including those who may have contact with high-risk groups. It is contraindicated in individuals who are pregnant, immunosuppressed, receiving aspirin or other salicylates (because of the association of Reye syndrome with wild-type influenza infection). LAIV is also contraindicated for AYAs with a history of Guillain–Barré syndrome within 6 weeks of previous influenza vaccination; hypersensitivity, including anaphylaxis, to eggs; taking influenza antiviral medications in the previous 48 hours. LAIV should not be used in those who will have close contact with severely immunocompromised persons within 7 days of vaccination. While not strict contraindications, the safety of LAIV in persons with asthma, reactive airways disease, or other chronic condition has not been established, and these conditions should be considered precautions for LAIV use. LAIV is administered only through the intranasal route, 0.25 mL in each nostril. Only a single dose is required for those older than 9 years.

Catch-Up Vaccines

Adolescents who have been partially vaccinated should have their vaccination series completed without restarting the series. Likewise, adolescents who begin a vaccination series can complete it at any time after the vaccination process is interrupted, even if there has been a substantial delay between doses. **Figure 5.4** is the CDC catch-up immunization schedule for adolescents.

Consent for Vaccination

Since 1994, all health care providers who administer measles, mumps, rubella (MMR), polio, diphtheria and tetanus toxoids and pertussis (DTP), and Td vaccines have been required to distribute vaccine information sheets each time a patient is vaccinated. The clinic should obtain a signature from the patient, parent, or guardian acknowledging that they have been provided with vaccine information. This should also be noted in the medical record. Appropriate documentation of vaccination includes consent for vaccination, immunization type, date of administration, injection site, manufacturer and lot number of vaccine, and name and address of the health care provider administering the vaccine. For example, in California, teens can consent for the HPV vaccine without a parent's permission.

Vaccine refusal by patients and their parents is becoming more common and has been associated with a rise in rates of measles, mumps, and pertussis in recent years (http://www.cfr.org/interactives/GH_Vaccine_Map/#map). The AAP recommends responding to parent concerns, but also asking them to sign a waiver if they refuse recommended vaccines. The waiver can be found at https://www2.aap.org/immunization/pediatricians/pdf/refusaltovaccinate.pdf.

Improving Vaccine Delivery

To improve vaccination rates, the ACIP has specifically addressed a variety of situations in which many practitioners have deferred or delayed vaccination. Situations that specifically *do not* represent contraindications to vaccination include the following:

1. Reaction to a previous dose of DTP vaccine with only soreness, redness, or swelling
2. Mild acute illness with low-grade fever
3. Current antimicrobial therapy
4. Pregnancy of a household contact
5. Recent exposure to an infectious disease
6. Breast-feeding
7. History of nonspecific allergies

8. Allergy to penicillin or other antimicrobials except anaphylactic reactions to neomycin or streptomycin
9. Allergies to duck meat or duck feathers
10. Family history of seizures

Furthermore, "minor illnesses" such as mild upper respiratory tract infections, with or without low-grade fever, are not contraindications to vaccination. Vaccine hesitancy in the setting of mild acute illness has contributed to many missed opportunities to protect children and adolescents from vaccine-preventable disease.

PREVENTIVE HEALTH COUNSELING

After completing the patient evaluation, the provider should provide anticipatory guidance regarding high-risk behavior, and support positive choices that the adolescent or young adult is already making. This preventive health counseling portion of the examination should be done with the patient alone if confidential topics will be reviewed.

Approaches to Preventive Health Counseling

Preventive health counseling requires active listening, explicit questioning, and generating specific strategies in collaboration with the AYAs. Providers also need to be able to efficiently and effectively communicate simple key preventive health messages to their patients. Commonly used messages on a range of topics have been developed by Bright Futures, the Adolescent Health Working Group (AHWG), and others. A listing of resources and Web sites is available at the end of this chapter.

There are various approaches to preventive health counseling. One brief office-based intervention model, originally developed by the National Cancer Institute and recently modified by the USPSTF as a framework for behavioral counseling interventions, is the 5 A's approach:

1. Ask about the behavior.
2. Advise a different course.
3. Assess willingness to change.
4. Assist in behavior change.
5. Arrange for follow-up.

A complementary approach developed for the AMA's GAPS offers a standardized method of assessment and intervention that embodies health education principles but remains practical for office practice.[26] The mnemonic GAPS refers to gather information, assess further, problem identification, and specific solutions. **Figure 5.5** from the AHWG summarizes the steps.[25]

G (Gather Initial Information): Obtain a complete psychosocial history (HEEADSSS) from the patient. This initial screening step may be facilitated by use of questionnaires, computers, or nonclinician personnel. If the screening result is negative and no increased risk is identified, basic information and positive reinforcement of the healthy behavior should be offered. If the result is positive, proceed to the next level.

A (Assess Further): Assess the level and nature of risk in the particular area. Identify the seriousness of the problem by assessing the patient's knowledge and involvement, predisposing and protective factors, the availability of family and other support, and the consequences for the patient's health and function (e.g., school, peer relationships). The intervention offered depends on the assessed risk. For the patient at low risk, the provision of health information, a few targeted suggestions, and positive reinforcement about what the patient is already doing to stay healthy is often sufficient.[31] If the patient is at high risk, he or she probably needs an in-depth evaluation that may be beyond the scope of a preventive services visit. A return visit for more intensive intervention, or referral, is warranted. Patients who are at intermediate risk also require an explicit intervention, such as that suggested in the next step. This can be begun within the context of the preventive services visit.

Catch-up immunization schedule for persons aged 4 months through 18 years who start late or who are more than 1 month behind —United States, 2015.

The figure below provides catch-up schedules and minimum intervals between doses for children whose vaccinations have been delayed. A vaccine series does not need to be restarted, regardless of the time that has elapsed between doses. Use the section appropriate for the child's age.

Vaccine	Minimum Age for Dose 1	Dose 1 to Dose 2	Children and adolescents age 7 through 18 years	
Tetanus, diphtheria; tetanus, diphtheria, and acellular pertussis[5]	7 years[4]	4 weeks	4 weeks if first dose of DTaP/DT was administered before the 1st birthday. / 6 months (as final dose) if first dose of DTaP/DT was administered at or after the 1st birthday.	6 months if first dose of DTaP/DT was administered before the 1st birthday.
Human papillomavirus[12]	9 years		Routine dosing intervals are recommended.[12]	
Hepatitis A[11]	Not applicable (N/A)	6 months		
Hepatitis B[1]	N/A	4 weeks	8 weeks and at least 16 weeks after first dose.	
Inactivated poliovirus[7]	N/A	4 weeks	4 weeks[7]	6 months[7]
Meningococcal[13]	N/A	8 weeks[13]		
Measles, mumps, rubella[9]	N/A	4 weeks		
Varicella[10]	N/A	4 weeks	3 months if younger than age 13 years. 4 weeks if age 13 years or older.	

FIGURE 5.4 Catch-up immunizations. (see Centers for Disease Control and Prevention. Available at http://www.cdc.gov/vaccines/schedules/downloads/child/catchup-schedule-pr.pdf for schedule and footnotes.)

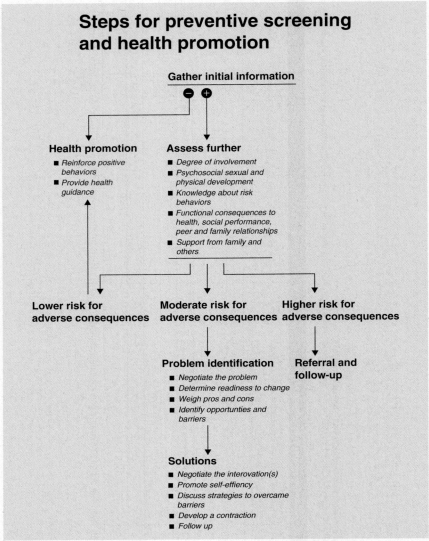

Steps for preventive screening and health promotion

Gather initial information

Health promotion
- *Reinforce positive behaviors*
- *Provide health guidance*

Assess further
- *Degree of involvement*
- *Psychosocial sexual and physical development*
- *Knowledge about risk behaviors*
- *Functional consequences to health, social performance, peer and family relationships*
- *Support from family and others*

Lower risk for adverse consequences

Moderate risk for adverse consequences

Higher risk for adverse consequences

Problem identification
- *Negotiate the problem*
- *Determine readiness to change*
- *Weigh pros and cons*
- *Identify opportunties and barriers*

Referral and follow-up

Solutions
- *Negotiate the interovation(s)*
- *Promote self-effiency*
- *Discuss strategies to overcame barriers*
- *Develop a contraction*
- *Follow up*

FIGURE 5.5 Steps for preventive screening and health promotions *AHWG.* (Simmons S, Shalwitz J, Pollock S, et al. *Adolescent Health Care 101: The Basics.* San Francisco, CA: Adolescent Health Working Group, 2003.

P (Problem Identification): This step involves working with the patient toward an agreement on the problem, helping the patient decide to make a change, and working with the patient to develop a specific plan for that change. The goal is to be "patient centered" in the approach—that is, to help the *patient* decide what is in his or her best interest, rather than assuming the patient will accept the clinician's view of the problem or behavior. Problem identification is an attempt to define the problem in terms that the patient recognizes (e.g., What is the difference between the way things are and the way I want them to be?).

When an adolescent or young adult is engaging in risky health behavior, clinicians often attempt to impart health knowledge rather than engaging the patient and obtaining specific information. For example, imagine a clinical encounter in which a sexually active adolescent patient is asked about condom use. The patient responds that she uses condoms "sometimes." While a clinician might talk about the importance and health benefits of condom use, the patient's inconsistency with condom use is likely not lack of knowledge but lies elsewhere—she cannot afford them, her partner refuses to use them, someone is allergic to latex, or there never seems to be a condom available when one is required. None of these potential barriers is likely to emerge if the clinician does not engage the adolescent. Productive advice for this particular patient rests in exploring the specific barriers that are getting in the way of condom use for this individual patient. It is important to move beyond barriers to a focus on how the adolescent or young adult is able to be successful in using a condom (e.g., What is the adolescent doing when they are able to use a condom "some of the time?").[32] A focus on strengths can be integrated into risk reduction discussions, with a clinician reinforcing positive behavior and building on successful experiences. If a sexually active teenager was having difficulty regularly using condoms, he might be asked about when he was last able to use a condom, thereby shifting the emphasis to what circumstances enabled him to be successful. Likewise, if a teenager was consistently using a condom, he should receive positive reinforcement for the healthy and safe behavior.[33]

If the patient does not agree that there is a problem with a specified behavior, look for areas of agreement and common ground. For example, a patient may not accept that his or her use of alcohol is problematic, but may acknowledge that binge drinking puts him or her at risk or is getting in the way of some goal (e.g., disapproval from friends or a romantic interest). Any problem that poses an immediate threat to the patient's safety warrants an immediate intervention or referral even if the patient does not agree that it is a problem or is not fully prepared for change.

S (Specific Solutions): Self-efficacy, Support, Solving Problems, and "Shaking on a Contract" *Self-efficacy* is assessed by asking the patient about his or her confidence to carry out the proposed plan. If the adolescent or young adult is not clear that they can be successful, revisit perceived barriers and attempt to redefine specific solutions. Plans should be concrete and achievable so that success becomes self-reinforcing. An overly ambitious plan may need to be modified.

Support in modifying behavior is important. Patients should be encouraged to identify people who can help them carry out their plan. Hopefully, they will be able to call on resources such as trusted adults or close friends. At times, AYAs may want advice on how best to recruit their support system. In addition to offering advice, the clinician may be helpful in facilitating the disclosure of information from patients to parents or others.

Solving problems reminds us to assess the barriers that the patient foresees and to work with the adolescent or young adult in developing specific strategies to overcome them. For example, if an adolescent recognizes that he will have difficulty not drinking at an upcoming party, he must have a plan for how to deal with that situation. It is usually most helpful if patients come up with their own solutions, identifying what has been helpful to them before and recognizing what they have been able to do to be successful.[32] The clinician can suggest modifications to the patient-derived solution, or suggest options that the adolescent or young adult might not have considered.

"Shaking on a contract" and/or writing down the agreed upon plan is a crucial step. It serves as a tangible reinforcement of the proposed plan and implies some commitment on the patient's part. It is important to specify the actions agreed to and the time frame in which the actions are to be taken. Make sure that the adolescent or young adult feels comfortable with the plan and understands it. If you are able to involve another party in the contract, such as a friend or parent, there is likely to be better follow-through. Follow-up is critical and should be arranged in some form—a visit, telephone contact, or e-mail—in the time frame agreed to in the contract.

ACKNOWLEDGMENTS

The authors wish to acknowledge David S. Rosen and Lawrence S. Neinstein for their contributions to previous versions of this chapter.

REFERENCES

1. Ozer EM, Irwin CE Jr. Adolescent and young adult health: from basic health status to clinical interventions. In: Lerner R, Steinberg L, eds. *Individual basis of adolescent development: Volume 1, Handbook of adolescent psychology.* 3rd ed. Hoboken, NJ: Wiley, 2009:618–641.
2. Mulye TP, Park MJ, Nelson CD, et al. Trends in adolescent and young adult health in the United States. *J Adolesc Health* 2009;45(1):8–24.
3. Centers for Disease Control and Prevention (CDC). *Injury prevention and control: data and statistics. WISQARS: leading causes of death [online database].* Available at http://www.cdc.gov/ncipc/wisqars/. Accessed on February 3, 2014.
4. Ozer EM, Urquhart JT, Brindis CD, et al. Young adult preventive health care guidelines: there but can't be found. *Arch Pediatr Adolesc Med* 2012;166(3):240–247.
5. Hagan JE SJ, Duncan PM. *Bright futures: guidelines for health supervision of infants, children, and adolescents.* 3rd ed. Elk Grove Village, IL: American Academy of Pediatrics, 2008.
6. US Preventive Services Task Force. *Homepage.* Available at http://www.uspreventiveservicestaskforce.org/. Accessed on July, 2013.
7. Cantor JC, Monheit AC, DeLia D, et al. Early impact of the Affordable Care Act on health insurance coverage of young adults. *Health Serv Res* 2012;47(5):1773–1790.
8. Irwin CE Jr, Adams SH, Park MJ, et al. Preventive care for adolescents: few get visits and fewer get services. *Pediatrics* 2009;123(4):e565–e572.
9. Jasik CB, Adams SH, Irwin CE Jr, et al. The association of BMI status with adolescent preventive screening. *Pediatrics* 2011;128(2):e317–e323.
10. Callahan ST, Cooper WO. Changes in ambulatory health care use during the transition to young adulthood. *J Adolesc Health* 2010;46(5):407–413.
11. Fortuna RJ, Robbins BW, Halterman JS. Ambulatory care among young adults in the United States. *Ann Intern Med* 2009;151(6):379–385.
12. Lau JS, Adams SH, Irwin CE Jr, et al. Receipt of preventive health services in young adults. *J Adolesc Health* 2013;52(1):42–49.
13. Adolescent Health Services. *Missing opportunities: committee on adolescent health services and models of care for treatment, prevention, and healthy development.* Washington, DC: National Academies Press, 2009.
14. Solberg LI, Nordin JD, Bryant TL, et al. Clinical preventive services for adolescents. *Am J Prev Med* 2009;37(5):445–454.
15. Tylee A, Haller DM, Graham T, et al. Youth-friendly primary-care services: how are we doing and what more needs to be done? *Lancet* 2007;369(9572):1565–1573.
16. Marcell AV, Klein JD, Fischer I, et al. Male adolescent use of health care services: where are the boys? *J Adolesc Health* 2002;30(1):35–43.
17. Tebb KP, Wibbelsman C, Neuhaus JM, et al. Screening for asymptomatic Chlamydia infections among sexually active adolescent girls during pediatric urgent care. *Arch Pediatr Adolesc Med* 2009;163(6):559–564.
18. Pastore DR, Murray PJ, Juszczak L, et al. School-based health center: position paper of the Society for Adolescent Medicine. *J Adolesc Health* 2001;29(6):448–450.
19. Ozer EM, Scott JT, Brindis CD. Seizing the opportunity: improving young adult preventive health care. *Adolesc Med State Art Rev* 2013;24(3):507–525.
20. Nakamura MM, Ferris TG, DesRoches CM, et al. Electronic health record adoption by children's hospitals in the United States. *Arch Pediatr Adolesc Med* 2010;164(12):1145–1151.
21. Ford C, English A, Sigman G. Confidential health care for adolescents: position paper for the society for adolescent medicine. *J Adolesc Health* 2004;35(2):160–167.
22. Anoshiravani A, Gaskin GL, Groshek MR, et al. Special requirements for electronic medical records in adolescent medicine. *J Adolesc Health* 2012;51(5):409–414.
23. Blythe MJ, Del Beccaro MA. Standards for health information technology to ensure adolescent privacy. *Pediatrics* 2012;130(5):987–990.
24. Ozer EM, Martin M, Jasik C, et al. The development of a clinic-based interactive behavioral health screening module for adolescents. Paper presented at the 2013 International Congress on Adolescent Health; 2013; Istanbul.
25. Simmons M, Shalwitz J, Pollock S, et al. *Adolescent health care 101: the basics.* San Francisco, CA: Adolescent Health Working Group, 2003. Available at http://www.anthem.com/ca/provider/f3/s1/t4/pw_a113103.pdf?refer=provider. Accessed on October 28, 2014.
26. Elster AB, Kuznets N. *Guidelines for Adolescent Preventive Services (GAPS): recommendations and rationale.* Chicago, IL: American Medical Association, 1994.
27. Zuckerbrot RA, Cheung AH, Jensen PS, et al. Guidelines for Adolescent Depression in Primary Care (GLAD-PC). I. Identification, assessment, and initial management. *Pediatrics* 2007;120(5):e1299–e1312.
28. Knight JR, Sherritt L, Shrier LA, et al. Validity of the CRAFFT substance abuse screening test among adolescent clinic patients. *Arch Pediatr Adolesc Med* 2002;156(6):607–614.
29. National Adolescent and Young Adult Health Information Center. *Summary of recommended guidelines for clinical preventive services for young adults ages 18–26: risk factors and recommended screening tests.* San Francisco, CA: National Adolescent and Young Adult Health Information Center, University of California, San Francisco, 2013. Available at http://nahic.ucsf.edu/wp-content/uploads/2014/04/FINAL-Screening-Guidelines-4.11.pdf. Accessed on October 28, 2014.
30. Rosen DS; American Academy of Pediatrics Committee on Adolescence. Identification and management of eating disorders in children and adolescents. *Pediatrics* 2010;126(6):1240–1253.
31. Ozer EM, Adams SH, Orrell-Valente JK, et al. Does delivering preventive services in primary care reduce adolescent risky behavior? *J Adolesc Health* 2011;49(5):476–482.
32. Ozer MN. *Management of persons with chronic neurological illness.* Woburn, MA: Butterworth-Heinemann, 2000.
33. Duncan PM, Garcia AC, Frankowski BL, et al. Inspiring healthy adolescent choices: a rationale for and guide to strength promotion in primary care. *J Adolesc Health* 2007;41(6):525–535.

ADDITIONAL RESOURCES AND WEBSITES ONLINE

Nutrition

Michael R. Kohn

Nutrition is an essential component of adolescent and young adult (AYA) health care. Optimal nutrition assists in reaching the potential for physical growth, development, and the prevention of illness. Two important transformations occur during adolescence that change nutritional needs. Growth and changes in body composition are greater and more rapid than at any other time in life, except infancy. In general, there is also a significant change in the adolescent's eating habits and food consumption. Adolescents typically reduce regular breakfast consumption, increase consumption of prepared foods, snacks, fried foods, nutrient-poor foods, and sweetened beverages, and have a significant increase in portion size at each meal. This is associated with a decrease in the consumption of dairy products, fruits, and vegetables. Sodium intake is far in excess of recommended levels, whereas calcium and potassium intakes are below recommended levels.[1] The nutritional needs of young adults differ from both adolescents and the average population values.[2,3]

Health care providers should assess nutritional status and provide appropriate nutritional counseling as part of health supervision visits. Information quantifying nutritional requirements and providing illustration of healthy eating information are available at http://circ.ahajournals.org/content/112/13/2061.full. Further assistance for families to provide nutritious, balanced meals is available from the US Department of Agriculture (USDA) MyPlate site (http://kidshealth.org/parent/nutrition_center/healthy_eating/myplate.html). MyPlate includes sections for vegetables, fruits, grains, and foods high in protein. MyPlate's user-friendly, interactive Web site provides simple messages for parents (Fig. 6.1).

POTENTIAL NUTRITIONAL PROBLEMS

The National Health and Nutrition Examination Survey (NHANES) (http://www.cdc.gov/nchs/nhanes/ about_nhanes.htm) concluded that the highest prevalence of unsatisfactory nutritional status occurs in the adolescent age-group. Of particular note were deficiencies in the intake of calcium, iron, riboflavin, thiamine, and vitamins A and C.

Risk Factors
1. Increased nutritional needs during adolescence are related to several factors.
   a. Adolescents gain 20% of their adult height.
   b. Adolescents gain 50% of their adult skeletal mass.

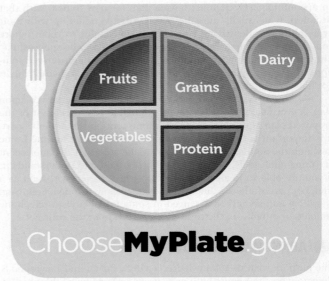

FIGURE 6.1 The My Plate site provides a range of healthy eating strategies and advice for professionals and consumers. (From the USDA Center for Nutrition Policy and Promotion's ChooseMyPlate.gov Web site.)

   c. Caloric and protein requirements are maximal.
   d. Specific nutrient needs—gender, chronic illness.
2. Increased physical activity of AYAs makes proper nutrition essential.
3. Poor eating habits of AYAs contribute to nutritional problems.[4,5]
   a. Missed meals are common.
   b. High-energy snacks of low nutritional value are popular.
   c. Peer pressure leads to changes in a range of eating behaviors, including restrictive and overeating patterns and purging behaviors.
   d. The adolescent's family may exhibit poor eating habits, and meal preparation may be inadequate.
   e. Inadequate financial resources to purchase food or to prepare nutritious meals.
4. In AYAs, dietary choices contribute to increased risk for cardiovascular disease.
   a. Low fruit and vegetable consumption and high sweetened beverage consumption are independently associated with the prevalence of metabolic syndrome in specific sex-ethnicity populations.
   b. High-fiber diets may protect against obesity and cardiovascular disease by lowering insulin levels.

NUTRITIONAL ASSESSMENT

Assessing the nutritional status of an adolescent or young adult should be part of a comprehensive health evaluation. This becomes even more important in AYAs who are identified as nutritionally at risk. Such young people include those with nutritionally related medical conditions, dietary deficiencies, or those with conditions that predispose them to inadequate nutrition. Nutritional assessment requires repeated measurements of nutritional status over time. Methods used in the nutritional assessment of adolescents include dietary and clinical evaluation, measurements of body composition, and obtaining laboratory data.

Dietary Data

There is a range of validated strategies used to obtain dietary data from AYAs. These include food records, 24-hour recall of all food consumed, food frequency questionnaires, and other questionnaires (http://appliedresearch.cancer.gov/assess_wc/review/agegroups/adolescents/validation.html?&url=/tools/children/review/agegroups/adolescents/validation.html).

An example of screening questions that are quick and easy to ask includes the following:

1. How many meals do you usually eat in a day? Any snacks?
2. Tell me everything you have eaten in the past 24 hours.
3. Are there any foods that you have eliminated from your diet?
4. Are you on a diet?
5. Are you comfortable with your eating habits?
6. Do you ever eat in secret? Do you ever feel you can't stop eating?
7. Have you recently lost or gained weight, or has your weight stayed the same?
8. Do you feel that your weight is too much, too little, or about right?
9. What is the most you have ever weighed, and what would you like to weigh?

Helpful screening questions for AYAs (followed by the associated sensitivity and specificity for disordered eating in adolescence) include the following[6]:

1. How many diets have you been on in the past year? (Two or three diets, 88% sensitivity and 63% specificity; four or five diets, 69% sensitivity and 86% specificity).
2. Do you feel you should be dieting? (Often, 94% sensitivity and 67% specificity; usually, 87% sensitivity and 82% specificity).
3. Do you feel dissatisfied with your body size? (Often, 96% sensitivity and 61% specificity; usually, 88% sensitivity and 74% specificity).
4. Does your weight affect the way you feel about yourself? (Often, 97% sensitivity and 61% specificity; usually, 91% sensitivity and 74% specificity).

Each of these questions appears to have a very high correlation with the score on the Eating Attitudes Test (EAT-26).[7] This screening test examines attitudes and behaviors regarding food, weight, and body image and has been validated for use in AYAs.

Clinical Signs of Nutritional Deficiencies

Please see **Table 6.1**.

Anthropometric Measurements

1. Weight and height: Weight-for-age and height-for-age charts can be obtained from the Centers for Disease Control Prevention (CDC) on their Web site at http://www.cdc.gov/growthcharts/.
2. Body mass index is a very useful screening tool, but it has its limitations. See Chapter 32 on Obesity.
3. Skin fold measurements and waist–hip ratio all provide valuable information in a nutritional assessment. These measurements can assist in quantifying obesity and have shown to have predictive value with respect to health outcomes such as cardiovascular disease and insulin resistance. They are

TABLE 6.1

Clinical Signs of Nutritional Deficiency

Body Parts	Nutritional Deficiency	Clinical Signs of Deficiency
Skin	Iron Vitamin A Hyperlipidemia Vitamin C Vitamin K, C, and folate	Pallor Follicular hyperkeratosis Xanthoma Petechiae Bruising and purpura
Eyes	Riboflavin, niacin Vitamin A	Angular palpebritis Night blindness
Lips	Riboflavin, niacin	Angular stomatitis Cheilosis
Tongue	Niacin, folic acid, vitamins B_6 and B_{12} Niacin, folic acid, vitamins B_6 and B_{12}, or iron Zinc	Glossitis Papillary atrophy Loss of taste
Gums	Vitamin C	Hypertrophy, bleeding
Teeth	Diet high in refined sugars	Cavities
Hair	Protein energy malnutrition	Dry, dull, brittle
Neck	Iodine	Goiter
Nails	Malnutrition, iron, or calcium Vitamin A	Brittle with frayed borders Concave or eggshell
Bones and Joints	Vitamin D Vitamin C	Rickets Scurvy

not, however, currently recommended for clinical use because they require specific training to perform accurately.

Laboratory Tests

Laboratory tests helpful in assessing nutritional status include hemoglobin, hematocrit, ferritin, serum protein, albumin, and vitamins D, B_{12}, and folate.

Nutritional Requirements

Dietary reference intakes (DRIs) represent quantitative estimates of nutrients used to plan and evaluate diets for healthy people, including AYAs. The DRIs are a set of four nutrient reference values.

1. Recommended dietary allowance (RDA): This is the dietary intake level that is sufficient to meet the nutrient requirements of almost all healthy individuals (97% to 98%) in the United States.
2. Adequate intake (AI): This is the value based on observed or experimentally determined approximations of nutrient intake by a group—used when RDA cannot be determined.
3. Estimated average requirement (EAR): This is the intake value that is estimated to meet the requirement defined by a specified indicator of adequacy in 50% of an age- and gender-specific group. At this level of intake, the remaining 50% of the specified group would not have its needs met.
4. Tolerable upper intake level (UL): This is the maximum level of daily nutrient intake that is unlikely to pose risks of adverse health effects to almost all of the individuals in the group for whom it is designed.

The DRIs cover the following groups of nutrients:

1. Calcium, vitamin D, phosphorus, magnesium, and fluoride
2. Folate and other B vitamins
3. Antioxidants (e.g., vitamin C, vitamin E, selenium)
4. Macronutrients (e.g., proteins, fats, carbohydrates)
5. Trace elements (e.g., iron, zinc)
6. Electrolytes and water
7. Other food components (e.g., fiber, phytoestrogens)

The requirements are reported to differ slightly between AYAs (between 19 and 30 years of age). Details of the recommended DRIs definitions are available at http://www.hc-sc.gc.ca/fn-an/alt_formats/hpfb-dgpsa/pdf/nutrition/dri_tables-eng.pdf.

Energy Requirements

Energy requirements are determined by basal metabolic rate, growth status, physical activity, and body composition. Energy requirements of adolescents vary depending on the timing of growth and pubertal development. As such, energy needs are based on height because it provides a better estimate of total daily caloric recommendations. Suggested caloric intakes are listed in **Table 6.2**.

Protein

Protein provides 4 kcal of energy in each gram. Protein requirements are based on the amount of protein needed to maintain existing lean body mass and the increase in additional lean body mass with growth and development. Protein requirements are highest during the peak height velocity. In the populations surveyed in the United States, most AYA diets exceed the RDA for protein.

Carbohydrates

Carbohydrates provide 4 kcal of energy in each gram. Carbohydrates should make up approximately 50% of the daily caloric intake. However, no more than 10% to 25% of calories should come from sweeteners (sucrose and high-fructose corn syrup). Nearly, 12% of carbohydrates consumed by AYAs come from the added sweeteners in soft drinks.

Carbohydrate-containing foods include grain products, fruits, and vegetables. Approximately 25 to 35 g of fiber should be consumed daily. Fiber is found in whole grain foods, fruits, vegetables, legumes, nuts, and seeds.

Glycemic index (GI) classifies carbohydrate foods on the basis of the effect on blood glucose. The index ranges from 0 to 100, with glucose or other reference standard being 100. Hence, the lower the GI, the lower the expected rise in blood sugar for a given food. In general, foods are classified into low GI (<40), moderate GI (40 to 70), and high GI (>70).

Alcohol provides 7 cal of energy in each gram and can also be a significant source of calories.

Fat

Fat provides 9 kcal of energy in each gram. AYAs require dietary fat and essential fatty acids for many vital functions in the body. An AYA diet should contain no more than 30% of calories from fat. Most AYAs' total and saturated fat intake is greater than that recommended. For AYAs, trans fatty acid (TFA) intake should be reduced as much as possible because of its adverse effects on lipids and lipoproteins. The replacement of TFA with other saturated and unsaturated fatty acids in foods beneficially affects low-density lipoprotein cholesterol, the primary target for cardiovascular disease risk reduction.

Minerals

Iron: There is an increased need for iron in both males and females during adolescence because of the rapid growth, and increase in muscle mass and blood volume. In addition, AYA females require increase in iron because of menstrual losses. High-iron foods include lean meats, fish, and eggs. Nonheme iron present in plant sources is less bioavailable, but its absorption can be enhanced by concurrent intake of vitamin C.

Calcium: Requirements for dietary calcium increase substantially during periods of peak velocity of growth and accrual of bone mineral content. AYAs tend to eat a diet deficient in calcium. The DRI for calcium for 9- to 18-year-olds is 1,300 mg/day (**Table 6.3**). Many AYAs have inadequate calcium intakes, in part due to the substitution of carbonated beverages for milk and increasing concern about lactose intolerance.

Those AYAs not taking in adequate calcium from food sources may need to take supplemental calcium such as calcium carbonate, citrate, lactate, or phosphate (absorption varies from 25% to 35%). Optimal absorption of the calcium supplements occurs when no more than 500 mg/dose is taken with food. In addition to dairy products, calcium is found in tofu, salmon and sardines, dark green leafy vegetables, and calcium-fortified foods (such as orange juice).

Zinc: Zinc is needed for adequate growth, sexual maturation, and wound healing. The RDA for zinc was set at 8 mg/day for adolescents

TABLE 6.2

Recommended Dietary Allowances for AYAs

Category	Male (y) 11–14	15–18	19–24	Female (y) 11–14	15–18	19–24	Pregnancy	Lactating (first 6 mo)	Lactating (second 6 mo)
Weight (kg)	45	66	72	46	55	58			
Height (cm)	157	176	177	157	163	164			
Energy (cal)	2,500	3,000	2,900	2,200	2,200	2,200	+300	+500	+500
Protein (g)	45	59	58	46	44	46	60	65	62
Minerals									
Iron (mg/d)	12	12	10	15	15	15	30	15	15
Zinc (mg/d)	15	15	15	12	12	12	15	19	16
Iodine (µg/d)	150	150	150	150	150	150	175	200	200
Vitamins									
Vitamin A (IU)	10	10	10	10	10	10	10	10	10

Adapted from Food and Nutrition Board, National Research Council. *Recommended dietary allowances.* 10th ed. Washington, DC: National Academy Press, 1989.

TABLE 6.3

Recommended Dietary Allowances (Light Face Type) and Adequate Intake (Bold Face Type) Values, by Age

Daily Amount	Male (y)			Female (y)			Pregnant (y)		Lactating (y)	
	9–13	14–18	19–30	9–13	14–18	19–30	<19	19–30	<19	19–30
Calcium (mg)	1,300	1,300	1,000	1,300	1,300	1,000	1,300	1,000	1,300	1,000
Phosphorus (mg)	**1,250**	**1,250**	**700**	**1,250**	**1,250**	**700**	**1,250**	**700**	**1,250**	**700**
Magnesium (mg)	**240**	**410**	**400**	**1,250**	**1,250**	**700**	**1,250**	**700**	**1,250**	**700**
Fluoride (mg)	2	3	4	2	3	3	3	3	3	3
Selenium (pg)	**40**	**55**	**55**	**40**	**55**	**55**	**60**	**60**	**70**	**70**
Vitamin C (mg)	45	75	90	45	65	75	80	85	115	120
Vitamin D (µg)	5	5	5	5	5	5	5	5	5	5
Vitamin E (mg)	**11**	**15**	**15**	**11**	**15**	**15**	**15**	**15**	**19**	**19**
Thiamine (mg)	1.2	1.2	1.2	0.9	1.0	1.1	1.4	1.4	1.5	1.5
Riboflavin (mg)	0.9	1.3	1.3	0.9	1.0	1.1	1.4	1.4	1.6	1.6
Niacin (mg)	12	16	16	12	14	14	18	18	17	17
Vitamin B$_6$ (mg)	1.0	1.3	1.3	1.0	1.2	1.3	1.9	1.9	2.0	2.0
Folacin (µg)	300	400	400	300	400	400	600	600	500	500
Vitamin B$_{12}$ (µg)	1.8	2.4	2.4	1.8	2.4	2.4	2.6	2.6	2.8	2.8
Pantothenic acid (B$_5$) (mg)	4	5	5	4	5	5	6	6	7	7
Biotin (µg)	20	25	30	20	25	30	30	30	35	35
Choline (mg)	375	550	550	375	550	550	450	450	550	550

Adapted from Food and Nutrition Board, National Academy of Sciences. US Department of Agriculture. Available at www.nalusda.gov/fnic/etext/000105.html. 1998.

9- to 13-years-old and 9 mg/day and 11 mg/day for females and males 11- to 14-years-old, respectively. Young adults have slightly decreased requirement. Good food sources of zinc include lean meats, seafood, eggs, and milk.

Vitamins

Vitamin requirements increase during adolescence, especially for vitamin B$_{12}$; folate; vitamins A, C, D, and E; thiamine; niacin; and riboflavin (**Table 6.3**). It has been shown that supplements of antioxidant vitamins (A, C, E, and β-carotene) probably reduce the risk of cardiovascular disease and certain cancers, but there is no current recommendation to prescribe them routinely.

GUIDELINES FOR NUTRITIONAL THERAPY

General Recommendations

1. Be aware of and sensitive to the family context, lifestyle, and cultural milieu.
2. Motivate lifestyle change by stressing the positive effects of dietary changes, for example, feeling good about oneself, feeling energetic.
3. Use the MyPlate Food Guide (Fig. 6.1) to recommend the appropriate number of daily servings from each food group.
4. Recommend that AYAs participate in a regular exercise program for at least 30 minutes, at least 4 days of the week. Balance dietary energy intake with physical activity to maintain normal growth and development.

5. Simplify good nutrition concepts by recommending the following to AYAs and their families:
   - Maintain a healthy weight.
   - Eat a wide variety of nutritious foods, including lean meat, fish, and poultry.
   - Limit solid fats (butter, margarine, shortening, lard) and choose foods low in saturated fat and TFA. Use more polyunsaturated fats.
   - Broil or bake instead of frying foods.
   - Use nonfat (skim) or low-fat milk and dairy products daily.
   - Eat plenty of vegetables, legumes, and fruits.
   - Eat plenty of cereals (including breads, rice, pasta, and noodles), preferably wholegrain.
   - Drink water instead of soft drinks or fruit drinks. Limit juice intake.
   - Eat meals and snacks regularly. Eating family meals is correlated with improved nutritional intake and reduces the likelihood that youth will develop eating disorders.[4,5]

Special Conditions

Vegetarian Diets

AYAs may be vegetarian because of ecological, economic, religious, or philosophical beliefs. AYAs who are vegetarians (but not choosing to be vegan) are likely to have an adequate nutritional intake. Nutritional counseling may be of benefit to ensure AI of energy, protein, and micronutrients as well as to assess the need for supplements.[8,9]

Types of Vegetarians (http://www.vrg.org/):

Semivegetarians eat milk products and limited seafood and poultry but no red meat.

Lactovegetarians consume milk products but no eggs, meat, fish, or poultry.

Ovolactovegetarians consume milk products and eggs but no meat, fish, or poultry.

Vegans consume vegetable foods only and no foods of animal origin (i.e., no eggs, milk products, meat, fish, or poultry).

Fruitarians consume raw fruit and seeds only. Examples of such fruits include pineapple, mango, banana, avocado, apple, melon, orange, all kinds of berries, and the vegetable fruits such as tomato, cucumber, olives, and nuts.

Supplemental Needs of Vegetarians:

Potential nutritional issues with vegetarian diets include macronutrient and micronutrient deficiencies such as protein, fat, vitamin B_{12}, iron, zinc, calcium, and vitamin D.

Vitamins: Semivegetarians, lactovegetarians, and ovolactovegetarians have no need for supplements if attention is paid to dietary composition. Vegans may need supplemental iron, calcium, riboflavin, and vitamins B_{12} and D.

Protein: Adequate protein intake has been a traditional concern for vegetarians; however, vegetarians usually meet or exceed protein requirements (except for vegans). There is also mounting evidence that the practice of eating complementary proteins in the same meal is unnecessary. However, it is recommended that the day's meals supply all of them.

Minerals: There is no uniform need for supplements, but vegetarians are at increased risk for iron and zinc deficiencies. Vegetarians may need up to 50% more zinc in their diet since phytate (found in plants) and calcium hinder zinc absorption.

Lactose Intolerance

AYAs with lactose intolerance are at risk of inadequate calcium intake. Some AYAs with lactose intolerance can tolerate small amounts of milk products, including aged cheese or yogurt with active cultures. There are many nondairy foods high in calcium, including green vegetables, such as broccoli and kale; fish with edible bones, such as salmon and sardines; calcium-fortified orange juice; and soymilk. There are a variety of lactose-reduced/free dairy products in the supermarket, including milk, cottage cheese, and processed cheese slices. AYAs often find lactase enzyme replacement pills or liquid helpful.[10]

Pregnancy

Energy requirements are greater for pregnant compared with nonpregnant AYAs. Adolescents may require higher energy intake than young adults. As indicated in **Table 6.2**, pregnant adolescents should not consume less than 2,000 kcal/day and in many cases their needs may be higher. The best gauge of adequate energy intake during pregnancy is satisfactory weight gain. Goals for weight gain are based on prepregnancy weight, height, age, stage of development, and usual eating patterns. Young pregnant women who are below an optimal weight are advised to gain more weight than overweight women.[11]

Folate is essential for nucleic acid synthesis and is required in greater amounts during pregnancy. Taking folic acid before and during early pregnancy can reduce the risk of spina bifida and other neural tube defects. Because these defects occur early in gestation, it is advised that women of childbearing age and those who are capable of becoming pregnant consume 400 µg/day of folic acid. The DRI for folate during pregnancy is 600 µg/day. Good sources of folate include leafy dark green vegetables, legumes, citrus fruits and juices, peanuts, whole grains, and some fortified breakfast cereals.

The calcium recommendation during pregnancy is 1,300 mg/day for adolescents and 1,000 mg/day for young adults. Since most nonpregnant AYA females consume significantly less than the recommended amount of calcium, pregnant AYAs should either add calcium-rich foods to their diet or take calcium supplementation.

Dietary counseling can be one of the most important interventions for a pregnant AYA to ensure a healthy pregnancy and a healthy baby. AYAs should be encouraged to obtain their nutrients from food. A low-dose vitamin–mineral supplement is recommended for pregnant adolescents who do not regularly consume a healthy diet. AYAs should be counseled against dieting during pregnancy.

Athletes

Risk for Iron and Zinc Deficiency: Both male and female AYA athletes are at risk for iron deficiency.[12] Athletes (especially menstruating females and those involved in endurance sports such as distance running) should be screened for low hemoglobin or hematocrit levels. Serum ferritin can be helpful in determining loss of iron stores and need for supplementation. A ferritin level of <16 µg/L corresponds with depleted iron stores. For the athlete who is not anemic but has low iron stores (latent iron deficiency), 50 to 100 mg of elemental iron daily (ferrous gluconate 240 or 325 mg twice daily or ferrous sulfate 325 mg daily or twice daily) should be recommended. For the anemic athlete, 100 to 200 mg of elemental iron daily (ferrous gluconate 325 mg three times daily or ferrous sulfate 325 mg twice daily) should be given. Laboratory measurements should be repeated after 2 to 3 months to document response to therapy. Athletes with iron deficiency anemia may also be zinc deficient. Education regarding good dietary sources of zinc and iron should be provided.[13]

Sodium and Potassium: Athletes need increased intake of sodium and potassium. This requirement will generally be met as they increase their calorie intake.[14]

Calories: The active athlete who engages in 2 hours/day of heavy exercise needs 800 to 1,700 extra calories/day beyond the recommended minimum for age, sex, height, and weight to maintain energy balance. The American Dietetic Association recommends the approximate distribution of calories should be carbohydrates, 55% to 60%; proteins, 12% to 15%; and fats, 25% to 30%.[15]

Hydration: Attention must be given to hydration before and during activity.[16]

- Athletes should drink 10 to 16 oz of cold water 1 to 2 hours before exercise.
- Repeat 20 to 30 minutes before exercise.
- Drink 4 to 6 oz of cold water every 10 to 15 minutes during exercise.
- Cold fluids are preferable because gastric emptying is more rapid.
- Plain water can be used for exercise periods of <2 hours.
- Sports drinks may be used to provide carbohydrates for longer events. Fructose-containing solutions should be avoided since they are not as well absorbed as solutions with sucrose or glucose and can cause gastrointestinal upset.

Weight Restrictions: Avoid any major weight restriction during the adolescent growth spurt. Alterations in diet to cause rapid weight gain or loss should be discouraged. Eating disorders are prevalent among athletes (largely female athletes), especially in those involved in running, swimming, diving, gymnastics, or dance (see Chapter 33). Therefore, it is important to carefully explore issues related to body image, desired weight, and menstrual function in all athletes. The female athlete triad (amenorrhea, disordered eating, and osteoporosis) should be suspected in an athlete with secondary amenorrhea.

Carbohydrate Loading: Diets that are chronically high in carbohydrate are not recommended. For optimal performance, the athlete should train lightly or rest 24 to 36 hours before competition. On the day of competition, the athlete may consider a high-carbohydrate, low-fat meal 3 to 6 hours before an event and an optional snack 1 to 2 hours before the event. Foods high in carbohydrates (60% to 70%) have also been recommended after competition to replace glycogen stores. However, Hawley et al.[17] pointed out that a diet of 5,000 kcal/day that is only 45% carbohydrate is sufficient to restore muscle glycogen within 24 hours. An initial "depletion phase" consisting of vigorous workouts and low-carbohydrate eating before competition is also no longer recommended.

Nutritional Supplements: The word "ergogenic" is derived from the Greek word *ergon*, which means "to increase work or potential for work." Anecdotal reports suggest that compounds such as bee pollen, caffeine, glycine, carnitine, lecithin, brewer's yeast, and gelatin improve strength or endurance. However, scientific research has failed to substantiate these claims.[18,19]

AYA athletes who are considering the use of nutritional supplements should be aware that the effects of long-term supplement use have not been studied. In addition, supplement use can be quite costly. Most athletes can maximize their performance through consistent, appropriate training and attention to adequate nutrition rather than relying on supplement use (http://www.drugfreesport.com/choices/supplements/). See Chapter 83 for further discussion on herbal therapies. Gains in muscle mass may best be sought by attempting to take advantage of timing of ingestion and composition of the proteins or amino acids ingested. Most athletes habitually ingest sufficient protein; so recommending greater protein intakes does not appear warranted. Current literature suggests that it may be too simplistic to rely on recommendations of a particular commercial formulation, given the metabolic response is dependent on other factors, including the timing of ingestion in relation to exercise and/or other factors, such as the composition of ingested amino acids. Excessive protein intakes are unlikely to be advantageous. Nevertheless, the popularity of protein supplements in the form of powders and shakes continues for AYAs involved in physical training. There remains much to be studied about the optimal protein intake and long-term studies on the impact of different amounts of protein on performance variables, body composition, as well as the metabolic and molecular mechanisms relevant to physical performance.

📶 **ADDITIONAL RESOURCES AND WEBSITES ONLINE**

REFERENCES

1. Bethene ER, Wang C-Y, Wright JD, et al. Dietary intake of selected minerals for the United States population: 1999–2000. In: *Advance data from vital and health statistics of the National Center for Health Statistics (0147–3956)*, Vol. 341. Hyattsville, MD: Centers for Disease Control and Prevention, 2004:1.
2. Kirkpatrick SI, Tarasuk V. Food insecurity is associated with nutrient inadequacies among Canadian adults and adolescents. *J Nutr* 2008;138:604–612.
3. U.S. Department of Agriculture; U.S. Department of Health and Human Services. *Dietary guidelines for Americans*, 7th ed. Washington, DC: US Government Printing Office, 2010.
4. Larson N, MacLehose R, Fulkerson JA, et al. Eating breakfast and dinner together as a family: associations with sociodemographic characteristics and implications for diet quality and weight status. *J Acad Nutr Diet* 2013;113(12):1601–1609.
5. Neumark-Sztainer D, Eisenberg ME, Fulkerson JA, et al. Family meals and disordered eating in adolescents: longitudinal findings from project EAT. *Arch Pediatr Adolesc Med* 2006;65:35–41.
6. Anstine D, Grinenko D. Rapid screening for disordered eating in college aged females in the primary care setting. *J Adolesc Health* 2000;26:338–342.
7. Gleaves DH, Pearson CA, Ambwani S, et al. Measuring eating disorder attitudes and behaviors: a reliability generalization study. *J Eat Disord* 2014;2:6–10.
8. Key TJ, Appleby PN, Rosell MS. Health effects of vegetarian and vegan diets. *Proc Nutr Soc* 2006;65:35–41.
9. Craig WJ, Mangels A; American Dietetic Association. Position of the American Dietetic Association: vegetarian diets. *J Am Diet Assoc* 2009;109(7):1266–1282.
10. Shaukat A, Levitt MD, Taylor BC, et al. Systematic review: effective management strategies for lactose intolerance. *Ann Intern Med* 2010;152(12):797–803.
11. Yin J, Quinn S, Dwyer T, et al. Maternal diet, breastfeeding and adolescent body composition: a 16-year prospective study. *Eur J Clin Nutr* 2012;66(12):1329–1334.
12. Cooper MJ, Cockell KA, L'Abbé MR. The iron status of Canadian adolescents and adults: current knowledge and practical implications. *Can J Diet Pract Res* 2006;67(3):130–138.
13. Domellöf M, Thorsdottir I, Thorstensen K. Health effects of different dietary iron intakes: a systematic literature review for the 5th Nordic Nutrition Recommendations. *Food Nutr Res* 2013;12;57–60.
14. Rodriguez NR, DiMarco NM, Langley S; American Dietetic Association; Dietitians of Canada; American College of Sports Medicine: Nutrition and Athletic Performance. Position of the American Dietetic Association, Dietitians of Canada, and the American College of Sports Medicine: Nutrition and Athletic Performance. *J Am Diet Assoc* 2009;109(3):509–527.
15. Shriver LH, Betts NM, Wollenberg G. Dietary intakes and eating habits of college athletes: are female college athletes following the current sports nutrition standards? *J Am Coll Health* 2013;61(1):10–16.
16. Desbrow B, McCormack J, Burke LM, et al. Sports Dietitians Australia position statement: sports nutrition for the adolescent athlete. *Int J Sport Nutr Exerc Metab* 2014; 24(5):570–584.
17. Hawley JA, Dennis SC, Lindsay FH, et al. Nutritional practices of athletes: are they sub-optimal? *J Sports Sci.* 1995 Summer;13:S75–81.
18. Hoyte CO, Albert D, Heard KJ. The use of energy drinks, dietary supplements, and prescription medications by United States college students to enhance athletic performance. *J Community Health* 2013;38(3):575–580.
19. Buckman JF, Farris SG, Yusko DA. A national study of substance use behaviors among NCAA male athletes who use banned performance enhancing substances. *Drug Alcohol Depend* 2013;131(1/2):50–55.

CHAPTER 7

Complementary and Alternative Medicine in Adolescents and Young Adults

Cora Collette Breuner

Complementary and alternative medicine (CAM) encompasses a wide spectrum of healing resources, modalities, and practices other than those fundamental to the conventional, traditional health system (Fig. 7.1).

CAM therapies may not be provided in some conventional medicine practices due to insufficient knowledge of efficacy, proof of safety, or lack of availability of specific therapies.

Those who choose CAM approaches may be searching for a way to improve their general health, to alleviate symptoms associated with chronic illnesses, or to ameliorate adverse effects of conventional treatments.[1]

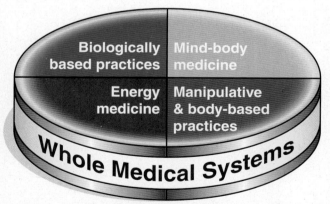

FIGURE 7.1 CAM Domains Whole (or alternative) Medical Systems are similar to the Western, allopathic model in that they are complete systems of theory and practice. They consist of a set of beliefs about the origin of diseases, ways to promote health, and types of treatment. Mind–body medicine uses a variety of techniques designed to enhance the mind's ability to affect bodily function and symptoms. Energy medicine involves the use of energy fields, such as magnetic fields or biofields (energy fields that some believe surround and penetrate the human body). Manipulative and body-based practices work with the structures and systems of the body, including bones and joints, soft tissues, and circulatory and lymphatic systems. Biologically based practices include the use of botanicals (herbs), animal-derived extracts, vitamins, minerals, fatty acids, amino acids, proteins, prebiotics and probiotics, whole diets, and functional foods. (From National Center for Complementary and Alternative Medicine, http://www.nccam.nih.gov.)

Data suggest that 16.4% of 12- to 17-year-olds and 36.3% of 18- to 29-year-olds are using some form of CAM (Fig. 7.2). CAM was more likely to be used by children and adolescents if parents used CAM and if they were between 12 and 17 years of age. For all children 0 to 17 years of age, CAM use was noted more among White children (12.8%) compared to Hispanic (7.9%) and Black youth (5.9%), in those whose parents reported higher education levels (14.7% >high school), in children with six or more health conditions (23.8%), and, importantly, in children whose families delayed conventional care because of cost (16.9%).[2]

CAM therapies most frequently used by adolescents and young adults (AYAs) include herbs, vitamins, supplements, chiropractic, homeopathy, massage, and acupuncture.[3] Medical conditions most frequently treated with CAM include respiratory and gastrointestinal (GI) ailments, musculoskeletal and skin complaints, and chronic conditions such as cystic fibrosis, cancer, autism, and arthritis.[3,4]

IMPORTANT ISSUES FOR THE CLINICIAN

Clinicians should ask AYAs about their use of any form of CAM, especially herbal products and supplements, during the initial visit and every subsequent office visit to learn of all therapies that a patient is taking or using, to screen for drug–herb interaction, and to provide information to the patient about safety and efficacy. A gentle and knowledgeable approach goes far with the AYA patient and can be quite effective to illustrate that "natural" may not mean safe and an endorsement on an Internet site does not guarantee efficacy. Open communication with the clinician leads to a more informed patient and family who is less likely to rely on erroneous and false information obtained from friends, family, or the Internet.[5]

An ethical and legal dilemma may present itself to the clinician when a patient wishes to utilize an alternative treatment where there may be a lack of sufficient evidence to support its use and a paucity of safety data. According to Cohen and Kemper,[6] important questions for AYAs and their families as health care providers who elect to use CAM include the following:

1. Will effective care be utilized when the patient's condition is life-threatening?
2. Will using a CAM treatment deflect from conventional treatment?
3. What is known about the safety and/or efficacy of the treatment?
4. Has the patient consented to the use of CAM?
5. Would this proposed CAM therapy be acceptable to another clinician?
6. Does this treatment have some support in the medical literature?[7,8]

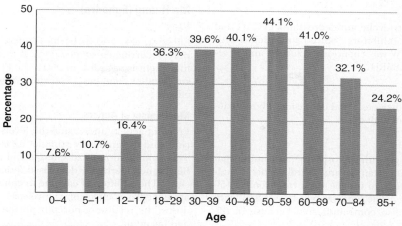

FIGURE 7.2 CAM use by age—2007. Percentage of persons in 2007 who used CAM during the past 12 months, by age. CAM use is greatest among those aged 30 to 69. (From Barnes PM, Bloom B, Nahin R. *Complementary and alternative medicine use among adults and children: United States, 2007*. CDC National Health Statistics Report #12. December 10, 2008. Courtesy of National Center for Complementary and Alternative Medicine, NIH, DHHS.)

HERBAL REMEDIES

Overview and Regulation

Herbal retail sales reached an all-time high of $6.4 billion in 2012; up almost 3% in 2011, a growth of 16% over the past five years.[8] The Dietary Supplement Health and Education Act (DSHEA) of 1994 defines herbal products as supplements because they are not tested according to the same scientific standards as conventional drugs. Packaging or marketing information does not need to be approved by the US Food and Drug Administration (FDA) before a product reaches the market. Supplements cannot be marketed for the diagnosis, treatment, cure, or prevention of disease, despite evidence to the contrary. They can only describe how the "structure and function" of the human body is affected. No protection is offered against misleading or fraudulent claims. The American Academy of Pediatrics Committee on Children with Disabilities has issued guidelines for discussing CAM use, specifically herbal therapies, with families.[9]

Herb–Drug Interactions and Toxicity

Important herb–drug interactions that clinicians should be aware of are outlined and easily accessible (www.standardprocess.com/MediHerb-Document-Library/Catalog-Files/herb-drug-interaction-chart.pdf). Antiplatelet activity and interaction with the cytochrome P450 (CYP) 3A4 enzyme system are two significant adverse effects noted in many herbs, in particular St. John's wort (SJW).[10] Patients suffering trauma who visit an emergency room or who are undergoing surgery should be questioned about use of herbal remedies. They should be counseled on the discontinuation of herbal remedies at least 2 weeks before surgery.[11,12]

A lack of quality control and regulation has resulted in contamination and misidentification of plant species. Herbal preparations may be contaminated with heavy metals or bacteria/fungal organisms while being manufactured or stored.

Dosing Issues and Active Compounds

In conventional medicine, clinicians have become accustomed to using pharmaceutical products standardized with the same strength and high quality; this is not always the case with herbal medicines. Because herbs represent complex entities containing hundreds of constituents, it is difficult to find one particular component representing the active agent. In many cases, particular herbal treatments have been evaluated with a focus on individual extracts and chemical entities such as *Ginkgo biloba* extract 761 (Egb 761).

Patients should be counseled on the use of a clinically studied specific extract in an herbal product. Manufacturers may have their products tested for contamination and standard strength/quality, and the results of these assays are available online with the purchase of a membership (www.consumerlab.com).

The dosage and length of treatment of various herbal remedies are also controversial. With most pharmaceutical agents, as the dosage is increased, there is an increased risk of adverse effects. It is therefore wise to recommend using the lowest dosages of an herbal remedy.

Long-term Use

Most studies involving herbal treatments do not evaluate long-term effects. Herbal remedies should only be used on a limited basis until more data are available regarding long-term safety. AYAs wishing to remain on herbal remedies should be monitored periodically for signs of toxicity and potential adverse effects. Periodic measurements of liver function tests and renal function may be prudent. Ultimately, patients should be advised not to take herbal treatments long-term without the supervision of a clinician.

Use in Pregnancy and Lactation

Women contemplating pregnancy, currently pregnant, or nursing should not use herbal remedies, given the lack of evidence and safety studies.

Common Herbal Remedies

AYAs are likely to use herbal remedies to treat a number of conditions, including obesity, depression and anxiety, sleep disorders, upper respiratory tract infections, and also to improve athletic performance.[13,14] AYAs with eating disorders may use herbal remedies to suppress appetite or induce vomiting.[15]

PSYCHOACTIVE HERBAL REMEDIES

St. John's Wort

Uses

SJW has historically been used for depression.

Mechanism of Action

The two active ingredients are hypericin and hyperforin which inhibit the reuptake of serotonin, norepinephrine, and dopamine as well as neurotransmitters.

Clinical Studies

Studies of SJW compared to tricyclic antidepressants (TCAs) and selective serotonin reuptake inhibitors (SSRIs) in patients with mild depression show that SJW was superior to placebo and as effective as low-dose TCAs and SSRIs.[16]

Adverse Effects

These include GI symptoms, dizziness, and confusion. Phototoxicity may occur with ingestion of high doses.

Drug Interactions

There is a significant interaction with cyclosporine, oral anticoagulants, oral contraceptives, and certain antiretroviral agents including indinavir due to SJW ability to induce the cytochrome P450 (CYP) 3A4 enzyme system.[17,18] The concomitant use of SJW with standard antidepressants is also contraindicated because of the risk of serotonin syndrome.

Valerian Root

Uses

Valerian root is used for insomnia and as a sedative. It is also used for migraine headaches, fatigue, and intestinal cramps.

Mechanism of Action

It is felt that valerian root has effects on γ-aminobutyric acid (GABA) receptors, leading to its effects on insomnia.

Clinical Studies

In a review of 18 randomized controlled trails, valerian was effective subjectively for insomnia, although quantitative or objective measurements did not demonstrate efficacy.[19]

Adverse Effects

These include headache, excitability, uneasiness, and cardiac disturbances.

Drug Interactions

Care should be exercised when combining valerian root with other sedative agents and alcohol.

Chamomile

Uses

Chamomile has been used historically for GI discomfort, peptic ulcer disease, pediatric colic, and mild anxiety.

Mechanism of Action

Chamomile may act via binding to central benzodiazepine receptors.

Clinical Studies

Several small human trials have noted chamomile to have hypnotic-sedative properties. However, none of these trials have been randomized or controlled.

Adverse Effects

Several cases of significant allergic reactions to chamomile have been reported; no significant toxicity has been reported.

Drug Interactions

No drug–herb interactions have been noted.

⬤ HERBS FOR WEIGHT LOSS

Multiple supplements advertised effectively on the Internet are touted for weight loss, lipolysis, and decrease in hunger; yet, none have been shown through standard research methods to be proven efficacious.[20]

Ma Huang (Ephedra)

Uses

Ephedra, also known by its Chinese name Ma Huang, is a naturally occurring substance derived from plants. Its principal active ingredient is ephedra. In 2004, the FDA banned the sale of dietary supplement containing ephedra owing to reported serious adverse effects.

Mechanism of Action

Ephedra acts by increasing the levels of norepinephrine, epinephrine, and dopamine by stimulating α- and β-adrenergic receptors. This combination of adrenergic and dopaminergic effects leads to heightened alertness, decreased fatigue, and a lessened desire for sleep. The addition of caffeine to ephedra appears to blunt the negative feedback effect on the release of norepinephrine. At higher doses, the release of norepinephrine causes anxiety, restlessness, and insomnia.

Clinical Studies

In one randomized, double-blind trial, 90 obese adult subjects received one of the three treatments for 24 weeks: 200 mg caffeine/20 mg ephedrine, leptin A-200 or a combination of the leptin A-200 and caffeine/ephedrine. The caffeine/ephedrine and leptin combination groups lost more weight than the leptin only group.[21]

Adverse Effects

It is well known that Ma Huang has the potential to cause adverse effects that may be serious and have led to a number of reported deaths. Adverse effects include increased blood pressure, palpitations, tachycardia, chest pain, coronary vasospasm, and even cardiomyopathy. The structural similarity of ephedrine to amphetamine raises concern about possible abuse.

Guarana (Paullinia cupana, P. cyrsan, P. sorbilis)

Uses

Guarana is a small climbing maple plant native to Venezuela and northern Brazil known for the high stimulant content of the fruit. Guarana acts as a stimulant and contains the caffeine-like product guaranine along with theobromine theophylline, xanthine, and other xanthine derivatives and acts as a stimulant.[22]

Mechanism of Action

The applicable part of the guarana is the seed. Guarana contains 3.6% to 5.8% caffeine compared with 1% to 2% in coffee.

Clinical Studies

No clinical studies have shown efficacy over placebo.[23]

Adverse Effects

Due to the similarity to caffeine, care should be taken to discuss possible overdose of caffeine as guarana has the same toxicity profile.

Garcinia cambogia/Hydroxycitric Acid

Uses

Garcinia is marketed as an herbal weight loss product.

Mechanism of Action

It is thought that hydroxycitric acid can increase fat oxidation by inhibiting citrate lyase, an enzyme that plays a crucial role in energy metabolism during de novo lipogenesis.

Clinical Studies

In vivo studies support the antiobesity effects via increase in serotonin level regulation while reducing de novo lipogenesis. However, results from clinical studies showed both negative and positive antiobesity effects of *Garcinia*/hydroxycitric acid without definitive positive findings.[24]

Adverse Effects

Higher dosages may lead to abdominal pain and vomiting.

Hoodia gordonii

Uses

H. gordonii is a succulent from the Kalahari Desert in southern Africa. Bushmen from the area have been using *Hoodia* for centuries to diminish hunger during lengthy trips in the desert.

Mechanism of Action

A steroidal glycoside with anorectic activity in animals, termed P57AS3 (P57), has been isolated from *H. gordonii* and may increase the content of adenosine triphosphate (ATP), causing a decrease in hunger.

Clinical Studies

Preliminary data suggest that overweight men who consume P57 have significantly lower calorie intake than those on placebo.[25]

Adverse Effects

None reported.

 HERBAL REMEDIES FOR SPORTS ENHANCEMENT

Ginseng (Panax ginseng)

Uses

Ginseng has been used for more than 2,000 years to strengthen both mental and physical capacity. Recently, ginseng has become popular as an "adaptogenic" (stress-protective) agent.

Mechanism of Action

Ginseng's active component is a saponin called ginsenoside which has immune-modulating effects, antioxidant attributes, and antitumor effects as well as an impact on glucose control via modification of insulin secretion.

Clinical Studies

Many earlier studies examining the pharmacological effects of ginseng on physical performance were not sufficiently robust in design or methodology. Despite attempts in more recent investigations to improve on the scientific rigor used in examining the ergogenic properties of ginseng, many of the same methodological shortcomings observed in past studies persist. Enhanced physical performance after ginseng administration in well-designed investigations remains to be demonstrated.[26]

Adverse Effects

These include nervousness, insomnia, and GI disturbance associated with prolonged use. Ginseng use has led to mastalgia and vaginal bleeding in some female patients due to estrogen-like effects.

Drug Interactions

Ginseng may interact with oral anticoagulants, antiplatelet agents, corticosteroids, and hypoglycemic agents.

 MISCELLANEOUS HERBAL REMEDIES

Echinacea (E. angustifolia, E. pallida, E. purpurea)

Uses

Echinacea has been used for centuries by Native Americans for aches, colds, and as a topical analgesic for snake bites, stings, and burns. It has become extremely popular as a natural immune booster.

Mechanism of Action

It is felt that *Echinacea* works by protecting the integrity of the hyaluronic acid matrix and by stimulating the alternate complement pathway. It also promotes nonspecific T-cell activation by binding to T cells and increasing interferon production. The polysaccharides arabinogalactan and echinacin are the active ingredients of *Echinacea* and are felt to have immune-modulating effects on the body. Other ingredients include glycosides, alkaloids, alkylamides, polyacetylenes, and fatty acids and are believed to inhibit viral replication, improve the motility of polymorphonuclear cells, and enhance phagocytosis.[26]

Clinical Studies

In a recent review, *Echinacea* preparations were found to be better than placebo in the treatment of upper respiratory symptoms.[28] Several studies have noted that *Echinacea* does not prevent upper respiratory infections. Patients with progressive systemic diseases such as multiple sclerosis, tuberculosis, systemic lupus erythematosus, autoimmune diseases, and HIV infection should not use *Echinacea* because of its possible effects on the immune system.

Adverse Effects

These include skin rash, GI upset, and diarrhea.

Drug Interactions

Echinacea should not be used in patients on immunosuppressant medications.

Feverfew

Uses

Feverfew is an often used herbal remedy for prevention and treatment of migraine headaches. Historically, it has also been used for upper respiratory infections, melancholy, and GI distress.

Mechanism of Action

Feverfew may inhibit prostaglandin, thromboxane, and leukotriene synthesis. It also reduces serotonin release from thrombocytes and polymorphonuclear leukocytes. The mechanism of action for preventing migraine headaches is unknown.

Clinical Studies

Randomized trials demonstrated benefit in use of feverfew for prevention of migraine.[29]

Adverse Effects

Adverse effects include occasional mouth ulcerations, contact dermatitis, dizziness, diarrhea, and heartburn.

Drug Interactions

Feverfew may interact with anticoagulants and antiplatelet agents due to its platelet aggregation inhibition.

Butterbur (Petasites hybridus)

Uses

Pain, stomach upset, gastric ulcers, headaches including migraine headaches, chronic cough, chills, anxiety, plague, fever, insomnia, whooping cough, asthma, allergic rhinitis, and for irritable bladder and urinary tract spasms.

Mechanism of Action

The active constituents of butterbur are the sesquiterpene compounds, petasin, and isopetasin. Butterbur is thought to have antispasmodic effects on smooth muscle and vascular walls and may have anti-inflammatory effects by inhibiting leukotriene synthesis.

Clinical Studies

Butterbur has been shown to be helpful as a prophylactic in decreasing migraine frequency in 68.2% of children between 6 and 17 years.[30] Butterbur was reported to be effective in 48% of adults using 75 mg twice daily for 4 months.[31]

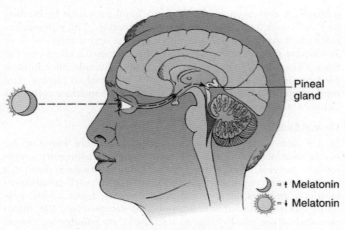

FIGURE 7.3 Melatonin (and subsequently serotonin) levels depend on exposure to sunlight. Melatonin induces sleep during dark hours and is suppressed by daylight. Dark months result in seasonal affective disorder for some people. (From Timby BK Smith NE. *Introductory medical-surgical nursing.* 10th ed. Philadelphia, PA: Lippincott Williams & Wilkins, 2009.)

Adverse Effects

Preparations containing hepatotoxic pyrrolizidine alkaloids are likely unsafe.

Melatonin

Uses

Jet lag, insomnia, shift work disorder, circadian rhythm disorders in the blind, and benzodiazepine and nicotine withdrawal (Fig. 7.3)

Mechanism of Action

In the brain, melatonin is considered a chronic biotic and appears to increase the binding of GABA to its receptors by affecting membrane characteristics, not by increasing the number of receptors

Clinical Studies

Benefits of melatonin for sleep disorders have been reported in AYAs with attention deficit hyperactivity disorder, in cancer patients, and in those with autism.[32] The studies have involved small numbers of subjects with a trial of short-term use of melatonin. No robust data have been reported on safety and efficacy of long-term melatonin use.

Adverse Effects

These include inhibition of ovulation, impair glucose utilization, and a decrease in prothrombin activity. Concomitant use of melatonin with alcohol, benzodiazepines, or other sedative drugs might cause additive sedation.

Horny Goat Weed (*Epimedium*)

Uses

Erectile dysfunction, impotence.

Mechanism of Action

The glycosides in horny goat weed might have hormonal effects although there is no reliable research.

Clinical Studies

None

Adverse Effects

It can interfere with the clotting cascade and can cause death in those with prolong QT syndrome.[33]

ACUPUNCTURE

Overview

Acupuncture is widely used in AYAs and is one of the most frequently recommended CAM therapies.

Theory

Originating in China more than 2,000 years ago, acupuncture is an ancient Chinese therapeutic treatment based on the premise that energy (*Qi*, Chi) flows through the body along channels known as meridians, connected by acupuncture points. The flow of *Qi* is manipulated by insertion of fine needles at acupuncture points along the involved meridians (Fig. 7.4). There is segmental inhibition of pain impulses at the local site of needle stimulation that are carried in the slower unmyelinated C fibers and sensory A delta fibers. Opioid peptides and other neurotransmitters are released, and naloxone has been shown to reverse the analgesic effects of acupuncture.

In assessing AYAs, an acupuncturist takes a history and then performs an examination, which includes the determination of the shape, color and coating of the tongue and the force, flow, and character of the radial pulse. The specific treatment is based on the diagnosis and may include solid sterile needle placement, moxibustion (the practice of burning dried herbs over the acupuncture needles), acupressure, or cupping (where cups are placed on skin

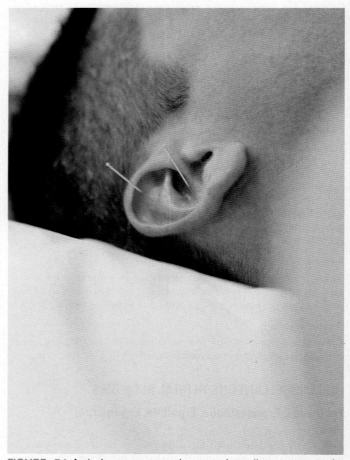

FIGURE 7.4 Auricular acupuncture is a growing adjunct treatment for chemical dependency. Practitioners place small needles under the skin of the outer ear to deliver an electrical impulse to the brain. Resulting relaxation may foster adherence to other substance abuse treatments and manage stress so that clients do not feel the need to engage in drinking or use of drugs. (From Mohr W. *Psychiatric-mental health nursing.* 8th ed. Philadelphia, PA: Lippincott Williams & Wilkins, 2012.)

to create suction, and this is believed to mobilize blood flow in order to promote healing).

Acupuncture may be effective for the following chronic pain conditions: back and neck pain, osteoarthritis, headache, and shoulder pain. In a systematic review to identify randomized controlled trials, acupuncture was superior to both sham and no-acupuncture control for each pain condition.[34] Patients receiving acupuncture had less back and neck pain, osteoarthritis, and chronic headache.

Evidence of Health Benefits[35]

* Dental Pain
* Postoperative nausea and vomiting
* Chemotherapy nausea and vomiting

Possible Health Benefits[35]

* Migraine/tension headaches
* Back pain
* Dysmenorrhea
* Acute and chronic pain
* Substance abuse

Complications

* Pneumothorax, angina, septic sacroiliitis, epidural, and temporomandibular abscess.

YOGA

Yoga is widely known for helping to build strength and flexibility through a combination of meditation, controlled breathing, and stretches. Extensive research has explored yoga's potential value as an adjunct treatment for such health problems as anxiety, hypertension, heart disease, depression, low back pain, headaches, and cancer. More studies are needed to evaluate the efficacy of this intervention.[35–37] Recent studies have shown efficacy among AYAs with eating disorders.[38]

BIOFEEDBACK

Biofeedback makes information about certain biological activities available to the mind. When the mind receives biologic information (pulse, temperature, muscle tension) and the patient uses cognitive reflection to the bodily reaction of stress, the AYA patient can use this information to restore the body to a state of balance, thus relieving the effects of stress. Modalities recorded include electromyograph, skin temperature, galvanic skin response or electrodermal response, respiratory rate, heart rate, heart rate variability, and in some brain centers (neurofeedback). Studies have shown efficacy for migraine and chronic daily headache.[39,40]

MASSAGE

Overview

Consumers in the United States spend over 3 billion dollars annually on massage therapy treatments, with over 135,000 trained massage therapists practicing in the United States. Employment of massage therapists is projected to grow 23% from 2012 to 2022.

Theory

Massage therapy is thought to release muscle tension, remove toxic metabolites, and facilitate oxygen transport to cells and tissues. Of the five forms of massage therapy, the most common is traditional European or Swedish. The focus is to relax the muscles and improve circulation (Fig. 7.5). The second form of massage is the deep muscle or deep tissue technique commonly used in sports. The third form is structural massage and movement integration, also called "bodywork." This technique utilizes deep tissue massage to correct posture problems and movement imbalances.

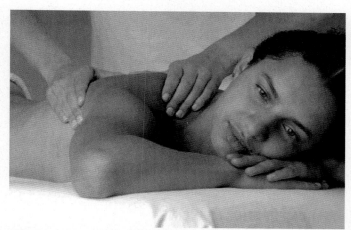

FIGURE 7.5 Wellness massage is massage to decrease stress, promote relaxation, and support the body's natural restorative mechanisms. (Image used with permission from Associated Bodywork & Massage Professionals [ABMP].)

Evidence of Health Benefits[41,42]

* Type I and II diabetes mellitus
* Juvenile rheumatoid arthritis

Possible Health Benefits[42,43]

* Atopic dermatitis
* Cystic fibrosis
* Eating disorders
* Depression
* Asthma

Complications

* None reported.

CHIROPRACTIC

Overview

Doctors of Chiropractic (DCs) are the most frequently visited CAM providers in the United States and treat many conditions, including low back pain, cervical pain, headache, otitis media, dysmenorrhea, and carpal tunnel syndrome.

Theory

Chiropractic, founded by Daniel David Palmer (1845 to 1961), is based on the theory that all disease could be traced to malpositioned bones in the spinal column called "subluxations," which lead to the entrapment of spinal nerves. Subluxations produce symptoms of disease because optimal functioning of tissues and organs are not allowed. Physical adjustment of the spine restores proper alignment of the spine by relieving nerve entrapments.

There are two theories underlying the practice of chiropractic medicine. The International Chiropractic Association focuses on the use of chiropractic adjustments for health promotion. Vertebral subluxations are thought to disrupt spinal nerves, which can result in a variety of problems with function. By correcting the subluxations, the bodies' self-healing powers may lead to optimal health. This organization comprises 5% to 10% of all DCs in the United States and is known for its opposition to mandatory immunizations and advancement of pediatric chiropractic care. The American Chiropractic Association uses a wide range of diagnostic tools, including laboratory tests and advanced imaging (magnetic resonance imaging and computed tomography). They may also recommend nutritional supplements and herbal remedies as treatment options.[45]

Evidence of Health Benefits[46]

- Acute back pain

Possible Health Benefits

- Acute otitis media

Complications

- Strokes, myelopathies, and radiculopathies after cervical manipulation
- Adverse outcomes most likely to occur with bleeding dyscrasia, when improper diagnosis is made, in the presence of a herniated disc or when an improper manipulative method is utilized.[47]

HOMEOPATHIC MEDICINE

Overview

Homeopathy is a medical discipline first promoted in the late 18th century by Dr. Samuel Hahnemann (1755 to 1843). In some European countries, up to 40% of physicians use homeopathy in their practice.

Theory

Three concepts embody the philosophy of homeopathic medicine: (1) finding the similum or similar substance, (2) treating the totality of symptoms, and (3) using the minimum dose through potentization. The "principle of similars," is that highly dilute preparations of substances causing specific symptoms in healthy volunteers are reported to stimulate healing in ill patients who have similar symptoms. For example, the homeopathic remedy *Allium cepa*, which is made from the red onion, could be used to treat the common cold in a person who has symptoms such as sneezing, lacrimation, and a clear nasal discharge.

Homeopathy is one of the most controversial of the CAM therapies. Many health care providers do not believe that infinitesimally diluted substances retain their biological effects, yet others believe that homeopathic remedies do retain their effects.

The preparation of homeopathic remedies requires serial dilution and succussion (shaking). A "30C potency" is a remedy that has been diluted by a factor of 1:100 thirty successive times. There are several theories for the mechanism of action of these highly dilute substances, most importantly the "memory of water" theory: Through the process of serial dilution and succussion, water molecules are altered and can therefore provide relief to the patient.

Results of randomized trials suggest that individualized homeopathy has some effect over placebo, but the evidence is not convincing because of methodological shortcomings and lack of scientific rigor.[48]

Possible Health Benefits

- Recurrent upper respiratory tract infections
- Otitis media
- Attention deficit disorder in which hyperactivity

Complications

- Aggravation of symptoms
- Contamination of remedy
- Delay in treatment

CONCLUSION

There are many CAM therapeutic health care options available to AYAs and their families. Open, honest, and nonjudgmental discussions with adolescents or young adults using or planning to use CAM will bring about a safe and rational use of these treatments for which there is evidence of efficacy and enable AYAs to make informed

TABLE 7.1
Talking with AYAs about CAM

Be open-minded. Most patients are reluctant to share information about their use of CAM therapies because they are concerned their physicians will disapprove. By remaining open-minded, you can learn a lot about your patients' use of unconventional therapies. These strategies will help foster open communication:

Ask the question. Ask every patient every patient about his or her use of alternative therapies during routine history taking. One approach is simply to inquire, "Are you doing anything else for this condition?" It is an open-ended question that gives the patient the opportunity to tell you about his or her use of other health care providers or therapies. Another approach is to ask, "Are you taking any over-the-counter remedies such as vitamins or herbs?"

Avoid using the words "alternative therapy," at least initially. This will help you to avoid appearing judgmental or biased.

Do not dismiss any therapy as a placebo. If a patient tells you about a therapy that you are unaware of, make a note of it in the patient's record and schedule a follow-up visit after you have learned more—when you will be in a better position to negotiate the patient's care. If you determine the therapy might be harmful, you will have to ask the patient to stop using it. If it is not harmful and the patient feels better using it, you may want to consider incorporating the therapy into your care plan.

Discuss providers as well as therapies. Another way to help your patients negotiate the maze of alternative therapies is by stressing that they see appropriately trained and licensed providers. Know who to refer to in your area. Encourage your patients to ask alternative providers about their background and training and the treatment modalities they use. By doing so, your patients will be better equipped to make educated decisions about their health care.

Discuss CAM therapies with your patients at every visit. Charting the details of their use will remind you to raise the issue. It may also help alert you to potential complications before they occur.

Breuner CC. Complementary medicine in pediatrics: a review of acupuncture, homeopathy, massage and chiropractic therapies. *Current Probs Pediatr Adolesc Health Care* 2002;32(10):347–384. Reprinted with permission.

choices.[49] Improved communication can be addressed by following the recommendations outlined in **Table 7.1**. Clinicians should inquire frequently and regularly about CAM use in their AYA patients and also need to communicate with CAM practitioners in their community.

REFERENCES

1. Committee on the Use of Complementary and Alternative Medicine by the American Public; Board on Health Promotion and Disease Prevention; Institute of Medicine of the National Academies. *Complementary and alternative medicine in the United States.* Washington, DC: The National Academies Press, 2005.
2. Barnes PM, Bloom B, Nahin R. Complementary and alternative medicine use among adults and children: United States, 2007. *Natl Health Stat Rep* 2008;12:1–23.
3. Braun CA, Bearinger LH, Halcon LL, et al. Adolescent use of complementary therapies. *J Adolesc Health* 2005;37:76.
4. Adams D, Dagenais S, Clifford T, et al. Complementary and alternative medicine use by pediatric specialty outpatients. *Pediatrics* 2013;131:225–232.
5. Valji R, Adams D, Dagenais S, et al. Complementary and alternative medicine: a survey of its use in pediatric oncology. *Evid Based Complement Alternat Med* 2013;2013:527163. doi: 10.1155/2013/527163.
6. Cohen MH, Kemper KJ. Complementary therapies in pediatrics: a legal perspective. *Pediatrics* 2005;115:774.
7. Cohen MH, Hrbek A, Davis RB, et al. Emerging credentialing practices, malpractice liability policies and guidelines governing complementary and alternative medical practices and dietary supplement recommendations. *Arch Intern Med* 2005;165:289–295.
8. Ekor M. The growing use of herbal medicines: issues relating to adverse reactions and challenges in monitoring safety. *Front Pharmacol* 2013;4:177.
9. American Academy of Pediatrics; Committee on Children with Disabilities. Counseling families who choose complementary and alternative medicine for their child with chronic illness or disability. *Pediatrics* 2001;107:598.
10. Gilmour J, Harrison C, Asadi L, et al. Natural health product-drug interactions: evolving responsibilities to take complementary and alternative medicine into account. *Pediatrics* 2011;128 (suppl 4):S155–S160.
11. Losier A, Taylor B, Fernandez CV. Use of alternative therapies by patients presenting to a pediatric emergency department. *J Emerg Med* 2005;28:267–271.
12. Posadzki P, Watson LK, Ernst E. Adverse effects of herbal medicines: an overview of systematic reviews. *Clin Med* 2013;13:7–12.

13. Sarris J, Panossian A, Schweitzer I, et al. Herbal medicine for depression, anxiety and insomnia: a review of psychopharmacology and clinical evidence. *Eur Neuropsychopharmacol* 2011;21:841–860.

14. Astell KJ, Mathai ML, Su XQ. A review on botanical species and chemical compounds with appetite suppressing properties for body weight control. *Plant Foods Hum Nutr* 2013;68:213–221.

15. Trigazis L, Tennankore D, Vohra S, et al. The use of herbal remedies by adolescents with eating disorders. *Int J Eat Disord* 2004;35:223.

16. Kim HL, Streltzer J, Goebert D. St. John's wort for depression: a meta-analysis of well-defined clinical trials. *J Nerv Ment Dis* 1999;187(9):532–538.

17. Rahimi R, Abdollahi M. An update on the ability of St. John's wort to affect the metabolism of other drugs. *Expert Opin Drug Metab Toxicol* 2012;8:691–708.

18. Mannel M. Drug interactions with St John's wort: mechanisms and clinical implications. *Drug Saf* 2004;27:773–797.

19. Fernández-San-Martín MI, Masa-Font R, Palacios-Soler L, et al. Effectiveness of Valerian on insomnia: a meta-analysis of randomized placebo-controlled trials. *Sleep Med* 2010;11(6):505–511.

20. Vaughan RA, Conn CA, Mermier CM. Effects of commercially available dietary supplements on resting energy expenditure: a brief report. *ISRN Nutr* 2014:650264.

21. Liu AG, Smith SR, Fujioka K, et al. The effect of leptin, caffeine/ephedrine, and their combination upon visceral fat mass and weight loss. *Obesity* 2013;21:1991–1996.

22. Heck CI, de Mejia EG. Yerba Mate Tea (Ilex paraguariensis): a comprehensive review on chemistry, health implications, and technological considerations. *J Food Sci* 2007;72(9):R138–R151.

23. Burke LM, Stear SJ, Lobb A, et al. A–Z of nutritional supplements: dietary supplements, sports nutrition foods and ergogenic aids for health and performance—part 19. *Br J Sports Med* 2011;45:456–458.

24. Astell KJ, Mathai ML, Su XQ. Plant extracts with appetite suppressing properties for body weight control: a systematic review of double blind randomized controlled clinical trials. *Complement Ther Med* 2013;21:407–416.

25. van Heerden FR. Hoodia gordonii: a natural appetite suppressant. *J Ethnopharmacol* 2008;119:434–437.

26. Blankson KL, Thompson AM, Ahrendt DM, Patrick V. Energy drinks: what teenagers (and their doctors) should know. *Pediatr Rev* 2013;34:55–62.

27. Shah SA, Sander S, White CM, et al. Evaluation of echinacea for the prevention and treatment of the common cold: a meta-analysis. *Lancet Infect Dis* 2007;7:473–480.

28. Karsch-Völk M, Barrett B, Kiefer D, et al. Echinacea for preventing and treating the common cold. *Cochrane Database Syst Rev* 2014; 2:CD000530.

29. Pareek A, Suthar M, Rathore GS, et al. Feverfew (*Tanacetum parthenium* L.): a systematic review. *Pharmacogn Rev* 2011;5:103–110.

30. Pothmann R, Danesch U. Migraine prevention in children and adolescents: results of an open study with a special butterbur root extract. *Headache* 2005;45(3):196–203.

31. Lipton RB, Göbel H, Einhäupl KM, et al. Petasites hybridus root (butterbur) is an effective preventive treatment for migraine. *Neurology* 2004;63(12):2240–2244.

32. Sanchez-Barcelo EJ, Mediavilla MD, Reiter RJ. Clinical uses of melatonin in pediatrics. *Int J Pediatr* 2011;2011:892624. doi:10.1155/2011/892624.

33. Phillips M, Sullivan B, Snyder B, et al. Effect of enzyte on QT and QTc intervals. *Arch Intern Med* 2010;170:1402–1404.

34. Linde K, Streng A, Jurgens S, et al. Acupuncture for patients with migraine. *JAMA* 2005;293:2118–2125.

35. Telles S, Joshi M, Dash M, et al. An evaluation of the ability to voluntarily reduce the heart rate after a month of yoga practice. *Integr Physiol Behav Sci* 2004; 39:119–125.

36. Evans S, Moieni M, Sternlieb B, et al. Yoga for youth in pain: the UCLA pediatric pain program model. *Holist Nurs Pract* 2012;26:262–271.

37. Carei TR, Fyfe-Johnson AL, Breuner CC, et al. Randomized controlled clinical trial of yoga in the treatment of eating disorders. *J Adolesc Health* 2010;46:346–351.

38. Perrin JM, Coury DL, Hyman SL, et al. Complementary and alternative medicine use in a large pediatric autism sample. *Pediatrics* 2012;130:S77–S82.

39. Nestoriuc Y, Martin A. Efficacy of biofeedback for migraine: a meta-analysis. *Pain* 2007;128:111–127.

40. Blume HK, Brockman LN, Breuner CC. Biofeedback therapy for pediatric headache: factors associated with response. *Headache* 2012;52:1377–1386.

41. Seburg EM, Horvath KJ, Garwick AW, et al. Complementary and alternative medicine use among youth with juvenile arthritis: are youth using CAM, but not talking about it. *J Adolesc Health* 2012;51(2):200–202.

42. McCarty RL, Weber WJ, Loots B, et al. Complementary and alternative medicine use and quality of life in pediatric diabetes. *J Altern Complement Med* 2010;16(2): 165–173.

43. Beider S, Mahrer NE, Gold JI. Pediatric massage therapy: an overview for clinicians. *Pediatr Clin North Am* 2007;54:1025–1041.

44. Beider S, Moyer CA. Randomized controlled trials of pediatric massage: a review. *Evid Based Complement Alternat Med* 2007;4:23–34.

45. Alcantara J, Ohm J, Kunz D. The safety and effectiveness of pediatric chiropractic: a survey of chiropractors and parents in a practice-based research network. *Explore* 2009;5:290–295.

46. Hawk C, Schneider M, Ferrance RJ, et al. Best practices recommendations for chiropractic care of infants children and adolescents: results of a consensus process. *J Manipulative Physiol Ther* 2009;32:639–647.

47. Vohra S, Johnston BC, Cramer K, et al. Adverse events associated with pediatric spinal manipulation: a systematic review. *Pediatrics* 2007;119:e275–e283.

48. Linde K, Scholz M, Ramirez G, et al. Impact of study quality on outcome in placebo-controlled trials of homeopathy. *Clin Epidemiol* 1999;52:631–636.

49. Canadian Pediatric Society. Children and natural health products: what every clinician should know. *Paediatr Child Health* 2005;10:227–232.

50. Gilmour J, Harrison C, Asadi L, et al. Informed consent: advising patients and parents about complementary and alternative medicine therapies. *Pediatrics* 2011;128 (suppl 4):S187–S192.

ADDITIONAL RESOURCES AND WEBSITES ONLINE

CHAPTER 8

Chronic Health Conditions in Adolescents and Young Adults

Susan M. Sawyer

KEY WORDS

- Adherence
- Adolescent development
- Adolescent-friendly health care
- Brain maturation
- Chronic health conditions
- Chronic illness
- Contraception
- Fertility
- Parents
- Puberty
- Sexual and reproductive health
- Special health care needs
- Transition to adult health care

Adolescents with chronic health conditions face the same challenges as their healthy peers in their transition to adulthood in terms of individuation and autonomy, relationships with family and peers, education and employment, and sexuality. Yet, the challenges they experience are commonly amplified by the complexity of their health condition in the context of the demands, expectations, and social roles that they assume as they mature. A major difference to their healthy peers is the extent to which adolescents and young adults (AYAs) with chronic health conditions need to engage more independently with the health care system as they mature, while continuing to rely on their families for support. Specific health conditions bring particular challenges, but the basis of this chapter is that AYAs face common issues as a result of the experiences they face growing up with a chronic health condition, which benefit from common responses from families and health care systems, as well as from education and other supportive systems (e.g., schools, employers, health insurance).

HOW ARE CHRONIC HEALTH CONDITIONS DEFINED?

In addition to diagnostic (e.g., asthma, diabetes) and functional definitions (e.g., intellectual disability), common features of the many different definitions of a chronic health condition include the following:

- The condition may have a complex etiology.
- There can be a lengthy period in which symptoms fluctuate in severity and functional impact.
- There is a prolonged course of illness in which other conditions or comorbidities may arise.
- There is associated impairment or disability.

As opposed to permanency, most chronic conditions are defined by a prolonged or episodic course and an impact that can change with growth and development. For example, cerebral palsy is the result of a static developmental insult, yet the requirement for orthopedic surgery in adolescence results from dynamic growth. Physical health conditions, behavioral and emotional disorders including neurodevelopmental conditions (e.g., attention deficit hyperactivity disorder [ADHD]), and related disorders (e.g., substance abuse) are all considered chronic health conditions, based on the presence of associated impairments or disability. In this regard, disability is viewed as an overarching term for impairments at the level of the body, the person, and the person in social situations, which result in limitation of activities or restrictions to full participation in age-appropriate activities.[1]

In contrast to a definition based on the presence of impairments or disabilities, the term "Children with Special Health Care Needs" refers to children with one or more chronic physical, emotional, developmental, and behavioral conditions who also require health and related services of a type or amount beyond that required by children generally.[2] This definition is equally inclusive of a wide variety of conditions, and is as relevant for AYAs as it is for children.

HOW PREVALENT ARE CHRONIC HEALTH CONDITIONS?

Over the past few decades, technical advances have resulted in dramatic improvements in the survival of children with conditions that were largely considered fatal in childhood, such as congenital heart disease, cystic fibrosis, and spina bifida. The majority of adolescents with such conditions now expect to survive into adulthood.[3]

Disease-specific surveys are able to describe the incidence and prevalence of conditions, and how this has changed over time. There is a real increase in the *incidence* of certain conditions, such as type 1 diabetes, allergies and anaphylaxis, and chronic inflammatory bowel disease. Other surveys demonstrate increasing prevalence in certain conditions over time, such as overweight and obesity with a resultant increase in hypercholesterolemia, hypertension, metabolic syndrome, and type 2 diabetes, especially in young adults. In many parts of the world, treatment of human immunodeficiency virus (HIV) infection has resulted in HIV/acquired immunodeficiency syndrome now being largely considered to be a chronic health condition.

The extent of emotional disorders in AYAs is increasingly appreciated, as is the effect of puberty on risk of onset.[4] One in four young people have experienced a mental health disorder over the past year.[5] The most common conditions are mood and anxiety disorders (e.g., depression), behavioural and neurodevelopmental disorders (e.g., ADHD, conduct disorder) and substance use disorders. Comorbidity between different mental health disorders is apparent in adolescence and young adulthood, as is the co-occurrence of chronic physical conditions with mental health conditions.[5]

However, even for the same condition, the use of different definitions of a condition within different surveys nationally and internationally can yield inconsistent estimates. The difficulty in obtaining a picture of the incidence and prevalence of chronic health conditions in adolescence and young adulthood is further compounded by poor assessment across adolescence and young adulthood. Many surveys span childhood and adolescence; however, data for adolescents are inconsistent due to the use of different age-cuts (e.g., 10 to 14 years, 15 to 19 years versus 11 to 13 years, 14 to 15 years, 16 to 17 years). Other surveys do not report adolescent data separately (e.g., 0 to 17 years). The prevalence of different chronic health conditions in young adulthood is not well appreciated as many age-cuts fail to bring visibility to this age group (e.g., 14 to 65 years, 18 to 40 years, 18 to 65 years).

Much advocacy around AYAs with chronic health conditions has successfully influenced policy by focusing on a specific condition or group of similar conditions (e.g., mental health conditions, cancers). In this regard, disease-specific surveys can be very valuable in measuring the changing incidence or prevalence of a particular condition, the presence and type of unmet health care needs, access (or lack of access) to health insurance, and particular educational or employment challenges. In addition to disease-specific advocacy, other policies are best advanced by understanding the issues affecting chronic health conditions in AYAs as a group. For example, the relative proportion of time that specialist medical training programs dedicate to AYA health would be better supported by surveys that describe the broad prevalence of chronic health conditions, rather than by individual conditions. Similarly, knowledge of the extent of comorbid physical and mental health conditions has the potential to alter models of health care delivery to AYAs. In this regard, the 2009 to 2010 National Survey of Children with Special Health Care Needs in the United States found that 18.4% of 12- to 17-year-olds had special health care needs in comparison to 9.3% of 0- to 5-year-old children.[6] That is, the prevalence of special health care needs increases with age across adolescence, and increases further again into young adulthood. Of these children, 66% had health conditions that consistently or moderately affected their daily activities, while 16% had missed 11 or more days of school in the past year. Such information can also help support more generic interventions, such as the concept of a "medical home" that is built on the notion of quality health care, continuity of care, and patient- and family-centered care together with expectations of comprehensive and accessible services.[7]

INTERACTION OF ADOLESCENT DEVELOPMENT AND CHRONIC HEALTH CONDITIONS

The two defining aspects of biological development in adolescence, namely puberty and neurocognitive maturation, can have even more profound implications for adolescents with chronic health conditions than their healthy peers. The interaction of chronic health conditions with adolescent development is complex and bidirectional; the health condition may affect development and/or development may affect the condition. For example, some chronic health conditions, such as chronic renal failure and anorexia nervosa, can cause pubertal delay, changing the timing and trajectory of peak height velocity. When extreme, these changes can result in stunting of adult height. For other conditions such as asthma, the onset of puberty can reduce the severity of the disease, while the reverse is more typical in diabetes mellitus, with onset of puberty a risk for poor metabolic control. Regular monitoring of growth and puberty is an important component of health care for all adolescents with chronic health conditions.

During adolescence, the fundamental cognitive and problem-solving skills acquired in earlier childhood undergo further development.[8] Cognitive maturation results in greater capacity for insights around the significance of life-limiting conditions, such as cystic fibrosis, which may contribute to anxiety and depression. A growing capacity to maintain attention, greater working memory, and inhibitory control of emotions promote the development of more goal-directed activities, which bring greater capacity for

self-management of chronic health conditions. Importantly, future planning skills continue to develop well into the mid-20s, with particular implications for adherence to treatment. Social cognition, or the ability to make sense of the world through the processing of signals from others, accelerates from puberty and is central to interpersonal functioning, mental health and well-being, educational attainment, and future employment.[9] The effects of deficits in such cognitive skills, that can occur in a range of neurodevelopmental and mental health conditions, are commonly amplified in late childhood and adolescence. Regardless of the cause (e.g., mobility limitations, parental overprotectiveness), fewer opportunities for peer engagement will reduce opportunities for social and emotional learning, social confidence, and self-esteem.

THE SOCIAL CONTEXT OF HEALTH-RELATED BEHAVIORS AND STATES

The social determinants of health influence health outcomes in AYAs with chronic health conditions.[10] Structural determinants such as national economic wealth will influence the availability of health insurance, education, and employment, which are all relevant for young people with chronic health conditions and their future health and life opportunities. More proximal determinants, also known as risk and protective factors, operate within the individual and their family, peers, school, and community. A chronic health condition is a risk factor within the individual domain that, when compounded by risks within other domains (e.g., family dysfunction, bullying, unsupportive schooling, high rates of youth unemployment), can influence adolescents' and young adults' engagement in health-related behaviors (e.g., tobacco use) and states (e.g., depression). For example, bullying increases the likelihood of a number of health-related behaviors and states, including substance misuse, unsafe sex, depression, antisocial and illegal activities, and dangerous driving.[11]

Given the importance of academic success for future employment, promoting school engagement by minimizing school absenteeism from illness and medical appointments is important. However, beyond academic achievement, schools are important social environments for adolescents with chronic health conditions that promote peer connections, emotional control, and well-being. Peer support groups, whether face-to-face or online, can be helpful in normalizing the differences young people with chronic health conditions can experience,[12] which may consequently promote well-being and continued engagement with schooling.

Many studies have explored the question of whether adolescents with chronic health conditions have a higher rate of mental health disorders. Most robust studies suggest that this group has an elevated risk[13] that is largely mediated by the same factors as in healthy young people such as family connectedness.[14] Youth with certain conditions, such as physical and intellectual disabilities, appear to be at even higher risk.

Many health professionals might assume that AYAs with chronic health conditions, especially when severe, would be less likely than their healthy peers to engage in health-related behaviors such as unsafe sex, or unsafe alcohol or drug use. However, there is little evidence to support this notion. Instead, studies suggest that young people with chronic health conditions are as likely, if not more likely, to engage in health-related behaviors.[15] The explanation for potentially higher rates is unclear. At least some of the increased risk is mediated through depression. Part of the explanation may reflect biological differences in cognitive processing that result in a different appreciation of the risk associated with particular behaviors (e.g., ADHD). However, a more simple explanation may be the greater challenge to feel "normal" experienced by many AYAs with chronic health conditions, which may render them more sensitive to perceived peer norms in order to fit in socially.

What is apparent is that the risks of certain health-related behaviors are greater for AYAs with particular chronic health condition.[3] For example, while smoking is unhealthy for all young people, it is even more damaging for AYAs with diabetes, due to its effect on microvascular and macrovascular disease. It is similarly more risky for young people with chronic lung or cardiac conditions. In the same way, while heavy alcohol use is unsafe for all, alcohol can lower the seizure threshold for young people with epilepsy, and make blood glucose control more challenging in those with diabetes.

AYA-FRIENDLY HEALTH CARE

Within many children's services, most support services and physical facilities remain oriented to young children as they constitute the age group that has historically been the major user of such facilities. Yet, around the world, as the upper age of specialist pediatrics increases and the proportion of adolescents managed by pediatricians and specialist children's services grows, services and facilities need to become better aligned to adolescents with chronic health conditions, because young people require different approaches from their health care providers and health services than those oriented to younger children.[16]

Young adults also require different approaches from adult services, which typically assume that the patient is responsible for managing their health care without the extent of reliance on family that typifies many young adults with chronic health conditions, even if they no longer live at home.[17] For different reasons, the notion of patient- and family-centered care is equally relevant in both settings, with its emphasis on respect, care coordination, appropriate provision of information, high-quality communication, patient involvement in decisions about care, and the ability of health care providers to listen to patient needs.[18]

The World Health Organization describes adolescent-friendly health care as an approach to better orienting health services to the needs of young people.[19] Also referred to as youth-friendly health care, this approach emerged out of concerns about the lack of developmentally appropriate primary health care for adolescents in low- and middle-income countries. The approach is equally relevant to adolescents in high-income countries, to specialist services as much as primary care and to young adults as much as adolescents.

A recently developed conceptual framework for adolescent-friendly health care in hospital settings has salience in providing quality health care to AYAs with chronic health conditions, in specialist settings and primary care.[16] As outlined in Figure 8.1, the provision of adolescent-friendly health care (a term used to refer to quality health care for adolescents) is embedded in the notion of patient- and family-centered care, and implemented through a strong focus on providing a positive experience of care for the young person and evidence-based care to treat the underlying condition. Both depend on the other; that is, evidence-informed care or guideline-based care will not be as effectively implemented unless young people and their parents (and carers) are actively engaged in their health care and have a positive experience of care with the health care provider and the health service. Engagement with care reflects both the quality of young people's experiences with individual staff as well as their wider experiences of the health service. This might include how welcome young people feel in attending a clinic or hospital, the age appropriateness of the physical spaces (e.g., waiting areas) and services it provides (e.g., educational supports), and the extent to which young people feel sufficiently involved in decisions about their health care. A critical element for adolescents with chronic health conditions is that active engagement by patients and families is required to set expectations around self-management practices (e.g., adherence with treatment), as well as future engagement with health services (e.g., transition to adult health care) (Fig. 8.1).

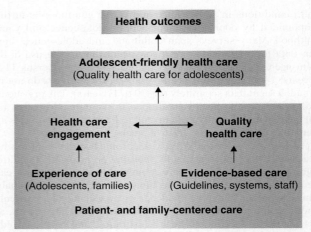

FIGURE 8.1 Conceptual framework of adolescent-friendly health care. (Reproduced with permission from Sawyer SM, Ambresin AE, Bennett KE, et al. A measurement framework for quality healthcare for adolescents in hospitals. *J Adolesc Health* 2014;55(4):484–490.)

PUTTING ADOLESCENT- AND YOUNG ADULT—FRIENDLY HEALTH CARE INTO PRACTICE

There are myriad elements for health care professionals to keep in mind in providing developmentally appropriate health care to AYAs with chronic health conditions, as portrayed in Figure 8.2. Putting this into practice can be simplified when the clinician *attends to the young person* with the health condition by applying the principles of AYA medicine, *works with the young person and their family* to promote the young person's growing capacity for self-management as they mature, and *understands health care delivery in the context of the health care system* in which they practice (Fig. 8.2).

One of the key differences in working with young people with chronic health conditions (as compared to managing more acute health care issues in AYAs) is that health care professionals need to explicitly attend to the AYA patient as well as to their parents or carers. Parents generally provide a high level of support to AYAs with chronic health conditions.[17] In the best of scenarios, parents can set appropriately high expectations for their children with chronic health conditions, and balance the care they provide while fostering their child's developing autonomy and independence. Supporting young people's emerging capacities is a critical role for parents of AYAs with chronic health conditions. Parents are particularly important in helping AYAs negotiate the health care system by accompanying their children to appointments, supervising treatments at home, supporting the actual transfer to adult health care, negotiating the complexity of health insurance and clarifying what questions to explore with health care providers.[17,20] At times, however, parents may inadvertently foster dependency, reduce opportunities for social learning, and undermine young people's social confidence and resilience. This can include unintentionally undermining the potential learning to be gained within the health consultation itself.[21]

Parents of AYAs, especially those with chronic conditions diagnosed during early childhood, often develop very close and trusting relationships with their child's health care professionals. During adolescence, it is especially important that health care visits include time during which the health care provider meets with the adolescent alone. There is no single "right" way to do this; some providers consult briefly with the adolescent and parent together, then spend the bulk of the consultation with the adolescent alone, and bring the parent back into the consultation to sum up. In this context, it is critical that the notion of confidentiality is carefully reviewed with both the adolescent and the parent.[21,22] This

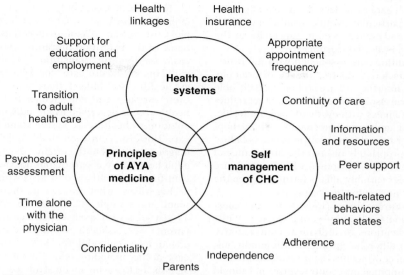

FIGURE 8.2 A Venn diagram that outlines the three major components for health care professionals to attend to in providing adolescent-friendly health care for AYAs with chronic health conditions (CHC). Developmentally appropriate care is provided by applying the principles of AYA medicine, working with the young person and their family to promote the young person's capacity for self-management, in the context of the health care system in which they practice (Modified from Kennedy A, Sawyer S. Transition from pediatric to adult services: are we getting it right? *Curr Opin Pediatr* 2008;20:403–409).

approach provides an opportunity for the health care provider to actively engage with the adolescent themselves (rather than the parent), to respectfully educate the adolescent about their condition and its treatment (rather than assume they know as much as their parents), and to set expectations about their engagement in self-management, including adherence behaviors. Typically, as time goes on, the proportion of the consultation spent with the young person increases.

The following section briefly highlights three specific issues to consider when managing AYAs with chronic health conditions: adherence with treatment; sexual and reproductive health care; and transition to adult health care.

Adherence with Treatment

The majority of AYAs with chronic health conditions struggle to adhere to their treatment regimen. Adherence with medication is problematic at all ages, with only about 50% of patients adhering to treatment recommendations.[23] The responsibility lies with health care providers to routinely address adherence to any aspect of recommended treatment. The challenge for health professionals (and parents) is that, compared to adults, AYAs have not yet developed the same extent of goal-directed behavior, remain less influenced by longer-term fears of health complications, need greater assistance to develop treatment routines, and are more price-sensitive if they have to pay for treatment.[24]

There is no "right" age by which adolescents can be expected to no longer rely on their parents to support adherence-promoting behaviors. Indeed, parents continue to play a critical role for many years in supporting some children with their medical treatments. The young adult years can be especially challenging in relation to poor adherence; parents are typically less influential at this time but young people's capacity to adhere does not magically improve on their 18th birthday. Rather, it continues to evolve across their 20s.

Given this, one responsibility for health care professionals is, as much as possible, to choose simple treatment regimens (e.g., twice rather than three times daily). Attending to adherence behaviors at every consultation is another important role for health professionals. In the first instance, establishing a ball-park understanding

of what is actually being adhered to—or not—is the goal. Consider the following principles:

- As adherence can differ for each medication or treatment, questions about adherence must be treatment specific.
- Make it easier for AYAs to be honest about poor adherence by asking questions that assume that adherence is poor rather than good. Empathize about the challenge of adherence.
- Respectfully use parents to confirm or challenge young people's feedback about their adherence behaviors.
- Congratulate positive adherence behaviors (and intentions) and seek clarification of why adherence is good for a particular medication/treatment at this time.
- Identify barriers to adherence behaviors, including social barriers (e.g., having to take medication at school).
- Be clear about the rationale for why every medication or treatment is prescribed.
- Be prepared to negotiate around alternative approaches, especially if the effect of a drug holiday can be tested with an objective measure of health.
- Engage with the adolescent or young adult about what they think might work for them (e.g., more or less support from parents, telephone alarms as reminders, adherence apps).
- Consider the contribution of poor mental health (e.g., depression) to poor adherence.
- When all else fails, be prepared to tolerate less than ideal adherence, but continue to have expectations for change with maturation.

Sexual and Reproductive Health Care

Adolescents with chronic health conditions, including disabilities, become sexually active at a similar age to their healthy peers.[25,26] For this group, the health risks of sexual activity may be exacerbated by the illness itself, the medications used to treat it, or by a maladaptive emotional response to illness. Many AYAs with chronic illness and disability have concerns about their sexual attractiveness, the normalcy of their reproductive system and sexual response, fertility, safety of contraception use, and genetic aspects of their disease. In this context, it is concerning how little information

AYAs receive from their health care providers about sexuality education that is specific to their particular chronic health condition.[27] The extent of sexual abuse and sexual assault, especially in the context of cognitive disability, is also concerning.[25]

Some chronic health conditions are associated with infertility, either related to the disease itself or to its treatment. For example, males with cystic fibrosis are infertile, yet are still biologically able to father children using sperm aspiration and assisted reproductive techniques. In contrast, females with cystic fibrosis are fertile, and experience high rates of unplanned pregnancy. While there may be many explanations for this, the most obvious one is failure by health care services to appropriately discuss the importance of contraception for sexually active young women who do not desire pregnancy. Treatment of cancer variably affects fertility, hence the importance of timely fertility preserving interventions.

Long-acting reversible contraceptives (LARC) are the most effective form of contraception for healthy young women. While there are multiple contraindications to individual contraceptive agents for young people with different chronic health conditions, LARC are safer than hormonal contraceptives for many health conditions.[28] For example, the combined oral contraceptive pill should be avoided in conditions having a greater risk of thrombosis, in the context of severe liver disease, or in the presence of indwelling intravenous access. Discussions about fertility, contraception, and pregnancy risks for the mother and fetus (e.g., teratogenicity of medication) are important to have throughout adolescence into adulthood with young people as well as their parents, when appropriate.

Given the risks of immunosuppression in AYAs with various conditions (e.g., transplantation), immunization with the human papillomavirus vaccine is an important element of preventive care for adolescent boys as well as girls.[27]

Transition to Adult Health Care

Transition to adult health care refers to the planned movement of AYAs with chronic health conditions from child-oriented to adult-oriented health services.[29] As such, transition is a *process* that is initiated by child health services and continues well after the actual *event* of transfer to the adult service.

Historically, the notion of transition to adult health care related to specialist services.[20] In the 1970s, 80s, and even the 90s, there were few adult specialist services interested in accepting the "survivors" of chronic illness in childhood and little planning by pediatric health services in developing closer linkages between pediatric and adult services. At that time, neither specialist pediatric nor adult services had much understanding of AYA development, and young people and their parents were poorly prepared to transfer to adult health care. In this context, it is not surprising that once adolescents transferred to adult services, negative experiences led to poor engagement with adult services and high rates of service "drop out" within the first year or so after transfer, sometimes with dire consequences for health outcomes.

Increasing attention is now paid to the needs of AYAs to better prepare them and their families prior to transfer, and to better support their engagement in adult health care once they have transferred to adult services. In addition, transition to adult health care is now appreciated to be as relevant for primary care as it is for specialist services. For those who transfer from specialist pediatric to adult services, primary care can function to support the continuity of care across the transition years, and be particularly valuable should lack of engagement with adult services occur. A greater role for primary care is in supporting the large cohort of young people whose care is coordinated by primary care rather than specialist pediatric services, but for whom a change in orientation to more independently focused care is still required. At this time, many older AYAs move away from home for education or employment, which will commonly necessitate a shift in the primary care provider as well as specialist services.

The critical aspect of transition to adult health care is that it is embedded in the knowledge that health care functions as a complex system that AYAs must negotiate to make it work for them.[20] Some of the transition literature, especially from subspecialist areas, uses the term "transition to adult health care" synonymously with "quality health care" for AYAs or "developmentally appropriate health care." Indeed, there is much blurring in the literature of these various terms and themes. In Figure 8.2, transition to adult health care is described as an individual element of particular orientation to health care systems and the principles of AYA health care. However, transition could equally sit at the very center of the diagram (as it did in the original diagram). Supporting transition to adult health care is part of, but not the totality of, providing adolescent-friendly health care to AYAs with chronic health conditions.

Regardless what we call it, there is still room for improvement. For example, in the 2009 to 2010 survey of parents of 12- to 17-year-olds with special health care needs in the United States,[30] parents were asked how often their child's health care providers encouraged their children to take responsibility for their health care needs, including taking medication, understanding their diagnosis, or following medical advice. While the majority were positive, 22% reported that this did not usually occur. More concerning was that only 40% of 12- to 17-year-olds met the standard to make an effective transition to adult health care. This was based on parents reporting that their children received anticipatory guidance on a number of key areas and that their providers usually or always encouraged them to take responsibility for their health. It was especially concerning that adolescents whose conditions more severely affected their daily activities were half as likely to achieve this objective as those whose conditions never affect their daily activities (26% versus 52%). Children living in poverty were also half as likely as those in the highest-income bracket to receive transition services (25% versus 52%).

The following points summarize some of the key elements of transition planning:

- Early planning helps prepare patients, families, and health care teams.
- Transition planning is an individualized, collaborative process between the adolescent and their family, and the various health care services including the primary health care provider.
- Tailored, written transition plans can help foster progressive development of disease-related knowledge and self-management skills. Transition plans can be used to set goals for adolescents and allow for regular review of progress by health care providers.
- While the timing of transfer to adult care might ideally be informed by patient readiness rather than age, in reality, all planning around transfer to adult health care is done in the context of the age limitations and policies of specialist health services that are typically based on age.
- Transfer to adult health care should be coordinated by both transferring and receiving physicians.
- Structured transition programs that allow young adults to meet with new providers before transfer increase clinic attendance within the adult health care system and increase patient satisfaction.
- It is better to transfer health care at a time of disease stability than in a crisis or period of instability.
- Transition coordinators act as liaisons between pediatric and adult health care systems. They can promote continuity of care during the transition process by supporting patients and their families to navigate complex health care systems.

Within child-oriented services, many complex health conditions are managed by multidisciplinary teams. Such teams often have a strong focus on internal communication between team members, which can support the delivery of coordinated, accessible care. Such teams have historically been less common within adult health care services. In their absence, many adolescents and their families, supported by their primary care provider, end up developing their individual "team." While such teams can be equally effective in the longer term, they risk being associated with delayed access to health care in the short term.

Some groups of patients continue to struggle to identify appropriate adult specialist services that provided the same intensity of support as offered through specialist pediatric services.[20] This is particularly the case for patients with developmental disorders such as intellectual disability, autism, and ADHD. Those with mental disorders can also struggle to identify and engage in appropriate services, especially in terms of ongoing care, rather than simply assessment. Identifying an appropriate adult specialist provider can also be difficult for those disorders that sit at the interface of specialist medical and mental health care within pediatric services, such as eating disorders. All too often, in the absence of specialist adult providers, the responsibility for care then lies with primary care providers.

REFERENCES

1. World Health Organization. *International classification of functioning, disability and health.* Geneva, Switzerland: World Health Organization, 2001.
2. McPherson M, Arango P, Fox H, et al. A new definition of children with special health care needs. *Pediatrics* 1998;102:137–140.
3. Sawyer SM, Drew S, Yeo MS, et al. Adolescents with a chronic condition: challenges living, challenges treating. *Lancet* 2007;369(9571):1481–1489.
4. Patton GC, Viner R. Pubertal transitions in health. *Lancet* 2007;369(9567):1130–1139.
5. Costello E, Mustillo S, Keeler G, et al. Prevalence of psychiatric disorders in childhood and adolescence. In: Levin B, Petrila J, Hennessy K, eds. *Mental health services: a public health perspective.* Oxford, UK: Oxford University Press, 2004:111–128.
6. http://www.childhealthdata.org/. Accessed on August 27, 2014.
7. http://www.pcmh.ahrq.gov/page/defining-pcmh. Accessed on August 27, 2014.
8. Blakemore SJ, Choudhury S. Development of the adolescent brain: implications for executive function and social cognition. *J Child Psychol Psychiatry* 2006;47(3/4):296–312.
9. Goddings AL, Burnett Heyes S, Bird G, et al. The relationship between puberty and social emotion processing. *Dev Sci* 2012;15(6):801–811.
10. Viner RM, Ozer EM, Denny S, et al. Adolescence and the social determinants of health. *Lancet* 2012;379(9826):1641–1652.
11. Sawyer SM, Afifi RA, Bearinger LH, et al. Adolescence: a foundation for future health. *Lancet* 2012;379(9826):1630–1640.
12. Olsson CA, Boyce M, Toumbourou JW, et al. Chronic illness in adolescents: the role of peer support groups. *Clin Child Psychol Psychiatry* 2005;10:78–87.
13. Cohen P, Pine DS, Must A, et al. Prospective associations between somatic illness and mental illness from childhood to adulthood. *Am J Epidemiol* 1998;147:232–239.
14. Wolman C, Resnick MD, Harris LJ, et al. Emotional well-being among adolescents with and without chronic conditions. *J Adolesc Health* 1994;15:199–204.
15. Suris JC, Michaud PA, Akre C, et al. Health risk behaviours in adolescents with chronic conditions. *Pediatrics* 2008;122:e1113–e1118.
16. Sawyer SM, Ambresin AE, Bennett KE, et al. A measurement framework for quality healthcare for adolescents in hospitals. *J Adolesc Health* 2014;55(4):484–490.
17. Beresford B, Stuttard L. Young adults as users of adult healthcare: experiences of young adult with complex or life-limiting conditions. *Clin Med* 2014;14(4):404–408.
18. Picker Institute. *Principles of patient-centred care.* Available at http://pickerinstitute.org/about/picker-principles/. Accessed on April 22, 2015.
19. World Health Organisation. *Adolescent friendly health services: an agenda for change.* Geneva, Switzerland: World Health Organisation, 2002.
20. Kennedy A, Sawyer S. Transition from pediatric to adult services: are we getting it right? *Curr Opin Pediatr* 2008;20:403–409.
21. Duncan RE, Jekel M, O'Connell M, et al. Balancing parental involvement with adolescent friendly health care in teenagers with diabetes: are we getting it right? *J Adolesc Health* 2014;55(1):59–64.
22. Ford C, English A, Sigman G. Confidential health care for adolescents: position paper of the Society for Adolescent Medicine. *J Adolesc Health* 2004;35(2):160–167.
23. World Health Organization. *Adherence to long-term therapies: evidence for action.* Geneva, Switzerland: World Health Organization, 2003. Available at http://www.who.int/chp/knowledge/publications/adherence_full_report.pdf. Accessed on April 22, 2015.
24. Sawyer SM, Aroni R. The sticky issue of adherence. *J Pediatr Child Health* 2003;39:2–5.
25. Cheng MM, Udry JR. Sexual behaviours of physically disabled adolescents in the United States. *J Adolesc Health* 2002;31:48–58.
26. Suris JC, Resnick MD, Cassuto N, et al. Sexual behavior of adolescents with chronic disease and disability. *J Adolesc Health* 1996;19(2):124–131.
27. Frayman K, Sawyer SM. Sexual and reproductive health in cystic fibrosis: a life-course perspective. *Lancet Respir Med* 2015;3(1):70–86.
28. World Health Organisation. *Medical eligibility criteria wheel for contraceptive use. 2008 Update.* Geneva, Switzerland: World Health Organisation, 2009.
29. Blum RW, Garell D, Hodgman CH, et al. Transition from child-centered to adult health-care systems for adolescents with chronic conditions. A position paper of the Society for Adolescent Medicine. *J Adolesc Health* 1993;14:570–576.
30. http://mchb.hrsa.gov/cshcn0910/more/pdf/co.pdf. Accessed on April 22, 2015.

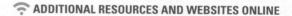 **ADDITIONAL RESOURCES AND WEBSITES ONLINE**

CHAPTER 9

Understanding Legal Aspects of Care

Abigail English, JD
Rebecca Gudeman, JD

KEY WORDS

- Confidentiality
- Consent
- Ethics
- Family Educational Rights and Privacy Act (FERPA)
- Health Insurance Portability and Accountability Act (HIPAA)
- Law
- Patient protection and Affordable Care Act (ACA)
- Payment

INTRODUCTION

Whenever a health care practitioner treats an adolescent or young adult, it is essential the practitioner have a clear understanding of the legal framework within which care is to be provided. The laws related to health care delivery differ based on age, legal status, and geography. This chapter will discuss the legal framework in the United States.

In the United States, the governing laws for adolescents and young adults (AYAs) who are aged 18 years or older are typically the same as those for other adults. For adolescents who are minors—younger than age 18 years in almost all states—the laws may be different. The legal issues that arise most frequently fall into three specific areas:

1. Consent: Who is authorized to give consent for the adolescent's or young adult's care and whose consent is required?
2. Confidentiality: Who has the right to control the release of confidential information about the care, including medical records, and who has the right to receive such information?
3. Payment: Who is financially liable for payment and is there a source of insurance coverage or is public funding available that the adolescent or young adult can access?

LEGAL FRAMEWORK

Over the past few decades, the legal framework that applies to the delivery of adolescent health care in the United States has evolved in several significant ways.

- Courts have recognized that minors, as well as adults, have constitutional rights although there has been considerable debate concerning the scope of these rights.
- All states in the United States have enacted statutes to authorize minors to give their own consent for health care in specific circumstances.
- The laws governing the confidentiality and disclosure of health care information have evolved in ways that affect AYAs.

- The financing of health care services for all age groups and income levels is undergoing major change, at an increasingly rapid pace, which has had and will continue to have a significant impact on adolescents' and young adults' access to health care.

Within this legal framework, the application of the law is shaped by ethics and policy. Health care practitioners may be bound to comply with certain ethical principles as part of their professional obligations and medical license or with certain policies as part of an employment contract. In addition, several important international documents that are not legally binding in the United States, such as the United Nations Convention on the Rights of the Child (http://www.unicef.org/crc/index_30160.html) and the European Convention on Human Rights (http://www.hri.org/docs/ECHR50. html), may provide guidance, particularly as awareness increases of health care as a human right. While often the ethical principles, policies, and other guidance reinforce the law, their intersection will influence application of law, particularly where the law allows for practitioner discretion or is open for interpretation.

Constitutional Issues

Beginning with *In re Gault* (1967), in which the US Supreme Court stated that "neither the Fourteenth Amendment nor the Due Process Clause is for adults alone,"[1] the court has held repeatedly that minors have constitutional rights. The *Gault* decision, which accorded minors certain procedural rights when they are charged by the state with juvenile delinquency offenses, was followed by others recognizing, in *Tinker v. Des Moines Independent School District* (1969),[2] that minors had rights of free speech under the First Amendment and, in *Planned Parenthood of Central Missouri v. Danforth* (1976)[3] and *Carey v. Population Services International* (1977),[4] that they also had privacy rights. Although the Supreme Court subsequently addressed a wide variety of constitutional issues affecting minors and rendered some decisions that were more equivocal about the scope of minors' constitutional rights, the basic principles articulated in the early cases still stand.

One area of frequent constitutional litigation has been the rights of minors with respect to reproductive health care, particularly abortion. The early cases, *Carey* and *Danforth*, clearly established that the right of privacy protects minors as well as adults and encompasses minors' access to contraceptives and the abortion decision. The subsequent history of constitutional litigation with respect to abortion has been complex. After the decision in the *Danforth* case, which held that parents cannot exercise an arbitrary veto with respect to the abortion decisions of their minor daughters, the US Supreme Court decided a series of cases—beginning with *Bellotti v. Baird* (1979),[5] and continuing more recently with *Planned Parenthood of Southeastern Pennsylvania v. Casey* (1992),[6] and *Ayotte v. Planned Parenthood of Northern New England* (2006)[7]—addressing parental notification and consent issues related to abortion. The collective import of these cases has been that although a state may enact a mandatory parental involvement requirement for minors who are seeking abortions, the laws must include an exception when necessary for the preservation of the adolescent's life or health and establish an alternative procedure whereby a minor may obtain authorization for an abortion without first notifying her parents.[7] This alternative most often takes the form of a court proceeding known as a *"judicial bypass."* In the bypass proceeding, a minor must be permitted, without parental involvement, to seek a court order authorizing an abortion. If the minor is mature enough to give an informed consent, the court must allow her to make her own decision; and, if she is not mature, the court must determine whether an abortion would be in her best interest.[5] Many, but not all, states have enacted such parental involvement or judicial bypass statutes, some of which have been implemented, although others have been enjoined by the courts. As of February 2014, at least 38 states have laws in effect that require either the consent or notification of at least one parent; all but 1 of these states provide for a judicial bypass; all but 3 have an exception for medical emergencies; 16 include exceptions for victims of abuse, assault, incest, or neglect; and several provide for consent or notification of an adult family member other than a parent.[8]

State and Federal Laws

Although the constitutional litigation concerning minors' rights in the reproductive health care arena has attracted significant attention, most of the specific legal provisions that affect adolescents' and young adults' access to health care are contained in state and federal statutes and regulations or in "common law" decisions of the courts. These provisions cover a broad range of issues related to consent, confidentiality, and payment, and are critical in defining the parameters of what providers are legally permitted and required to do. Therefore, practitioners providing services to AYAs must develop a familiarity not only with the general constitutional principles that have evolved in recent decades but also with federal laws and state laws, including court decisions, that apply in their own states.

● CONSENT

The law generally requires the consent of a parent before medical care can be provided to a minor. There are, however, numerous exceptions to this requirement. In many situations, someone other than a biological parent—such as a guardian, caretaker relative, foster parent, juvenile court, social worker, or probation officer—may be able to give consent in the place of the parent. State law typically dictates which adults may provide substitute consent. Moreover, in emergency situations, care may be provided without prior consent to safeguard the life and health of the minor, although typically parents must be notified as soon as possible thereafter.

Other exceptions to the parent consent requirement that are highly significant for the AYA health care practitioner authorize minors themselves to give consent for their care. These provisions typically authorize minors to consent for their own care based on either the type of services sought or the status of the minor.

All states have enacted one or more provisions that authorize minors to consent to certain health services.[9,10] These specific areas may include the following:

- Emergency situations where care may be provided without prior consent to safeguard the life and health of the minor
- Contraceptive care
- Pregnancy-related care
- Diagnosis and treatment for sexually transmitted infections, sometimes referred to in statutes as venereal disease

- Diagnosis and treatment of either human immunodeficiency virus, or acquired immunodeficiency syndrome
- Diagnosis and treatment of reportable or contagious diseases
- Examination and treatment related to sexual assault
- Counseling and treatment for drug or alcohol problems
- Counseling and treatment for mental health issues

Few states have statutes covering all of these services. In many cases, the statutes contain minimum age requirements, which most frequently fall between the ages of 12 and 15 years.[9,10]

Similarly, all states have enacted one or more provisions that authorize minors who have attained a specific status to give consent for their own health care.[9,10] The groups of minors most frequently given this authority include the following[9,10]:

- Emancipated minors
- Minors living apart from their parents
- Married minors
- Minors in the armed services
- Minors who are the parent of a child
- High school graduates
- Minors who have attained a certain age
- "Mature minors" who are explicitly authorized by statute to consent for care in a few states.[9]

Few states have enacted all of these provisions, and laws are frequently amended. Therefore, practitioners are advised to have current information about their state laws.

The Mature Minor Doctrine and Informed Consent

"Mature minor" is generally understood to mean a minor who, in the eyes of the medical professional, exhibits the maturity to authorize his or her own health care. Even in the absence of a specific statute, "mature minors" may have the legal capacity to give consent for their own care. The mature minor doctrine emerged from court decisions addressing the circumstances in which a physician could be held liable in damages for providing care to a minor without parental consent.[9,11] In a few states, courts explicitly have chosen not to hold practitioners liable for delivering care to a "mature" minor capable of providing informed consent. The basic criteria for determining whether a patient is capable of giving an informed consent are that the patient must be able to understand the risks and benefits of any proposed treatment or procedure and its alternatives, and must be able to make a voluntary choice among the alternatives. These criteria for informed consent apply to minors, as well as adults. During the past few decades, diligent searches have found no reported decisions holding a physician liable in such circumstances solely on the basis of failure to obtain parental consent when nonnegligent care was provided to a mature minor who had given informed consent, although a few states have rejected application of the "mature minor" doctrine in particular circumstances. In most states, this suggests that unless a state has explicitly rejected the mature minor doctrine, there may be little likelihood a practitioner will incur liability for failure to obtain parental consent for care provided that the minor consents and the minor is an older adolescent (typically at least 15 years old) who is capable of giving an informed consent and the care is not of high risk, is for the minor's benefit, and is within the mainstream of established medical opinion. Again, however, laws do vary from state to state; practitioners must be familiar with local requirements and should consider consulting with local legal counsel to obtain legal advice on this issue.

Note that state-by-state analysis of consent and confidentiality are available at:

- http://www.cahl.org/state-minor-consent-laws-a-summary-third-edition/ (for purchase)
- http://www.guttmacher.org/statecenter/spibs/spib_PIMA.pdf

Young Adults and Capacity to Consent

The law generally allows adults aged 18 years and older to consent to their own health care. One exception is the rare circumstance in which an adult lacks the capacity to provide informed consent. "Capacity" is typically defined in state law and addressed by ethical principles, but generally it means the capacity to understand the risks and benefits of a proposed treatment or procedure and its alternatives, and make a voluntary choice.[12] If a practitioner believes an adult patient does not have the capacity to consent either in a particular context or in general, state law typically provides alternative mechanisms to ensure patients receive appropriate and adequate health care. At the extreme, this may include asking a court to appoint a health care conservator to make medical decisions for the patient. A practitioner treating an incapacitated adolescent should not assume that a parent can simply continue to consent for the child's care once the child turns 18 years old. Practitioners with questions about their obligations in this type of situation or about local law and practice in this area should consult local legal counsel.

● PRIVACY AND CONFIDENTIALITY

There are numerous reasons why it is important to maintain confidentiality in the delivery of health care services to AYAs. The most compelling is to encourage these young people both to seek necessary care on a timely basis and to provide a candid and complete health history when they do so.[13] Additional reasons include supporting their growing sense of privacy and autonomy as well as protecting them from the humiliation and discrimination that could result from disclosure of confidential information.[13]

The confidentiality obligation has numerous sources in law and policy. They include the federal and state constitutions; federal statutes and regulations such as the HIPAA Privacy Rule issued under the Health Insurance Portability and Accountability Act, Medicaid, family planning programs, and federal drug and alcohol programs; state statutes and regulations such as medical confidentiality and medical records laws, doctor–patient privilege statutes, professional licensing laws, and funding programs; court decisions; and professional ethical standards. Many health care professional organizations also have policy statements and codes of ethics that require confidentiality protections.[14-18]

In any given situation, one or several of the above laws and policies may apply depending upon the funding source, the location of service delivery, the type of practitioner, and the type of service delivered. For this reason, practitioners must develop their own understanding of what is confidential and how to handle confidential information. In reviewing relevant confidentiality provisions, practitioners should look for what *may be* disclosed (based on their discretion and professional judgment), what *must be* disclosed, and what *may not be* disclosed, as confidentiality protections are rarely, if ever, absolute. Practitioners may want to consider the following questions:

- What information *is* confidential (because it is considered private and is protected against disclosure)?
- What information *is not* confidential (because such information is not protected)?
- What *exceptions* are there in the confidentiality requirements?
- What information can be released *with consent*?
- What other mechanisms allow for *discretionary* disclosure without consent?
- What *mandates* exist for reporting or disclosing confidential information?

Across the numerous confidentiality obligations, there are commonalities. Generally, personal health information is confidential but may be disclosed pursuant to an authorization obtained from the patient or another appropriate person. Usually, when minors have the legal right to consent to their own care, they also have the right to control disclosure of confidential information about that care. This is not always the case—there are a number of circumstances in which disclosure over the objection of the minor might be required—if a specific legal provision requires disclosure to parents; if a mandatory reporting obligation applies, as in the case of suspected physical or sexual abuse; or if the minor poses a severe danger to himself or herself or to others that ethical principles or legal provisions require to be reported.[14,15,19-22]

When the minor does not have the legal right to consent to care or to control disclosure, the release of confidential information usually must be authorized by the minor's parent or the person (or entity) with legal custody or guardianship. In these cases, there are often exceptions that allow the practitioner to restrict parent authority to access or authorize disclosure of health records when the minor is a victim of abuse or is at risk.[19,20]

When parent authorization is necessary, it is still advisable—from an ethical perspective—for the practitioner to seek the agreement of the minor to disclose confidential information and certainly, at minimum, to advise the minor at the outset of treatment of any limits to confidentiality.[15]

Practitioners can never promise absolute confidentiality to a minor patient nor can they promise absolute disclosure to a parent or guardian. Fortunately, in many circumstances, issues of confidentiality and disclosure can be resolved by discussion and informal agreement between a physician, the adolescent patient, and the parents without reference to legal requirements.

The HIPAA Privacy Rule

In 2002, the final provisions of the HIPAA Privacy Rule were issued. These federal medical confidentiality regulations apply to general health information and protect the health care information of both adolescent minors and young adults. States may adopt more protective confidentiality provisions but cannot waive the minimum protections established by the HIPAA Privacy Rule. The provisions of the HIPAA Privacy Rule that affect the health care information of minors were built on the framework of consent and confidentiality laws developed over the past several decades. Specifically, when minors are authorized to consent for their own health care and do so, the Rule treats them as "individuals" who are able to exercise rights over their own protected health information. Also, when parents have acceded to a confidentiality agreement between a minor and a health professional, the minor is considered an "individual" under the Rule.[19,20]

Generally, the HIPAA Privacy Rule gives parents access to the health information of their unemancipated minor children, including adolescents. However, on the issue of when parents may have access to protected health information for minors who are considered "individuals" under the Rule and who have consented to their own care, it defers to "state and other applicable law."[19,20]

Therefore, the laws that allow minors to consent for their own health care acquired increased significance with the advent of the HIPAA Privacy Rule. The Rule must also be understood in the broader context of other laws that affect disclosure of adolescents' confidential health information to their parents. Specifically, if state or other law explicitly requires information to be disclosed to a parent, the regulations allow a health care provider to comply with that law and disclose the information. If state or other law explicitly permits, but does not require, information to be disclosed to a parent, the regulations allow a health care provider to exercise discretion to disclose or not. If state or other law prohibits the disclosure of information to a parent without the consent of the minor, the regulations do not allow a health care provider to disclose it without the minor's consent. If state or other law is silent or unclear on the question, an entity covered by the Rule has discretion to determine whether to grant access to a parent to the protected health information, as long as the determination is made by a health care professional exercising professional judgment.[19,20]

Providing Health Care in School Settings

The legal framework for consent to treatment for AYAs remains the same when services are provided in a school setting; however, health care providers should be aware that different confidentiality rules may apply when delivering health care in either secondary schools or student health centers on college and university campuses. While the HIPAA Privacy Rule typically would control release of health information created by practitioners, the HIPAA Privacy Rule explicitly excludes from its purview health records that are part of an "education record" as that is defined under the Family Educational Rights and Privacy Act (FERPA).[23] FERPA is a federal statute that controls the disclosure of the educational records of students at most primary, secondary, and postsecondary schools. FERPA defines "education record" in a way that can include health records created by health care providers employed or acting on behalf of a school or university. Thus, health records created by medical professionals employed by a school or university may be part of an "education record" and subject to FERPA rather than HIPAA.

There is an exception to this, however, that is particularly relevant for health providers who work in school settings with AYAs who are aged 18 years or older. FERPA specifically states that the term "education records" does *not* include "records on a student who is 18 years of age or older, or is attending an institution of postsecondary education, which are made or maintained by a physician, psychiatrist, psychologist, or other recognized professional or paraprofessional acting in his professional or paraprofessional capacity, or assisting in that capacity, and which are made, maintained, or used only in connection with the provision of treatment to the student, and are not available to anyone other than persons providing such treatment, except that such records can be personally reviewed by a physician or other appropriate professional of the student's choice."[24] If FERPA does not apply, then these records are subject to HIPAA and relevant state confidentiality law.

The privacy protections in HIPAA and FERPA, including who may authorize release of records and who may access records without need of authorization, are different. For this reason, it is important for practitioners in school settings to understand which regulations apply to and control release of their patient information.

Often, which regulation applies will be fact and situation specific. In light of the important ramifications, health care practitioners who provide care in school settings should consult with their legal counsel about whether their student health records are governed by HIPAA, FERPA, or state privacy laws.

🔴 PAYMENT

There is an integral relationship among the legal provisions that pertain to consent, confidentiality, and payment in the delivery of health care services to AYAs. A source of payment is essential whether an adolescent or young adult needs care on a confidential basis or not. The issue is particularly critical for youth from economically disadvantaged families or those who have no family to support them, especially when a young person needs confidential care.

If an adolescent does not have available a source of free care or access to insurance coverage, legal provisions that allow adolescents to give consent for care and to expect confidentiality protections to apply to that care do not guarantee access. Some of the state minor consent laws specify that if a minor is authorized to consent to care, it is the minor rather than the parent who is responsible for payment. In reality, however, few, if any, adolescents are able to pay for health care "out of pocket," unless there is a sliding fee scale with very minimal payments required. Financing for the care is therefore an essential element of both confidentiality and access.

There are some federal and state health care funding programs that enable AYAs to obtain confidential care with little or no cost to them. Most notable is the federal Family Planning program funded under Title X of the Public Health Services Act.[22] As significant a role as these programs play, they do not ensure access to the full array of comprehensive health services needed by adolescents or young adults. The financing available through insurance is therefore all the more important.

Adolescents have been uninsured and underinsured at higher rates than other groups in the population, and young adults have been uninsured at the very highest rates. Those AYAs living below the poverty level are at the greatest risk for lacking health insurance. Private employer-based coverage for adolescents has declined in recent decades, but coverage through public insurance programs such as Medicaid and the Children's Health Insurance Program has increased.[25]

With the advent of the Patient Protection and Affordable Care Act of 2010 (ACA), increasing numbers of AYAs have been and will be covered by private health insurance or Medicaid.[25] Beginning in 2010, more than 3 million young adults under age 26 have been able to remain on a parent's health insurance policy who would not otherwise have had coverage.[26] As of late January 2014, 26 states have expanded Medicaid to provide coverage for individuals up to 133% of the federal poverty level (FPL), enabling many previously uninsured young adults to qualify.[27] AYAs with family incomes between 100% and 400% FPL are also able to receive subsidized coverage in the form of premium tax credits—and other cost sharing assistance if their family incomes are between 100% and 250% FPL—if they enroll in private health insurance plans through health insurance marketplaces operated by the states and the federal government.[25,26] The ACA requires health plans to cover without cost sharing a wide range of preventive services that are important for AYAs.[25,26] The ACA also has potential to expand coverage for vulnerable groups of youth such as those exiting foster care, those in or leaving the juvenile or criminal justice system, and homeless youth.[28]

Even when adolescents have health insurance coverage, confidentiality is not guaranteed. Particularly for those who are covered as dependents on a family policy, confidentiality is often compromised through the billing and health insurance claims process. A small number of states have begun to implement policies to enable covered dependents to receive confidential services without forfeiting payment by the insurer. Nevertheless, the limits on confidentiality that exist in the insurance arena remain a challenge that health care practitioners should be aware of and inform their AYA patients about.[29,30]

It is only through a comprehensive understanding by practitioners of the legal framework for adolescent health services, including the relationships among consent, confidentiality, and payment issues, that adolescents' and young adults' access to the health care they need can be ensured. Extensive resources are available on Web sites and in peer-reviewed journals to assist practitioners in becoming familiar with this legal framework.

🔴 DISCLAIMER

Please note that this information does not represent legal advice. Health care practitioners are reminded that laws change and that statutes, regulations, and court decisions may be subject to differing interpretations. It is the responsibility of each health care professional to be familiar with the current relevant laws that affect the health care of AYAs. In difficult cases involving legal issues, advice should be sought from someone with state-specific expertise.

The information in this chapter applies to the United States. All health care professionals should consult with their local legal counsel.

REFERENCES

1. In re Gault, 387 US 1 (1967).
2. *Tinker v. Des Moines Independent School District,* 393 US 503 (1969).
3. *Planned Parenthood of Central Missouri v. Danforth,* 428 US 52 (1976).
4. *Carey v. Population Services International,* 431 US 678 (1977).
5. *Bellotti v. Baird,* 443 US 622 (1979).
6. *Planned Parenthood of Southeastern Pennsylvania v. Casey,* 505 US 833 (1992).
7. *Ayotte v. Planned Parenthood of Northern New England,* 546 US 320 (2006).
8. Guttmacher Institute. State policies in brief: parental involvement in minors' abortions. Available at http://www.guttmacher.org/statecenter/spibs/spib_PIMA.pdf. Accessed on February 1, 2014.
9. English A, Bass L, Boyle AD, et al. *State minor consent laws: a summary.* 3rd ed. Chapel Hill, NC: Center for Adolescent Health & the Law, 2010.
10. Guttmacher Institute. State policies in brief: an overview of minors' consent laws. Available at http://www.guttmacher.org/statecenter/spibs/spib_OMCL.pdf. Accessed on February 1, 2014.
11. Steinberg L. Does recent research on adolescent brain development inform the mature minor doctrine? *J Med Philos* 2013;38(3):256–267.
12. Post LF, Blustein J, Dubler NN. *Handbook for health care ethics committees.* Baltimore, MD: Johns Hopkins University Press, 2007.
13. Ford CA, English A. Limiting confidentiality of adolescent health services: what are the risks? *JAMA* 2002;288:752.
14. Morreale MC, Dowling EC, Stinnett AJ, eds. *Policy compendium on confidential health services for adolescents.* 2nd ed. Chapel Hill, NC: Center for Adolescent Health & the Law, 2005. Available at http://www.cahl.org/policy-compendium-2005/. Accessed on April 22, 2015.
15. Ford CA, English A, Sigman G. Position paper of the Society for Adolescent Medicine: confidential health care for adolescents. *J Adolesc Health* 2004;35:160.
16. American Academy of Pediatrics. *Confidentiality in adolescent health care.* Policy Statement RE9151. April 1989; Reaffirmed January 1993, November 1997, May 2000, and May 2004.
17. American College of Obstetricians and Gynecologists. Confidentiality in adolescent health care. In: *Guidelines for adolescent health care.* 2nd ed. Washington, DC: American College of Obstetricians and Gynecologists, 2011.
18. American Medical Association. *Confidential health services for adolescents.* Policy H-60.965. CSA Rep. A, A-92; Reaffirmed by BOT Rep. 24, A-97; Reaffirmed by BOT Rep. 9, A-98.
19. English A, Ford CA. The HIPAA privacy rule and adolescents: legal questions and clinical challenges. *Perspect Sex Reprod Health* 2004;36:80.
20. Gudeman, R. Adolescent confidentiality and privacy under the health insurance portability and accountability Act. *Youth Law News,* Jul–Sep 2003. Available at http://www.youthlaw.org/publications/yln/00/july_september_2003/adolescent_confidentiality_and_privacy_under_the_health_insurance_portability_and_accountability_act/. Accessed on April 22, 2015.
21. Gudeman, R. Federal privacy protection for substance abuse treatment records. *Youth Law News,* Jul–Sep 2003. Available at http://www.youthlaw.org/publications/yln/00/july_september_2003/federal_privacy_protection_for_substance_abuse_treatment_records_protecting_adolescents/. Accessed on April 22, 2015.
22. Gudeman R, Madge S. The federal title X family planning program: privacy and access rules for adolescents. *Youth Law News,* Jan–Mar 2011. Available at http://www.youthlaw.org/publications/yln/2011/jan_mar_2011/the_federal_title_x_family_planning_program_privacy_and_access_rules_for_adolescents/. Accessed on April 22, 2015.
23. 45 C.F.R. § 160.103.
24. 20 U.S.C. § 1232g; 34 C.F.R. § 99.3.
25. English A. *The Patient Protection and Affordable Care Act of 2010: how does it help adolescents and young adults.* Chapel Hill, NC: Center for Adolescent Health & the Law, 2010. Available at http://nahic.ucsf.edu/wp-content/uploads/2011/02/HCR_Issue_Brief_Aug2010_Final_Aug31.pdf. Accessed on April 22, 2015.
26. English A, Park MJ. *The Supreme Court ACA decision: what happens now for adolescents and young adults.* Chapel Hill, NC: Center for Adolescent Health & the Law, 2012. Available at http://nahic.ucsf.edu/wp-content/uploads/2012/11/Supreme_Court_ACA_Decision_Nov29.pdf. Accessed on April 22, 2015.
27. Henry J. Kaiser Family Foundation. *Status of state action on Medicaid expansion decisions,* 2014. Available at http://kff.org/health-reform/state-indicator/state-activity-around-expanding-medicaid-under-the-affordable-care-act/. Accessed on April 22, 2015.
28. English A, Scott J, Park MJ. *Implementing the ACA: how much will it help vulnerable adolescents & young adults?* Chapel Hill, NC: Center for Adolescent Health & the Law, 2014. Available at http://nahic.ucsf.edu/wp-content/uploads/2014/01/VulnerablePopulations_IB_Final.pdf. Accessed on April 22, 2015.
29. English A, Gold R, Nash E, et al. *Confidentiality for individuals insured as dependents: a review of state laws and policies.* New York, NY: Guttmacher Institute and Public Health Solutions, 2012. Available at http://www.guttmacher.org/pubs/confidentiality-review.pdf. Accessed on April 22, 2015.
30. Gold R. A new frontier in the era of health reform: protecting confidentiality for individuals insured as dependents. *Guttmacher Policy Rev* 2013;16(4):2–7. Available at http://www.guttmacher.org/pubs/confidentiality-review.pdf. Accessed on April 22, 2015.

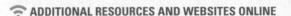

ADDITIONAL RESOURCES AND WEBSITES ONLINE

Technology and Social Media

Megan A. Moreno

"OMG." "TTYL." "LOL." It may look and sound like a strange new language, and in some ways, it is. These acronyms represent popular terms used by adolescents and young adults (AYAs), terms that have emerged as a result of communicating via the Internet and texting. Translation of these terms includes "Oh my God," "talk to you later," and "laugh out loud," respectively. Adolescents today have grown up immersed in technology, with iPads, smart phones, and social networking sites (SNSs) at their fingertips. The rapid advancements in technology over the past decade have provided AYAs with numerous benefits, including expansive access to knowledge and far-reaching communication tools. Adolescents have been dubbed the "digital generation" or "digital natives" given that they have grown up with access to computers and the Internet from an early age.[1] However, there are concomitant risks to technology use that include balancing online and offline lives, and exposure to risky health behaviors via social media. This chapter provides an overview of technology and social media use—the most popular form of Internet use, reviews benefits and risks, and considers opportunities to use these tools to improve health for AYAs.

WHAT IS SOCIAL MEDIA?

The first iteration of the Web was known as Web 1.0 and its purpose was to provide information to consumers. Technological advancements led to Internet 2.0, a new web that both provided information to consumers and empowered users to view, create, and share multimedia data with peers and the public. Web 2.0 led to what has been called social media, also called immersive or interactive media.[2] Social media represent a set of Web 2.0 tools that are centered on interaction and sharing of content with others.

The idea of interacting and sharing content via media is a remarkable concept in the areas of media studies. Traditional media, such as television, typically featured a corporation creating the content and the viewer consuming this content. Messages were unidirectional, easily represented by a single arrow pointing from the corporation to the consumer. In the new world of social media, Internet users became both creators and consumers of content. Messages could now flow in all directions, from corporations to users, among users, and back to corporations through a seemingly endless array of potential paths. Thus, today's AYAs have increased capacity to interact with each other and the larger world using media,

enhanced opportunities to explore and experiment via media, and an increased likelihood of being influenced by media.

Popular Social Media Sites

The most common type of social media use is through a SNS profile. The majority of AYAs report ownership of at least one SNS profile.[3] There are different types of SNS available on the Internet. The most common SNSs used by AYAs include Facebook and Twitter.

Facebook

The mission of Facebook, as posted on the Web site, is "to give people the power to share and make the world more open and connected." Facebook achieved remarkable popularity among teens and has also drawn adult populations in recent years.[3] Facebook's ongoing popularity may be related to its ability to combine functions from other sites such as photo sharing, email communication, games, blogs, and really simple syndication feeds.

Twitter

Twitter users are able to post "tweets," 140-character posts, about recent events, ideas, or even random thoughts. Tweets are typically labeled with "hashtags," a word or unspaced phrase with the number sign (#) as a prefix, which incorporate that tweet into a particular topic or content area. Content from others can also be "retweeted." In addition to generating one's own tweets, Twitter users can choose to "follow" the Twitter posts of other Twitter users.

Other Social Media and Online Gaming Sites

Other social media sites present different activities and varied cultures within each site that draws those whose interests match. Pinterest is a site that can best be described as an online bulletin board that includes fashion, crafts, and recipes. Users can identify items they link and "pin" them to their own boards. YouTube is a Web site for users to view and upload videos. Some videos are made by companies and uploaded onto YouTube, such as old sitcom episodes. Many other videos are user generated, meaning created and uploaded by users. Reddit is a platform for discussion of specific topics where user votes shape what stories or news items are most prominent. Finally, LinkedIN, is another popular site which is intended for professional networking that often appeals to older AYAs as they prepare to enter the job market.

Other types of social media include online gaming, in which players are connected across the globe while playing immersive games such as World of Warcraft. Social media can also include music sharing such as through sites like Spotify or Pandora. Many social media Web sites are linked to apps, while other apps are freestanding and only available on mobile phones. Each year sites change in popularity, new sites emerge and older sites die out, leading to a constantly changing landscape of social media.

Social Media and Technology Use Rates

Social media use has surged over the past decade and this exponential growth is expected to continue.[4] The rate of social media use is especially high among AYAs.[3] Adolescents report that 77% use Facebook and 24% use Twitter. Young adults report similar rates: 84% use Facebook and 31% use Twitter. Many young adults also use the professional, job-related site LinkedIn (15%).[4]

Texting is an increasingly common form of communication among AYAs using mobile devices. Current estimates include that approximately three-quarters of adolescents have a cell phone, and almost half of teens own smartphones.[3] Among older adolescent females who own smartphones, over half report they access and use the Internet mostly from their phones. Among college students, a 2013 study found that 88% reported owning a smartphone, with rates up from 67% in 2012 and 56% in 2011.[5]

Internet and computer access among AYAs is commonplace. The vast majority of adolescents have computer access at home.[4] Among young adults, nearly all college students (99%) report using a personal laptop.[5] Tablet computers are owned by almost a quarter of adolescents, a comparable rate to tablet ownership among adults.[4] Among young adult college students, use of tablets has received increased focus with proposed possibilities that tablets could enhance the collegiate learning experience. A recent study reported that approximately one-quarter of college students owned a tablet computer; however, only 58.3% reported using it for schoolwork.[5]

In recent years, the digital divide in Internet access between high and low socioeconomic groups has narrowed. Adolescents who fall into lower socioeconomic groups are now just as likely, and in some cases more likely, to use their cell phones for primary access to the Internet compared to teens from higher socioeconomic groups.[4]

How SNSs Are Used

Adolescents who own an SNS profile are able to choose and modify its content on a moment-to-moment basis. SNS content may include audio, images (e.g., pictures and video), and text (e.g., blogs and personal descriptions). A widely used feature of some SNSs such as Facebook is called "status updates," which allow users to share a short text description of their current location, emotion, or activity. Examples of status updates include "Jay is excited for Friday's game!" or "Emily is loving the new Lady Gaga album!" SNSs often allow profile owners to create online photo albums and to share photographs with other profile owners. Facebook also provides a venue for profile owners to describe their favorite sports, movies, music, and other activities, and link via these interests to other profiles with similar interests. Thus, SNSs allow AYAs with opportunities for self-expression and identity development through what they choose to display and communicate on their profiles.

SNSs typically provide a venue for communication with other profile owners in three formats: messaging, instant messaging, and publicly displayed comments. First, AYAs can use Facebook messaging to communicate privately. These messages are similar to email; messages are sent from profile to profile as asynchronous communication. Second, AYAs can send instant messages to other profile owners, whose profiles are linked as "friends" if they are also online at that moment, leading to synchronous communication. Third, AYAs can publicly comment on the content of their peers' profiles and thus leave a digital record of their opinions about events, as well as content displayed by peers.

Finally, SNSs provide opportunities to link one's profile into a social network via "friending." When two profile owners accept each other as online "friends," the two profiles become linked and content is mutually accessible. In summary, these sites allow individual many opportunities for self-expression, a means of peer communication and feedback, as well as connection to an online social network.

Influence of Social Media

Previous work, rooted in observational theory, has established strong links between what AYAs see and how they act.[6] Observation of peers is a major source of influence on AYA health attitudes, intentions, and behaviors.[7] For example, adolescents who perceive that their peers are sexually active are more likely to report intention to become sexually active themselves.[8] Studies of college students have illustrated that alcohol consumption patterns are highly influenced by one's peer group.[9] Many studies of adolescents have illustrated links between traditional media and health behaviors. For example, previous work has illustrated that younger adolescents exposed to tobacco use through media such as movies are more likely to initiate this behavior themselves.[10]

Social media combine peer and media effects and thereby represent a powerful motivator of behavior whether it is by content created by the individual or content she or he finds and shares with peers. It has been argued that Facebook may have greater influence than traditional media, as Facebook combines the power of interpersonal persuasion with the reach of mass media.[11] Facebook has been described as "the most significant advance in persuasion since the radio was invented in the 1890s" and initiated a new form of persuasion labeled "mass interpersonal persuasion."[11]

A previous study examined the potential ways in which Facebook may influence AYAs and found four distinct constructs.[12] Those areas include (**Table 10.1**): (1) *Connection*: Facebook provides and enhances peer communication, networking, and connection; (2) *Comparison*: Facebook allows comparison between peers to take place using tangible information such as photos, stated behaviors, and the ability to note peer comments on these information; (3) *Identification*: Facebook allows a profile owner to develop an online identity through a profile. Profile owners can then reflect and revise that identity via feedback from peers' comments and "likes," or by personal perusal through the Facebook "timeline." The ability to develop one's identity in real time provides a unique multimedia view of the self; and, (4) *Immersive experience:* Facebook provides a Web site that provides positive, negative, tool-based and distracting features toward an immersive and powerful experience for users.

Benefits of Social Media

There are many areas in which use of social media and technology provides benefits to today's AYAs. Described below are some of the key features of social media, particularly of SNSs, that may provide unique benefits to this population.

Social Support and Social Capital

Virtual communities play an increasing role in the lives of today's youth. Previous work illustrates that adolescents who experienced a greater number of positive reactions to their SNS profile also experienced higher self-esteem and satisfaction with their life.[13] Comparably, a study of young adults demonstrated that Facebook usage was positively correlated with life satisfaction, social trust, and civic engagement.[13] Epidemiological studies over the years have repeatedly demonstrated that as the size of one's social network increases, so does their physical and mental health.[14] The varied social media sites available allow AYAs to develop several new arenas in which social support can be built and cultivated.

Identity Development

One of the most important milestones in adolescence is the development of an identity. SNSs in particular provide adolescents a technological canvas on which they can explore and shape their identity, by choosing what information about themselves to display to the public and how the information they display changes in response to new experiences as well as related to feedback from peers. For young adults, feedback from peers may reinforce

TABLE 10.1

Areas of Influence Adapted from the Facebook Influence Model

Area of Influence	Cluster Topics within This Area	Example Items That Represent the Cluster
Connection	Connection to people	—Allows people to constantly stay updated with other's lives —Way to get to know acquaintances almost instantly —Keep in touch with people you would not call or text
	Far reaching	—Ability to reach many people with one Web site —Can reach anyone, young and old, rich and poor —Bonding across cultures and distances
	Fast communication	—Feel connected and in the loop constantly —Puts everyone you know and what they are doing in one place —Updates on people's lives faster than with a cell phone
	Business and promotion	—Ability to plan influential events such as protests or sit-ins —Statuses provide a way to blog instantly about events or political topics —Every company uses it to promote business or provide deals
	Accessible and adaptable	—Largest network in human history —Easy to use and navigate —Widely known and talked about
	Data and Information	—Huge database of information —Compiled data from millions of individuals —News feature
Identification	Identity expression	—Freedom to express things and let it be heard —Present the best side of yourself —Show off accomplishments to everyone you are friends with on Facebook, not just close friends
	Influence on identity	—Provides others with pictures that can influence perceptions —Display aspects of yourself that you would not share in offline life (sexuality, substance use) —Wonder if you should be doing what you see everyone doing in pictures
Comparison	Curiosity about others	—Can know what people are up to without asking them about it and without them knowing you know —Creep culture/stalking —See who associates with whom with pictures and comments
	Facebook establishing social norms	—Reinforces beliefs or opinions by seeing that others hold same beliefs or opinions —Can see what is popular by observation —Can follow norms
Facebook as an experience	Distractions	—Procrastination —Addictive —Huge distraction
	Positive experiences	—Facebook is referenced in daily life —Provides entertainment at any time —Status updates can promote a good mood
	Negative experiences	—Changes the nature of communication from face-to-face to screen-to-screen —People willing to sacrifice privacy —Inspires competition in people

Moreno MA, Kota R, Schoohs S, et al. The Facebook influence model: a concept mapping approach. *Cyberpsychol Behav Soc Netw* 2013;16(7):504–511.

particular aspects of their identity. One study of African American college students found that Facebook provided a platform to use both photographs and text to signal racial identity.[15] For those AYAs with interests outside the mainstream culture, SNSs provide an outlet to meet new people who share their interests. These online peer groups may provide AYAs with the support they need to develop and reinforce one's identity.

Education and Civic Engagement

There are several ways in which technology use can contribute to education. Youth in high school, technical school, and colleges/

universities can use the Internet to seek information sources for reports, or augment learning on classroom topics. The Internet can provide audio, video, or multimedia sources to expand the learning found in traditional textbooks. One of the more common uses of SNS in schools is using blogging to help increase skills in creative writing.[13] Further, technology can be used as a means of communication between students as well as between students and teachers to discuss homework assignments and projects.

Technology and social media can also contribute to AYAs' civic engagement. One feature of SNS such as Facebook is the ability to create groups and events, which can be private or publicly available to others. Many of the existing groups on Facebook are dedicated to political, religious, or community purposes. This provides AYAs' opportunities for exposure to new ideas and information. A national survey of AYAs found that those who used the Internet more often were more politically aware and civically engaged compared to those who used the Internet less often.[16]

Health Access and Illness Support

Social media allow AYAs to access health information for questions that may be embarrassing or stigmatizing, such as sexual behavior or substance use.[17] A key issue is to ensure that AYAs have knowledge of and access to sites that provide accurate and reliable information. Toward that end, numerous health organizations, such as Planned Parenthood, maintain a social media presence. Many of these social media sites allow real-time interactions to answer questions or provide resources. Technology and social media also allow opportunities for AYAs with chronic illnesses, or their parents, to connect to support groups to find support during challenging times or share stories with others. Some patients use technology or social media to interact with classmates, or even virtually attend classes, during prolonged hospital stays.

Risks of Social Media

While many AYAs are quite savvy when it comes to using technology, their knowledge of Internet safety is lacking and many are unaware of the ramifications of their actions in cyberspace. One study found that one-third (32%) of participants have given their password to friends and one-fourth (25%) were unaware that content uploaded online cannot be deleted.[18] AYAs may not consider the potential consequences that sharing this information has if their relationships with people change. Further, in a recent study of female college students, participants believed that sharing too much information online was considered both a safety risk, as well as a risk to one's public image. Some participants commented that as a young adult, risks to one's personal reputation from "oversharing" were more salient compared to risks related to online safety.[19]

Risks Related to Posted Content

Adolescence is frequently a time of behavioral experimentation, which, for some adolescents, includes experimentation with health-risk behaviors. As SNSs such as Facebook give adolescents the opportunity to post information about their personal lives, such as likes, dislikes, and activities, they also present the opportunity for adolescents to display information about risky behaviors, both in text and picture format. Approximately half of adolescent SNS profiles feature references to one or more health-risk behaviors.[20] One study found that approximately 41% of 18-year-old's profiles displayed references to substance use, 24% displayed references to sex, and 14% displayed references to substance use.[20] Studies of young adult college students have found that up to 85% of college students' SNS profiles include references to alcohol use.[21]

Future Employers: Displaying health-risk behavior information on a personal Web profile, such as information about sexual activity or substance use, makes this information available in a globally public venue. Content displayed on an SNS profile can be copied, downloaded, or distributed by any profile viewer. Therefore, this information is published, public, permanent, and persuasive. This information may then become accessible to people whom the profile owner would prefer not to view it, such as potential employers, teachers, or other adults. Many employers currently screen potential job candidates using social media tools like Facebook. Though many AYAs understand these risks, many remain unclear about or unmotivated to maintain security settings that protect their displayed content on social media.[22,23] A recent study of female college students found that young adults frequently believe in "urban myths" about how outside individuals or companies could access displayed online information despite privacy protections on

sites such as Facebook and Twitter.[19] While it seems unlikely that every university or company is conducting surreptitious hacking into Facebook profiles, the recent news about National Security Association's access to personal online data is unlikely to mitigate young adults' beliefs in these urban myths.[24] These urban myths may explain some adolescent or young adults' reluctance to take the time to learn or maintain online privacy settings,[23] as they may believe that these are futile in the face of hackers and companies.

Influencing Others: Regardless of whether displayed content on an SNS is real, AYAs may respond to another's disclosures as if they were real and this in turn may influence intentions and behaviors. A previous study found that adolescents viewed displayed alcohol references on SNS profiles as accurate and influential representations of alcohol use.[25] Further, display of sexual content by females has been linked to increased sexual expectations by young adult males who view these profiles.[26] Content promoting eating disorders, known as pro-anorexia or "pro-ana" and pro-bulimia or "pro-mia," are also present on social media sites.[27]

Sexting: The term "sexting" refers to sending, receiving, or forwarding sexually explicit messages or pictures over cell phone, computer, or other digital device. A recent study of adolescents found that 60% reported having been asked for a sext, 31.4% reported asking for a sext, and 27.6% reported having sent a sext. Further, sending a sext was associated with being sexually active one year later.[28] Among young adults, a previous study reported that 38% of college-aged participants reported that exchanging sexts makes "hooking up with others more likely."[29] Sexting by AYAs can have unintended negative consequences. Consequences include embarrassment, regret, or being harassed as a result of sending a sext. The sext can also be distributed beyond the target recipient. A previous survey revealed that 40% of adolescents had been shown a message of a sexual nature that had been intended for someone else.[30] There are also potential legal consequences, which can include prosecution under child pornography statutes, a potentially devastating consequence. Some states have adapted specific status that apply to sexting but these laws remain rare.[31] Finally, previous studies have linked sexting to other risky behaviors involving impulsivity, such as substance use.[32]

Cyberbullying: Cyberbullying is often defined as the deliberate use of technology including social media to communicate false, embarrassing, or hostile information about another individual. It can include name calling, spreading rumors, pretending to be someone else, sending unwanted pictures or texts, distributing pictures without consent, making threats, or asking someone to do something sexual.[33] Though cyberbullying can have similar consequences as traditional offline bullying, such as depression and anxiety, there are some unique aspects of cyberbullying that may increase the potential severity of these consequences. For instance, because it occurs online, cyberbullying can occur at any time, not just when one is face-to-face. Additionally, given the wide use of SNS, cyberbullying has the potential to reach a large audience.[33]

Among adolescents, cyberbullying is less common compared to traditional forms of bullying, and is commonly associated with other traditional bullying behaviors.[34] A challenge in understanding the prevalence of cyberbullying is the varied definitions that have been used in research studies. One study of younger Canadian adolescents defined cyberbullying as "harassing using technology such as email, computer, cell phone, video cameras, etc." In this study, the prevalence rate of cyberbullying victimization was 25%.[35] A second study of adolescents defined cyberbullying broadly as "mean things" or "anything that someone does that upsets or offends someone else." This study found that 72% of adolescents considered themselves victims of cyberbullying.[36] While much attention has been paid to bullying behaviors of younger teens, less is known about young adult college students. Current data suggest that up to 20% of college students have experienced cyberbullying.[37] Risk factors and prevalence of cyberbullying among college students is an area in need of further study. If left unchecked, young adult bullies may continue their behavior into adulthood and the workplace. Workplace bullies have been characterized as manipulating others to gain power or privilege, often through subtle techniques that do not involve being directly hostile.[38] These techniques share similarities with participants' descriptions of cyberbullying. Thus, the college years may represent the last opportunity to identify or intervene with bullies, as well as victims, before patterns and consequences are established that may impact the years ahead.

Problematic Use and Multitasking

Problematic Internet use (PIU) is a new and growing health concern for AYAs. PIU may be defined as Internet use that is risky, excessive, or impulsive in nature leading to adverse life consequences, specifically physical, emotional, social, or functional impairment.[39] A previous study worked with older adolescents and health professionals to develop a concept map towards understanding PIU which included 7 distinct constructs as components of PIU. The psychosocial risk factors construct may provide insight into key risk factors for PIU. The clusters of impulsive and risky use may describe potential pathways to the development of PIU. Several clusters describe potential consequences of PIU, including emotional, social, and functional impairment. Several studies in the US and internationally suggest links between Internet overuse and negative mental and physical health consequences.[40] Finally, the cluster of dependent Internet use is of great interest as it relates PIU to other conditions involving addictive behaviors.

Media multitasking is defined as using more than one media device, or program, concurrently. One study of young adults texted participants at random intervals throughout the day and asked them to report their current Internet use time and activities. Study findings illustrated that young adults reported frequent multitasking, and across all times in which young adults were online, over half the time they were multitasking.[41] Media multitasking is an area in need of further study, as it is unclear what impact multitasking has on brain development during the AYA stage of life. It has been argued that the fragmentary nature of attention while multitasking may impact a teen's ability to hold concentration for a necessary period of time, such as studying. Conversely, some have argued that in today's modern media society, multitasking is a necessary strategy to get work completed.

ROLE OF THE AYA PROVIDER REGARDING SOCIAL MEDIA USE

Fortunately, there are strategies available for health care providers, educators, and parents to help AYAs avoid risks associated with technology use. One approach is through focusing on three key concepts: balance, boundaries, and communication.[42]

Balance

The balance between online and offline time is a critical concept to discuss with AYAs. Spending time offline, including hanging out with friends, exercising, or spending time outside, is critical to AYA development. Further, achieving balance provides protection against concerns such as PIU.

Boundaries

Boundaries refers to setting limits around what AYAs are willing to display about themselves online or on social media, as well as setting limits in where adolescents spend their time online. Discussing guidelines on what types of personal information are not appropriate to post on social media sites with teens can help prevent them from several online safety risks. These risks include being targets of bullying, unwanted solicitation, or embarrassment.

Communication

Just as with many tenets of adolescent health, parents should discuss social media and technology with their adolescents early and often. Establishing home rules for social media and technology use as soon as the child begins using these tools is an important way to promote healthy technology use from the beginning.

AYA providers can consider these core constructs in their efforts toward prevention, education, screening, and intervention. Specific strategies to consider include the following.

Prevention

- Supervision
  - Encourage parents to take an active role in supervising and providing guidance regarding technology use during the early adolescent years
  - Learning to engage in technology should involve a period of time in which sessions are supervised and guidance is offered, followed by a gradual progression to independent use once skills have been learned and demonstrated.
- Balance
  - There are many approaches to promote balance with teens, and one example is setting a "media curfew" to establish times after which no technology is used, such as after 9 p.m. at night.
  - Some families establish "media-free times," such as family dinners, to provide time and space for families to interact without technological interruptions.
  - Among young adults, anecdotal reports suggest that some college professors ask students to engage in media-free periods, such as a "screen-free week" or avoiding social media for a time period to promote increased awareness of their offline environment.
- Boundaries
  - Among younger adolescents, it is important for families to discuss setting boundaries around what types of sites are appropriate for teens, as well as what actions to take if an adolescent stumbles onto a site with concerning content.
  - Promoting boundaries often involves helping AYAs see connections between their online and offline persona and audience. One proposed guideline suggested by a teen is "If what you're going to post is something you wouldn't want your grandmother to see, don't post it."
- Media multitasking
  - Encourage AYAs to avoid media multitasking, particularly when doing homework or academic tasks as multitasking is associated with lower academic performance.
  - For the high school student heading to college, providers can provide a timely reminder of the importance of avoiding media multitasking during study periods.
- Communication
  - Providers can encourage parents to take opportunities or schedule times to check in on an adolescent's social media presence and to revisit house rules as an adolescent gets older.
  - For the older adolescent or young adult living outside the home, parents can still play a role in prompting their child to take care in how much personal information they display online, and in maintaining a healthy balance of offline and online time.

Education

- Adolescent providers may consider working with schools or community groups to offer talks or educational sessions on these topics, and to share resources. Concerns regarding social media and technology use by youth are shared concerns among health care providers, educators, the legal and law enforcement community, and other youth-oriented community groups.

Screening

- Balance
  - Ask AYAs about their media and technology use, as well as how much time they spend each day without media.
  - Ask AYAs about what rules, if any, they or their family use to regulate or monitor media use.
- Boundaries
  - Ask AYAs about their privacy settings on social media sites, and how often they update or check these settings to ensure they are current.
- Communication
  - Ask AYAs about how often they discuss their social media and technology use with their parents, other family members, or other adults.
- Problematic Internet Use
  - Among AYAs who express concerns with overuse or overengagement with the Internet, screening for PIU may be indicated. The Problematic and Risky Internet Use Screening Scale[43] has been validated for use in AYAs.
- Ask patients directly about risk behaviors such as sexting
  - Studies suggest that sexting is associated with offline sexual behaviors, and screen for sexual behaviors among teens who engage in sexting.
- Ask patients about experiences with online harassment or cyberbullying
  - Since older AYAs may not consider cyberbullying a form of "bullying," consider using other terms such as "cyberbullying," "online harassment," or "electronic harassment." Among teens who have engaged as bullies or victims in cyberbullying provide support and offer counseling as needed to address the common consequences including negative self-esteem and depression.

Intervention

- Balance: Providers can engage with participants to develop media use plans or media-free times during the day, for AYAs struggling with balance or showing early signs of PIU. For some AYAs who have a more impaired relationship with the Internet or technology, counseling may be indicated.
  - While there are currently no validated interventions for PIU, counseling may assist AYAs in developing ways to reduce their use and cope with associated symptoms and signs such as social isolation or impulsivity.
- Boundaries: Encourage families to have scheduled check-ins with their adolescents to view social media profiles together. This practice can ensure that security settings are up to date and that displayed information does not endanger the adolescent. Among young adults who live outside the home, this type of approach is more problematic, though providers can emphasize the impact that displayed personal information may have on the young adults' employment prospects.

ELECTRONIC HEALTH RECORDS

While not a form of social media, electronic health records (EHRs) are digital health records that can be shared electronically across providers.[44] Some EHRs also provide patient portals that allow a patient, or a patient proxy, to communicate with the health care provider and access personal health information. Thus, EHRs may share characteristics with social media in allowing AYAs increased opportunities to communicate, connect, and share information. AYAs frequently go online to access health information, including information about sexually transmitted infections, nutrition, exercise, and sexuality.[45] Given AYA's comfort with seeking health information online, and high rates of Internet access and use, this group is poised to uniquely benefit from increasing rates of EHR use.[3,46]

EHRs are now a national expectation for hospitals. Key characteristics of EHR systems include providing "lifelong, integrating information, controlled by the patient or family, private, secure and can facilitate communication between family and providers."[47] In 2007, only 1% of the population had access to an Internet-based EHR,[48] yet by 2011, up to 20% of physician offices provided EHR access.[49]

There are many potential benefits for AYAs having access to personal EHR portals. Studies have consistently shown health literacy benefits among adult patients who use online health systems, including obtaining prescription refills, asking nonurgent questions, and obtaining lab results.[50-59] Further, studies in adult patients have shown improved physician access, patient–physician relationship, and continuity of care.[54,59-63]

However, there are also barriers to access to EHR patient portals, particularly for adolescents. Many health care systems allow parents to have proxy access to their children's EHR during childhood. Often, access is blocked to both parents and patients when adolescents are between the ages of 13 and 17 due to concerns about confidentiality and consent.[64] In the US, adolescents who are legally considered minors may only consent to their own health care in certain circumstances, such as reproductive health or substance use treatment.[65,66] Release of information and access to such information for patients under age 18 is complicated and may vary state by state. In many cases, when a minor can legally provide consent for care, the adolescent minor may also be entitled to access medical records regarding that care.[67] Thus, for reproductive health care, an adolescent may have access to medical records and a parent may not because confidential adolescent health information may be legally protected from parent access. However, parents can access standard nonconfidential health information such as information about an ankle sprain, while it is unclear whether an adolescent has legal rights to access this information since the adolescent is not the individual consenting to care. These legal issues complicate the issue of adolescent access to their own standard health care records, as well as parental access to the teens' confidential health care records. Protecting adolescent privacy in large health care organizations that may provide coverage to multiple states with varying laws about adolescent privacy also presents a challenge.[64] Consulting with experts on this topic is critical in deciphering these issues.

Distinguishing standard medical information from protected or confidential adolescent health information remains a major challenge. At present, there is no widely available technology that can distinguish between confidential and standard medical record information. Addressing this concern may require creative solutions, such as allowing AYA patients to review their online medical information and sequester any information that can be legally protected as confidential; this could be done in the clinic setting or from a home computer.[64]

Given the rise of EHRs and the potential benefits in improving health care access and engagement by AYAs, the Society for Adolescent Health and Medicine published a position paper.[44] Key recommendations from this paper include that EHR design, implementation, and use need to address the needs of AYAs for access to health information and protection of confidentiality. Thus, EHR vendors need to develop systems that meet regulatory requirements and address the unique privacy needs of AYAs by building privacy settings into all aspects of their products. Further, health care systems implementing EHRs must provide training to all staff in techniques to protect confidential patient information as per national and state laws, as well as institutional policies.

- Providers working with AYAs should act as advocates for privacy in the implementation of EHRs used within their institutions. As AYAs are not typically advocates within health systems, it falls to their providers to advocate for systems that provide them the best quality care.
- Providers should also provide guidance to AYAs and their families on how to use an EHR including discussions about confidentiality.

⬤ CONCLUSION

In conclusion, technology and social media are an integral part of AYAs' lives. These tools are accessible, influential, and used in many ways throughout AYAs' daily life. Social media and technologies offer AYAs a new world of opportunities, as well as novel risks to their health and safety. Providers can apply a framework of balance, boundaries, and communication to counsel patients regarding their social media and technology use to maximize the benefits and minimize the risks of these novel tools. EHRs with patient portals offer many potential benefits to engage and involve AYAs in their health care; however, barriers exist in providing confidential care in the EHR realm.

REFERENCES

1. Palfrey J, Gasser U. *Born digital*. New York, NY: Basic Books, 2012.
2. O'Reilly T. *What is Web 2.0. 2005*. Available at http://oreilly.com/web2/archive/what-is-web-20.html. Accessed on April 23, 2015.
3. Madden M, Lenhart A, Duggan M, et al. *Teens and technology*. Washington, DC: Pew Research Center, 2013.
4. Duggan M, Smith A. *Social media update 2013*. Washington, DC: Pew Research Center, 2013.
5. Division of Information Technology. *Student computing survey report*. Madison, WI: University of Wisconsin, 2013.
6. Bandura A. *Social foundations of thought and action: a social cognitive theory*. Englewood Cliffs, NJ: Prentice Hall, 1986.
7. Borsari B, Carey KB. How the quality of peer relationships influences college alcohol use. *Drug Alcohol Rev* 2006;25(4):361–370.
8. Kinsman SB, Romer D, Furstenberg FF, et al. Early sexual initiation: the role of peer norms. *Pediatrics* 1998;102(5):1185–1192.
9. Reifman A, Watson WK. Binge drinking during the first semester of college: continuation and desistance from high school patterns. *J Am Coll Health* 2003;52(2):73–81.
10. Titus-Ernstoff L, Dalton MA, Adachi-Mejia AM, et al. Longitudinal study of viewing smoking in movies and initiation of smoking by children. *Pediatrics* 2008;121(1):15–21.
11. Fogg BJ. Mass interpersonal persuasion: an early view of a new phenomenon. In: *Third international conference on persuasive technology*. Berlin, Germany: Springer, 2008:23–34.
12. Moreno MA, Kota R, Schoohs S, et al. The Facebook influence model: a concept mapping approach. *Cyberpsychol Behav Soc Netw* 2013;16(7):504–511.
13. Ahn J. The effect of social network sites on adolescents' social and academic development: current theories and controversies. *J Am Soc Inf Sci Technol* 2011;62(8):1435–1445.
14. Rajani R, Berman DS, Rozanski A. Social networks—are they good for your health? The era of Facebook and Twitter. *QJM* 2011;104:819–820.
15. Lee EB. Young, black, and connected: Facebook usage among African American college students. *J Black Stud* 2012;43(3):336–354.
16. Beaumont E, Colby A, Erhrlich T, et al. Promoting political competence and engagement in college students: an empirical study. *J Polit Sci Educ* 2006;2(3):249–270.
17. Selkie EM, Benson M, Moreno M. Adolescents' views regarding uses of social networking websites and text messaging for adolescent sexual health education. *Am J Health Educ* 2011;42(4):205–212.
18. Rideout VJ, Foehr UG, Roberts D. *Generation M2: media in the lives of 8 to 18 year olds*. Menlo Park, CA: Kaiser Family Foundation, 2010.
19. Moreno MA, Kelleher E, Rastogi S, et al. Young adult females' views regarding online privacy protection at two time points. *J Adolesc Health* 2014; 55(3):347–51.
20. Moreno MA, Parks MR, Zimmerman FJ, et al. Display of health risk behaviors on MySpace by adolescents: prevalence and associations. *Arch Pediatr Adolesc Med* 2009;163(1):35–41.
21. Egan KG, Moreno MA. Alcohol references on undergraduate males' Facebook profiles. *Am J Mens Health* 2011;5(5):413–420.
22. Debatin B, Lovejoy JP, Horn AK, et al. Facebook and online privacy: attitudes, behaviors, and unintended consequences. *J Comput-Mediat Commun* 2009;15(1):83–108.
23. Moreno MA, Grant A, Kacvinsky L, et al. Older adolescents' views regarding participant in Facebook research. *J Adolesc Health* 2012;51:439–444.
24. Lichtblau E, Risen J. Officials say US Wiretaps exceeded law. *New York Times*. 2009.
25. Moreno MA, Briner LR, Williams A, et al. Real use or "real cool": adolescents speak out about displayed alcohol references on social networking websites. *J Adolesc Health* 2009;45(4):420–422.
26. Moreno M, Swanson M, Royer H, et al. Sexpectations: male college students' views about displayed sexual references on females' social networking web sites. *J Pediatr Adolesc Gynecol* 2011;24:85–89.
27. Peebles R, Wilson JL, Litt IF, et al. Disordered eating in a digital age: eating behaviors, health, and quality of life in users of websites with pro-eating disorder content. *J Med Internet Res* 2012;14(5):e148.
28. Temple JR, Choi H. Longitudinal association between teen sexting and sexual behavior. *Pediatrics* 2014;134(5):X15.
29. National Campaign to Prevent Teen and Unplanned Pregnancy. *Sex and tech: results of a survey of teens and young adults*. Washington, DC: National Campaign to Prevent Teen and Unplanned Pregnancy, 2008.
30. Dowdell EB, Burgess AW, Flores JR. Online social networking patterns among adolescents, young adults, and sexual offenders. *Am J Nurs* 2011;111(7):28–36.
31. Hinduja S, Patchin JW. *State sexting laws*. Cyberbullying Research Center, 2014. http://cyberbullying.us/state-cyberbullying-laws-a-brief-review-of-state-cyber-bullying-laws-and-policies/
32. Temple JR, Le VD, van den Berg P, et al. Brief report: teen sexting and psychosocial health. *J Adolesc* 2014;37(1):33–36.
33. Mishna F, Cook C, Gadalla T, et al. Cyber bullying behaviors among middle and high school students. *Am J Orthopsychiatry* 2010;80:362–374.
34. Perren S, Dooley J, Shaw T, et al. Bullying in school and cyberspace: associations with depressive symptoms in Swiss and Australian adolescents. *Child Adolesc Psychiatry Ment Health* 2010;4:28.
35. Li Q. A cross-cultural comparison of adolescents' experience related to cyberbullying. *Educ Res* 2008;50(2):223–234.
36. Juvonen J, Gross EF. Extending the school grounds?—Bullying experiences in cyberspace. *J Sch Health* 2008;78(9):496–505.
37. Molluzzo JC, Lawler J. A study of the perceptions of college students on cyberbullying. *Inf Syst Educ J* 2012;10(4):84.
38. Zapf D, Einarsen S, Hoel H, et al. Empirical findings on bullying in the workplace. In: Einarsen S, Hoel H, Zapf D, Cooper C, eds. *Bullying and emotional abuse in the workplace: international perspectives on research and practice*. London, UK: Taylor and Francis, 2003.
39. Moreno MA, Jelenchick LA. Problematic internet use among older adolescents: a conceptual framework. *J Adolesc Health* 2013;52(2):S86–S86.
40. Moreno MA, Jelenchick LA, Young H, et al. Problematic internet use among US youth: a systematic review. *Arch Pediatr Adolesc Med* 2011;165(9):797–805.
41. Moreno MA, Jelenchick L, Koff R, et al. Internet use and multitasking among older adolescents: an experience sampling approach. *Comp Hum Behav* 2012;28:1097–1102.
42. Moreno MA. *Sex, drugs 'n Facebook*. Alameda, CA: Hunter House, 2013.
43. Jelenchick LA, Eickhoff J, Christakis DA, et al. The problematic and risky internet use screening scale (PRIUSS) for adolescents and young adults: development and refinement. *Comput Hum Behav* 2014;35:171–178.
44. Haryden Gray S, Pasternake R, Gooding H, et al. Recommendations for electronic health record use for delivery of adolescent health care. *J Adolesc Health* 2014;54(4):487–490.
45. Borzekowski D, Rickert V. Adolescent cybersurfing for health information: a new resource that crosses barriers. *Arch Pediatr Adolesc Med* 2001;155(7):813–817.
46. Anoshiravani A, Gaskin G, Groshek M, et al. Special requirements for electronic medical records in adolescent medicine. *J Adolesc Health* 2012;51:409–414.
47. Britto MT, Wimberg J. Pediatric personal health records: current trends and key challenges. *Pediatrics* 2009;123 (suppl 2):S97–S99.
48. Bright B. Benefits of electronic health records seen as outweighing privacy risks. *Wall Street J*. November 29, 2007.
49. Wynia MK, Torres GW, Lemieux J. Many physicians are willing to use patients' electronic personal health records, but doctors differ by location, gender, and practice. *Health Aff (Millwood)* 2011;30(2):266–273.
50. Couchman GR, Forjuoh SN, Rascoe TG. E-mail communications in family practice: what do patients expect? *J Fam Pract* 2001;50(5):414–418.
51. Couchman GR, Forjuoh SN, Rascoe TG, et al. E-mail communications in primary care: what are patients' expectations for specific test results? *Int J Med Inform* 2005;74(1):21–30.
52. Ferguson T. Digital doctoring—opportunities and challenges in electronic patient-physician communication. *J Am Med Assoc* 1998;280(15):1361–1362.
53. Fridsma DB, Ford P, Altman R. A survey of patient access to electronic mail: attitudes, barriers, and opportunities. *Proc Annu Symp Comput Appl Med Care* 1994:15–19.
54. Hassol A, Walker JM, Kidder D, et al. Patient experiences and attitudes about access to a patient electronic health care record and linked web messaging. *J Am Med Inform Assoc* 2004;11(6):505–513.
55. Honeyman A, Cox B, Fisher B. Potential impacts of patient access to their electronic care records. *Inform Primary Care* 2005;13(1):55–60.
56. Neill RA, Mainous AG, Clark JR, et al. The utility of electronic mail as a medium for patient-physician communication. *Arch Fam Med* 1994;3(3):268–271.
57. Neinstein L. Utilization of electronic communication (E-mail) with patients at university and college health centers. *J Adolesc Health* 2000;27(1):6–11.
58. Sittig DF. Results of a content analysis of electronic messages (email) sent between patients and their physicians. *BMC Med Inform Decis Mak* 2003;3:11.
59. Ralston JD, Carrell D, Reid R, et al. Patient web services integrated with a shared medical record: patient use and satisfaction. *J Am Med Inform Assoc* 2007;14(6):798–806.
60. Taylor H, Leitman R. *Study reveals big potential for the internet to improve doctor-patient relations*. 2001 [cited December 14, 2007]. Available at http://www.harrisinteractive.com/news/newsletters/healthnews/HI_HealthCareNews-V1-Issue1.pdf.
61. Liederman EM, Lee JC, Baquero VH, et al. Patient-physician web messaging: the impact on message volume and satisfaction. *J Gen Intern Med* 2005;20(1):52–57.
62. Katz SJ, Nissan N, Moyer CA. Crossing the digital divide: evaluating online communication between patients and their providers. *Am J Manag Care* 2004;10(9):593–598.
63. Balas EA, Jaffrey F, Kuperman GJ, et al. Electronic communication with patients. Evaluation of distance medicine technology. *J Am Med Assoc* 1997;278(2):152–159.
64. Moreno MA, Ralston JR, Grossman DC. Adolescent access to online health services: perils and promise. *J Adolesc Health* 2009;44:244–251.
65. English A, Kenney KE. *State minor consent laws: a summary*. Chapel Hill, NC: Center for Adolescent Health and the Law, 2003.
66. Boonstra H, Nash E. *Minors and the right to consent to health care*. 2000 [cited 2008 January 14]; Available at www.guttmacher.org. Accessed on April 23, 2015.
67. Health Insurance Portability and Accountability Act of 1996 (HIPAA). Federal Register, 1996.

📶 ADDITIONAL RESOURCES AND WEBSITES ONLINE

Endocrine Problems

11

Abnormal Growth and Development

M. Joan Mansfield
Jonathan M. Swartz

This chapter focuses on the adolescent whose growth and/or development falls outside the range of normal. These issues are usually of enormous concern to adolescents and their family, and the health care provider must have a clear understanding of how to evaluate and manage these problems. In evaluating growth during adolescence, it is necessary to assess whether a teen has reached puberty, whether puberty is proceeding normally, and whether the bony epiphyses are still open to permit further growth.

SHORT STATURE WITHOUT DELAYED PUBERTY

Adolescents who are progressing normally through puberty may present with concerns about short stature. Most of these teens have genetic or familial short stature with other major categories including chronic disease, constitutional delay of growth and development, and endocrine diseases. Girls who are short may seek medical attention for this complaint when they have just reached menarche and worry that future growth in height will be limited. Boys may present as their pubertal growth spurt slows and they are still shorter than they had hoped. Most hormonal deficiencies, chronic diseases, and malabsorptive states that slow growth will also cause at least some delay in puberty or failure to progress normally through puberty; these are less likely causes for the short stature in teens who have normal puberty.

Definition of Short Stature

Adult height is strongly dictated by genetic factors; therefore, evaluation of short stature must be assessed considering the heights of family members. Generally, 2 standard deviation (SD) (2.3 percentile) below the mean height on a cross-sectional growth chart is used as the lower limit of normal.

Criteria for Evaluation An adolescent should be considered for an evaluation of short stature if:

1. Linear growth rate is <4 cm/year during the years prior to the normal age for peak linear growth velocity.
2. No evidence of a peak linear growth velocity by age 16 years in boys and 14 years in girls.
3. Deceleration below an individual's established growth velocity occurs.
4. The adolescent's height is more than 2 SDs below the calculated midparental height (see Chapter 2).

5. The adolescent's height is more than 3 SDs below the mean. Consideration should be given to carrying out a full evaluation if an adolescent's height is between 2 and 3 SDs below the mean; at a minimum, a careful history and physical examination, screening laboratory tests, and observation of growth for 6 months are warranted.

Differential Diagnosis

1. Familial short stature
2. Chronic illness—can include diseases such as cystic fibrosis, human immunodeficiency virus (HIV) infection, severe asthma, congestive heart failure, renal failure, inflammatory bowel disease, celiac disease, among others
3. Constitutional delay of puberty
4. Endocrine—can include hypothyroidism, isolated growth hormone (GH) deficiency, hypercortisolism, adrenal insufficiency, and poorly controlled diabetes mellitus
5. Congenital syndromes including Down syndrome (trisomy 21), Turner syndrome (45X), Noonan, Hurler, Silver–Russell syndrome, Laron syndrome (GH receptor gene mutations), short stature homeobox gene (SHOX) deficiency
6. Intrauterine growth retardation or small for gestational age
7. Skeletal dysplasias—including chondrodysplasias (often have abnormally short extremities)

Evaluation

History

1. Maternal pregnancy history—medical illnesses and medication use
2. Birth weight and length, and estimate of gestational age—important because premature infants with appropriate small weight tend to have a normal growth potential, whereas infants with intrauterine growth retardation who are inappropriately small for gestational age may not have catch-up growth
3. Complete review of systems:
   a. Renal—polyuria and polydipsia for hypothalamic and/or pituitary disorders
   b. Cardiac—peripheral edema, murmurs, and cyanosis
   c. Gastrointestinal—diarrhea, flatulence (malabsorption), vomiting, and/or abdominal pain
   d. Pulmonary—sleep apnea, asthma, or symptoms suggestive of cystic fibrosis
   e. Neurological—headaches, visual field defects suggesting pituitary neoplasms
4. Growth history—review of symptoms and growth charts
5. Family history—adult height, and patterns of growth and puberty in first- and second-degree relatives
6. Dietary history

Physical Examination

A complete physical examination is the next step in the evaluation and should include:

1. Height and weight (including growth measurements that are plotted on appropriate developmental charts for height, weight, and body mass index [BMI])
2. Arm span and upper-to-lower (U/L) body-segment ratio
3. Sexual maturity ratings (SMRs)—specifically breast and genital development, and not pubic hair only
4. A general physical examination, with special attention to the thyroid gland, ophthalmological examination, neurological examination, and stigmata of congenital syndromes

Laboratory/Radiologic Evaluation

The laboratory evaluation of short stature should include the following:

1. Routine laboratory screening: Includes complete blood cell (CBC) count with differential, sedimentation rate, urinalysis (under age 3), chemistry profile including serum creatinine, insulin-like growth factor-1 (IGF-1), and thyroid-stimulating hormone (TSH) and free thyroxine (free T_4). Screening for celiac disease with total immunoglobulin A and anti-tissue transglutaminase is also advised in asymptomatic short children.
2. Bone age: X-ray of the left hand and wrist for bone age (since the bone age can determine if there is more potential for growth and be used to estimate predicted final height).[1]
3. Midparental height calculation: It is also useful to obtain the parents' heights and calculate a midparental height (formula provided in Chapter 2). Although there are many genes involved in stature, and an offspring's height frequently varies considerably from midparental height, the midparental or target height can still give a good clue that the short stature is genetic.
4. Karyotype: A karyotype is useful when signs of Turner syndrome are present, as well as in girls with unexplained short stature and otherwise normal labs. It can also be useful in boys with genital anomalies.
5. Other tests: Other tests may be indicated depending on the history and physical examination and may include:
   a. Central imaging studies—cranial magnetic resonance imaging (MRI) with contrast
   b. Gastrointestinal studies
   c. Endocrine studies:
      (1) Serum levels of IGF-1 and insulin-like growth factor-binding protein 3 (IGFBP-3) are often assessed when the growth pattern is concerning for GH deficiency. IGFBP-3 can be useful in underweight or nutritionally deficient children who have low IGF-1 levels.
      (2) GH stimulation testing is usually done by a pediatric endocrinologist using one of several protocols (insulin, glucagon, arginine, L-dopa, or clonidine). Two tests are usually carried out together and the patient is considered GH deficient if the GH response is <7 to 10 ng/mL on both tests. In prepubertal adolescents, priming with estrogen (in males and females) before stimulation testing should be considered for maximal GH release.
   d. Genetic testing: SHOX testing may be considered when a constellation of typical features are present such as short stature, increased upper/lower segment ratio, reduced arm span-to-forearm length ratio, cubitus valgus, Madelung wrist deformity, forearm bowing, short metacarpals or metatarsals, apparent muscular hypertrophy, increased BMI, high arched palate, abnormal auricular development, micrognathia, or short neck.[2]

Suggestions for Diagnosis

1. Constitutional delay of puberty: Most short stature in adolescents is the result of either constitutional delay of puberty or familial short stature. Guidelines for diagnosis are outlined later in this chapter.
2. Genetic or familial short stature: Genetic or familial stature is suggested by the following:
   a. Normal history and physical examination findings
   b. Family history of short stature
   c. Growth curve that generally parallels the 3rd percentile
   d. Bone age that is appropriate for chronological age
3. Chronic illness: Chronic renal disease and Crohn's disease are additional causes of short stature. These diseases are usually diagnosed by an abnormal history, physical examination findings, or results of tests including screening CBC, sedimentation rate, urinalysis, and chemistry studies. Renal tubular acidosis can be overlooked as a cause of short stature, especially in children under 3. This process may be suggested by family history, urine pH level, or serum bicarbonate values.
4. Endocrine causes: Endocrine causes of short stature, such as hypothyroidism, GH deficiency, adrenal insufficiency, and adrenocortical excess, are less common. Hypothyroidism and adrenocortical excess can usually be detected by the patient's history, physical examination including a growth chart, or screening laboratory tests. Adolescents with classic GH deficiency can be difficult to differentiate from those with constitutional delay of puberty. This is particularly difficult during the time of expected peak linear growth velocity, when the growth of an adolescent with constitutional delay of puberty slows from the normal growth curve as other adolescents accelerate their growth velocities. Individuals with classic GH deficiency have normal body proportions and often a high-pitched voice, a tendency toward hypoglycemia, a microphallus in boys, a child-like face, soft and finely wrinkled skin, and a large prominent forehead.

Treatment of Short Stature with GH

GH Deficiency

Patients with classic GH deficiency have marked benefit in statural outcome as the result of GH treatment. In addition, those with complete GH deficiency benefit from treatment (from the metabolic effects of GH) with regard to improving bone density, decreasing fat mass, and improving muscle strength, even if epiphyseal fusion has been achieved. It appears that these subjects should continue GH treatment at a markedly reduced dose, compared with that used for growth augmentation, throughout life.

Bioengineered human GH has been available since the 1980s. Patients with classical GH deficiency usually present with extreme short stature and slow growth (<4 cm/year) well before adolescence, although acquired GH deficiency, sometimes due to head trauma or tumors, may present in adolescence with slow growth and relatively delayed puberty.[3]

Other Conditions

Turner Syndrome: GH has been used to increase height velocity and increase final adult height in patients who do not have GH deficiency by GH stimulation tests. GH is approved for use in patients with short stature due to Turner syndrome using a higher dose than is recommended for GH deficiency (0.05 mg/kg/day subcutaneously or 0.35 mg/kg/week for Turner syndrome). IGF-1, thyroid screens, and bone ages by x-ray are monitored during therapy. Patients with Turner syndrome should have baseline renal ultrasonography and periodic cardiac MRI and echocardiograms to screen for aortic root enlargement. Aortic dissection is a rare but potentially fatal cause of severe chest pain in patients with Turner syndrome. GH treatment should ideally be initiated early in childhood when growth rate begins to fall off. Estrogen replacement is usually delayed to age 12 to 14 or sometimes later to maximize height gain in patients with Turner syndrome. GH can also be used similarly in Noonan syndrome.

Intrauterine Growth Retardation: GH is also approved by the US Food and Drug Administration (FDA) for use in patients with short stature due to intrauterine growth retardation without catch-up growth, Prader–Willi syndrome, and chronic renal failure before transplantation. GH has also been approved for treatment of children and adolescents with idiopathic short stature who are more than 2.25 SD below the mean in height and who are unlikely to catch up in height.[4-7] Patients who qualify for a trial of treatment with human GH for idiopathic short stature must have open epiphyses permitting further height gain. Patients with severe short stature who desire treatment with GH should be referred to a pediatric endocrinologist.

 DELAYED PUBERTY

Review of Normal Development

The pattern of normal puberty is discussed in detail in Chapter 2.

Definition

In general, 2 SDs above and below the mean are used to define the range of normal variability. Chapter 2 is helpful in determining guidelines for evaluation, and further guidelines are discussed subsequently.

Delayed development is defined by the absence of breast budding by age 13 in girls or the lack of testicular enlargement by age 14 in boys, both 2.5 SD beyond the average age at onset of these changes. Alterations in the chronological relationship of pubertal events are also common causes for evaluation. These include phallic enlargement in the absence of testicular enlargement in boys or the absence of menarche by age 16, or 4 years after the onset of breast development, in girls. If puberty is interrupted, there is a regression or failure to progress in the development of secondary sexual characteristics, accompanied by a slowing in growth rate.

General Guidelines for Evaluating Puberty
In Males

A male adolescent may be considered to have delayed puberty if:

1. Genital stage 1 persists beyond the age of 13.7 years, or pubic hair stage 1 (PH1) persists beyond the age of 15.1 years.
2. More than 5 years have elapsed from initiation to completion of genital growth.

In Females

A female adolescent may be considered to have delayed maturation if:

1. Breast stage 1 persists beyond the age of 13.4 years, PH1 persists beyond the age of 14.1 years, or there is failure to menstruate beyond the age of 16 years.
2. More than 5 years have elapsed between initiation of breast growth and menarche.

These general guidelines must be considered in the context of the teen's family history as to growth and pubertal development, his or her previous growth pattern, and with regard to the review of systems and physical examination.

Differential Diagnosis

Delayed development occurs more commonly in boys than in girls. Most patients who present for an evaluation of slow growth and delayed development are high school–aged boys who are concerned about their short stature, as well as their lack of muscular and secondary sexual development, which puts them at a disadvantage among their peers. Most of these boys have constitutionally delayed development; however, the clinical presentation of the patient with constitutional delay may be indistinguishable from that of the patient whose pubertal delay is the result of an organic lesion.

Constitutional Delay of Puberty

Adolescents with constitutional delay of puberty have often been slow growers throughout childhood. In the absence of sex steroids of puberty, growth may slow even further to <5 cm/year as these children reach an age when puberty would normally occur. Growth velocity increases into the normal range when these teens finally enter puberty. Adolescents with constitutional delay of puberty often have a family history of delayed growth and development in relatives. Teens with constitutional delay of puberty eventually enter puberty on their own. Although they have a longer time to grow before their epiphyses close, they tend to have a less exuberant growth spurt than earlier developers so that their final height is often shorter than average.

Functional Causes of Delayed Puberty

Gonadotropin-releasing hormone (GnRH) secretion can be inhibited centrally by the following:

1. Inadequate nutrition, including eating disorders
2. Chronic disease including chronic heart disease, severe asthma, inflammatory bowel disease, celiac disease, rheumatoid arthritis, chronic renal failure, renal tubular acidosis, sickle cell anemia, diabetes mellitus, systemic lupus erythematosus, cystic fibrosis, and infection with HIV
3. Severe environmental stress
4. Intensive athletic training
5. Hypothyroidism and excess cortisol states
6. Drugs such as opiates and stimulants

Eating disorders associated with self-imposed restriction of caloric intake can delay or interrupt the progression of puberty. Anorexia nervosa most often develops in girls in early to middle adolescence, who have already entered puberty. Young adolescent boys or girls who are dieting because of fear of obesity may present with the complaint of delayed development. Crohn's disease or celiac disease may also present with delayed development and poor growth as the major symptoms. Since adolescence is normally a period of rapid growth and weight gain, failure to gain or small amounts of weight loss may be manifestations of significant nutritional insufficiency. Poor growth and delayed puberty are common in cystic fibrosis, thalassemia major, renal tubular acidosis, renal failure, cyanotic congenital heart disease, sickle cell anemia, systemic lupus erythematosus, acquired immune deficiency syndrome, or very poorly controlled asthma or type 1 diabetes mellitus. Patients who are on stimulants such as methylphenidate (Ritalin) for treatment of attention deficit disorder may have decreased appetite because of the medication and slower growth rates as a result of nutritional insufficiency.

Hypothyroidism may present in an adolescent with slowing of height velocity (height-dropping percentiles on the growth chart) whose weight is well preserved for height or who is mildly overweight, sometimes with delayed or interrupted pubertal development. The classic signs include dull dry skin, perhaps with scalp hair loss, decrease in pulse rate and blood pressure, constipation, and cold intolerance. A goiter is not always present. Autoimmune thyroiditis is the most common cause of hypothyroidism in teens. There may be a family history of hypothyroidism or autoimmune issues.

Cushing syndrome (endogenous glucocorticoid overproduction) or chronic exposure to high doses of glucocorticoids for medical treatment causes excessive weight gain, slowing of height velocity, and may interrupt or delay puberty or, if endogenous sex steroid production is also increased, may present with precocious puberty without a growth spurt (Fig.11.1).

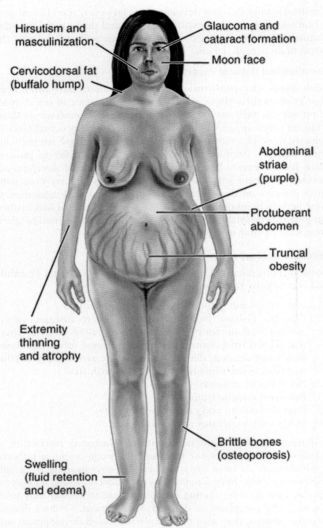

Hirsutism and masculinization

Glaucoma and cataract formation

Moon face

Cervicodorsal fat (buffalo hump)

Abdominal striae (purple)

Protuberant abdomen

Truncal obesity

Extremity thinning and atrophy

Brittle bones (osteoporosis)

Swelling (fluid retention and edema)

FIGURE 11.1 Typical features consistent with Cushing syndrome including central and cervical adiposity, moon face, thin extremities, along with violaceous striae. Hirsutism can be noted in females. (From Diane SA, Samantha JV. *Drug therapy in nursing.* 4th ed. Philadelphia, PA: Lippincott Williams & Wilkins, 2011.)

Hypothalamic Causes of Delayed or Absent Puberty

The ability of the hypothalamus to secrete GnRH may be damaged by:

1. Local tumors (germinomas, craniopharyngiomas, astrocytomas, or gliomas)
2. Infiltrative lesions such as central nervous system (CNS) leukemia or histiocytosis X
3. CNS irradiation
4. Traumatic gliosis
5. Mass lesions such as brain abscesses or granulomas due to sarcoidosis or tuberculosis
6. Congenital defects in the ability to secrete GnRH (including isolated hypogonadotropic hypogonadism and Kallman syndrome). Recent studies have confirmed a number of genes involved in cases of hypogonadotropic hypogonadism including but is not limited to GNRHR, KISS1R, TAC3, TACR3, GnRH1, KAL1, FGFR1, PROK2, PROKR2, FGF8, CHD7, WDR11, and NELF.[8]
7. Congenital brain malformations associated with inability to secrete GnRH include septooptic dysplasia.

Pituitary Causes of Delayed Puberty

Puberty may not begin or may fail to proceed if the pituitary cannot respond to GnRH stimulation with luteinizing hormone (LH) and follicle-stimulating hormone (FSH) production. This may be due to:

1. Pituitary tumor
2. Selective impairment of gonadotrope function by hemochromatosis
3. Congenital hypopituitarism, which is usually diagnosed either in the neonatal period or with poor growth during childhood; causes include genetic defects that interfere with pituitary formation and empty sella syndrome.
4. Acquired hypopituitarism
5. Prolactinoma—excessive prolactin production by a pituitary adenoma (prolactinoma) or other tumor may interrupt or prevent puberty by interfering with gonadotropin production. Patients with prolactinomas most often present with secondary amenorrhea often with galactorrhea, but may present with stalled puberty. Headaches are sometimes present. Prolactinomas are more common in girls than boys, but can occur in both. Psychotropic drugs such as antipsychotics are a frequent cause of hyperprolactinemia.

Gonadal Failure

If the gonads are unable to respond to LH and FSH, puberty will not proceed.

The causes of gonadal failure with abnormal karyotype include:

1. Gonadal dysgenesis: The most common cause of gonadal failure is gonadal dysgenesis, which occurs in association with abnormalities of sex chromosomes. The gonads fail to develop and become rudimentary streaks. These patients are phenotypic females with normal immature female genitalia. The most common phenotype is Turner syndrome, which is caused by absence of part or all of a second sex chromosome. These patients are typically short with a final untreated height averaging 143 cm. Other identifying features of Turner syndrome are low-set ears, a webbed neck, widely spaced nipples, a trident hairline, an increased carrying angle of the lower arms, and short fourth and fifth fingers and toes. Renal abnormalities such as duplications and horseshoe kidney, and left-sided cardiovascular abnormalities such as bicuspid aortic valve, dilatation of the aortic root and coarctation of the aorta are also associated with Turner syndrome. Half of these patients have 45, X karyotypes, whereas the rest are mosaics or have various X chromosome abnormalities or deletions.
2. Klinefelter syndrome: Males with Klinefelter syndrome (47, XXY) may present with poorly progressing puberty caused by partial gonadal failure. Their testes can make some testosterone when driven by high levels of gonadotropins (LH and FSH) and they tend to have significantly impaired sperm production.[9] In the 47, XXY patient with pubertal development, the testes become small and firm because they become fibrotic. Gynecomastia and eunuchoid body habitus are often seen.

The causes of gonadal failure with normal karyotype include:

1. Acquired gonadal disorders
   a. Infection—viral or tubercular orchitis or oopheritis
   b. Trauma—bilateral testicular torsion resulting in anorchia is another cause of gonadal failure in males
   c. Postsurgical removal
   d. Radiation, chemotherapy with agents such as cyclophosphamide
   e. Autoimmune oophoritis or orchitis (sometimes with multiple autoimmune endocrine abnormalities)
   f. The resistant ovary syndrome
   g. Sarcoidosis

h. Fragile X may present as secondary amenorrhea in females with ovarian failure

i. Cryptorchidism—in males who are cryptorchid, the testes may fail to function, particularly if they remain intra-abdominal beyond infancy

2. Congenital gonadal disorders
   a. Anorchism: In the "vanishing testis syndrome," the testes are absent in a phenotypic male, presumably as a result of destruction in utero.
   b. Pure gonadal dysgenesis: This presents as absent puberty in patients with a normal karyotype (46, XX or 46, XY), normal stature, and a female phenotype.
   c. Enzyme defects in androgen and estrogen production: Enzymatic defects, such as 17α-hydroxylase or 20,22-desmolase deficiency, which render the gonad unable to produce estrogens or androgens, are other rare causes of primary gonadal failure. No specific cause for gonadal failure can be found in many cases.
   d. Gonadal failure is associated with other diseases such as congenital galactosemia in girls and ataxia telangiectasia.

3. Androgen-receptor defects
   a. Complete androgen insensitivity (previously referred to as "testicular feminization") presents as a patient who is a phenotypic female with tall stature, absence of sexual hair, normal breast development and timing of puberty, but absence of menarche. The vagina is a short pouch and there is no uterus. The karyotype is 46, XY, and testosterone levels are elevated.
   b. Partial androgen insensitivity (previously referred to as a variety of syndromes, including Reifenstein syndrome).

Syndromes Associated with Pubertal Delay

There are several syndromes that are characterized by extreme obesity, short stature, and delayed puberty. These include the following:

1. Prader–Willi (extreme obesity, developmental delay, small hands and feet, and chromosome 15 deletion) (Fig. 11.2)
2. Bardet–Biedl syndrome (obesity, polydactyly, retinitis pigmentosa, genital hypoplasia, developmental delay) (Fig. 11.3)
3. Borjeson–Forseeman–Lehman (obesity, severe mental deficiency, microcephaly, epilepsy, and skeletal anomalies)

Another congenital syndrome is congenital absence of the uterus and upper vagina (Mayer–Rokintansky–Kuster–Hauser syndrome). This is associated with normal puberty, but absent menses.

WORK-UP OF DELAYED PUBERTY

Most adolescents with delayed maturation have constitutional delay of puberty. However, this diagnosis is made by excluding other causes of delayed puberty. Following is a discussion of the evaluation of the adolescent with delayed puberty, including criteria for a provisional diagnosis of constitutional delay of puberty. A detailed history and physical examination will help focus and minimize the laboratory testing needed to evaluate an adolescent with delayed development.

History

1. Neonatal history: The neonatal history should include birth weight, history of previous maternal miscarriages, and congenital lymphedema (Turner syndrome). The past medical history should focus on any history of chronic disease, congenital anomalies, previous surgery, radiation exposure, chemotherapy, or drug use.
2. Growth records: Past growth measurements that are plotted on appropriate developmental charts for height, weight, and BMI are important in evaluating the adolescent with delayed puberty. The overall pattern of growth and changes in that

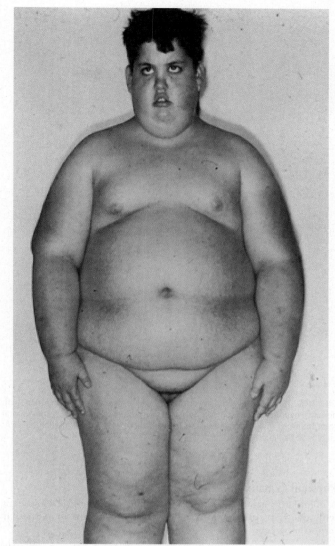

FIGURE 11.2 Some of the features of Prader–Willi syndrome include severe obesity, hypogonadism, and developmental delay. (From Sadler TW. *Langman's medical embryology*. 12th ed. Philadelphia, PA: Lippincott Williams & Wilkins, 2011.)

pattern often lead to a diagnosis. The child whose delayed puberty is associated with a nutritional deficiency due to an eating disorder, inflammatory bowel disease, celiac disease, or other chronic disease will show a greater decline in weight gain than in height and be underweight for height. In contrast, the child who has delayed puberty on the basis of an endocrinopathy such as acquired hypothyroidism or gonadal dysgenesis will have a greater slowing in height gain than in weight gain, and have weight well preserved for height, often being mildly overweight.

3. Review of systems: Special attention should be paid to weight changes, dieting, environmental stress, exercise and athletics, gastrointestinal symptoms, headache, neurological symptoms (including abnormal peripheral vision and anosmia), and symptoms suggestive of thyroid disease.
4. Nutritional history and eating habits: This helps to discount a problem of chronic malnutrition.
5. Family history: The family history should include the heights, and timing of secondary sexual development and fertility of family members, a history of anosmia, and a history of endocrine disorders.

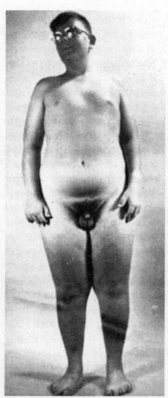

FIGURE 11.3 Bardet–Biedl syndrome. Nineteen-year-old young man with obesity, hypogonadism, polydactyly (toes), retinitis pigmentosa, and mental retardation. (From Lewis PR. *Merritt's neurology.* 11th ed. Philadelphia, PA: Lippincott Williams & Wilkins, 2005.)

Physical Examination

A complete physical examination is indicated for the adolescent with delayed puberty, but the following areas are of particular importance:

1. Overall nutritional status and measurements of height, weight, and vital signs
2. Body measurements including the following:
   a. Arm span
   b. Upper-to-lower segment ratio: This can be measured by measuring symphysis pubis to floor for lower, subtracting lower from total height for upper. This measurement can be useful for patients who have either short extremities (short bone syndromes, congenital short stature syndromes) or long extremities (eunuchoid appearance). The normal U/L ratio is 1.7 at birth, 1.0 at age 10 years, and 0.9 to 1.0 in adulthood in Caucasians, and 0.85 to 0.9 in African Americans. Untreated hypothyroidism will cause a U/L ratio to remain greater than 1.0, which would also be the case in most patients with chondrodysplasia. Hypogonadism will usually have a U/L ratio close to 0.9 or less. A normal ratio is often found in those with GH deficiency, constitutional delay of puberty, and chronic disease states.
3. Congenital anomalies, including midline facial defects
4. Staging of sexual maturity: The patient should be examined for a delay in pubertal development as assessed by staging of breast and pubic hair in girls, and genitalia and pubic hair in boys (see Chapter 2). Pubic hair may be present, although the genitalia are prepubertal in a boy who had normal adrenarche, but lacks gonadal activation. Any evidence of heterosexual development, such as clitoromegaly or hirsutism in girls or gynecomastia in boys, should be noted.

5. Thyroid: Check for evidence of goiter. Absence of goiter can be seen with hypothyroidism.
6. Chest: Check for evidence of chronic pulmonary disease.
7. Cardiac: Check for evidence of congenital heart disease.
8. Abdomen: Check for abdominal distension as a sign of a malabsorptive disease and check for evidence of liver or spleen enlargement as a sign of a chronic systemic disorder.
9. Genital examination: The examination of the external genitalia in girls should focus on obvious congenital anomalies and an assessment of estrogen effect. A pale pink vaginal mucosa with white secretion indicates the current presence of estrogen. A pelvic examination is not necessary as a part of the initial evaluation of a girl with delayed secondary sexual development, but an assessment of the depth of the vagina should be done if possible to rule out gynecological congenital anomalies in a girl who has normal pubertal development but delayed menarche. The examination should be carried out by a practitioner who is familiar with the techniques used for examining nonsexually active teen girls such as assessing the depth of the vagina with a saline-moistened cotton-tipped applicator, and considering a one-finger bimanual vaginal–abdominal examination if the vaginal introitus comfortably permits. If amenorrhea is a problem, then pelvic ultrasonography can be performed if needed to determine the presence of müllerian structures (uterus and tubes) and to visualize ovaries.[10]
10. Neurological examination: Ophthalmoscopic examination and visual field assessment are done to look for abnormalities of the optic nerves and signs of intracranial hypertension.

Laboratory Tests

Laboratory evaluation should be focused according to the clinical impression. In the patient who is underweight for height, studies would include screening tests for chronic disease or malabsorptive states such as celiac disease.

Bone Age

The most useful initial examination in delayed puberty and slow growth is often an x-ray of the left hand and wrist for a bone age assessment. This information can be used to assess how much height growth potential remains in the patient with short stature and delayed development. A predicted adult height can be obtained using the Bayley–Pinneau tables in the Atlas of Skeletal Maturation by Gruelich and Pyle.[11]

1. Constitutional delay of puberty: The patient with constitutional delay of puberty will usually have an equal delay of height age and bone age. Caution should be used in height predictions in patients with constitutional delay of puberty since boys with constitutional delay and short stature frequently reach a final height short of the final adult height predicted by the tables.
2. Delayed bone age: Patients with GH deficiency, hypothyroidism, and chronic disease usually have bone ages that are delayed several years behind their chronological age.
3. Normal bone age: Typically seen with familial short stature. Bone age may also be used in conjunction with height age and chronological age to give clues about a diagnosis as indicated below. Height age is determined by locating the corresponding age at which the patient's height would be equal to the 50th percentile.

Routine Laboratory Tests: Initial laboratory studies to be considered in the adolescent with delayed puberty include a CBC count, erythrocyte sedimentation rate (useful as a screening test for chronic illness such as inflammatory bowel disease) electrolytes, blood urea nitrogen, creatinine, glucose, calcium, phosphorus, albumin, liver enzymes, and urinalysis.

Evaluation for Celiac Disease: Evaluation for celiac disease (anti-tissue transglutaminase and total IgA) should be considered. More extensive testing for inflammatory bowel disease includes an upper gastrointestinal tract series with small bowel follow through and barium enema.

Central Imaging Studies: If there is a suspicion of a CNS tumor, cranial magnetic imaging with contrast is the best way to evaluate the hypothalamus and pituitary. A computed tomography scan is a less sensitive alternative.

Hormonal Tests: Hormonal tests to be considered include thyroid function tests (free T_4, TSH), prolactin, LH and FSH, dehydroepi-androsterone sulfate (DHEAS), testosterone or estradiol, and IGF-1 and IGFBP-3.

In the early stages (SMR 2) of puberty, breast budding and vaginal maturation in girls and penile and testicular enlargement in boys are more sensitive indicators of pubertal neuroendocrine-gonadal func-tion than a single daytime measurement of gonadotropin (LH and FSH) levels, estradiol, or testosterone. LH, FSH, and testosterone or estradiol may be in the prepubertal range on a daytime sample even though these hormones are actively being secreted at night. A first morning value to catch overnight activity is often more valuable in early puberty. Testosterone or estradiol levels may be valuable in following the patient whose puberty is not progressing normally by clinical assessment of growth and secondary sexual development.

GH is secreted primarily during sleep, so daytime levels are expected to be low. IGF-1 and IGFBP-3 are used to assess GH suffi-ciency. IGF-1 levels should be compared with normals for SMR stage or bone age rather than chronological age since the levels increase during puberty. IGF-1 levels are low in patients with nutritional insufficiency. Patients with delayed puberty and slow growth often have temporarily decreased GH secretion simply due to pubertal delay, which increases to normal as puberty begins. If GH deficiency is suspected, the patient should be referred to a pediatric endocri-nologist for GH stimulation testing. Patients with constitutional delay of puberty who are prepubertal may appear GH deficient on GH stimulation testing unless primed with estrogen before the test.

LH and FSH determinations are only useful if they are ele-vated since these hormones are secreted primarily during sleep in the early phases of puberty. Early to mid-pubertal levels (SMR B2) are indistinguishable from prepubertal levels, usually with a very low LH and FSH higher than LH. Elevated LH and FSH levels are suggestive of primary gonadal failure. If LH and FSH levels are elevated, further laboratory evaluation would include blood karyotyping in search of a chromosomal abnormality such as 45, X. Patients with gonadal dysgenesis who have Y chromosomal material present should have their gonads removed surgically because of an increased risk for gonadoblastoma. If the chromo-somes are normal in the patient with gonadal failure, anti-adrenal (21OHase) and anti-thyroid antibodies may be obtained to look for autoimmune issues associated with gonadal insufficiency. Pelvic ultrasonography may be used to visualize the uterus and ovaries, but should be interpreted with caution since the prepu-bertal uterus is small and may be missed on ultrasonography. A vaginal ultrasonography is usually postponed until adulthood.

If the initial prolactin level is elevated, it should be repeated without a breast examination on the day of the testing, and ideally in a fasting state. Patients with significantly elevated prolactin lev-els should have a cranial MRI with contrast.

Neuroendocrine Pharmacological Testing: If there is a question of multiple pituitary hormone defects, the patient may be referred to an endocrinologist for pharmacological and physiological tests of neuroendocrine function.

Constitutional Delay of Puberty

The chief diagnostic challenge in the patient with pubertal delay is to distinguish between constitutional delay and true GnRH

TABLE 11.1

Criteria for Provisional Diagnosis of Constitutional Delay of Puberty

Required Features

Detailed negative review of systems
Evidence of appropriate nutrition
Linear growth of at least 3.7 cm/y
Normal findings on physical examination, including genital anatomy, sense of smell, and U/L body-segment ratio
Normal CBC, sedimentation rate, urinalysis results, adjusted T_4 concentration, and prepubertal levels of serum LH and FSH
Bone age delayed 1.5–4.0 y compared with chronological age

Supportive Features

Family history of constitutional delay of puberty
Height between 3rd and 25th percentiles for chronological age

U/L, upper-to-lower; CBC, complete blood cell; LH, luteinizing hormone; FSH, follicle-stimulating hormone.

From Barnes HV. Recognizing normal and abnormal growth and development during puberty. In: Moss AV, ed. *Pediatrics update: reviews for physicians.* New York, NY: Elsevier–North Holland Publishing, 1979:103, with permission.

deficiency. About 90% to 95% of delayed puberty is constitutional delay of puberty. No single test reliably separates patients with constitutional delay from those with idiopathic hypogonadotropic hypogonadism.[12] This diagnosis is made by excluding the other causes, as discussed. However, using the guidelines in **Table 11.1**, one can confidently make a provisional diagnosis (**Table 11.1**).

Clues to Other Diagnoses

1. Gonadotropin deficiency
   a. Low serum FSH and LH levels, particularly if bone age is more than 13 years
   b. Low response to GnRH
   c. Abnormal central imaging study results
   d. History of neurological symptoms, CNS infections, radia-tion, or disease
   e. Possible anosmia (Kallmann syndrome)

The presence of midline facial defects, anosmia, cryptorchi-dism, or microphallus strongly suggests idiopathic hypogonado-tropic hypogonadism; however, the diagnosis cannot be firmly established until the patient reaches the age of 18 years and is still prepubertal. Genes for hypothalamic hypogonadism have been identified, as have some genes for familial pubertal delay.

2. Gonadal disorder
   a. History of gonadal radiation, surgery, infection, or trauma
   b. Significantly elevated FSH and LH
   c. Abnormal karyotype, such as 46, XY in a phenotypic girl
   d. Low U/L body-segment ratio
   e. Arm span may exceed height by >2 in
   f. Significant gynecomastia in a boy
   g. Testes that are small for a given stage of puberty can be associated with 47, XXY (Klinefelter syndrome) (Fig. 11.4)
3. Turner syndrome: Excluding constitutional delay of puberty, one of the more common causes of maturation delay is Turner syndrome. The patient may have a 45, X karyotype, a mosaic karyotype such as 45, X/46, XX or ring or isochromosomes. Patients with Turner syndrome usually have some of the fol-lowing characteristics:
   • Short stature
   • Streak gonads
   • Absent pubertal growth spurt
   • Poor development of secondary sexual characteristics, with less breast development than pubic hair development
   • Lymphedema

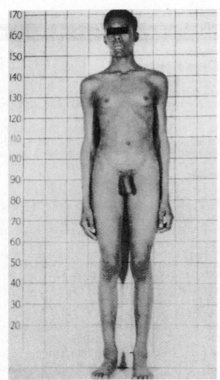

FIGURE 11.4 Klinefelter syndrome. Young man displaying typical features including gynecomastia, low U/L body-segment ratio, and normal phallic development. (From Theresa K, Susan C. *Essentials of pediatric nursing*. 2nd ed. Philadelphia, PA: Lippincott Williams & Wilkins, 2012.)

- Nail dysplasia
- High arched palate
- Strabismus
- Hearing deficit due to chronic otitis
- Cubitus valgus
- Webbing of the neck
- Low hairline
- Shield-shaped chest
- Coarctation of the aorta
- Horseshoe kidneys
- Short fourth metacarpal
- Multiple pigmented nevi
- Normal vagina, cervix, and uterus
- Poor space-form perception with normal overall intelligence

A karyotype is recommended in all girls with unexplained short stature, delayed puberty, webbed neck, lymphedema, or coarctation of the aorta.[13] Karyotype should also be considered for girls with a height below the 5th percentile and two or more features of Turner syndrome, such as high palate, nail dysplasia, short fourth metacarpal, and strabismus (Fig. 11.5).

4. Chronic illness
   a. Abnormal findings on review of systems or physical examination
   b. Falling off height and weight curves at onset of disease
   c. Abnormal CBC count, sedimentation rate, urinalysis results, or chemistry panel results

MANAGEMENT OF DELAYED PUBERTY

Observation every 6 months is appropriate before age 14 years in girls and age 16 years in boys, as long as there is no evidence of an underlying disease or neurological abnormality and the initial evaluation reveals normal prepubertal hormone levels. The young

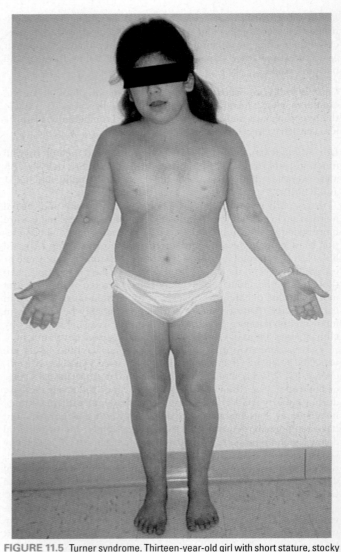

FIGURE 11.5 Turner syndrome. Thirteen-year-old girl with short stature, stocky build, crest chest, widely spaced nipples, lack of breast development, and cubitus valgus. (From Shulman D, Bercu B. *Atlas of clinical endocrinology: neuroendocrinology and pituitary disease*. Philadelphia, PA: Current Medicine, 2000.)

person should have interval measurements of growth, assessment of pubertal status by physical examination, and reassurance if progression of secondary sexual development is evident. There is no clinically available lab test that distinguishes constitutional delay from isolated hypogonadotropic hypogonadism, and close monitoring remains the best approach. After the first signs of testicular or breast enlargement are observed, follow-up at regular intervals is desirable to reassure the patient and parents that puberty is progressing. Since the testes begin to enlarge in males before increased testosterone production and increased growth velocity occur, support and guidance in dealing with the frustrations of delayed puberty are important, even after there is evidence that secondary sexual development has begun.

If the evaluation reveals primary gonadal failure, cyclic estrogen and progestin therapy in girls or testosterone therapy in boys will be necessary. Adolescents with hypogonadotropic hypogonadism or hypopituitarism will also need estrogen or testosterone replacement, often with replacement of other hormones as well. Short courses of estrogen or testosterone can also be used to initiate development in constitutional delay of puberty if there is no sign of development by age 14 in girls or 15 in boys.

Treatment for Girls

In girls, there are several regimens for replacing estrogen and progesterone. If growth is desired, estrogen is begun at a low dose, since height velocity is greater at low estrogen doses, and higher doses cause more rapid epiphyseal closure. The three phases of estrogen replacement are:

1. Induction of breast development and increase in height velocity in the patient with no secondary sexual development
2. Establishment of normal menses and increase in bone mineralization
3. Long-term maintenance of a normal estrogen state

Induction of Breast Development

In the first phase, a number of low-dose estrogen preparations have been used: oral estrogen regimens include conjugated estrogens (Premarin) 0.3 mg tablet or less (1/2 tablet) daily by mouth or 0.5 mg micronized estradiol (Estrace) for the first 6 to 12 months of treatment or until linear growth slows. Transdermal estradiol (6.25 to 25 µg) changed twice weekly is now the preferable option available for pubertal induction.[14,15] Certain patches (Vivelle dot) can be cut into ½ or ¼ size patches to deliver small initial doses of estrogen. Other patches cannot be cut.

Induction of Menses

In the second phase, the daily dose of estrogen is increased to 25 to 50 µg transdermal estradiol patch, or if oral estrogens are used 0.625 mg conjugated estrogens, or 1 mg micronized estradiol. After 2 to 3 months, a progestin such as medroxyprogesterone (Provera) 10 mg or micronized progesterone 200 mg is added initially 5 days each month.

Long-term Estrogen Replacement

In the third phase, 10 mg of medroxyprogesterone or other progestin is given 12 to 14 days a month to decrease the risk of endometrial hyperplasia. Estrogen regimens for long-term replacement include transdermal estradiol 75 to 100 µg 2×/week, oral conjugated estrogens 0.625 to 1.25 mg daily, ethinyl estradiol 20 to 35 µg daily, conjugated estrogens 0.625 to 1.25 mg daily, or micronized estradiol 1 to 2 mg daily. Once growth is complete, replacement can be given as a combined estrogen–progestin preparation.

Oral estrogens pass first through the liver, which could theoretically increase side effects. Transdermal alternatives include estradiol patches (Vivelle dot, Climera, Alora, and Estraderm), which are changed once or twice a week depending on the preparation. An oral progestin (medroxyprogesterone 10 mg or micronized progesterone 200 mg) is added for 12 to 14 days each month.

Many patients with delayed puberty have decreased bone density for age. The optimal dose of estrogen replacement for increasing bone density in adolescents remains to be established, but it is probably higher than in menopausal women. A bone density by dual-energy x-ray absorptiometry (DXA) of the hip and spine at baseline and every 2 years is sometimes carried out in adolescents on estrogen or testosterone replacement. Bone density is compared with age-matched norms. The importance of appropriate calcium (1,300 mg/day) intake by diet or supplements and at least 600 IU vitamin D to support bone calcification should be stressed on each visit. The timing of initiation of sex steroid therapy to achieve maximum height depends on the patient's chronological and skeletal age and current height velocity.

Treatment for Boys

In boys with constitutional delay of puberty, 3- to 6-month courses of intramuscular (IM) testosterone enanthate or cypionate 25 to 50 mg every 2 to 4 weeks can be used to initiate secondary sexual development. Exposure to testosterone may speed the onset of the patient's own puberty. Since sex steroids cause fusion of epiphyses, care must be taken in the timing and monitoring of these therapies

so that final height is not compromised. These patients should therefore be referred to an endocrinologist for treatment. The timing of such an intervention must take into account such complex issues as psychosocial stress, self-image, and school performance, which appear to be more affected by pubertal delay than by short stature alone. Males with gonadal failure, hypopituitarism, or hypothalamic hypogonadism are maintained on long-term testosterone replacement using testosterone gel or IM testosterone replacement. They should receive dietary adequate calcium and vitamin D and should have DXA scans for spinal and hip bone density measurements since they are at risk for a low bone mass. In both males and females whose delayed puberty is due to abnormalities in hypothalamic GnRH secretion that do not correct with time, fertility can be achieved using a small pump to deliver pulses of GnRH intravenously or subcutaneously for weeks or months. Some GnRH-deficient males will achieve spermatogenesis with human chorionic gonadotropin (hCG) alone or in combination with FSH. Ovulation can be induced by FSH and hCG in GnRH-deficient females.

Treatment of Specific Conditions

Hypothyroidism

Treatment is begun with levothyroxine (see Chapter 12). Thyroid function tests are repeated in 6 weeks and the dose is adjusted to maintain the TSH concentration in the midnormal range. The final dose is usually 75 to 100 µg in females and 100 to 125 µg in males. Noncompliance with medication is often the underlying issue in teens whose TSH is elevated despite receiving unusually high doses of thyroid replacement. A 7-day pill package and adult supervision of doses may be helpful. Once the dose is established, thyroid tests are repeated at 6-month intervals. Catch-up growth is expected when thyroid hormone replacement is initiated, but patients who have been untreated for several years will lose some adult height.

Turner Syndrome and Gonadal Dysgenesis

Short stature associated with Turner syndrome can be treated with human growth hormone (hGH). The FDA and other worldwide regulatory agencies have approved the use of hGH for statural improvement in Turner syndrome. The hGH therapy should be started before the adolescent years and before beginning estrogen therapy for feminization.[16] The dose used is approximately double that used for subjects with classic GH deficiency. Data from the National Cooperative Growth Study from Genentech have shown GH to be effective in improving the final height of girls with Turner syndrome and that GH is safe for these patients. Estrogen replacement is usually initiated around age 12 to 13 (by age 14) unless the patient is predicted to be extremely short, in which case some delay of estrogen administration can be appropriate.

If there is a Y chromosome present on the karyotype to diagnose Turner syndrome, the patient will require gonadectomy. However, Y chromosomal material, rather than a full Y chromosome, may be present in girls who are virilized, either at birth or with puberty. These girls should have fluorescent in situ hybridization for the Y chromosome to ensure that no Y chromosomal material has been translocated. The presence of any Y material is an indication for gonadectomy, to prevent potential malignant neoplasias. Surgery should be followed by hormonal replacement therapy during and after puberty.

Chronic Illness

Treatment of pubertal delay caused by chronic illness necessitates treating the underlying disorder. For example, enzyme replacement in cystic fibrosis, gluten-free diet in celiac disease, corrective surgery for congenital heart disease, and hyperalimentation in inflammatory bowel disease usually result in catch-up growth and maturity. Medications such as steroids or antimetabolites can inhibit growth. Catch-up growth can be observed after discontinuation of treatment with these drugs. In patients with chronic renal failure, there may be some growth after improved nutrition and hemodialysis or transplantation. However, many patients with chronic renal failure remain short. GH can be administered to subjects with chronic renal failure before transplantation to improve height, without causing deterioration of underlying renal function.

 ## PATIENT EDUCATION

Young adolescents are preoccupied with their physical appearance. Any variation from the normal timing of sexual development is a major source of embarrassment to them and evokes feelings of personal inadequacy. A review of a patient's progress on their individual pubertal growth and growth chart can help reassure him or her that growth is proceeding in a pattern that is appropriate. For patients who have a permanent defect in reproductive function, counseling and support from both the primary health provider and medical specialist can be helpful in enabling the patient to establish a positive self-image of himself or herself as a capable adult. Further counseling by a mental health professional may be necessary. Questions about fertility should be answered as they arise, with emphasis on the patient's ability to function normally as a marriage partner and parent of adopted children. With current technology, pregnancies are possible using in vitro fertilization with donor eggs in patients with ovarian insufficiency.

EXCESSIVE GROWTH: TALL STATURE

Tall stature is seldom a complaint in males, but is occasionally a source of concern in adolescent females. This is less common than in the past since the role models of athletes and fashion models have made tall stature more socially acceptable in women now than in the past. Most commonly, tall stature is genetic and one or both parents are also tall.

Differential Diagnosis

1. Constitutional tall stature
2. Excess GH (e.g., GH-secreting tumors)
3. Anabolic steroid excess (exogenous, adrenal tumor, gonadal tumor, congenital adrenal hyperplasia—classic or nonclassical, precocious puberty, premature adrenarche)
4. Hyperthyroidism
5. Miscellaneous
   a. Marfan syndrome
   b. Neurofibromatosis
   c. Hypogonadism in boys
   d. Androgen-receptor deficiency in boys
   e. Estrogen deficiency in boys
   f. Homocystinuria
   g. Hereditary abnormalities of the skeleton
   h. Soto syndrome

Evaluation

Obese girls tend to be taller than average, perhaps due to higher levels of insulin. Many genetically tall girls who are above the 95th percentile for height in the early adolescent period are experiencing an early pubertal growth spurt, but will have a final adult height in the normal range. Review of the growth chart and a bone age is useful. If growth rate is excessive, evaluation might include thyroid function tests looking for hyperthyroidism, and an IGF-1, IGFBP-3, and random GH to exclude GH excess. If GH is low, acromegaly is unlikely. Elevated GH may be a random pulse and should be repeated. IGF-1 is elevated in acromegaly. Marfan syndrome is usually diagnosed clinically and can be confirmed with genetic testing for variants of fibrillin-1. The phenotype is characterized by tall stature, lean body habitus, and elongated extremities. A slit lamp examination by an ophthalmologist may detect lens dislocation in 50% of patients. Echocardiogram may reveal a dilated aortic root.

Treatment

In the past, high doses of estrogen were used to limit height gain in girls whose predicted height would be more than 6 ft (183 cm). Estrogen affects growth by suppressing IGF-1 and accelerating epiphyseal fusion. This is no longer done currently since female tall stature has become more socially acceptable and the long-term risks are unacceptable. High-dose estrogen treatment in girls is associated with side effects, which include nausea, breast soreness, hypertension, and, rarely, blood clots.

 ## PRECOCIOUS PUBERTY

Definition

In boys, development before age 9 years or 2.5 SD earlier than average is considered precocious. Early development in boys is rare. There are 10 times as many girls with precocious puberty as boys. There has been controversy over the definition of precocious puberty in North American girls. In girls, the cutoff has traditionally been 8 years or 2.5 SD below the average of breast development. However, a 1997 study of 17,000 American girls found a mean age of breast development of just below 10 years in Caucasian girls and 9 years in African American girls; 15% of African American girls having the appearance of breast development by 7 to 8 years and 5% of Caucasian girls having breast development by 7 to 8 years.[17] Pubic hair was present in 3% of Caucasian girls and 18% of African American girls by age 7 to 8 years. This has led to a revision of the definition of precocious puberty by the Lawson Wilkins Pediatric Endocrine Society as the presence of breast or pubic hair before age 7 in Caucasian and before age 6 years in African American girls.[18] Since then, numerous reports have pointed out that cases of true pathology such as CNS tumors may be missed by excluding 7- to 8-year-old girls from evaluation. Girls who have both pubic hair and breast development at ages 7 to 8 should have at least a bone age for height prediction, a review of growth and history, and consideration of further testing. Girls with rapid progression or unusual progression of puberty, a predicted height below 150 cm or –2 SD below target midparental height, those with neurological symptoms, or girls who are having psychological difficulty due to early puberty should be referred for further evaluation and consideration of possible suppression of puberty with GnRH analog therapy. Puberty is normally held back in humans during childhood by inhibitory connections to the hypothalamus, which suppress GnRH pulsations. If these inhibitory connections are damaged, GnRH pulse amplitude increases and central puberty ensues. There is often a family history of early puberty in girls with precocious puberty; some studies suggest an autosomal dominant or imprinted pattern with variable penetrance.

The vast majority of girls with central precocious puberty have idiopathic precocious puberty. Boys are much more likely to have a specific lesion causing their precocity.

Causes

Central causes of precocious puberty include the following:

1. CNS tumors (optic gliomas, craniopharyngiomas, dysgerminomas, ependymoma)
2. CNS malformations (hamartomas, arachnoid and suprasellar cysts, hydrocephalus, septooptic dysplasia)
3. Infiltrative lesions (histiocytosis, granulomas, abscess)
4. CNS damage (irradiation, trauma, meningitis, encephalitis)

Gonadotropin-independent causes of precocity in girls include the following:

1. Ovarian cysts, sometimes with McCune–Albright syndrome
2. Ovarian or adrenal estrogen-secreting tumors
3. Severe hypothyroidism
4. Exposure to exogenous estrogen

In boys, in addition to the central causes listed above, precocious puberty can be caused by androgen exposure, congenital adrenal hyperplasia, gonadal and adrenal tumors secreting androgens, and familial activating mutations of the LH receptor.

Incomplete Forms of Precocious Puberty
Premature Thelarche

Premature thelarche occurs often in female infants and toddlers. Self-limited breast budding, which is also transient, occurs in girls aged 6 and above. There is no sustained growth spurt or bone age advancement in these girls. Breast budding may appear and recede several times before sustained puberty ensues.

Premature Adrenarche

Benign premature adrenarche presents with underarm odor, and pubic and/or axillary hair development usually at ages 6 to 8 years. Bone age is often slightly advanced (1 year) and adrenal androgens are in the pubertal range. Twenty percent of the girls with benign premature adrenarche will go on to have polycystic ovary syndrome as teens. Patients with a history of intrauterine growth retardation followed by excessive weight gain and insulin resistance in childhood may present with premature adrenarche. They are at increased risk for polycystic ovary syndrome and sometimes glucose intolerance as teens. Virilization in girls is rare and can be due to an androgen-secreting adrenal or ovarian tumor, topical androgen exposure, or congenital adrenal hyperplasia. Symptoms of virilization include rapid growth and bone age advancement, deepening of the voice, clitoromegaly, or muscular development. A thorough evaluation is required.

Evaluation of Precocious Puberty
History

History includes a review of family history of endocrine or pubertal disorders, timing of puberty in family members, use of estrogen- or androgen-containing gels by family members, and heights of family members. The patient's past history should be reviewed for evidence of predisposing medical conditions. The growth chart should be obtained.

Physical Examination

The physical examination includes careful measurement of height and weight, vital signs, examination of the skin for large irregular café au lait spots suggestive of McCune–Albright syndrome, examination of the fundi, assessment for thyroid enlargement, abdominal examination, and examination of SMR (measurement of breast or testicular and phallic dimensions, and pubic hair staging). The vaginal introitus can be examined for signs of estrogen effect on the labia minora and presence of leukorrhea in the frog-leg position. Internal examination is not necessary unless unexplained vaginal bleeding is present in which case an experienced observer can often visualize the vagina and cervix in the knee chest position without instrumentation. In boys, the testicular examination should focus on any testicular asymmetry or masses, or phallic enlargement without testicular enlargement suggesting a source of androgens outside of the testes, such as congenital adrenal hyperplasia.

Laboratory Evaluation

A bone age x-ray of the left hand and wrist is useful. If the bone age is 2 years advanced, more evaluation is usually indicated. A baseline prediction of adult height can be made using the average charts from the Bayley–Pinneau table at the back of the Gruelich and Pyle Atlas of Skeletal maturation (see Chapter 1 for details).

Laboratory evaluation might include an 8 a.m. LH, FSH, estradiol, DHEAS, 17-OH progesterone, and TSH in girls, and a testosterone and 8 a.m. 17-OH progesterone and DHEAS, hCG, LH, and FSH in boys. The LH and FSH will be in the prepubertal range in the early stages of central puberty, with an LH level typically less than 0.1 to 0.3 IU/L depending on the assay.[19] By the time breast or gonadal development is in SMR stage 3, LH and FSH are often in the pubertal range. To confirm central puberty, it is sometimes necessary to do a GnRH or GnRH analog stimulation test (GnRH itself is now unavailable) using 20 µg/kg up to 500 µg leuprolide acetate and obtaining an LH, FSH, and estradiol or testosterone 1, 2, and 3 hours after the injection. If estradiol is markedly elevated (more than 100 pg/mL) and LH and FSH are suppressed, an ovarian cyst or more rarely tumor is suspected. A pelvic ultrasonography can be done in girls if an ovarian cyst or tumor is thought to be the cause of the precocity. In boys, an hCG level should be checked to rule out a hCG-producing tumor that could be causing testosterone production. A cranial MRI with contrast should be done to rule out CNS lesion in all boys with central precocious puberty, in all girls younger than 6 years, and should be considered in girls between 6 and 8 years of age depending on the clinical history. An adrenocorticotropic hormone stimulation test may be needed if congenital adrenal hyperplasia is suspected as a cause of androgen excess.

Treatment of Precocious Puberty

If the evaluation has not revealed a specific treatable cause of precocious puberty and the child has central precocious puberty, GnRH analog treatment should be considered. Most girls in the 7- to 9-year range do not require treatment for suppression of puberty.[20]

Many girls in this age range have a slow intermittent progression of their puberty and reach a final height that is not short. Early developers take longer on average to reach menarche than later developers. Often, parents are most worried about how they will handle menses in a grade school child, and can be reassured that menarche is not imminent in most cases and that menses can be suppressed if necessary using GnRH analog therapy. Untreated girls should be followed up at 6-month to 1-year intervals. If the child has an initial predicted adult height below 62 in (157 cm), bone age may need to be repeated in 6 months to 1 year because the predicted height can decline with rapid bone age advancement, and therapy may be required to preserve height potential. Depot leuprolide at an initial dose of 0.2 to 0.3 mg/kg can be given q28 days intramuscularly. A 3-month leuprolide formulation is also available and can be given every 12 weeks in 11.25 or 30 mg dosing forms. LH, FSH, and estradiol in girls or testosterone in boys can be obtained 1 to 2 hours after the depot leuprolide to document adequate suppression of puberty on therapy after 2 to 3 months of treatment.[21] Annual placement of 50-mg histrelin-acetate implants are also available and achieve pubertal suppression. Partial suppression of puberty has been achieved in girls with gonadotropin-independent puberty (McCune–Albright syndrome) with aromatase inhibitors. Similar regimens with anti-androgens and aromatase inhibitors have been used in boys with familial LH-activating mutations.

REFERENCES

1. Gruelich WW, Pyle SI. *Atlas of skeletal development of the hand and wrist*. 2nd ed. Stanford, CA: Stanford University Press, 1959.
2. De Sanctis V, Tosetto I, Iughetti L, et al. The SHOX gene and the short stature. Roundtable on diagnosis and treatment of short stature due to SHOX haploinsufficiency: how genetics, radiology and anthropometry can help the pediatrician in the diagnostic process Padova (April 20th, 2011). *Pediatr Endocrinol Rev* 2012;9(4):727–733. Available at http://www.ncbi.nlm.nih.gov/pubmed/23304810. Accessed on April 24, 2015.
3. Wilson TA, Rose SR, Cohen P, et al. Update of guidelines for the use of growth hormone in children: the Lawson Wilkins Pediatric Endocrinology Society Drug and Therapeutics Committee. *J Pediatr* 2003;143(4):415–421. Available at http://www.ncbi.nlm.nih.gov/pubmed/14571209. Accessed on April 24, 2015.
4. Kemp SF, Kuntze J, Attie KM, et al. Efficacy and safety results of long-term growth hormone treatment of idiopathic short stature. *J Clin Endocrinol Metab* 2005;90(9):5247–5253. doi:10.1210/jc.2004-2513.
5. Cuttler L. Safety and efficacy of growth hormone treatment for idiopathic short stature. *J Clin Endocrinol Metab* 2005;90(9):5502–5504. doi:10.1210/jc.2005-1676.
6. Lee MM. Clinical practice. Idiopathic short stature. *N Engl J Med* 2006;354(24):2576–2582. doi:10.1056/NEJMcp060828.
7. Wit JM, Clayton PE, Rogol AD, et al. Idiopathic short stature: definition, epidemiology, and diagnostic evaluation. *Growth Horm IGF Res* 2008;18(2):89–110. doi:10.1016/j.ghir.2007.11.004.
8. Young J. Approach to the male patient with congenital hypogonadotropic hypogonadism. *J Clin Endocrinol Metab* 2012;97(3):707–718. doi:10.1210/jc.2011-1664.

9. Aksglaede L, Juul A. Testicular function and fertility in men with Klinefelter syndrome: a review. *Eur J Endocrinol* 2013;168(4):R67–R76. doi:10.1530/EJE-12-0934.

10. Emans SJ, Laufer MR GD, eds. *Pediatric and adolescent gynecology.* 6th ed. Philadelphia, PA: Lippincott Williams and Wilkins, 2011.

11. Bayley N, Pinneau SR. Tables for predicting adult height from skeletal age: revised for use with the Greulich–Pyle hand standards. *J Pediatr* 1952;40(4):423–441. Available at http://www.ncbi.nlm.nih.gov/pubmed/14918032. Accessed on April 24, 2015.

12. Harrington J, Palmert MR. Clinical review: distinguishing constitutional delay of growth and puberty from isolated hypogonadotropic hypogonadism: critical appraisal of available diagnostic tests. *J Clin Endocrinol Metab* 2012;97(9):3056–3067. doi:10.1210/jc.2012-1598.

13. Sävendahl L, Davenport ML. Delayed diagnoses of Turner's syndrome: proposed guidelines for change. *J Pediatr* 2000;137(4):455–459. doi:10.1067/mpd.2000.107390.

14. DiVasta AD, Gordon CM. Hormone replacement therapy and the adolescent. *Curr Opin Obstet Gynecol* 2010;22(5):363–368. doi:10.1097/GCO.0b013e32833e4a35.

15. Ankarberg-Lindgren C, Elfving M, et al. Nocturnal application of transdermal estradiol patches produces levels of estradiol that mimic those seen at the onset of spontaneous puberty in girls. *J Clin Endocrinol Metab* 2001;86(7):3039–3044. doi:10.1210/jcem.86.7.7667.

16. Reiter EO, Blethen SL, Baptista J, et al. Early initiation of growth hormone treatment allows age-appropriate estrogen use in Turner's syndrome. *J Clin Endocrinol Metab* 2001;86(5):1936–1941. doi:10.1210/jcem.86.5.7466.

17. Herman-Giddens ME, Slora EJ, Wasserman RC, et al. Secondary sexual characteristics and menses in young girls seen in office practice: a study from the Pediatric Research in Office Settings network. *Pediatrics* 1997;99(4):505–512. Available at http://www.ncbi.nlm.nih.gov/pubmed/9093289. Accessed on April 24, 2015.

18. Kaplowitz PB, Oberfield SE. Reexamination of the age limit for defining when puberty is precocious in girls in the United States: implications for evaluation and treatment. Drug and Therapeutics and Executive Committees of the Lawson Wilkins Pediatric Endocrine Society. *Pediatrics* 1999;104 (4, Part 1):936–941. Available at http://www.ncbi.nlm.nih.gov/pubmed/10506238. Accessed on April 24, 2015.

19. Neely EK, Wilson DM, Lee PA, et al. Spontaneous serum gonadotropin concentrations in the evaluation of precocious puberty. *J Pediatr* 1995;127(1):47–52. Available at http://www.ncbi.nlm.nih.gov/pubmed/7608810. Accessed on April 24, 2015.

20. Carel J-C, Eugster EA, Rogol A, et al. Consensus statement on the use of gonadotropin-releasing hormone analogs in children. *Pediatrics* 2009;123(4):e752–e762. doi:10.1542/peds.2008-1783.

21. Bhatia S, Neely EK, Wilson DM. Serum luteinizing hormone rises within minutes after depot leuprolide injection: implications for monitoring therapy. *Pediatrics* 2002;109(2):E30. Available at http://www.ncbi.nlm.nih.gov/pubmed/11826240. Accessed on April 24, 2015.

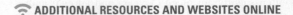 **ADDITIONAL RESOURCES AND WEBSITES ONLINE**

12

Thyroid Function and Disease in Adolescents and Young Adults

Cecilia A. Larson

KEY WORDS

- Goiter
- Graves disease
- Hyperthyroidism
- Hypothyroidism
- Thyroid cancer
- Thyroid nodules
- TSH

The thyroid is both affected by and contributes to diverse aspects of development including physical and intellectual growth and sexual development. There are thyroid receptors throughout the body that mediate the effects of thyroid hormone that is itself regulated by pituitary thyroid-stimulating hormone (TSH), which in turn is regulated by the hypothalamic hormone thyroid-releasing hormone (TRH). Disruption of the normal process of thyroid regulation affects thyroid function, causing either underactivity (hypothyroidism) or overactivity (hyperthyroidism) of the thyroid gland. In addition to disorders of thyroid function, the adolescents and young adults (AYAs) is susceptible to structural disorders of the thyroid including thyromegaly and nodular thyroid disease. Timely detection and treatment of thyroid disease during adolescence and early adulthood is essential for normal growth and development. This chapter discusses both functional and growth disorders of the thyroid and presents an approach to detection, evaluation, and management of these disorders. The framework for recognition of thyroid disorders relies on an understanding of thyroid development, a complete medical history, physical examination, and laboratory and imaging evaluations.

THYROID MIGRATION, GROWTH, AND FUNCTION DURING DEVELOPMENT

- The thyroid gland forms during the first trimester of fetal development from the medial and lateral anlagen and follows a complex migratory path.
- Insufficient migration can lead to a lingual thyroid. Lingual thyroids may cause obstruction of the upper airway or develop thyroid cancer, but are not routinely removed if these complications do not develop.
- Partial nonclosure of the migratory tract can lead to a thyroglossal duct cyst; thyroglossal duct cysts are usually benign and not of clinical significance unless infection of the cyst occurs, which may require surgical intervention.
- Postnatally to age 8 years, thyroid growth is similar and steady in males and females.
- During puberty, there is a more than four-fold increase in thyroid volume, which correlates not only with age and gender, but also with weight, height, body mass index, and pubertal stage.[1]

- By the end of puberty, the average weight of the female thyroid is 14.4 g, and for the male, it is 16.4 g.[2]
- Despite the significant increased growth of the thyroid during puberty, levels of free thyroxine (fT_4) and TSH decrease from age 1 year to adulthood.
- There is an increase in thyroid disorders of both structure and function during puberty.

FOCUSED MEDICAL HISTORY

Medical conditions and genetic syndrome that are associated with an increased risk of thyroid functional disorders:

- Trisomy 21
- Turner syndrome
- Klinefelter syndrome
- Autoimmune disorders (personal or family history)
  - Rheumatoid arthritis
  - Diabetes mellitus type 1
  - Celiac disease
  - Autoimmune polyglandular syndrome

Iodine exposure increases risk of thyroid functional disorders

- Computerized axial tomogram (CT) scan with iodinated contrast
- Kelp or seaweed supplements
- Amiodarone which contains iodine

Medications that can affect thyroid function

- Lithium
- Valproate
- Amiodarone
- Interferon
- Thionamides
- Interleukin-2
- Tyrosine kinase inhibitors
- Dopamine
- Dobutamine
- Glucocorticoids
- Bexarotene

Thyroid cancer risk is increased in certain syndromes and with positive family history of certain types of thyroid cancer:

- Cowden syndrome
- Bannayan–Riley–Ruvalcaba syndrome
- Gardner syndrome
- Multiple endocrine neoplasia (MEN) type 2
- Familial medullary thyroid cancer

TABLE 12.1
Clinical Effects of Thyroid Hormone

Clinical Effect	Hyperthyroidism	Hypothyroidism
Height velocity	Increased	Decreased
Weight	Decreased	Increased
Temperature	Increased in extreme cases	Decreased in extreme cases
Hair and skin	Oily and hair loss diffusely Pretibial myxedema[a]	Dry Myxedema generalized
Fingernails	Ridges	Brittle
Bowels	Increased frequency	Constipation
Cardiac	Increased heart rate Atrial fibrillation	Decreased heart rate
Menstruation	Lighter flow, irregular menses	Heavier flow, irregular menses
Skeleton	Bone loss Advanced bone age	Normal bone density Delayed bone age
Blood pressure	Systolic hypertension Increased mean arterial pressure	Diastolic hypertension
Eyes	Stare, lid lag, dry eye exophthalmos[a]	Periorbital edema
Reflexes	Normal	Delayed relaxation
Cognition	Decreased school performance	Decreased school performance

[a]Associated specifically with Graves Hyperthyroidism.

- Familial papillary thyroid cancer (PTC)
- Carney complex type 1

Ionizing radiation exposure increases risk of both functional (hypothyroidism) and structural disorders, increasing the risk of both benign nodule and cancer formation.

- Radiation treatment for childhood cancers
- Fallout from nuclear reactor accidents

The review of symptoms is especially relevant since thyroid hormone affects so many different tissues and organ systems. For a list of functional symptoms associated with thyroid activity, see **Table 12.1**

Structural symptoms such as airway or esophageal obstruction and hoarseness are less common than functional symptoms, although structural signs such as an enlarged thyroid commonly lead to thyroid evaluation.

While thyroid function and gland size and structure are sometimes related, it is important to recognize that hypo-, hyper-, and eu-thyroidism can exist in normal, small, enlarged (goitrous), or nodular thyroid glands. Thus, it is critical to assess both structure and function of the thyroid.

PHYSICAL EVALUATION OF THYROID STRUCTURE

- Inspection, palpation, and imaging by ultrasound, CT, or magnetic resonance imaging all provide information about the physical aspects of the thyroid gland.
- Inspection (see **Fig. 12.1**) and palpation are best evaluated while the patient swallows, causing the thyroid to elevate. Ultrasound

of the thyroid is the preferred imagine modality to assess thyroid gland structure. It allows for quantification of the size of the gland or a lesion, so it can be monitored and compared with a subsequent ultrasound. In addition, it can also identify features that aid in clarifying the diagnosis of thyroid enlargement:
- Autoimmune thyroiditis
  - Diffuse heterogeneity is present.
- Nodule(s)
  - Low risk for cancer:
    - Hyperechoic
    - Peripheral vascularity
    - Spongiform appearance
    - Resembles puff or Napoleon Pastry
    - Comet-tail shadowing
  - Increased risk for cancer:
    - Hypoechoic
    - Microcalcifications
    - Central vascularity
    - Irregular margins
    - Incomplete halo
    - Nodule is taller than wide
    - Significant growth of nodule

LABORATORY EVALUATION OF THYROID FUNCTION

Thyroid function is typically assessed by measuring blood tests associated with thyroid activity, and can aid in determining whether the signs and symptoms that the individual displays are indeed related to thyroid status. The most useful test is TSH, followed by fT_4. In selected situations, total triiodothyronine (T_3), reverse T_3 (rT_3), and thyroid antibody testing is necessary and helpful in establishing a diagnosis and/or monitoring response to therapy.

- TSH is the most sensitive assay of thyroid function in steady-state situations.
- When TSH is abnormal, or if a central (hypothalamic or pituitary) abnormality is suspected, fT_4 is also measured.
- Total T_3 is helpful when TSH is suppressed to identify and monitor response to antithyroid treatment in Graves disease.
- In inflammatory thyrotoxicosis due to release of preformed thyroid hormone, the ratio of T_4:T_3 is preserved (4:1).
- When acute illness is a factor, rT_3 levels can be measured, which if elevated suggests that the changes observed in TSH, early suppression followed by elevation, are associated with the acute illness and recovery phases. A "sick-euthyroid" pattern may also be reflected by a low total T_3, a pattern common in AYAs with eating disorders.
- The most specific thyroid antibody is thyroid-stimulating antibody (TSAb), which is typically measured in hyperthyroid patients to confirm Graves disease.
- Thyroid peroxidase (TPO) antibody is the most sensitive antibody to detect autoimmune thyroid disease and can be elevated in patients with either hypo- or hyperthyroidism. It is most helpful in subclinical hypothyroidism where fT_4 is normal and there is a mild TSH elevation <10 mU/L, where the presence of elevated TPO antibodies is associated with higher risk for overt hypothyroidism and can be an indication for thyroid hormone treatment.

RADIOLOGIC EVALUATION OF THYROID FUNCTION

The nuclear medicine thyroid scans allow the use of a small dose of a radioactive tracer whose thyroid and whole-body uptake can be imaged and quantified. There are three main uses of nuclear medicine studies for thyroid disorders:

1. Quantification of uptake in hyperthyroidism where increased uptake is consistent with Graves disease, while decreased uptake suggests either exogenous thyroid ingestion or release of preformed thyroid hormone associated with inflammatory thyroiditis

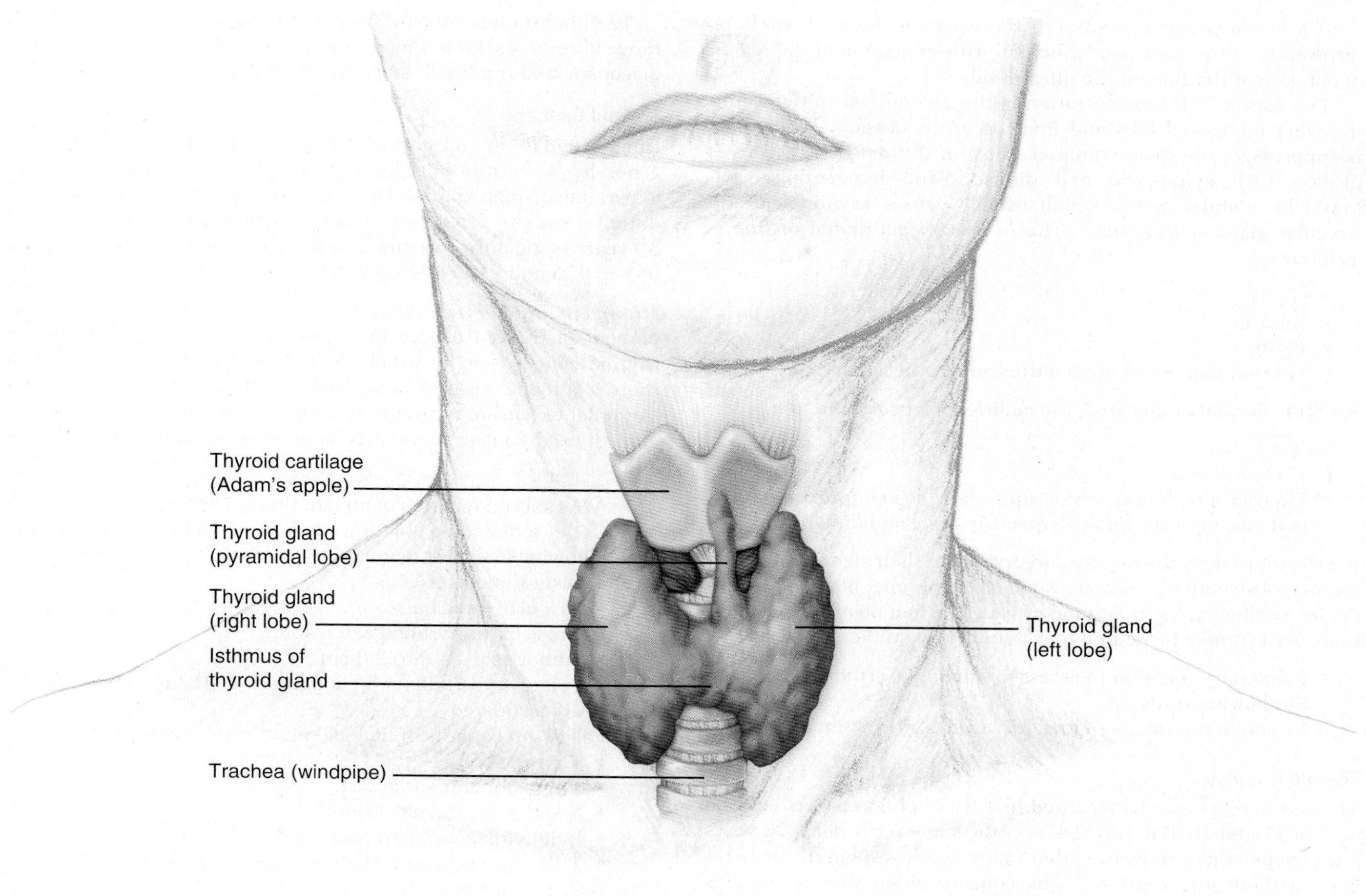

FIGURE 12.1 Location of the thyroid. (Asset provided by Anatomical Chart Co.)

2. Assessment of pattern of uptake to determine if a nodule takes up tracer and suppresses the rest of the gland, uptake indicating a toxic nodule, or if a nodule takes up less tracer than the rest of the gland indicating that the nodule requires further evaluation by fine-needle aspiration
3. Determination if iodine-avid thyroid tissue exists after complete thyroidectomy for thyroid cancer

ROLE OF GENETIC TESTING IN THYROID DISEASE

Many genes have been identified that affect thyroid development and function, as well as the risk of thyroid cancer.

- The paired box gene (PAX-8), tissue transcription factor (TTF-2), and connexin genes are associated with abnormally located or absent thyroid glands in neonates.[3]
- Rearrangements in peroxisome proliferator-activated receptor gamma and PAX-8 genes are found in follicular thyroid cancers (FTCs).[4]
- Rearranged during transfection (RET) oncogene rearrangements are common in PTC in children.[5]
- Mutations in the v-raf murine sarcoma viral oncogene homolog B1 (BRAF) are common in adults with PTC.[6]
- MEN2 and familial medullary thyroid carcinoma syndromes are associated with RET oncogene mutations.

There are currently two specific situations where genetic testing has led to improved outcomes:

1. Screening at-risk individuals for the presence of specific RET mutations has helped identify and guide timing for prophylactic thyroidectomy even prior to the development of medullary thyroid cancer and has improved outcome.[7]
2. In adults, the testing of fine-needle aspiration specimens with atypia of unknown significance for the presence of gene expression classifiers can be useful for identifying nodules with higher risk of cancer.[8]

It is likely that additional genetic testing will be developed to aid in risk stratification for individuals with nodules and for individuals with positive family history of thyroid cancer.

THYROID DISORDERS

Thyroid Structural Disorders

Thyromegaly

- Worldwide, the leading cause of an enlarged thyroid (goiter) is *iodine deficiency* leading to hypothyroidism with TSH-stimulated thyroid growth in an attempt to better capture the limited iodine in the diet.
- In *iodine-sufficient* areas such as the US, the leading cause of an enlarged gland is inflammatory thyroiditis.
- Thyroid size is a function of gender, weight, body mass index, and age. A simplified formula for estimation of normal size of the gland is $T = 1.48 + 0.054A$ where T is weight of the thyroid in grams and A is the age in months.[9]
- It is important to distinguish thyroid enlargement from other causes of neck swelling such as:
  - Neck fold fatty tissue
  - Increased strap muscle tissue
  - Lymph node or other glandular or soft tissue swelling

If it is not possible to discern the cause of the neck swelling, ultrasound of the neck can be helpful with indication of the region of concern at the time of the ultrasound.

The serum TSH concentration is the pivotal test in determining what additional labs and imaging are necessary. When TSH is suppressed, the most common cause of thyromegaly is Graves disease with symmetric and diffuse gland hypertrophy, followed by nodular goiter, which usually causes asymmetric and irregular gland enlargement. The necessary additional testing is as follows:

- fT_4
- Total T_3
- TSAb
- Thyroid scan followed by ultrasound, if necessary.

If TSH is normal or elevated, the additional labs needed are:

- fT_4
- TPO antibodies
- Thyroid ultrasound, which may show signs of inflammation, nodules, or cysts, and will quantify the gland dimensions.

Rarely, thyroid glands require surgery due to their size and location causing obstructive symptoms such as dysphonia, hoarseness, difficulty swallowing or breathing, or cough. When obstructive symptoms exist, it may be helpful to get additional studies such as:

- Pulmonary function to assess for airway obstruction,
- Swallowing study, or
- Direct laryngoscopy to look for vocal cord dysfunction.

Thyroid Nodules

Thyroid nodules can be palpated in 1.8% of children between the ages of 11 and 18, but only 0.45% of the same individuals 20 years later have nodules indicating that many nodules spontaneously regress without intervention.[10] The concern about thyroid nodules is the potential for malignancy. While malignancy is rare (0.5% of nodules), morbidity and mortality are increased in later detected cancers. Nodules that are associated with change in voice such as hoarseness, difficulty swallowing, or other obstructive symptoms are more likely to be cancerous.

After detecting a nodule, the next step is measurement of TSH. There is a correlation between TSH and risk of thyroid cancer with increases in TSH carrying higher cancer risk, which may relate to the pathogenic role of TSH elevation in carcinogenesis. Furthermore, toxic thyroid nodules carry a low risk of thyroid cancer, so if TSH is suppressed, the thyroid should next be imaged by nuclear thyroid scanning with I-123. If the nodule concentrates iodine, it can be managed as a toxic thyroid nodule, but such nodules are rare in adolescence. If the TSH is suppressed and the nodule does not concentrate iodine, or if the TSH is elevated or normal, thyroid ultrasound is indicated. Nodules greater than 0.9 cm are generally biopsied, especially if other concerning ultrasound findings are present. Biopsy can be performed by fine-needle aspiration typically done with ultrasound guidance. There are numerous potential pathological results detected by fine-needle aspiration, with varying positive predictive values for the presence of malignancy. The spectrum of results includes the following:

1. Nondiagnostic specimens with insufficient material for diagnosis
2. Benign, consistent with macrofollicular adenoma
3. Atypical cells of unknown significance
4. Consistent with follicular neoplasm
5. Suspicious for PTC
6. Suspicious for other malignancy
   i. Medullary thyroid cancer
   ii. Intrathyroidal lymphoma
   iii. Metastases from another primary tumor

It is important to prepare the patient and the family for this wide range of results prior to biopsy and to guide them through the next diagnostic and treatment steps based on the pathological findings.

Thyroid Cancers

Differentiated thyroid cancers (PTC and FTC) and MTC should generally be treated initially with complete thyroidectomy by an experienced, high-volume thyroid surgeon. Long-term outcomes differ for the two categories of cancer with survival rates at 15 and 30 years being only 86% and 15% for MTC compared with rates of 95% to 97% and 91% to 92% for PTC and FTC.[11]

Management of Differentiated Thyroid Cancer: Ninety-five percent of thyroid cancer in adolescents is of the differentiated thyroid cancer type, of which the vast majority is PTC. Although there is a higher risk for multifocal disease and presence of extrathyroidal extension of tumor at diagnosis, prognosis for differentiated thyroid cancer survival is as good as or better than that of adults.

- AYAs should undergo complete thyroidectomy.
- Use of radioiodine ablation can be reserved for those with the following high-risk features[12]:
  - Distant metastases
  - Vascular invasion
  - Gross extrathyroidal extension
  - Tumor size >1.0 to 2.0 cm
  - Tumor type tall cell, columnar cell, insular or poorly differentiated
- Follow-up consists of lifelong monitoring of the following:
  - Thyroglobulin
  - Thyroglobulin antibodies
  - Neck exam and ultrasound
  - Iodine imaging when necessary
  - TSH (aim to keep at the lower range of normal)

Management of Medullary Thyroid Cancer: In individuals with history of MTC, monitoring includes the following:

- Calcitonin
- Carcinoembryonic antigen
- Ultrasound follow-up

Thyroglobulin levels and iodine scanning/treatment are not indicated since the cell of origin for medullary thyroid cancer is the neuroendocrine C cell, which does not take up iodine or produce thyroglobulin. In kindreds with MTC, the RET gene is autosomal dominant with high penetrance and there is a strong genotype–phenotype correlation such that there is age-specific guidelines for RET testing and, if necessary, prophylactic thyroidectomy.[13,14]

Functional Thyroid Disorders

The thyroid gland produces the two thyroid hormones T_4 and T_3 in a 4:1 ratio. The overabundance of T_4 (relative to T_3) serves as a reservoir of available thyroid hormone that can quickly be upregulated or downregulated, depending on the need for active thyroid hormone.

In addition to making thyroid hormones, the thyroid also produces thyroglobulin, which binds to the thyroid hormones within the thyroid follicles.

Peripherally, the thyroid hormones are principally bound to thyroid-binding globulin and albumin and other serum proteins made in the liver.

The thyroid gland is regulated by the hypothalamic and pituitary hormones TRH and TSH in a negative feedback loop system as shown in **Figure 12.2.** Excess amounts of thyroid hormone downregulate production of TRH and TSH, which in turn leads to reduced production of the thyroid hormones, T_3 and T_4, as well as thyroglobulin.

- Thyroglobulin levels are not elevated.
- The duration of excess thyroid hormone levels is limited by the amount of preformed, stored thyroid hormone, and usually lasts a few weeks to a couple of months.
- The thyrotoxic phase can be followed by a late and sometimes permanent hypothyroidism.
- It occurs as a consequence of trauma to or inflammation of the thyroid.
  - Types of inflammatory thyrotoxicosis include the following:
    - Painful subacute thyroiditis
    - Postpartum thyroiditis
    - Painless sporadic thyroiditis

Hyperthyroidism

Hyperthyroidism is a specific subset of thyrotoxicosis where there is ongoing overproduction of thyroid hormone, which can be due to (in declining frequency in AYAs):

- Graves disease
- Excessive iodine load
- Autonomous nodular thyroid disease
- Inappropriate TSH overproduction by a pituitary tumor
- Overactive ectopic thyroid tissue (e.g., struma ovarii)

Graves Disease: Graves disease is the most common cause of hyperthyroidism in AYAs. While the prevalence of Graves disease in children is 1:5,000, between the ages of 15 and 25 there is a dramatic increase in Graves disease, especially in women. Graves' is an autoimmune disease caused by the production of TSAbs, which are capable of directly stimulating thyroid tissue to overproduce thyroid hormones T_3 and T_4. There is lymphocytic infiltration of the thyroid and when glycosaminoglycans and lymphocytes accumulate in the orbital connective tissue and pretibial skin it can lead to exophthalmos, as shown in Figure 12.3, and pretibial myxedema, which are pathognomonic for Graves disease. The other symptoms and signs of Graves disease are the same as for other thyrotoxicoses as shown in Table 12.1. The female-to-male ratio is approximately 5:1 for Graves' in AYAs.

The diagnosis of Graves disease can be made when there is (are):

- Pathognomonic findings are present (thyrotoxicosis with pretibial myxedema and/or exophthalmous and/or thyroid bruit) or
- T_3 hormone predominant thyrotoxicosis, or by
- Thyroid nuclear medicine scan demonstrating diffuse increased thyroid uptake in the context of a suppressed TSH.

Initial treatment of Graves disease can include the use of a beta blocker such as daily atenolol to control adrenergic hyperthyroid symptoms (palpitations and tremor especially) as well as more specific antithyroid therapy, which can be used as a bridge to definitive therapy or for 1 to 2 years in an attempt to achieve remission. Antithyroid therapy with methimazole (MMI) to decrease

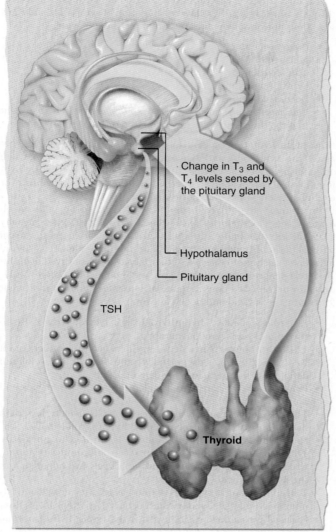

FIGURE 12.2 Feedback loop for thyroid hormone production. (Asset provided by Anatomical Chart Co.)

Thyroid hormone T_4 contains four iodine molecules, and a deiodinase removes one iodine and converts T_4 to T_3. It is the free T_3 that binds to the thyroid receptor to mediate thyroid hormone effects.

The signs and symptoms of too much thyroid hormone (thyrotoxicosis) or underactivity (hypothyroidism) of the thyroid gland are manifested in the thyroid-responsive organs such as the skin, brain, heart, skeletal system, and intestinal and reproductive tracts (see Table 12.1).

Excess thyroid hormone can be either TSH or non-TSH mediated. In the case of TSH mediated, the TSH and thyroid hormones are both elevated, and this is due to central (secondary or tertiary) hyperthyroidism, an extremely rare entity usually associated with a pituitary tumor or hypothalamic lesion.

However, most of the time TSH is appropriately suppressed in response to elevated thyroid hormone levels. Elevated thyroid hormones can be released from preformed, stored thyroid hormone, or be due to *de novo* thyroid hormone production (hyperthyroidism).

Excess thyroid hormone levels occurring as a consequence of excessive release of already synthesized, stored T_4 and T_3 are characterized by the following:

- The ratio of T_4 to T_3 is 4:1.

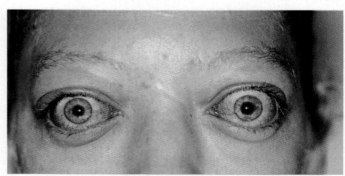

FIGURE 12.3 Patient with Graves' ophthalmopathy. (From Penne RB. *Wills Eye Institute—oculoplastics.* 2nd ed. Philadelphia, PA: Lippincott Williams & Wilkins, 2011.)

thyroid hormone production is usually highly effective, though some patients can develop adverse reactions, which limit its use such as severe skin allergy, hepatitis (much less common than with propylthiouracil (PTU) use), or rarely agranulocytosis. If a severe adverse reaction is suspected (rash, fever or sore throat, or right upper quadrant pain or jaundice), the MMI (or PTU) should be discontinued and definitive therapy with radioiodine or surgery is indicated.

Some experts recommend radioiodine ablation therapy routinely for Graves disease due to high rates of relapse after antithyroid therapy is discontinued. Others favor a trial of antithyroid therapy before definitive (surgery or radioiodine ablation) therapy of Graves disease. There is consensus that definitive therapy is indicated when:

- Serious adverse response to antithyroid therapy occurs.
- Relapse after withdrawal of antithyroid medication occurs.
- Patient prefers individualized therapy based on availability (high-volume thyroid surgeon and/or radioiodine) and advantages/disadvantages of each type of treatment.
- Coexistence of concerning nodular thyroid disease, or severe Graves eye disease when thyroid surgery may be indicated.

When initiating antithyroid therapy, the dose is based on:

- Degree of thyroid overactivity and gland size
- In patients with a small goiter and a milder degree of hyperthyroid symptoms and free T_4 and total T_3 concentrations, a dose of 0.25 mg/kg/day MMI is used.
- The higher range of 0.5 to 1.0 mg/kg/day is reserved for those with a large goiter and higher fT_4 and total T_3 levels.

Thyroid function tests are monitored every 4 to 6 weeks initially and dose is titrated in 0.25 mg/kg increments to achieve normal thyroid levels with dosage reduction beginning when fT_4 drops (even if TSH is still suppressed). Once TSH has stabilized and is normal, monitoring can be every 3 to 4 months.

Predictors of remission include the following:

- Smaller gland size,
- Rapid restoration of euthyroidism (<3 months) and low dose of antithyroid medication, and
- Higher body mass index.

Risk of relapse is greatest in the first year following discontinuation of antithyroid therapy, but can occur much later and lifelong thyroid function monitoring is indicated.

Autonomous nodule(s) that overproduce thyroid hormone independent of TSH are rare in younger patients and risk for such nodules increases with age. Such nodules are usually >2 cm in size if they are producing sufficient thyroid hormone such that TSH is suppressed. Treatment of toxic nodules can be with antithyroid medication, radioiodine, or surgery.

Hypothyroidism

The vast majority, >99%, of hypothyroidism occurs due to primary failure of the thyroid gland to make sufficient thyroid hormone. Abnormally located and partial thyroid glands are usually detected in the newborn period, mostly by mandatory heelstick newborn screening thyroid hormone levels. Hypothyroidism in the AYAs is usually acquired underactivity of the thyroid gland. When the gland itself is unresponsive to the stimulatory signal TSH, it is termed primary hypothyroidism. However, sometimes, the regulatory signal is deficient causing secondary (TSH) or tertiary (TRH) hypothyroidism. The common factor for all types of hypothyroidism is a reduced and falling level of thyroid hormone (fT_4). The symptoms and signs of primary hypothyroidism (**Table 12.1**) are the same as seen in secondary and tertiary hypothyroidism.

Because thyroid receptors are located in virtually all tissues throughout the body, there is a constellation of symptoms and signs seen in hypothyroidism and these include the following:

- Decreased energy
- Sluggishness
- Constipation
- Dry skin and hair
- Decreased heart rate
- Decreased rate of linear growth despite increase in body weight
- In girls, there can be delayed, missed or heavy menses

None of the symptoms specifically signals hypothyroidism, and because the symptoms and signs are common symptoms that can arise for a variety of reasons, thyroid function evaluation by testing fT_4 and TSH levels is generally required to make/confirm or exclude the diagnosis of hypothyroidism.

In primary hypothyroidism, there is reduced fT_4 and an elevated TSH. The majority of the time, thyroid antibodies (usually TPO and thyroglobulin antibodies) are also positive, as the usual pathogenesis of hypothyroidism is autoimmune-mediated thyroid failure, or Hashimoto disease. Other causes of hypothyroidism include surgical resection of the gland, radioiodine ablation by I-131, or as an unintended consequence of ionizing radiation treatment for treatment of head and neck cancers.

- Regardless of cause, hypothyroidism is treated with T_4 (levothyroxine) replacement therapy.
- T_3 (liothyronine) is not necessary because the conversion of T_4 to T_3 still proceeds normally unless there is a selenium deficiency or other cause for deiodinase inactivity.
- Usual doses of T_4 are 2 to 4 µg/kg in 10- to 15-year-olds and 1.6 µg/kg in adulthood.[15]
- The dose of thyroid hormone necessary is usually less than needed for patients with congenital hypothyroidism.
- Dosing in primary hypothyroidism is titrated to normalize TSH and target TSH is between 0.5 µL/mL and 3.0 µL/mL, which is usually associated with an fT_4 in the upper half of the normal range.
- TSH monitoring is typically 4 to 6 weeks after dosage adjustments. (Note: in secondary and tertiary hypothyroidism dose is based on achieving fT_4 levels in the upper half of normal without monitoring TSH.)
- Monitoring should be every 4 to 6 months in growing individuals, and yearly in those who have attained maximal height.
- Levels should additionally be monitored if symptoms of hypo- or hyperthyroidism develop and if diseases involving the gastrointestinal tract such as celiac disease, gastric bypass, or diabetes-associated diarrhea develop and/or if medications that affect thyroid hormone requirements are added. In most cases, treatment is lifelong.

Nonthyroidal Illness

The thyroid axis has a complex response to acute illness, including sustained malnutrition, which includes a reduction in thyroid hormone production, and in recovering from acute illness, there is a stage where the TSH is elevated to prompt restoration of normal thyroid levels. If testing occurs at this time, it may appear to represent primary hypothyroidism, but thyroid antibodies are typically negative, and if the patient improves clinically, the TSH and fT_4 typically normalize. Another feature of recovery from acute illness is that the reverse T_3 (rT_3) is usually elevated early in the process, and this can be measured when it is difficult to distinguish hypothyroidism from recovery from acute illness. Low T_3 levels in nonthyroidal illness predict worse clinical outcome, and it is not clear whether T_4 and or T_3 treatment has an effect on outcome. Measurement of total T_3 levels can be especially helpful in the care of AYAs with eating disorders as a low level of this hormone can indicate a more significant energy deficit.

PREGNANCY AND THYROID DISORDERS

While it is not routine to screen for thyroid disease in asymptomatic young women who are (or are contemplating becoming) pregnant, the symptoms of thyroid disorders are nonspecific and common, so that many reproductive-aged women undergo thyroid testing. If thyroid tests are obtained, the appropriate TSH reference range for such women is <2.5 µL/mL.

Young women with preexisting hypothyroidism typically need a 30% to 40% increase in thyroid dose during pregnancy and can be instructed to increase their thyroid dose by two pills per week (for example, continue one pill daily Monday to Friday and two pills on Saturday and Sunday) as soon as they know they are pregnant. Monthly monitoring allows appropriate adjustment of maternal thyroid dose with an aim of keeping the TSH <2.5 µL/mL.

In women with a history of Graves disease, there is a risk of hyperthyroidism in the fetus and newborn, even if the mother has had definitive treatment for the Graves disease and is on thyroid hormone replacement therapy. This occurs because the maternal TSAbs mediate the fetal effects—rapid fetal heart rate, poor growth, goiter, and exophthalmous. If the fetus shows signs of hyperthyroidism such as intrauterine growth retardation, tachycardia, and reduced amniotic fluid, the mother is typically treated with the antithyroid medication PTU that crosses the placenta and can treat the fetus. If only the fetus has hyperthyroidism and the mother is euthyroid or hypothyroid, the mother needs to be treated with thyroid hormone (to maintain/restore her euthyroidism) and antithyroid medication (for the fetus).

Radioactive iodine, even tracer doses, is not used during pregnancy or during breast-feeding, and ultrasound is the only imaging used during and shortly after pregnancy.

Postpartum thyroid disorders occur in 5% to 10% of US pregnancies, and also may occur after pregnancy loss or termination. These thyroid issues can manifest any time during the first-year postpartum and can cause transient hyperthyroidism (which must be distinguished from newly detected Graves disease in the postpartum period) or hypothyroidism, which can be transient or permanent. Women who have had postpartum thyroid issues in prior pregnancies are at increased risk for recurrence of thyroid issues with subsequent pregnancies.

Thyroid nodules detected during pregnancy are evaluated the same way as nodules detected in nonpregnant individuals with the exception that nuclear medicine thyroid scans are not obtained in pregnant women. Thyroid cancers detected during pregnancy can be surgically removed in the second trimester or after the pregnancy.

REFERENCES

1. Fleury Y, Van Melle G, Woringer V, et al. Sex-dependent variations and timing of thyroid growth during puberty. *J Clin Endocrinol Metab* 2001;86:750.
2. Pankow BG, Michalak J, McGee MK. Adult human thyroid weight. *Health Phys* 1985;49:1097.
3. Polak M, Sura-Trueba S, Chauty A, et al. Molecular mechanisms of thyroid dysgenesis. *Horm Res* 2004;62 (suppl 3):14–21.
4. Foukakis T, Au AY, Wallin G, et al. The Ras effector NORE1A is suppressed in follicular thyroid carcinomas with a PAX8-PPARgamma fusion. *J Clin Endocrinol Metab* 2006;91:1143–1149.
5. Fenton CL, Lukes Y, Nicholson D, et al. The ret/PTC mutations are common in sporadic papillary thyroid carcinoma of children and young adults. *J Clin Endocrinol Metab* 2000;85:1170–1175.
6. Penko K, Livezey J, Fenton C, et al. BRAF mutations are uncommon in papillary thyroid cancer of young patients. *Thyroid* 2005;15:320–325.
7. Kloos RT, Eng C, Evans DB, et al. Medullary thyroid cancer: management guidelines of the American Thyroid Association. *Thyroid* 2009;19:565–612.
8. Alexander EK, Kennedy GC, Baloch ZW, et al. Preoperative diagnosis of benign thyroid nodules with indeterminate cytology. *N Engl J Med* 2012;367(8):705.
9. Kay C, Abrahams S, McClain P. The weight of normal thyroid glands in children. *Arch Pathol* 1966;82:349.
10. Rallison ML, Dobyns BM, Keating FR Jr, et al. Thyroid nodularity in children. *JAMA* 1975;233(10):1069–1072.
11. Hogan AR, Zhuge Y, Perez EA, et al. Pediatric thyroid carcinoma: incidence and outcomes in 1753 patients. *J Surg Res* 2009;156(1):167.
12. American Thyroid Association Guidelines Task Force on Thyroid Nodules and Differentiated Thyroid Cancer, Cooper DS, Doherty GM, Haugen BR, et al. Revised ATA management guidelines for patients with thyroid nodules and differentiated thyroid cancer. *Thyroid* 2009;19(11):1167.
13. American Thyroid Association Guidelines Task Force, Kloos RT, Eng C, Evans DB, et al. Medullary thyroid cancer: management guidelines of the American Thyroid Association. *Thyroid* 2009;19(6):565.
14. Romei C, Tacito A, Molinaro E, et al. Twenty years of lesson learning: how does the RET genetic screening test impact the clinical management of medullary thyroid cancer? [published online ahead of print December 2, 2014]. *Clin Endocrinol* doi:10.1111/cen.12686.
15. LaFranchi S. Thyroiditis and acquired hypothyroidism. *Pediatr Ann* 1992;21:29.

ADDITIONAL RESOURCES AND WEBSITES ONLINE

CHAPTER 13

Diabetes Mellitus

Laura M. Kester
Donald P. Orr
Tamara S. Hannon

KEY WORDS

- Diabetic ketoacidosis
- Hemoglobin A1C
- Hyperglycemia
- Insulin resistance
- Type 1 diabetes
- Type 2 diabetes

Diabetes mellitus (DM) constitutes a group of metabolic diseases, characterized by hyperglycemia due to defects in insulin secretion, insulin action, or both. The metabolic derangements associated with untreated or undertreated diabetes lead to acute complications, including diabetic ketoacidosis (DKA) and nonketotic hyperosmolar coma. Chronic hyperglycemia is associated with long-term microvascular (retinopathy, nephropathy, and neuropathy), accelerated macrovascular (coronary artery disease and stroke), and neurocognitive complications. Data obtained from the Diabetes Control and Complications Trial (DCCT)[1] and Epidemiology of Diabetes Interventions and Complications study[2] indicate that intensive blood glucose (BG) control in individuals with type 1 diabetes cost-effectively reduces the risk of diabetes-related complications. Comparable clinical trials of intensified treatment and glycemic control for individuals with type 2 diabetes have also demonstrated a significant reduction in risk for microvascular complications. In aggregate, the available evidence supports initiating intensive, multidisciplinary therapy in persons with diabetes at the onset of diagnosis with the goal of treating evidence-based recommended glycemic, blood pressure, and lipid targets.

CLASSIFICATION AND ETIOLOGY

DM (or more commonly, diabetes) includes a spectrum of disorders with overlapping characteristics, making classification difficult in some cases, especially in the face of the obesity epidemic. Currently, classification of diabetes is based on the presumed etiology, rather than the mode of treatment.[3] The more common types of diabetes include the following (see **Table 13.1**):

1. **Type 1 diabetes** is the result of pancreatic β-cell destruction, leading to absolute insulin deficiency. Adolescents and young adults (AYAs) are typically symptomatic (i.e., have polyuria, polydipsia, and weight loss) at presentation, and are at risk for DKA.
   a. *Immune-mediated type 1A diabetes:* The most common form of diabetes in AYAs, type 1A diabetes, is linked to genetic susceptibility associated with the major histocompatibility genes, most notably human leukocyte antigen class II immune recognition molecules (DR and DQ) located on chromosome 6. One or more environmental factors are likely necessary to trigger the onset of the disease. Autoimmune-mediated destruction of the β-cells involves T cells that recognize β-cell-specific antigens resulting in insulitis and circulating immune markers. Associated immune markers may be detected many months to years before the onset of diabetes and include antibodies directed against islet cells (islet cell antibody), insulin, glutamate decarboxylase (anti-GAD$_{65}$), receptor-linked tyrosine phosphatases (IA-2, IA-2$_\beta$), and zinc transporter ZnT8. Antibodies are present in 85% to 90% of children and adolescents with type 1 diabetes at the time of diagnosis.
   b. *Ketosis-prone, idiopathic, or type 1B:* Persons with insulin deficiency without evidence of autoimmunity and no other cause of β-cell destruction are described as having ketosis-prone diabetes.[4]
   c. *Latent autoimmune diabetes in adults:* Approximately 10% of phenotypic type 2 diabetic patients are positive for at least one of the islet autoantibodies.[5] This form of diabetes is characterized by circulating autoantibodies against β-cell antigens and progressive β-cell failure to insulin dependence after several months to years of relatively mild diabetes.

2. **Type 2 diabetes** comprises a spectrum of disorders characterized by varying degrees of hyperglycemia associated with insulin resistance in combination with relative impairment in insulin secretion in the absence of circulating immune markers.[6] Type 2 diabetes disproportionally affects people of minority race and ethnicity; genetic susceptibility is an important risk factor and represents complex interaction among numerous genes and environmental factors.[7,8] It is characterized by decreased muscle glucose uptake, increased hepatic glucose production, impaired and progressively deteriorating insulin secretion, and overproduction of free fatty acids. Prevalence has increased dramatically mirroring the increase in obesity throughout the world.

3. **Congenital genetic defects** (leading to various forms of diabetes):
   a. *Monogenic diabetes* (also known as maturity-onset diabetes) of the young, or MODY, comprises a group of autosomal dominantly inherited disorders associated with disordered β-cell function, impaired insulin secretion, with minimal or no defects in insulin action, and lack of autoantibodies.[9] It represents <5% of cases of diabetes and is seen in all racial/ethnic groups. Six specific types of gene defect have been characterized as forms of MODY.
      - Hepatocyte nuclear factor-4-alpha (MODY 1)—Insulin secretory defect with good initial response to treatment with sulfonylureas.[10]
      - Glucokinase (MODY 2)—Reduced or delayed glucose sensing leads to a higher threshold for glucose-stimulated insulin secretion. Results in mild diabetes, which can be controlled with diet.[9]

TABLE 13.1

Characteristics of Common Forms of Diabetes

	Type 1A	Type 2, Ketosis-Prone	Type 2	Monogenic[a]
Age	Childhood	Pubertal	Pubertal	Usually <age 25
Onset	Acute; severe	Acute; severe	Mild to severe; often insidious	Mild; insidious
Insulin secretion	Very low	Moderately low	Variable	Variable
Insulin sensitivity	Normal	Normal	Decreased	Normal
Insulin dependence	Permanent	Variable	Progression from variable to permanent	Usually no, until late
Groups at increased risk	Non-Hispanic Whites	Non-Hispanic Blacks	Minority race/ethnicity	All
Genetics	Polygenic	Autosomal dominant	Polygenic	Autosomal dominant
Association with obesity	No	Variable	Strong	No
Acanthosis nigricans	No	Variable	Yes	No
Autoimmune etiology	Yes	No	No	No

[a]Maturity-onset diabetes of youth (MODY).

- Hepatocyte nuclear factor-1-alpha (MODY 3)—Insulin secretory defect with good initial response to treatment with sulfonylureas. Mutations also result in a low renal threshold for glucose leading to detectable glycosuria after a glucose load.[11]
- Insulin promoter factor 1 (MODY 4)—Reduced binding of the protein to the insulin gene promoter leads to disordered β-cell function.[9]
- Hepatoctye nuclear factor-1-beta (MODY 5)—Results in pancreatic atrophy, abnormal renal development progressive renal insufficiency, hypomagnesemia, elevated serum aminotransferases, and genital abnormalities.[12]
- Neurogenic differentiation factor-1 (MODY 6)—Faulty pancreatic development, also associated with permanent neonatal diabetes.[13]

b. **Mitochondrial:** This very rare form of diabetes is caused by a rare sporadic or maternally inherited mitochondrial genetic mutation at position 3243 in transfer RNA.[14] It is almost always associated with other symptoms—deafness, neurological disorders, cardiac failure, renal failure, and myopathy.

c. **Various genetic defects of insulin action** include type A insulin resistance, leprechaunism, Rabson–Mendenhall syndrome, and lipoatrophic diabetes.[15]

4. **Diseases of the exocrine pancreas** leading to destruction of endocrine function include pancreatitis, trauma/pancreatectomy, neoplasia, hemochromatosis, and cystic fibrosis-related diabetes (CFRD). CFRD is associated with decreased pulmonary function, protein catabolism, poor growth, and weight loss.[16] It results primarily from insulinopenia, although insulin resistance may be observed during periods of infection and with glucocorticoid therapy. Insulin treatment is associated with increased body weight and improvement in pulmonary function.

5. **Genetic syndromes that may be associated with diabetes include** Down syndrome, Klinefelter syndrome, Turner syndrome, Wolfram syndrome, Friedreich ataxia, Huntington chorea, Laurence–Moon syndrome, myotonic dystrophy, and Prader–Willi syndrome.

6. **Gestational DM:** Pregnancy leads to both insulin resistance and increased insulin requirements, which results in diabetes in women whose pancreatic function is insufficient to withstand these requirements for the growing fetus.[17]

EPIDEMIOLOGY

1. Prevalence
   a. **Type 1 diabetes**: The prevalence of type 1 diabetes varies by race/ethnicity and country, with the highest rates in areas most distant from the equator. Prevalence estimates indicate that there are nearly 500,000 children under the age of 15 years with type 1 diabetes worldwide, the largest numbers being in Europe (129,000) and North America (108,700).[18] In the US, approximately 1 in every 400 children and adolescents has diabetes, with the majority of these being cases of type 1 diabetes.[19,20]
   b. **Type 2 diabetes**: Type 2 diabetes accounts for up to 20% of the diabetes cases diagnosed in AYAs in some large diabetes centers.[21] Type 2 diabetes rarely occurs among youth aged <10 years, and more than 80% of AYAs with type 2 diabetes have a family history of the disease in a first- or second-degree relative. Native American, non-Hispanic Black, and Hispanic youth are at significantly increased risk as compared with non-Hispanic White youth. Socioeconomically disadvantaged youth and females are disproportionately affected.[22]

2. Emergence of diabetes during adolescence

Normal physiologic insulin resistance occurs during pubertal growth and development, as insulin is an important growth-permissive anabolic hormone. Insulin sensitivity decreases significantly at sexual maturity rating (SMR) 2, remains constant from SMR 2 to 4, and returns almost to prepubertal levels by SMR 5.[23]

SCREENING AND DIAGNOSTIC CRITERIA

1. **Type 1 diabetes:** No screening is recommended unless in the context of a clinical trial.

2. **Type 2 diabetes:** The American Diabetes Association and the American Academy of Pediatrics have endorsed use of fasting plasma glucose (FPG) for screening of overweight youth (BMI ≥85th percentile) who have at least two additional risk factors for type 2 diabetes (see below).[24] FPG was chosen for its specificity for diabetes and has been shown to be both reproducible and reliable for detecting diabetes. The use of hemoglobin (Hb) A1C has also been endorsed as a screening test; however, adolescent data have not strongly supported this recommendation.[25]

TABLE 13.2

American Diabetes Association Criteria for the Diagnosis of DM

A1C ≥6.5%[a] OR	Method should be NGSP certified and standardized to the DCCT assay.
FPG ≥126 mg/dL (7.0 mmol/L)[a] OR	Fasting is defined as no caloric intake for at least 8 h.
OGTT 2-h PG ≥200 mg/dL (11.1 mmol/L)[a] OR	OGTT with a glucose load containing the equivalent of 1.75 g/kg up to a maximum of 75 g anhydrous glucose dissolved in water
Random PG ≥200 mg/dL (11.1 mmol/L)	This criterion is applicable for a patient with classic symptoms of hyperglycemia or hyperglycemic crisis.

[a]In the absence of unequivocal hyperglycemia, this should be confirmed by repeat testing. FPG, fasting plasma glucose; PG, plasma glucose; OGTT, oral glucose tolerance test. American Diabetes Association. Diagnosis and classification of diabetes mellitus. *Diabetes Care* 2013;36 (suppl 1):S67–S74.

a. **Screening:** Screen with FPG testing or HbA1c every other year, starting at 10 years or at onset of puberty, if puberty occurs first.
b. **Risk factors for type 2 diabetes:** Family history of type 2 diabetes in first- or second-degree relative, or mother with gestational diabetes; minority race/ethnicity; signs of insulin resistance or conditions associated with insulin resistance, such as acanthosis nigricans, hypertension, dyslipidemia, and polycystic ovary syndrome (**Table 13.2**).

EVALUATION

At initial presentation, patient hydration and acid–base balance must be evaluated to determine the presence or absence of DKA as well as the need for fluids and insulin administration. Once the acute presentation has been addressed, the following should be evaluated.

1. **Medical history:** Duration and presentation of symptoms, family history of diabetes and other autoimmune-mediated disease (i.e., thyroid disease) and medication history. Type 2 diabetes may present with history of obesity, hypertension, dyslipidemia, and/or strong family history of diabetes. However, obesity does not rule out a diagnosis of type 1 diabetes.
2. **Physical examination:** In addition to routine examinations, pubertal status, presence or absence of acanthosis nigricans, and the thyroid exam should be noted.
3. **Laboratory:** HbA1c will provide appropriate information on average blood sugar over the prior 2- to 3-month period. Venous pH and urinary ketones will detect ketoacidosis. Measurement of diabetes-related autoantibodies may be useful if the etiology is unclear. Up to 10% of adolescents who

clinically appear to have type 2 diabetes will have positive antibodies.[26]

TREATMENT

The treatment of diabetes should incorporate a multidisciplinary team, including the health care provider, certified diabetes educator, dietitian, and medical social worker. The team should have access to consultation from a mental health provider familiar with diabetes in AYAs.

1. **Education:** Diabetes education is ongoing. Initial diabetes education should be developmentally appropriate and specific to the type of diabetes. It should minimally include pathophysiology, BG testing, insulin dosing and administration, detection and treatment of hypoglycemia and hyperglycemia, meal planning and carbohydrate counting, and sick-day management.
2. **Insulin:** Insulin therapy is always necessary for type 1 diabetes, and for other types of diabetes when adequate glycemic control is not achieved on other regimens. See **Table 13.3** for a summary of commonly used insulins.
   a. *Rapid-acting preparations* are given before or immediately after meals.
   b. *Extended-acting analogs* are utilized as "basal" insulins. Extended-acting analogs *should not be mixed* with other insulin preparations (**Table 13.3**).
   c. *Continuous subcutaneous insulin infusion (CSII) (insulin pumps)* deliver short-acting insulin only (basal rate insulin plus boluses through the pump). Pumps permit added flexibility in designing an insulin regimen, compensating for exercise, variations in carbohydrate intake including delayed meals, and the dawn phenomenon, which presents as an increase in early morning fasting glucose due to a surge of hormones produced around 4:00 to 5:00 a.m. each morning. CSII is particularly useful for individuals who experience severe, recurrent nocturnal hypoglycemia and erratic day-to-day schedules with respect to meal times and exercise. Individuals with poor adherence to diabetes self-care are generally poor candidates for pump therapy, due to the rigor of the management skills involved. AYAs who wish to use CSII should be referred to an experienced diabetes team.
3. **Insulin regimens:** Multiple daily injection (MDI) regimens or pump therapy is most common and offers flexibility to accommodate variations in food intake, exercise schedules, and meal times in addition to offering the potential for improved glycemic control. Contemporary MDI insulin regimens are based on the use of a long-acting insulin or continuous subcutaneous insulin (pump) to provide *basal* insulin requirements (suppression of hepatic glucose production in the fasting state) and premeal *boluses* of rapid-acting insulin to cover the amount of carbohydrate consumed (food dose) and to correct for fluctuations in premeal BG (corrective dose). See Online Resources at the end of this chapter for information on insulin dosing.

TABLE 13.3

Characteristics of Insulin Preparations

Description	Proprietary Name	Onset (h)	Peak (h)	Effective Duration (h)	Max Duration (h)
Rapid acting	Lispro, aspart, glulisine	0.25	1–2	2–3	4
Short acting	Regular	0.5–1.0	2–3	3–6	4–6
Intermediate acting	Neutral protamine hagedorn	2–4	4–10	10–16	14–18
Long acting	Detemir	1–2	8–11	12–20	14–22
	Glargine	2–4	None	>24	24–36

4. **Treatment of type 2 diabetes and MODY:** Treatment should be based on the known pathophysiology—insulin resistance, hepatic overproduction of glucose, and relative insulin deficiency associated with known genetic defects.

   a. *Acute management of newly diagnosed, symptomatic patients:* Individuals who are ketotic and those with significant hyperglycemia at diagnosis (BG >250 mg/dL) initially require insulin therapy to achieve metabolic control. Metformin therapy is generally started when the patient is no longer ketotic. Insulin can be gradually withdrawn as good glycemic control is achieved. Insulin is necessary at any time when glycemic goals are unable to be met with other medications. Modifications in diet and exercise are a mainstay of treatment and complication prevention.[27]

   b. *Medication management:* Oral hypoglycemic agents (metformin) and/or insulin therapy should be maintained to achieve target glycemic goals (HbA1c ≤7%). When a single medication has not achieved the desired degree of control after 6 months, consider adding insulin.[27] Combining oral agents has not been well studied in AYAs. Biguanide (metformin) is the first-line oral hypoglycemic agent. It lowers FPG primarily by reducing hepatic glucose output, and may improve insulin sensitivity. The major side effects are mild gastrointestinal symptoms that generally resolve; side effects may be minimized by increasing the dose slowly. Hypoglycemia is uncommon, and lactic acidosis, a potentially serious condition associated with the predecessor biguanide (phenformin), is extremely rare with the only available agent in this class, *metformin*. Discontinue and ensure adequate hydration prior to contrast studies that may impair renal function and with illness associated with dehydration.

5. Assessing glycemic control

   a. *Capillary BG testing:* For any patient on multiple daily doses of insulin, it is recommended that they test BG before meals, at bedtime, as well as prior to exercise and driving. Additionally, testing is recommended whenever hypoglycemia is suspected, as well as after treating the hypoglycemic episode. Testing blood sugars at 2 to 3 a.m. is useful for evaluating nighttime hypoglycemia and fasting hyperglycemia. If there is a goal to lower HbA1c, then frequent BG monitoring must be incorporated.

   b. *HbA1c:* It should be measured quarterly. Based on the DCCT, the target HbA1c level for AYAs to avoid microvascular complications is 7.5%.

ASSOCIATED CONDITIONS AND FOLLOW-UP CARE

1. **Autoimmune disorders (type 1 diabetes):** Approximately 10% to 15% of patients with type 1 diabetes develop autoimmune thyroiditis. Because presentation is usually asymptomatic, routine annual screening to detect hypothyroidism is recommended; thyroid-stimulating hormone is generally sufficient.

2. **Microvascular complications:** Microvascular complications are directly correlated with the level of glycemic control, duration of diabetes, and are exacerbated by hypertension.

   a. *Retinopathy:* Initial exam should be performed shortly after diagnosis of type 2 diabetes and within 5 years of diagnosis of type 1 diabetes. A yearly dilated fundoscopic examination is recommended.

   b. *Nephropathy:* Annual screening for urinary albumin is recommended. The level of random urinary microalbumin:creatinine ratio is highly correlated with timed specimens. Angiotensin-converting enzyme (ACE) inhibitors or angiotensin receptor antagonists and improved blood pressure control are recommended for persistent microalbuminuria to delay the progression of nephropathy.

   c. *Neuropathy* has been shown to be more common with increase in age, longer duration of diabetes diagnosis and

diabetes type (type 2 > type 1).[28] Additional examination of the feet for pulses, sensation, deep tendon reflexes, hygiene, calluses, and evidence of infection is indicated. The monofilament test for sensation is a rapid, sensitive screening test for distal sensory neuropathy. Symptomatic autonomic neuropathy (heart rate invariability and/or postural hypotension) and gastroparesis (postprandial nausea or vomiting, postprandial hypoglycemia, and diarrhea or constipation) are also rare in this age group.

3. **Dyslipidemia:** Dyslipidemia is common in type 2 and poorly controlled type 1 diabetes. It increases the risk for cardiovascular disease and reflects various degrees of insulin resistance, obesity, diet, and poor glycemic control. The typical pattern is elevated triglycerides and decreased HDL-C. If LDL-C levels of less than 100 mg/dL have not been attained with adequate glycemic control, and reduced intake of saturated fat, treatment with lipid-lowering medications is indicated. New-generation "statin" drugs are generally preferred. Yearly measurement of fasting lipid profiles is recommended among those with previously abnormal profiles or ongoing poor glycemic control. Measurement every 5 years is sufficient if initial LDL-C is <100 mg/dL in children and every 2 years in young adults.[29,30]

4. **Hypertension:** Hypertension even with mild elevations of blood pressure (>130/80 mm Hg) is associated with an increased risk of microvascular complications. The appearance often coincides with the onset of persistent microalbuminuria. ACE inhibitors/receptor antagonists are the drugs of choice.

5. **Gluten sensitivity:** Gluten sensitivity is estimated to be present in 5% of individuals with type 1 diabetes. Evaluate with immunoglobulin A anti-tissue transglutamase antibodies if symptoms are suggestive of malabsorption or unexplained postprandial hypoglycemia.

6. **Eating disorders:** Disordered eating (including underdosing or omission of insulin) may be present in up to 30% of women with type 1 diabetes. The coexistence of eating disorders and diabetes is associated with noncompliance with treatment for diabetes and an increased risk of retinopathy.[31]

7. **Hypoglycemia:** Severe hypoglycemia is common with intensified regimens targeting euglycemia. An episode of severe hypoglycemia increases the risk for additional hypoglycemia because it is associated with a reduced magnitude of autonomic and neuroglycopenic symptoms, counterregulatory hormone responses, and cognitive dysfunction during subsequent hypoglycemia.

8. **Alcohol use:** Alcohol inhibits gluconeogenesis and interferes with the counterregulatory responses to insulin-induced hypoglycemia. Anticipatory guidance should include moderation, eating additional carbohydrates at the time of alcohol consumption, and informing others that they have diabetes.

9. **Pregnancy:** Education should be provided on the importance of preconception counseling to decrease risk for unplanned pregnancy and pregnancy complications. All pregnant diabetics should be referred to a high-risk obstetrical program.

SPECIAL CONSIDERATIONS FOR COMPLIANCE WITH AYAs[32,33]

- Identify the reason(s) for poor control and develop a strategy for remediation. Serious psychopathology (including eating disorders), recurrent DKA, and mental health disorders are indications for a mental health referral and evaluation.
- Identify one reasonable and measurable target behavior for action.
- Identify short-term relevant reinforcers—fewer symptoms (hypoglycemia or nocturia), improved physical performance, more flexibility in timing and content of meals, rewards from parents, and greater independence.

- Establish a realistic time frame for accomplishment based on behavior and provide frequent feedback; see the adolescent more frequently.
- For all adolescents, examine the extent of parental support; more support and monitoring by parents of mid-adolescents is associated with lower HbA1c.[34]
- Group coping-skill training improves long-term glycemic control and quality of life.[35]
- Consider referral to a diabetes specialist if control has not improved within 6 months.

REFERENCES

1. The Diabetes Control and Complications Trial Research Group. The effect of intensive treatment of diabetes on the development and progression of long-term complications in insulin-dependent diabetes mellitus. *N Engl J Med* 1993;329(14):977–986.
2. Nathan DM, Cleary PA, Backlund JY, et al. Intensive diabetes treatment and cardiovascular disease in patients with type 1 diabetes. *N Engl J Med* 2005;353(25):2643–2653.
3. American Diabetes Association. Diagnosis and classification of diabetes mellitus. *Diabetes Care* 2014;37 (suppl 1):S81–S90.
4. Balasubramanyam A, Nalini R, Hampe CS, et al. Syndromes of ketosis-prone diabetes mellitus. *Endocr Rev* 2008;29(3):292–302.
5. Naik RG, Brooks-Worrell BM, Palmer JP. Latent autoimmune diabetes in adults. *J Clin Endocrinol Metab* 2009;94(12):4635–4644.
6. Stumvoll M, Goldstein BJ, van Haeften TW. Type 2 diabetes: pathogenesis and treatment. *Lancet* 2008;371(9631):2153–2156.
7. Valdez R, Yoon PW, Liu T, et al. Family history and prevalence of diabetes in the U.S. population: the 6-year results from the National Health and Nutrition Examination Survey (1999–2004). *Diabetes Care* 2007;30(10):2517–2522.
8. Cowie CC, Rust KF, Byrd-Holt DD, et al. Prevalence of diabetes and impaired fasting glucose in the U.S. population: National Health and Nutrition Examination Survey 1999–2002. *Diabetes Care* 2006;29(6):1263–1268.
9. Thanabalasingham G, Owen KR. Diagnosis and management of maturity onset diabetes of the young (MODY). *BMJ* 2011;343:d6044.
10. Gupta RK, Vatamaniuk MZ, Lee CS, et al. The MODY1 gene HNF-4alpha regulates selected genes involved in insulin secretion. *J Clin Invest* 2005;115(4):1006–1015.
11. Stride A, Ellard S, Clark P, et al. Beta-cell dysfunction, insulin sensitivity, and glycosuria precede diabetes in hepatocyte nuclear factor-1alpha mutation carriers. *Diabetes Care* 2005;28(7):1751–1756.
12. Bellanne-Chantelot C, Chauveau D, Gautier JF, et al. Clinical spectrum associated with hepatocyte nuclear factor-1beta mutations. *Ann Intern Med* 2004;140(7):510–517.
13. Sagen JV, Baumann ME, Salvesen HB, et al. Diagnostic screening of NEUROD1 (MODY6) in subjects with MODY or gestational diabetes mellitus. *Diabet Med* 2005;22(8):1012–1015.
14. Donovan LE, Severin NE. Maternally inherited diabetes and deafness in a North American kindred: tips for making the diagnosis and review of unique management issues. *J Clin Endocrinol Metab* 2006;91(12):4737–4742.
15. Vatier C, Bidault G, Briand N, et al. What the genetics of lipodystrophy can teach us about insulin resistance and diabetes. *Curr Diab Rep* 2013;13(6):757–767.
16. Moran A, Becker D, Casella SJ, et al. Epidemiology, pathophysiology, and prognostic implications of cystic fibrosis-related diabetes: a technical review. *Diabetes Care* 2010;33(12):2677–2683.
17. Sullivan SD, Jablonski KA, Florez JC, et al. Genetic risk of progression to type 2 diabetes and response to intensive lifestyle or metformin in prediabetic women with and without a history of gestational diabetes. *Diabetes Care* 2014;37(4):909–911.
18. Patterson C, Guariguata L, Dahlquist G, et al. Diabetes in the young—a global view and worldwide estimates of numbers of children with type 1 diabetes. *Diabetes Res Clin Prac* 2014;103(2):161–175.
19. Centers for Disease Control and Prevention. *National diabetes fact sheet: national estimates and general information on diabetes and prediabetes in the United States, 2011.* Atlanta, GA: U.S. Department of Health and Human Services, Centers for Disease Control and Prevention, 2011.
20. Pettitt DJ, Talton J, Dabelea D, et al. Prevalence of diabetes mellitus in U.S. Youth in 2009: The SEARCH for diabetes in youth study. *Diabetes Care* 2014;37(2):402–408.
21. Rosenbloom AL, Silverstein JH, Amemiya S, et al. Type 2 diabetes in children and adolescents. *Pediatr Diabetes* 2009;10 (suppl 12):17–32.
22. Copeland KC, Zeitler P, Geffner M, et al. Characteristics of adolescents and youth with recent-onset type 2 diabetes: the TODAY cohort at baseline. *J Clin Endocrinol Metab* 2011;96(1):159–167.
23. Moran A, Jacobs DR Jr, Steinberger J, et al. Changes in insulin resistance and cardiovascular risk during adolescence: establishment of differential risk in males and females. *Circulation* 2008;117(18):2361–2368.
24. Type 2 diabetes in children and adolescents. American Diabetes Association. *Diabetes Care* 2000;23(3):381–389.
25. Hanas R, John G. 2010 consensus statement on the worldwide standardization of the hemoglobin A1C measurement. *Clin Chem Lab Med* 2010;48(6):775–776.
26. Klingensmith GJ, Pyle L, Arslanian S, et al. The presence of GAD and IA-2 antibodies in youth with a type 2 diabetes phenotype results from the TODAY study. *Diabetes Care* 2010;33(9):1970–1975.
27. Copeland KC, Silverstein J, Moore KR, et al. Management of newly diagnosed type 2 diabetes mellitus (T2DM) in children and adolescents. *Pediatrics* 2013;131(2):364–382.
28. Eppens MC, Craig ME, Cusumano J, et al. Prevalence of diabetes complications in adolescents with type 2 compared with type 1 diabetes. *Diabetes Care* 2006;29(6):1300–1306.
29. Silverstein J, Klingensmith G, Copeland K, et al. Care of children and adolescents with type 1 diabetes a statement of the American Diabetes Association. *Diabetes Care* 2005;28(1):186–212.
30. Funnell MM, Brown TL, Childs BP, et al. National standards for diabetes self-management education. *Diabetes Care* 2011;34 (suppl 1):S89–S96.
31. Rydall AC, Rodin GM, Olmsted MP, et al. Disordered eating behavior and microvascular complications in young women with insulin-dependent diabetes mellitus. *N Engl J Med* 1997;336(26):1849–1854.
32. Orr DP. Contemporary mangement of adoelscents with diabetes mellitus 1:type 1 diabetes. *Adolesc Health Update* 2000;12(2):2.
33. Orr DP. Contemporary mangement of adoelscents with diabetes mellitus 1:type 2 diabetes. *Adolesc Health Update* 2000;12(3):2.
34. Anderson B, Ho J, Brackett J, et al. Parental involvement in diabetes management tasks: relationships to blood glucose monitoring adherence and metabolic control in young adolescents with insulin-dependent diabetes mellitus. *J Pediatr* 1997;130(2):257–265.
35. Grey M, Boland EA, Davidson M, et al. Coping skills training for youth with diabetes mellitus has long-lasting effects on metabolic control and quality of life. *J Pediatr* 2000;137(1):107–113.

🛜 ADDITIONAL RESOURCES AND WEBSITES ONLINE

Cardiovascular Problems

Cardiac Risk Factors and Hyperlipidemia

Michael R. Kohn
Marc S. Jacobson

An important goal of adolescent and young adult (AYA) health care is early intervention to prevent diseases that occur during adulthood. Atherosclerosis, as conceptualized in the "injury hypothesis," results from chronic inflammation and healing responses of the arterial wall to endothelial damage beginning in childhood, accelerating during adolescence and causing clinical disease in early- to mid-adulthood. Lesions progress to cause cardiovascular disease (CVD) through the interaction of lipoproteins, cholesterol, and a range of white blood cells, with cellular constituents of the arterial wall. Delaying or preventing this progression is critical to successful management. CVD can be prevented through primordial prevention strategies.[1] Screening and lifestyle modification (i.e., adhering to a heart-healthy diet, regular exercise habits, avoidance of tobacco products, and maintenance of a healthy weight) remain critical components of health promotion and CVD risk reduction.[2] These modifications alone are not sufficient for those AYAs who have genetic abnormalities of lipid metabolism, which significantly elevate risk and shorten their healthy lifespan. For this group of patients, early recognition and aggressive management are paramount.[3] The cost effectiveness of CVD reduction by preventive strategies has been established for the statins, a group of 3-hydroxy-3-methylglutaryl-coenzyme A reductase inhibitor medications.

Understanding the pivotal role of lipids in evaluating cardiovascular risk is essential. These concepts are reviewed in this chapter, which describes lipid physiology and classification of lipid disorders. Resources tabling epidemiological data for indices of screening and risk are referenced throughout the text. The latter sections of the chapter discuss screening and management of CVD risk and draw upon pediatric, adolescent, and adult guidelines for assessment and treatment. In 2011, the National Heart, Lung, and Blood Institute (NHLBI) released the Expert Panel on Integrated Guidelines for Cardiovascular Health and Risk Reduction in Children and Adolescents.[4] Guidelines on the detection, evaluation, and treatment of high cholesterol in adults were released by the NHLBI as the Adult Treatment Panel (ATP) III guidelines in 2001.[5,6] The ATP IV was convened to update the guidelines and was renamed the American College of Cardiology (ACC)/American Heart Association (AHA) Expert Panel. In late 2013, this panel released the 2013 ACC/AHA Guideline on the Treatment of Blood Cholesterol to Reduce

Atherosclerotic Cardiovascular Risk in Adults.[7,8] Compared to the ATP III, the 2013 ACC/AHA Blood Cholesterol Guideline is more limited in scope, focusing upon evidence in randomized control trials (RCTs) and disease outcomes wherever possible. Because the transition from ATP III to the new guideline is ongoing (and because the newer guidelines reference some recommendations from the ATP III), the ATP III-recommended targets are also included in this chapter. The links for the guidelines relevant to AYAs are:

Integrated Guidelines for Cardiovascular Health and Risk Reduction in Children and Adolescents—http://www.nhlbi.nih.gov/health-pro/guidelines/current/cardiovascular-health-pediatric-guidelines

Third Report of the Expert Panel on Detection, Evaluation, and Treatment of High Blood Cholesterol in Adults (Adult Treatment Panel [ATP] III)—http://www.nhlbi.nih.gov

2013 ACC/AHA Guideline on the Treatment of Blood Cholesterol to Reduce Atherosclerotic Cardiovascular Risk in Adults

Practice Guideline—http://content.onlinejacc.org/article.aspx?articleID=1879710

Full Panel Report Supplement—http://circ.ahajournals.org/content/suppl/2013/11/07/01.cir.0000437738.63853.7a.DC1

LIPID PHYSIOLOGY

Cholesterol and triglycerides are the major blood lipids. Cholesterol is a key constituent of cell membranes and a precursor of bile acids and steroid hormones. Cholesterol circulates in the bloodstream in spherical particles called *lipoproteins* containing both lipids and proteins called *apolipoproteins*. These particles consist of a core of triglycerides, cholesterol, and cholesterol esters, in varying amounts, surrounded by an outer shell of cholesterol and phospholipids. The apolipoproteins are embedded in the outer lipid layers (Fig. 14.1).

1. Classification of lipoproteins: Five major classes of lipoproteins act as transport systems for cholesterol and triglycerides. They differ in physical and chemical characteristics and function, as well as in amounts of cholesterol, triglyceride, phospholipid, and protein. The lipoproteins can be separated by ultracentrifugation or electrophoresis, on the basis of differences in densities and surface properties. Ultracentrifugation yields chylomicrons, very-low-density lipoprotein (VLDL), low-density lipoproteins (LDLs), and high-density lipoproteins (HDLs).

2. Estimation of lipoproteins: Non-HDL Cholesterol (non-HDL-C) represents the cholesterol content of all plasma lipoproteins and may soon replace LDL-C in risk assessment, particularly when non fasting lipids are used. NonHDL-C

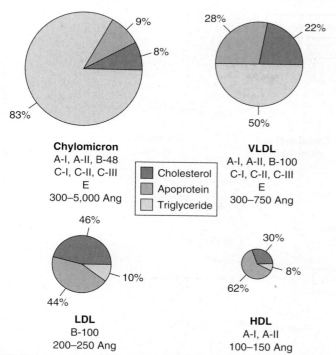

Chylomicron
A-I, A-II, B-48
C-I, C-II, C-III
E
300–5,000 Ang

9%
8%
83%

Cholesterol
Apoprotein
Triglyceride

VLDL
A-I, A-II, B-100
C-I, C-II, C-III
E
300–750 Ang

28%
22%
50%

LDL
B-100
200–250 Ang

46%
10%
44%

HDL
A-I, A-II
100–150 Ang

30%
8%
62%

FIGURE 14.1 Characteristics of lipoproteins. Apoproteins and volume are detailed below each lipoprotein. Ang, angstroms; VLDL, very-low-density lipoprotein; LDL, low-density lipoprotein; HDL, high-density lipoprotein. (Adapted from Hardoff D, Jacobson MS. Hyperlipidemia. *Adolesc Med State Arts Rev* 1992;3:475.)

is calculated as follows: Total cholesterol minus HDL-C = nonHDL-C.

The calculation of the proportion of LDL is made with the following formula:

$$\text{Total cholesterol} = \text{LDL} + \text{HDL} + \text{VLDL}$$

HDL is measured directly, and VLDL is estimated by dividing the fasting triglyceride concentration by 5 (true, so long as the triglyceride concentration is <400 mg/dL). Therefore,

$$\text{LDL} = \text{Total cholesterol} - \text{HDL} - (\text{triglycerides}/5)$$

Each lipoprotein has a characteristic apolipoprotein profile. These apolipoproteins serve as cofactors for enzymes involved in lipoprotein metabolism, they help in the binding of lipoproteins to cellular receptors, and they facilitate lipid transfer between lipoproteins. Apolipoprotein B-100 (apoB-100) is an important component of VLDL and is the only apolipoprotein in LDL cholesterol (LDL-C). Uptake of LDL by cells is dependent on its binding to the LDL receptor, which is regulated by apoB-100. Abnormalities in both quality and quantity of these proteins, even in the absence of an elevated cholesterol concentration, may contribute to atherosclerosis.

3. Lipoprotein circulation and sources: (Fig. 14.2)
   a. Exogenous: Chylomicrons are formed after absorption of dietary fat. They are secreted into the lymph. Fatty acids are stored in adipose tissue, or are used in skeletal muscle and myocardium, where they release diet-derived triglycerides. This reaction is catalyzed by lipoprotein lipase. The chylomicron remnants are rapidly absorbed in the liver by specific receptors for these particles. In liver cells, the remnants are degraded to free cholesterol, which is excreted into bile.

   b. Endogenous: The endogenous transport system includes VLDL, intermediate-density lipoprotein (IDL), LDL, and HDL. Excess calories from carbohydrates and fatty acids are metabolized in the liver into triglycerides. The lipoproteins carrying these triglycerides are primarily VLDL, which moves to adipose tissue; the result is the formation of IDL and LDL. The IDL particles are rapidly removed from circulation by LDL receptors in the liver.
   • LDL transports cholesterol to peripheral tissues. In addition to the lipid component, LDL particles contain a single apoB-100 molecule, the protein that binds to LDL receptors. After binding to LDL cell-surface receptors, the LDL particles deliver cholesterol for synthesis of cell membranes in all cells; for steroid hormones in the adrenal glands, ovary, and testes, and for bile acids in the liver. The LDL-C found in macrophages and smooth muscle cells of atherosclerotic lesions enters by additional mechanisms. This LDL-C is modified by intravascular oxidation and is taken up in lesions by oxy-LDL receptors and scavenger receptors. This process may provide alternative pathways for therapeutic intervention.
   • HDL is secreted from the liver or intestine in a lipid-poor form or is made de novo in the plasma. As it matures, HDL accumulates cholesterol from tissues, including blood vessel walls, and therefore has a major role in removing excess cholesterol and delivering it to the liver by means of the triglyceride-rich lipoproteins and cholesterol ester transfer protein.

LIPID PATHOPHYSIOLOGY AND CVD

1. Epidemiological evidence:
   a. In populations throughout the world, there is a direct correlation between serum cholesterol levels and CVD rates. The prevalence of hyperlipidemia has been well documented.[9] Traditional risk factor assessment has focused on parameters derived from the Bogalusa[10,11] and Framingham Heart Study[12] (age, hypertension, cholesterol, family history, and cigarette smoking). New emerging risk factors, both biological and genetic, are reshaping the understanding of heart disease and the approach to risk stratification. The Pathobiological Determinants of Atherosclerosis in Youth Study described the relationship between atherosclerosis and serum lipoprotein cholesterol concentrations and smoking in AYA males.[13]
2. Genetic evidence (characteristics of inherited hyperlipoproteinemias are listed in **Table 14.1**):
   a. Familial hypercholesterolemia (FH): In its most common form, FH is an autosomal dominant condition resulting in defects in the LDL receptor and elevated levels of LDL-C. About 1 in 300 to 500 AYAs in the US is heterozygous for the abnormality; these individuals account for 15% of cases of premature CVD. Homozygous individuals (~1 in 1,000,000) lack LDL cell-surface receptor activity, have very high cholesterol levels, and may develop severe atherosclerosis in the first two decades of life. Clinical manifestations such as xanthomas and other signs of cutaneous lipid deposition are generally seen in the fourth decade of life in heterozygotes and during adolescence in homozygotes (Fig. 14.3).[14]
   b. Familial combined hyperlipidemia (FCHL): It is the autosomal dominant syndrome that affects approximately 1% to 2% of the population. Most, if not all, patients with this condition have elevated levels of LDL apoB. Abnormal metabolism of VLDL and partial lipoprotein lipase deficiency have also been described in association with this syndrome. Individuals with FCHL account for a significant proportion of cases of early-onset CVD.

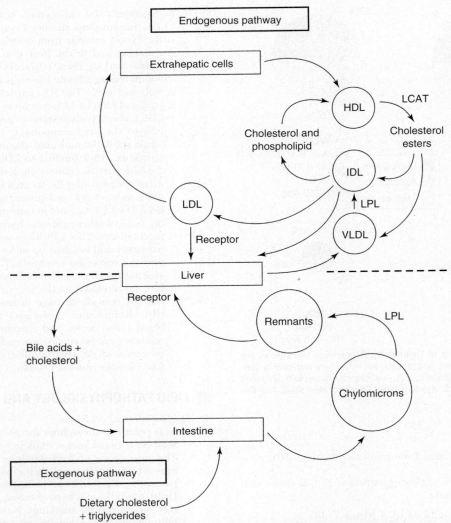

FIGURE 14.2 Pathways of lipoprotein metabolism. LCAT, lecithin-cholesterol acyltransferase; LPL, lipoprotein lipase; HDL, high-density lipoprotein; LDL, low-density lipoprotein; IDL, intermediate-density lipoprotein; VLDL, very-low-density lipoprotein. (From Weis S, Lacko AG. Role of lipoproteins in hypercholesterolemia. *Pract Cardiol* 1988:12–18.)

c. Apolipoprotein E (apoE)[15]: Three common alleles of apoE, at a single-gene locus on chromosome 19, code for three isoforms of apoE: designated as apoE-II, apoE-III, and apoE-IV. Increased cardiovascular risk is associated with apoE-IV, in comparison with the more common apoE-III.

3. Novel biomarkers:
a. High-sensitivity C-reactive protein (hs-CRP) assays: Inflammation is an important risk factor for atherogenesis. C-reactive protein (CRP), the most studied biomarker of inflammation in CVD, is secreted by foam cells in the arterial wall. CRP is implicated in the development of CVD through its actions: induction of a prothrombotic state, increasing leukocyte adhesion, and promotion of intimal damage. CRP has been shown to be a lipid-independent risk factor for CVD. CRP assays have traditionally been used to detect inflammation and/or infection. Hs-CRP assays detect low levels of CRP and may have utility in predicting a healthy person's risk of CVD. While guidelines have been proposed for the use of hs-CRP in asymptomatic adults at intermediate risk of CVD, there are currently no clear guidelines for the use of hs-CRP assays to predict CVD risk among AYAs.

b. Apolipoprotein-associated phospholipase A2 (Lp-PLA2)[16]: The enzyme Lp-PLA2 is a member of the phospholipase A family. It is actively expressed in unstable atherosclerotic plaques, suggesting its role in increasing plaque vulnerability. Lp-PLA2 is both less variable than CRP and a more specific marker of vascular inflammation.
c. Myeloperoxidase (MPO) and oxidized LDL[17]: Products of the MPO pathway may be good markers of CVD, and possibly therapeutic targets as well.

4. Interventional trials: Interventional trials support the conclusion that lowering total and LDL-C concentrations reduces the incidence of CVD events. The degree of benefit is greatest in individuals who have other associated risk factors, such as cigarette smoking, diabetes, and hypertension.

5. Relationship of particular lipoproteins to cardiovascular risk:
a. LDL-C: Studies show a positive relationship between the level of cholesterol, and the frequency of CVD.
b. HDL-C: Population studies suggest an inverse relation between HDL-C and CVD. An HDL-C level of <30 mg/dL carries a significantly increased risk of CVD. A level >50 mg/dL is associated with low risk, and >75 mg/dL is associated with very low risk. The Framingham Heart Study demonstrated a 10% increase in CVD for each 4 mg/dL decrease

TABLE 14.1

Characteristics of Inherited Hyperlipoproteinemias

Hyperlipoproteinemia	Phenotype	Cholesterol	Triglyceride	Xanthomas	Frequency (%)	Risk of CVD
Familial lipoprotein lipase deficiency	I	Normal	↑	Eruptive	Very rare	0
Familial hypercholesterolemia	IIa	↑	↑	Tendon	0.1–0.5	4+
	IIb			Tuberous xanthelasma		
Polygenic hypercholesterolemia	II	↑	Normal	Tuberous	5	2+
Familial dysbetalipoproteinemia	III	↑	↑	Palmar	Rare	4+
				Planar tuberous tendon		
Familial combined hyperlipoproteinemia	IIa	↑	↑	Any type	1–2	3+
	IIb					
	IV					
	Rarely V					
Familial hypertriglyceridemia	IV	Normal	↑	Eruptive	1	1+
	Rarely V					

CVD, coronary artery disease; NL, normal.
From Arky RA, Perlman AJ. Hyperlipoproteinemia. In: Rubenstein E, Federman DD, eds. *Scientific American medicine.* New York, NY: Scientific American, 1988, with permission.

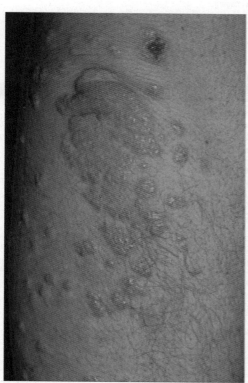

FIGURE 14.3 Xanthoma. (Courtesy of Dr. Steven Gammer.)

in HDL. In addition, low HDL-C levels have been correlated with an increased number of diseased coronary arteries. There also appears to be a higher rate of restenosis after angioplasty in individuals with low HDL-C levels. HDL has two components, HDL_2 and HDL_3. The former is considered a better indicator of negative CVD risk than total HDL. Exercise raises the level of cardioprotective HDL_2, whereas ethanol raises the level of HDL_3. Unfortunately, raising

HDL-C is not currently a therapeutic option. Pharmaceutical trials have so far failed to show reduction in CVD and some have been discontinued because of higher CVD in drug-treated than placebo groups.

c. Apolipoproteins: Apolipoproteins A-I (apoA-I), A-II (apoA-II), and apoB are used in predicting the risk of CVD. Elevated concentrations of apoA-I and apoA-II are associated with a lower risk, and an elevated apoB concentration is associated with a higher risk of CVD. Isoforms of apoE have also been implicated in cardiovascular risk, as noted previously. In addition, the measurement of the apoB-100 to apoA-I ratio may provide another assessment of cardiovascular risk.

d. Ratios: CVD risk rises sharply when the LDL:HDL ratio exceeds 3.0. Another ratio predictive of CVD risk is that of total cholesterol to HDL-C. A ratio of <4.5 denotes below-average risk, whereas the optimum ratio is 3.5:1. The AHA recommends that the absolute numbers for total blood cholesterol, LDL-C, HDL-C, and non-HDL-C be used. The AHA suggests that these numbers are more useful than ratios to the physician determining appropriate treatment for patients.

6. Other experimental work: Proprotein convertase subtilisin/kinexin type 9 (PCSK9)[16]: PCSK9 is a serine protease. It binds the low-density lipoprotein receptor (LDL-R) in circulation and promotes LDL-R degradation. A missense mutation in PCSK9 leads to higher circulating LDL. Several, new therapeutic options targeting PCSK9, including monoclonal antibody–based therapies, have entered trials with promising results in subjects with both familial and nonfamilial forms of hypercholesterolemia.

CLASSIFICATION OF HYPERLIPIDEMIAS

Patients with hyperlipidemia are classified based on lipid pathways, phenotype, pathophysiology, and genetics.[14] The three pathways are the exogenous (intestinal), the endogenous (hepatic), and the reverse cholesterol pathway. Metabolic characteristics of the clinically important derangements in lipid metabolism are summarized in **Table 14.2**.

Metabolic Classification of Dyslipoproteinemia in Children and Adolescents

1. Disorders of LDL metabolism/disorders with increased LDL
   a. Decreased LDL removal
      —Familial hypercholesterolemia
      —Defective apoB-100
   b. Increased LDL production
      —Familial combined hypercholesterolemia
      —Hyperapobetalipoproteinemia
   c. Other
      —Polygenic hypercholesterolemia

2. Disorders of triglyceride-rich lipoproteins
   a. Decreased removal (type I dyslipoproteinemia)
      —Lipoprotein lipase deficiency
      —ApoC-II deficiency (cofactor for lipoprotein lipase)
   b. Production of abnormal VLDL
      —Familial hypertriglyceridemia (AD)
   c. Decreased removal/increased production
      —Type V dyslipoproteinemia (AD)
      —Dysbetalipoproteinemia

3. Deficiency in HDL
   a. Increased HDL removal
   b. Decreased HDL production

LDL, low-density lipoprotein; VLDL, very-low-density lipoprotein; AD, autosomal dominant; HDL, high-density lipoprotein.
From Kwiterovich PO Jr. Diagnosis and management of familial dyslipoproteinemia in children and adolescents. *Pediatr Clin North Am* 1990;37:1489, with permission.

TABLE 14.3
Screening Elements for Cardiovascular Risk Assessment

1. Clinical evaluation: history, including medical conditions leading to dyslipidemia and accelerated atherosclerosis; e.g., insulin resistance (obesity, metabolic syndrome, polycystic ovary syndrome (PCOS), diabetes), chronic inflammatory diseases, endocrine diseases (hypothyroidism, renal disease, organ transplantation)
2. Family history: cardiovascular events prior to 55 y of age, history of risk factors in parents
3. Physical examination: including anthropometric measurement, blood pressure, presence of stigmata of hyperlipidemia; e.g., xanthoma, xanthelasma, corneal arcus
4. Global Risk Scoring (FRS, SCORE, Reynolds; http://www.reynolds riskscore.org/)
5. Bloods: Established markers LDL-C, non-HDL cholesterol (=Total cholesterol minus HDL-C can be assessed fasting or nonfasting)
   Emerging markers—apolipoprotein B, HDL-C, lipoprotein "little a" (Lp(a)), lipoprotein fractionation and particle (VAP, NMR)*, hsC-reactive protein (CRP) >2 mg/dL, lipoprotein-associated phospholipase A2 (Lp-PLA2)
   Homocysteine (clinical significance if >10 nmol/L)
6. Noninvasive assessment of subclinical atherosclerosis
   Carotid intima-media thickness using ultrasound
   CT for coronary calcium
   Flow-mediated dilatation

FRS, Framingham Risk Score; LDL-C, low-density lipoprotein cholesterol; HDL-C, high-density lipoprotein cholesterol; CT, computerized tomography; MRI, magnetic resonance imaging.

CARDIOVASCULAR RISK ASSESSMENT

Risk factors for CVD have genetic, physiologic, behavioral, and environmental components and may be determined by history, physical examination, laboratory, and other assessments (detailed in **Table 14.3**). The relationship between cardiovascular risk factors and CVD has been demonstrated in longitudinal studies.[13,18] Risk factors can be identified prior to adulthood and track into adult life.[19] Nonmodifiable risk factors include genetics, parent with elevated total cholesterol (>240 mg/dL), and gender. Modifiable major risk factors include hypertension, smoking, diet, weight, diabetes/insulin resistance (with metabolic syndrome), and dyslipidemia. Interventions exist for the management of this latter group of risk factors, once they are identified. Several medical conditions also confer increased risk for CVD.

- **Table 14.4** lists elements of the family history and risk factors.
- **Table 14.5** lists special risk conditions that confer high- and moderate risk for CVD in the Integrated Guidelines for Cardiovascular Health and Risk Reduction in Children and Adolescents.
- **Table 14.6** lists major risk factors that modify LDL-C goals in the ATP III guidelines.

Screening recommendations for modifiable risk factors are detailed below. Historical factors and patient report alone will lead to identification of only a minority of those with hyperlipidemia; therefore, identification of AYAs with hyperlipidemia requires universal lipid assessment. Non-HDL cholesterol (non-HDL-C) is the best predictor of atherosclerosis, and is elevated in both FH and FCHL—see section Classification of Hyperlipidemia. It is calculated as:

$$\text{Non-HDL-C} = \text{Total cholesterol} - \text{HDL-C}$$

A practical advantage of non-HDL-C is that it can be measured in nonfasting patients.

TABLE 14.4
Risk Factor Definitions for Dyslipidemia Algorithms

(+) Family history:
- Myocardial infarction, angina, coronary artery bypass graft/stent/angioplasty, sudden cardiac death in parent, grandparent, aunt, or uncle, male <55 y, female <65 y

High level risk factors:
- Hypertension requiring drug therapy (BP ≥ 99th percentile + 5 mm Hg)
- Current cigarette smoker
- BMI ≥ 97th percentile
- Presence of high-risk conditions (Table 14.5)

(Diabetes mellitus [DM] is also a high level risk factor, but it is classified here as a high-risk condition to correspond with *Adult Treatment Panel III* recommendations for adults that DM is considered a CVD equivalent.)

Moderate-level RFs:
- Hypertension not requiring drug therapy
- BMI ≥ 95th percentile, < 97th percentile
- HDL-C < 40 mg/dL
- Presence of moderate risk conditions (Table 14.5)

Hypertension

For AYAs with asymptomatic, Stage 1 hypertension and no other risk factors, nonpharmacologic interventions should be recommended, including a low-salt diet, weight reduction, and aerobic exercise. Classification, assessment, and intervention for hypertension are covered in detail in Chapter 17.

Cigarette Smoking

Most cigarette smoking begins early in adolescence. Effective education programs, such as those reviewed by the World Health Organization (http://www.euro.who.int/document/e82993.pdf), must

TABLE 14.5

Assessment and management algorithm for Cardiovascular Risk—targeting LDL-C

High Risk	Moderate Risk
• Diabetes mellitus, type 1 and type 2	• Kawasaki disease with regressed coronary aneurysms
• Chronic kidney disease/end-stage renal disease/postrenal transplant	• Chronic inflammatory disease (systemic lupus erythematosus, juvenile rheumatoid arthritis)
• Postorthotopic heart transplant	• Human immunodeficiency virus infection (HIV)
• Kawasaki disease with current aneurysms	• Nephrotic syndrome

TABLE 14.6

Assessment and management algorithm for Cardiovascular Risk—targeting Triglycerides

- Cigarette smoking
- Hypertension (blood pressure ≥140/90 mm Hg or on antihypertensive medication)
- Low HDL cholesterol (<40 mg/dL)[b]
- Family history of premature CHD (CHD in first-degree male relative <55 y; CHD in first-degree female relative <65 y)
- Age (men ≥45 y; women ≥55 y)

[a]Diabetes is regarded as a coronary heart disease (CHD) risk equivalent.
[b]High-density lipoprotein (HDL) cholesterol ≥60 mg/dL counts as a "negative" risk factor; its presence removes one risk factor from the total count.
From Expert Panel on Detection, Evaluation, and Treatment of High Blood Cholesterol in Adults. Executive summary of the third report of the National Cholesterol Education Program Expert Panel on detection, evaluation, and treatment of high blood cholesterol in adults (ATP III). *JAMA* 2001;285(19):2486–2497, with permission

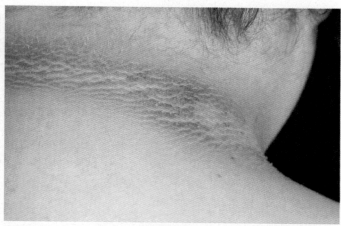

FIGURE 14.4 Acanthosis Nigricans. (From Baranoski S, Ayello EA. *Wound care essentials.* 3rd ed. Philadelphia, PA: Lippincott Williams & Wilkins, 2011.)

be developed and implemented at the national level, at the local school level, and in the practitioner's office.

Obesity

Obesity is a strong risk factor for CVD. The best therapy for obesity is to prevent it. This requires early recognition and management, ideally prior to and during the adolescent growth spurt. The waist–hip ratio is also an important predictor of lipoprotein levels. A waist circumference of >40 in. (102 cm) in men or 35 in. (80 cm) in women is considered abdominal obesity, a part of the metabolic syndrome. In adolescents, the metabolic syndrome is best managed with lifestyle changes aimed at overweight and obesity.

Nonlipid (Novel) Risk Factor Assessment

Insulin resistance is suspected when high triglycerides and low HDL-C occur in conjunction with central adiposity with or without acanthosis nigricans (Fig. 14.4). Various cutoffs and ratios for glucose and insulin levels have been proposed but none are yet definitive. Insulin resistance is associated with accelerated atherosclerosis through various mechanisms including lipid oxidation, endothelial dysfunction, and thrombogenic abnormalities. It is associated with the metabolic syndrome (syndrome X), which consists of at least three of the following five: central adiposity, hypertension, elevated triglyceride levels, decreased HDL-C levels, impaired glucose tolerance.[20]

ATP III recognizes metabolic syndrome as a secondary target of cardiovascular risk reduction after LDL lowering. Routine screening of fasting insulin is not recommended; rather, it should be reserved for individuals with risk factors for type 2 diabetes (such as family history, obesity, or acanthosis nigricans).

Other potential emerging risk factors include inflammatory markers such as CRP, coagulation factors (such as fibrinogen and factors VIII and VII), deficiency of antioxidant vitamins, and chlamydia infections.

SCREENING FOR DYSLYPIDEMIA

Dyslipidemias place AYAs at increased risk for accelerated early atherosclerosis.[21] Selective screening of children and adolescents for FH has been recommended for over three decades. FH is strongly suggested by a nonfasting test of non-HDL-C that is ≥190 mg/dL or a fasting test of LDL-C that is >160 mg/dL on two occasions. Screening for dyslipidemia in the context of evaluating cardiovascular risk should include the following:

- Family history of premature CVD (younger than 55 years for male and 65 for female relatives) such as myocardial infarction or other sequelae of atherosclerosis
- Family history of dyslipidemia
- Signs of peripheral lipid deposition, on physical examination (xanthoma, xanthelasma, corneal arcus)

The Expert Panel Integrated Guidelines for Cardiovascular Health and Risk Reduction in Children and Adolescents

These guidelines stress the importance of initial screening for FH beginning at 2 years of age if there is a positive family history of early cardiovascular event, or diagnosis of FH in a parent.[4] Relative to screening in AYAs, the guidelines recommend the following (Fig. 14.5):

- 9- to 11-year-olds: Universal lipid screening with nonfasting lipid panel and calculation of non-HDL-C.
- 12- to 16-year-olds: Routine screening is *not* recommended because the sensitivity and specificity for predicting adult levels of LDL-C are reduced in this age group. Fasting lipids should be obtained for 12- to 16-year-olds if they have diabetes, hypertension, BMI ≥85th percentile, or close family member with evidence of early atherosclerotic CVD.
- 17- to 21-year-olds: Universal lipid screening once during this time period with nonfasting lipid panel and calculation of non-HDL-C.

If non-HDL-C ≥145 mg/dL and/or HDL-C <40 mg/dL, fasting lipids should be measured on two occasions (at least 2 weeks apart within a 3-month period). The results from these two measurements should be averaged to guide treatment.

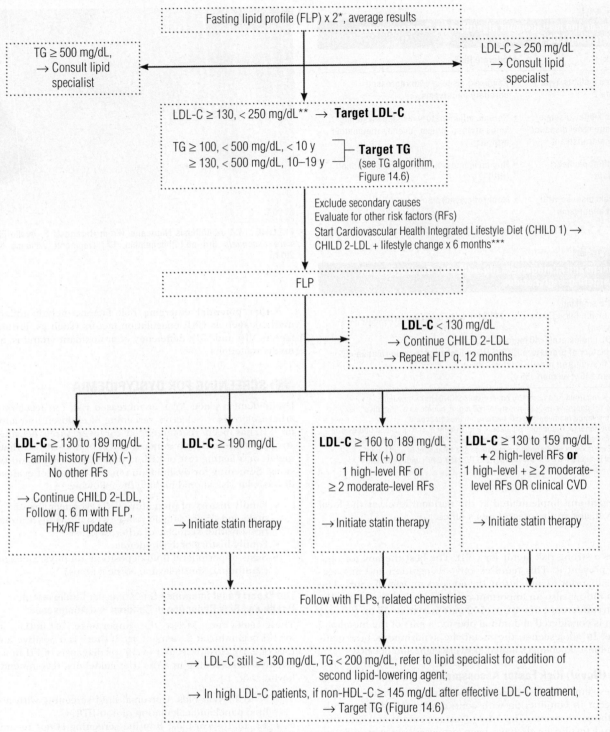

FIGURE 14.5 Dyslipidemia algorithm: target LDL-C (low-density lipoprotein cholesterol)

(From National Institutes of Health. *Expert Panel on Integrated Guidelines for Cardiovascular Health and Risk Reduction in Children and Adolescents* (Summary report). Washington, DC: US Department of Health and Human Services, October 2012. http://www.nhlbi.nih.gov/files/docs/peds_guidelines_sum.pdf)

Screening in Young Adults

2013 ACC/AHA Blood Cholesterol Guideline

1. The 2013 Guideline, consistent with the ATP III guideline, recommends that all adults have a fasting lipid panel measured by age 20 and that screening for FH should be undertaken in first-degree relatives (including children) of patients with LDL-C >190 mg/dL.
2. Evaluate for secondary causes of hyperlipidemia in individuals with LDL-C >190 mg/dL OR triglycerides >500 mg/dL.

ATP III Recommendations

ATP III recommendations for young adults aged 20 to 35 years are:

1. Fasting lipid profile is the preferred method of assessing lipid risk and should be determined in every young adult regardless of family history at least once every 5 years.
2. The number of risk factors is counted (**Table 14.6**). For those with two or more risk factors, Framingham scoring is then used to assign 10-year risk of a coronary event.
3. The lipid profile is interpreted by the following guidelines:

- LDL-C

Optimal	<100 mg/dL
Near optimal	100–129 mg/dL
Borderline high	130–159 mg/dL
High	160–189 mg/dL
Very high	190 mg/dL

- Total cholesterol

Desirable	<200 mg/dL
Borderline	200–239 mg/dL
High risk	>240 mg/dL

- HDL-C

Low	<40 mg/dL
High	>60 mg/dL

Screening for Hypertriglyceridemia

Moderate hypertriglyceridemia alone is not independently correlated with CVD. Severe hypertriglyceridemia (≥1,000 mg/dL) is associated with an increased incidence of acute life-threatening pancreatitis and must be aggressively treated with diet, weight loss, and pharmacotherapy. The Framingham study has found that a triglyceride concentration of >150 mg/dL, in combination with a HDL level of <35 mg/dL, is as good a predictor of CVD as an elevated LDL level.[22]

The Expert Panel on Integrated Guidelines for Cardiovascular Health and Risk Reduction in Children and Adolescents (2 to 20 years) defines hypertriglyceridemia as follows: "acceptable" <90 mg/dL, "borderline" 90 to 129 mg/dL, and "high" >130 mg/dL (**Fig. 14.6** and **Table 14.7**).[4] The 2013 ACC/AHA Blood Cholesterol Guideline notes that the Expert Panel did not conduct a systematic review of the management of severe hypertriglyceridemia. The guideline refers to the ATP III guideline and recommends evaluation for secondary causes of hyperlipidemia in individuals with LDL-C ≥190 mg/dL OR triglycerides ≥500 mg/dL.

The ATP III strictly defines hypertriglyceridemia as follows:

Normal triglycerides	<150 mg/dL
Borderline-high triglycerides	150–199 mg/dL
High triglycerides	200–499 mg/dL
Very high triglycerides	>500 mg/dL

THERAPY FOR HYPERLIPIDEMIA

Lifestyle Interventions

Heart-healthy lifestyle habits (referred to as therapeutic lifestyle changes (TLCs) in ATP III) are the cornerstone of therapy for hyperlipidemia and should be recommended to all individuals. These include healthy dietary patterns, regular physical exercise, maintenance of healthy body weight, and abstinence and cessation of tobacco use.

Heart-Healthy Diet

The principal treatment of hyperlipidemia in AYAs is a diet with modified amounts of fat, saturated fat, and cholesterol without increased simple carbohydrates. As specified by the 2013 ACC/AHA Blood Cholesterol Guideline, a heart-healthy diet is rich in vegetables, fruits, low-fat dairy, whole grains, poultry, fish, legumes, nuts, and vegetable oil with limited intake of red meat, sweets, and sugar-containing beverages, *trans* fat, and sodium. In general, this diet should limit intake of saturated fat to 5% to 6% of calories.

Recommendations from the Integrated Guidelines for Cardiovascular Health and Risk Reduction in Children and Adolescents differ from those for adults because of the careful consideration and monitoring of energy and micronutrient consumption required to support normal growth and development. This is particularly important during the adolescent growth years, when energy, protein, mineral, and vitamin requirements are increased. Nutritional counseling is needed that focuses on meeting fat and cholesterol recommendations while ensuring adequate macronutrient and micronutrient intake. The Committee on Nutrition of the American Academy of Pediatrics recently set lower limits on the recommended fat intake of children and adolescents at no more than 30% of the average daily caloric intake and no less than 20% of the average daily caloric intake. Evidence-based recommendations for 11- to 21-year-olds include the following:

- Limiting total fat to 25% to 30% of daily kcal
- Saturated fat 8% to 10% of daily kcal
- Avoidance of *trans* fat as much as possible
- Monounsaturated/polyunsaturated fat up to 20% of daily kcal
- Cholesterol <300 mg/day
- Encourage high dietary fiber intake from foods

In addition, these guidelines recommend limiting naturally sweetened juice and sugar-sweetened beverages, limiting sodium intake, and encouraging eating meals as a family. Please see the complete guidelines for specific recommendations for adolescents and adults.

Pharmacologic Treatment of Hyperlipidemia

The use of pharmacologic agents to treat AYAs with high cholesterol levels is the subject of interest and debate because little is known about the long-term risks and benefits of drug treatment in this population. Several studies have demonstrated the short-term (1 to 2 years) safety and efficacy of statins in children and adolescents with FH so that the US Food and Drug Administration (FDA) has now approved atorvastatin, lovastatin, pravastatin, rosuvastatin, and simvastatin for use in 8- to 18-year-olds with FH.[4] Statins, the primary therapy for hypercholesterolemia particularly in FH, are contraindicated in pregnancy; therefore, AYA females using statins must be counseled accordingly. It is important to have a frank discussion and full disclosure of risks.

General Principles of Pharmacologic Therapy

1. Diagnose and treat secondary causes of hyperlipidemia.
2. Implement and assess for adherence to healthy lifestyle interventions.
3. Reduce risk factors. Intervene when there are risk factors that can be modified, including smoking, hypertension, and diabetes.

2013 ACC/AHA Blood Cholesterol Guideline

The 2013 Guideline notes that there were no primary-prevention RCT data available for individuals 21 to 39 years of age. Given the focus on evidence from RCTs, the 2013 ACC/AHA Blood Cholesterol Guideline is narrower in scope, particularly regarding treatment in the AYA population.

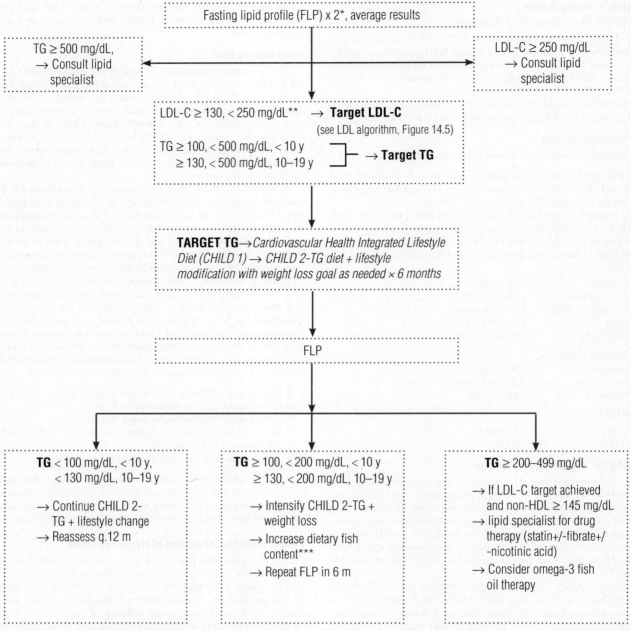

Fasting lipid profile (FLP) x 2*, average results

TG ≥ 500 mg/dL,
→ Consult lipid
specialist

LDL-C ≥ 250 mg/dL
→ Consult lipid
specialist

LDL-C ≥ 130, < 250 mg/dL**   → **Target LDL-C**
(see LDL algorithm, Figure 14.5)

TG ≥ 100, < 500 mg/dL, < 10 y
≥ 130, < 500 mg/dL, 10–19 y   → **Target TG**

TARGET TG→*Cardiovascular Health Integrated Lifestyle
Diet (CHILD 1) → CHILD 2-TG diet + lifestyle
modification with weight loss goal as needed × 6 months*

FLP

TG < 100 mg/dL, < 10 y,
< 130 mg/dL, 10–19 y

→ Continue CHILD 2-
TG + lifestyle change
→ Reassess q.12 m

TG ≥ 100, < 200 mg/dL, < 10 y
≥ 130, < 200 mg/dL, 10–19 y

→ Intensify CHILD 2-TG +
weight loss
→ Increase dietary fish
content***
→ Repeat FLP in 6 m

TG ≥ 200–499 mg/dL

→ If LDL-C target achieved
and non-HDL ≥ 145 mg/dL
→ lipid specialist for drug
therapy (statin+/-fibrate+/
-nicotinic acid)
→ Consider omega-3 fish
oil therapy

*   Obtain FLPs at least 2 wk but no more than 3 mo apart.

**   Use of drug therapy is limited to children ≥ 10 y with defined risk profiles.

*** The Food and Drug Administration (FDA) and the Environmental Protection Agency are advising women of childbearing age who may become pregnant,
pregnant women, nursing mothers, and young children to avoid some types of fish and shellfish and eat fish and shellfish that are lower in mercury.
For more information, call the FDA's food information line toll free at 1-888-SAFEFOOD or visit www.fda.gov/Food/FoodSafety/Product-specificinformation/
Seafood/FoodbornePathogensContaminants/Methylmercury/ucm115644.htm.

CHILD = Cardiovascular Health Integrated Lifestyle Diet - Available in the reference document: Section 5. Nutrition and Diet

Note: Values given are in mg/dL. To convert to SI units, divide results for total cholesterol (TC), low-density
lipoprotein cholesterol (LDL-C) high-density lipoprotein cholesterol (HDL-C), and non-HDL-C by 38.6; for
triglycerides (TG), divide by 88.6.

FIGURE 14.6 Dyslipidemia algorithm: target TG (triglycerides)

(From National Institutes of Health. *Expert Panel on Integrated Guidelines for Cardiovascular Health and Risk Reduction in Children and Adolescents* (Summary
report). Washington, DC: US Department of Health and Human Services, October 2012. http://www.nhlbi.nih.gov/files/docs/peds_guidelines_sum.pdf)

TABLE 14.7

Acceptable, Borderline, and Abnormal Plasma Lipid, Lipoprotein, and Apolipoprotein Concentrations in Adolescents

	Acceptable (mg/dL)	Borderline (mg/dL)	High (mg/dL)[a]
Total cholesterol	<170	170–199	>200
LDL cholesterol	<110	110–129	>130
Non-HDL cholesterol	<120	120–144	>145
Apolipoprotein B	<90	90–109	>110
Triglycerides (10–19 yr)	<90	90–129	>130
HDL cholesterol	>45	40–45	<40
Apolipoprotein A-1	>120	115–120	<115

[a]Low cut points for HDL and apolipoprotein A-1 represent approximately the 10th percentile. Cut points for high and borderline represent approximately the 95th and 75th percentiles, respectively.
LDL, low-density lipoprotein; HDL, high-density lipoprotein.
Values for plasma lipid and lipoprotein levels are from the NCEP Expert Panel on Cholesterol Levels in Children. Non-HDL cholesterol values from the Bogalusa Heart Study are equivalent to the NCEP Pediatric Panel cut points for LDL cholesterol. Values for plasma apolipoprotein B and apolipoprotein A-1 are from the National Health and Nutrition Examination Survey III.
Adapted from Expert Panel on Integrated Guidelines for Cardiovascular Health and Risk Reduction in Children and Adolescents; National Heart, Lung, and Blood Institute. Expert panel on integrated guidelines for cardiovascular health and risk reduction in children and adolescents: summary report. *Pediatrics* 2011;128(suppl 5):S213–S256.

The ACC/AHA Guideline Expert Panel (2013) was unable to find RCT evidence to support titrating cholesterol-lowering drug therapy to achieve target LDL-C or non-HDL-C levels, as recommended by ATP III. However, the Expert Panel did find extensive RCT evidence that the appropriate intensity of statin therapy should be used to reduce CVD risk. On the basis of these findings, the 2013 ACC/AHA Blood Cholesterol Guideline has abandoned the use of the LDL targets utilized in ATP III and focused on intensity of statin therapy in four patient groups for which there is evidence that therapy exceeds risk:

- Adults (including young adults) with clinical atherosclerotic CVD
- Adults (including young adults) with LDL-C ≥190 mg/dL
- Adults aged 40 to 75 years with diabetes and LDL-C 70 to 189 mg/dL
- Adults aged 40 to 75 years with 10-year atherosclerotic CVD risk between 5% and 7.5% (as determined by NHLBI's Pooled Cohort Equations (based on age, sex, smoking status, total cholesterol and HDL-C levels, systolic blood pressure, and use of antihypertensive medications). A CVD risk calculator is available at http://my.americanheart.org/cvriskcalculator.

The 2013 ACC/AHA Blood Cholesterol Guideline recommends the following for young adults without clinical CVD or diabetes:

1. Heart-healthy lifestyle habits should be recommended to and encouraged of all individuals.
2. Adults ≥21 years with primary elevations of LDL-C ≥190 mg/dL should be treated with statins.
   a. High-intensity statins (atorvastatin at 40 to 80 mg or rosuvastatin at 20 to 40 mg) are preferred.
   b. Regularly monitor adherence to lifestyle habits.
   c. Monitor adherence and response to drug therapy with lipid assessments (4 to 12 weeks after initiation of a statin or change in dose).
   d. The Expert Panel found insufficient evidence from RCTs to support titration of statin therapy to specific LDL-C or non-HDL-C target values. Rather, the goal of therapy is to achieve at least 50% reduction in LDL-C level.
   e. The Expert Panel recommends against routinely monitoring ALT, AST, or creatinine kinase (CK) in the absence of symptoms.
3. The Expert Panel found insufficient evidence from RCTs to recommend the use of nonstatin cholesterol-lowering medications. Based on expert opinion, the Expert Panel noted that it is reasonable to consider the addition of a nonstatin drug to further lower LDL-C:
   a. In adults with untreated primary LDL-C ≥190 mg/dL who have inadequate response after the maximum intensity of statin therapy has been administered.
   b. In adults who are candidates for statin treatment but who are completely statin intolerant.

When used, the clinician should weigh the potential benefits in CVD risk reduction versus the risk of adverse effect and drug–drug interactions.

ATP III Recommendations

In young adults without CVD (the vast majority of 20- to 35-year-olds), the ATP III guidelines recommend the following[2]:

- If LDL-C is <160 mg/dL, TLCs are indicated.
- If LDL-C >190 mg/dL, lipid-lowering medications should be considered.
- If LDL-C is 160 to 189 mg/dL, LDL-C lipid-lowering drugs are optional and their use should be guided by clinical judgment, taking into account the presence or absence of two broad classes of additional factors: *life habits* (e.g., obesity, sedentary lifestyle, and atherogenic diet) and *emerging risk factors* (e.g., Lp[a], homocysteine, prothrombotic and proinflammatory plasma factors, as well as impaired glucose tolerance).

As noted previously, the ATP III emphasized treating to specific LDL-C targets.

- In high-risk persons, the recommended target LDL-C goal is <100 mg/dL, but when risk is very high, an LDL-C goal of <70 mg/dL is a therapeutic option (that is, a reasonable clinical strategy on the basis of available clinical trial evidence). This therapeutic option extends also to patients at very high risk who have a baseline LDL-C <100 mg/dL.
- In a high-risk patient with high triglycerides or low HDL-C, consideration should be given in combining a fibrate or nicotinic acid with an LDL-lowering drug.
- For moderately high-risk persons (≥2 risk factors and 10-year risk of 10% to 20%), the recommended LDL-C goal is <130 mg/dL, but an LDL-C goal <100 mg/dL is a therapeutic option on the basis of trial evidence. This option is also applicable to moderately high-risk persons with a baseline LDL-C of 100 to 129 mg/dL.
- When LDL-lowering drug therapy is used in high-risk or moderately high-risk persons, intensity of therapy should be sufficient to achieve at least a 30% to 40% reduction in LDL-C levels.
- Any person at high- or moderately high risk who has lifestyle-related risk factors (e.g., obesity, physical inactivity, elevated triglycerides, or metabolic syndrome) should institute TLCs to modify these risk factors regardless of LDL-C level.

TABLE 14.8

Drug Therapy for Hyperlipidemia

Type of Drug	Mechanism of Action	Major Effects	Example	Starting Dose	Adverse Reactions
Statin	Inhibits cholesterol synthesis in hepatic cells, resulting in increased LDL-receptor activity	Lowers LDL cholesterol and triglyceride, raises HDL-C	Atorvastatin, lovastatin, pravastatin, simvastatin, rosuvastatin	5–20 mg depending on which drug is used	Raised hepatic enzymes, muscle soreness possibly progressing to myolysis
Bile acid sequestrants	Binds intestinal bile acids interrupting enterohepatic recirculation, which in turn results in LDL-receptor upregulation	Lowers LDL-C; raises triglycerides	Cholestyramine, colesevelam	One to two packs of powder or four tablets (1 g) daily, with 8 oz water	Limited to GI tract; gas, bloating, constipation, cramps, fat-soluble vitamin deficiency
Fibric acid	Probably inhibits hepatic synthesis of VLDL	Mainly lowers triglycerides and raises HDL-C, with less effect on LDL-C	Gemfibrozil, fenofibrate	Varies with preparation	Dyspepsia, constipation, raised liver enzymes, myositis, rhabdomyolysis, anemia
Nicotinic acid	Upregulates hepatic LDL receptors, decreases hepatic LDL and VLDL production	Lowers triglycerides LDL-C and Lp(a), raises HDL-C	Niaspan	500 mg begin slowly to minimize side effects	Flushing, hepatic toxicity, hyperglycemia
Cholesterol absorption inhibitor	Inhibits cholesterol absorption in small intestine, interferes with enterohepatic recirculation	Lowers LDL-C	Ezetimibe	10 mg	Hepatitis, pancreatitis, cholecystitis, diarrhea, abdominal pain, athralgia

LDL, low-density lipoprotein; HDL-C, high-density lipoprotein cholesterol; LDL-C, low-density lipoprotein cholesterol; VLDL, very-low-density lipoprotein; GI, gastrointestinal.

TABLE 14.9

High-, Moderate-, and Low-Intensity Statin Therapy (Used in the RCTs Reviewed by the Expert Panel)[a]

High-intensity statin therapy	Moderate-intensity statin therapy	Low-intensity statin therapy
Daily dose lowers LDL-C, on average, by approximately <50%	Daily dose lowers LDL-C, on average, by approximately 30% to <50%	Daily dose lowers LDL-C, on average, by <30%
Atorvastatin (40[b])–80 mg **Rosuvastatin 20 (40) mg**	**Atorvastatin 10 (20) mg** **Rosuvastatin (5) 10 mg** **Simvastatin 20–40 mg[c]** **Pravastatin 40 (80) mg** **Lovastatin 40 mg** *Fluvastatin XL 80 mg* **Fluvastatin 40 mg b.i.d.** *Pitavastatin 2–4 mg*	*Simvastatin 10 mg* **Pravastatin 10–20 mg** **Lovastatin 20 mg** *Fluvastatin 20–40 mg* *Pitavastatin 1 mg*

[a]Individual responses to statin therapy varied in the RCTs and should be expected to vary in clinical practice. There might be a biologic basis for a less-than-average response.

[b]Evidence from 1 RCT only: down-titration if unable to tolerate atorvastatin 80 mg in the IDEAL (Incremental Decrease through Aggressive Lipid Lowering) study.

[c]Although simvastatin 80 mg was evaluated in RCTs, initiation of simvastatin 80 mg or titration to 80 mg is not recommended by the FDA because of the increased risk of myopathy, including rhabdomyolysis.

Boldface type indicates specific statins and doses that were evaluated in RCTs included in CQ1, CQ2, and the Cholesterol Treatment Trialists 2010 meta-analysis included in CQ3. All of these RCTs demonstrated a reduction in major cardiovascular events. *Italic type* indicates statins and doses that have been approved by the FDA but were not tested in the RCTs reviewed.

b.i.d. indicates twice daily; CQ, critical question; FDA, Food and Drug Administration; LDL-C, low-density lipoprotein cholesterol; RCTs, randomized controlled trials.

From Stone NJ, Robinson JG, Lichtenstein AH, et al. 2013 ACC/AHA guideline on the treatment of blood cholesterol to reduce atherosclerotic cardiovascular risk in adults: a report of the American College of Cardiology/American Heart Association Task Force on practice guidelines. *J Am Coll Cardiol* 2014;63 (25, Pt B):2889–2934.

TABLE 14.10

Characteristics of Statin Drugs

Characteristic	Lovastatin	Pravastatin	Simvastatin	Atorvastatin	Fluvastatin	Rosuvastatin
Maximum dose (mg/d)	80	40	80	80	80	40
Maximal LDL cholesterol reduction (%)	40	34	47	60	24	63
Serum triglyceride reduction produced (%)	16	24	18	29	10	n/a
Serum HDL cholesterol elevation produced (%)	8.6	12	12	6	8	10
Plasma half-life (h)	2	1–2	1–2	14	1.2	19
Optimal time of administration	With meals (morning and evening)	Bedtime	Evening	Evening	Bedtime	Evening
CNS penetration	Yes	No	Yes	No	No	n/a
Hepatic metabolic mechanism	Cytochrome P-450 3A4	Sulfation	Cytochrome P-450 3A4	Cytochrome P-450 3A4	Cytochrome P-450 2C9	Cytochrome P-450 2C9

LDL, low-density lipoprotein; HDL, high-density lipoprotein; CNS, central nervous system.
Adapted from Knopp RH. Drug treatment of lipid disorders. *N Engl J Med* 1999;341:498, with permission.

Pharmacologic Agents

Table 14.8 summarizes mechanisms of action and major effects and lists recommended doses and side effects of the drugs used for hyperlipidemic conditions.

1. Inhibitors of HMG-CoA reductase (statins)
   The 2013 ACC/AHA Blood Cholesterol Guideline classifies therapy with statins as high-, moderate-, and low-intensity based on their ability to lower LDL-C in RCTs (**Table 14.9**).
   a. Lovastatin (Mevacor):
      * Action: Competitively inhibits the rate-limiting enzyme in cholesterol biosynthesis. LDL-R activity is also increased, leading to an increase in the rate of removal of LDL.
      * Effects: Causes an average reduction in the LDL-C concentration of 25% to 45%.
      * Side effects: Usually well tolerated. The most common side effects include gastrointestinal (GI) upset, muscle aches, and hepatitis. There is an increase in aminotransferase levels in 1.9% of patients. Careful monitoring of liver function is essential. Myalgias occur in approximately 2.4% of individuals. Other side effects include headaches, nausea, fatigue, insomnia, skin rashes, and myositis. Transient mild elevations in CK are commonly seen; in the few patients in whom markedly elevated CK levels and myositis develop, the drug should be discontinued. Results from the lovastatin adolescent trial on 132 male adolescents with FH show efficacy similar to that seen in adults, with normal growth and development.
      * Dose: Usually, the starting dose is 20 mg once daily with the evening meal, with increases to 40 mg and then 80 mg as a single evening dose or in divided doses. Liver function should be checked at the start of therapy at 4 to 6 weeks, 6 months, and then yearly.
   b. Pravastatin (Pravachol):
      * Action, effects, and side effects: Similar to those of lovastatin
      * Dose: 10 to 40 mg
   c. Simvastatin (Zocor):
      * Action, effects, and side effects: Similar to those of lovastatin
      * Dose: 5 to 80 mg

   d. Atorvastatin (Lipitor):
      * Action, effects, and side effects: Similar to those of lovastatin, with the additional effect of lowering triglycerides
      * Dose: 5 to 80 mg

   Simvastatin and atorvastatin have now been included in several randomized clinical trials in adolescents with FH. They are the recommended statins for use in young adults ≥21 years with primary elevations of LDL-C ≥190 mg/dL.[21]

   e. Rosuvastatin (Crestor):
      * Action, effects, and side effects: Similar to those of lovastatin, with the additional effect of lowering triglycerides
      * Dose: 5 to 40 mg
   f. Drugs that interfere with statin metabolism: As indicated in **Table 14.10**, the cytochrome P-450 CYP3A4 and CYP2C9 pathways are involved in metabolism of some of the statins. This can cause problems with the following medications:
      * Inhibits CYP3A4 (raises serum drug concentrations): erythromycin, clarithromycin, cyclosporine, ritonavir, fluconazole, verapamil, grapefruit juice
      * Induces CYP3A4 (lowers serum drug concentrations): barbiturates, carbamazepine, nafcillin, phenytoin, primidone, rifampin
      * Inhibits CYP2C9 (may raise serum fluvastatin concentrations): amiodarone, cimetidine, trimethoprim-sulfamethoxazole, fluoxetine, isoniazid, ketoconazole, metronidazole
      * Induces CYP2C9 (may lower serum fluvastatin concentrations): barbiturates, carbamazepine, phenytoin, primidone, rifampin
2. Bile acid sequestrants:
   a. Cholestyramine (Questran), colesevelam (Welchol), and colestipol (Colestid) are hydrophilic, insoluble anion-exchange resins that are available as powder for suspension in liquid or as pills.
      * Action: Interrupts the enterohepatic circulation of bile acids and binds bile acids in the intestine to form an insoluble complex, which is excreted in feces and thereby increases hepatic synthesis of bile acids from cholesterol. The advantage of these drugs in the treatment of AYAs is that there is no systemic absorption or toxic effects. However, the GI side effects may lead to problems in compliance.

- Effects: Lowering of both total cholesterol and LDL-C levels by 15% to 30% at 16 to 24 g/day
- Side effects
  - GI effects include nausea, bloating, and constipation.
  - Powder is difficult to take because it must be suspended in a liquid vehicle. If water is unsatisfactory, an unsweetened juice may improve palatability. Rapid ingestion may cause air swallowing.
  - Bleeding tendencies, osteoporosis, or iron deficiency may result from poor absorption of vitamin K, calcium, or iron, but these complications are rare.
- Dose: Available in powder form (16 to 24 g). Should be started at 4 g/day twice a day and gradually increased over a month to the full dose. The average dose is two or three packs (8 to 12 g) or two pills taken orally, twice daily with meals.

3. Nicotinic acid (niacin):
   a. Action: Reduces VLDL production by inhibiting lipoprotein synthesis in the liver. It also has effects on lipoprotein lipase in the adipocyte. Niacin is an effective drug but requires considerable patient education because of flushing. Proprietary forms of extended-release niacin have increased efficacy and reduced flushing.
   b. Effects: Primarily reduces triglyceride levels but also lowers LDL-C levels and causes a rise in HDL-C. A dose of 1 to 2 g/day can result in a 40% decrease in triglyceride and VLDL levels, a 20% decrease in LDL levels, and a 30% increase in HDL levels. Nicotinic acid is particularly valuable in combination therapy with a bile acid sequestrant because of the complementary modes of action—niacin inhibiting LDL and VLDL production and the bile acid sequestrant increasing LDL excretion. Statin plus niacin is also effective in mixed dyslipidemias.
   c. Side effects: The vitamin preparation is poorly tolerated in the dose needed for lipid lowering.
      - Gastritis, peptic ulcer disease, vomiting, and diarrhea can occur.
      - Liver function abnormalities can occur.
      - Vasodilatation with flushing is also a troublesome side effect.
   d. Dose: The side effects can be reduced by using the sustained-release product and starting with a dose of 500 mg with meals or at bed time and gradually increasing for 1 month to 6 weeks. The average daily dose is 1 to 2 g. The possibility of flushing as a side effect should be discussed in advance with the patient and parent. Because the flushing is due to prostaglandin effects, it can be ameliorated by taking one aspirin (81 mg) 30 minutes before each dose. Individuals taking niacin should have regular monitoring of aminotransferase, glucose, alkaline phosphatase, and uric acid values.

4. Fibric acid derivatives:
   a. Gemfibrozil (Lopid):
      - Action: Increases lipoprotein lipase activity, decreases hepatic triglyceride production, and inhibits peroxisome proliferator-activated receptor gamma.
      - Effects: Reduces both VLDL and triglyceride levels. In some individuals, cholesterol levels may decrease and HDL levels may rise. The drug is primarily used for lowering high levels of triglycerides.
      - Side effects: Biliary tract disease, and contraindicated in liver or kidney disease. Abdominal discomfort, diarrhea, muscle ache, and increased appetite can occur. Not used in combination with statins due to increased risk of myositis.
      - Dose: 600 to 1,200 mg/day in two doses.
   b. Fenofibrate (Tricor, Trilipix, several others):
      - Action, effects, and side effects: Similar to those of gemfibrozil, but can be used in combination with a statin
      - Dose: 48 or 145 mg/day

5. Ezetimibe (Zetia):
   - Action: Blocks cholesterol absorption at the intestinal brush border. Interferes with the enterohepatic reabsorption of cholesterol.
   - Effects: Lowers LDL-C and is synergistic with statins allowing for a lower statin dose with increased efficacy and fewer side effects.
   - Side effects: Hepatitis, pancreatitis, cholecystitis, diarrhea, abdominal pain, and arthralgia are reported but rarely seen in clinical practice. Currently, ezetimibe is FDA approved as an adjunct to dietary therapy in combination with simvastatin in patients with heterozygous FH (adolescent males and postmenarchal females aged 10 to 17 years).
   - Dose: 10 mg/day

In the past, the bile acid sequestrants used together with nicotinic acid have been considered first-line agents. Fibrates have been used as a second step. However, they are less effective in lowering LDL-C. Now, inhibitors of HMG-CoA reductase, statins, have become first-line agents. Statins are even more effective when used in conjunction with a bile acid sequestrant, niacin, or ezetimibe.

Adherence to Drug Therapy

1. Drug therapy should be considered an adjunct and not a replacement for TLCs. Many AYAs, once they are able to make healthier food choices and engage in regular vigorous physical activity, can lower their lipids into the target range without medications.
2. The adolescent or young adult must be well informed about the goals of drug treatment and the side effects.
3. It is important to start with small doses of drugs, particularly with sequestrants or nicotinic acid.
4. The frequency of use of the medication and the impact on lifestyle must be discussed.
5. It is important to maintain regularly scheduled follow-up with the AYAs.

⬤ CONCLUSION

In conclusion, the future looks bright for CVD prevention. The 124,000 or more US AYAs with heterozygous FH can now be identified and treated using current universal screening guidelines. This can result in healthy life extension of a decade or more for them with minimal risk. In the process of identifying these most virulent forms of premature atherosclerosis, we will also identify risk factors among the 9 million plus obese individuals who can be made aware of their risk and begun on treatment. While this optimistic view ignores the considerable social and political barriers to this primordial prevention, at last we have a scientific basis to focus research on how to overcome the significant individual barriers to behavioral change. A multipronged intensive approach to CVD risk reduction using many techniques is the goal.

REFERENCES

1. Kones R. Low-fat versus low-carbohydrate diets, weight loss, vascular health, and prevention of coronary artery disease: the evidence, the reality, the challenge, and the hope. *Nutr Clin Pract* 2010;25(5):528–541.
2. Stone NJ, Bilek S, Rosenbaum S. Recent National Cholesterol Education Program Adult Treatment Panel III update: adjustments and options. *Am J Cardiol* 2005; 96(4):53e–59e.
3. Yancy CW. Is ideal cardiovascular health attainable? *Circulation* 2011;123(8):835–837.
4. Expert Panel on Integrated Guidelines for Cardiovascular Health and Risk Reduction in Children and Adolescents; National Heart, Lung, and Blood Institute. Expert panel on integrated guidelines for cardiovascular health and risk reduction in children and adolescents: summary report. *Pediatrics* 2011;128 (suppl 5): S213–S256.
5. Lloyd-Jones DM, Hong Y, Labarthe D, et al. Defining and setting national goals for cardiovascular health promotion and disease reduction: the American Heart Association's strategic Impact Goal through 2020 and beyond. *Circulation* 2010;121(4):586–613.
6. National Cholesterol Education Program (NCEP) Expert Panel on Detection, Evaluation, and Treatment of High Blood Cholesterol in Adults (Adult

Treatment Panel III). Third report of the National Cholesterol Education Program (NCEP) Expert Panel on detection, evaluation, and treatment of high blood cholesterol in adults (Adult Treatment Panel III) final report. *Circulation* 2002;106(25):3143–3421.

7. Stone NJ, Robinson JG, Lichtenstein AH, et al. 2013 ACC/AHA guideline on the treatment of blood cholesterol to reduce atherosclerotic cardiovascular risk in adults: a report of the American College of Cardiology/American Heart Association Task Force on practice guidelines. *J Am Coll Cardiol* 2014;63 (25, Pt B):2889–2934.

8. Stone NJ, Robinson JG, Lichtenstein AH, et al. Treatment of blood cholesterol to reduce atherosclerotic cardiovascular disease risk in adults: synopsis of the 2013 American College of Cardiology/American Heart Association cholesterol guideline. *Ann Int Med* 2014;160(5):339–343.

9. Centers for Disease Control and Prevention (CDC). Prevalence of abnormal lipid levels among youths—United States, 1999–2006. *MMWR Morb Mortal Wkly Rep* 2010;59(2):29–33.

10. Berenson GS, Srinivasan SR, Bao W, et al. Association between multiple cardiovascular risk factors and atherosclerosis in children and young adults. The Bogalusa Heart Study. *N Engl J Med* 1998;338(23):1650–1656.

11. Li S, Chen W, Srinivasan SR, et al. Childhood cardiovascular risk factors and carotid vascular changes in adulthood: the Bogalusa Heart Study. *JAMA* 2003;290(17):2271–2276.

12. Levy D, Wilson PW, Anderson KM, et al. Stratifying the patient at risk from coronary disease: new insights from the Framingham Heart Study. *Am Heart J* 1990;119 (3, pt 2):712–717.

13. McMahan CA, Gidding SS, Malcom GT, et al. Comparison of coronary heart disease risk factors in autopsied young adults from the PDAY Study with living young adults from the CARDIA study. *Cardiovasc Pathol* 2007;16(3):151–158.

14. Kwiterovich PO Jr. Diagnosis and management of familial dyslipoproteinemias. *Curr Cardiol Rep* 2013;15(6):371.

15. Burman D, Mente A, Hegele RA, et al. Relationship of the ApoE polymorphism to plasma lipid traits among South Asians, Chinese, and Europeans living in Canada. *Atherosclerosis* 2009;203(1):192–200.

16. Stein EA, Swergold GD. Potential of proprotein convertase subtilisin/kexin type 9 based therapeutics. *Curr Atheroscler Rep* 2013;15(3):310.

17. Shao B, Oda MN, Oram JF, et al. Myeloperoxidase: an oxidative pathway for generating dysfunctional high-density lipoprotein. *Chem Res Toxicol* 2010;23(3):447–454.

18. Morrison JA, Friedman LA, Gray-McGuire C. Metabolic syndrome in childhood predicts adult cardiovascular disease 25 years later: the Princeton Lipid Research Clinics Follow-up Study. *Pediatrics* 2007;120(2):340–345.

19. Bambs C, Kip KE, Dinga A, et al. Low prevalence of "ideal cardiovascular health" in a community-based population: the heart strategies concentrating on risk evaluation (Heart SCORE) study. *Circulation* 2011;123(8):850–857.

20. Reaven G. Metabolic syndrome: pathophysiology and implications for management of cardiovascular disease. *Circulation* 2002;106(3):286–288.

21. Kohn M, Jacobson MS. Cholesterol (and cardiovascular risk) in adolescence. *Curr Opin Pediatr* 2004;16(4):357–362.

22. Miller M, Stone NJ, Ballantyne C, et al. Triglycerides and cardiovascular disease: a scientific statement from the American Heart Association. *Circulation* 2011;123(20):2292–2333.

23. Kuryan RE, Jacobson MS, Frank GR. Non-HDL-cholesterol in an adolescent diabetes population. *J Clin Lipidol* 2014;8(2):194–198.

24. Urbina EM Williams RV, Alpert BS, et al. Noninvasive assessment of subclinical atherosclerosis in children and adolescents: recommendations for standard assessment for clinical research: a scientific statement from the American Heart Association. *Hypertension* 2009;54(5):919–950.

🛜 ADDITIONAL RESOURCES AND WEBSITES ONLINE

CHAPTER 15

Syncope, Vertigo, and Sudden Cardiac Arrest

Amy D. DiVasta
Mark E. Alexander

KEY WORDS

- Conversion Reaction
- Fainting
- Long QT Syndrome
- Palpitations
- Sudden Cardiac Arrest
- Supraventricular tachycardia
- Syncope
- Vertigo
- Wolf Parkinson White

SYNCOPE

Cardiac symptoms in adolescents and young adults (AYAs) are very common; true cardiac disease is not. Syncope is a frequent complaint, often raising concerns of future sudden cardiac arrest (SCA).[1] The clinician's critical task is to distinguish between benign and significant syncope. The epidemiology almost always favors innocent causes.

Etiology

Syncope is a sudden, transient loss of consciousness and postural tone, lasting several seconds to a minute, followed by spontaneous recovery. Syncope is common, particularly among adolescent females aged 13 to 18 years.[1,2] Any condition that leads to decreased cerebral perfusion may cause syncope.

Classification

There are three major categories of syncope: (1) neurocardiogenic, including vasovagal/reflex and postural orthostatic tachycardia; (2) cardiovascular, including structural and arrhythmogenic; and (3) noncardiovascular, including epileptic and psychogenic. Vertigo or seizures are generally obvious on initial evaluation, though the symptoms can overlap.

Syncope of unknown origin (i.e., *simple syncope*) and neurocardiogenic syncope account for 85% to 90% of events.[3–5] Ineffective cerebral blood flow, resulting from inadequate cardiac output, leads to loss of consciousness. Only 1% to 5% of patients have significant cardiac disease. Seizures or psychiatric diagnoses account for a small minority of episodes.

History and Physical Examination

An accurate diagnosis stems from a detailed history (including family history) and thorough physical examination. Key elements of the history include (1) onset and frequency of episodes; (2) circumstances, such as exercise, posture, or other precipitating factors; (3) prodromal symptoms, including dizziness, diaphoresis, nausea, pallor, palpitations, chest pain, dyspnea; (4) complete or incomplete loss of consciousness, duration, time to recovery; (5) abnormal movements, incontinence, or injury; (6) past medical history and medications; and (7) family history of sudden death

(particularly if <40 years old), similar episodes, or early onset of heart disease.

"Warning signs" that suggest a more serious etiology include syncope during exercise, syncope in a supine position, family history of sudden death, personal history of cardiac disease, or an event precipitated by a loud noise, intense emotion, or fright. The physical examination should include at least a brief neurologic assessment and a dynamic cardiac examination performed with the patient in multiple positions to evaluate for a pathologic murmur.

Table 15.1 presents a differential diagnosis for a syncopal event. Common etiologies are discussed below.

Neurocardiogenic Syncope

Neurocardiogenic syncope (i.e., *vasovagal syncope*) is the most common form of syncope.

1. Duration: Few seconds to minutes.
2. Onset: Gradual, typically with a prodrome.
3. Etiology: Precipitating factors (fear, anxiety, pain, hunger, overcrowding, fatigue, injections, sight of blood, prolonged upright posture) are usually identifiable.
4. Prodromal symptoms: Nausea, dizziness, visual spots or dimming, feelings of apprehension, pallor, yawning, diaphoresis, and feelings of warmth.
5. Syncopal event: Brief loss of consciousness with gradual loss of muscle tone.
6. Syncopal seizures: Rarely, a brief period of opisthotonus will occur following syncope.
7. Recovery: Rapid (<1 minute to consciousness), though residual fatigue, malaise, weakness, nausea, and headache are common
8. Pathophysiology: Neurally mediated syncope results from a combination of inappropriate peripheral vasodilation and cardiac slowing, resulting in a transient period of inadequate cerebral (and other organ) blood flow. Fainting restores cerebral blood flow and permits the reflexes to return to normal.
9. Specific situational syncope syndromes including needle phobia, hair brushing syncope, stretch syncope, micturition syncope, and post-tussive syncope require minimal investigation.
10. There is likely some decline in the preponderance of neurocardiogenic syncope and a small increase in the frequency of "adult" causes of syncope as AYAs age into their mid- to later 20s. This shift in disease frequency is subtle, but will influence diagnostic approaches.

Diagnostic Evaluation of Neurocardiogenic Syncope

AYAs with a true syncopal event should undergo a thorough history, physical examination, and electrocardiogram (ECG).[6] A normal diagnostic screen (reassuring history, benign examination, and

TABLE 15.1

Differential Diagnosis of a Syncopal Event

	Typical/Vasovagal	Cardiac	Atypical/Conversion	Vertigo
Position	Upright	Supine or upright	Either	Change in position
Prodrome	Frequent	None	Variable	Rare
Duration	<1 min	<1 min longer really aborted arrest	Minutes	Brief, may cluster
Color	Pale	May be normal	Flushed/normal	Normal
Visual symptoms	Gradual dimming	Abrupt dimming	Variable	Room spinning
Exercise	Post exertional or no relationship	Peak exercise	Variable	Uncommon
Palpitations	Hard	Rapid, precedes faints	Variable	Uncommon
Injury/incontinence	Rare	Moderately frequent	Rare	Rare
Frequency	Isolated or episodic	Isolated or episodic	Often very frequent	Episodic
School disability	Rare	Rare	Frequent	Rare
Family history	Possibly "fainting" but otherwise negative	Often positive		Rare
ECG	Normal or nonspecific PR < 220 QTc < 460 Right atrial enlargement Borderline LVH	T wave inversion QTc > 480 WPW QRS > 120, bundle branch block	Normal or nonspecific	Normal or nonspecific
Comments	Borderline ECG findings likely nonspecific though consultation appropriate	Often established cardiac diagnosis	Typical event as a trigger	

normal ECG) is generally sufficient to exclude cardiac disease.[7] Further testing is needed only if concerns of cardiac or neurologic disease continue.

1. Routine laboratory investigation, electroencephalogram (EEG), or intracranial imaging is not needed.
2. Echocardiogram has very low yield for routine evaluation; it should be utilized to evaluate exertional syncope or syncope with high-risk features. There will be a 5% to 10% incidence of incidental, unrelated findings.[8]
3. Exercise testing is required if syncopal episodes occur during exercise.
4. Tilt table testing: Specificity is poor (35% to 100%) and sensitivity is variable (75% to 85%); 40% of healthy AYAs have a positive tilt test. Head-up tilt testing has fallen out of favor because of these poor test characteristics.
5. Ambulatory ECG monitoring can be useful for correlating symptoms and rhythm. The choice of monitoring (Holter monitor, external loop recorder, implantable loop recorder) requires consideration of symptom frequency, severity, and a need for more precise data.
6. When situational triggers are identified, either behavioral or medical therapies aimed at those triggers are appropriate. Common examples include syncope triggered by dysmenorrhea/crampy abdominal pain or events following phlebotomy.

Management of Neurocardiogenic Syncope

Management includes (1) reassurance; (2) hydration and caffeine/alcohol avoidance; (3) recognition of prodromal symptoms and preventative techniques, including assumption of supine position or postural tone (isometric contractions of the extremities, folding the arms, or crossing the legs); (4) upright, weight-bearing exercise; (5) drug therapy for refractory cases that do not respond to supportive therapy (**Table 15.2**). Generally, a 12-month symptom-free interval is considered a reasonable duration of treatment; subsequently, a trial off medication is warranted.

Postural Orthostatic Tachycardia Syndrome

Postural orthostatic tachycardia syndrome (POTS) is a heterogeneous disorder of autonomic regulation. Patients complain of fatigue, dizziness, and exercise intolerance with upright position. POTS is characterized by a marked pulse change (>40 bpm) or excessive tachycardia (>120 bpm) with upright position. AYAs have sufficient tachycardia that there is typically little or no blood pressure change. POTS is likely a result of both ineffective vascular constriction with standing (hence an appropriate tachycardia) and exaggerated sympathetic response. This physiology is created in normal subjects with spaceflight or even modest periods of bed rest. Chronic fatigue syndrome and POTS overlap considerably.[9] Treatment includes fluids and vasoconstrictors for symptom relief. β-Blockers are also commonly used. The heterogeneity of therapy options reflects the variable physiology and diagnostic criteria utilized in POTS, and the lack of clear "best practice" treatment for the condition. Though often difficult to implement, slowly progressive physical reconditioning may be the most important therapy.[10]

Orthostatic Hypotension

Orthostatic hypotension (drop in systolic blood pressure >20 mm Hg or drop in diastolic blood pressure >10 mm Hg with upright posture) is less common in AYAs. Etiologies of orthostatic hypotension include pregnancy, malnutrition, volume depletion, medication side effects, or neurologic disorders.

TABLE 15.2
Pharmacologic Treatment Options for Neurocardiogenic Syncope

Drug	Dose	Proposed Mechanism of Action	Side Effects	Quality of Data
Fludrocortisone	0.1–0.2 mg/d	↑ Renal Na⁺ absorption	Bloating or edema	
		↑ Circulating blood volume	Hypokalemia	+
			Hypertension	
Midodrine	5–10 mg q4h	α-Agonist	Piloerection	
	Maximum four doses/d	↑ Peripheral vascular resistance	Scalp pruritus	
			Hypertension	++
			Urinary retention	
			Difficult adherence to treatment	
β-Blockers		Blocks excess sympathetic response (paradoxical effect)	Fatigue	
Atenolol	25–50 mg daily		Depression	±
Metoprolol	25–50 mg b.i.d.			
SSRIs		↑ Extracellular serotonin leads to downregulation of receptor density	Headache	
Fluoxetine	20 mg daily		Insomnia	±
Sertraline	50 mg daily		GI effects	

+, moderate data to support efficacy; ++, strong data to support efficacy; ±, mixed data to support efficacy.
SSRIs, serotonin reuptake inhibitors; GI, gastrointestinal.

Cardiovascular Syncope

Cardiovascular syncope is an acute collapse with few premonitory symptoms, often in association with exercise or exertion. It occurs secondary to arrhythmia, obstructed left ventricular (LV) filling, obstructed LV outflow, or ineffective myocardial contraction (Table 15.3). When this persists for more than a minute or so, it represents a SCA. Cardiac syncope should be suspected with a personal history of significant cardiac disease and when any of the "warning signs" are present (Table 15.4). Important historical details include a history of prior episodes, exercise intolerance, exertional chest discomfort, and a family history of premature coronary artery disease, sudden death, syncope, or hypertension.[11] Clues to cardiac disease on examination include hypertension, abnormal cardiac rhythm, heart murmur, or features suggestive of Marfan syndrome. Many patients with cardiac syncope will have previously recognized cardiac conditions; the clinician should seek rapid cardiology input for these patients. However, the majority of patients with new cardiac etiologies (and those at risk of SCA) will have a completely normal physical examination. The ECG is a convenient screening tool, but is often normal. Exercise electrocardiography is useful in a patient with exertional chest discomfort, syncope, exercise intolerance, or worrisome palpitations. Patients should be referred to a cardiologist if cardiac disease is suspected. Strenuous activity, competitive athletics, and operation of a motor

TABLE 15.3
Differential Diagnosis of Cardiac Syncope

Structural/Functional	Electrical	Acquired
HCM	LQTS (inherited or	Commotio cordis
Dilated cardiomyopathy	secondary)	Drugs (cocaine,
Coronary artery	Brugada syndrome	stimulants, inhalants)
anomalies	WPW syndrome	Atherosclerotic
Arrhythmogenic right	Short QT syndrome	coronary artery disease
ventricular dysplasia	Heart block	Myocarditis
Aortic stenosis	(congenital or	Postoperative
Aortic dissection/	acquired)	congenital heart
Marfan syndrome	Catecholamine-	disease
Pulmonary	exercise ventricular	Tetralogy of Fallot
hypertension	tachycardia	Transposition of the
Pulmonic stenosis		great arteries
		Fontan surgery
		Hypoplastic left heart
		syndrome
		Coarctation of the aorta

TABLE 15.4
"Warning Signs" of Syncope That May Be due to Cardiovascular Causes

Historical Signs	Examination/ECG Signs
Event in supine position	Abnormal cardiac rhythm
Event during exertion	Hypertension
Event precipitated by noise, strong emotion, stress	Pathologic murmur or click
Lack of prodromal symptoms	Abnormal QTc interval
Family history of sudden death or heart failure in relative aged <50 y	Heart block

vehicle should be restricted until evaluation by the cardiologist is complete.

Palpitations, Arrhythmias, and Wolff–Parkinson–White

Palpitations can result from sustained or nonsustained arrhythmias or from symptomatic sinus tachycardia. The typical history for supraventricular tachycardia (SVT) is an abrupt onset of palpitations, often with a rapid position change such as standing up after tying a shoe or a sudden jump. These palpitations are sensed as being quite rapid, may be associated with dizziness and lightheadedness at onset, and can last for minutes to hours. When palpitations persist and are present during the medical evaluation, the diagnosis is usually obvious. When palpitations self-terminate, the classic history is that they stop abruptly, though in practice the history is often unclear. Sustained SVT usually results from either an accessory pathway or atrioventricular node reentry. SVT is bothersome but not life-threatening, unless the patient has Wolff–Parkinson–White (WPW) syndrome, an arrhythmia identified by the typical delta wave on resting ECG (Fig. 15.1). While the 50% of WPW that is identified in those with unrelated symptoms is in many ways a "low-risk" condition, the most extensive experience suggests that most patients, early adolescent or older, warrant referral for possible catheter ablation.[12,13]

Isolated atrial and ventricular premature beats can produce a sense of skipped heart beats, but usually these beats are asymptomatic and recognized during a physical examination. Infrequent, isolated ectopy is a variant of normal, and may not require more evaluation than an examination and ECG. More frequent or sustained ectopy warrants further evaluation.

An ECG is a good first step in the evaluation of palpitations. A normal ECG early in the evaluation permits triaging of any further cardiac evaluation. In the absence of associated cardiac symptoms or family history of cardiomyopathy, an adolescent or young adult with infrequent, self-limited palpitations, a normal ECG, and reasonable access to medical care can be managed via an expectant approach. For more worrisome cases, further investigation may be needed. Ambulatory monitoring techniques each have advantages and limitations and can be chosen depending on the frequency and duration of symptoms. Traditional Holter monitors are best for documenting the frequency of clinically apparent or occult arrhythmias. Smartphone-enabled recorders or injectable long-term event monitors are required for correlating symptoms, especially if they occur less frequently than every week or so.

Noncardiovascular Syncope

Hyperventilation frequently causes dizziness, but true syncope is rare. The history may include details of peripheral tingling and anxiety that may be reproduced in the office. Metabolic disturbances can lead to syncope.

Psychogenic or "hysterical" syncope is typically characterized by a gradual slump to the floor, without injury, anxiety, or vital sign instability. The history is often difficult to refine, and the frequency of the episodes may cluster and increase.

Rare etiologies include subclavian steal syndrome and cerebral occlusive disease. Migraine sufferers can have syncope, vertigo, or dizziness preceding or accompanying the headaches.

● VERTIGO

Vertigo is a sensation of rotary movement/spinning, rather than dizziness. Causes of true vertigo (Table 15.5) may be either peripheral (accompanied by tinnitus and/or hearing loss) or central (accompanied by ataxia or other motor signs).

History

Historical details allow differentiation of vertigo from syncope and seizures, and may also be helpful in identifying the specific etiology for the vertigo. In most cases, the diagnosis is established by history and negative physical and neurologic examination findings.

1. Descriptions of the episode and any previous attacks
2. Circumstances preceding the attack
3. Precipitating factors
4. Alleviating factors: recumbence; food, fresh air, and sudden movements

Physical Examination

General physical examination with special emphasis on the following:

1. Neurologic examination:
   a. Evidence of cranial nerve deficits, particularly III, IV, VI, VII, and VIII; funduscopic examination
   b. Focal motor deficits
   c. Tendon reflexes: loss, asymmetry, and hyperreflexia
   d. Cerebellar function: Truncal or appendicular ataxia
   e. Nystagmus with straight gaze. Horizontal nystagmus suggests peripheral etiology, whereas a vertical and diagonal nystagmus is more suggestive of central etiology.

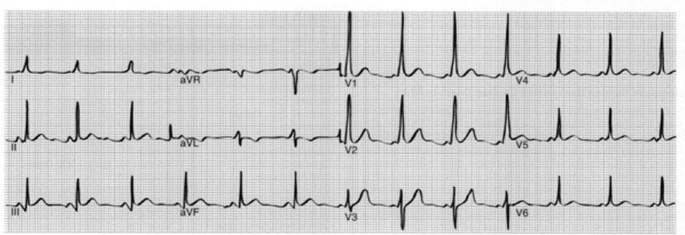

FIGURE 15.1 Wolff–Parkinson–White syndrome. The PR interval is very short and prominent delta waves are present. Delta waves are easily seen in the precordial leads but are less prominent in the frontal plane (I, II, III, avR, avL, avF). This suggests the common left sided location of the accessory pathway. The pre-excitation and abnormal ventricular activation results in prominent anterior (V1, V2) voltages and somewhat wider QRS than normal for age. Right sided and septal pathways are typically more obvious. From Woods SL, Froelicher ES, Motzer SA, Bridges EJ. Cardiac Nursing. 6th edition. Philadelphia, PA: Lippincott Williams & Wilkins, 2009.

TABLE 15.5

Etiologies of Vertigo

Peripheral	Central
Vestibular neuritis (acute labyrinthitis)	Tumors of the brainstem and cerebellum
Benign positional vertigo	Demyelinating diseases
Ototoxic drugs	Vasculitis
Acoustic neuromas	Cerebral infarctions
Meniere disease	Infections of the nervous system
Perilymphatic fistulas	Postinfectious inflammatory demyelination
Otitis media	Basilar migraine
Motion sickness	Brain injury due to head trauma
Ear obstruction	

   f. Sensory abnormalities. Peripheral sensory loss suggests neuropathy.
   g. Skin color, temperature, response to "scratch" to check for evidence of autonomic neuropathy
2. Special examination procedures for vertigo:
   a. Quick head turn
   b. The Valsalva maneuver
   c. Sudden turn while walking
   d. Nylen–Bárány test: Have the adolescent or young adult sit at the edge of a table. Holding on to the patient's head, have him or her abruptly lie back as you place his or her head 45 degrees below the table and at a 45-degree angle to one side. Repeat the test with the head at a 45-degree angle to the opposite side. Elicitation of nystagmus indicates a "positive" test result, suggesting benign positional vertigo.

For sustained vertigo or vertigo that seems positional in origin, referral to a neurologist or otolaryngologist is advisable for further evaluation and testing. An otolaryngologist should promptly evaluate patients with abrupt onset of vertigo and auditory symptoms. Treatment of vertigo is difficult. Short-term therapy for vertigo and vomiting may include antihistamines such as meclizine, antiemetics, or mild sedatives.

SUDDEN CARDIAC ARREST IN AYAs

SCA accounts for only about 10% of the overall sudden death rate in the AYA population, with an incidence of 1 to 2/100,000 patient-years.[14,15] Hypertrophic cardiomyopathy (HCM) is the most common cause of SCA in the US for ages 15 to 35 years.[16] Competitive athletes are likely at minimally higher risk for SCA than sedentary peers or recreational athletes.[17] Most SCA occurs at rest or even with sleep.[18]

Etiologies of Sudden Unexpected Cardiac Death in AYAs

Structural anomalies, electrical abnormalities, sequelae of congenital heart disease, and acquired conditions can all lead to SCA, and mirror the etiologies of cardiac syncope (Table 15.4). Many of these conditions may be familial. Any patient with a suspected cardiac condition should be referred to a cardiologist for a full evaluation and determination of appropriate athletic and recreational activities. Many common medications such as stimulants have recently been implicated in the etiology of SCA; however, large case-control studies have not shown a link between stimulant use and cardiac events.[19] Common SCA etiologies are reviewed below.

Hypertrophic Cardiomyopathy

1. Definition: An inherited cardiac muscle disorder, leading to myocardial hypertrophy. The prevalence is 1 in 500 in the general population.

2. Natural history and prognosis: Genetically and phenotypically heterogeneous. Most patients are asymptomatic. If symptoms develop, usual complaints include exertional chest pain, exercise intolerance, shortness of breath, and syncope.
3. Diagnostic findings in HCM:
   a. Systolic ejection murmur at the left lower sternal border (increasing with standing and decreasing with squatting) and a prominent LV lift.
   b. ECG: LV hypertrophy, ST-T wave changes, or atrial enlargement; ECG abnormal in up to 25% of patients with HCM.
   c. Echocardiogram: Close to the "gold standard." Key findings include thickened interventricular septum and LV free wall, asymmetric septal hypertrophy, and dynamic LV outflow tract obstruction.
4. Sudden death: Rare in HCM, but HCM is the most common cause of SCA in 15–35 year old athletes. The mechanism of cardiac arrest is ventricular fibrillation. Risk factors for sudden death include previous cardiac arrest, positive family history of sudden death, and exertion-related syncope. Since HCM may be inherited in autosomal dominant manner, all family members should be screened. Even asymptomatic patients should avoid athletic participation. For patients at high risk of SCA, implantable defibrillator therapy is recommended.

Long QT Syndrome

1. Definition: Long QT syndrome (LQTS) is a disorder of delayed ventricular repolarization, leading to risk for arrhythmias (torsades de pointes, ventricular fibrillation), syncope, seizure, and SCA. Patients may be asymptomatic.
2. Familial LQTS: Estimated frequency 1/2,000. While traditionally described as both an autosomal recessive (Jervell and Lange-Nielsen syndrome) and autosomal dominant disease (Romano–Ward), modern genetic investigations have demonstrated more than a dozen important ion channels, which contribute to the final phenotype. With this understanding, familial LQTS represents a spectrum from homozygous and compound heterozygous disease to latent mutations. The majority of these disorders represent potassium and sodium channel defects.
3. Acquired LQTS: May be related to underlying disease state, or secondary to drug effect (Table 15.6).
4. Diagnosis: The diagnosis of LQTS begins with an ECG, but requires careful patient-specific and family investigation. Acute illness, multiple drugs (and neurally mediated syncope)

TABLE 15.6

Conditions/Medications Associated with QT Interval Prolongation

Conditions	Medications
Electrolyte abnormality[a]	Antiarrhythmic drugs
Recent syncope	Tricyclic antidepressants
Coronary artery disease	Azole antifungals
Myocarditis	Terfenadine[b]
Alcoholism	Macrolide antibiotics
Eating disorders	Arsenic
Liquid protein diets	Diuretics (via electrolyte changes)
Hypothyroidism	Antipsychotics
CVA	Fluoroquinolones
Encephalitis	Methadone
Traumatic brain injury	Antimalarials
Subarachnoid hemorrhage	Trazodone

[a]Electrolyte abnormality: hypokalemia, hypocalcemia, hypomagnesemia
[b]Removed from market.
CVA, cerebrovascular accident.
For a frequently updated list, please visit crediblemeds.org.

may transiently prolong the QT. LQTS is rare when QTc <450 msec, and frequently confirmed when QTc >480 to 500 msec. The diagnosis is most challenging for QTc values between 450 and 480 msec.

5. Treatment: To decrease the mortality rate, all patients should be referred to a cardiologist and be counseled about treatment. Treatment includes the following:
   a. Avoidance of drugs/medications known to prolong the QT interval (http://crediblemeds.org) and emotional stressors or vigorous activity that may precipitate a syncopal episode
   b. Restriction from competitive athletics and prudent changes in recreational activities. This practice is evolving but requires detailed discussions with the family.
   c. Cascade screening beginning with an ECG should be obtained in first-degree relatives of patients diagnosed with LQTS.
   d. β-Blockers: The initial treatment of choice, β-blockers decrease cardiac events, but do not change the QT interval nor provide absolute protection against SCA. Medication compliance is essential; life-threatening arrhythmia can occur if the medication is suddenly discontinued.
   e. Implantable cardioverter-defibrillators are being used less frequently for most LQTS, but remain important for those with cardiac arrest or recurrent syncope.
   f. Left cervical sympathectomy is a thoracoscopic procedure that offers significant benefit in selected patients.

Other Ion Channel Defect Disorders

Brugada syndrome is a distinctive mutation of the cardiac sodium channel gene that leads to dynamic right ventricular conduction delays; patients often present with syncope or cardiac arrest. Other ion channel defects include catecholaminergic ventricular tachycardia and a short QT syndrome.

SCA and Genetic Screening

Increasingly, familial heart diseases are being recognized. This is almost certainly the result of both better care of those with the disorders and increased recognition of less severely affected family members. The details of significant heart disease of first-degree relatives (parents, siblings) allow for more informed care of the adolescent or young adult. An affected family member will more frequently have a genetic diagnosis, because precise genetic testing is now technically feasible in 50% to 80% of families. Genetic testing also allows for relatively prompt identification of unaffected family members. For those families without a clear genetic marker, regular follow-up is warranted to track the potential phenotype. Given the significant costs and sometimes ambiguous results of current genetic testing, referral for cardiology consultation is a more efficient approach for the adolescent or young adult with a family history of these disorders but no signs/symptoms and no familial genetic marker.[20]

Prevention: To Screen or Not to Screen?

There continues to be controversy surrounding universal cardiac screening programs targeting either high school athletes or all adolescents. The epidemiology of SCA is relatively clear. Most developed countries report approximately 1 to 2 deaths per 100,000 patient-years, which corresponds to 1 to 2 high school students/year in most states. When SCA occurs in athletes, it results in significant local press coverage and appropriately heightened concern and anxiety. HCM, the most common cause of SCA for AYAs, will usually result in an abnormal ECG. The second most common cause of athletic SCA is anomalous coronary arteries. These patients will have a normal ECG and examination; diagnosis can be difficult, even with echocardiogram. Arrhythmias contributing to SCA (WPW, LQTS) will also typically have an abnormal ECG.

The risk of SCA may be elevated in athletes compared to other AYAs. Among athletes, SCA is most prevalent in Black basketball players, and is less common in both females and in athletes

competing in other sports. In many schools, more than 70% of students participate in sports, at least at the level that requires a signed "clearance." The rarity of SCA and the large numbers of youth participating in athletics create challenging ethical questions about where to focus screening efforts. Universal screening efforts in other countries have had mixed results. The success of screening in Italy has been challenged by multiple contradictory experiences. Those observations, combined with the need to potentially screen 3 to 5 million students/year, have informed current US recommendations against using routine ECGs for primary care or school-based screening. Those youth with significant family history, abnormal examination, or symptoms of palpitations, chest pain, or syncope should be referred for further evaluation. Several small to moderate efforts have incorporated ECGs into systematic screening. When ECG screening is performed, approximately 4% to 8% of the ECGs are abnormal. Recent efforts, focused on reducing the number of false positives, have decreased the referral rate to <3%.[21] These efforts have been of insufficient scale to provide accurate estimates for discovering HCM or LQTS. In one demonstration project in Texas that used ECGs and immediate performance of a limited echocardiogram, 19% of those with potentially critical diagnoses never returned to follow-up or therapy.[22]

While the ECG can identify some heart disease, it is a marginal screening test for previously unrecognized heart disease in AYAs. Specificity is quite poor, given the rarity of the relevant diseases and the number of borderline ECGs that occur. The significant costs associated with ECG are drawbacks to universal screening. There is also concern that universal screening may create barriers to youth participation in athletics and other physical activity. Thus, universal screening could have the unintended consequence of contributing to morbidity and mortality from obesity, diabetes, and hypertension in adulthood. In contrast, the supporters of universal screening maintain that utilizing both ECGs and echocardiograms can substantially reduce the false positive rate. Supporters argue that these studies can be performed at very high volume, high quality, and minimal cost.

Primary care and adolescent medicine clinicians can reduce morbidity and mortality by preventing heat injury, increasing the availability of school-based AEDs (Automated External Defibrillators), and assuring that there are reasonable emergency action plans in place. In addition, given the frequency of premonitory symptoms in youth with subsequent SCA, prompt investigation of patients with syncope, palpitations, and similar symptoms remains important.

REFERENCES

1. Kenny RA, Bhangu J, King-Kallimanis BL. Epidemiology of syncope/collapse in younger and older western patient populations. *Prog Cardiovasc Dis* 2013;55(4):357–363.
2. Anderson JB, Czosek RJ, Cnota J, et al. Pediatric syncope: National Hospital Ambulatory Medical Care Survey results. *J Emerg Med* 2012;43(4):575–583.
3. Driscoll DJ, Jacobsen SJ, Porter JC, et al. Syncope in children and adolescents. *J Am Coll Cardiol* 1997;29(5):1039–1045.
4. Ritter S, Tani L, Etheridge P, et al. What is the yield of screening echocardiography in pediatric syncope? *Pediatrics* 2000;105(5):E58.
5. Steinberg LA, Knilans TK. Syncope in children: diagnostic tests have a high cost and low yield. *J Pediatr* 2005;146(3):355–358.
6. Strickberger SA, Benson DW, Biaggioni I, et al. AHA/ACCF scientific statement on the evaluation of syncope: from the American Heart Association Councils on Clinical Cardiology, Cardiovascular Nursing, Cardiovascular Disease in the Young, and Stroke, and the Quality of Care and Outcomes Research Interdisciplinary Working Group; and the American College of Cardiology Foundation in collaboration with the Heart Rhythm Society. *J Am Coll Cardiol* 2006;47(2):473–484.
7. Friedman KG, Alexander ME. Chest pain and syncope in children: a practical approach to the diagnosis of cardiac disease. *J Pediatr* 2013;163(3):896–901, e1–3.
8. Angoff GH, Kane DA, Giddins N, et al. Regional implementation of a pediatric cardiology chest pain guideline using SCAMPs methodology. *Pediatrics* 2013;132(4):e1010–e1017.
9. Stewart JM, Gewitz MH, Weldon A, et al. Patterns of orthostatic intolerance: the orthostatic tachycardia syndrome and adolescent chronic fatigue. *J Pediatr* 1999;135(2, Pt 1):218–225.
10. Shibata S, Fu Q, Bivens TB, et al. Short-term exercise training improves the cardiovascular response to exercise in the postural orthostatic tachycardia syndrome. *J Physiol* 2012;590 (Pt 15):3495–3505.
11. Drezner JA, Fudge J, Harmon KG, et al. Warning symptoms and family history in children and young adults with sudden cardiac arrest. *J Am Board Fam Med* 2012;25(4):408–415.

12. Pediatric and Congenital Electrophysiology Society, Heart Rhythm Society, American College of Cardiology Foundation, et al. PACES/HRS Expert Consensus Statement on the management of the asymptomatic young patient with a Wolff-Parkinson-White (WPW, Ventricular Preexcitation) electrocardiographic pattern: developed in partnership between the Pediatric and Congenital Electrophysiology Society (PACES) and the Heart Rhythm Society (HRS). Endorsed by the governing bodies of PACES, HRS, the American College of Cardiology Foundation (ACCF), the American Heart Association (AHA), the American Academy of Pediatrics (AAP), and the Canadian Heart Rhythm Society (CHRS). *Heart Rhythm* 2012;9(6):1006–1024.

13. Pappone C, Vicedomini G, Manguso F, et al. Wolff-Parkinson-White syndrome in the era of catheter ablation: insights from a registry study of 2169 patients. *Circulation* 2014;130(10):811–819.

14. Driscoll DJ, Edwards WD. Sudden unexpected death in children and adolescents. *J Am Coll Cardiol* 1985;5 (suppl):118B–121B.

15. Cross BJ, Estes NA III, Link MS. Sudden cardiac death in young athletes and non-athletes. *Curr Opin Crit Care* 2011;17(4):328–334.

16. Wren C. Sudden death in children and adolescents. *Heart* 2002;88(4):426–431.

17. Asif IM, Rao AL, Drezner JA. Sudden cardiac death in young athletes: what is the role of screening? *Curr Opin Cardiol* 2013;28(1):55–62.

18. Pilmer CM, Kirsh JA, Hildebrandt D, et al. Sudden cardiac death in children and adolescents between 1 and 19 years of age. *Heart Rhythm* 2014;11(2):239–245.

19. Olfson M, Huang C, Gerhard T, et al. Stimulants and cardiovascular events in youth with attention-deficit/hyperactivity disorder. *J Am Acad Child Adolesc Psychiatry* 2012;51(2):147–156.

20. Ackerman MJ, Priori SG, Willems S, et al. HRS/EHRA expert consensus statement on the state of genetic testing for the channelopathies and cardiomyopathies: this document was developed as a partnership between the Heart Rhythm Society (HRS) and the European Heart Rhythm Association (EHRA). *Europace* 2011;13(8):1077–1109.

21. Drezner JA, Ackerman MJ, Anderson J, et al. Electrocardiographic interpretation in athletes: the 'Seattle criteria'. *Br J Sports Med* 2013;47(3):122–124.

22. Zeltser I, Cannon B, Silvana L, et al. Lessons learned from preparticipation cardiovascular screening in a state funded program. *Am J Cardiol* 2012;110(6):902–908.

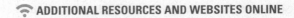 **ADDITIONAL RESOURCES AND WEBSITES ONLINE**

16

Heart Murmurs, Congenital Heart Disease, and Acquired Heart Disease

Amy D. DiVasta
Mark E. Alexander

Cardiac murmurs occur in at least 50% of all normal children and often persist into adolescence and young adulthood. Murmurs are the most frequent reason for referral to a cardiologist.[1] The vast majority are considered to be "innocent" or "physiologic" in origin. In most patients with a cardiac murmur, a careful history and physical examination establish a diagnosis and/or guide further referral and evaluation.

HISTORY

Murmurs first heard in childhood or adolescence are more likely to be innocent murmurs. Complaints of fatigue, decreased exercise tolerance, exertional chest pain, or palpitations are suggestive of pathologic heart disease.[2] Any adolescent or young adult with syncope or near-syncope during exercise merits a cardiac evaluation. A thorough family history should also be obtained, including a history of sudden death or a structural cardiac abnormality in a first-degree relative.

PHYSICAL EXAMINATION

A careful, stepwise examination is crucial, including performance of a dynamic cardiac exam.

1. General appearance, including assessment of growth and maturation
2. Pulses in upper and lower extremities
3. Blood pressures in arm and leg with an appropriate-size blood pressure cuff
4. Palpation: (a) A thrill, heave, or lift over the precordium or suprasternal notch is usually pathologic; (b) Increased intensity and/or lateral displacement (away from the midclavicular line) of the point of maximal impulse suggests left ventricular (LV) enlargement.
5. Auscultation (see individual diagnoses for details):
   a. First heart sound (S_1): S_1 is produced by closure of the mitral and then the tricuspid valve and is best heard at the cardiac apex. Splitting of S_1 can be a normal finding. However, auscultation of another sound close to S_1 is usually either a fourth heart sound (S_4) or an ejection click.
   b. Second heart sound (S_2): The first component (aortic valve closure, A_2) and the second component (pulmonary valve closure, P_2) of S_2 should be of equal intensity. Normally, there is respiratory variation or physiological splitting of the S_2, with widening of the separation with inspiration and narrowing or disappearance of the split with exhalation. Wide, fixed splitting suggests right ventricular (RV) volume overload such as seen with an atrial septal defect (ASD). A single S_2 is also abnormal.
   c. Third heart sound (S_3): S_3 may be a normal finding in adolescents and young adults (AYAs), and is more prominent in hyperdynamic states.
   d. Fourth heart sound (S_4): S_4 may be normal in older adults, but is almost always pathologic in AYAs. Practically, the distinctions can be challenging and influenced by heart rate and clinical context.
   e. Clicks: Sharp, high-frequency sounds that are important clues to organic disease
   f. Murmurs: Assess murmur characteristics, including timing, loudness, length, tonal quality, and location. All diastolic murmurs, except venous hums, should be considered pathologic.

DIAGNOSTIC CLUES SUGGESTIVE OF INNOCENT (NORMAL) MURMURS

1. History: Asymptomatic, no family history of cardiac disease
2. Physical examination: Normal, other than the presence of the murmur
3. Timing of murmur: Early systolic; almost never diastolic or holosystolic
4. Intensity: Usually grade 1 to 3/6, and often changing with position (louder in supine position and quieter with sitting or standing)
5. Quality: Vibratory; no clicks. There is physiological splitting of S_2.
6. Location: May vary, but frequently at lower or upper left sternal border (LSB), without extensive radiation

TYPES OF INNOCENT (NORMAL) MURMURS

Still's Murmur

- A grade 1 to 3/6 low-to-medium-pitched midsystolic murmur with a vibratory or musical quality best heard at lower LSB. The murmur decreases with sitting or standing.
- Still's murmur is differentiated from hypertrophic cardiomyopathy (HCM) because the murmur decreases with standing,

and is less harsh than a murmur associated with a ventricular septal defect (VSD).

Pulmonary Flow Murmur

- A grade 1 to 3/6 short crescendo–decrescendo midsystolic murmur best heard at the upper LSB, between the second and third left intercostal spaces. The murmur is decreased by inspiration and sitting and is often heard in the setting of tachycardia due to fever, anxiety, or exertion.
- A pulmonary flow murmur is differentiated from valvular pulmonary stenosis by the absence of a click and from an ASD because S_2 splits normally.

Cervical Venous Hum

- A medium-pitched, soft, blowing continuous murmur heard best above the sternal end of clavicle, at the base of the neck
- The murmur is increased by rotating the head away from the side of the murmur. The murmur is decreased by jugular venous compression or supine position—unique for a normal murmur.

Supraclavicular (Carotid) Bruit

- This is a short, high-pitched early systolic murmur, usually grade 2/6, heard best above the clavicles with radiation to the neck while the adolescent or young adult is sitting. The murmur is decreased by hyperextending the shoulders (bringing the elbows behind the back).

⬭ DIAGNOSTIC CLUES SUGGESTIVE OF PATHOLOGIC MURMURS

1. History: Growth failure, decreased exercise tolerance, exertional syncope or near-syncope, exertional chest pain[3]
2. Physical examination: Clubbing, cyanosis, decreased or delayed femoral pulses, apical heave, palpable thrill, tachypnea, inappropriate tachycardia
3. Murmur: Diastolic, holosystolic, loud or harsh, extensive radiation, increases with standing, associated with a thrill, abnormal S_2 (Table 16.1)

⬭ MURMURS ASSOCIATED WITH STRUCTURAL HEART DISEASE

Mildly symptomatic congenital heart disease may not be recognized until adolescence, particularly in underserved populations (Table 16.2).

Atrial Septal Defect

1. Physical examination: Signs and symptoms depend on shunt size.
   a. Hyperdynamic precordium with RV lift with sizable shunt; no thrill
   b. Widely split and fixed S_2
   c. Pulmonary flow murmur: Grade 2 to 3/6 systolic ejection murmur at upper LSB
   d. Mid-diastolic rumble at lower LSB
2. Further evaluation
   a. Electrocardiogram (ECG): Right axis deviation, RV conduction delay (rSR′ pattern), right atrial enlargement, or RV hypertrophy
   b. Chest x-ray: Mild to moderate cardiomegaly with increased pulmonary vascularity
   c. Echocardiogram: Diagnostic with visualization of location and size of defect
   d. Cardiac magnetic resonance imaging allows excellent imaging of the atrial septum and RV volume.

TABLE 16.1

Types of Pathologic Murmurs

Murmur Type	Characteristics	Common Defects
Systolic ejection	Crescendo–decrescendo Begins after S_1; ends before S_2 Best heard with diaphragm	Aortic stenosis Pulmonary stenosis Coarctation of the aorta ASD
Holosystolic	Begins with and obscures S_1 Ends at S_2 Heard at LSB or apex	VSD Mitral regurgitation
Early diastolic	Decrescendo Begins immediately after S_2 High–medium pitch	Aortic insufficiency Pulmonary insufficiency
Mid-diastolic	Low pitch Rumble Best heard with bell	ASD VSD Mitral stenosis
Continuous	Extend up to and through S_2 Continue through all/part of diastole Best heard with diaphragm	PDA

ASD, atrial septal defect; LSB, left sternal border; VSD, ventricular septal defect; PDA, patent ductus arteriosus.

3. Management: Both surgical closure and transcatheter device closure are safe, effective, and popular management choices.

Ventricular Septal Defect

1. Physical examination: Shunt volume determines findings.
   a. With increasing shunt size, the precordium becomes increasingly hyperdynamic. A thrill may be present with either a large or small shunt.
   b. S_2 is normal with small shunts, accentuated with larger shunts. An S_3 may be present. A loud P_2 (suggesting pulmonary hypertension) is a worrisome finding.
   c. Grade 2 to 3/6 holosystolic murmur at lower LSB
   d. Mid-diastolic rumble at the apex with large shunts
2. Further evaluation
   a. ECG: Normal in small defects; LV hypertrophy with large defects
   b. Chest x-ray: Normal in small defects; cardiomegaly with increased pulmonary vascularity in large defects
   c. Echocardiogram: Provides anatomical detail of location and size of defect; color Doppler permits visualization of very small defects.
3. Management: Depends on RV pressure and may require catheterization to make appropriate therapeutic decisions. Prophylaxis for subacute bacterial endocarditis (SBE) is no longer recommended for VSD.

Patent Ductus Arteriosus

1. Physical examination: Shunt volume determines findings.
   a. Normal precordium with small shunt; hyperdynamic with a thrill with large shunt
   b. Grade 2 to 4/6 continuous murmur at upper LSB
   c. Wide pulse pressure and bounding pulses with large shunt
2. Further evaluation
   a. ECG: Often normal. LV hypertrophy seen if left-to-right shunting is significant

TABLE 16.2

Clues to Specific Organic Cardiac Lesions

Diagnosis	Auscultation	Other Findings	Chest X-ray	ECG
Patent ductus arteriosus	Continuous murmur LUSB and subclavicular area	Wide pulse pressure Bounding pulses	Prominent pulmonary artery	Normal LAE/LVH
ASD	Fixed, widely split S_2 Systolic ejection murmur at LUSB Mid-diastolic rumble at LLSB	RV lift	Prominent RV outflow	Incomplete RBBB (rSR' pattern)
Pulmonary stenosis	Systolic ejection click (mild PS) P_2 delayed and soft SEM at LUSB	RV lift Thrill at LUSB	Prominent RV outflow Poststenotic dilation	RVH RAE
Aortic stenosis	Early systolic murmur RUSB, transmitted to neck Systolic ejection click (mild AS) Soft A_2	LV lift Decreased pulses	LVE	LVH
Mitral regurgitation	Holosystolic murmur with radiation to axilla; soft S_1	LV lift	Large LA and LV	Bifid P waves Left axis deviation
MVP	Midsystolic click; mid- or late systolic murmur			Abnormal T waves Arrhythmias
Hypertrophic cardiomyopathy	Midsystolic murmur at LLSB, increased with standing and decreased with Valsalva maneuver	Rapid carotid upstroke	±LVE ±LAE	LVH ±Q waves
VSD	High-pitched, harsh holosystolic murmur at LLSB	Thrill at LLSB	Normal	Normal (if small VSD)
Pulmonary hypertension	Loud P_2 No murmur or regurgitant murmur at LLSB	Clubbing	Variable	RAE RVH
Coarctation of aorta	Continuous/systolic precordial murmur Systolic ejection click from bicuspid aortic valve	SBP lower in legs than arms Decreased/delayed femoral pulses	Rib notching Increased pulmonary markings	LVH

ECG, echocardiogram; LUSB, left upper sternal border; LAE, left atrial enlargement; LVH, left ventricular hypertrophy; LLSB, left lower sternal border; RV, right ventricular; RBBB, right bundle-branch block; PS, pulmonic stenosis; RVH, right ventricular hypertrophy; RAE, right atrial enlargement; SEM, systolic ejection murmur; RUSB, right upper sternal border; AS, aortic stenosis; LV, left ventricular; LA, left atrium; LVE, left ventricular enlargement; VSD, ventricular septal defect.

b. Chest x-ray: Cardiomegaly and increased pulmonary vascularity with large shunt

c. Echocardiogram: Visualization with two-dimensional and color Doppler imaging

3. Management: Cardiac catheterization is rarely required for diagnosis but is commonly done for coil or device occlusion.

Valvular Pulmonary Stenosis

1. Physical examination: Severity of obstruction determines findings.

a. RV lift with systolic thrill at upper LSB in more severe forms

b. Systolic ejection click at upper LSB, which is louder with expiration (more difficult to hear with severe stenosis)

c. S_2 normal or widely split S_2, depending on severity of stenosis

d. Grade 2 to 4/6 harsh systolic ejection murmur at upper LSB; may radiate to the lung fields and back

2. Further evaluation

a. ECG: Normal, with progression to RV hypertrophy (upright T wave in lead V1) as stenosis increases

b. Chest x-ray: Prominent pulmonary artery segment with normal vascularity

c. Echocardiogram: Permits evaluation of valve morphology

d. Cardiac catheterization is rarely required for diagnosis.

3. Management: Treatment of choice is balloon pulmonary valvuloplasty.

Valvular Aortic Stenosis

1. Physical examination: Severity of obstruction determines findings.

a. Prominent apical impulse and systolic thrill (at upper RSB or suprasternal notch)

b. Intensity of S_1 may be diminished due to poor ventricular compliance.

c. Systolic ejection click at lower LSB/apex that radiates to aortic area at upper RSB; no respiratory variation
    d. Grade 2 to 4/6 long, harsh systolic crescendo–decrescendo ejection murmur at upper RSB
    e. High-frequency early diastolic decrescendo murmur of aortic regurgitation
    f. Careful assessment for features of associated Turner or Williams syndrome
2. Further evaluation
    a. ECG: Normal to LV hypertrophy, with strain pattern (ST segment depression and T wave inversion in left precordium) indicating severe stenosis
    b. Chest x-ray: Normal heart size with prominent ascending aorta
    c. Echocardiogram: Permits evaluation of valve morphology and determination of level of stenosis; 70% to 85% of stenotic valves are bicuspid.
    d. Cardiac catheterization is rarely required for diagnosis.
3. Management: In select cases, aortic balloon valvuloplasty may be an initial palliative procedure.

Hypertrophic Cardiomyopathy (Fig. 16.1)

1. Physical examination
    a. Careful assessment for features of skeletal myopathy
    b. Normal to hyperdynamic precordium with increased LV impulse, dynamic thrill
    c. Auscultation may be normal. Dynamic examination demonstrates systolic ejection murmur at the lower LSB with *increasing* intensity in standing position and *decreasing* intensity with squatting or Valsalva maneuver.
    d. Dynamic murmur of mitral insufficiency or LV outflow obstruction
2. Further evaluation
    a. ECG: Normal in some cases. LV and/or septal hypertrophy, ST-T wave changes, and atrial enlargement may be seen.
    b. Chest x-ray: May show cardiomegaly, but is rarely indicated.
    c. Echocardiogram: Diagnostic, with excessive LV wall thickness, impaired ventricular filling, variable degrees of LV outflow tract obstruction, and variable systolic anterior motion of the mitral valve
3. Management: Management of HCM remains problematic, but may include implantable defibrillators, surgical or catheter treatment, or drug therapy. The adolescent or young adult is restricted from competitive sports. Prophylaxis for SBE is no longer recommended.

Mitral Valve Prolapse

Mitral valve prolapse (MVP) is a heterogeneous disorder, with a wide spectrum of pathologic, clinical, and echocardiographic manifestations. The modern understanding of MVP identifies the mitral valve involvement as either part of global connective tissue abnormalities—such as Marfan syndrome, Ehlers–Danlos syndrome (EDS), or osteogenesis imperfecta—or as an isolated finding. MVP has also been found to be more common in malnourished AYAs with anorexia nervosa. Weight loss decreases the size of the LV muscle mass, but the valvular connective tissue does not change in size. This mismatch leads to a large, redundant valve and MVP. Most AYA patients with MVP have an excellent prognosis. Those with other connective tissue disease are at increased risk for the development of mitral regurgitation, infective endocarditis (IE), cerebral embolism, life-threatening arrhythmia, and sudden death. This important distinction helps the clinician to alleviate unnecessary anxiety and to avoid activity limitations or antibiotic prophylaxis in otherwise healthy young people.

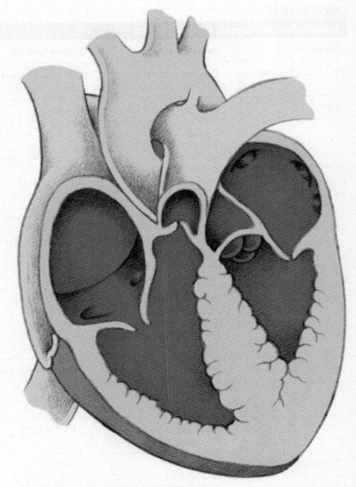

FIGURE 16.1 Hypertrophic cardiomyopathy. (From Cardiomyopathy, hypertrophic. In Lippincott's Nursing Advisor 2011. Philadelphia: Lippincott Williams & Wilkins, 2011.)

The prevalence of MVP in the general population is estimated at 2% to 3%, with equal gender distribution.[4] Although the diagnosis of MVP is common, clinically important MVP occurs infrequently.[5] MVP may be diagnosed at any age. Like HCM, the frequency of MVP and symptomatic MVP increases as adolescents age into adulthood; therefore, symptoms are more likely among older AYAs.

Many cardiac symptoms (including chest pain, palpitations, exercise intolerance, and syncope) that were historically attributed to the presence of MVP are no more common than in the general population and are unrelated to MVP.[6]

1. Physical Examination: (a) Dynamic mid-to-late systolic click that moves later into systole with supine position or squatting and earlier into systole with standing or Valsalva; (b) high-pitched, late systolic murmur, heard best at the apex of the heart. Some AYA patients have no click and only a late systolic murmur; (c) associated physical abnormalities including scoliosis, pectus excavatum, decreased anteroposterior diameter, and stigmata of associated connective tissue disorders.
2. Further Evaluation: (a) ECG is normal; (b) chest x-ray is normal; (c) ambulatory ECGs (Holter or event monitoring) may be indicated to evaluate for arrhythmia if the adolescent or young adult patient has palpitations that disrupt activities of daily living or cause serious symptoms (syncope, dizziness); (d) echocardiogram allows visualization of the

mitral valve, assessment for mitral regurgitation, and confirmation of the diagnosis of MVP. Mild bowing of a mitral leaflet, a normal variant, should not be misdiagnosed as frank prolapse.

3. Management: (a) Asymptomatic AYAs without mitral regurgitation need reassurance but do not need activity restriction, antibiotic prophylaxis, or follow-up echocardiography; (b) AYAs with mitral insufficiency, ventricular arrhythmias, history of cardiac syncope, or family history of premature sudden death may require activity restriction and careful consideration of athletic choices.[7] (c) Routine prophylaxis for IE is no longer recommended for MVP. (d) β-Blocking agents may be indicated for either symptomatic relief or to target a specific arrhythmia; there is no evidence that β-blockade decreases the already low risk of sudden death[8]; (e) mitral regurgitation is generally well tolerated during pregnancy and delivery[9]; (f) first-degree relatives of patients with myxomatous MVP should be considered for evaluation and echocardiogram because of the high prevalence of the diagnosis within families.

4. Complications: Complications of MVP are rare unless significant disease is present[10]; however, (a) arrhythmias are the most frequent complication, including premature ventricular contractions, supraventricular tachyarrhythmia, ventricular tachycardia, and bradyarrhythmia; (b) increased risk of bacterial endocarditis (BE) in patients with MVP and mitral regurgitation; (c) progressive mitral regurgitation, which is rare in otherwise healthy AYAs; (d) very low risk of sudden cardiac death, but the incidence is still greater than that in the general population, likely due to ventricular arrhythmia; and there remains (e) a controversial risk of stroke.

Mitral Valve Regurgitation

1. Physical Examination: Findings depend on severity of regurgitation. (a) Normal to hyperdynamic precordium; (b) grade 2 to 4/6 high-frequency holosystolic apical murmur; may radiate toward the base (upper LSB); (c) low-frequency apical mid-diastolic rumble with severe regurgitation.

2. Further evaluation: (a) ECG: bifid P wave of left atrial enlargement if regurgitation is chronic and severe; (b) chest x-ray is normal or shows cardiomegaly; (c) echocardiogram demonstrates the cause of valve abnormality and severity of regurgitation.

3. Management: (a) AYA patients no longer require BE prophylaxis; (b) AYAs are followed to determine the need for afterload reducing agents or for surgery.

SYSTEMIC CONNECTIVE TISSUE DISEASE AND THE HEART

Marfan Syndrome

Marfan syndrome is an autosomal dominant global connective tissue disorder with specific ocular, musculoskeletal, and cardiac involvement (Fig. 16.2). Cardiac management of MVP in patients with Marfan syndrome is based upon the aortic root dilation.[11] β-Blockers are used as prophylaxis to try to slow dilation, which may progress rapidly during pregnancy.[9] AYAs with Marfan syndrome are generally restricted from high intensity and collision sports.[12]

Ehlers–Danlos Syndromes

EDSs are a range of connective tissue disorders characterized by abnormalities in collagen and musculoskeletal involvement (Fig. 16.3). MVP is relatively common in the classic subtype of EDS. Aortic root dilation is less severe and less frequent than in Marfan syndrome. Patients with EDS may experience palpitations, presyncope, and syncope associated with the autonomic

dysregulation and neurally mediated hypotension of postural orthostatic tachycardia.[13]

Fragile X Syndrome

This alteration in the *FMR1* gene is associated with mental retardation, joint laxity, and some incidence of aortic root dilation and MVP. The cardiac involvement may not be apparent until adolescence.[14] Periodic cardiac screening may be warranted.

ACQUIRED INFECTIOUS AND INFLAMMATORY HEART DISEASE

Bacterial Endocarditis: Recognition and Prophylaxis

AYAs with significant valvular heart disease, unrepaired or residual VSD, prosthetic valves, and many other forms of congenital heart disease are at increased risk of acute or subacute BE. BE can be a devastating infection resulting in stroke or acute valve failure, and may require extended therapy. While many of these infections are the result of oral flora, the most important protective maneuvers are maintaining good oral hygiene and recognizing the potential for infection. The routine use of antibiotics prior to dental cleaning did not reliably prevent either acute or subacute BE, but may have interfered with regular care. Current recommendations from the American Heart Association significantly reduce the indications for antibiotic prophylaxis of IE (Tables 16.3–16.6).[15] The complete guidelines are available at http://circ.ahajournals.org/content/116/15/1736.full.pdf and a wallet card is available at http://www.heart.org/HEARTORG/Conditions/More/ToolsForYourHeartHealth/Infective-Bacterial-Endocarditis-Wallet-Card_UCM_311659_Article.jsp. This shift in preventative strategy does not eliminate the need to be vigilant about potential BE. Appropriate testing with blood cultures and consultation for persistent unexplained fever in the at-risk patient remain the key to recognize these infections.[15]

Inflammatory Heart Disease
Lyme Carditis

Lyme disease is an epidemic infection in many areas caused by the tick-borne spirochete *Borrelia burgdorferi*. Cardiac involvement occurs during the early disseminated phase concurrent with potential neurologic manifestations. The carditis ranges from asymptomatic first-degree block to advanced heart block to a fulminant myocarditis with hemodynamic collapse. An ECG is not warranted for localized Lyme disease with only a target lesion or for late Lyme arthritis. With early disseminated disease (such as facial palsy or meningitis), an ECG allows for rapid triage. PR intervals >220 msec should raise suspicion for some cardiac involvement. PR intervals >300 msec are associated with progression to more advanced heart block; these patients should have inpatient monitoring while intravenous therapy is initiated.

Myopericarditis

Viral or idiopathic myopericarditis is a spectrum of diseases ranging from relatively benign inflammation localized to the pericardium to catastrophic involvement with large effusions, arrhythmias, or hemodynamic collapse. Myopericarditis can be occult and nearly asymptomatic or present as acute and quickly life-threatening "fulminant" myocarditis. When chest pain is a presenting symptom, the pain is usually more severe and lasts longer than "typical" musculoskeletal pain. ECG typically demonstrates diffuse ST-T wave changes. Cardiac auscultation frequently reveals abnormalities including tachycardia, arrhythmia, or pericardial rubs. Serum troponin levels are usually elevated. Urgent cardiology consultation is warranted when significant chest pain is associated with any suggestion of syncope, arrhythmia, or hemodynamic instability.

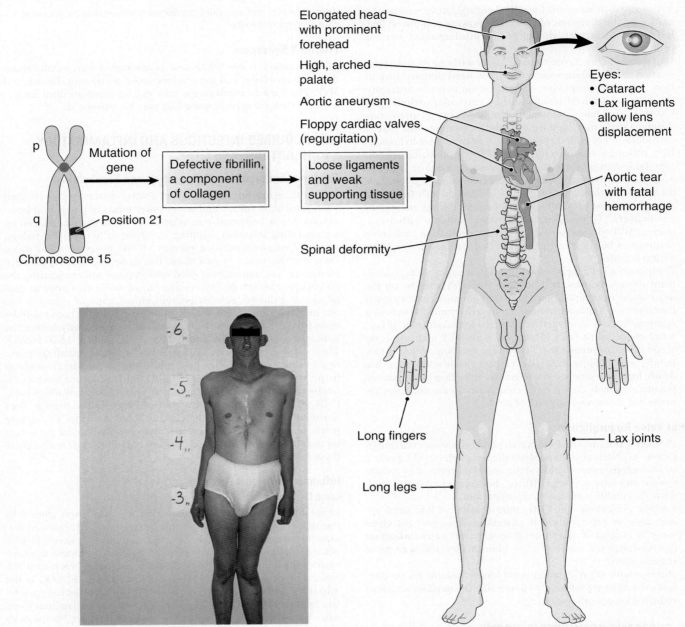

FIGURE 16.2 Marfan syndrome. (From McConnell TH. *Nature of disease*. 2nd ed. Philadelphia, PA: Lippincott Williams & Wilkins, 2013.)

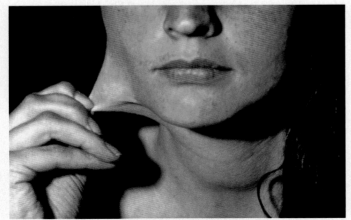

FIGURE 16.3 Ehlers–Danlos syndrome. (Courtesy of V. Voigtländer, Klinikum Ludwigshafen.)

GENERAL CONSIDERATIONS IN THE EVALUATION OF HEART LESIONS

By adolescence and young adulthood, most patients with significant congenital heart disease have been previously identified. New disease is most likely to be diagnosed in underserved populations, or to be as a result of an acquired process (acute myocarditis, acquired cardiomyopathy). Slowly progressive valvular disease (e.g., bicommissural aortic valve disease, MVP, and mitral insufficiency) may become apparent. The identification of arrhythmias and complex ion channel disorders clearly increases during later adolescence and young adulthood.

A careful history and examination should allow differentiation of normal from pathologic murmurs. ECGs and chest radiographs do not add to the accuracy of diagnosis. Echocardiography adds little to the diagnosis of a "normal" murmur. The cost-effective choice between referring to a pediatric cardiologist (which often includes an echocardiogram) and directly obtaining an echocardiogram

TABLE 16.3
Cardiac Conditions Associated with Endocarditis

Endocarditis Prophylaxis Recommended	Endocarditis Prophylaxis Not Recommended
Prosthetic cardiac valve	Innocent murmurs
Previous IE	MVP
Congenital heart disease (CHD)[a]	Hypertrophic cardiomyopathy
Unrepaired cyanotic CHD, including palliative shunts and conduits	
Completely repaired congenital heart defect with prosthetic material or device, whether placed by surgery or by catheter intervention, during the first 6 mo after the procedure[b]	
Repaired CHD with residual defects at the site or adjacent to the site of a prosthetic patch or prosthetic device (which inhibits endothelialization)	
Cardiac transplantation recipients who develop cardiac valvulopathy	

[a]Except for the conditions listed above, antibiotic prophylaxis is no longer recommended for any other form of CHD.
[b]Prophylaxis is recommended because endothelialization of prosthetic material occurs within 6 mo after the procedure.
Adapted from Wilson W, Taubert KA, Gewitz M, et al. Prevention of infective endocarditis: guidelines from the American Heart Association. *Circulation* 2007;115:1.

TABLE 16.4
Summary of Major Changes in New 2007 AHA Guidelines on Prevention of IE

Bacteremia resulting from daily activities is much more likely to cause IE than bacteremia associated with a dental procedure

Only an extremely small number of cases of IE might be prevented by antibiotic prophylaxis even if prophylaxis is 100% effective

Antibiotic prophylaxis is not recommended based solely on an increased lifetime risk of acquisition of IE

Recommendations for IE prophylaxis is recommended only to those with conditions listed in Table 16.3

Antibiotic prophylaxis is no longer recommended for any other form of CHD, except for the conditions listed in Table 16.3

Antibiotic prophylaxis is recommended for all dental procedures that involve manipulation of gingival tissues or periapical region of teeth or perforation of oral mucosa only for patients with underlying cardiac conditions associated with the highest risk of adverse outcome from IE (Table 16.3)

Antibiotic prophylaxis is recommended for procedures on respiratory tract or infected skin, skin structures, or musculoskeletal tissue only for patients with underlying cardiac conditions associated with the highest risk of adverse outcome from IE (Table 16.3)

Antibiotic prophylaxis solely to prevent IE is not recommended for genitourinary or gastrointestinal tract procedures

The writing group reaffirms the procedures noted in the 1997 prophylaxis guidelines for which endocarditis prophylaxis is not recommended and extends this to other common procedures, including ear and body piercing, tattooing, and vaginal delivery and hysterectomy

Adapted from Wilson W, Taubert KA, Gewitz M, et al. Prevention of infective endocarditis: guidelines from the American Heart Association. *Circulation* 2007;115:1.

TABLE 16.5
Dental Procedures and Recommendations for Endocarditis Prophylaxis (for Patients in Table 16.3)

Prophylaxis Is Recommended for:	Prophylaxis *Is Not* Recommended for:
• Manipulation of gingival tissue	• Routine anesthetic injection through noninfected tissue
• Manipulation of periapical region of teeth	• Dental radiographs
• Perforation of the oral mucosa	• Placement of removable prosthodontic or orthodontic appliances
	• Adjustment of orthodontic appliances
	• Placement of orthodontic brackets
	• Shedding of deciduous teeth
	• Bleeding from trauma to lips or oral mucosa

TABLE 16.6
Regimens for Dental Procedures

Situation	Agent	Regimen: Single Dose 30 to 60 min Before Procedure	
		Adults	Children
Oral	Amoxicillin	2 g	50 mg/kg
Unable to take oral medication	Ampicillin **OR**	2 g IM or IV	50 mg/kg IM or IV
	Cefazolin **OR**	1 g IM or IV	50 mg/kg IM or IV
	Ceftriaxone		
Allergic to penicillins or Ampicillin—oral	Cephalexin[a,b] **OR**	2 g	50 mg/kg
	Clindamycin **OR**	600 mg	20 mg/kg
	Azithromycin **OR**	500 mg	15 mg/kg
	Clarithromycin		
Allergic to penicillins or ampicillin and unable to take oral medication to take oral medication	Cefazolin **OR**	1 g IM or IV	50 mg/kg IM or IV
	Ceftriaxone[b] **OR**	600 mg IM or IV	20 mg/kg IM or IV
	Clindamycin		

[a]Or other first- or second-generation oral cephalosporin in equivalent adult or pediatric dosage.
[b]Cephalosporins should not be used in an individual with a history of anaphylaxis, angioedema, or urticaria with penicillins or ampicillin.
IM, intramuscular; IV, intravenous.

depends on the relative cost of the test, the accessibility of consultation, and the skill of the individual practitioner in identifying pathologic murmurs.[16] If the murmur is deemed innocent, the clinician should emphasize that the heart is normal. This helps prevent healthy AYAs from being labeled with cardiac diagnoses, and reduces needless patient, parental, and provider anxiety.

CONGENITAL HEART DISEASE IN AYAs

Because of advances in surgical and medical management, many types of congenital heart disease have very low early and late mortality rates. As a result, an increasing number of youth with congenital heart disease survive to adulthood. Over a million Americans currently have a history of repaired or palliated heart disease.

For all but the most serious disorders, adolescence is often a period of medical quiescence. Youth feel well, and are coping with the usual tasks of adolescence with little to remind them of their need for medical care. However, though the quantitative risks vary substantially, many of these repairs carry long-term risks of arrhythmias, myocardial failure, and valve dysfunction (**Table 16.7**).

Even without progression of hemodynamic or "cardiac" concerns, a history of neonatal and childhood cardiac surgery is associated with a nearly dose-dependent decline in health-related well-being.[17] Somewhat paradoxically, patients systematically report that they have good exercise performance and feel well; thus, very specific questioning about daily activities and well-being is a critical part of understanding their true cardiac status. For most complicated defects, peak exercise capacity is clearly decreased, while submaximal exercise capacity is relatively preserved.[4] Accurate knowledge of expected and actual exercise capacity may help in choosing appropriate recreational and vocational activities.[18]

For the primary care provider, the most critical tasks are to ensure routine health maintenance including immunizations, counseling regarding risk-taking behaviors, and effective transition to adulthood, while also facilitating continued specialized cardiac care. Children with significant heart disease are often lost to follow-up toward the end of elementary school and again during the transition to adulthood. Even in a publicly funded health system, over a quarter had lapsed follow-up by age 12, with over 50% having minimal follow-up by age 22.[19] The medical home is an ideal place to evaluate and optimize school and social function for patients with established heart disease. Deficits in cognitive testing at the start of school have been associated with each of the following: a history of cardiac bypass, complex cardiac repair, or long stays in the ICU.[20] The impact of these deficits on school performance during adolescence is not yet known. A history of prior cardiac surgery is almost always a reasonable indication for Individualized Educational Program testing when there are concerns. Many congenital heart programs can facilitate that evaluation.

There are also guidelines for participation in competitive and recreational athletic activities for youth with known heart disease.[7,12] These guidelines provide a reasonable starting point for discussing athletic participation and can help the clinician to determine when specialty consultation may be needed prior to clearance for participation in athletic endeavors.

Transition to Adult Care for Youth with Congenital Heart Disease

Specialized care during the transition to adulthood may take a variety of forms, and is influenced by the severity of the underlying disease, the locally available resources, and clinician or patient/family preference. Some youth may remain with the cardiologist who cared for them during childhood, while others may transition to an adult cardiologist or to a specialized adult congenital center (if available).

Congenital heart disease in the young adult can be broadly categorized by the ability of the initial intervention to cure or palliate the disease, by the number of initial interventions, and by the expected need for future interventions. The American College of Cardiology/American Heart Association 2008 Consensus document regarding the adult with congenital heart disease provides a useful framework.[21] Three classifications from simple to complex congenital disease are used:

- **Simple congenital heart disease** includes such lesions as mild valvar pulmonary stenosis and repaired ASD or VSD. These "nearly normal" patients will require little to no activity restriction, no endocarditis prophylaxis, and infrequent follow-up. Most can be cared for in the general medical community.

TABLE 16.7

Common Forms of Congenital Heart Disease antd Potential Issues in Adolescence

	Common Issues	Rare Concerns
Simple CHD		
Repaired ASD		Atrial tachycardia Heart block
Repaired VSD	Residual VSD Right bundle branch block	Arrhythmias
Mild pulmonary stenosis		
Moderate complexity		
Tetralogy of Fallot	Pulmonary insufficiency Atrial tachycardia RV dysfunction	Ventricular tachycardia LV dysfunction
Ebsteins disease	Arrhythmias Exercise intolerance	Cyanosis
Aortic valve disease	Widely variable	
Aortic coarctation	Additional aortic/mitral valve disease Hypertension	
Arterial switch for d-transposition	Neo-aortic valve disease Mild coronary insufficiency Branch pulmonary artery stenosis	
AV canal defects	Arrhythmias Mitral insufficiency	
High complexity		
Complex tetralogy of Fallot	Conduit obstruction Branch pulmonary artery stenosis	
Single ventricular-Fontan	Sinus node dysfunction Exercise intolerance Arrhythmias Fluid retention	Protein-losing enteropathy Ventricular failure
Truncus arteriosus	Conduit obstruction Truncal valve dysfunction	
Atrial switch for d-TGA	Arrhythmias Systemic RV failure	

ASD, atrial septal defect; VSD, ventricular septal defect; AV, arterioventricular; d-TGA, dextro-transposition of the great arteries.

- The young adult with **congenital heart disease of moderate complexity** often feels well but has significant risk of requiring additional interventions. Tetralogy of Fallot and aortic coarctation are two examples where the residual disease may be very slowly progressive or occult. Also included in this category is the patient with moderate but asymptomatic valve disease who may require future intervention. These young adults should be seen periodically at regional adult congenital heart centers.

- The young adults with **congenital heart disease of great complexity**—characterized by repairs involving conduits, functional single ventricle physiology, and/or pulmonary hypertension—require regular, often intensive, support from specialized adult congenital heart disease centers.

Clinicians caring for youth with congenital heart disease should be preparing for the transition to adulthood during early and middle adolescence. The goal is to facilitate a planned, purposeful transition to adult-oriented care for youth and families rather than an abrupt transfer to adult care during a time of crisis. Pregnancy (and prepregnancy planning) is an example of one of many times during the transition to adulthood that resources for youth and families will be needed.

REFERENCES

1. Geggel RL. Conditions leading to pediatric cardiology consultation in a tertiary academic hospital. *Pediatrics* 2004;114(4):e409–e417.
2. Biancaniello T. Innocent murmurs. *Circulation* 2005;111(3):e20–e22.
3. Frank JE, Jacobe KM. Evaluation and management of heart murmurs in children. *Am Fam Physician* 2011;84(7):793–800.
4. Mueller GC, Stark V, Steiner K, et al. Impact of age and gender on cardiac pathology in children and adolescents with Marfan syndrome. *Pediatr Cardiol* 2013;34(4):991–998.
5. Freed LA, Levy D, Levine RA, et al. Prevalence and clinical outcome of mitral-valve prolapse. *N Engl J Med* 1999;341(1):1–7.
6. Hayek E, Gring CN, Griffin BP. Mitral valve prolapse. *Lancet* 2005;365(9458):507–518.
7. Maron BJ, Zipes DP. Introduction: eligibility recommendations for competitive athletes with cardiovascular abnormalities-general considerations. *J Am Coll Cardiol* 2005;45(8):1318–1321.
8. Priori SG, Aliot E, Blomstrom-Lundqvist C, et al. Task force on sudden cardiac death of the European Society of Cardiology. *Eur Heart J* 2001;22(16):1374–1450.
9. Lerman TT, Weintraub AY, Sheiner E. Pregnancy outcomes in women with mitral valve prolapse and mitral valve regurgitation. *Arch Gynecol Obstet* 2013;288(2):287–291.
10. Nishimura RA, McGoon MD, Shub C, et al. Echocardiographically documented mitral-valve prolapse. Long-term follow-up of 237 patients. *N Engl J Med* 1985;313(21):1305–1309.
11. Taub CC, Stoler JM, Perez-Sanz T, et al. Mitral valve prolapse in Marfan syndrome: an old topic revisited. *Echocardiography* 2009;26(4):357–364.
12. Maron BJ, Chaitman BR, Ackerman MJ, et al. Recommendations for physical activity and recreational sports participation for young patients with genetic cardiovascular diseases. *Circulation* 2004;109(22):2807–2816.
13. Rowe PC, Barron DF, Calkins H, et al. Orthostatic intolerance and chronic fatigue syndrome associated with Ehlers-Danlos syndrome. *J Pediatr* 1999;135(4):494–499.
14. Crabbe LS, Bensky AS, Hornstein L, et al. Cardiovascular abnormalities in children with fragile X syndrome. *Pediatrics* 1993;91(4):714–715.
15. Wilson W, Taubert KA, Gewitz M, et al. Prevention of infective endocarditis: guidelines from the American Heart Association: a guideline from the American Heart Association Rheumatic Fever, Endocarditis and Kawasaki Disease Committee, Council on Cardiovascular Disease in the Young, and the Council on Clinical Cardiology, Council on Cardiovascular Surgery and Anesthesia, and the Quality of Care and Outcomes Research Interdisciplinary Working Group. *J Am Dent Assoc* 2007;138(6):739–745, 747–760.
16. Danford DA. Cost-effectiveness of echocardiography for evaluation of children with murmurs. *Echocardiography* 1995;12(2):153–162.
17. Mellion K, Uzark K, Cassedy A, et al. Health-related quality of life outcomes in children and adolescents with congenital heart disease. *J Pediatr* 2014;164(4):781–788.e1.
18. Kempny A, Dimopoulos K, Uebing A, et al. Reference values for exercise limitations among adults with congenital heart disease. Relation to activities of daily life—single centre experience and review of published data. *Eur Heart J* 2012;33(11):1386–1396.
19. Mackie AS, Rempel GR, Rankin KN, et al. Risk factors for loss to follow-up among children and young adults with congenital heart disease. *Cardiol Young* 2012;22(3):307–315.
20. McGrath E, Wypij D, Rappaport LA, et al. Prediction of IQ and achievement at age 8 years from neurodevelopmental status at age 1 year in children with D-transposition of the great arteries. *Pediatrics* 2004;114(5):e572–e576.
21. Warnes CA, Williams RG, Bashore TM, et al. ACC/AHA 2008 guidelines for the management of adults with congenital heart disease: a report of the American College of Cardiology/American Heart Association Task Force on Practice Guidelines (Writing Committee to Develop Guidelines on the Management of Adults with Congenital Heart Disease). Developed in Collaboration With the American Society of Echocardiography, Heart Rhythm Society, International Society for Adult Congenital Heart Disease, Society for Cardiovascular Angiography and Interventions, and Society of Thoracic Surgeons. *J Am Coll Cardiol* 2008;52(23):e143–e263.

ADDITIONAL RESOURCES AND WEBSITES ONLINE

Systemic Hypertension

Joseph T. Flynn

Hypertension is one of the most common chronic diseases in adults, affecting about 30% of adults of all ages and 7.3% of young adults 18 to 39 years of age.[1,2] In children <18 years of age, however, hypertension is much less common, with recent screening studies demonstrating a 3% to 4% prevalence of persistent hypertension. Some studies have reported a higher prevalence of up to 5% in obese minority adolescents,[3] reflecting a similar impact of the obesity epidemic as seen in adults.[2,4] Other recent analyses have demonstrated an increase in prevalence of hypertension in children and adolescents ≤18 years of age, again likely because of the obesity epidemic.[5] On the other hand, the prevalence of hypertension in those ≥18 years of age has remained stable over time.[2]

Most adolescents and adults with hypertension have primary hypertension—that is, no identifiable underlying cause can be found for their blood pressure (BP) elevation. Since most hypertensive adolescents and young adults (AYAs), particularly those with primary hypertension, are asymptomatic, it is imperative to measure BP whenever an adolescent or young adult is seen for health care in order to detect hypertension and institute appropriate measures to reduce cardiovascular risk.

DEFINITION OF HYPERTENSION

The cardiovascular end points used to define hypertension in adults (e.g., myocardial infarction, stroke) do not occur in children and adolescents. Therefore, the definition of hypertension in those <18 years of age is a statistical one derived from analysis of a large database of BPs obtained from healthy children.[6] The resulting normative BP values for adolescents ≤17 years of age are listed in **Tables 17.1** and **17.2**. To use these tables, height should first be obtained and plotted on a standard growth curve to determine the height percentile. Then, the gender-appropriate chart should be used to determine the BP percentile. BP readings ≥95th percentile are considered hypertensive in this age group, and should be staged (see below) and repeated as appropriate (see **Table 17.3**). Elevated BP readings ≥95th percentile on three or more occasions are required to make a diagnosis of hypertension.[5]

For young adults ≥18 years, any BP reading ≥140/90 is considered hypertensive, regardless of age or gender. Individuals with BP values of this magnitude on two or more occasions are considered to have hypertension.[7]

Prehypertension

Common to both the pediatric (<18 years of age) and adult BP classification schemes is the concept of "prehypertension," referring to BPs between the normal and hypertensive ranges. Although the term has proved to be controversial, it is meant to serve as an alert to patients and physicians to the potential for future development of hypertension and of the need to make lifestyle changes that might prevent this from occurring. The same BP value of >120/80 mm Hg is used in both adolescents and adults to designate prehypertension.

Staging

Also common to both the pediatric and adult BP classification schemes is the concept of "staging" the severity of hypertension. The staging system helps to determine how rapidly a hypertensive patient should be evaluated and when antihypertensive drug therapy should be initiated. The currently accepted staging systems for hypertension in AYAs[6,7] are compared in **Table 17.3**.

FACTORS THAT INFLUENCE BP

Height and Weight

Height is part of the definition of normative BP in patients ≤17 years of age[6]; its inclusion was based on statistical analysis of the childhood BP database. Others hold that weight is the most important factor in determining BP. Weight has long been shown to have a positive relationship with BP, as demonstrated in a study of adolescent Minneapolis school children.[8] Increased body mass index (BMI) is also one of the most important influences on BP in adults ≥18 years old.[2]

Age

BP increases with age in a nonlinear manner through adolescence; this is likely related to growth. Beyond adolescence, BP, especially systolic BP (SBP), continues to increase in a significant percentage of individuals as the result of genetic and environmental factors, as well as age-associated vascular changes.

Sodium and Other Dietary Constituents

Numerous studies have done little to settle the controversy concerning the relationship of sodium intake to BP. For most individuals, little correlation exists. However, in certain salt-sensitive individuals, sodium restriction appears beneficial.[9] Decreased sodium intake on a population basis might be more beneficial[10]; a recent study demonstrated that reducing dietary sodium intake in England was accompanied by a reduction in population BP levels.[11]

TABLE 17.1

BP Values for Adolescent Boys 17 Years or Younger

Age (y)	BP Percentile	Systolic BP (mm Hg) ← Percentile of Height →							Diastolic BP (mm Hg) ← Percentile of Height →						
		5th	10th	25th	50th	75th	90th	95th	5th	10th	25th	50th	75th	90th	95th
10	50th	97	98	100	102	103	105	106	58	59	60	61	61	62	63
	90th	111	112	114	115	117	119	119	73	73	74	75	76	77	78
	95th	115	116	117	119	121	122	123	77	78	79	80	81	81	82
	99th	122	123	125	127	128	130	130	85	86	86	88	88	89	90
11	50th	99	100	102	104	105	107	107	59	59	60	61	62	63	63
	90th	113	114	115	117	119	120	121	74	74	75	76	77	78	78
	95th	117	118	119	121	123	124	125	78	78	79	80	81	82	82
	99th	124	125	127	129	130	132	132	86	86	87	88	89	90	90
12	50th	101	102	104	106	108	109	110	59	60	61	62	63	63	64
	90th	115	116	118	120	121	123	123	74	75	75	76	77	78	79
	95th	119	120	122	123	125	127	127	78	79	80	81	82	82	83
	99th	126	127	129	131	133	134	135	86	87	88	89	90	90	91
13	50th	104	105	106	108	110	111	112	60	60	61	62	63	64	64
	90th	117	118	120	122	124	125	126	75	75	76	77	78	79	79
	95th	121	122	124	126	128	129	130	79	79	80	81	82	83	83
	99th	128	130	131	133	135	136	137	87	87	88	89	90	91	91
14	50th	106	107	109	111	113	114	115	60	61	62	63	64	65	65
	90th	120	121	123	125	126	128	128	75	76	77	78	79	79	80
	95th	124	125	127	128	130	132	132	80	80	81	82	83	84	84
	99th	131	132	134	136	138	139	140	87	88	89	90	91	92	92
15	50th	109	110	112	113	115	117	117	61	62	63	64	65	66	66
	90th	122	124	125	127	129	130	131	76	77	78	79	80	80	81
	95th	126	127	129	131	133	134	135	81	81	82	83	84	85	85
	99th	134	135	136	138	140	142	142	88	89	90	91	92	93	93
16	50th	111	112	114	116	118	119	120	63	63	64	65	66	67	67
	90th	125	126	128	130	131	133	134	78	78	79	80	81	82	82
	95th	129	130	132	134	135	137	137	82	83	83	84	85	86	87
	99th	136	137	139	141	143	144	145	90	90	91	92	93	94	94
17	50th	114	115	116	118	120	121	122	65	66	66	67	68	69	70
	90th	127	128	130	132	134	135	136	80	80	81	82	83	84	84
	95th	131	132	134	136	138	139	140	84	85	86	87	87	88	89
	99th	139	140	141	143	145	146	147	92	93	93	94	95	96	97

To use the table, first plot the child's height on a standard growth curve (www.cdc.gov/growthcharts). The child's measured SBP and DBP are compared with the numbers provided in the table according to the child's age and height percentile.

BP, blood pressure; SBP, systolic blood pressure; DBP, diastolic blood pressure.

Adapted from National High Blood Pressure Education Program Working Group on High Blood Pressure in Children and Adolescents. *The fourth report on the diagnosis, evaluation, and treatment of high blood pressure in children and adolescents.* NIH Publication 05-5267. Bethesda, MD: National Heart, Lung, and Blood Institute, 2005.

TABLE 17.2

BP Values for Adolescent Girl 17 Years or Younger

Age (y)	BP Percentile	Systolic BP (mm Hg) ← Percentile of Height →							Diastolic BP (mm Hg) ← Percentile of Height →						
		5th	10th	25th	50th	75th	90th	95th	5th	10th	25th	50th	75th	90th	95th
10	50th	98	99	100	102	103	104	105	59	59	59	60	61	62	62
	90th	112	112	114	115	116	118	118	73	73	73	74	75	76	76
	95th	116	116	117	119	120	121	122	77	77	77	78	79	80	80
	99th	123	123	125	126	127	129	129	84	84	85	86	86	87	88
11	50th	100	101	102	103	105	106	107	60	60	60	61	62	63	63
	90th	114	114	116	117	118	119	120	74	74	74	75	76	77	77
	95th	118	118	119	121	122	123	124	78	78	78	79	80	81	81
	99th	125	125	126	128	129	130	131	85	85	86	87	87	88	89
12	50th	102	103	104	105	107	108	109	61	61	61	62	63	64	64
	90th	116	116	117	119	120	121	122	75	75	75	76	77	78	78
	95th	119	120	121	123	124	125	126	79	79	79	80	81	82	82
	99th	127	127	128	130	131	132	133	86	86	87	88	88	89	90
13	50th	104	105	106	107	109	110	110	62	62	62	63	64	65	65
	90th	117	118	119	121	122	123	124	76	76	76	77	78	79	79
	95th	121	122	123	124	126	127	128	80	80	80	81	82	83	83
	99th	128	129	130	132	133	134	135	87	87	88	89	89	90	91
14	50th	106	106	107	109	110	111	112	63	63	63	64	65	66	66
	90th	119	120	121	122	124	125	125	77	77	77	78	79	80	80
	95th	123	123	125	126	127	129	129	81	81	81	82	83	84	84
	99th	130	131	132	133	135	136	136	88	88	89	90	90	91	92
15	50th	107	108	109	110	111	113	113	64	64	64	65	66	67	67
	90th	120	121	122	123	125	126	127	78	78	78	79	80	81	81
	95th	124	125	126	127	129	130	131	82	82	82	83	84	85	85
	99th	131	132	133	134	136	137	138	89	89	90	91	91	92	93
16	50th	108	108	110	111	112	114	114	64	64	65	66	66	67	68
	90th	121	122	123	124	126	127	128	78	78	79	80	81	81	82
	95th	125	126	127	128	130	131	132	82	82	83	84	85	85	86
	99th	132	133	134	135	137	138	139	90	90	90	91	92	93	93
17	50th	108	109	110	111	113	114	115	64	65	65	66	67	67	68
	90th	122	122	123	125	126	127	128	78	79	79	80	81	81	82
	95th	125	126	127	129	130	131	132	82	83	83	84	85	85	86
	99th	133	133	134	136	137	138	139	90	90	91	91	92	93	93

To use the table, first plot the child's height on a standard growth curve (www.cdc.gov/growthcharts). The child's measured SBP and DBP are compared with the numbers provided in the table according to the child's age and height percentile.

BP, blood pressure; SBP, systolic blood pressure; DBP, diastolic blood pressure.

Adapted from National High Blood Pressure Education Program Working Group on High Blood Pressure in Children and Adolescents. *The fourth report on the diagnosis, evaluation, and treatment of high blood pressure in children and adolescents.* NIH Publication 05-5267. Bethesda, MD: National Heart, Lung, and Blood Institute, 2005.

TABLE 17.3

Classification of BP in AYAs

BP classification	Adolescents <18 y of age[a]	Young Adults ≥18 y of age[b]
Normal	SBP and DBP <90th percentile	SBP <120 mm Hg and DBP <80 mm Hg
Prehypertension	SBP or DBP 90–95th percentile; or if BP is >120/80 even if <90th percentile	SBP 120–139 mm Hg or DBP 80–89 mm Hg
Stage 1 hypertension	SBP or DBP ≥95th to 99th percentile plus 5 mm Hg	SBP 140–159 mm Hg or DBP 90–99 mm Hg
Stage 2 hypertension	SBP or DBP >99th percentile plus 5 mm Hg	SBP ≥160 mm Hg or DBP ≥100 mm Hg

[a]Adapted from National High Blood Pressure Education Program Working Group on High Blood Pressure in Children and Adolescents. *The fourth report on the diagnosis, evaluation, and treatment of high blood pressure in children and adolescents.* NIH Publication 05-5267. Bethesda, MD: National Heart, Lung, and Blood Institute, 2005.
[b]Adapted from Chobanian AV, Bakris GL, Black HR, et al. The seventh report of the joint national committee on prevention, detection, evaluation, and treatment of high blood pressure: the JNC 7 report. *JAMA* 2003;289:2560.

Other studies have found a link between potassium intake and both elevated and low BP, although the preponderance of evidence appears to show a protective effect of increased potassium intake.[10] However, efforts to correlate calcium and other divalent cations with BP have been equivocal. Similarly, suggested correlations between BP and vitamins A, C, and E remain to be proved. Falkner et al.[12] noted that dietary modification of certain nutrients when instituted at an early age could contribute to the prevention of hypertension in urban minority adolescents at risk for hypertension.

Stress

Both physical and mental stressors evoke changes in BP. Indeed, the degree of change has been thought by some to be useful in predicting later-life hypertension. Early studies have demonstrated that hypertensive adolescents had significantly greater increases in heart rate, SBP, and diastolic BP (DBP) during mental stress (performance of difficult arithmetic problems) than normotensive adolescents.[13] It has been proposed that impaired renal sodium handling is the mechanism underlying stress-induced increases in BP in adolescents.[14] In adults, occupational stress has been shown to contribute to the development of hypertension and other cardiovascular diseases,[15] suggesting that stress may have lifelong adverse cardiovascular effects.

Race

As recent survey data have shown, there are substantial racial differences in the prevalence of hypertension in adults ≥18 years of age, with non-Hispanic Blacks having the highest rates of hypertension.[1] While race is felt to be less of a factor in adolescents, it should be noted that the recent increase in hypertension prevalence in those <18 has been more pronounced among Blacks and Mexican Americans than in Whites,[5] suggesting differential susceptibility to the development of hypertension by race at all ages. Additionally, in one recent study, Black AYAs 13 to 20 years old had higher BPs than non-Black AYAs.[16] Ethnicity and socioeconomic status have also been related to BP and cardiovascular reactivity.[17]

Genetics

Both familial aggregation BP studies and twin studies indicate a strong positive correlation between hereditary influences and BP measurements. Family history has been shown to be an important determinant of overall cardiovascular risk.[18] It is estimated that about one-third of variations in BP among individuals are heritable, most likely from several genes.[19] Additionally, several single-gene defects have been described,[20] which account for hypertension in a small number of patients, especially those with a family history of severe, early-onset hypertension.

Birth Weight and Other Perinatal Factors

The "fetal origins" hypothesis maintains that low birth weight is a risk factor for the subsequent development of primary hypertension in adulthood.[21] This hypothesis stems from findings of large population studies that demonstrate an inverse correlation between birth weight and adult BP.[22,23] Proposed explanations for this effect include deficient maternal nutrition, possibly leading to development of a reduced number of nephrons in utero. Studies suggest that maternal smoking during pregnancy and bottle-feeding of newborns may also lead to hypertension later in life.[24,25] Other epidemiologic studies have found that adult BP is more closely related to early childhood growth[21,26] than to birth weight. More research is needed; however, available evidence suggests that perinatal and early childhood factors may play an important role in the later development of hypertension in some individuals.

ETIOLOGY

At least 80% to 90% of hypertensive adolescents have no known cause for their disorder and are labeled as having primary or essential hypertension. As in younger children, renal parenchymal diseases are the most common secondary cause in the adolescents. Primary hypertension in adolescents is frequently characterized by isolated SBP elevation,[27] whereas DBP elevation is more likely to be present in secondary hypertension. Obesity and a positive family history of hypertension are also common in adolescents with primary hypertension.

Primary or essential hypertension accounts for at least 95% of all cases of hypertension in adults ≥18 years of age.[28] Unfortunately, there are no data available on specific etiologies of hypertension in young adults 18 to 25 years of age compared to other age groups. A high index of suspicion in the clinician caring for hypertensive young adults is therefore needed for detection of cases of secondary hypertension.

DIAGNOSIS

BP Measurement

There are several important points regarding measurement of BP that should be considered in patients of any age. They are as follows:

1. Although various methods are available to measure BP, auscultation is the method of choice because it is most accurate. Because of the removal of mercury sphygmomanometers from most health care settings, aneroid devices should be utilized. The stethoscope bell should be used for auscultation, as it is better suited to detect the soft, low-pitched Korotkoff sounds than the diaphragm.
2. Proper cuff bladder size is critical. The length of the cuff bladder should be at least 80% of the mid-arm circumference.[3] For practical purposes, use the largest cuff that fits the arm while leaving the antecubital fossa free for auscultation. Given the obesity epidemic, many AYAs will require large adult or even thigh-sized cuffs because of increased arm circumferences.
3. BP measurements should be taken while the patient is seated with feet on the floor and the arm at heart level. The arm (preferably the right) used for the measurement should be

recorded in the chart. Ideally, the patient should have rested for several minutes and should not have smoked or ingested caffeine within 30 minutes before measurement.

4. For apprehensive patients, BP measurements obtained outside of the office setting, such as by a school nurse or at home using a calibrated over-the-counter device, may provide insight as to the existence of "white coat" hypertension. However, ambulatory BP monitoring, in which BP measurements are obtained over a 24-hour period with an automated device, is the preferred technique for diagnosing white coat hypertension.[29,30]

Confirmation of Hypertension Diagnosis

In adolescents <18 years of age, three BP determinations on different days must show a high (≥95th percentile) systolic or diastolic pressure or both before a diagnosis of hypertension is made. This is because BP in this age group has been shown to be quite labile, leading to the possibility of overdiagnosis if only one or two BP readings are relied upon.[6] As stated above, assessment for white coat hypertension, ideally with ambulatory BP monitoring,[29] is increasingly advocated. Studies suggest that white coat hypertension may actually be a prelude to permanent hypertension, and others have shown that adolescents with white coat hypertension have early evidence of target-organ damage.[31]

Confirmation of hypertension in adults requires documentation of elevated BP (≥140/90) on just two occasions.[7] Twenty-four-hour ambulatory BP monitoring or home measurement of BP is often recommended to evaluate for possible white coat hypertension.[30] Interestingly, the prevalence of white coat hypertension in young adult patients aged 18 to 30 years has recently been shown to be <4%,[32] compared to nearly 30% in a recently published referral series of children and adolescents aged 15.6 ± 3.7 years.[33] This difference would suggest that the recommendation for a greater number of elevated readings in patients <18 years before confirming a diagnosis of hypertension is warranted.

Diagnostic Evaluation

Once the diagnosis of hypertension is made, a diagnostic evaluation and management plan can be initiated. The diagnostic evaluation must be tailored to the individual, taking into account age, sex, race, family history, and level of hypertension. For example, a 12-year-old White female with a past medical history of recurrent urinary tract infections, no family history of hypertension, and a BP of 150/115 mm Hg would be a candidate for an aggressive evaluation for secondary causes (particularly renal parenchymal disease, specifically reflux nephropathy). In contrast, invasive studies to identify a secondary cause are unlikely to be helpful in a 21-year-old obese, Black male with a family history of hypertension and a BP of 150/78 mm Hg.

1. History: A detailed history should assess for possible secondary causes, target-organ damage, and other cardiovascular risk factors. Ask about (1) symptoms of urinary tract infections or renal disease; (2) family history of hypertension or other cardiovascular disease; (3) activity, dietary, and other habits; and (4) alcohol, tobacco, and substance use. Substances that may elevate BP are listed in **Table 17.4**, and historical clues suggestive of secondary hypertension are in **Table 17.5**.

2. Physical examination: A thorough examination is also an essential part of the diagnostic study. The examination should evaluate for evidence of a secondary cause or end-organ damage and include the following:
   a. Height, weight, and calculated BMI
   b. BP in both arms and a lower extremity
   c. Femoral pulses
   d. Neck: Carotid bruits or an enlarged thyroid gland
   e. Fundi: Arteriolar narrowing, arteriovenous nicking, hemorrhages, exudates
   f. Abdomen: Bruits, hepatosplenomegaly, flank masses

TABLE 17.4
Substances That May Elevate BP

Prescription Medications	Nonprescription Medications	Others
Calcineurin inhibitors (cyclosporine, tacrolimus)	Caffeine	Cocaine
Dexedrine[a]	Ephedrine	Ethanol
Erythropoietin	Nonsteroidal anti-inflammatory drugs[a]	Heavy metals (lead, mercury)
Glucocorticoids	Pseudoephedrine	MDMA ("Ecstasy")
Methylphenidate[a]		Tobacco
Oral contraceptives		Herbal preparations (*Ephedra, Glycyrrhiza*)
Phenylpropanolamine		
Pseudoephedrine		
Tricyclic antidepressants[a]		

[a]These cause elevated blood pressure relatively infrequently compared with the other agents in the table.

   g. Heart: Rate, precordial heave, clicks, murmurs, arrhythmias
   h. Extremities: Pulses, edema
   i. Nervous system
   j. Skin: Striae, acanthosis nigricans, café au lait spots, neurofibromas

Physical examination findings suggestive of secondary causes of hypertension are listed in **Table 17.5**. In addition, the clinician should remember that severe hypertension in an adolescent or young adult suggests a secondary cause, particularly renal disease. Acute onset may also be due to acute renal disease.

3. Laboratory testing: Basic/screening studies should be performed in all patients with confirmed BP elevation. Specific testing is indicated when secondary hypertension is suspected or for those with stage 2 hypertension.
   a. *Screening tests*—should be done in all patients:
      • Electrolytes, blood urea nitrogen, and creatinine
      • Urinalysis (Urine cultures should be obtained if history or urinalysis suggests infection.)
      • Lipid profile (Initial test does not have to be fasting.)
      • Complete blood cell count
      • Fasting glucose with or without fasting insulin in obese patients to screen for impaired glucose tolerance/hyperinsulinemia
   b. *Specific laboratory tests* should be directed by findings on history and physical examination, or from the screening test results. Examples include (1) antinuclear antibody test and sedimentation rate in a hypertensive female adolescent with a malar rash, and (2) thyroid studies if there is history suggestive of thyroid dysfunction (e.g., heat/cold intolerance).
   c. *Echocardiogram* is recommended for all adolescents <18 years old with confirmed hypertension to detect left ventricular hypertrophy (LVH).[6] LVH occurs commonly in hypertensive adolescents and is a risk factor for sudden cardiac death.[34] While LVH may be present in up to 20% of unselected hypertensive adults, routine echocardiography is not recommended for hypertensive patients ≥18 years of age.[35]
   d. *Advanced testing* should only be done when secondary causes of hypertension are suspected. For example, obtain plasma normetanephrine if pheochromocytoma is suspected or a 24-hour urine collection for protein if there is persistent proteinuria.
   e. *Imaging studies* are indicated only in specific circumstances. Renal ultrasonography should be obtained for all

TABLE 17.5

History and Physical Examination Findings Suggestive of Secondary Causes of Hypertension

Present in History	Suggests
Known UTI/UTI symptoms	Reflux nephropathy
Joint pains, rash, fever	Vasculitis, SLE
Acute onset of gross hematuria	Glomerulonephritis, renal thrombosis
Renal trauma	Renal infarct, RAS
Abdominal radiation	Radiation nephritis, RAS
Renal transplant	Transplant RAS
Precocious puberty	Adrenal disorder
Muscle cramping, constipation	Hyperaldosteronism
Excessive sweating, headache, pallor, and/or flushing	Pheochromocytoma
Known illicit drug use	Drug-induced HTN
Present on Examination	**Suggests**
BP >140/100 mm Hg at any age	Secondary hypertension
Leg BP < arm BP	Aortic coarctation
Poor growth, pallor	Chronic renal disease
Turner syndrome	Aortic coarctation
Café au lait spots	Renal artery stenosis
Delayed leg pulses	Aortic coarctation
Precocious puberty	Adrenal disorder
Bruits over upper abdomen	Renal artery stenosis
Edema	Renal disease
Excessive sweating	Pheochromocytoma
Excessive pigmentation	Adrenal disorder
Striae in a male	Drug-induced HTN

UTI, urinary tract infection; BP, blood pressure; SLE, systemic lupus erythematosus; RAS, renal artery stenosis; HTN, hypertension.

adolescents <18 years with stage 2 hypertension, or for those with stage 1 hypertension and an abnormal urinalysis.[6] As with echocardiography, routine renal imaging is not currently recommended for evaluation of hypertensive patients ≥18 years of age. Chest x-ray should only be obtained if the cardiac examination is abnormal. More advanced imaging studies such as nuclear medicine scans or angiography are useful in a small percentage of hypertensive patients and should only be obtained under the direction of a subspecialist.

THERAPY

Prevention

Optimally, measures to prevent or minimize the effects of hypertension should be applied to all patients at risk for developing hypertension. The difficulty lies in identifying those at risk and deciding what measures to apply. Though prevention studies for AYAs with long-term follow-up are lacking, a reasonable starting point is to consider patients with the characteristics listed below as being at risk. They should be counseled about nonpharmacologic approaches to maintain lower BP and should be periodically monitored:

1. Prehypertension (BP >120/80 mm Hg)
2. BMI >85th percentile, particularly if parents are obese
3. Hyperlipidemia or a family history of the disorder, particularly if there is a family history of coronary artery disease or stroke
4. Two or more family members with treated hypertension, particularly Black and Latino individuals

Nonpharmacologic Interventions

Weight loss, aerobic exercise, and dietary modifications have all been shown to successfully reduce BP in hypertensive patients of all ages. These interventions should be part of the treatment plan for all AYAs with hypertension:

1. Weight reduction: Excess body weight is correlated closely with increased BP. Weight reduction reduces BP in a large proportion of hypertensive individuals who are >10% above ideal weight.
2. Dietary changes: Moderate sodium restriction in hypertensive individuals has been shown to reduce SBP, on average, by 4.9 mm Hg and DBP by 2.6 mm Hg. Although there has been some evidence to suggest that potassium, calcium, or magnesium supplementation might be beneficial, studies have not consistently confirmed this effect. On the other hand, the so-called "DASH (Dietary Approaches to Stop Hypertension) diet," which is lower in sodium and higher in potassium and calcium content, has been demonstrated to be of benefit in hypertensive adults[36] and adolescents.[37]
3. Regular physical exercise: Regular aerobic physical activity, adequate to achieve at least a moderate level of physical fitness, may be beneficial for both prevention and treatment of hypertension. Regular aerobic physical activity (≥30 minutes/session, 4 to 5 days/week) can reduce SBP in hypertensive patients by approximately 10 mm Hg.
4. Other lifestyle changes: Smoking cessation and avoidance of alcohol excess, medications (except as directed by health care providers), and drugs (e.g., cocaine, amphetamines). Cigarette smoking increases BP and is a major risk factor for cardiovascular disease. Excessive alcohol intake can raise BP and cause resistance to antihypertensive therapy.

Pharmacologic Treatment—Adolescents <18 Years

1. Antihypertensive medications are definitely indicated for patients with[6]:
   a. Symptoms of hypertension
   b. Stage 2 hypertension
   c. Evidence of hypertensive end-organ damage
   d. Type 1 or type 2 diabetes
   e. Secondary hypertension
   f. Persistent hypertension despite lifestyle changes
2. If none of these indications are present, drug treatment can be withheld. The lifestyle modifications discussed earlier should be recommended. If BP remains elevated after a reasonable trial of these measures (usually 6 to 12 months), then medication should be prescribed.
3. Once-daily medications should be used if possible to improve adherence for what may be a lifelong but asymptomatic problem.
4. Explicit education should be provided about hypertension and the reasons for therapy using language the adolescent understands.

5. The adolescent should generally be responsible for taking his or her own medication, but parents should be encouraged to help the adolescent maintain adherence.
6. Antihypertensive agents should be chosen to obtain the maximum benefit and minimize side effects. The ideal hypertensive agent would
   a. Lower BP in almost all hypertensive individuals
   b. Address specific pathogenic mechanisms
   c. Be associated with few biochemical changes
   d. Be associated with few or no adverse reactions
   e. Be dosed once or, at most, twice daily
   f. Be inexpensive
7. Unfortunately, the ideal antihypertensive agent does not exist.[38] The National High Blood Pressure Education Program Working Group[6] has stated that a variety of agents are acceptable for use in children and adolescents. Recently published reviews may help guide the clinician selecting from among these agents.[39]
8. As illustrated in Figure 17.1, a stepped-care approach should be followed when prescribing antihypertensive agents in patients <18 years. In this approach, a monotherapy drug regimen is superimposed on nonpharmacologic therapy as initial treatment.[6,39]
9. Suggested initial and maximum doses of various antihypertensive agents for patients <18 years are given in Table 17.6. Many have pediatric-specific Food and Drug Administration (FDA)-approved labeling as a result of recent trials in children and adolescents.[39]
10. For adolescents <18 years with uncomplicated primary hypertension, target BP should be the 95th percentile for age, gender, and height; for those with secondary hypertension, diabetes, or chronic kidney disease, target BP should be the 90th percentile.[6]
11. After an extended course of drug therapy and sustained BP control, a gradual reduction in or withdrawal of medication can be attempted with close observation and continuation of nonpharmacologic therapy. This will probably be successful only in the adolescent who has been successful with lifestyle modification.

Pharmacologic Treatment—Young Adults ≥18 Years

1. Drug therapy is generally initiated for SBP ≥140 mm Hg and/or DBP ≥90 mm Hg in adults <60 years of age.[40,41] This is based on epidemiologic evidence of reduction in stroke, myocardial infarction, and other cardiovascular disease with effective antihypertensive treatment.
   a. Several months of nonpharmacologic measures should be implemented before drug therapy is begun in patients with stage 1 hypertension.
   b. Patients with stage 2 hypertension, secondary hypertension, diabetes, or underlying kidney disease warrant immediate initiation of drug therapy.
2. The general comments made above about the ideal antihypertensive agent for adolescents apply also to young adult patients.
3. Initial therapeutic regimens have been debated. In adults, the most recent report from the Joint National Committee panelists recommends choosing from several classes of antihypertensive medications, with preferred classes for Black patients (see below) and those with kidney disease or diabetes.[41]
4. Combination preparations are acceptable as first-line therapy, and may improve both adherence and the ability to reach treatment goals.
5. Similar to the stepped-care approach illustrated in Figure 17.1, medication doses should be titrated to achieve goal BP, and additional medications added as needed if BP control cannot be achieved with the initial regimen chosen.
6. In young adults, SBP should be lowered to <140 mm Hg for those with uncomplicated primary hypertension, and SBP/DBP lowered to <140/90 in those with chronic kidney disease or diabetes.[41]
7. Withdrawal of antihypertensive medications after a period of drug treatment may be attempted if the patient is motivated to continue lifestyle changes.[42]

Pharmacologic Treatment—Special Populations

1. Black AYAs: In Black AYAs, diuretics have been proven to reduce hypertensive morbidity and mortality rates; so diuretics should be seriously considered for use in the absence of other conditions that prohibit their use. Angiotensin-converting enzyme (ACE) inhibitors are often less effective in Black than in White patients. Calcium channel blockers and α-receptor blockers have similar efficacy in both populations.
2. Females who take oral contraceptives: Most females who take oral contraceptives have small increases in SBP and DBP but usually within the reference range. Hormonal contraceptives, mainly those that contain estrogen, can increase angiotensinogen in some individuals, with resultant increases in angiotensin II and BP. The risk of overt hypertension appears to increase with age, duration of use, and body mass. Many of the studies of BP and oral contraceptive agents involved

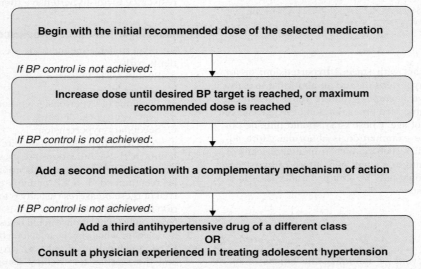

FIGURE 17.1 Stepped-care approach to antihypertensive therapy in adolescents <18 years of age. BP, blood pressure.

TABLE 17.6

Antihypertensive Agents for Use in Chronic Treatment of Hypertension in Adolescents <18 years old[a]

Class	Drug	Starting Dose	Interval	Maximum Dose[b]
ACE inhibitors	Benazepril	0.2 mg/kg/d up to 10 mg/d	q.d.	0.6 mg/kg/d up to 40 mg q.d.
	Captopril	0.3–0.5 mg/kg/dose	b.i.d.–t.i.d.	6 mg/kg/d up to 450 mg/d
	Enalapril	0.08 mg/kg/d	q.d.	0.6 mg/kg/d up to 40 mg/d
	Fosinopril	0.1 mg/kg/d up to 10 mg/d	q.d.	0.6 mg/kg/d up to 40 mg/d
	Lisinopril	0.07 mg/kg/d up to 5 mg/d	q.d.	0.61 mg/kg/d up to 40 mg/d
	Quinapril	5–10 mg/d	q.d.	80 mg/d
	Ramipril	2.5 mg/d	q.d.	20 mg/d
Angiotensin receptor blockers α- and β-Antagonists	Candesartan	4 mg/d	q.d.	32 mg q.d.
	Losartan	0.75 mg/kg/d up to 50 mg/d	q.d.–b.i.d.	1.44 mg/kg/d up to 100 mg/d
	Olmesartan	20–35 kg: 10 mg/d ≥35 kg: 20 mg/d	q.d.	20–35 kg: 20 mg q.d. ≥35 kg: 40 mg q.d.
	Valsartan	6–17 y: 1.3 mg/kg/d up to 40 mg/d	q.d.	6–17 y: 2.7 mg/kg/d up to 160 mg/d
	Labetalol	2–3 mg/kg/d	b.i.d.	10–12 mg/kg/d up to 1.2 g/d
	Carvedilol	0.1 mg/kg/dose up to 6.25 mg b.i.d.	b.i.d.	0.5 mg/kg/dose up to 25 mg b.i.d.
β-Antagonists	Atenolol	0.5–1 mg/kg/d	q.d.–b.i.d.	2 mg/kg/d up to 100 mg/d
	Bisoprolol/HCTZ	2.5/6.25 mg/d	q.d.	10/6.25 mg q.d.
	Metoprolol	1–2 mg/kg/d	b.i.d.	6 mg/kg/d up to 200 mg/d
	Propranolol	1 mg/kg/d	b.i.d.–t.i.d.	16 mg/kg/d
Calcium channel blockers	Amlodipine	0.10 mg/kg/d	q.d.	0.6 mg/kg/d up to 10 mg/d
	Felodipine	2.5 mg/d	q.d.	10 mg/d
	Isradipine	0.05–0.15 mg/kg/dose	t.i.d.–q.i.d.	0.8 mg/kg/d up to 20 mg/d
	Extended-release nifedipine	0.25–0.5 mg/kg/d	q.d.–b.i.d.	3 mg/kg/d up to 120 mg/d
Central α-agonists	Clonidine	5–10 µg/kg/d	b.i.d.–t.i.d.	25 µg/kg/d up to 0.9 mg/d
	Methyldopa	10 mg/kg/d	b.i.d.–q.i.d.	65 mg/kg/d up to 3 g/d
Diuretics	Amiloride	5–10 mg/d	q.d.	20 mg/d
	Chlorthalidone	0.3 mg/kg/d	q.d.	2 mg/kg/d up to 50 mg/d
	Furosemide	0.5–2.0 mg/kg/dose	q.d.–b.i.d.	6 mg/kg/d
	HCTZ	1 mg/kg/d	b.i.d.	3 mg/kg/d up to 50 mg/d
	Spironolactone	1 mg/kg/d	q.d.–b.i.d.	3.3 mg/kg/d up to 100 mg/d
	Triamterene	1–2 mg/kg/d	b.i.d.	3–4 mg/kg/d up to 300 mg/d
Peripheral α-antagonists	Doxazosin	1 mg/d	q.d.	4 mg/d
	Prazosin	0.05–0.1 mg/kg/d	t.i.d.	0.5 mg/kg/d
	Terazosin	1 mg/d	q.d.	20 mg/d
Vasodilators	Hydralazine	0.25 mg/kg/dose	t.i.d.–q.i.d.	7.5 mg/kg/d up to 200 mg/d
	Minoxidil	0.1–0.2 mg/kg/d	b.i.d.–t.i.d.	1 mg/kg/d up to 50 mg/d

[a]Consult comprehensive reviews or other references for specific side effects
[b]The maximum recommended adult dose should never be exceeded. Note that for some drugs, the maximum adult dose may be higher than what is listed in this table.
q.d., once daily; b.i.d., twice daily; t.i.d., three times daily; q.i.d., four times daily; HCTZ, hydrochlorothiazide.

higher doses of both estrogen and progesterone than are used currently. If concurrent treatment with an oral contraceptive and antihypertensive medication is needed, consideration should be given to using a low-estrogen or progestin-only contraceptive.

3. Adolescents with asthma: β-Blocking drugs can worsen bronchoconstriction and are therefore relatively contraindicated for patients with asthma and hypertension. Newer, more cardioselective β_1 receptor selective agents such as metoprolol or bisoprolol may be tried, especially in those with mild asthma.

4. Diabetes: The diagnosis of hypertension or even prehypertension in an adolescent or young adult with either type 1 or type 2 diabetes is an indication to initiate antihypertensive drug therapy. ACE inhibitors or angiotensin receptor blockers should be used as the initial agent in hypertensive diabetic patients because of their potential benefit in slowing or preventing diabetic nephropathy.

HYPERTENSIVE EMERGENCIES

Rarely, an adolescent or young adult will have signs of encephalopathy or heart failure at presentation and be found to have extraordinarily high BP, at levels well above stage 2 hypertension. This constitutes a true emergency and may have disastrous consequences unless efforts to lower the BP are begun at once. Assistance from an expert in hypertension should be sought. Meanwhile, the patient should be hospitalized and an intravenous line placed. Usually, a continuous infusion of either nicardipine or labetalol should be started at a low dose and then titrated as needed to slowly reduce the BP. The initial reduction should be no more than 25% over the first 8 hours in order to prevent cerebral, cardiac, or renal ischemia from overly rapid BP reduction.[43,44] BP can then be lowered to the 95th percentile over the next 24 hours. When adequate pressure control has been achieved, oral antihypertensive agents can be gradually introduced and the intravenous agents discontinued. A thorough evaluation to determine the cause of the hypertension must be made once the patient's condition has been stabilized.

REFERENCES

1. Nwankwo T, Yoon SS, Burt V, et al. *Hypertension among adults in the United States: National Health and Nutrition Examination Survey, 2011–2012.* NCHS data brief, no 133. Hyattsville, MD: National Center for Health Statistics, 2013.
2. Egan BM, Li J, Hutchison FN, et al. Hypertension in the United States, 1999 to 2012: progress toward healthy people 2020 goals. *Circulation* 2014;130:1692–1699.
3. Sorof JM, Lai D, Turner J, et al. Overweight, ethnicity, and the prevalence of hypertension in school-aged children. *Pediatrics* 2004;113:475.
4. Flynn J. The changing face of pediatric hypertension in the era of the childhood obesity epidemic. *Pediatr Nephrol* 2013;28:1059–1066.
5. Din-Dzietham R, Liu Y, Bielo MV, et al. High blood pressure trends in children and adolescents in national surveys, 1963 to 2002. *Circulation* 2007;116:1488–1496.
6. National High Blood Pressure Education Program Working Group on High Blood Pressure in Children and Adolescents. *The fourth report on the diagnosis, evaluation, and treatment of high blood pressure in children and adolescents.* NIH Publication 05-5267. Bethesda, MD: National Heart, Lung, and Blood Institute, 2005.
7. Chobanian AV, Bakris GL, Black HR, et al. The seventh report of the Joint National Committee on prevention, detection, evaluation, and treatment of high blood pressure: the JNC 7 report. *JAMA* 2003;289:2560.
8. Luepker RV, Jacobs DR, Prineas RJ, et al. Secular trends of blood pressure and body size in a multi-ethnic adolescent population: 1986 to 1996. *J Pediatr* 1999;134:668.
9. Weinberger MH. Pathogenesis of salt sensitivity of blood pressure. *Curr Hypertens Rep* 2006;8(2):166–170.
10. Aaron KJ, Sanders PW. Role of dietary salt and potassium intake in cardiovascular health and disease: a review of the evidence. *Mayo Clin Proc* 2013;88:987–995.
11. He FJ, Pombo-Rodrigues S, Macgregor GA. Salt reduction in England from 2003 to 2011: its relationship to blood pressure, stroke and ischaemic heart disease mortality. *BMJ Open* 2014;4:e004549.
12. Falkner B, Sherif K, Michel S, et al. Dietary nutrients and blood pressure in urban minority adolescents at risk for hypertension. *Arch Pediatr Adolesc Med* 2000;154:918.
13. Falkner B. Blood pressure response to mental stress. *Am J Hypertens* 1991;4:621S–623S.
14. Harshfield GA, Dong Y, Kapuku GK, et al. Stress-induced sodium retention and hypertension: a review and hypothesis. *Curr Hypertens Rep* 2009;11:29–34.
15. Backé EM, Seidler A, Latza U, et al. The role of psychosocial stress at work for the development of cardiovascular diseases: a systematic review. *Int Arch Occup Environ Health* 2012;85:67–79.
16. Brady TM, Fivush B, Parekh RS, et al. Racial differences among children with primary hypertension. *Pediatrics* 2010;126:931–937.
17. Barnes VA, Treiber FA, Musante L, et al. Ethnicity and socioeconomic status: impact on cardiovascular activity at rest and during stress in youth with a family history of hypertension. *Ethn Dis* 2000;10:4.
18. Giussani M, Antolini L, Brambilla P, et al. Cardiovascular risk assessment in children: role of physical activity, family history and parental smoking on BMI and blood pressure. *J Hypertens* 2013;31:983–992.
19. Colhoun H. Commentary: confirmation needed for genes for hypertension. *Lancet* 1999;353:1200.
20. Lifton RP, Gharavi AG, Geller DS. Molecular mechanisms of human hypertension. *Cell* 2001;104:545.
21. Edvardsson VO, Steinthorsdottir SD, Eliasdottir SB, et al. Birth weight and childhood blood pressure. *Curr Hypertens Rep* 2012;14:596–602.
22. Barker DJP, Gluckman PD, Godfrey KM, et al. Fetal nutrition and cardiovascular disease in adult life. *Lancet* 1993;341:941.
23. Zureik M, Bonithon-Kopp C, Lecomte E, et al. Weights at birth and in early infancy, systolic pressure and left ventricular structure in subjects aged 8 to 24 years. *Hypertension* 1996;27 (pt 1):339.
24. Beratis NG, Panagoulias D, Varvarigou A. Increased blood pressure in neonates and infants whose mothers smoked during pregnancy. *J Pediatr* 1996;128:806.
25. Singhal A, Cole TJ, Lucas A. Early nutrition in preterm infants and later blood pressure: two cohorts after randomized trials. *Lancet* 2001;357:413.
26. Falkner B, Hulman S, Kushner H. Birth weight versus childhood growth as determinants of adult blood pressure. *Hypertension* 1998;31 (pt 1):145.
27. Flynn JT, Alderman MH. Characteristics of children with primary hypertension seen at a referral center. *Pediatr Nephrol* 2005;20:961.
28. Carretero OA, Oparil S. Essential hypertension, Part I: definition and etiology. *Circulation* 2000;101:329–335.
29. Flynn JT, Urbina EM. Pediatric ambulatory blood pressure monitoring: indications and interpretations. *J Clin Hypertens (Greenwich)* 2012;14:372–382.
30. Ghuman N, Campbell P, White WB. Role of ambulatory and home blood pressure recording in clinical practice. *Curr Cardiol Rep* 2009; 11:414–421.
31. Kavey RE, Kveselis DA, Atallah N, et al. White coat hypertension in childhood: evidence for end-organ effect. *J Pediatr* 2007;150:491–497.
32. Conen D, Aeschbacher S, Thijs L, et al. Age-specific differences between conventional and ambulatory daytime blood pressure values. *Hypertension* 2014;64:1073–1079.
33. Davis ML, Ferguson MA, Zachariah JP. Clinical predictors and impact of ambulatory blood pressure monitoring in pediatric hypertension referrals. *J Am Soc Hypertens* 2014;8:660–667.
34. Kavey RE. Left ventricular hypertrophy in hypertensive children and adolescents: predictors and prevalence. *Curr Hypertens Rep* 2013;15:453–457.
35. Kaplan NM. Primary hypertension: natural history and evaluation. In: Kaplan NM, Victor RG, eds. *Kaplan's clinical hypertension*, 10th ed. Philadelphia, PA: Lippincott-Williams and Wilkins, 2009:108–140.
36. Appel LJ, Moore TJ, Obarzanek E, et al. A clinical trial of the effects of dietary patterns on blood pressure. *N Engl J Med* 1997;336:1117.
37. Couch SC, Saelens BE, Levin L, et al. The efficacy of a clinic-based behavioral nutrition intervention emphasizing a DASH-type diet for adolescents with elevated blood pressure. *J Pediatr* 2008;152:494–501.
38. Batisky DL. What is the optimal first-line agent in children requiring antihypertensive medication? *Curr Hypertens Rep* 2012;14:603–607.
39. Ferguson MA, Flynn JT. Rational use of antihypertensive medications in children. *Pediatr Nephrol* 2013;29(6):979–988.
40. Weber MA, Schiffrin EL, White WB, et al. Clinical practice guidelines for the management of hypertension in the community: a statement by the American Society of Hypertension and the International Society of Hypertension. *J Clin Hypertens (Greenwich)* 2014;16:14–26.
41. James PA, Oparil S, Carter BL, et al. 2014 evidence-based guideline for the management of high blood pressure in adults: report from the panel members appointed to the Eighth Joint National Committee (JNC 8). *JAMA* 2014;311:507–520.
42. Nelson M, Reid C, Krum H, McNeil J. A systematic review of predictors of maintenance of normotension after withdrawal of antihypertensive drugs. *Am J Hypertens* 2001;14:98–105.
43. Flynn JT, Tullus K. Severe hypertension in children and adolescents: pathophysiology and treatment. *Pediatr Nephrol* 2009;24:1101–1112.
44. Sarafidis PA, Georgianos PI, Malindretos P, et al. Pharmacological management of hypertensive emergencies and urgencies: focus on newer agents. *Expert Opin Investig Drugs* 2012;21:1089–1106.

🛜 **ADDITIONAL RESOURCES AND WEBSITES ONLINE**

PART IV

Musculoskeletal Problems and Sports Medicine

Common Musculoskeletal Problems

Keith J. Loud
Blaise A. Nemeth

Musculoskeletal problems, including injury, are among the most common reasons for adolescents and young adults (AYAs) to seek medical attention. Appropriate management of these concerns cannot only decrease morbidity and prevent sequelae but also earn the confidence of the patient.

This chapter outlines a general approach to all musculoskeletal complaints, highlighting those conditions that are frequently seen or are unique to AYAs, with special attention to spinal deformities.

GENERAL PRINCIPLES OF MUSCULOSKELETAL INJURY CARE

Triage and Initial Management of Common Complaints

Health care providers for AYAs can provide most of the initial care for orthopedic problems. When patients present with pain in the ankle, knee, hip, and spine, the health care provider should be able to prioritize the most likely diagnoses and develop an initial management plan on the basis of the description of the (1) mechanism of injury or onset of symptoms, (2) factors that worsen or improve the pain, and (3) physical examination findings. Resources that are likely to be helpful to the health care provider include the following:

1. Reference materials to manage specific diagnoses:
   a. *Essentials of Musculoskeletal Care*, 4th Edition, published jointly by the American Academy of Pediatrics (AAP) and American Academy of Orthopedic Surgeons (AAOS)—a comprehensive, practical guide to the diagnosis and treatment of virtually all orthopedic problems encountered in primary care practice.
   b. *Care of the Young Athlete*, 2nd Edition, an encyclopedic textbook also published jointly by the AAP and AAOS.
   c. *Sports Medicine in the Pediatric Office*, by Jordan Metzl—a text and DVD that demonstrates hands-on examination techniques
   d. *The Sports Medicine Patient Advisor*, by Pierre Rouzier—a thorough compilation of patient education materials including handouts with rehabilitative exercises
2. Rehabilitation specialists: A strong working relationship with local rehabilitation specialists, such as physical therapists and athletic trainers, in practice and in schools is essential because formal supervised rehabilitation is a mainstay in the treatment of many conditions.
3. Musculoskeletal specialists: Ready consultation with orthopedic surgeons and primary care sports medicine physicians when needed.

General Indications for Radiographs in Patients with Acute Trauma of an Extremity

In general, plain radiographs (x-rays) should be considered for any:

1. Significant unilateral complaint (with greater urgency for pain, which awakens a patient from sleep)
2. Unexplained or persistent bilateral complaints

General Indications for Referral to a Musculoskeletal Specialist for Patients with Acute Trauma of an Extremity

General criteria for immediate consultation regardless of the injury site include any of the following:

1. Obvious deformity
2. Acute locking (joint cannot be moved actively or passively past a certain point) or other concern for osteochondritis dissecans (OCD)
3. Penetrating wound of major joint, muscle, or tendon
4. Neurological deficit
5. Joint instability perceived by the adolescent or young adult or elicited by the health care provider or other concern for internal joint derangement
6. Bony crepitus

Treatment and Rehabilitation of Injuries—General Concepts

The prevention of long-term sequelae of injury depends on complete rehabilitation, characterized by full, pain-free range of motion (ROM) and normal strength, endurance, and proprioception.

There are four phases of rehabilitation:

1. Limit further injury and control pain and swelling.
2. Improve strength and ROM of injured structures.
3. Achieve near-normal strength, ROM, endurance, and proprioception of injured structures.
4. Return to activity (exercise, sport, or work) free of symptoms.

Since AYAs progress through these phases at different rates, avoid predicting time frames for return to participation

Phase 1: Limit Further Injury and Control Pain and Swelling

1. The affected part must be rested and protected, using appliances (e.g., wrap, splint, crutches, sling) as necessary to achieve pain relief. Reevaluate frequently to avoid extended use of crutches or bracing without indication.

2. Elevation, compression, and ice should be applied as often as possible during waking hours. Ice should be applied continuously for 20 minutes, directly to the skin and 3 to 4 times a day for the first few days.
3. Nonsteroidal anti-inflammatory drugs (NSAIDs), if prescribed, should be dosed regularly (rather than "as needed") to achieve therapeutic steady-state levels, but limited to 5 to 10 days.
4. Uninjured structures should be exercised to maintain fitness and psychological health.

Phase 2: Improve Strength and ROM of Injured Structures

1. *Relative rest* is the cardinal principle, allowing activity as long as it does not cause pain within 24 hours of the activity.
2. Specific exercises should be done within a pain-free ROM. Isometric exercises can be started on the first day if there is little pain-free ROM but the patient is able to contract the muscles.
3. NSAIDs may be continued to interrupt the cycle of pain, muscle spasm, inflexibility, weakness, and decreased endurance; however, they should not be used to mask pain and allow premature return to play. In addition to reducing swelling, ice is also a good analgesic.
4. General fitness maintenance should continue, as described for Phase 1.

Phase 3: Achieve Near-Normal Strength, ROM, Endurance, and Proprioception of Injured Structures

1. Exercise is increased as long as the subject follows the *relative rest* principle.
2. Healing is characterized by minimal discomfort or laxity with provocative testing, normal ROM, no tenderness along the ligament or pain with stretching, and progressively less pain with activities of daily living.

Phase 4: Return to Exercise or Sport Free of Symptoms

1. Functional rehabilitation should be sport-specific, practicing components at a decreased level and advancing gradually to full-force execution.
2. Premature return is likely to result in further injury or another injury.
3. Successful rehabilitation minimizes the risk of reinjury and returns the injured structures to baseline ROM, strength, endurance, and proprioception.

In the clinician's office, safe return to participation in physical activities can be advocated when the patient demonstrates:

1. Absolutely no residual deformities or edema in the injured body part. An exception to this rule is the ankle, which may demonstrate soft tissue swelling (not effusion) long after functional restoration has been achieved.
2. Full and equal ROM compared to the uninjured, paired joint
3. At least 90% muscle strength compared with the uninjured paired extremity
4. No pain at rest or with activity. If there is post-activity discomfort, it should resolve completely before the next activity session (practice or competition), without regular use of analgesics. Discomfort after subsequent activity sessions should not be greater in intensity than the initial session, even if it completely resolves in between.

ANKLE INJURIES

Ankle injuries—sprains and fractures—are the single most common acute injury in adolescent athletes. The diagnosis and treatment of ankle injuries in adolescents are the same as in young adults, with the exception that early teens may have open growth plates that may be fractured, whereas in a young adult the primary injury is likely to be a sprain of ligaments.

Historical Clues

In the majority of acute ankle injuries, the mechanism of injury is inversion (turning the ankle under or in). Injuries resulting from eversion are generally more serious because of the higher risk of fracture and "high ankle sprains" (syndesmosis injury).

Physical Examination

1. Acute injury: The best and most informative time to examine any musculoskeletal injury is immediately after the injury. However, patients commonly present hours to days after the injury with diffuse swelling, tenderness, and decreased ROM. At this point, the physical examination will be limited in terms of diagnosing specific lesions. At a minimum, the examination should include the following:
   a. Inspect for gross abnormalities, asymmetry, and vascular integrity.
   b. Palpate for bony tenderness specifically at the distal/posterior 6 cm of the tibia (medial malleolus) or fibula (lateral malleolus), the tarsal navicular, and base of the fifth metatarsal (Fig. 18.1).
   c. Assess ability to bear weight.
2. Three to four days after injury: The physical examination may be more informative at this time, as the patient may have had an opportunity to use rest, ice, compression, and elevation.
   a. Inspect for swelling and ecchymosis.
   b. Assess active ROM in six directions:
      • Plantarflexion; plantarflexion and inversion; plantarflexion and eversion
      • Dorsiflexion; dorsiflexion and inversion; dorsiflexion and eversion
   c. Assess resisted ROM in the same six directions.
   d. Palpate again for bony tenderness.
   e. Attempt passive ROM—plantarflexion, dorsiflexion, and inversion, which will provoke discomfort with the most common lateral ankle injury.
   f. Assess ligamentous stability—see reference texts to perform talar tilt and anterior drawer tests.
   g. Assess for pain-free weight bearing with normal gait and then with heel-and-toe walking.
3. Associated injuries: Complications associated with ankle sprains:
   a. Fractures are common in ankle injuries that cause complete ligament tears. The most common sites are the talus, fifth metatarsal, fibula, and tibia. If there is bony tenderness in an adolescent with open physes, assume that a fracture is present even if the radiography results are negative. Immobilize without weight bearing for 1 week; if tenderness persists, casting for 2 weeks is recommended. An exception is the distal fibular physis. Many authorities will manage and monitor a presumed Salter–Harris I fracture (normal radiographs) like a lateral ankle sprain. Similarly, a small avulsion fracture at the tip of the distal fibula or tibia may be treated conservatively.
   b. "High ankle sprains"—tibiofibular syndesmosis injury accounts for 6% of ankle sprains. These are more serious injuries than the typical lateral ligament sprain. On examination, there is tenderness proximal to the joint line along the syndesmosis. Pressing the midshaft together and then releasing the pressure may worsen the pain.

Diagnosis

Radiographic Examination: Ottawa Ankle Rules

The Ottawa Ankle Rules are a well-validated set of clinical decision rules that suggest that an ankle or foot plain radiograph is indicated if there is bone tenderness at (1) the distal/posterior 6 cm of the tibia or fibula (ankle series); (2) at the tarsal navicular; (3) at the base of the fifth metatarsal (foot series); or (4) if the patient

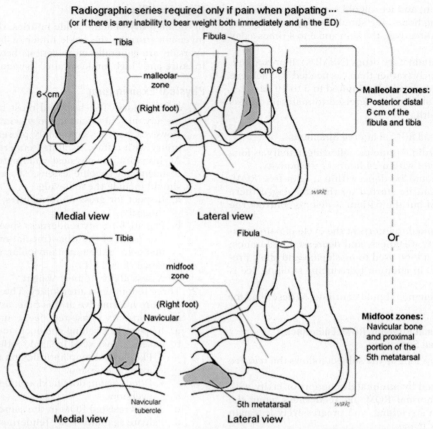

Radiographic series required only if pain when palpating ...
(or if there is any inability to bear weight both immediately and in the ED)

Medial view   Lateral view

Medial view   Lateral view

Malleolar zones:
Posterior distal
6 cm of the
fibula and tibia

Midfoot zones:
Navicular bone
and proximal
portion of the
5th metatarsal

FIGURE 18.1 Ottawa ankle rules for suspected fracture. (From Chila A; American Osteopathic Association. *Foundations of osteopathic medicine.* 3rd ed. Philadelphia, PA: Lippincott Williams & Wilkins, 2010.)

is unable to take four steps both immediately after the injury AND during the examination, regardless of limping (Fig. 18.1).[1] Stress views are typically not indicated in the evaluation of the acute or chronically injured ankle.

Treatment—Acute Phase

The goal is to limit disability. Successful treatment is defined by the absence of pain and by return to full ROM, strength, and proprioception. Mainstays of initial treatment are:

1. *Relative rest*, ice, compression, and elevation: Used in the same manner as described earlier
2. Compression and stability can be provided by an air stirrup type ankle brace, which should be used for all acute sprains not complicated by fracture. Casting is not indicated. The brace provides stability to inversion and eversion, allowing for active dorsiflexion and plantarflexion, which includes weight-bearing gait, a key to successful rehabilitation.
3. Stirrup braces should spare the use of crutches. If crutches are needed for significant pain, the patient should be instructed in partial weight-bearing techniques. Patients should be advised to discontinue use of crutches as soon as possible by using the brace consistently and aggressively increasing the proportion of weight bearing, guided by their discomfort.

Rehabilitation

Rehabilitation should start on the first day of evaluation.

1. Stretching: Primarily soleus and gastrocnemius, by doing calf stretches
2. Strengthening: Band exercises, toe–heel walking, pain free, and progressive (can be done with the air stirrup on)

3. Proprioceptive retraining: Raising on toes with little support (one or two fingers on a chair) and eyes closed for 5 minutes a day
4. Functional progression of exercise: For instance, toe walking → walking at a fast pace → jogging → jogging and sprinting → sprinting and jogging on curves → figure-of-eight running → back to sports participation
5. The stirrup or lace-up-type ankle brace should be worn in competition sports for 6 months after the injury.

THE KNEE

Knee injuries and pain syndromes are among the most common chief complaints seen by musculoskeletal specialists who work with AYAs. Primary care clinicians can develop a working diagnosis and initiate treatment for the majority of these patients.

Historical Clues

1. Knee pain that occurs while running straight, without direct trauma or fall.
   a. Chronic pain: Likely to be patellofemoral pain syndrome (PFS).
   b. Acute pain: Consider OCD and pathological fracture. Any adolescent with knee pain without a history of trauma who has an examination that does not pinpoint the diagnosis should have a radiographic examination of the knee. If the hip examination is abnormal, radiographs of the hip are also needed to rule out slipped capital femoral epiphysis (SCFE) manifesting as knee pain. Osgood–Schlatter disease and PFS do not require radiographs to establish a diagnosis.
2. Knee injury that occurs during weight bearing, cutting while running, or an unplanned fall: Consider internal derangement

including ligamentous and meniscal tears and fracture, especially if there is hemarthrosis within 24 hours of the injury. A patient who injures the knee while cutting, without being hit or having direct trauma, has a high likelihood of having an anterior cruciate ligament (ACL) tear or patellar dislocation.

3. A valgus injury to the knee (i.e., a force delivered to the outside of the knee, directed toward the midline) is likely to tear the medial collateral ligament, possibly the ACL, and either the medial or lateral meniscus.

4. Chronic anterior knee pain that is worse when going up stairs and/or after sitting for prolonged periods, or after squatting or running, is likely to be PFS. *In general*, if the patient does not give a history of the knee giving out or locking, sharp pain, effusion, the sensation of something loose in the knee, or the sensation that something tore with the initial injury, then the injury will probably not require surgical intervention or referral. At the activity site, the ability to bear weight and walk without pain is the best indicator that the injury is probably not major and does not need immediate referral.

Physical Examination

Knee anatomy is shown in Figure 18.2. The physical examination should include the following:

1. Observation of gait (weight bearing? antalgic gait?)
2. Inspection for swelling and discoloration
3. Observation of vastus medialis obliquus contraction, looking for reduced bulk and tone
4. Peripatellar palpation (tenderness over the tibial tuberosity is diagnostic of Osgood–Schlatter disease; peripatellar pain is characteristic of patellofemoral dysfunction)
5. Observation of quadriceps and hamstring flexibility
6. Examination for evidence of ligamentous instability, including valgus and varus testing (for medial collateral and lateral collateral ligaments, respectively)
7. Examination for evidence of meniscal tears (McMurray and modified McMurray tests), ACL tears (Lachman and pivot shift tests), and posterior cruciate ligament tears (sag sign and posterior drawer test) requires practice and experience; the reference materials demonstrate examination techniques for readers who wish to learn these skills.

Diagnosis

Radiographic Evaluation of Knee Injuries

According to the *Ottawa Knee Rule*, another validated clinical decision rule, a radiograph is indicated after an acute knee injury if any one of the following criteria is present:

1. Inability to bear weight
2. Fibular head tenderness
3. Isolated tenderness of the patella
4. Inability to flex the knee beyond 90 degrees

These decision rules have been shown to have a sensitivity of 100% in detecting knee fractures in adults and could potentially reduce the use of plain radiographs by 28%.[2]

Anteroposterior and lateral views are standard. The sunrise view details the patellofemoral joint and should be ordered if patellar dislocation is suspected, while the tunnel view should be ordered if suspicious for OCD, ACL injury, or other intra-articular pathology. Magnetic resonance imaging (MRI) evaluation is not routinely indicated in the acute or chronically injured knee. MRI should be reserved for diagnostic dilemmas and for patients who do not respond to conservative management, as it adds little to a history and physical examination performed by an experienced clinician in the diagnosis of knee injuries.

Acute Traumatic Knee Injuries—General Principles of Treatment

1. Establish a working diagnosis.

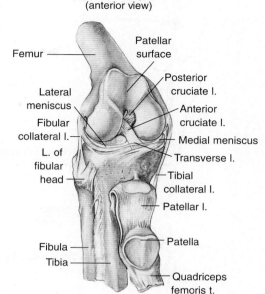

Right knee joint
(anterior view)

FIGURE 18.2 Right knee joint (anterior view). (Courtesy of the Anatomical Chart Company, 2015.)

2. Use the Ottawa Knee Rule.
3. Relative rest: Prescribe use of crutches if the patient cannot bear weight without pain or there is suspicion of fracture. An elastic wrap is adequate in the initial phase of treatment or until there is a definitive diagnosis and treatment plan. Knee immobilizers have a limited role in the management of acute knee injuries because they are bulky and awkward, and limit return of ROM. However, if a fracture has been ruled out and the clinician is concerned about patellar or joint instability, a brace can allow for safer weight-bearing gait.
4. Start isometric quadriceps contractions on the first day if possible. If the patient cannot contract the quadriceps and it is anticipated that he or she will be unable to do so for several days, consider an electrical stimulation unit to contract the quadriceps until the patient can do so.

Anterior Knee Pain Syndromes—Differential Diagnosis and Approach to Management

Anterior knee pain syndromes are among the most common diagnoses in sports medicine clinics that serve AYAs.

Patellofemoral Pain Syndrome

Definition: PFS, patellar malalignment syndrome, or patellofemoral dysfunction is a frequent cause of knee pain among AYAs, accounting for as much as 70% to 80% of knee pain problems in females and 30% in males. It is also the leading cause of knee problems in athletes. The condition had traditionally been known as chondromalacia patellae. However, this term has largely been abandoned because it implies softening and damage to the patellar articular cartilage, which is infrequently demonstrated on MRI or arthroscopy. The term patellofemoral pain syndrome is a better descriptive term for part of the pathophysiology of the condition.

Etiology: PFS is often a result of abnormal biomechanical forces that occur across the patella. Even in an individual with normal anatomy, the force that occurs in this area is tremendous, especially when the body is supported with one leg and the knee is partially flexed. Abnormal forces can result from the following:

1. Quadriceps femoris muscle imbalance or weakness or abnormality in the attachment of the vastus medialis

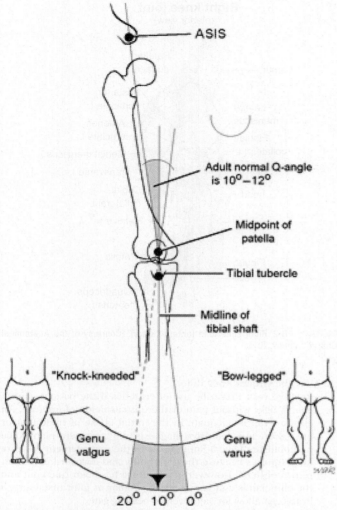

FIGURE 18.3 Q-angle. Q-angle (quadriceps angle) normally measures 10 to 12 degrees. Key landmarks for establishing the Q-angle are the ASIS, the patella, and the tibial tuberosity. Note the change in the Q-angle in genu valgus and varus. (From Chila A; American Osteopathic Association. *Foundations of osteopathic medicine*. 3rd ed. Philadelphia, PA: Lippincott Williams & Wilkins, 2010.)

2. Altered patellar anatomy, such as a small- or high-riding patella
3. Increased femoral neck anteversion, with associated knee valgus and external tibial torsion, which increases lateral stress on the patella
4. Increased Q-angle—the angle found between a line drawn from the anterosuperior iliac spine through the center of the patella and a line from the center of the patella to the tibial tubercle (normal, <15 degrees) (Fig. 18.3)
5. Variations in the patellar facet anatomy

Epidemiology: PFS is common in both male and female athletes. There is a higher prevalence among females in the general population but a higher prevalence among males in athletic populations.

Clinical Manifestations:
1. The pain of PFS is characterized by the following:
   a. Peripatellar or retropatellar location
   b. Relation to activity: The pain usually increases with activities such as running, squatting, or jumping, and decreases with rest. Often, the pain is worst immediately on getting up to start an activity after sitting.
   c. Insidious onset
2. Positive movie or theater sign: Prolonged sitting with flexed knee is uncomfortable.

3. Pain is often severe on ascending or descending stairs.
4. Knees may seem to buckle, especially when going up or down stairs, but do not give way.
5. Crepitus or a grating sensation may be felt, especially when climbing stairs.
6. History of injury to the patella area may be present.
7. Symptoms are bilateral in one-third of AYAs.
8. Two-thirds of patients have at least a 6-month history of pain.
9. Physical examination
   a. Inspection of the patient with PFS may reveal anatomical abnormalities, but often does not.
   b. Dynamic patellar compression test, or "grind sign," may be performed by compressing the superior aspect of the patella between thumb and index finger as the patient actively tightens the quadriceps in 10 degrees of flexion. Pain is elicited if retropatellar PFS is present. Direct compression of the patella against the femur with the knee flexed will also elicit pain. This is not a sensitive test because it can also elicit pain in the normal knee.
   c. Active knee ROM is usually normal but hamstrings are often tight.
   d. Joint effusion usually does not occur but can be present in severe cases. Swelling, when appreciated, is related to peripatellar bursitis.
   e. Decreased bulk of the area around the vastus medialis on the affected side may be present.

Diagnosis: The diagnosis is usually made by compatible history and physical examination. Radiographs usually are of little help but are important in excluding other conditions. They should include anteroposterior, lateral, tunnel (to rule out OCD), and tangential views (also known as skyline or Merchant views). Hip disorders often manifest as vague knee or thigh pain, especially SCFE.

Treatment:
1. Control of symptoms as described earlier
2. Muscle strengthening: Most patients benefit from a formal physical therapy evaluation and can then be moved to a home program. As soon as tolerated, muscle-strengthening exercises should be performed at least once a day. Initially, these should be isometric quadriceps exercises (straight-leg raises). Strengthening of the vastus medialis is particularly important. Stretching of the hamstrings is an essential component of most therapy programs.
3. Graduated running: After symptoms are controlled and 6 to 10 lb of weight are held in straight-leg raises, a graduated running program can be instituted. Ice may be helpful immediately after exercise.
4. Maintenance: When the condition is under control, a maintenance program of quadriceps and hamstring exercises should be done 2 to 3 times a week. Most patients respond to nonoperative management.
5. Knee braces: Use of knee braces in patients with PFS is controversial. Theoretically, they keep the patella from moving too far laterally. However, because the patella moves in various planes, knee braces are best used in patients with lateral subluxation visible on examination. *The knee brace is not a substitute for muscle-strengthening exercises.*
6. Taping the knee: Although this may reduce friction, results are also controversial.
7. Footwear: Athletic shoes are in a near constant state of evolution, but the quality and age of the athletic shoes are more important than a particular brand name.
8. Over-the-counter arch supports or custom orthotics: These can be helpful to some patients. Custom orthotics are expensive and are generally not required, but in some patients these may be more helpful than over-the-counter supports.
9. Surgery: This is considered as a last resort for patellofemoral pain.

Osgood–Schlatter Disease

Definition: Osgood–Schlatter disease is a painful enlargement of the tibial tubercle at the insertion of the patellar tendon. It is a common problem, especially among active adolescent males.

Etiology: During development of the anterior tibial tubercle, a small ossification center develops in the largely cartilaginous tubercle. With puberty, developing muscle mass places this small area under great traction stress from the patellar tendon. Small fragments of cartilage or of the ossification center can be avulsed. The problem is often aggravated by activities that involve quadriceps femoris contraction, such as running and jumping.

Epidemiology:
1. Prevalence is higher in males than females.
2. Mean age at onset: Onset usually coincides with the period of rapid linear growth.
   a. Females: 10 years, 7 months
   b. Males: 12 years, 7 months

Clinical Manifestations:
1. Point tenderness and soft tissue swelling over the tibial tubercle
2. Normal knee joint with full ROM
3. Unilateral involvement more common than bilateral involvement
4. Duration usually lasts several months but can last longer.

Diagnosis:
1. History: Pain at the tibial tubercle, aggravated by activity and relieved by rest
2. Physical examination: Tenderness and swelling of the tibial tubercle
3. Radiograph: Not essential for diagnosis but generally done only to eliminate the possibility of other processes. The radiograph may reveal soft tissue swelling anterior to the tibial tubercle and/or fragmentation of the tibial tubercle.

Therapy: Since this is also an anterior knee pain syndrome, rehabilitation proceeds as for PFS. In addition:

1. Explanation: Careful explanation of the condition to the adolescent and parents is essential to alleviate fears and misconceptions.
2. Restriction of activity: If symptoms are mild, the patient may continue in the chosen sport. If symptoms are more severe, limiting running and jumping activities for 2 to 4 weeks is usually sufficient.
3. Immobilization: If symptoms are severe or fail to respond to restriction of activity, immobilization with a knee immobilizer for a few weeks is effective. Immobilization should also be strongly considered when the patient has difficulty actively bringing the knee to full extension.
4. Knee pads: Knee pads should be used for activities in which kneeling or direct knee contact might occur.
5. Surgery: Surgery is rarely indicated. If the patient continues to have symptoms after skeletal maturity, there may be a persistent ossicle that has not united with the rest of the tibial tubercle. Simple excision of this fragment may bring relief.

Prognosis: The prognosis is excellent, but adolescents should be informed that the process might recur if excessive activity is performed. When growth is completed, the problem usually stops, leaving only a prominent tubercle. The patient may still have difficulty kneeling on the prominent tubercle, even into adulthood. Rarely, patients with Osgood–Schlatter disease may fracture through the tibial tubercle.

Osteochondritis Dissecans

OCD is an important idiopathic condition of focal avascular necrosis in which bone and overlying articular cartilage separate from the medial femoral condyle, or less commonly, from the lateral femoral condyle. The peak incidence is in the preadolescent age-group. The clinical course and treatment vary according to the age at onset, with children and young adolescents having a better prognosis than older adolescents and adults. Insidious onset of intermittent, nonspecific knee pain that does not respond to PFS treatment should raise suspicion for OCD, especially if associated with intermittent effusion or a sensation of knee locking. Diagnosis of OCD should prompt referral to a musculoskeletal specialist.

THE HIP

Hip pain is a less common reason for AYAs to seek musculoskeletal care, but the differential diagnosis includes a true orthopedic surgical emergency, SCFE, which must be recognized by clinicians caring for this population.

Slipped Capital Femoral Epiphysis

Definition

SCFE is a disease in which the anatomic relationship between the femoral head and neck is altered secondary to a disruption at the level of the physis. A "stable" slip progresses slowly with insidious onset of pain. "Unstable" slips present acutely with inability to bear weight and represent a surgical urgency.

Etiology

The femoral head slips posteriorly, inferiorly, and medially on the femoral metaphysis. This occurs through the hypertrophic cell layer of the epiphysis that widens during the accelerated growth of puberty. Obesity may alter the mechanics, increasing the vector of shear force acting at the physis, in addition to the increased forces caused by excess body weight itself.

Most cases of SCFE are unrelated to an endocrine disorder, although the disease has been associated with hypopituitarism, hypogonadism, and hypothyroidism, all having increased risk for bilateral slips. Endocrine abnormalities should be considered in patients at the extremes of the adolescent age-group (before age 9 or after age 16).

Epidemiology

1. Sex: The prevalence is 2 to 4 times higher in males than in females.
2. Average age at onset: Usually, symptoms occur shortly before or during the period of accelerated growth (10 to 13 years in girls, 12 to 15 years in boys).
3. Weight: Nearly 90% occur in patients who are overweight or obese.

Clinical Manifestations

Pain is localized to the hip or groin in most patients, although pain may occur in the thigh or knee, referred from the obturator nerve. Some patients present with a painless limp. Motion around the hip is decreased, including internal rotation, adduction, and flexion. The affected leg is often held in slight external rotation both at rest and with ambulation, as well as in abduction at rest. A limp is present in 50% of patients, although the adolescent with an unstable slip refuses to bear weight.

Diagnosis

The condition should be considered in any adolescent with hip or knee pain or a limp, especially those with body mass index >85% for age and sex. Anteroposterior and lateral (frog-leg or cross-table) radiographs of the pelvis should be taken. In a normal anteroposterior radiograph of the hip, a line drawn on the superior edge of the femoral neck intersects the epiphysis; in a slip, the epiphysis falls below this line (Fig. 18.4). Frog-leg lateral views better display early and more subtle slips. In suspected early cases that have normal radiographs, MRI may be helpful, demonstrating edema around the physis on T2-weighted images.

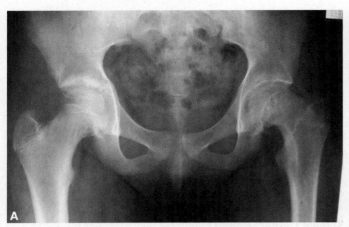 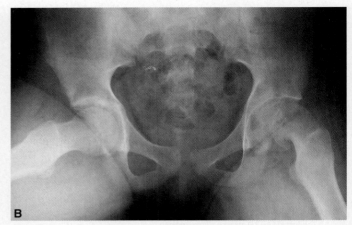

FIGURE 18.4 A: In the normal hip on the right, a line drawn on the superior femoral neck intersects the proximal femoral epiphysis. In the hip on the left with a slipped epiphysis, the epiphysis lies completely below a line drawn on the superior femoral neck. **B:** This is better visualized on the frog-lateral views.

Treatment

Orthopedic referral for surgery should occur immediately to prevent further slip. Patients should be made non–weight bearing, either on crutches or in a wheelchair. Further slip can be prevented by the introduction of threaded screws across the epiphyseal plate in situ, although anatomic reduction via surgical dislocation of the hip has been advocated to decrease sequelae of SCFE. Avascular necrosis occurs more commonly in unstable slips and persists as a complication of open dislocation with reduction.[3] Premature degenerative joint disease is a frequent late development in many patients with severe, chronic slips, after fixation in situ, presenting as early as late adolescence and young adulthood. For moderate and severe cases, corrective osteotomies can be performed after the growth plate has closed to improve gait and ROM.

Chronic Hip Pain

Pain around the hip that develops insidiously presents a common diagnostic dilemma.

Clinical Manifestations

Patients describe anterior hip or groin pain and occasionally a snapping sensation deep within the hip and/or catching or locking with increased pain. Specific positions may exacerbate symptoms.

Differential Diagnosis

1. SCFE (skeletally immature—this is the most urgent diagnosis to exclude)
2. Iliopsoas tendinosis or bursitis
3. Femoro-acetabular impingement (FAI)
4. Hip labral tear

Iliopsoas-Related Hip Pain

Etiology: Theorized to develop when the iliopsoas tendon rubs over the pelvic brim during internal and external rotation of the hip, which may occur in adolescents and also in young adults. Potential biomechanical factors include:

1. Muscle imbalances
   a. Relatively weak hip external rotators
   b. Tight iliopsoas, hamstrings, and/or iliotibial band
2. Hypermobility
3. Foot hyperpronation

Diagnosis: Diagnosis is difficult due to the deep location of the tendon and the frequent dynamic component. Imaging, including ultrasound, is often equivocal.[4] MRI does not demonstrate abnormalities but may be helpful in excluding other causes of pain.

Treatment: Physical therapy improves symptoms by improving hip and pelvis mechanics. Injection of the iliopsoas bursa with local anesthetic and corticosteroids under ultrasound guidance assists in both diagnosis and treatment, improving ability to perform physical therapy.[4] Immediate pain relief confirms the area of involvement and steroids provide longer-term relief; lack of improvement should lead the clinician to consider other diagnoses. Surgical release of the iliopsoas tendon is rarely necessary.

Femoro-acetabular Impingement and Labral Tears

Definition: FAI occurs if the femoral head is not round or if the acetabulum is too deep, resulting in abnormal contact between the femoral head and the rim of the acetabulum. Impingement of the bony structures can cause pain and predispose to tears of the labrum. The labrum of the hip, like that of the shoulder, deepens the socket. Both circumstances can occur in adolescents but are more common in young adults.

Etiology:
1. The cause of an abnormally shaped femoral head in most patients is unknown.
2. FAI can occur following childhood orthopedic disorders, such as SCFE, Legg–Calvé–Perthes disease, hip dysplasia, or hip trauma.
3. Labral tears occur as a result of acute or chronic trauma.
4. Labral tears are noted incidentally in asymptomatic individuals who come to MRI and/or surgery for other indications, so many are of no concern, especially in adolescents.

Symptoms: Patients with FAI usually present with limitations in hip ROM or pain at the end of ROM. Labral tear-related pain may be experienced deep in the hip anteriorly, in the groin, or even in the back.[5]

Diagnosis: Radiographs are usually sufficient to diagnose FAI. Labral tears require MRI, usually with intra-articular contrast.[6]

Treatment:
1. Physical therapy to adjust hip and pelvic mechanics
2. Alterations in symptom-producing activities
3. Intra-articular injection of local anesthetic and steroid assists in localizing the pain to an intra-articular location and provide indication for arthroscopy.
4. Both FAI and labral tears may be treated surgically via arthroscopic techniques, although occasionally open procedures are used for FAI.

SPINAL DISORDERS

Several abnormalities of the spine, including scoliosis and kyphosis, present during adolescence and young adulthood. Differentiating the causes requires a systematic approach to the physical examination and utilization of appropriate radiographs.

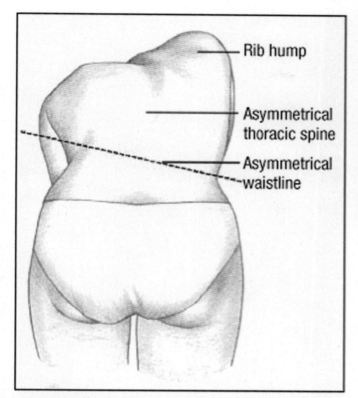

FIGURE 18.5 Testing for scoliosis. When assessing the patient for an abnormal spinal curve, use this screening test for scoliosis. Have the patient remove her shirt and stand as straight as she can with her back to you. Instruct her to distribute her weight evenly on each foot. While the patient does this, observe both sides of her back from neck to buttocks. Look for these signs: uneven shoulder height and shoulder blade prominence, unequal distance between the arms and the body asymmetrical waistline, uneven hip height, a sideways lean. With the patient's back still facing you, ask the patient to do the "forward-bend" test. In this test, the patient places her palms together and feet shoulder-width apart. She slowly bends forward keeping her head down and her hands midline. As she complies, check for these signs: asymmetrical thoracic spine or prominent rib cage (rib hump) on either side asymmetrical waistline. (From *Lippincott's Nursing Advisor 2009.* Philadelphia, PA: Lippincott Williams & Wilkins, 2009.)

Physical Examination of the Spine

Physical examination should include evaluation of the patient while standing and observation from behind to identify:

1. Shoulder asymmetry suggestive of an upper thoracic scoliotic curve
2. Alignment of the head over the pelvis (coronal balance). If off-center, suspect scoliosis, abnormality of the central nervous system (CNS), or muscle disease.
3. Leg-length discrepancy by placing fingers on the iliac crests to better identify asymmetry
4. Adam's forward-bend test—The patient bends forward at the waist with feet shoulder-width apart and hands palm-to-palm in the midline. Prominences along the spine on one or both sides at different levels suggest scoliosis (Fig. 18.5), although abnormalities in chest wall shape or a leg-length discrepancy appear similarly. Importantly, the Adam's forward-bend test should be performed to screen for scoliosis at every well-child check until the adolescent reaches skeletal maturity.
5. ROM of the spine involves not only forward flexion, but also extension, lateral flexion, and rotation.

Examination from the lateral position:

1. Sagittal-plane balance, including relative amount of thoracic kyphosis and lumbar lordosis. Slumped posture and shoulder protraction suggest altered mechanics and poor postural awareness.
2. On forward bending, the normal smooth arc of the spine or presence of a gibbus deformity of Scheuermann kyphosis (Fig. 18.6).

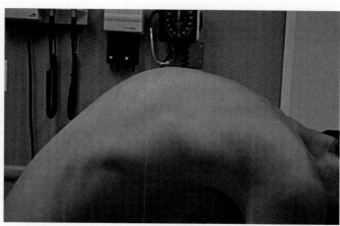

FIGURE 18.6 The more acute (gibbus) angulation of Scheuermann kyphosis seen from the side on Adam's forward-bend test.

Sitting or supine examination:

1. Straight-leg raise: The straight-leg raise may be performed supine or sitting. Raising the leg may elicit symptoms of radiculopathy from a disc protrusion on the involved side.
2. Neuromuscular examination: Evaluation of the patient with spinal complaints requires a thorough neuromuscular examination, assessment of muscle strength, deep tendon reflexes, and sensation over the upper and lower extremities to localize pathology to a specific nerve root level (Table 18.1), cauda equina, or the entire spine (myelopathy).

Additional examination findings to note include the shape of the chest wall (pectus excavatum or carinatum may suggest Marfan syndrome), joint hypermobility and/or hyperextensible skin (Ehler–Danlos), café au lait spots and/or axillary freckling (neurofibromatosis), and appearance of the feet (high arches and hammertoes may be seen in spinal dysraphism or peripheral neuropathy; flat feet accompany Marfan and Ehler–Danlos syndromes).

Low Back Pain Syndromes

Spondylolysis/Spondylolisthesis

Definition:

1. *Spondylolysis* represents a stress fracture through the pars interarticularis of the vertebral body (Fig. 18.7A), most commonly at L5 and with decreasing frequency moving cephalad. Spondylolysis occurs primarily in adolescents.
2. *Spondylolisthesis* occurs when one vertebral body is anteriorly positioned relative to the one below (Fig. 18.7B).
   a. *Isthmic spondylolisthesis* develops in many cases of bilateral spondylolysis as the fractures free the vertebral body from the stabilization that normally occurs posteriorly and will be the only type of spondylolisthesis discussed in the remaining sections. Progression typically occurs prior to skeletal maturity, but patients may develop occult spondylolysis and progression to listhesis that is not detected until young adulthood when pain or other symptoms develop.
   b. Other types include congenital, degenerative, and traumatic.

Etiology:

1. Increased stress on the pars interarticularis due to repetitive hyperextension such as in ballet, gymnastics, figure skating, and playing on the line in football

TABLE 18.1

Neurologic Evaluations of Nerve Root Levels

Nerve Root Level	Sensory	Motor	Reflex
C4	Lateral shoulder/ deltoid		
C5	Lateral elbow	Deltoid (shoulder abduction), biceps	Biceps
C6	Thumb	Wrist extension	Bracioradialis
C7	Middle finger	Wrist flexion/elbow extension	Triceps
C8	Little finger	Finger flexors	
T1	Medial elbow	Interossei (finger abduction)	
T10	Abdomen at level of umbilicus		Abdominal
L2	Anterior thigh	Hip flexion	
L3	Medial knee	Knee extension	Patellar
L4	Medial calf	Ankle dorsiflexion	Patellar
L5	Lateral calf/ dorsum of foot	Great toe extension	
S1	Lateral heel	Ankle plantarflexion	Achilles
S2	Posterior thigh		

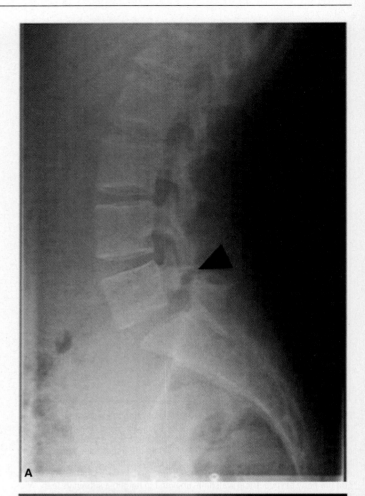

2. Biomechanical factors that may contribute to excess stress include increased lordosis in the lumbar spine; tight hamstrings; and/or Scheuermann kyphosis. These same factors may also contribute to the progression of spondylolysis to spondylolisthesis.

Clinical Manifestations:
1. Insidious onset of pain with activity, but the pain becomes more pervasive when left untreated.
2. On clinical examination, patients demonstrate loss of lumbar lordosis and pain with back extension (**Table 18.2**).
3. Radicular symptoms and findings are rare in spondylolysis and more concerning for higher grades of spondylolisthesis with tethering of the nerve root.
4. Often patients demonstrate tight hamstrings.

Diagnosis:
Initial radiographs should include postero-anterior (PA) and lateral views of the lumbar spine to identify an obvious fracture, evidence of spondylolisthesis, or other diagnoses (destructive lesions, congenital vertebral anomalies). Bilateral oblique films of the lumbar spine have been recommended in the past for cases of suspected spondylolysis with normal AP and lateral radiographs but add little additional information in most cases,[7] so advanced imaging, if available, is preferable.

Advanced imaging is best left to the specialist. Bone scan with single-photon emission computed tomography and CT carry the highest sensitivity, but utilize high radiation doses. MRI possesses lower sensitivity for detection of spondylolysis but may be utilized if there is concern for associated pathology.

Prognosis:
Bilateral spondylolysis rarely heals, but unilateral lesions may undergo bony union.[8] Fibrous nonunion usually provides enough

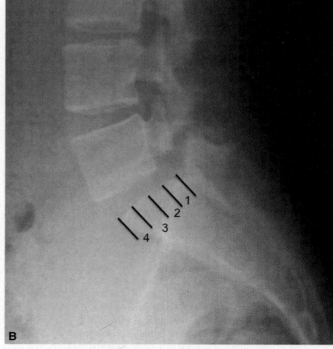

FIGURE 18.7 A: Spondylolysis (arrow) seen on a lateral lumbar x-ray as a lucency in the pars interarticularis of L5. **B:** Spondylolisthesis (same patient). The amount of slip is graded based on how far anteriorly the superior vertebral body has moved on the inferior one. This patient has Grade 1 spondylolisthesis (0% to 25%). Further progression is classified as Grade 2 (26% to 50%), Grade 3 (51% to 75%), and Grade 4 (76% to 100%).

TABLE 18.2

Clinical Findings of Causes of Low Back Pain

	Spondylolysis	Discogenic	Nonspecific/ Muscular
Pain at rest	+/–	+	+/–
Pain with activity	+	+	+/–
Pain on forward bending	–	+	+/–
Pain on backward bending	+	–	+/–
Radiating pain	– (rarely +)	+	–

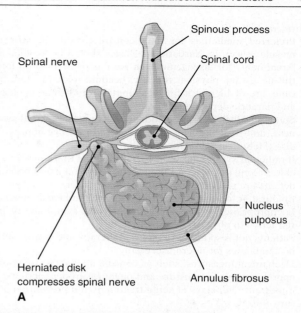

A

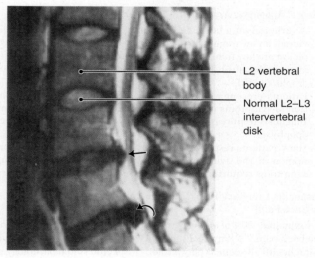

B

FIGURE 18.8 Herniated disk. **A:** The central mass of the disk protrudes into the spinal canal, putting pressure on the spinal nerve. **B:** MRI of the lumbar spine, sagittal section, showing herniated disks at multiple levels. There is a bulging L3–L4 disk (*straight arrow*) and an extruded L4–L5 lumbar disk (*curved arrow*). (From Cohen BJ, DePetris A. *Medical terminology.* 7th ed. Philadelphia, PA: Lippincott Williams & Wilkins, 2013.)

stability to resolve symptoms and prevent progressive listhesis. As a result, advanced imaging to document healing is rarely indicated.

Spondylolisthesis may be measured on radiographs and graded (Fig. 18.7B) to follow progression. Isthmic spondylolisthesis may progress over time, but rarely after skeletal maturity. Progression to a high-grade slip (Grades 3 or 4) is rare (<5% of patients).

Treatment: The goals of treatment are resolution of symptoms and decreasing risk of progression. Most patients with spondylolysis require:

1. *Relative rest,* including restriction from participation in sport and other activity until pain resolves (typically 4 to 6 weeks)
2. Subsequently, a physical therapy program of similar duration to correct functional deficits (e.g., hamstring tightness, unbalanced core strength, and/or postural mechanics)
3. Progressing to return-to-play over a similar span of time
4. *Bracing:* Patients refractory to activity restriction, or who have pain outside of sport, often respond to bracing. Controversy over type and duration of bracing abounds, ranging from elastic lumbar corsets to restrict activity to anti-lordotic lumbosacral orthosis or thoracolumbosacral orthosis (TLSO) to decompress the area(s) of spondylolysis.
5. Surgery may be indicated for pain refractory to nonoperative management, for cases of progressive high-grade spondylolisthesis, fusing the spine at the levels of involvement to stabilize the spine and prevent further progression.

Discogenic Back Pain

Definition:
1. Herniation of the nucleus pulposus (Fig. 18.8A)
2. Mass effect in the neural foramina causes radicular symptoms over the distribution of the nerve root exiting below the level of involvement (e.g., L5-S1 disc herniation typically results in symptoms involving the distribution of S1).

Epidemiology:
Less common in AYAs than in older populations, but prevalence may be increasing.

Clinical Manifestations:
1. Acute onset of back pain.
2. Exacerbation of symptoms with Valsalva/coughing and forward flexion.
3. Positive straight-leg raise (supine or sitting) (Table 18.2).
4. Occasionally, discogenic pain may develop insidiously.
5. The presence of radicular pain requires careful neuromuscular evaluation to identify any deficits.

Diagnosis:
1. Clinical history and examination are usually sufficient for diagnosis.

2. Radiographs are usually negative but may be indicated because spondylolysis can cause similar findings on history and examination.
3. MRI is rarely indicated in the primary care setting.
   a. MRI confirmation is not necessary, since degenerative disc disease and disc bulges on MRI are seen in nearly half of asymptomatic young adults and identification of a herniation does not change treatment[9] (Fig. 18.8B).
   b. MRI should be reserved for those whose back pain fails to improve after 6 weeks of physical therapy to look for other etiologies or to guide more invasive treatment.
   c. MRI is indicated for patients with neurologic deficits. Such patients should be referred to a spine specialist for further management. Some specialists prefer to obtain their own MRIs while others prefer the MRI to be performed prior to consultation.

Treatment:

1. Preferred medicines for pain control include NSAIDs and muscle relaxants. Narcotic analgesics should be avoided as a "treatment" for discogenic back pain as patients often forego the necessary physical therapy, become tolerant, and, over time, are at high risk for development of chronic back pain and narcotic dependence.
2. Spine physical therapy to address mechanics, postural awareness, and institution of other modalities to decompress the disc (McKenzie exercises, traction)
3. If radicular symptoms are present, physical therapy is reasonable as long as there are no deficits noted on examination or deficits are resolving following an acute onset.
4. Epidural or foraminal injection of steroid and local anesthetic is appropriate for patients with radicular symptoms or pain refractory to physical therapy.
5. Patients not responsive to physical therapy and injection may be candidates for microdiscectomy.
6. Mechanical measures, such as corsets, appliances to assist in appropriate sitting posture and ongoing physical activity, are important mainstays of acute treatment and prevention of future episodes.

Vertebral Apophysis Avulsion

1. A variation on a herniated disc in a skeletally immature individual, an awareness of the diagnosis, and a high index of suspicion are key in making the diagnosis of a vertebral apophysis avulsion because the avulsion is rarely visible on plain radiographs or MRI.
2. Patients present with acute onset of back pain and exacerbation of symptoms with Valsalva/coughing and forward flexion.
3. Diagnosis requires CT scan to identify the avulsion of the bony apophysis.
4. Many patients respond well to physical therapy, but callus formation at the avulsion may lead to persistent or worsening symptoms requiring resection of the avulsed apophysis.

Nonspecific Low Back Pain ("Mechanical" or "Muscular" Low Back Pain)

Approximately 20% of adolescents and 40% of young adults experience back pain.[10,11] Physical inactivity, psychosocial stressors, and mental health all seem to play a role.[9-11] Specific spinal pathology is not present, although most patients display features that suggest a muscular component and relationship to altered mechanics.

Clinical Manifestations:

1. Insidious onset of back pain, although occasionally an acute strain can cause more abrupt onset of symptoms.
2. Pain worsens with inactivity, although intermittent activity may worsen pain (Table 18.2).
3. Movement may be slow, but not as limited and antalgic as in an acute disc herniation. Other than mild ROM limitations due to discomfort, neuromuscular examination is unremarkable.
4. Pain often occurs with both spine flexion and extension.
5. Tenderness localizes more to the paraspinous muscles. This is a nonspecific finding given that paraspinous spasm and tenderness also occur in spondylolysis, discogenic pain, and lumbar Scheuermann disease.
6. Patients often have tight hip flexors and hamstrings with increased or decreased lumbar lordosis.[12]

Diagnosis:

Plain radiographs are usually sufficient to evaluate for spondylolysis or other pathologic cause of back pain. Advanced imaging is indicated for those with suspected pathology as discussed in other sections. Since the most likely MRI findings are incidental disc bulges, MRI is reserved for patients with an otherwise normal examination who fail to improve after 6 to 8 weeks of appropriate physical therapy to look for insidious pathologic causes of back pain.

Treatment:

1. Physical therapy should focus on postural awareness, spinal mobility, hamstring, and hip flexor stretching and improving strength and muscular balance throughout the core, including in the gluteal and periscapular muscles. An awareness of mechanical factors contributing to pain onset is important to prevent exacerbations and persistent symptoms.
2. Narcotic analgesics should never be used for muscular back pain. NSAIDs are helpful in relieving acute flares, but prolonged use should be discouraged due to potential renal and gastrointestinal side effects.
3. Elastic lumbar corset bracing may provide temporary relief and improve postural mechanics while awaiting physical therapy.
4. Some patients with chronic low back pain may benefit from cognitive behavioral therapy.

Spinal Deformities
Scoliosis

Definition:

1. A spinal curve of >10 degrees in the coronal plane as measured by the Cobb angle (Fig. 18.9A) on a full-length PA radiograph
2. Adolescent idiopathic scoliosis (AIS) occurs in patients >10 years old. AIS is the most common form of scoliosis and will be the focus of this section.
3. Scoliosis may involve the thoracic spine, lumbar spine, or both. Scoliotic curves do not resolve and will remain present throughout one's life.
4. Curves <10 degrees are more appropriately called "spinal asymmetry" and represent variations in postural alignment that frequently resolve, whereas true scoliosis persists into adulthood.
5. Curve onset prior to 10 years old is considered "early-onset" scoliosis and carries a high risk of progression. A history of early-onset scoliosis in an adolescent presenting with spinal or lower-extremity complaints warrants attention because of higher rates of underlying conditions such as CNS disease, genetic syndrome, or neuromuscular disorder. The clinician should consider additional consultation and/or spine MRI.
6. Congenital scoliosis involves vertebral body malformations and defects of segmentation, such as hemivertebrae and/or bars (Fig. 18.10). Congenital scoliosis is often diagnosed incidentally on radiographs performed for other reasons. Congenital scoliotic curves often progress during child and adolescent growth and require annual monitoring.
   a. Vertebral malformations and spinal dysraphism frequently occur together, so advanced spinal imaging with MRI may be indicated.[13]
   b. Association with malformation of other systems (as seen in VATER/VACTERL) should prompt the clinician to consider evaluating for other anomalies with cardiac Echo and renal ultrasound.
   c. Treatment for progressive curves involves surgical fusion or excision of the abnormal vertebral segment(s).

Etiology:

The cause of AIS is likely multifactorial. Genetics seem to play a role as the risk of scoliosis is higher in first-degree relatives. Suspected causative factors include muscle, connective tissue, and bone disorders, as well as minor abnormalities of the CNS and hormone expression.

AIS actually represents a three-dimensional deformity of the spine, rather than the simple "side-to-side" curve as appears on radiographs. One theory of progression implicates asymmetric vertebral body growth resulting in rotation of the spine, such that the sagittal kyphosis and lordosis develop a coronal-plane orientation, to maintain overall postural alignment.

Epidemiology:

AIS occurs in 1% to 3% of adolescents, at similar rates in males and females.

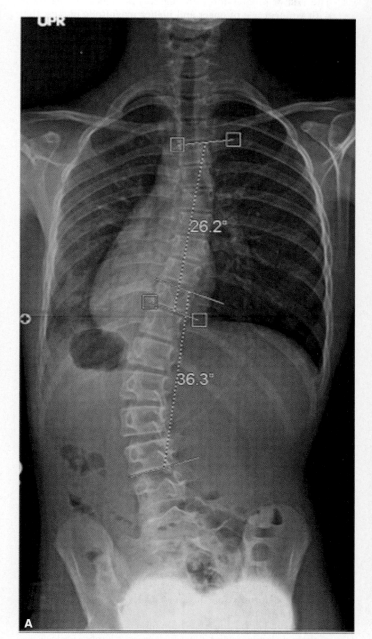
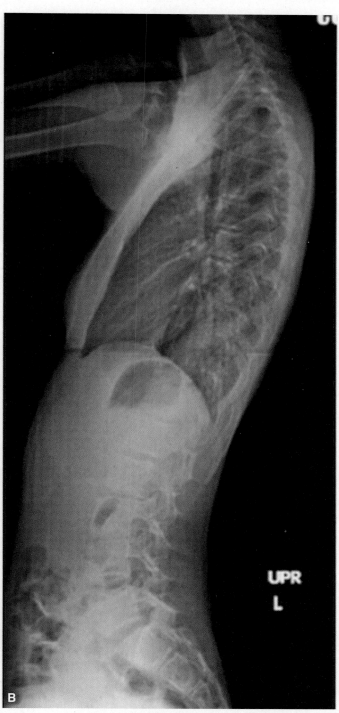

FIGURE 18.9 For patients with concerns regarding spinal alignment, including scoliosis and kyphosis, full-length spinal x-rays should be obtained. **A:** The PA view identifies scoliosis and allows measurement of the angulation of the curves using the Cobb method (lines). **B:** The lateral view visualizes the sagittal alignment that should include thoracic kyphosis and lumbar lordosis, both of which are decreased in this patient with scoliosis.

Clinical Manifestations:
1. Patients may present with concerns regarding an asymmetric appearance to the shoulders or hips/waist, or be identified on Adam's forward-bend screening tests at schools and well-child checks.
2. Rotation of the spine results in the characteristic rib hump of scoliosis seen on Adam's forward-bend test that may become more prominent as progression occurs (Fig. 18.5), although obesity frequently masks detection. An inclinometer more

precisely measures trunk rotation and assists in following progression if radiographs are not used; referral should occur at 5 to 7 degrees of trunk rotation.[14]
3. Leg-length discrepancies result in a tilted pelvis, so the spine bends to correct the patient's alignment (Fig. 18.11). Unlike true structural scoliosis, curves related to leg-length discrepancies do not involve rotation and resolve when the patient's leg-length difference is corrected by having them sit or by placing a block or lift of appropriate height under the shorter

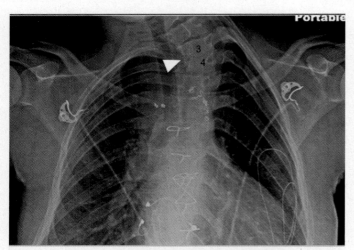

FIGURE 18.10 Congenital scoliosis due to right-sided fusion (*arrowhead*) of T3 and T4, noted incidentally on a chest x-ray. Notice the sternotomy wires indicative of cardiac surgery, reinforcing the association between vertebral anomalies and congenital heart disease.

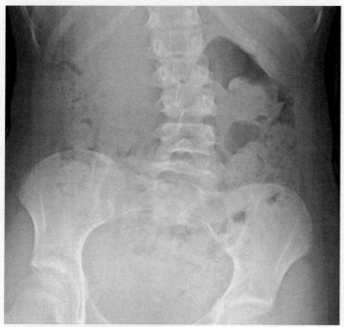

FIGURE 18.11 A leg-length difference resulting in a compensatory curve of the lumbar spine.

leg. Note that some patients have scoliosis and a leg-length discrepancy.
4. Right-sided and double curves are common.
5. Left-sided thoracic curves are "atypical" and carry a higher association with Chiari malformation and syringomyelia.[15]

Diagnosis:
1. Radiographs confirm and characterize scoliosis.
   a. Appropriate imaging of a patient with clinically significant scoliosis includes both PA and lateral images obtained on a 36-inch cassette while the patient is standing so that the entire spine is imaged in continuity and overall balance may be assessed in both planes (Fig. 18.9A and B).
   b. If the patient cannot stand, then images may be performed while sitting.

2. Advanced imaging is only indicated if there is concern for spinal dysraphism, tumor, or another etiology of the curve; for evaluation of causes of back pain; or for surgical planning.

Prognosis:
1. The risk of progression (>5 degrees) is higher among those with younger age of onset and higher magnitude curves, that is, during adolescence.
2. Progression after skeletal maturity is rare for smaller curves, but curves >50 degrees after skeletal maturity often progress slowly, starting in young adulthood.
3. Cardiorespiratory symptoms develop around 80 degrees, but many adults do well despite seemingly significant curves.[16]
4. Patients with scoliosis occasionally experience achy back discomfort, but scoliosis should not be considered a cause of more significant pain. Pathologic etiologies of back pain occur in patients with scoliosis, so appropriate evaluation should be performed as in any patient with back pain.

Treatment:
1. Many adolescents require no treatment, as the ultimate goal of treatment is to prevent progression to a symptomatic magnitude. Young adults with scoliosis do not require treatment unless their curves progress over time.
2. Bracing utilizing a rigid TLSO (Fig. 18.12A) decreases the risk of progression to surgery in children with progressive curves that reach 20 to 25 degrees and who still possess a significant amount of remaining growth.[17] Greatest success occurs with brace-wear exceeding 12 to 16 hours/day, allowing for removal during activity. Bracing is discontinued as the patient approaches skeletal maturity.
3. Research on other nonsurgical interventions is insufficient to support widespread recommendations at this time.
4. Surgery is reserved for skeletally immature patients with curves over 40 to 50 degrees or progressive curves in AYAs who are skeletally mature. Surgery involves spinal fusion, utilizing internal hardware to correct the curve and maintain alignment while fusion occurs (Fig. 18.2B). Following surgery, most patients have few activity limitations after 6 months, once the spine completely fuses. Complications of surgery include blood loss and spinal cord injury. Removal of hardware is rare, typically occurring only if there is prominence that causes pain due to irritation. Minimally invasive surgery is being explored at certain centers as a means to control growth of the spine and decrease curve magnitudes without utilizing fusion.

Scheuermann Disease

Definition
1. A deformity of the spine in the sagittal plane with increased thoracic kyphosis or decreased lumbar lordosis accompanied by deformity of the vertebral bodies and endplates (Fig. 18.13A and B)
2. In the sagittal plane, the spine normally contains 25 to 45 degrees of thoracic kyphosis and 30 to 70 degrees of lumbar lordosis.
3. Schmorl's nodes, a characteristic radiographic abnormality, represent eruptions of the intervertebral discs through the endplates (Fig. 18.13C).
4. Scheuermann kyphosis typically refers to deformity of the thoracic spine.
5. "Lumbar" or "atypical" Scheuermann disease occurs in the lumbar spine.

Etiology
The etiology of Scheuermann disease is unknown, but genetic and structural disorders, as in scoliosis, have been proposed.

Epidemiology
Scheuermann disease develops primarily in the peripubertal period. Reported prevalence rates vary, but appear to be similar to scoliosis at

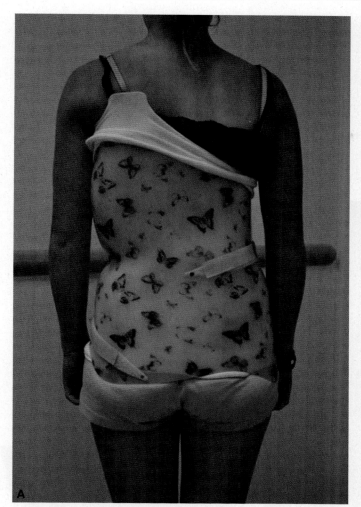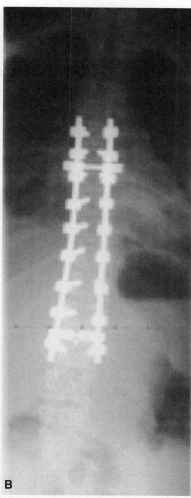

FIGURE 18.12 A: A thoracolumbosacral orthosis (TLSO) worn by a patient with AIS to improve alignment and decrease risk of curve progression. **B:** For curves >50 degrees in skeletally immature patients, spinal fusion is used to correct the curve and prevent further progression. Internal hardware (*white lines*) is used to de-rotate and then stabilize the spine while awaiting bony fusion following surgery.

1% to 3%. Scheuermann disease can occur concomitantly with scoliosis. Most patients are identified during late adolescence or early young adulthood.

Clinical Manifestations
Scheuermann kyphosis must be differentiated from poor posture.

1. Typical "poor posture" presents with protracted (rounded) shoulders, increased thoracic kyphosis, and/or flattened lower back with loss of lumbar lordosis. These kyphotic curves retain flexibility and resolve once the patient lies down.
2. Scheuermann kyphosis appears more severe and the kyphosis persists in the supine position. On forward bending, the spine displays an acute angulation when viewed from the side rather than the normal smooth curve (Fig. 18.6).
3. Scheuermann disease of the lumbar spine differs in that patients have loss of normal lumbar lordosis (and thus could be considered to be "relatively kyphotic") with flattening of the lower back and decreased ROM on back extension.
4. Pain occurs commonly in Scheuermann disease, usually during development of the endplate abnormalities and progression of the disorder. The pain is more severe when there is lumbar or thoracolumbar involvement.

Diagnosis
1. PA and lateral radiographs including the entire spine should be performed on 36-inch cassettes.
2. Radiographic criteria for thoracic Scheuermann kyphosis include kyphosis >45 degrees with the presence of three consecutive vertebral bodies with at least 5 degrees of anterior wedging (Fig. 18.13A). Abnormalities of the vertebral body endplates, Schmorl's nodes, and narrowing of the disc spaces may also be evident (Fig. 18.13A–C).
3. Lumbar Scheuermann disease is also characterized by abnormalities at the disc and vertebral endplates, including Schmorl's nodes. Instead of a kyphotic appearance, the lumbar spine displays loss of lordosis with a more vertical orientation of the vertebral bodies (Fig. 18.13B). Vertebral body wedging is rare other than at the first or second lumbar vertebrae when the kyphosis is situated at the thoracolumbar junction.

Prognosis
Scheuermann disease, like scoliosis, typically progresses during skeletal growth, requiring regular radiographic monitoring. The risk of progression during adulthood remains unknown. Kyphosis of the thoracic spine rarely results in cardiorespiratory compromise (unlike scoliosis), but obvious effects on posture may contribute to

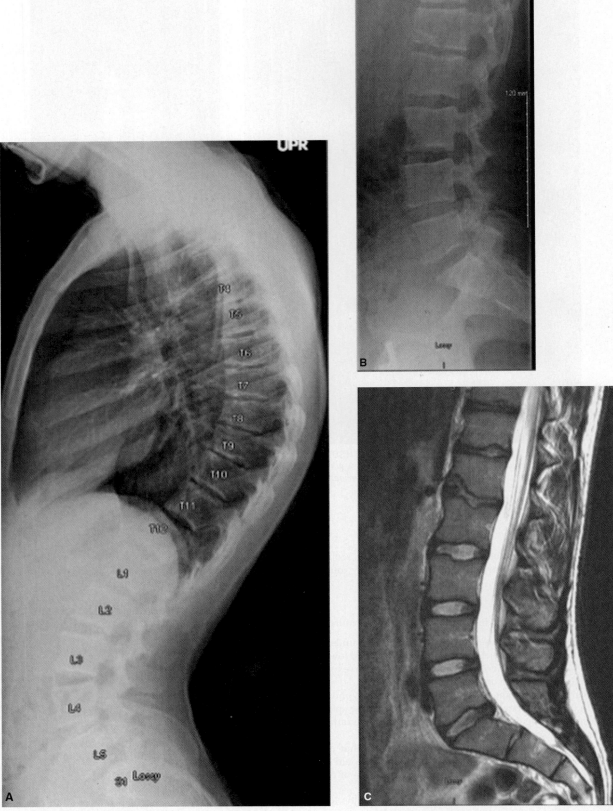

FIGURE 18.13 A: Thoracic Scheuermann kyphosis, with wedging of the vertebral bodies, irregularities of the endplates (top and bottom) of the wedged vertebral bodies, and narrowing of the disc spaces. **B:** Lumbar Scheuermann disease demonstrating loss of lumbar lordosis and Schmorl nodes. **C:** Schmorl nodes, as seen on MRI, represent eruptions of the disc through the endplate of the vertebral body (B and C are from the same patient as in Figure 18.6).

the development of neck pain. Pain can persist after skeletal maturity due to muscular dysfunction related to the decreased ROM at involved levels.

Treatment

1. Physical therapy targeting postural awareness, core strength, spinal mobility, and overall muscular balance assists in pain relief but does not improve the degree of kyphosis.
2. Bracing does slow progression of thoracic kyphosis, requiring a relatively flexible curve. Bracing is initiated once curves exceed 55 degrees, although many patients refuse bracing because it may require a high anterior extension up the chest or to the chin.
3. Surgery includes correction of the hyperkyphosis and fusion. Surgery is reserved for patients with pain not amenable to physical therapy and/or kyphosis >80 degrees.
4. Lumbar Scheuermann disease rarely requires bracing or surgery. Physical therapy is the mainstay of treatment.

OTHER CAUSES OF MUSCULOSKELETAL PAIN

Bone Tumors

While malignancy can occur among AYAs, it is important to remember that it is rare. A thorough history and physical examination will raise suspicion. Radiographic imaging and laboratory analysis usually result in appropriate diagnosis.

Clinical Manifestations

Tumors present with pain or as a painless mass. When present, pain is often worse at night. Tumors that are near or that involve the spine cause abnormalities in posture and mobility.

Nonmetastatic Neoplasms: **Osteoid osteoma** commonly presents in the diaphysis of long bones and the spine. Pain usually worsens at night and is relieved by NSAIDs. In long bones, callus formation with sclerosis around a central lucency is seen on x-ray. In the spine, radiographs are usually negative.

Histiocytosis (eosinophilic granuloma) is a locally aggressive lesion that can be multifocal, but without metastasis, and is the most common cause of vertebral body collapse (vertebra plana) from tumor infiltration.

Malignant Neoplasms: The most common malignancies among AYAs include leukemia and lymphoma, Ewing sarcoma, and osteosarcoma. The peak incidence for leukemia and Ewing sarcoma is in childhood and adolescence while that of osteosarcoma is during adolescence and young adulthood. While bone pain from leukemia may be generalized, other tumors usually present with focal symptoms. Pain is progressive, usually at rest and often with nighttime awakening.

Infection

1. *Osteomyelitis* occurs primarily through hematogenous spread in skeletally immature children, but direct infection is more common after skeletal maturity. Patients may present only with pain, although osteomyelitis can occur simultaneously with septic arthritis.
2. *Septic arthritis* occurs at all ages, but gonococcal arthritis should be considered in sexually active AYAs. Diagnosis should be suspected in patients with pain in which there is redness and warmth and refusal to move the joint, although only the latter may be present when the hip is involved.
3. Discitis presents as severe back pain while pyomyositis presents as acute, severe, atraumatic pain occurring almost anywhere, but frequently around the pelvis.

Diagnosis

1. Radiographs should be obtained to identify other causes of pain but rarely show any abnormalities in infection except in advanced cases. Because the diagnosis of discitis is often

delayed, radiographs frequently demonstrate loss of disc space height.
2. Complete blood count (CBC) typically reveals an elevated white blood cell count (WBC) with a prevalence of neutrophils.
3. C-reactive protein is elevated in the first 3 to 5 days of onset, followed by an elevation in erythrocyte sedimentation rate (ESR), usually >40 mm/hour.
4. Blood culture should be performed in all suspected cases of infection.
5. Joint aspiration is crucial for diagnosis in cases of a swollen joint as synovial fluid WBC >50,000/mm^3 indicates likely infection and culture often reveals a causative organism. The WBC count of synovial fluid in inflammatory arthritis and Lyme disease is usually <50,000/mm^3.
6. MRI with and without contrast assists in diagnosis of osteomyelitis and pyomyositis; however, septic, inflammatory, and traumatic arthritis all appear similar on MRI.
7. Lyme disease should be considered in endemic areas, and positive screening tests should be confirmed with Western blot testing.

Treatment

1. Osteomyelitis and discitis usually require only antibiotics (intravenous, followed by oral). Surgery is reserved for abscesses, infection causing mass effect, or infection that is refractory to antibiotics.
2. Pyomyositis and septic arthritis require surgical irrigation and debridement in addition to antibiotic treatment; equivocal cases of septic arthritis based on joint aspiration often undergo surgical irrigation to avoid the potential catastrophic sequelae of osteonecrosis related to untreated infection.

Inflammatory Arthropathies

1. Diagnosis requires >6 weeks of symptoms and no other apparent causes. Fever or fatigue may be present.
2. Patients experience stiffness more than pain, and warm, swollen joints are evident in the appendicular skeleton. Involvement of the sacroiliac joints of the pelvis or spine (spondyloarthropathy) is harder to diagnosis, but can occur in combination with inflammatory bowel disease.
3. Radiographic changes usually do not occur except in advanced disease.
4. Laboratory evaluation is indicated in the assessment of swollen joints to look for signs of infection.
   a. A CBC should be normal. ESR may be normal or elevated.
   b. Antinuclear antibody, cyclic-citrullinated peptide, and rheumatoid factor testing is not helpful in the diagnosis of juvenile idiopathic arthritis and should not be routinely obtained.[18]
   c. Human leukocyte antigen B27 may be useful in cases of suspected spondyloarthropathy but may also be present in asymptomatic individuals.
5. MRI with and without intravenous contrast usually confirms synovitis or sacroiliitis.
6. Treatment usually requires use of disease-modifying antirheumatic drugs and/or intra-articular steroid injection.
7. Physical therapy assists in recovery of muscle dysfunction associated with abnormal mechanics.

REFERENCES

1. Steill IG, Greenberg GH, McKnight RD, et al. The "real" Ottawa ankle rules. *Ann Emerg Med* 1996;27:103.
2. Steill IG, Greenberg GH, Wells GA, et al. Prospective validation of a decision rule for the use of radiography in acute knee injuries. *JAMA* 1996;275:611.
3. Sankar WN, Vanderhave KL, Matheney T, et al. The modified Dunn procedure for unstable slipped capital epiphysis: a multicenter perspective. *J Bone Joint Surg Am* 2013;95(70):585–591.
4. Blankenbaker DG, De Smet AA, Keene JS. Sonography of the iliopsoas tendon and injection of the iliopsoas bursa for diagnosis and management of the painful snapping hip. *Skeletal Radiol* 2006;35(8):565–571.

5. Clohisy JC, Baca G, Beaulé PE, et al. Descriptive epidemiology of femoroacetabular impingement: a North American cohort of patients undergoing surgery. *Am J Sports Med* 2013;41(6):1348–1356.

6. Sutter R, Zubler V, Hoffman A, et al. Hip MRI: how useful is intraarticular contrast material for evaluating surgically proven lesion of the labrum and articular cartilage? *Am J Roentgenol* 2014;201(1):160–169.

7. Beck NA, Miller R, Baldwin K, et al. Do oblique views add value in the diagnosis of spondylolysis in adolescents? *J Bone Joint Surg Am* 2013;95(10):e65.

8. Miller SF, Congeni J, Swanson K. Long-term functional and anatomical follow-up of early detected spondylolysis in young athletes. *Am J Sports Med* 2004;32(4):928–933.

9. Takatalo J, Karppinen J, Niinaimäki J, et al. Prevalence of degenerative imaging findings in lumbar magnetic resonance imaging among young adults. *Spine* 2009;34(16):1716–1721.

10. Masiero S, Carraro E, Celia A, et al. Prevalence of nonspecific low back pain in schoolchildren aged between 13 and 15 years. *Acta Paediatr* 2008;97(2):212–216.

11. Gilkey DP, Keefe TJ, Peel JL, et al. Risk factors associated with back pain: a cross-sectional study of 963 college students. *J Manipulative Physiol Ther* 2010;33(2):88–95.

12. Handrakis JP, Friel K, Hoeffner F, et al. Key characteristics of low back pain and disability in college-aged adults: a pilot study. *Arch Phys Med Rehabil* 2012;93(7):1217–1224.

13. Basu PS, Elsebaie H, Noordeen MHH. Congenital spinal deformity—a comprehensive assessment at presentation. *Spine* 2002;27(20):2255–2259.

14. Labelle H, Richards SB, De Kleuver M, et al. Screening for adolescent idiopathic scoliosis: an information statement by the Scoliosis Research Society International Task Force. *Scoliosis* 2013;8(1):17.

15. Spiegel DA, Flynn JM, Stasikelis PJ, et al. Scoliotic curve patterns in patients with Chiari I malformation and/or syringomyelia. *Spine* 2003;28(18):2139–2146.

16. Weinstein SL, Dolan LA, Spratt KF, et al. Health and function of patients with untreated idiopathic scoliosis: a 50-year natural history study. *JAMA* 2003;289(5):559–567.

17. Weinstein SL, Dolan LA, Wright JG, et al. Effects of bracing in adolescents with idiopathic scoliosis. *N Engl J Med* 2013;369(16):1512–1521.

18. Wong KO, Bond K, Homik J, et al. *Antinuclear antibody, rheumatoid factor and cyclic-citrullinated peptide tests for evaluating musculoskeletal complaints in children. Comparative Effectiveness Review No. 50* [Prepared by the University of Alberta Evidence-based Practice Center under Contract No. HHSA 290 2007 10021 I]. AHRQ Publication No. 12-EHC015-EF. Rockville, MD: Agency for Healthcare Research and Quality, 2012. Available at Effectivehealthcare.ahrq.gov/reports/final.cfm. Accessed March 3, 2014.

🛜 **ADDITIONAL RESOURCES AND WEBSITES ONLINE**

Guidelines for Promoting Physical Activity and Sports Participation

Keith J. Loud

WHY PROMOTE ATHLETIC ACTIVITY?

As noted by the US government's Healthy People 2020 initiative (www.healthypeople.gov), physical activity in adolescence and young adulthood can:

- Improve bone health
- Improve cardiorespiratory and muscular fitness
- Decrease levels of body fat
- Reduce symptoms of depression

In adults, physical activity can decrease the risk of the following:

- Early death
- Coronary heart disease
- Stroke
- High blood pressure
- Type 2 diabetes
- Breast and colon cancer
- Falls
- Depression

Moreover, adolescent boys participating in team sports have lower rates of overweight and obesity,[1] and adolescent girls participating in team sports have lower rates of pregnancy and greater self-esteem than peers who do not participate in team sports.[2]

All health care professionals caring for adolescents and young adults (AYAs) should therefore be prepared to promote safe physical activity and/or sports participation ("athletics") for all youth by:

- Assessing the risks associated with athletic participation for individual AYAs
- Prescribing exercise and advising on sports participation to improve fitness while minimizing athletic injury and illness

WHY DO WE NEED TO GUIDE ATHLETIC ACTIVITIES?

Despite its benefits, athletic activity entails both perceived risks, such as concerns over stunting growth, and real risk of injury, including death and disability.

Maturational Issues

It has been suggested that adolescents should not play contact sports before midpuberty and that adolescents playing contact sports should be segregated based on early, middle, or late puberty to reduce the risk of injury; however, there are no data to show that these interventions decrease injury rates. Injury rates increase with pubertal maturation. In contact sports (Table 19.1), this finding is consistent with the understanding that injury is related to the force of impact, which increases with the speed and body mass of the athletes involved. For noncontact sports, this finding may reflect greater force generation related to greater body mass and greater fat-free mass, as well as the increase in training intensity that tends to occur with the age-associated increase in level of competition.

Another concern is that adult stature could be compromised by excessive sports activities and exercise in the prepubertal and pubertal years, as suggested by the finding of short stature among adolescent gymnasts. However, there is a significant confounder in that the short stature in gymnastics may be related to selection bias rather than intense training. The argument for selection bias is strengthened by the observation that runners, figure skaters, and ballet dancers may train as hard as gymnasts without adverse effects on adult stature, timing of peak height, or rate of growth.

Morbidity and Mortality

Although football has been associated with a high incidence of injuries, the number of injury events resulting in permanent disability or death has been on the decline since the 1970s. While football is still associated with the greatest number of catastrophic injuries among all sports, the incidence of injury per 100,000 high school participants is higher for both gymnastics and ice hockey. A full report is available at the Web site for the National Center for Catastrophic Sports Injury Research (http://nccsir.unc.edu/). This site includes the breakdown of injuries and fatalities stratified by high school and college and by type of sport and by year. For the 1982 to 1983 through 2011 to 2012 seasons, the high school sports with the highest incidence of fatalities from direct injuries per 100,000 participants were gymnastics for males and cheerleading for females. Nonfatal injuries were also similar in regard to the common sports involved.

Catastrophic injuries to female athletes have increased over the years from one in 1982 to 1983 to an average of 8.7/year in the last 30 years. A major factor in this increase has been the change in cheerleading which increasingly involves gymnastic stunts. Cheerleading now accounts for 63.3% of all catastrophic injuries to female high school athletes and 71.2% of catastrophic injuries to females at the college level.

TABLE 19.1

Classification of Sports by Contact

Contact or Collision	Limited Contact	Noncontact
Basketball	Adventure racing[a]	Badminton
Boxing[b]	Baseball	Bodybuilding[c]
Cheerleading	Bicycling	Bowling
Diving	Canoeing or kayaking	Canoeing or kayaking
Extreme sports[d]	(white water)	(flat water)
Field hockey	Fencing	Crew or rowing
Football, tackle	Field events	Curling
Gymnastics	High jump	Dance
Ice hockey[e]	Pole vault	Field events
Lacrosse	Floor hockey	Discus
Martial arts[f]	Football, flag or touch	Javelin
Rodeo	Handball	Shot-put
Rugby	Horseback riding	Golf
Skiing, downhill	Martial arts[f]	Orienteering[g]
Ski jumping	Racquetball	Power lifting[c]
Snowboarding	Skating	Race walking
Soccer	Ice	Riflery
Team handball	In-line	Rope jumping
Ultimate Frisbee	Roller	Running
Water polo	Skiing	Sailing
Wrestling	Cross-country	Scuba diving
	Water	Swimming
	Skateboarding	Table tennis
	Softball	Tennis
	Squash	Track
	Volleyball	
	Weight lifting	
	Windsurfing or surfing	

[a]Adventure racing has been added since the previous statement was published and is defined as a combination of 2 or more disciplines, including orienteering and navigation, cross-country running, mountain biking, paddling, and climbing and rope skills.
[b]The American Academy of Pediatrics opposes participation in boxing for children, adolescents, and young adults.
[c]The American Academy of Pediatrics recommends limiting bodybuilding and power lifting until the adolescent achieves sexual maturity rating 5.
[d]Extreme sports has been added since the previous statement was published.
[e]The American Academy of Pediatrics recommends limiting the amount of body checking allowed for hockey players 15 years and younger, to reduce injuries.
[f]Martial arts can be subclassified as judo, jujitsu, karate, kung fu, and tae kwon do; some forms are contact sports, and others are limited-contact sports.
[g]Orienteering is a race (contest) in which competitors use a map and a compass to find their way through unfamiliar territory.
From Committee on Sports Medicine and Fitness. Medical conditions affecting sports participation. *Pediatrics* 2008;121:841–848, with permission.

Overuse Injuries

Repetitive strain, or overuse, injuries are far more common than catastrophic or acute traumatic injuries in AYAs; however, the true burden of injury is unknown, given a lack of robust epidemiologic surveillance systems in high school, youth, and recreational sports. A 2011 consensus panel report identified the sheer volume of repetitive use—measured as distance traveled in running or swimming, number of overhead pitches thrown, or time participating in physical activities—as the most consistent risk factor for athletic injury among AYAs.[3] The report stressed the importance of preparticipation physical evaluation (PPE) to screen for conditions that may predispose to injury or illness and called for more research and better surveillance systems.

HOW TO PROMOTE SAFE ATHLETIC PARTICIPATION

The consensus monograph entitled *The Preparticipation Physical Evaluation, 4th Edition*, also known as "The Monograph," is a collaboration of six leading medical societies[4]:

- American Academy of Family Physicians (AAFP)
- American Academy of Pediatrics (AAP)

- American College of Sports Medicine (ACSM)
- American Medical Society for Sports Medicine (ASSM)
- American Orthopaedic Society for Sports Medicine (AOSSM)
- American Osteopathic Academy of Sports Medicine (AOASM)

The Monograph is the definitive guide for physicians and other health professionals who evaluate athletes before training or competition—an essential tool for promoting the health and safety of athletes. *The Monograph* provides the medical background for decisions by the individual athlete's physician or the team physician. As of the second edition in 1997, it specifically includes the American Heart Association's (AHA's) recommendations concerning cardiovascular screening.

Objectives and Components of the PPE

The primary objectives of the PPE, as stated in *The Monograph*, include the following[4]:

- Screening for conditions that may be life-threatening or disabling
- Screening for conditions that may predispose to injury or illness

Because the PPE may "serve as an entry point to the health care system for adolescents," and may also do so for some young adults, the objectives listed in the fourth edition also include determining general health and providing opportunity to initiate discussion on health-related topics. The inclusion of these objectives acknowledges and emphasizes the central role of the adolescent primary care provider (PCP) in the PPE.

The AAP and Maternal and Child Health Bureau's *Bright Futures* Guidelines for Health Promotion (www.brightfutures.org) recommend a comprehensive health evaluation at least yearly during adolescence. Ideally, an adolescent athlete would have an annual comprehensive health evaluation performed by his or her PCP, with additional sport-specific PPEs performed by a team physician who is responsive to the sponsoring athletic body and knowledgeable about the sport in question. In reality, *The Monograph* acknowledges that the PPE, which is performed primarily to meet legal requirements in 49 of 50 states, is often the only interaction that many adolescents (particularly male adolescents) have with the health care system. Therefore, it is recommended that the PPE be incorporated into a more general health maintenance visit with an established PCP. A multi-examiner, private station-based setup is a less desirable, but acceptable alternative. Mass screenings in large rooms such as gymnasiums are no longer considered appropriate. Details of how to structure a PPE outside the office setting can be found in *The Monograph*; the remainder of this section highlights the important elements of a history and physical examination to be performed for a PPE within a health maintenance visit. Chapter 5 details the other components of a thorough health maintenance evaluation.

History—Screening for Conditions That May Be Life-Threatening or Disabling

A medical history form from *The Monograph* is shown in Figure 19.1. A partnership between the athlete and the parent in completing the form is strongly recommended. The PPE form incorporates the AHA's recommended questions for cardiovascular screening:

1. Family history of premature death (sudden or otherwise).
2. Family history of heart disease in surviving relatives; significant disability from cardiovascular disease in close relatives younger than 50 years; or specific knowledge of the occurrence of certain conditions (hypertrophic cardiomyopathy [HCM], long-QT syndrome, Marfan syndrome, or clinically important arrhythmias).
3. Personal history of heart murmur.
4. Personal history of systemic hypertension.
5. Personal history of excessive fatigability.
6. Personal history of syncope, excessive or progressive shortness of breath, or chest pain or discomfort, particularly with exertion.

■ PREPARTICIPATION PHYSICAL EVALUATION
HISTORY FORM

(Note: This form is to be filled out by the patient and parent prior to seeing the physician. The physician should keep this form in the chart.)

Date of Exam _____

Name _____   Date of birth _____

Sex _____ Age _____ Grade _____ School _____ Sport(s) _____

Medicines and Allergies: Please list all of the prescription and over-the-counter medicines and supplements (herbal and nutritional) that you are currently taking

_____

_____

_____

Do you have any allergies?   ☐ Yes   ☐ No   If yes, please identify specific allergy below.
☐ Medicines   ☐ Pollens   ☐ Food   ☐ Stinging Insects

Explain "Yes" answers below. Circle questions you don't know the answers to.

GENERAL QUESTIONS	Yes	No
1. Has a doctor ever denied or restricted your participation in sports for any reason?		
2. Do you have any ongoing medical conditions? If so, please identify below: ☐ Asthma ☐ Anemia ☐ Diabetes ☐ Infections Other: _____		
3. Have you ever spent the night in the hospital?		
4. Have you ever had surgery?		

HEART HEALTH QUESTIONS ABOUT YOU	Yes	No
5. Have you ever passed out or nearly passed out DURING or AFTER exercise?		
6. Have you ever had discomfort, pain, tightness, or pressure in your chest during exercise?		
7. Does your heart ever race or skip beats (irregular beats) during exercise?		
8. Has a doctor ever told you that you have any heart problems? If so, check all that apply: ☐ High blood pressure ☐ A heart murmur ☐ High cholesterol ☐ A heart infection ☐ Kawasaki disease Other: _____		
9. Has a doctor ever ordered a test for your heart? (For example, ECG/EKG, echocardiogram)		
10. Do you get lightheaded or feel more short of breath than expected during exercise?		
11. Have you ever had an unexplained seizure?		
12. Do you get more tired or short of breath more quickly than your friends during exercise?		

HEART HEALTH QUESTIONS ABOUT YOUR FAMILY	Yes	No
13. Has any family member or relative died of heart problems or had an unexpected or unexplained sudden death before age 50 (including drowning, unexplained car accident, or sudden infant death syndrome)?		
14. Does anyone in your family have hypertrophic cardiomyopathy, Marfan syndrome, arrhythmogenic right ventricular cardiomyopathy, long QT syndrome, short QT syndrome, Brugada syndrome, or catecholaminergic polymorphic ventricular tachycardia?		
15. Does anyone in your family have a heart problem, pacemaker, or implanted defibrillator?		
16. Has anyone in your family had unexplained fainting, unexplained seizures, or near drowning?		

BONE AND JOINT QUESTIONS	Yes	No
17. Have you ever had an injury to a bone, muscle, ligament, or tendon that caused you to miss a practice or a game?		
18. Have you ever had any broken or fractured bones or dislocated joints?		
19. Have you ever had an injury that required x-rays, MRI, CT scan, injections, therapy, a brace, a cast, or crutches?		
20. Have you ever had a stress fracture?		
21. Have you ever been told that you have or have you had an x-ray for neck instability or atlantoaxial instability? (Down syndrome or dwarfism)		
22. Do you regularly use a brace, orthotics, or other assistive device?		
23. Do you have a bone, muscle, or joint injury that bothers you?		
24. Do any of your joints become painful, swollen, feel warm, or look red?		
25. Do you have any history of juvenile arthritis or connective tissue disease?		

MEDICAL QUESTIONS	Yes	No
26. Do you cough, wheeze, or have difficulty breathing during or after exercise?		
27. Have you ever used an inhaler or taken asthma medicine?		
28. Is there anyone in your family who has asthma?		
29. Were you born without or are you missing a kidney, an eye, a testicle (males), your spleen, or any other organ?		
30. Do you have groin pain or a painful bulge or hernia in the groin area?		
31. Have you had infectious mononucleosis (mono) within the last month?		
32. Do you have any rashes, pressure sores, or other skin problems?		
33. Have you had a herpes or MRSA skin infection?		
34. Have you ever had a head injury or concussion?		
35. Have you ever had a hit or blow to the head that caused confusion, prolonged headache, or memory problems?		
36. Do you have a history of seizure disorder?		
37. Do you have headaches with exercise?		
38. Have you ever had numbness, tingling, or weakness in your arms or legs after being hit or falling?		
39. Have you ever been unable to move your arms or legs after being hit or falling?		
40. Have you ever become ill while exercising in the heat?		
41. Do you get frequent muscle cramps when exercising?		
42. Do you or someone in your family have sickle cell trait or disease?		
43. Have you had any problems with your eyes or vision?		
44. Have you had any eye injuries?		
45. Do you wear glasses or contact lenses?		
46. Do you wear protective eyewear, such as goggles or a face shield?		
47. Do you worry about your weight?		
48. Are you trying to or has anyone recommended that you gain or lose weight?		
49. Are you on a special diet or do you avoid certain types of foods?		
50. Have you ever had an eating disorder?		
51. Do you have any concerns that you would like to discuss with a doctor?		
FEMALES ONLY		
52. Have you ever had a menstrual period?		
53. How old were you when you had your first menstrual period?		
54. How many periods have you had in the last 12 months?		

Explain "yes" answers here

_____

_____

_____

_____

_____

_____

_____

_____

I hereby state that, to the best of my knowledge, my answers to the above questions are complete and correct.

Signature of athlete _____ Signature of parent/guardian _____ Date _____

©2010 American Academy of Family Physicians, American Academy of Pediatrics, American College of Sports Medicine, American Medical Society for Sports Medicine, American Orthopaedic Society for Sports Medicine, and American Osteopathic Academy of Sports Medicine. Permission is granted to reprint for noncommercial, educational purposes with acknowledgment.

HE0503   9-2681/0410

FIGURE 19.1 Preparticipation physical evaluation form. (From the Council on Sports Medicine and Fitness, American Academy of Pediatrics. Available at http://www.aap.org/en-us/about-the-aap/Committees-Councils-Sections/Council-on-sports-medicine-and-fitness/Documents/PPE-4-forms.pdf, with permission.)

■ PREPARTICIPATION PHYSICAL EVALUATION
PHYSICAL EXAMINATION FORM

Name _____   Date of birth _____

PHYSICIAN REMINDERS
1. Consider additional questions on more sensitive issues
   - Do you feel stressed out or under a lot of pressure?
   - Do you ever feel sad, hopeless, depressed, or anxious?
   - Do you feel safe at your home or residence?
   - Have you ever tried cigarettes, chewing tobacco, snuff, or dip?
   - During the past 30 days, did you use chewing tobacco, snuff, or dip?
   - Do you drink alcohol or use any other drugs?
   - Have you ever taken anabolic steroids or used any other performance supplement?
   - Have you ever taken any supplements to help you gain or lose weight or improve your performance?
   - Do you wear a seat belt, use a helmet, and use condoms?
2. Consider reviewing questions on cardiovascular symptoms (questions 5–14).

EXAMINATION				
Height		Weight	☐ Male ☐ Female	
BP / (/) Pulse			Vision R 20/ L 20/	Corrected ☐ Y ☐ N

MEDICAL	NORMAL	ABNORMAL FINDINGS
Appearance • Marfan stigmata (kyphoscoliosis, high-arched palate, pectus excavatum, arachnodactyly, arm span > height, hyperlaxity, myopia, MVP, aortic insufficiency)		
Eyes/ears/nose/throat • Pupils equal • Hearing		
Lymph nodes		
Heart[a] • Murmurs (auscultation standing, supine, +/- Valsalva) • Location of point of maximal impulse (PMI)		
Pulses • Simultaneous femoral and radial pulses		
Lungs		
Abdomen		
Genitourinary (males only)[b]		
Skin • HSV, lesions suggestive of MRSA, tinea corporis		
Neurologic[c]		
MUSCULOSKELETAL		
Neck		
Back		
Shoulder/arm		
Elbow/forearm		
Wrist/hand/fingers		
Hip/thigh		
Knee		
Leg/ankle		
Foot/toes		
Functional • Duck-walk, single leg hop		

[a]Consider ECG, echocardiogram, and referral to cardiology for abnormal cardiac history or exam.
[b]Consider GU exam if in private setting. Having third party present is recommended.
[c]Consider cognitive evaluation or baseline neuropsychiatric testing if a history of significant concussion.

☐ Cleared for all sports without restriction

☐ Cleared for all sports without restriction with recommendations for further evaluation or treatment for _____
_____

☐ Not cleared
    ☐ Pending further evaluation
    ☐ For any sports
    ☐ For certain sports _____
       Reason _____
Recommendations _____

I have examined the above-named student and completed the preparticipation physical evaluation. The athlete does not present apparent clinical contraindications to practice and participate in the sport(s) as outlined above. A copy of the physical exam is on record in my office and can be made available to the school at the request of the parents. If conditions arise after the athlete has been cleared for participation, the physician may rescind the clearance until the problem is resolved and the potential consequences are completely explained to the athlete (and parents/guardians).

Name of physician (print/type) _____   Date _____

Address _____   Phone _____

Signature of physician _____ , MD or DO

HE0503   9-2681/0410

FIGURE 19.1 (*Continued*)

The remainder of the sport-specific history can be relatively brief and should assess for the following factors:

1. Past injuries that caused the athlete to miss a game or practice.
2. Any loss of consciousness or memory occurring after a head injury.
3. Previous exclusion from sports for any reason.
4. Allergies, asthma, or exercise-induced bronchospasm.
5. Medications and supplements, used currently or in the last 6 months.
6. The menstrual history in females.
7. A history of relatively rapid increase or decrease in body weight and the athlete's perception of current body weight.

Physical Examination—Screening for Conditions That May Predispose to Injury or Illness

The PPE requires a directed physical examination that augments the *Bright Futures* health maintenance examination with the goals of identifying medical problems or deficits that could worsen the athlete's performance or conditions that might be worsened by athletic participation.

Many conditions that preclude participation in sports are identified in the preadolescent age-group and are not subtle. For example, congenital heart disease and hemophilia are typically detected before adolescence. However, subtle presentations of congenital defects or acquired diseases may go undetected. The most commonly detected abnormalities on PPEs are musculoskeletal injuries that were previously unrecognized and/or have not been rehabilitated. The annual PPE should serve as "quality control" for the diagnosis and rehabilitation of injuries, particularly for adolescents. With this in mind, the physical examination should include assessment of the following:

1. Height, weight, and body mass index (BMI): Obesity, by itself, is not a reason for exclusion. However, the increased risk of heat illness and how that risk might be reduced must be discussed with the athlete, parent, and coach.
2. Blood pressure and pulse: Blood pressure should be taken in the right arm with the athlete sitting. Athletes with hypertension should be evaluated but not excluded from participation unless the hypertension is severe. Bradycardia in the 40- to 50-bpm range occurs commonly in the highly conditioned athlete and does not need evaluation if the athlete is asymptomatic.
3. Visual acuity and pupil equality: AYAs with corrected visual acuity worse than 20/40 in one or both eyes should be referred for further evaluation but are not excluded from participation if protective eyewear is worn. It is important to document the presence of baseline anisocoria before any closed head injury occurs.
4. Skin: Infections that are highly contagious (e.g., varicella, impetigo) should be identified. Identified athletes should not be allowed to return to sports in which skin-to-skin contact is possible until they are determined to be noninfectious (**Table 19.2**).
5. Teeth and mouth: These are examined only if the history suggests an acute problem.
6. Cardiac examination: AHA recommendations for PPE cardiac examination include the following:
   a. Perform precordial auscultation in supine and standing positions to identify heart murmurs consistent with dynamic left ventricular outflow obstruction.
   b. Assess femoral artery or lower extremity pulses to exclude coarctation of the aorta.
   c. Recognize the physical stigmata of Marfan syndrome; refer for further evaluation if a male is taller than 6 ft or a female taller than 5 ft 10 in *and* has
      • a family history of Marfan syndrome
      or
      • two of the following:
        – Kyphosis
        – High-arched palate
        – Pectus excavatum
        – Arachnodactyly
        – Arm span > height
        – Murmur (mitral valve prolapse or aortic)
        – Myopia
        – Lens dislocation
        – Thumb or wrist signs
   d. Assess brachial artery blood pressure in the sitting position.
   e. Document the presence of murmurs, clicks, or rubs (see Chapter 16). Normal or physiologic murmurs are characteristically <4/6 systolic murmurs that decrease in intensity from supine to standing with no diastolic component and with a normal physiologic split second heart sound (S_2). In contrast, the murmur of HCM (when a murmur is present) may sound like a normal murmur except that it *increases* in intensity when the patient moves from the supine to the standing position.
7. Abdomen: Organomegaly is a disqualifying condition for collision/contact or limited-contact sports until definitive evaluation and individual assessment for clearance has been completed.
8. Genitalia: An undescended testicle is not a contraindication to participation in contact sports; however, the athlete should wear a protective cup to protect the other, descended testis. An evaluation for the unidentified testis is necessary.
9. Sexual maturation stage: Sexual maturity rating assessment is part of the adolescent physical examination, but it has no role in determining whether the athlete should play a given sport.
10. Musculoskeletal screening: General musculoskeletal screening should include muscle strength, range-of-motion and joint-stability testing, and evaluation for structural abnormalities of major joints (e.g., ankle, knee, shoulder, elbow, back). An efficient musculoskeletal screening examination is demonstrated in **Figures 19.2 to 19.11**. A more in-depth examination of the specific body parts should be performed if there are concerns from the history or general screening examination (listed in parentheses are diagnoses to consider if the examination finding is abnormal):
    a. Body symmetry (**Figs. 19.2 to 19.11**): Observe the adolescent or young adult standing with arms at the sides, dressed in shorts and a shirt that allows inspection of the distal quadriceps muscles and acromioclavicular joints, respectively. Look for the following:
       • Head tilted or turned to side (consider primary cervical spine injury, primary or secondary trapezius, or cervical muscle spasm)
       • Asymmetry of shoulder heights (trapezius spasm, shoulder injury, scoliosis)
       • Enlarged acromioclavicular joint (previous acromioclavicular joint sprain, shoulder separation)
       • Asymmetrical iliac crest heights (scoliosis or leg-length difference, back spasm)
       • Swollen knee; prominent tibial tuberosity (any knee injury, Osgood–Schlatter disease). Ask the athlete to contract ("tighten") the quadriceps muscles, and look for atrophy of the vastus medialis obliquus, a characteristic of any knee or lower extremity injury in which the athlete avoids normal use of that leg.
       • Swollen ankle (ankle sprain that has not been rehabilitated)
    b. Neck examination (**Fig. 19.3**): This is especially important in players with a previous history of neck injury and brachial plexopathy (referred to as *stingers* or *burners*).
       • Have the athlete perform the following maneuvers:
         Look at the floor (cervical flexion).
         Look at the ceiling (cervical extension).
         Look over the left shoulder, then over the right shoulder (left and right rotation, respectively).

TABLE 19.2

Medical Conditions and Sports Participation

Condition	May Participate
Atlantoaxial instability (instability of the joint between cervical vertebrae 1 and 2) Explanation: Athlete (particularly if he or she has Down syndrome or juvenile rheumatoid arthritis with cervical involvement) needs evaluation to assess the risk of spinal cord injury during sports participation, especially when using a trampoline.	Qualified yes
Bleeding disorder Explanation: Athlete needs evaluation.	Qualified yes

Cardiovascular disease
  Carditis (inflammation of the heart)
  Explanation: Carditis may result in sudden death with exertion.
	No

Hypertension (high blood pressure) Explanation: Those with hypertension >5 mm Hg above the 99th percentile for age, gender, and height should avoid heavy weight lifting and power lifting, bodybuilding, and high-static component sports. Those with sustained hypertension (>95th percentile for age, gender, and height) need evaluation. The National High Blood Pressure Education Program Working Group report defined prehypertension and stage 1 and stage 2 hypertension in children and adolescents younger than 18 years of age.	Qualified yes
Congenital heart disease (structural heart defects present at birth) Explanation: Consultation with a cardiologist is recommended. Those who have mild forms may participate fully in most cases; those who have moderate or severe forms or who have undergone surgery need evaluation. The 36th Bethesda Conference defined mild, moderate, and severe disease for common cardiac lesions.	Qualified yes

Dysrhythmia (irregular heart rhythm)
        Long-QT syndrome
        Malignant ventricular arrhythmias
        Symptomatic Wolff–Parkinson–White syndrome
        Advanced heart block
        Family history of sudden death or previous sudden cardiac event
        Implantation of a cardioverter-defibrillator
Explanation: Consultation with a cardiologist is advised. Those with symptoms (chest pain, syncope, near-syncope, dizziness, shortness of breath, or other symptoms of possible dysrhythmia) or evidence of mitral regurgitation on physical examination need evaluation. All others may participate fully.
	Qualified yes

Heart murmur Explanation: If the murmur is innocent (does not indicate heart disease), full participation is permitted. Otherwise, athlete needs evaluation (see structural heart disease, especially HCM and mitral valve prolapse).	Qualified yes

Structural/acquired heart disease
        HCM
        Coronary artery anomalies
        Arrhythmogenic right ventricular cardiomyopathy
        Acute rheumatic fever with carditis
        Ehlers–Danlos syndrome, vascular form
        Marfan syndrome
        Mitral valve prolapse
        Anthracycline use
Explanation: Consultation with a cardiologist is recommended. The 36th Bethesda Conference provided detailed recommendations. Most of these conditions carry a significant risk of sudden cardiac death associated with intense physical exercise. HCM requires thorough and repeated evaluations, because disease may change manifestations during later adolescence. Marfan syndrome with an aortic aneurysm can also cause sudden death during intense physical exercise. Athlete who has ever received chemotherapy with anthracyclines may be at increased risk of cardiac problems because of the cardiotoxic effects of the medications, and resistance training in this population should be approached with caution; strength training that avoids isometric contractions may be permitted. Athlete needs evaluation.
	Qualified no
	Qualified no
	Qualified no
	Qualified no
	Qualified no
	Qualified yes
	Qualified yes
	Qualified yes

Vasculitis/vascular disease
        Kawasaki disease (coronary artery vasculitis)
        Pulmonary hypertension
Explanation: Consultation with a cardiologist is recommended. Athlete needs individual evaluation to assess risk on the basis of disease activity, pathologic changes, and medical regimen.
	Qualified yes

Cerebral palsy Explanation: Athlete needs evaluation to assess functional capacity to perform sports-specific activity.	Qualified yes
Diabetes mellitus Explanation: All sports can be played with proper attention and appropriate adjustments to diet (particularly carbohydrate intake), blood glucose concentrations, hydration, and insulin therapy. Blood glucose concentrations should be monitored before exercise, every 30 min during continuous exercise, 15 min after completion of exercise, and at bedtime.	Yes

TABLE 19.2

Medical Conditions and Sports Participation (*Continued*)

Condition	May Participate
Diarrhea, infectious Explanation: Unless symptoms are mild and athlete is fully hydrated, no participation is permitted, because diarrhea may increase risk of dehydration and heat illness (see fever).	Qualified no
Eating disorders Explanation: Athlete with an eating disorder needs medical and psychiatric assessment before participation.	Qualified yes

Eyes
    Functionally 1-eyed athlete
    Loss of an eye
    Detached retina or family history of retinal detachment at young age
    High myopia
    Connective tissue disorder, such as Marfan or Stickler syndrome
    Previous intraocular eye surgery or serious eye injury
Explanation: A functionally 1-eyed athlete is defined as having best-corrected visual acuity worse than 20/40 in the poorer-seeing eye. Such an athlete would suffer significant disability if the better eye were seriously injured, as would an athlete with loss of an eye. Specifically, boxing and full-contact martial arts are not recommended for functionally 1-eyed athletes, because eye protection is impractical and/or not permitted. Some athletes who previously underwent intraocular eye surgery or had a serious eye injury may have increased risk of injury because of weakened eye tissue. Availability of eye guards approved by the American Society for Testing and Materials and other protective equipment may allow participation in most sports, but this must be judged on an individual basis.
	Qualified yes

Conjunctivitis, infectious Explanation: Athlete with active infectious conjunctivitis should be excluded from swimming.	Qualified no
Fever Explanation: Elevated core temperature may be indicative of a pathologic medical condition (infection or disease) that is often manifest by increased resting metabolism and heart rate. Accordingly, during athlete's usual exercise regimen, the presence of fever can result in greater heat storage, decreased heat tolerance, increased risk of heat illness, increased cardiopulmonary effort, reduced maximal exercise capacity, and increased risk of hypotension because of altered vascular tone and dehydration. On rare occasions, fever may accompany myocarditis or other conditions that may make usual exercise dangerous.	No

Gastrointestinal
    Malabsorption syndromes (celiac disease or cystic fibrosis)
Explanation: Athlete needs individual assessment for general malnutrition or specific deficits resulting in coagulation or other defects; with appropriate treatment, these deficits can be treated adequately to permit normal activities.
 	
    Short-bowel syndrome or other disorders requiring specialized nutritional support, including parenteral or enteral nutrition
Explanation: Athlete needs individual assessment for collision, contact, or limited-contact sports. Presence of central or peripheral, indwelling, venous catheter may require special considerations for activities and emergency preparedness for unexpected trauma to the device(s).
	Qualified yes

Heat illness, history of Explanation: Because of the likelihood of recurrence, athlete needs individual assessment to determine the presence of predisposing conditions and behaviors and to develop a prevention strategy that includes sufficient acclimatization (to the environment and to exercise intensity and duration), conditioning, hydration, and salt intake, as well as other effective measures to improve heat tolerance and to reduce heat injury risk (such as protective equipment and uniform configurations).	Qualified yes
Hepatitis, infectious (primarily hepatitis C) Explanation: All athletes should receive hepatitis B vaccination before participation. Because of the apparent minimal risk to others, all sports may be played as athlete's state of health allows. For all athletes, skin lesions should be covered properly, and athletic personnel should use universal precautions when handling blood or body fluids with visible blood.	Yes
HIV infection Explanation: Because of the apparent minimal risk to others, all sports may be played as athlete's state of health allows (especially if viral load is undetectable or very low). For all athletes, skin lesions should be covered properly, and athletic personnel should use universal precautions when handling blood or body fluids with visible blood. However, certain sports (such as wrestling and boxing) may create a situation that favors viral transmission (likely bleeding plus skin breaks). If viral load is detectable, then athletes should be advised to avoid such high-contact sports.	Yes
Kidney, absence of one Explanation: Athlete needs individual assessment for contact, collision, and limited-contact sports. Protective equipment may reduce risk of injury to the remaining kidney sufficiently to allow participation in most sports, providing such equipment remains in place during activity.	Qualified yes
Liver, enlarged Explanation: If the liver is acutely enlarged, then participation should be avoided because of risk of rupture. If the liver is chronically enlarged, then individual assessment is needed before collision, contact, or limited-contact sports are played. Patients with chronic liver disease may have changes in liver function that affect stamina, mental status, coagulation, or nutritional status.	Qualified yes

(*Continued*)

TABLE 19.2

Medical Conditions and Sports Participation (*Continued*)

Condition	May Participate
Malignant neoplasm Explanation: Athlete needs individual assessment.	Qualified yes
Musculoskeletal disorders Explanation: Athlete needs individual assessment.	Qualified yes

Neurologic disorders
    History of serious head or spine trauma or abnormality, including craniotomy, epidural bleeding, subdural hematoma, intracerebral hemorrhage, second-impact syndrome, vascular malformation, and neck fracture
  Explanation: Athlete needs individual assessment for collision, contact, or limited-contact sports.
	Qualified yes

History of simple concussion (mild traumatic brain injury), multiple simple concussions, and/or complex concussion Explanation: Athlete needs individual assessment. Research supports a conservative approach to concussion management, including no athletic participation while symptomatic or when deficits in judgment or cognition are detected, followed by graduated return to full activity.	Qualified yes
Myopathies Explanation: Athlete needs individual assessment.	Qualified yes
Recurrent headaches Explanation: Athlete needs individual assessment.	Yes
Recurrent plexopathy (burner or stinger) and cervical cord neuropraxia with persistent defects Explanation: Athlete needs individual assessment for collision, contact, or limited-contact sports; regaining normal strength is important benchmark for return to play.	Qualified yes
Seizure disorder, well controlled Explanation: Risk of seizure during participation is minimal.	Yes
Seizure disorder, poorly controlled Explanation: Athlete needs individual assessment for collision, contact, or limited-contact sports. The following noncontact sports should be avoided: archery, riflery, swimming, weightlifting, power lifting, strength training, and sports involving heights. In these sports, occurrence of a seizure during activity may pose a risk to self or others.	Qualified yes
Obesity Explanation: Because of the increased risk of heat illness and cardiovascular strain, obese athlete particularly needs careful acclimatization (to the environment and to exercise intensity and duration), sufficient hydration, and potential activity and recovery modifications during competition and training.	Yes
Organ transplant recipient (and those taking immunosuppressive medications) Explanation: Athlete needs individual assessment for contact, collision, and limited-contact sports. In addition to potential risk of infections, some medications (e.g., prednisone) may increase tendency for bruising.	Qualified yes
Ovary, absence of one Explanation: Risk of severe injury to remaining ovary is minimal.	Yes
Pregnancy/postpartum Explanation: Athlete needs individual assessment. As pregnancy progresses, modifications to usual exercise routines will become necessary. Activities with high risk of falling or abdominal trauma should be avoided. Scuba diving and activities posing risk of altitude sickness should also be avoided during pregnancy. After the birth, physiologic and morphologic changes of pregnancy take 4 to 6 weeks to return to baseline.	Qualified yes

Respiratory conditions
    Pulmonary compromise, including cystic fibrosis
  Explanation: Athlete needs individual assessment but, generally, all sports may be played if oxygenation remains satisfactory during graded exercise test. Athletes with cystic fibrosis need acclimatization and good hydration to reduce risk of heat illness.
	Qualified yes

Asthma Explanation: With proper medication and education, only athletes with severe asthma need to modify their participation. For those using inhalers, recommend having a written action plan and using a peak flowmeter daily. Athletes with asthma may encounter risks when scuba diving.	Yes
Acute upper respiratory infection Explanation: Upper respiratory obstruction may affect pulmonary function. Athlete needs individual assessment for all except mild disease (see fever).	Qualified yes

TABLE 19.2

Medical Conditions and Sports Participation (*Continued*)

Condition	May Participate

Rheumatologic diseases
    Juvenile rheumatoid arthritis
Explanation: Athletes with systemic or polyarticular juvenile rheumatoid arthritis and history of cervical spine involvement need radiographs of vertebrae C1 and C2 to assess risk of spinal cord injury. Athletes with systemic or HLA-B27-associated arthritis require cardiovascular assessment for possible cardiac complications during exercise. For those with micrognathia (open bite and exposed teeth), mouth guards are helpful. If uveitis is present, risk of eye damage from trauma is increased; ophthalmologic assessment is recommended. If visually impaired, guidelines for functionally 1-eyed athletes should be followed.
 	
    Juvenile dermatomyositis, idiopathic myositis
    Systemic lupus erythematosis
    Raynaud phenomenon
Explanation: Athlete with juvenile dermatomyositis or systemic lupus erythematosis with cardiac involvement requires cardiology assessment before participation. Athletes receiving systemic corticosteroid therapy are at higher risk of osteoporotic fractures and avascular necrosis, which should be assessed before clearance; those receiving immunosuppressive medications are at higher risk of serious infection. Sports activities should be avoided when myositis is active. Rhabdomyolysis during intensive exercise may cause renal injury in athletes with idiopathic myositis and other myopathies. Because of photosensitivity with juvenile dermatomyositis and systemic lupus erythematosis, sun protection is necessary during outdoor activities. With Raynaud phenomenon, exposure to the cold presents risk to hands and feet.
	Qualified yes

Sickle cell disease Explanation: Athlete needs individual assessment. In general, if illness status permits, all sports may be played; however, any sport or activity that entails overexertion, overheating, dehydration, or chilling should be avoided. Participation at high altitude, especially when not acclimatized, also poses risk of sickle cell crisis.	Qualified yes
Sickle cell trait Explanation: Athletes with sickle cell trait generally do not have increased risk of sudden death or other medical problems during athletic participation under normal environmental conditions. However, when high exertional activity is performed under extreme conditions of heat and humidity or increased altitude, such catastrophic complications have occurred rarely. Athletes with sickle cell trait, like all athletes, should be progressively acclimatized to the environment and to the intensity and duration of activities and should be sufficiently hydrated to reduce the risk of exertional heat illness and/or rhabdomyolysis. According to National Institutes of Health management guidelines, sickle cell trait is not a contraindication to participation in competitive athletics, and there is no requirement for screening before participation. More research is needed to assess fully potential risks and benefits of screening athletes for sickle cell trait.	Yes
Skin infections, including herpes simplex, molluscum contagiosum, verrucae (warts), staphylococcal and streptococcal infections (furuncles [boils], carbuncles, impetigo, methicillin-resistant *Staphylococcus aureus* [cellulitis and/or abscesses]), scabies, and tinea Explanation: During contagious periods, participation in gymnastics or cheerleading with mats, martial arts, wrestling, or other collision, contact, or limited-contact sports is not allowed.	Qualified yes
Spleen, enlarged Explanation: If the spleen is acutely enlarged, then participation should be avoided because of risk of rupture. If the spleen is chronically enlarged, then individual assessment is needed before collision, contact, or limited-contact sports are played.	Qualified yes
Testicle, undescended or absence of one Explanation: Certain sports may require a protective cup.	Yes

This table is designed for use by medical and nonmedical personnel.

"Needs evaluation" means that a physician with appropriate knowledge and experience should assess the safety of a given sport for an athlete with the listed medical condition. Unless otherwise noted, this need for special consideration is because of variability in the severity of the disease, the risk of injury for the specific sports listed in Table 19.1

From Committee on Sports Medicine and Fitness. Medical conditions affecting sports participation. Pediatrics 2008;121:841.

Put right ear on right shoulder, then left ear on left shoulder (right and left lateral flexion).

- Look for limited or asymmetrical motion with the maneuvers listed (neck injury, congenital cervical abnormalities). Any athlete with limitation of range of motion (ROM), weakness or pain on neck examination is excluded from contact or collision sports, pending further evaluation.

c. Shoulder examination (Fig. 19.4)
- Have the athlete raise the arms from the side and touch the hands above the head, keeping elbows extended (full abduction). Look for the following:
  Asymmetric elevation of shoulder before arms reach 90 degrees (shoulder weakness due to a brachial plexopathy, shoulder instability, impingement syndrome).

Inability to raise arms to full abduction position (shoulder weakness due to brachial plexopathy, impingement syndrome, or apprehension from subluxation or dislocation).

- Have athlete hold the arms in front of the body (forward flexion) and then to the side (90 degrees abduction); examiner should push the hands down. Look for asymmetrical atrophy or fasciculations of anterior and middle deltoid muscles and pain and/or weakness (may be indicative of a variety of shoulder problems).
- Have athlete put hands behind head (maximal external rotation/abduction). Look for the following:
  Inability to get hand behind head (i.e., lack of external rotation of shoulder).

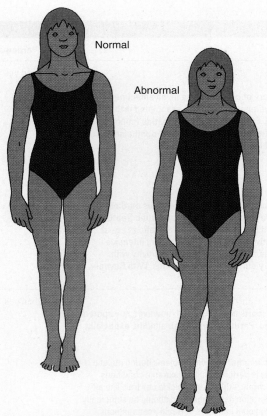

Normal

Abnormal

FIGURE 19.2 Body symmetry. (From Ross Laboratories. *For the practitioner: orthopedic screening examination for participation in sports*. Columbus, OH: Ross Products Division, Abbott Laboratories, 1981, with permission, copyright 1981 Ross Products Division, Abbott Laboratories.)

Apprehension or inability to pull the elbows, symmetrically, posterior to the shoulder (anterior subluxation or dislocation).

An athlete with limitation of motion should be evaluated further before clearance is granted for further participation.

d. Elbow and hand
  • Have athlete extend and flex elbows with arms to the side (90 degrees abduction) (Fig. 19.5). Look for asymmetrical elbow extension or flexion (prior dislocation or fracture, osteochondritis dissecans).
  • With arms at sides and elbows flexed 90 degrees, have the athlete pronate and supinate forearms (Fig. 19.6). Look for asymmetrical loss of motion (residual of forearm fractures, Little League elbow, osteochondritis dissecans of elbow). The cause of a limitation in ROM of the elbow should be established before a young athlete is cleared for participation, especially in throwing sports.
  • In the same position, have the athlete spread fingers and then make a fist (Fig. 19.7). Look for lack of finger flexion, swollen joints, and finger deformities (residuals of sprains, fractures). Hand injuries should be evaluated, and recommendations for sports participation should be based on the severity of the injury and the specific sport the athlete desires to play. Typically, the athlete is not excluded from participation unless there is a complication of a previous fracture or tendon rupture that needs further assessment.

e. Back and leg observation
  • Have the patient stand facing away from the examiner (Fig. 19.8). Look for the following:

Asymmetry of waist (scoliosis, leg-length difference)
Elevated shoulder (scoliosis or trapezius spasm from shoulder or neck injury)
Depressed shoulder (scoliosis, muscle weakness)
Prominent rib cage (scoliosis)
Increased lordosis (spondylolysis, tight hip flexors, weak hamstrings)
Idiopathic scoliosis is not usually a contraindication for sports participation, unless the angle is severe (i.e., a Cobb angle >45 degrees). If pain is present or there is a left major thoracic or lumbar scoliosis, then the diagnosis may not be idiopathic scoliosis and a definitive diagnosis should be established. This should include a neurologic examination and magnetic resonance imaging (MRI) of the spine.
  • Have athlete bend forward at waist/hips (lumbar flexion) to touch toes (Fig. 19.9). Look for the following:
Twisting or deviating of side (paraspinous muscle spasm)
Asymmetrical prominence of rib cage (scoliosis)
Inability to reverse the lumbar lordosis (spondylolysis, paraspinous muscle spasm caused by a chronic inflammatory condition such as ankylosing spondylitis)
  • Have athlete stand straight and rise onto toes (Fig. 19.10). Look for the following:
Asymmetry of heel elevation (calf weakness, restricted ankle motion from sprain or fracture)
Asymmetry of gastrocnemius (atrophy from incompletely rehabilitated ankle or leg injury)
  • Have athlete rise onto heels. Look for the following:
Asymmetry of elevation of forefoot or toes (weakness of ankle dorsiflexors, limitation of ankle motion from ankle fracture or sprain)
If asymmetry on toe or heel raising is detected, further evaluation and treatment are indicated before the athlete is cleared for full sports participation.

f. Hip, knee, and ankle screening: Have athlete slowly assume a painless squatting position (buttocks on heels) (Fig. 19.11). If the athlete cannot do this, then further evaluation is indicated. Ask athlete to take four steps forward in this squatting position ("duck walk"), then turn 180 degrees in this squatting position and take four more steps. Look for the following:
  • Asymmetry of heel height off ground (limited ankle motion or Achilles tendon tightness from tendonitis or injury).
  • Asymmetrical knee flexion, that is, difference in heel-to-buttock height from the rear view or inability to get down as far on one side as on the other (knee effusion, residual limitation of motion from sprain, torn meniscus, quadriceps tightness or weakness, patellofemoral pain, Osgood–Schlatter disease).
  • Pain at any point in the range of knee flexion. The cause of the pain should be established and the patient rehabilitated before allowing return to participation without restrictions.

g. Ankle screening: Have the athlete hop five times as high as possible on each foot. Inability to do so suggests an undiagnosed or unrehabilitated lower leg, ankle, or foot injury. The ankle should be evaluated and fully rehabilitated before full participation is allowed.

Laboratory Tests

Blood for hemoglobin and a dipstick of the urine for protein, glucose, and blood have been recommended as screening tests for athletic participation. Although the hemoglobin test may be indicated for general health maintenance evaluation, it is not recommended for asymptomatic adolescents or young adults. The diagnosis of anemia in highly trained aerobic athletes may be problematic, because some will have a reduced hematocrit due to intravascular volume

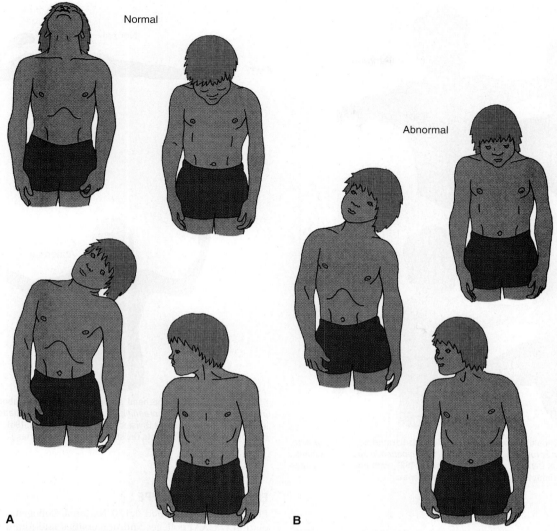

Normal

Abnormal

A   B

FIGURE 19.3 Neck symmetry. (From Ross Laboratories. *For the practitioner: orthopedic screening examination for participation in sports.* Columbus, OH: Ross Products Division, Abbott Laboratories, 1981, with permission, copyright 1981 Ross Products Division, Abbott Laboratories.)

expansion but a normal oxygen-carrying capacity. The urine dipstick test is not indicated in the absence of symptoms suggesting genitourinary tract dysfunction. Screening for iron deficiency in menstruating female athletes, especially those who participate in long-distance events, by measurement of serum ferritin is advocated by some experts. However, empirical iron therapy in the form of a daily multivitamin with iron may be the most cost-effective approach to preventing iron deficiency in healthy female athletes.

Estimating body composition with the use of anthropometric measurements (i.e., skin folds) is indicated in wrestling because prediction equations for minimum wrestling weights have been established. Use of skin-fold measurements as screening tests is not indicated for most athletes. Body weight measurement and BMI calculation are sufficient for tracking patients who choose to gain or lose weight.

Determining Clearance for Activity

Table 19.2 lists disqualifying medical conditions for sports participation as recommended by the AAP. These are only guidelines and may not apply in specific cases. However, it is notable that all except three (carditis or cardiomyopathy, diarrhea, and fever) allow for individualized or modified athletic participation after further

evaluation. The goal of the PPE, once again, is promotion of *safe* physical activity for all AYAs.

After the PPE, the patient should be given one of the following recommendations:

1. Cleared without restriction
2. Cleared, with recommendations for further evaluation or treatment
3. Clearance withheld pending further evaluation, treatment, or rehabilitation
4. Not cleared for certain types of sports or for all sports

If there are restrictions to participation, these restrictions should be discussed with the athlete and a parent or guardian, with clearly documented recommendations transmitted to a certified athletic trainer or coach. Otherwise, the message to the athlete may be misinterpreted. If clearance for athletic participation is not recommended, the clinician should be prepared to discuss the risks associated with continued participation, balancing the medical problem with the demands placed on the athlete in that sport. The clinician must also consider the importance of this sport compared to another activity; some young athletes may be willing to switch to an activity with a lower risk of reinjury.

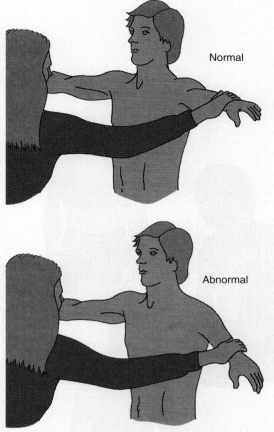

FIGURE 19.4 Shoulder symmetry. (From Ross Laboratories. *For the practitioner: orthopedic screening examination for participation in sports.* Columbus, OH: Ross Products Division, Abbott Laboratories, 1981, with permission, copyright 1981 Ross Products Division, Abbott Laboratories.)

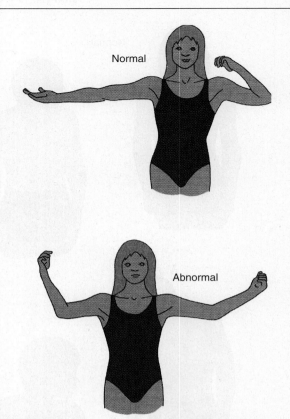

FIGURE 19.5 Elbow and hand symmetry. (From Ross Laboratories. For the *practitioner: orthopedic screening examination for participation in s*ports. Columbus, OH: Ross Products Division, Abbott Laboratories, 1981, with permission, copyright 1981 Ross Products Division, Abbott Laboratories.)

Medical–Legal Issues and Exclusion from Sports Participation

Athletes and their parents may seek to participate in a sport against medical advice, citing the Americans with Disabilities Act of 1990 or section 504(a) of the Rehabilitation Act of 1973, which prohibits discrimination against an athlete who is disabled if that person has the capabilities and skills required to play a competitive sport. Athletes with physical disabilities have successfully argued to retain their right to participate in professional athletics using these legal statues. However, an amateur athlete does not have an absolute right to decide whether to participate in competitive sports. Competition in sports is generally considered a privilege, not a right. The case of *Knapp versus Northwestern University* established that "difficult medical decisions involving complex medical problems can be made by responsible physicians exercising prudent judgment (which will be necessarily conservative when definitive scientific evidence is lacking or conflicting) and relying on the recommendations of specialist consultants or guidelines established by a panel of experts."[5] Clinicians should make decisions about athletic participation according to generally agreed-upon guidelines for participation with known medical conditions. As **Table 19.2** indicates, each decision must be made on an individual basis, and there may not be expert panel guidelines for all conditions. However, such guidelines do exist in many instances, an example being the 36th Bethesda Conference guidelines (discussed below).[6]

Effectiveness of the PPE

Pfister et al.[7] examined 1,110 National Collegiate Athletic Association (NCAA) colleges and universities and found that only 25% had forms that contained at least 9 of the recommended 12 AHA screening guidelines, while 24% contained 4 or fewer of these parameters. Authors of *The Monograph* acknowledge that there is need for national standardization of preparticipation screening to better assess its effectiveness and have called for Internet-based information sharing. Even with perfect implementation, however, Bundy and Feudtner[8] cogently argue that the prevalence of sports-related mortality is too low for the PPE to ever qualify as an effective screening program unless the focus is shifted to and systems created for appropriate rehabilitation of identified musculoskeletal deficits.

Addressing Other Important Conditions Identified on PPE
Risk for Anterior Cruciate Ligament (ACL) Tear

In general, female athletes have injuries and injury rates similar to those of male athletes in the same sport. The exception to this rule is the 2 to 8 times higher rate of ACL sprain among female athletes compared to their male counterparts in sports such as basketball and soccer. Definitive reasons for this difference are not established. Unfortunately, prophylactic bracing does not appear to be effective. In research settings, reductions in the incidence of acute knee injuries in female athletes after neuromuscular training courses have been reported suggesting a role for improved neuromuscular control in stabilizing the knee and preventing ACL injuries.[9] Specific neuromuscular training programs to replicate the research outcomes, specifically to strengthen the hamstrings and core muscles around the hips and buttocks which control the femur, have

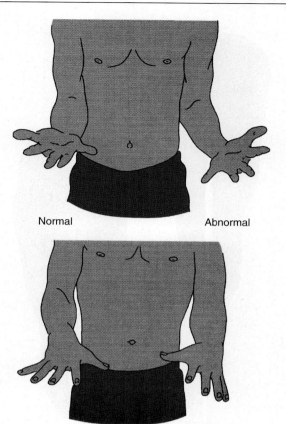

FIGURE 19.6 Elbow and hand symmetry, continued. (From Ross Laboratories. *For the practitioner: orthopedic screening examination for participation in sports.* Columbus, OH: Ross Products Division, Abbott Laboratories, 1981, with permission, copyright 1981 Ross Products Division, Abbott Laboratories.)

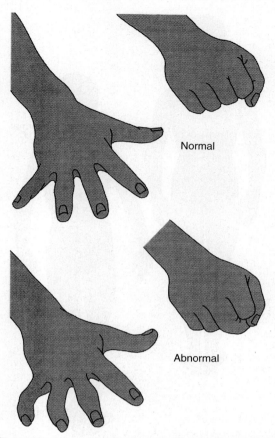

FIGURE 19.7 Elbow and hand symmetry, continued. (From Ross Laboratories. *For the practitioner: orthopedic screening examination for participation in sports.* Columbus, OH: Ross Products Division, Abbott Laboratories, 1981, with permission, copyright 1981 Ross Products Division, Abbott Laboratories.)

been developed and are available from the AAP online (http://www.aap.org/en-us/about-the-aap/Committees-Councils-Sections/Council-on-sports-medicine-and-fitness/Pages/ACL-Resources.aspx). However, the dynamic analysis of lower extremity biomechanics required to identify deficiencies entails a degree of expertise typically found only in rehabilitative specialists, to whom referral of AYA female athletes in these sports may be warranted.

Cardiac Conditions

Mortality during athletic participation is an extraordinarily rare (7.8 deaths per million athletes per year), but devastating event for the athlete's family, team, and community.[8] Most young athletes who die during sports participation die from sudden cardiac events; most of these athletes are asymptomatic before the event. Therefore, identifying cardiovascular risk conditions is a major focus of the PPE screening.

Any athlete complaining of true angina, syncope, presyncope, or palpitations while exercising, independent of the physical examination, should be excluded from participation, pending further evaluation. In consultation with a cardiovascular specialist, full evaluation may include a 12-lead electrocardiogram, a continuous ambulatory (Holter) or event capture monitor, a maximal stress test, and a two-dimensional echocardiogram.

The best reference for counseling individual athletes with known cardiac conditions is the 36th Bethesda Conference, 2005 Report: Eligibility Recommendations for Competitive Athletes With Cardiovascular Abnormalities,[6] accessed at http://www.cardiosource.org/~/media/Files/Science%20and%20Quality/Guidelines/Clinical_Documents/BethesdaConference36.ashx.

Hypertension and elevated blood pressure should be evaluated and managed as described in Chapter 17. AYAs with prehypertension or stage 1 hypertension should not be limited from athletics unless they are symptomatic, or have left ventricular hypertrophy (LVH) or other end-organ damage. In the absence of symptoms, LVH, or other end-organ damage, athletes with stage 2 hypertension may be restricted from high-static sports (classes IIIA to IIIC in Fig. 19.12) until their blood pressure is controlled stably in the normal range. In the presence of other cardiovascular diseases, guidelines for the specific additional condition from the 36th Bethesda Conference should be consulted.[6,10]

Concussion History

Sports-related mild traumatic brain injury (MTBI) or *concussion* is defined as "a complex pathophysiologic process affecting the brain, induced by traumatic biomechanical forces."[11] There are at least 300,000 sports-related traumatic brain injuries in the US annually, with increasing appreciation that the true incidence of this injury may be at least 10-fold greater. Since each concussion should be managed individually and independently, there is no threshold number of lifetime concussions that automatically disqualify a patient from sports participation. Nonetheless, repeat concussions which seem triggered by progressively smaller force impacts or require increasing duration for resolution should prompt a discussion with the patient and/or family about curtailing collision sports (Table 19.1). Concussion is discussed in Chapter 21.

Drug Use and Ergogenic Aids in Athletes

Studies suggest that in some groups, substance use may be more common among high school and college athletes than in nonathletes, with important differences depending on gender and the drug being studied. Specifically, there is evidence that marijuana and alcohol use are higher in male students who compete in competitive

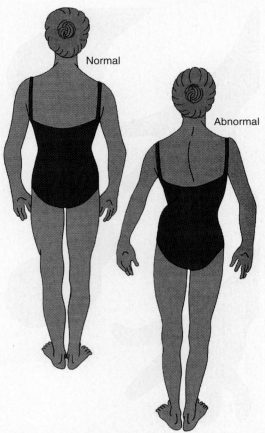

FIGURE 19.8 Back and leg symmetry. (From Ross Laboratories. *For the practitioner: orthopedic screening examination for participation in sports.* Columbus, OH: Ross Products Division, Abbott Laboratories, 1981, with permission, copyright 1981 Ross Products Division, Abbott Laboratories.)

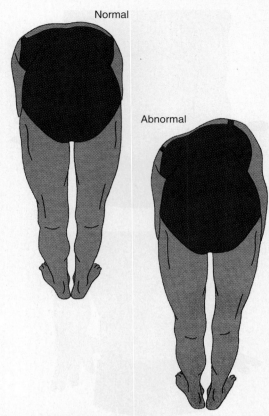

FIGURE 19.9 Back symmetry. (From Ross Laboratories. *For the practitioner: orthopedic screening examination for participation in sports.* Columbus, OH: Ross Products Division, Abbott Laboratories, 1981, with permission, copyright 1981 Ross Products Division, Abbott Laboratories.)

sports than in male peers not competing in sports; the reverse is true for female athletes.[12,13] Neither marijuana nor alcohol has ergogenic effects on athletic performance. Cigarettes tend to be used less by athletes.[12] Anabolic steroids are used more by athletes.

The major categories of drugs used to improve performance by athletes include anabolic steroids, stimulants, and pain relievers. In addition, the use of dietary supplements as ergogenic aids has become more common. These supplements include creatine, androstenedione and dehydroepiandrosterone (DHEA), and protein powders. For more information about drugs of abuse, access the National Clearinghouse for Alcohol and Drug Information online at www.samhsa.gov and see Chapters 63 to 67.

Therapeutic Drugs

Over-the-counter analgesics, decongestants, antihistamines, laxatives, antidiarrheal agents, and weight-loss medications are commonly used by AYAs. Athletes should be asked specifically about use of these medications during office visits, because they may not perceive them to be as important as prescription drugs and may not report their use. These medications have important side effects that may affect performance. Some are even banned by sports governing bodies (NCAA and US Olympic Committee). Clinicians are encouraged to consult the US (www.usantidoping.org) and World Anti-Doping Agencies (www.wada-ama.org) when advising athletes, especially college and elite athletes, about medication and prescription drug use.

Performance-Enhancing Drugs

Stimulants: Stimulants have been used extensively to combat psychological and muscular fatigue. These substances are banned by

the International Olympic Committee (IOC) and can be detected by urine tests.

Amphetamines: Fine motor coordination and performance on tasks requiring prolonged attention have been shown to improve with amphetamine use. Side effects include anxiety, restlessness, tremors, tachycardia, irritability, confusion, and poor judgment. Side effects occur more commonly at higher doses.

Cocaine: The effects of cocaine have not been shown to be ergogenic. These effects include increases in heart rate, reflexes, and blood pressure, with accompanying euphoria. In the inexperienced user, reflexes are often more rapid but dyssynchronous, leading to a decrement in athletic performance. Lethal toxicity can occur unexpectedly, particularly with intravenous use, because the doses of cocaine available on the street vary widely. Symptoms of acute overdose are difficult to treat and sometimes fatal, including arrhythmias, seizures, and hyperthermia. Metabolites can be found in the urine within 24 to 36 hours of ingestion and for up to 4 days after acute ingestion.

Caffeine: Caffeine is probably the most commonly used stimulant. Several studies have documented increased muscle work output for endurance activities. Significant side effects mimic those of other stimulants. Caffeine has a direct diuretic effect, potentially complicating fluid and electrolyte status in prolonged exercise activities. Caffeine is banned by the IOC in quantities >12 µg/mL (approximately equivalent to 4 to 8 cups of coffee or 8 to 16 cups of cola). Many currently popular "energy drinks" contain high doses of caffeine, prompting the AAP to counsel against their use.[14]

Anabolic Steroids

Anabolic steroid use is associated with increased muscle size and strength, especially in athletes who are weight training when the

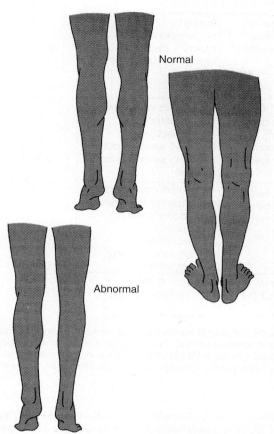

FIGURE 19.10 Leg symmetry. (From Ross Laboratories. *For the practitioner: orthopedic screening examination for participation in sports.* Columbus, OH: Ross Products Division, Abbott Laboratories, 1981, with permission, copyright 1981 Ross Products Division, Abbott Laboratories.)

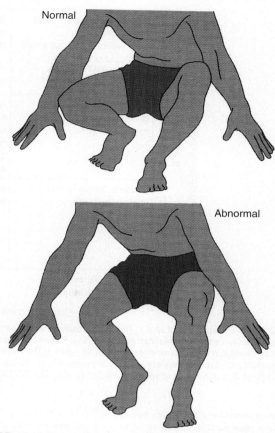

FIGURE 19.11 Leg symmetry, continued. (From Ross Laboratories. *For the practitioner: orthopedic screening examination for participation in sports.* Columbus, OH: Ross Products Division, Abbott Laboratories, 1981, with permission, copyright 1981 Ross Products Division, Abbott Laboratories, with permission.)

steroid use is initiated and in those who are consuming a high-calorie diet. Animal models demonstrate that anabolic steroids result in muscle hypertrophy in nonexercising muscle. There is no evidence that steroid use enhances aerobic power. There is evidence that anabolic steroids may aid the healing of muscle injury, in contrast to corticosteroids, which may account for their apparent efficacy in coordination sports such as baseball. Food and Drug Administration (FDA)-approved uses of anabolic steroids include weight gain in patients with acquired immunodeficiency syndrome, severe anemia, hereditary angioedema, metastatic breast cancer, or male adrenal insufficiency.

Anabolic steroids may be injected or taken orally, and they are often readily available from peers and coaches. Buckley et al.[15] reported 21% of 12th grade male adolescents who had used anabolic steroids indicated that their primary source was a health professional. In the Monitoring the Future study of 12th graders, the lifetime prevalence rates were 2.3% in 1995, 2.9% in 1999, 3.5% in 2003, 2.6% in 2005, and 2.1% in 2013 (www.monitoringthefuture.org). Among 8th graders, the lifetime prevalence rates rose from 2.0% in 1995 to 3.5% in 2003, but fell dramatically to 1.1% in 2013.[16] It would appear that the use of anabolic steroids has been substantially lower after high school than during 12th grade. The annual prevalence rates are very low for respondents in all young adult age groups (age 19 and older) and range from 0.05% to 0.7%. In the spring 2013, the American College Health Association National College Health Assessment (ACHA-NCHA) survey, approximately 1% of students reported using anabolic steroids (www.acha-ncha.org/docs/ACHA-NCHA-II_ReferenceGroup_DataReport_Spring2013.pdf).

Side effects of anabolic steroids include the following:

1. Alteration of myocardial textural properties (as detected by ultrasound). These changes are not seen in weight lifters who develop increased left ventricular mass with weight training but do not use anabolic steroids. The clinical and prognostic significance of these changes is unknown.
2. Altered myocardial function: 17α-Methyl testosterone has been associated with reduced myocardial compliance and reduced myocardial function in rats.
3. Risk of hepatic damage (manifested as elevated liver-specific enzymes): There are anecdotal reports, but the risk of developing hepatic neoplasm is unknown.
4. Decreased high-density lipoprotein (HDL) and increased low-density lipoprotein (LDL) cholesterol levels.
5. Oligospermia and azoospermia with decreased testicular size.
6. Premature epiphyseal closure in pubertal athletes.
7. Acne.
8. Masculinization in women: Presents as deepening of the voice, acne, and hair loss.
9. Feminization in men: Presents as gynecomastia and a high voice.
10. Adverse psychological effects, including increased aggressiveness and rage in some athletes.
11. Association with the use of other illicit drugs.

Injected steroids are detectable in the urine for six months or longer. Orally administered anabolic steroids disappear from the urine after days to weeks.

Narcotic Analgesics

Narcotic analgesics may allow an athlete to perform despite pain and/or injury, but they do not enhance athletic performance. In

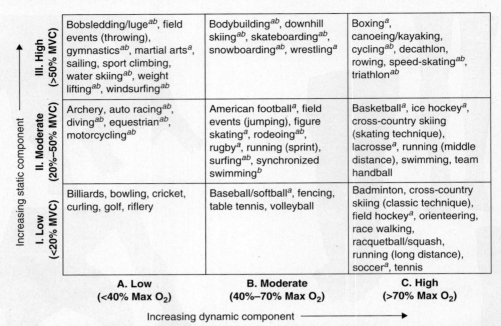

	A. Low (<40% Max O₂)	B. Moderate (40%–70% Max O₂)	C. High (>70% Max O₂)
III. High (>50% MVC)	Bobsledding/luge[ab], field events (throwing), gymnastics[ab], martial arts[a], sailing, sport climbing, water skiing[ab], weight lifting[ab], windsurfing[ab]	Bodybuilding[ab], downhill skiing[ab], skateboarding[ab], snowboarding[ab], wrestling[a]	Boxing[a], canoeing/kayaking, cycling[ab], decathlon, rowing, speed-skating[ab], triathlon[ab]
II. Moderate (20%–50% MVC)	Archery, auto racing[ab], diving[ab], equestrian[ab], motorcycling[ab]	American football[a], field events (jumping), figure skating[a], rodeoing[ab], rugby[a], running (sprint), surfing[ab], synchronized swimming[b]	Basketball[a], ice hockey[a], cross-country skiing (skating technique), lacrosse[a], running (middle distance), swimming, team handball
I. Low (<20% MVC)	Billiards, bowling, cricket, curling, golf, riflery	Baseball/softball[a], fencing, table tennis, volleyball	Badminton, cross-country skiing (classic technique), field hockey[a], orienteering, race walking, racquetball/squash, running (long distance), soccer[a], tennis

Increasing static component ↑

Increasing dynamic component →

FIGURE 19.12 Classification of sports. This classification is based on peak static and dynamic components achieved during competition. It should be noted, however, that higher values may be reached during training. The increasing dynamic component is defined in terms of the estimated percent of maximal oxygen uptake (Max O₂) achieved and results in an increasing cardiac output. The increasing static component is related to the estimated percent of maximal voluntary contraction (MVC) reached and results in an increasing blood pressure load. [a]Danger of bodily collision. [b]Increased risk if syncope occurs. (From Mitchell JH, Haskel W, Snell P, et al. Task force 8: classification of sports. *J Am Coll Cardiol* 2005;45:1364, with permission.)

standard doses, there also does not appear to be a detriment. However, they may be abused in an attempt to return to play prematurely. Their effects include psychomotor retardation, sedation, dysphoria, and nausea and vomiting.

Dietary Supplements as Ergogenic Aids

The potency, purity, and long-term effects of most dietary supplements are not known because they are not regulated by the FDA. Unfortunately, the 1994 Dietary Supplement Health and Education Act, which removed the FDA regulation, led to a rapid increase in the availability and use of these products among adolescents. Reputable information about dietary supplements can be found at http://ods.od.nih.gov/, but our awareness of the "latest" agents typically lags far behind their actual use by our patients. None of these supplements are recommended for use by AYAs.

Androstenedione: Androstenedione is an androgen produced by the gonads and adrenal glands. It is a precursor to estradiol and testosterone, yet it is marketed as a nutritional supplement and is not regulated by the FDA. Individuals taking androstenedione experience no beneficial effect on strength compared to controls. Use of androstenedione has been associated with increased serum estradiol levels, no change in serum testosterone levels, and an increased LDL:HDL ratio. There is no medically approved use for androstenedione, and its use is banned by the IOC, the NCAA, the National Football League, and other athletic organizations. However, because of its perceived benefit and because testing for androstenedione is not possible, its use is likely to continue.

Dehydroepiandrosterone: DHEA is an adrenal androgen marketed as a food supplement. It is a precursor of androgens and estradiol. Ergogenic effects have not been demonstrated in athletes. DHEA has been reported to increase insulin-like growth factor (IGF). The side effects are androgenic, including hair loss and irreversible deepening of the voice in females. Androgens can hasten the growth of prostatic cancer, and estrogens can similarly affect the growth of breast and endometrial cancer; however, the effects of DHEA on the growth of these tumors are unknown.

Creatine: Creatine is synthesized in the liver, kidney, and pancreas. Creatine is supplied in the diet in the form of meat and fish. The usual US diet supplies approximately 1 to 2 g of creatine daily to replenish that which is lost in the urine. Theoretically, creatine works as an ergogenic aid by increasing the cellular concentration of high-energy phosphocreatine, the immediate transport entity in the synthesis of adenosine triphosphate (ATP) from adenosine diphosphate (ADP). It has been suggested that those with lower intracellular creatine concentration may benefit most from creatine supplementation, yet there is no current method to assay for low intracellular concentration. There may be some benefit for short-duration (i.e., <30 seconds), high-intensity exercise, but this effect has been demonstrated in laboratory settings and has not translated into improved performance on the athletic field. In addition, there have been case reports of renal injury with the use of creatine and long-term safety has not been established.

Testing for Performance-Enhancing Drugs

Given that many jurisdictions that sponsor sports may be limited financially, it may be more cost-effective to advocate for balanced educational programs that increase student-athletes' knowledge than to mount an expensive testing program, particularly at the high school and youth sports levels. Readers who desire guidance on how to institute testing programs are encouraged to contact the NCAA (telephone 1-913-339-1906) or the US Olympic Committee (1-800-233-0393, Drug Control Hotline).

FEMALE ATHLETE TRIAD

The effects of excessive exercise on the reproductive system in young females deserve special mention. Female athletes with amenorrhea or oligomenorrhea have lower bone mineral density (BMD) and higher rates of stress fracture than eumenorrheic athletes. Recognizing this, the female athlete triad was defined in 1992 to describe the observed correlation of disordered eating, amenorrhea, and osteoporosis among athletes engaged in sports that emphasize low weight or lean physique. A long-term consequence of amenorrhea and osteopenia during the second decade may also be an increased risk of postmenopausal osteoporosis. Nichols and colleagues[17] examined the prevalence rate for the female athlete triad among high schools athletes. They found that among female athletes studied ($N = 170$), 18.2%, 23.5%, and 21.8% met the criteria for disordered eating, menstrual irregularity, and low bone mass, respectively. Ten girls (5.9%) met the criteria for two components of the triad, and two girls (1.2%) met criteria for all three components. Acknowledging that the triad is relatively rare in adolescent girls and young women, and that participation in athletics has benefits as well as risks for bone health, in 2007 the ACSM recast the female athlete triad to describe the interrelatedness of energy availability (dietary energy intake minus physical activity energy expenditure), menstrual function, and BMD, emphasizing that all three exist along a spectrum from deleterious to optimal.[18] While some athletes may intentionally limit their dietary intake, other athletes may have inadequate intake because they do not recognize the amount of energy required for intense physical activity.

Evaluation and Treatment

The first step in addressing hypothalamic amenorrhea/oligomenorrhea in female athletes is to detect it. The PPE history form has three questions to screen for menstrual irregularity. Clinicians caring for AYAs should obtain a comprehensive menstrual history, considering the many causes of amenorrhea/oligomenorrhea in this population. A thorough evaluation is important because the diagnosis of hypothalamic amenorrhea associated with inadequate caloric intake in the context of exercise (athletic energy deficit) is essentially a diagnosis of exclusion.

If a diagnosis of hypothalamic amenorrhea or oligomenorrhea associated with athletic energy deficit is made, reductions in training intensity and/or enhanced caloric intake are warranted. Amenorrheic athletes who gain weight through reduced training and improved diet may resume menses spontaneously and their BMD may increase. If the athlete has disordered eating or an eating disorder, then treatment should include coordinated medical, nutritional, and psychological therapy.

Changes in nutritional intake and exercise should be made in consultation with a dietitian and should seek to correct the energy deficit. An individualized approach is necessary given that there is variability in healthy body weight ranges and in the sensitivity of the hypothalamic–pituitary–ovarian axis to energy deficit and weight loss. If the athlete is <85% of her estimated healthy body weight, she should not exercise unless she is eumenorrheic and her weight is increasing weekly.

Appropriate Follow-up: The athlete should be assessed weekly until weight increases consistently. The visits can then be reduced to once every 2 weeks assuming the patient's weight continues to trend toward the estimated healthy body weight. The support of the coach is essential. Permission to collaborate with the athlete's coach and athletic trainers should be sought from the athlete and/or her caregivers when appropriate.

Evaluating BMD: A dilemma for practicing clinicians who care for this population is the indications for and utility of testing for BMD. Populations at risk for impairments in skeletal health, including AYAs with frank eating disorders and/or amenorrhea, are discussed elsewhere in this text. In 2007, the International Society for Clinical Densitometry developed guidelines to help identify children and adolescents who might warrant skeletal assessment by dual emission x-ray absorptiometry (DXA). These guidelines defined "clinically significant fractures" as:

- Any long bone fracture of the lower extremities
- Vertebral compression fractures
- Two or more long bone fractures of the upper extremities

The guidelines did not specifically address stress fractures,[19] which may be an indicator of low BMD. Although stress fractures

sustained with greater than 12 to 16 hours of weekly moderate-to-vigorous physical activity may represent fatigue failure of structurally normal bone, the following factors should increase suspicion for skeletal insufficiency and prompt consideration of DXA scanning:

- Family history of osteoporosis, osteopenia, or low BMD in first- or second-degree relatives
- Other comorbidities known to decrease BMD
- Any stress fracture of the upper extremity in an athlete who does not impact load the upper extremities. Only gymnasts and cheerleaders commonly perform maneuvers that load their arms in this way.
- Vertebral compression fractures
- Two or more stress fractures in the lower extremity
- Fractures in bones with a high proportion of cancellous bone, such as the
  - Calcaneus
  - Tarsal navicular
  - Talus
  - Femoral neck
  - Pelvic ring and sacrum
  - Pars interarticularis of the vertebral bodies (acquired spondylolysis)

Identification of low BMD requires a densitometrist skilled in the interpretation of DXA scans in children, adolescents, and young adults. Further evaluation of low BMD is described elsewhere in this text.

Calcium and vitamin D intake: Athletes, like all adolescent females, have a recommended daily intake of 1,300 to 1,800 mg of elemental calcium and at least 600 IU of vitamin D. It should be noted that in a cohort of healthy adolescents, longitudinal changes in BMD did not correlate with calcium intake, which ranged from 500 to 1,500 mg/day.[20]

HOW TO PRESCRIBE ATHLETIC ACTIVITY

Healthy People 2020 identifies improving "health, fitness, and quality of life through daily physical activity" as an overarching goal, with the following specific objectives (*Physical Activity Guidelines for Americans*, www.health.gov/PAGuidelines):

Reduce the proportion of adults who engage in no leisure-time physical activity

Increase the proportion of adults who meet current Federal physical activity guidelines for aerobic physical activity and for muscle-strengthening activity

- For substantial health benefits, adults should do at least 150 minutes (2 hours and 30 minutes) a week of moderate-intensity, or 75 minutes (1 hour and 15 minutes) a week of vigorous-intensity aerobic physical activity, or an equivalent combination of moderate- and vigorous-intensity aerobic activity. Aerobic activity should be performed in episodes of at least 10 minutes, and preferably, it should be spread throughout the week.
- For additional and more extensive health benefits, adults should increase their aerobic physical activity to 300 minutes (5 hours) a week of moderate-intensity, or 150 minutes a week of vigorous-intensity aerobic physical activity, or an equivalent combination of moderate- and vigorous-intensity activity. Additional health benefits are gained by engaging in physical activity beyond this amount.
- Adults should also do muscle-strengthening activities that are moderate or high intensity and involve all major muscle groups on 2 or more days a week, as these activities provide additional health benefits.

Increase the proportion of adolescents who meet current Federal physical activity guidelines for aerobic physical activity and for muscle-strengthening activity from 18.4% in 2009 to at least 20.2%

- Children and adolescents should do 60 minutes (1 hour) or more of physical activity daily.
  - Aerobic: Most of the 60 or more minutes a day should be either moderate- or vigorous-intensity aerobic physical activity, and should include vigorous-intensity physical activity at least 3 days a week.
  - Muscle-strengthening: As part of their 60 or more minutes of daily physical activity, children and adolescents should include muscle-strengthening physical activity on at least 3 days of the week.
  - Bone-strengthening: As part of their 60 or more minutes of daily physical activity, children and adolescents should include bone-strengthening physical activity on at least 3 days of the week.
- It is important to encourage young people to participate in physical activities that are appropriate for their age, that are enjoyable, and that offer variety.

Physical activity is defined as any bodily movement produced by skeletal muscles, which results in energy expenditure above the basal level. Exercise is physical activity that is planned, structured, repetitive, and purposeful in the sense that improvement in components of physical fitness and conditioning is the objective. Prescribing exercise entails specifying frequency, intensity, time, and type of athletic activity (FITT).

Physical Fitness and Conditioning

Fitness has four principal components:

1. Body composition
2. Cardiovascular fitness—maximum oxygen consumption (Vo_2 max) being the gold standard
3. Strength
4. Flexibility

Body Composition

Although a common notion is that the fitness of today's youth is poor, the only component of fitness that has been documented to have declined in the past three decades is body composition: Obesity has increased among AYAs.

With respect to reducing obesity while promoting nutritional adequacy for growth, adolescents need both reduced caloric intake and increased energy expenditure. Unfortunately, dieting often receives more attention in popular media than exercise.

Cardiovascular Fitness

If the goal is to improve cardiovascular fitness, a recommended training program should include *aerobic exercise* (continuous large muscle contractions that involve maintenance of 50% to 85% of the maximum heart rate) for more than 30 minutes, at least three or four times a week.

As an alternative to a structured exercise program that may hold little appeal for some sedentary AYAs, there has been increasing advocacy for a lifestyle approach to increasing activity. The objective is to incorporate moderate physical activity into the lifestyle of those who are sedentary. The Centers for Disease Control and Prevention and the ACSM guidelines recommend moderate-intensity physical activity on most days—either in a single session or in accumulated multiple bouts, each lasting 8 to 10 minutes.[21] This includes common activities such as climbing stairs (rather than taking the elevator), brisk walking, doing more house and yard work, and engaging in active recreational pursuits.

For those who desire more intensive training, an exercise prescription should be tailored to the AYA current level of fitness, desired level of fitness, motivation, and discipline to adhere to a training regime. More detailed goals and practical suggestions for reaching them can be found in the *Physical Activity Guide for All Americans* and the *Bright Futures in Practice: Physical Activity Online Guide* (http://www.brightfutures.org/physicalactivity).

Muscle-Strengthening

Regarding strength training, it is established that prepubescent and pubescent subjects, such as adults, can increase strength safely by resistance training. The training program should include close adult supervision, a PPE, and the use of well-maintained equipment (including sturdy shoes). Resistance training is associated with strength gains and neuromuscular adaptation in *preadolescents*, but it is not associated with muscle hypertrophy. Short-term resistance training has no effect on somatic growth or body composition and is not associated with increased injury rate or recovery or improved sports performance. Muscle hypertrophy will occur with resistance training in pubertal subjects. The AAP endorses strength training for children and adolescents, if done properly[22]; a suggested resistance training program could include the following:

1. Establish a 10-repetition maximum (i.e., the maximum weight that can be lifted 10 times), called the *10-rep max*.
2. To start resistance training, perform one set of 10 repetitions at 50% to 75% of the 10-rep max.
3. Then perform a second set of 10 repetitions at 75% of the 10-rep max.
4. Perform a third set at 100% of the 10-rep max, doing as many repetitions as possible.

When 15 repetitions are easily performed during the third set, the weight can be increased by no more than 10% each week. The weight should be lifted through the entire ROM of the joint to avoid loss of flexibility. Warm-up and cooldown periods, which could include stretching exercises, should accompany each session. Three sessions per week on alternate days is all that is recommended, allowing for a day of rest in between weight training sessions. *One-repetition maximum weight lifting should be avoided because it is a mechanism of injury.* Gains in strength from resistance training are more resistant to detraining than are gains in aerobic fitness, with up to 50% of the strength capacity retained for 1 year or longer in a person who is no longer training.

Bone-Strengthening

Adolescence is a particularly important time window for increasing lifelong BMD, with peak bone mass achieved by the early 20s and 50% of all calcium accrued in the skeleton in the 2 years before and after peak height velocity. Impact loading physical activity is the most significant modifiable factor for improving BMD. For developing bone, choose weight- or load-bearing activities such as running and jumping. Skeletal response is greatest at the sites of maximal stress; so adolescents should vary targets and perform activities that increase muscle strength in all or many muscle groups. Training stimulus must be greater than level habitually encountered and deconditioning is rapid; even brief daily weight-bearing can help reduce bone loss.

In terms of an exercise prescription,[23]

Frequency = numerous distributed sessions over the day are better than one prolonged bout, at least 3 days/week
Intensity: High strain rates (running and jumping) are more effective than low-intensity endurance exercises such as walking, biking, or swimming
Time: Durations of 10 to 20 minutes are effective
Type: No clear optimum recommendation

Flexibility

There is no study demonstrating that stretching in healthy, previously uninjured subjects prevents injuries. However, improving flexibility and strength in previously injured athletes decreases the likelihood of subsequent injuries. Flexibility programs for injured joints should not cause discomfort. If a healthy adolescent or young adult desires a stretching program, yoga classes, DVDs, or online instruction are good options.

AYAs with Special Health Care Needs

In addition to identifying the sports appropriate for the adolescent or young adult with special health care needs, the physician should assess current physical fitness activities for these young people. If the fitness activities are inadequate, and the individual and family are interested in more sports or fitness opportunities, the clinician should write an exercise prescription for more fitness activities. The clinician may decide to refer the adolescent or young adult to a physical therapist, physiatrist, exercise physiologist, or sports medicine clinic to design appropriate fitness activities. This should be done in conjunction with the youth's subspecialty clinicians. Youth with special health care needs may have limited access to exercise facilities, and health care providers should advocate on their behalf.

Avoiding Overuse and Burnout

Clinicians prescribing athletic activity must counsel the adolescent or young adult to avoid overuse injuries, which can undermine efforts to achieve greater physical fitness. The 2011 consensus panel failed to identify specific anatomic risk factors for injury. In addition to quality PPEs and expanded and improved injury surveillance systems, recommendations focus on limiting total training volumes (duration and intensity) by

- Starting a general fitness program at least 2 months before any competitive athletic seasons
- Increasing total volume of athletic activity by no more than 10% in any given week
- Limiting total athletic activity to no more than 12 to 16 hours per week. Some authorities suggest that the maximum hours per week should be the same as age in years.
- Participating in a variety of structured and unstructured athletic activities over the year
- Participating in only 1 structured athletic activity at a time
- Ensuring at least 1 to 2 days off each week from structured athletic activities
- Ensuring at least 2 to 3 months off each year from structured athletic activities

The latter four points are referred to as "delaying specialization" by the AAP.[24] These are among the strategies to decrease overtraining syndrome or "burnout, a series of psychological, physiologic, and hormonal changes that result in decreased sports performance." In young adults, burnout may present as chronic muscle or joint pain, personality changes, and elevated resting heart rate. In younger adolescents, burnout may present as fatigue, lack of enthusiasm about practice or competition, or difficulty with successfully completing usual routines.

📶 **ADDITIONAL RESOURCES AND WEBSITES ONLINE**

REFERENCES

1. Drake KM, Beach ML, Longacre MR, et al. Influence of sports, physical education, and active commuting to school on adolescent weight status. *Pediatrics* 2012;130(2):e296–e304.
2. Sabo DF, Miller KE, Farrell MP, et al. High school athletic participation, sexual behavior and adolescent pregnancy: a regional study. *J Adolesc Health* 1999;25(3):207–216.
3. Valovich McLeod TC, Decoster LC, Loud KJ, et al. National Athletic Trainers' Association Position Statement: prevention of pediatric overuse injuries. *J Athl Train* 2011;46(2):206–220.
4. American Academy of Family Physicians, American Academy of Pediatrics, American College of Sports Medicine, American Orthopedic Society for Sports Medicine and the American Osteopathic Academy of Sports Medicine. *Preparticipation physical evaluation.* 4th ed. Elk Grove, IL: American Academy of Pediatrics, 2010.
5. Maron BJ, Mitten Matthew J, Quandt EF, et al. Competitive athletes with cardiovascular disease: the case of Nicholas Knapp. *N Engl J Med* 1998;339:1634.
6. Maron BJ, Zipes DP. 36th Bethesda Conference. Eligibility recommendations for competitive athletes with cardiovascular abnormalities. *J Am Coll Cardiol* 2005;45:1313.
7. Pfister GC, Puffer JC, Maron BJ. Preparticipation cardiovascular screening for U.S. collegiate student-athletes. *JAMA* 2000;283:1597.
8. Bundy DG, Feudtner CF. Preparticipation physical evaluations for high school athletes: time for a new game plan. *Ambul Pediatr* 2004;4:260.
9. LaBella CR, Hennrikus W, Hewett TE. Anterior cruciate ligament injuries: diagnosis, treatment, and prevention. *Pediatrics* 2014;133;e1437–e1450.
10. American Academy of Pediatrics, Committee on Sports Medicine and Fitness. Athletic participation by children and adolescents who have systemic hypertension. *Pediatrics* 2010;125:1287–1294.
11. McGrory PR, Johnston K, Meeuwisse W, et al. Summary and agreement statement of the 2nd International Conference on Concussion in Sport, Prague 2004. *Br J Sports Med* 2005;39:196–204.
12. Aaron DJ, Dearwater SR, Anderson R, et al. Physical activity and the initiation on high-risk health behaviors in adolescents. *Med Sci Sports Exerc* 1995;27:1639.
13. Ewing BT. High school athletes and marijuana use. *J Drug Educ* 1998;28:147.
14. American Academy of Pediatrics, Committee on Nutrition and the Council on Sports Medicine and Fitness. Sports drinks and energy drinks for children and adolescents: are they appropriate? *Pediatrics* 2011;127:1182–1189.
15. Buckley WE, Yesalis CE, Friedl KE. Estimated prevalence of anabolic steroid use among male high school seniors. *JAMA* 1988;260:3441.
16. Johnston LD, O'Malley PM, Bachman JG, et al. *Monitoring the future national survey results on drug use, 1975–2005: Volume I, secondary school students* (NIH Publication No. 06–5883). Bethesda, MD: National Institute on Drug Abuse, 2006.
17. Nichols JF, Rauh MJ, Lawson MJ, et al. Prevalence of the female athlete triad syndrome among high school athletes. *Arch Pediatr Adolesc Med* 2006;160:137.
18. Nattiv A, Loucks AB, Manore MM, et al. American College of Sports Medicine position stand: the Female Athlete Triad. *Med Sci Sports and Exerc* 2007;39:1867–1882.
19. Bianchi ML, Baim S, Bishop NJ, et al. Official positions of the International Society for Clinical Densitometry (ISCD) on DXA evaluation in children and adolescents. *Pediatr Nephrol* 2010;25(1):37–47.
20. Lloyd T, Chinchilli VM, Hohnson-Rollings N, et al. Adult female hip bone density reflects teenage sports-exercise patterns but not teenage calcium intake. *Pediatrics* 2000;106:40.
21. Pate RR, Pratt M, Blair SN, et al. Physical activity and public health: a recommendation from the Centers for Disease Control and Prevention and the American College of Sports Medicine. *JAMA* 1995;273:402.
22. American Academy of Pediatrics, Committee on Sports Medicine and Fitness. Strength training by children and adolescents. *Pediatrics* 2008;121:835–840.
23. Kohrt WM, Bloomfield SA, Little KD, et al. American College of Sports Medicine position stand: physical activity and bone health. *Med Sci Sports Exerc* 2004;36(11):1985–1996.
24. Brenner JS; American Academy of Pediatrics Council on Sports Medicine and Fitness. Overuse injuries, overtraining, and burnout in child and adolescent athletes. *Pediatrics* 2007;119:1242–1245.

CHAPTER 20

Concussion

Michael A. Beasley
Cynthia J. Stein
William P. Meehan III

DEFINITION

Concussion has been known by many names, including mild traumatic brain injury (TBI) and *commotio cerebri*. In 2001, the Concussion in Sports Group created a broad definition of concussion at the 1st International Symposium on Concussion in Sport.[1] This definition has been revised in subsequent meetings, culminating in the current definition of concussion from the 4th International Conference in 2012:[2]

Concussion is a complex, pathophysiological process affecting the brain, induced by biomechanical forces. Several common features that incorporate clinical, pathologic, and biomechanical injury constructs that may be utilized in defining the nature of a concussive head injury include:

1. Concussion may be caused either by a direct blow to the head, face, neck, or elsewhere on the body with an "impulsive" force transmitted to the head.
2. Concussion typically results in the rapid onset of short-lived impairment of neurological function that resolves spontaneously. However, in some cases, symptoms and signs may evolve over a number of minutes to hours.
3. Concussion may result in neuropathological changes, but the acute clinical symptoms largely reflect a functional disturbance rather than a structural injury and, as such, no abnormality is seen on standard structural neuroimaging studies.
4. Concussion results in a graded set of clinical symptoms that may or may not involve loss of consciousness (LOC). Resolution of the clinical and cognitive symptoms typically follows a sequential course. However, it is important to note that in some cases symptoms may be prolonged.

PATHOPHYSIOLOGY

An important aspect of this definition is the recognition of concussion as primarily a *functional*, rather than a structural injury.

While the pathophysiology of concussion is incompletely understood, an underlying "acute metabolic cascade" has been suggested.[3] According to the current hypothesis, mechanical forces from rotational injury cause disruptive stretching of axons and neuronal cell membranes. A variety of changes have been described, including cell depolarization, ionic shifts, release of neurotransmitters, alteration of glucose metabolism, and changes in blood flow patterns. Although concussion grading scales were used extensively in the past, their reliance on LOC and amnesia at the time of injury had little prognostic value. Therefore, grading scales have been abandoned, and replaced by more individualized assessment and management.[1,4]

EPIDEMIOLOGY

Over the last decade, there has been an increase in the percentage of high school students participating in team sports,[5] with a concurrent increase in reported concussions sustained by both high school and collegiate athletes.[6] From 2001 to 2009, emergency department (ED) visits for sports and recreation-related (including falls due to skateboarding, bicycling, etc.) TBIs sustained by those aged 19 and younger rose by 62%.[7] However, there was no significant rise in hospitalizations from these ED visits. The increase in ED visits is likely related to both true incidence of concussion as well as heightened awareness leading to increased reporting and diagnosis.[7,8] The Centers for Disease Control and Prevention (CDC) estimates that as many as 3.8 million sport-related TBIs occur each year in the US.[9] Concussion represents between 9% and 15% of all high school sport-related injuries and over 90% of injuries to the head and face.[10,11] However, studies show that as many as 47% of high school athletes fail to report concussions.[12] In collegiate sports, concussion has been reported as 5.8% of all injuries,[10] with one study of NCAA Division I football players showing 23.4% of players indicating that they did not intend to report potential concussion symptoms.[13]

Sports and recreational activities are a common cause of head injury throughout childhood, adolescence, and into young adulthood.[7]

- For male high school athletes, football, ice hockey, and lacrosse have the highest incidences of concussion.
- For female high school athletes, the risk is highest in lacrosse, soccer, and field hockey.[14]
- Rates of concussion tend to be higher in collegiate sports than in high school sports.
- American football produces the largest overall number of concussions because of its large number of participants and frequent collisions.[7,11]

- Concussion generally occurs more often in competition than in practice.[6]
- Player–player contact is the most common mechanism of sport-related concussions (SRCs), representing 70%, followed by player–surface contact and player–equipment contact.[14]

While males suffer a greater overall number of sports- and recreation-related TBIs,[6] some studies suggest that females may be at higher risk for diagnosis of concussion in gender-comparable sports, such as soccer and basketball.[6,11,14] It has also been reported that female athletes have a larger number and greater severity of symptoms after injury, in addition to an increased risk of prolonged recovery.[15] A variety of hypotheses have been proposed to explain these findings, such as increased vulnerability for females due to smaller head size, weaker neck muscles, or limited dynamic head and neck stabilization compared to male athletes.[16] Increased reporting among female athletes has also been proposed as an explanation; however, this would not account for the greater deficits seen on neuropsychological testing observed in female athletes after concussion.[15]

DIAGNOSIS

As concussion is primarily a functional injury, the diagnosis remains clinical. The variability of concussion symptoms makes concussion a difficult and sometimes controversial diagnosis (Table 20.1).

- The most common symptom of concussion, both acutely and chronically, is headache.
- Dizziness or imbalance, cognitive slowing, difficulty concentrating, and fatigue are all reported by a majority of concussed athletes.[11,17]
- LOC and amnesia have previously been emphasized in the evaluation of concussion, but have been proven only to occur in a minority (4% and 24%, respectively) of SRCs.[11,17]
- Because LOC and amnesia are uncommon, concussions are often overlooked.

On-Field Assessment

Any athlete suspected of having sustained a concussion should be immediately removed from play. Initial evaluation should include assessment of airway, breathing, and heart function followed by an examination for cervical spine injury. If cervical spine injury cannot be ruled out, the athlete should be immobilized and transferred to an advanced emergency center immediately. A thorough neurological screening exam is necessary to rule out critical injury such as intracranial bleeding. After emergent cervical or neurological injury has been addressed or ruled out, the athlete should be evaluated further for concussion off the field. In the setting of confirmed or presumed concussion, the athlete should not be allowed to return to play on the same day and should be monitored for potential deterioration.[15]

Sideline Assessment

Several sideline tools have been developed to help evaluate signs and symptoms of concussion. The most recent Sport Concussion Assessment Tool (SCAT), the SCAT3™, was released as part of the consensus statement from the 4th International Conference on Concussion in Sport.[2] Previous editions of the SCAT had limited applicability in younger athletes; thus, the Child-SCAT3, designated for athletes 5 to 12 years old, was published simultaneously with the SCAT3 for athletes aged 13 or older.[2] Printable forms of both the SCAT3 (http://bjsm.bmj.com/content/47/5/259.full.pdf) and Child-SCAT3 (http://bjsm.bmj.com/content/47/5/263.full.pdf) are available online. The SCAT3 and similar tools are not designed to exclude or confirm the diagnosis of concussion independent of clinical judgment; thorough clinical evaluation remains necessary to properly assess a suspected concussion. Utilizing pre-injury or baseline scores for comparison may improve their use.[18]

Advanced Diagnostics

Standard imaging like computed tomography and magnetic resonance imaging (MRI) does not establish or exclude the diagnosis of concussion, but may help rule out structural injury (e.g., skull fractures, intracranial bleeding). Advanced imaging techniques like functional MRI, diffusion tensor imaging, and MR spectroscopy are being studied and may represent the future of concussion imaging. Similarly, standard electroencephalography (EEG) has been of limited use in concussion, but computer-aided analysis in quantitative EEG has shown promise.[19]

The use of accelerometers on sporting equipment has gained interest. While clinical "thresholds" for the force or acceleration required for concussion have not been established, collective data may someday prove useful in tracking the cumulative forces or "hit count" throughout an athlete's season or career.[20,21]

With increased availability of computerized assessments, the use of neurocognitive testing has grown dramatically. These tests allow for standardized, objective measures, which can be monitored over time and injury, and may detect decreased cognitive function even after self-reported resolution of symptoms.[22] These assessments, however, should only be used as an adjunct to a comprehensive concussion evaluation, and should be interpreted by

---

TABLE 20.1

Common Signs and Symptoms of Concussion

Physical	Cognitive	Emotional	Sleep
Headache	Feeling "foggy"	Irritable	Drowsiness
Nausea	Feeling "slowed down"	Sadness	Sleeping more than usual
Vomiting	Difficulty concentrating	More emotional	Sleeping less than usual
Balance problems	Difficulty remembering	Nervousness	Difficulty falling asleep
Dizziness	Forgets recent information		
Visual problems	Confusion		
Fatigue	Answers questions repeatedly		
Sensitivity to light	Confusion		
Sensitivity to noise	Answers questions slowly		
Numbness/tingling	Repeats questions		
Dazed			
Stunned			

Reprinted from Harmon KG, Drezner J, Gammons M, et al. American Medical Society for Sports Medicine position statement: concussion in sport. *Br J Sports Med* 2013;47(1):15–26, with permission.

health care professionals who have experience with their use and limitations. While neuropsychological testing has gained popularity and is now used frequently at the professional, collegiate, and youth levels, it should not be used as a stand-alone tool for diagnosis or for clearance.

 ## MANAGEMENT

The majority (80% to 90%) of concussions among adolescents and young adults (AYAs) resolve within 7 to 10 days, and well over 90% resolve within the first 4 weeks.[2,11,23] Therefore, the management of concussion typically involves supportive care and management of symptoms. This begins with educating the adolescent or young adult and family on the pathophysiology, natural history, and management of concussion, including current knowledge of potential short- and long-term effects of concussion. Physical and cognitive rest is the mainstay of therapy.[1,2] Current recommendations support a gradual return to both physical and cognitive activity after a brief period of near-complete rest, with activity remaining below the level of symptom exacerbation.[2,24,25]

Return to Play

Adolescents or young adults diagnosed with a concussion should not return to play on the day of the injury.[2,15] Once symptoms have resolved, a graduated return-to-play protocol can be used to progressively test the athlete with additional activity (**Table 20.2**).[2] Each stage requires a minimum of 24 hours, and if symptoms recur, the young person should return to the preceding symptom-free level for at least 24 hours before attempting to progress. In more prolonged recoveries and when caring for younger patients, longer symptom-free waiting periods between stages may be prudent.

Return to Academics

After a concussion, AYA students may have difficulty with cognitive activity and academic work. Symptoms and cognitive dysfunction

TABLE 20.2

Recommended Graduated Return-to-Play Protocol

Stage	Functional Exercise	Objective
1. No activity	Symptom limited physical and cognitive rest	Recovery
2. Light aerobic exercise	Walking, swimming, stationary bike Intensity <70% max heart rate No resistance training	Increase heart rate
3. Sport-specific exercise	Hockey—skating drills Soccer—running drills No head impact activities	Add movement
4. Noncontact training drills	More complex training drill; e.g., passing drills in football/hockey Begin progressive resistance training	Exercise, coordination, and cognitive load
5. Full-contact practice	Only after clearance in normal training	Restore confidence Assess functional skills
6. Return to play	Normal game play	

Reprinted from McCrory P, Meeuwisse WH, Aubry M, et al. Consensus statement on concussion in sport: the 4th International Conference on Concussion in Sport held in Zurich, November 2012. *Br J Sports Med* 2013;47:250–258, with permission.

are often magnified by the fatigue and sleep disturbances associated with concussion. When students are able to return to classes, they may require academic accommodations.[26] AYA students who have prolonged symptoms (>3 to 4 weeks) may benefit from a more formalized return strategy such as an individualized education plan or 504 plan, a federally recognized plan in public schooling systems designed to accommodate students with disabilities. Sports participation, full physical activity, and extracurricular activities are not recommended until the adolescent or young adult has returned to full academics at their baseline level of performance.[26] The American Academy of Pediatrics Councils on Sports Medicine and Fitness and School Health have developed recommendations for the return to learning.[26] Additionally, the CDC provides free online resources for students, parents, school officials, and managing health care professionals.

Pharmacologic Therapy

Medication use in the management of concussion is typically directed at alleviating symptoms, rather than treating the underlying pathophysiology. Initially, patients are managed solely with physical and cognitive rest. For those who suffer symptoms beyond the first few weeks, treatment for headaches, sleep disturbance, dizziness, and cognitive function are considered.[27,28] While acetaminophen may offer headache and pain relief, nonsteroidal anti-inflammatories are generally not recommended because of theoretical increased bleeding risk.[15] Patients with underlying secondary diagnoses (e.g., migraines, anxiety, sleep disturbance) are more likely to benefit from treatment of these specific disorders.[24] There is limited evidence for use of medications to treat concussion symptoms; these are typically experimental or "off-label" uses.[2,15] Medication should be reserved for adolescents or young adults with prolonged recoveries, whose symptoms are negatively impacting their quality of life, and should be administered by clinicians experienced in concussion management. Any patient being considered for return to play should be symptom-free while off of any medications initiated to treat symptoms believed to be solely concussion-related.[2,15,24] Anxiety, depression, and other mood disturbances may occur after a concussion as symptoms of the injury, an exacerbation of underlying disturbance, or adjustment reaction to the limitations associated with injury. Standard therapies aimed at these symptoms may benefit patients, especially those with prolonged recoveries.[2,15,24]

 ## COMPLICATIONS AND CHRONIC EFFECTS

There is growing concern that sustaining multiple concussions may lead to devastating effects, both acutely and in the long term. What was once thought to be a self-limited, mild injury has now been linked to increased risk of additional injury and chronic changes, including cognitive impairment, dementia, mood disorders, and memory difficulties. While uncommon for amateur athletes, the potential risk of these complications must be made clear to athletes who have suffered multiple concussions as they consider return to sport.

Second Impact Syndrome

Described in 1984 after the death of a 19-year-old football player,[29] second impact syndrome refers to a catastrophic injury involving an athlete who, while still suffering symptoms from an initial concussion, receives a secondary injury to the head. The secondary injuries may not be severe, and may involve blows to the chest or trunk with forces transmitted to the brain.[30] After this secondary injury, a loss of autoregulation of cerebral blood flow is believed to cause rapid vascular engorgement, increased intracranial pressure, herniation of the uncus of the temporal lobe or cerebellar tonsils, and eventual coma or death.[15,30] There is some debate about whether these cases may require only a single blow and represent malignant cerebral edema, a separate pathophysiology causing diffuse cerebral swelling.[15] Regardless of the specific diagnosis, the risk of severe injury while symptomatic from concussion is a major reason for the recommendation to restrict athletes from returning to play until they are entirely asymptomatic.

Chronic Traumatic Encephalopathy

Chronic traumatic encephalopathy (CTE) describes the pathology found in cases of retired professional athletes who developed emotional, cognitive, and somatic problems.[31,32] CTE represents a tauopathy (type of neurodegenerative disease) resulting in early onset of neuropsychiatric and behavioral syndromes with progression to gait disorders, slowed speech, and extrapyramidal signs.[31] While the association between recurrent head injury and the pathology of CTE appears clear, a true causal relationship remains to be proven. Current evidence consists of case reports and may be affected by confounding variables. The consensus statement from the 4th International Conference on Concussion in Sport called on clinicians to inform families of potential long-term effects of concussion, but to remain cautious of interpreting causation in CTE.[2]

Disqualification and Retirement from Sport

There are no evidence-based guidelines for clinicians to recommend disqualification or retirement from sport, nor is there an accepted number of concussions prohibiting further participation. Because of variability in symptoms, recovery time, exposure risk, and acceptance of risk by the patient or family, retirement or disqualification must be individualized to the athlete.

PREVENTION

Advanced personal protection, rule changes, and legislation have all been proposed as potential methods of preventing SRCs and their sequelae. Although critical in prevention of structural injuries, there is no reliable evidence that protective equipment in the form of helmets or mouth guards prevents SRCs.[33] Moreover, there are concerns that the use of protective equipment may provide a false sense of protection, leading to an increase in dangerous behavior.[15]

Reducing forces to the head by strengthening the neck and shoulder musculature has been proposed as a possible preventative measure. While no studies have shown a clear decreased risk of SRC associated with a strengthening program, overall neck strength has been shown to be at least a predictor of concussion.[34] Additionally, concussion frequently occurs when an athlete is unaware of, or unable to brace for the oncoming impact, which may limit the usefulness of any gains made from neck strengthening. Collision anticipation itself, however, is associated with a decreased risk of concussion.[35,36] Rule changes to minimize high-risk situations in sport may reduce concussion rates. Limiting exposure to collision certainly has potential to reduce injury, and many sports are currently decreasing the number of full-contact practices in an effort to minimize SRC. Consistent enforcement of rule changes is imperative for them to be effective.

CONCLUSION

Sports-related concussions are common in AYA sports. While most recover quickly and without complication, some suffer prolonged recovery. Any adolescent or young adult suspected of having a concussion should be removed from play immediately and should be evaluated and cleared by a medical professional before return to play is allowed. The foundation of concussion management is physical and cognitive rest, but a variety of other treatment options are available when needed. Research is ongoing to identify improved methods of preventing, diagnosing, and treating concussion.

REFERENCES

1. Aubry M, Cantu R, Dvorak J, et al. Summary and agreement statement of the 1st International Symposium on Concussion in Sport, Vienna 2001. *Clin J Sport Med* 2002;12:6–11.
2. McCrory P, Meeuwisse WH, Aubry M, et al. Consensus statement on concussion in sport: the 4th International Conference on Concussion in Sport held in Zurich, November 2012. *Br J Sports Med* 2013;47:250–258.
3. Shrey DW, Griesbach GS, Giza CC. The pathophysiology of concussion in youth. *Phys Med Rehabil Clin N Am* 2011;22(4):577–602.
4. Halstead ME, Walter KD, the Council on Sports Medicine and Fitness. Sport-related concussion in children and adolescents. *Pediatrics* 2010;126(3):597–615.
5. Center for Disease Control and Prevention. Youth risk behavior surveillance—United States, 2011. *MMWR* 2012;61(4).
6. Daneshvar DH, Nowinski CJ, McKee A, et al. The epidemiology of sport-related concussion. *Clin J Sports Med* 2011;30(1):1–17.
7. Gilchrist J, Thomas KE, Xu L, et al. Nonfatal traumatic brain injuries related to sports and recreation activities among persons aged ≤19 years—United States, 2001–2009. *MMWR* 2011;60(39):1337–1342.
8. Bakhos LL, Lockhart GR, Myers R, et al. Emergency department visits for concussion in young child athletes. *Pediatrics* 2010;126(3):e550–e556.
9. Centers for Disease Control and Prevention. Nonfatal traumatic brain injuries from sports and recreation activities—United States 2001–2005. *MMWR* 2007;56:733–737.
10. Gessel LM, Fields SK, Collins CL, et al. Concussions among United States High School and Collegiate Athletes. *J Athl Train* 2007;42(4):495–503.
11. Meehan WP III, d'Hemecourt P, Collins CL, et al. Assessment and management of sport-related concussions in United States high schools. *Am J Sports Med* 2011;39(11):2304–2310.
12. McCrea M, Hammeke T, Olsen G, et al. Unreported concussion in high school football players: implication for prevention. *Clin J Sports Med* 2004;14:13–17.
13. Baugh CM, Kiernan PT, Kroshus E, et al. Frequency of head impact related outcomes by position in NCAA Division I collegiate football players. *J Neurotrauma* 2015;32(5):314–326.
14. Marar M, McIlvain NM, Fields SK, et al. Epidemiology of concussions among United States high school athletes in 20 sports. *Am J Sports Med* 2012;40(4):747–755.
15. Harmon, KG, Drezner J, Gammons M, et al. American Medical Society for Sports Medicine position statement: concussion in sport. *Br J Sports Med* 2013;47(1):15–26.
16. Tierney RT, Sitler MR, Swanik B, et al. Gender differences in head-neck segment dynamic stabilization during head acceleratin. *Med Sci Sports Exerc* 2005;37:272–279.
17. Guskiewicz KM, McCrea M, Marshall SW, et al. Cumulative effects associated with recurrent concussion in collegiate football players: the NCAA Concussion Study. *JAMA* 2003;290(19):2549–2555.
18. Guskiewicz KM, Register-Mihalik J, McCrory P, et al. Evidence-based approach to revisiting the SCAT2: introducing the SCAT3. *Br J Sports Med* 2013;47:289–293.
19. Arciniegas DB. Clinical eletrophysiologic assessments and mild traumatic brain injury: state-of-the-science and implications for clinical practice. *Int J Psychophysiol* 2011;82:41–52.
20. Kutcher JS, McCrory P, Davis G, et al. What evidence exists for new strategies or technologies in the diagnosis of sports concussion and assessment of recovery? *Br J Sports Med* 2013;47:299–303.
21. Greenwald RM, Chu JJ, Beckwith JG, et al. A proposed method to reduce under-reporting of brain injury in sports. *Clin J Sports Med* 2012;22:83–85.
22. Lovell MR, Collins MW, Iverson GL, et al. Recovery from mild concussion in high school athletes. *J Neurosurg* 2003;98(2):296–301.
23. Meehan WP III, d'Hemecourt P, Comstock RD. High school concussions in the 2008–2009 academic year: mechanism, symptoms, and management. *Am J Sports Med* 2010;38(12):2405–2409.
24. Schneider KJ, Iverson GL, Emery CA, et al. The effects of rest and treatment following sports-related concussion: a systematic review of the literature. *Br J Sports Med* 2013;47:304–307.
25. Brown NJ, Mannix RC, O'Brien MJ, et al. Effect of cognitive activity level on duration of post-concussion symptoms. *Pediatrics* 2014;133(2):1–6.
26. Halstead ME, McAvoy K, Devore CE, et al. Returning to learning following a concussion. *Pediatrics* 2013;132(5):948–957.
27. Kinnaman KA, Mannix RC, Comstock RD, et al. Management strategies and medication use for treating paediatric patients with concussions. *Acta Paediatr* 2013;102(9):e424–e428.
28. Meehan WP III, Mannix RC, O'Brien MJ, et al. The prevalence of undiagnosed concussion in athletes. *Clin J Sports Med* 2013;23:339–342.
29. Saunders RL, Harbaugh RE. The second impact in catastrophic contact-sports head trauma. *JAMA* 1984;252(4):538–539.
30. Cantu RC, Gean AD. Second-impact syndrome and a small subdural hematoma: an uncommon catastrophic result of repetitive head injury with a characteristic imaging appearance. *J Neurotrauma* 2010;27(9):1557–1564.
31. McCrory P, Meeuwisse WH, Kutcher JS, et al. What is the evidence for chronic concussion-related changes in retired athletes: behavioural, pathological and clinical outcomes? *Br J Sports Med* 2013;47:327–330.
32. McKee AC, Cantu RC, Nowinski CK, et al. Chronic traumatic encephalopathy in athletes: progressive tauopathy after repetitive head injury. *J Neuropath Exp Neurol* 2009;68:709–735.
33. Benson BW, McIntosh AS, Maddocks D, et al. What are the most effective risk-reduction strategies in sport concussion? *Br J Sports Med* 2013;47:321–326.
34. Collins CL, Fletcher EN, Fields SK, et al. Neck strength: a protective factor reducing risk for concussion in high school sports. *J Prim Prev* 2014;35(5):309–319.
35. Mihalik JP, Blackburn JT, Greenwald RM, et al. Collision type and player anticipation affect head impact severity among youth ice hockey players. *Pediatrics* 2010;125:e1394–e1401.
36. Viano DC, Casson IR, Pellman EJ. Concussion in professional football: biomechanics of the struck player—part 14. *Neurosurgery* 2007;61(2):313–327.

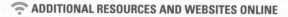 ADDITIONAL RESOURCES AND WEBSITES ONLINE

Skin Disorders

Acne

Daniel P. Krowchuk

ETIOLOGY

Acne is a disease of pilosebaceous units, composed of a follicle, sebaceous gland, and vellus hair. These structures are concentrated on the face, chest, and back, explaining the occurrence of acne in these areas. Although the pathophysiology of acne is not fully understood, several factors contribute:

1. Androgens and sebum production: At adrenarche, rising levels of dehydroepiandrosterone sulfate (DHEAS), likely after conversion to testosterone and dihydrotestosterone, cause sebaceous glands to enlarge and produce more sebum. Increased sebum production contributes to obstruction within follicles and correlates with acne severity.
2. Bacteria and the innate immune response: *Propionibacterium acnes* is an anaerobic gram-positive rod that colonizes pilosebaceous follicles following increases in sebum production. *P. acnes* elaborates lipases that can damage the follicle wall and releases a number of chemotactic factors and proinflammatory mediators.
3. Abnormal keratinization: Epithelial cells lining the follicle proliferate more rapidly and become more cohesive. The result is a collection of cells and sebum that leads to the development of the primary acne lesion, the microcomedo.[1] As obstruction increases, the follicle may rupture with spread of its contents into surrounding tissues, an event that contributes to inflammation.

CLINICAL MANIFESTATIONS

Acne Lesions

1. Obstructive lesions (comedones): Obstruction within follicles initially is microscopic (i.e., microcomedones) but ultimately becomes apparent as open and closed comedones. Open comedones (blackheads) have a dilated follicular orifice and a black color (thought to be due to oxidized melanin, altered transmission of light through epithelial cells, or the presence of certain lipids in sebum) (Fig. 21.1). Closed comedones (whiteheads) are small (1 mm in diameter) white to skin-colored papules (Fig. 21.2).
2. Inflammatory lesions: Rupture of obstructed follicles leads to the formation of erythematous papules (<5 mm in diameter),

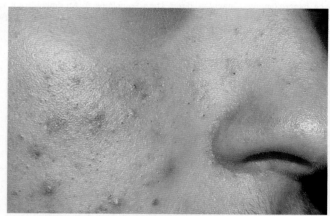

FIGURE 21.1 This patient has moderate mixed (inflammatory and comedonal) acne. He has inflammatory papules and pustules, erythematous macules (resolving inflammatory lesions), and open comedones. (From Jensen S. *Nursing health assessment*. Philadelphia, PA: Lippincott Williams & Wilkins, 2010.)

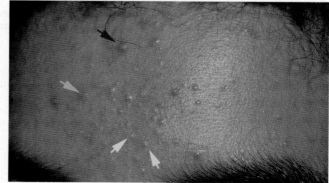

FIGURE 21.2 In this patient who has moderate mixed acne (inflammatory and comedonal), there are closed comedones (*yellow arrows*), papules (*green arrow*), and pustules (*blue arrow*).

pustules, and nodules (≥5 mm in diameter) (Fig. 21.1). As inflammatory lesions resolve, they often leave erythematous (Fig. 21.1), violaceous, or hyperpigmented (Fig. 21.3) macules that may persist for as long as a year. Patients often mistake these lesions for scars.

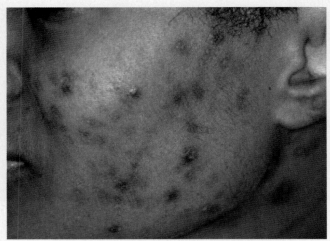

FIGURE 21.3 In persons of color, resolving inflammatory lesions may produce hyperpigmented macules. (From Lugo-Somolinos A, McKinley-Grant L, Goldsmith LA, et al. *Essential dermatology in pigmented skin*. Philadelphia, PA: Lippincott Williams & Wilkins, 2011.)

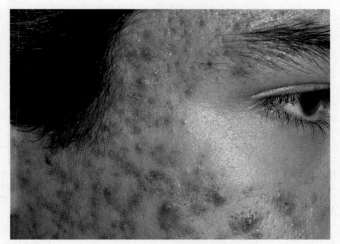

FIGURE 21.4 On the face, acne scars appear as small pits seen here in the temporal fossa. Based on the presence of scars and numerous inflammatory lesions, this patient has severe acne. (From Burkhart C, Morrell D, Goldsmith LA, et al. *Essential pediatric dermatology*. Philadelphia, PA: Lippincott Williams & Wilkins, 2009.)

3. Scars: Scarring is most likely to occur in those who have large inflammatory lesions (i.e., nodules). On the face, scars appear as small pits (Fig. 21.4), while on the trunk they are hypopigmented macules. Occasionally, patients develop hypertrophic scars (i.e., keloids) or cysts (compressible nodules that lack overlying inflammation).

Acne Variants

1. Pomade acne: Caused by physical obstruction of follicles, most often from inadvertent application of hair styling products (e.g., pomades, greases) to facial skin. Comedones are concentrated on the forehead near the scalp and in the temporal fossae.
2. Acne conglobata: A severe form of acne in which cysts, abscesses, and draining sinuses develop on the face, chest, or back (e-Fig. 21.1). Extensive scarring and keloid formation are common.
3. Acne fulminans: This severe acne variant is characterized by the abrupt onset of painful nodules and cysts that become hemorrhagic and ultimately suppurate. Ulcers form and heal

slowly, often leaving extensive scarring. Fever, chills, weight loss, myalgias, or arthritis may be present. Patients may have leukocytosis, anemia, elevated inflammatory markers and transaminases, and periosteal reaction suggestive of osteomyelitis.
4. Gram-negative folliculitis: Infection with gram-negative bacteria that complicates long-term oral antibiotic treatment of acne. The organisms most often responsible include *Escherichia coli*, *Enterobacter* spp, *Serratia marcescens*, and *Klebsiella* spp. Patients exhibit inflammatory papules and pustules concentrated around the nose.

⬤ EVALUATION

Elements of the history that may be helpful are presented in **Table 21.1**. At a minimum, the physical examination should include the face, chest, and back. To aid in assessing the effect of treatment, one can document the approximate number and types of acne lesions present on the face (forehead, each cheek, and chin), chest, and back. Including photographs in an electronic health record is especially helpful.

An assessment of acne severity serves to inform the development of a treatment plan. The method presented here focuses on the face, but involvement of the trunk should be considered.[1]

1. Mild acne: A minority of the face is involved; a few papules and pustules are present, but there are no nodules or scars.
2. Moderate acne: Approximately one-half of the face is involved; papules and pustules are more numerous, but nodules are few (Fig. 21.1).
3. Severe acne: The majority of the face is involved; papules and pustules are numerous, and there are several nodules; scarring may be present (Fig. 21.4).

Although androgens play an important role in acne, most patients have normal hormone concentrations. As a result, measuring concentrations of DHEAS, free testosterone, and 17-hydroxyprogesterone should be reserved for young women who have acne and other evidence of androgen excess (e.g., oligo- or amenorrhea, hirsutism, female-pattern alopecia, clitoromegaly).

⬤ DIFFERENTIAL DIAGNOSIS

Some conditions that mimic acne and differentiating features are presented below. In each of these disorders, comedones are absent.

1. Keratosis pilaris (KP): Small skin-colored papules located on the cheeks. A keratin plug emanating from the follicular orifice may be seen or palpated (differentiating the lesions from those of acne) (e-Fig. 21.2). KP often also affects the upper outer arms, thighs, and buttocks, areas not involved by acne.
2. Periorificial dermatitis: Erythematous papules, pustules, and scaling concentrated around the mouth, nose, or eyes. Unlike in acne, lesions are not present on the forehead or cheeks (e-Fig. 21.3).
3. Rosacea: Erythematous papules, pustules, and scaling involve the central face. Unlike in acne, flushing and telangiectasias are present (e-Fig. 21.4).
4. *Pityrosporum* folliculitis: Folliculitis caused by *Pityrosporum ovale* results in pruritic erythematous papules and pustules on the back, chest, and shoulders. In contrast to acne, the face is spared (e-Fig. 21.5). A potassium hydroxide preparation performed on a pustule roof may reveal spores and short hyphae.
5. Facial angiofibromas (adenoma sebaceum): Erythematous papules or nodules involving the nasolabial folds, nose, and medial cheeks (e-Fig. 21.6). Lesions typically appear in childhood, earlier than would be anticipated for acne.

TABLE 21.1
Key Elements of the History

Questions For All Patients	Rationale
When did your acne begin?	Early- or late-onset acne may indicate the presence of androgen excess.
What medications have you tried, and how did they work for you?	If the patient has used a medication you're planning to prescribe, was it effective? If not, is it possible that failure was the result of improper use or the occurrence of adverse effects?
Are you taking other medications?	—Are there potential drug interactions? —Could the medication be exacerbating acne (as might occur with depot medroxyprogesterone acetate, an oral corticosteroid, lithium, diphenylhydantoin, phenobarbital, or isoniazid)
Do you have "sensitive" skin or eczema?	Individuals who have sensitive skin or atopic dermatitis may be less likely to tolerate medications that are irritating or drying (e.g., topical retinoids)
What skin or hair care products do you use?	—Occlusive preparations placed on the skin may physically obstruct follicles and worsen acne. Advise the use of products that are labeled "nonacnegenic," "noncomedogenic," or "won't block pores." —Hair greases used for hair styling may obstruct follicles if inadvertently applied to facial skin.
Are there other factors that may worsen acne?	Pressure applied by athletic gear (especially pads or chin straps) or tight clothing may worsen acne.
Questions For Young Women	**Rationale**
Are you having menstrual periods and, if so, how often?	—Oligo- or amenorrhea may suggest androgen excess as might occur in polycystic ovary syndrome or late-onset congenital adrenal hyperplasia. —Premenstrual acne flares may occur.
Are you using birth control? If so, what form?	—Progestin-containing long-acting reversible contraceptives may worsen acne. —Combined oral contraceptives (COCs) (even those without a specific FDA indication for acne) likely result in improvement. —Young women using an oral contraceptive may need a secondary form of contraception (e.g., condom) if receiving an oral antibiotic for acne.

TABLE 21.2
Options for Managing Mild Acne

Face

- Inflammatory or mixed
  - Benzoyl peroxide (BPO) once daily
  - Alternatives (once daily):
    - BPO/antibiotic fixed-dose combination product
    - BPO/topical retinoid fixed-dose combination product
    - Topical antibiotic/topical retinoid fixed-dose combination product
- Comedonal
  - Topical retinoid (as single agent) or topical retinoid-containing fixed-dose combination product once daily

Chest and back

- Inflammatory or mixed: BPO wash once daily in shower
- Comedonal: Salicylic acid wash once daily in shower

If no improvement, proceed to Table 21.3 "Options for Managing Moderate Acne"

TABLE 21.3
Options for Managing Moderate Acne

Only the face is involved

- Topical retinoid at bedtime
  - Individual product (such as tretinoin cream 0.025% or adapalene cream 0.1%) *or*
  - Fixed-dose combination product (such as BPO/adapalene or clindamycin/tretinoin)
- Topical antimicrobial each morning
  - BPO (if topical retinoid alone prescribed), *or*
  - BPO/topical antibiotic fixed-dose combination product (if topical retinoid alone prescribed)

Face and chest or back involved

- Topical retinoid at bedtime to the face (as above) *and*
- Oral antibiotic (such as doxycycline or minocycline, 50–100 mg once or twice daily)
- Consider adding BPO wash once daily in the shower to the chest and back

If no improvement, proceed to Table 21.4 "Options for Managing Severe Acne" or refer to a dermatologist.

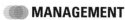 **MANAGEMENT**

Managing acne requires an understanding of the pathophysiology of the disease, its severity, the mechanisms of action and adverse effects of various medications. Evidence-based guidelines for acne management exist,[2] but treatment should be individualized taking into consideration the patient's perception of the severity of their disease, past experiences with medications, and the ability to adhere to a therapeutic plan. Suggested treatment plans for mild, moderate, and severe disease are presented in **Tables 21.2** to **21.4**, respectively. Ideally, one will develop a plan that is as simple as possible and employs medications that target various disease mechanisms.

Patient Education

The key components of patient education are outlined below. During the initial visit (and at return visits if needed), one should attempt to:

1. Dispel myths.
   a. Acne is not caused by dirt, and frequent washing will not be beneficial. In fact, washing too often or using harsh cleansers or applying toners (designed to remove oil, cosmetics, and dirt) may irritate the skin and limit one's ability

Options for Managing Severe Acne

Consider referral to a dermatologist *or* maximize the treatment plan

- Topical retinoid at bedtime to the face: If a low-potency agent was prescribed previously, consider increasing the potency (e.g., tretinoin micro gel 0.04% or 0.1%)
- High-dose oral antibiotic (such as doxycycline or minocycline 100 mg twice daily)
- Add BPO once daily to the face (if not being used as part of a fixed-dose combination product)
- For women, consider a COC

If no improvement, consider isotretinoin therapy (which usually involves referral to a dermatologist).

to tolerate topical medications.[2] Advise washing the face twice daily with a mild nonsoap cleanser (e.g., a synthetic detergent such as Cetaphil or Dove bar, or a lipid-free cleanser such as Cetaphil, CeraVe, or Aquanil).

b. Diet: The role of diet in causing or worsening acne is an issue of ongoing debate. Recent studies have suggested associations between acne and both a high-glycemic-load diet and the intake of milk.[1,2] At present, however, there is insufficient evidence to support dietary manipulation as an adjunct to acne management.[1–5]

2. Educate about the disease and its management.
   a. Describe the causes of acne.
   b. Discuss the role of aggravating factors: pressure applied by helmet chin straps, application of occlusive substances to the skin (such as hair greases or thick emollients), occupational exposure to oils or greases
   c. Advise the use of skin care products (moisturizers, cosmetics, sunscreens) that are labeled "nonacnegenic," "noncomedogenic," or "won't block pores."
   d. Discuss expectations for therapy: Advise the patient that
      • Eight weeks or longer may be required to see improvement once treatment is begun.
      • Currently available medications (with the possible exception of oral isotretinoin) are not curative. As a result, most patients require sustained therapy to control the disease.
      • The goal of treatment is to reduce the number and severity of lesions and prevent scarring. Although many patients desire skin that is free of acne, for many this is not possible.
   e. Advise against picking at acne lesions. Doing so can prolong the healing process, lead to secondary infection, or cause scarring.
   f. Provide guidance about using medications, and prepare the patient for possible adverse effects. Topical agents should be applied as a thin coat to all acne-prone areas, not only to lesions. When the entire face is to be treated, dispense an amount the size of a pea onto a fingertip (some products employ a pump to dispense an appropriate amount). Touch the medication to each side of the forehead, each cheek, and the chin. Use the fingertips to spread the medication, covering the entire face while avoiding the angles of the mouth, eyes, and alar folds (areas prone to irritation).

Topical Medications
Benzoyl Peroxide

1. Mechanism of action: Primarily bactericidal and somewhat comedolytic
2. Dosing
   a. Benzoyl peroxide (BPO) is considered by the US Food and Drug Administration (FDA) to be generally safe and

effective. Therefore, it is available without a prescription in concentrations ranging from 2.5% to 10% in a variety of vehicles (gels, creams, lotions, washes, and soaps). Some prescription forms remain, but they are often more expensive and may not be covered by insurance.
   b. For the face, consider using a gel in a 5% concentration applied once daily (gels are more effective than other vehicles). Increasing the concentration to 10% does not greatly enhance the therapeutic effect but increases the likelihood of drying and irritation.
   c. For the chest and back, consider a 10% wash that can be used once daily in the shower. Washes are convenient for treating large areas, although their efficacy is less than that of products applied to the skin and left on for several hours.
3. Adverse effects
   a. Redness, drying, and peeling: Can be moderated by applying a moisturizer, decreasing the concentration of BPO, or changing the vehicle (if, e.g., the patient is using a gel, consider prescribing one that is water based or changing to a cream or lotion)
   b. Bleaching: BPO bleaches fabrics (including clothing, wash cloths, towels, pillowcases) and hair
   c. Contact dermatitis: Uncommon occurrence that produces a pruritic eruption composed of erythema, small papules, or vesicles

Topical Antibiotics

1. Mechanism of action: Reduce concentrations of *P. acnes*, inflammatory mediators and, possibly, free fatty acids. As a result, these agents are useful in the management of mild to moderate inflammatory facial acne.
2. Dosing: Most products are designed to be used twice daily. However, if used in conjunction with another topical agent (e.g., a retinoid at bedtime), it may be applied once daily (in the morning).
   a. Single agents: Clindamycin, erythromycin, dapsone, and sodium sulfacetamide (with or without sulfur). Using a topical antibiotic as monotherapy is discouraged because of the potential for the development of antibiotic resistance.[2] For this reason, consider adding BPO in the form of a fixed-dose combination product (below) or as a separate agent.
   b. Fixed-dose combination products: Products that combine a topical antibiotic and BPO have greater efficacy than either of the individual components; the inclusion of BPO reduces the likelihood of antibiotic resistance. Fixed-dose combination products are convenient and likely increase adherence.[6] Cost may be a significant disadvantage. Available products include BPO 5%/erythromycin 3% (generic, Benzamycin), BPO 5%/clindamycin 1% (generic, Benzaclin, Duac), and BPO 2.5%/clindamycin 1% (Acanya).
3. Adverse effects: As single agents, topical antibiotics are well tolerated. When combined with BPO, the adverse effects discussed previously may occur.

Topical Retinoids

1. Mechanism of action: Normalize keratinization within follicles, thereby reducing obstruction and the risk of follicular rupture and enhancing the penetration of other topical medications. Also have anti-inflammatory properties.
2. Dosing: Available as single agents or in fixed-dose combination products (**Table 21.5**). Factors to consider in selecting an agent include the following:
   a. Determine if your patient would benefit from a single agent (retinoid alone) or a fixed-dose combination product. Factors to consider include the following:

TABLE 21.5

Topical Retinoids

Product	Vehicle/Concentration
Single agents	
• Tretinoin (generic, Retin-A [and other brands])[a]	• Cream: 0.025%, 0.0375%, 0.05%, 0.1% • Gel: 0.01%, 0.025% • Micro gel: 0.04%, 0.1%
• Adapalene (generic and Differin)	• Cream: 0.1% • Gel: 0.1%, 0.3% • Lotion: 0.1%
• Tazarotene (Tazorac, Avage)	• Cream: 0.05%, 0.1% • Gel: 0.05%, 0.1%
Fixed-dose combinations	
• Adapalene/BPO (Epiduo)	• Gel: adapalene 0.1%/BPO 2.5%
• Tretinoin/clindamycin (Ziana, Veltin)	• Gel: tretinoin 0.025%/clindamycin 1.2%

[a]Tretinoin (but not adapalene) is inactivated by benzoyl peroxide. Therefore, the two agents should not be applied simultaneously.

• Cost: Is the fixed-dose combination product on the patient's medication formulary, can she or he access and use a manufacturer's discount card or certificate?
• Severity of inflammatory acne: Will topical BPO or clindamycin (the agents contained in fixed-drug combination products) be sufficient to control the inflammatory component of acne? Will BPO be beneficial to manage bacterial antibiotic resistance?

b. If a retinoid-only product is desired, to reduce the likelihood of adverse effects, select a low-potency agent (such as tretinoin cream 0.025% or adapalene cream 0.1%). If the patient advises you that he or she has dry or sensitive skin, use a cream vehicle; if he or she has oily skin, consider a gel (such as tretinoin micro gel 0.04% or adapalene 0.1%).
c. With any topical retinoid, apply every second or third night and progress to nightly application as tolerated over 2 to 3 weeks.

3. Adverse effects:
a. Dryness, redness, and peeling are most common. In addition to the strategies described previously, to prevent drying, advise the regular use of a noncomedogenic emollient, especially during cold weather months. Using a product that contains a sunscreen will protect against retinoid-induced photosensitivity. Temporary worsening of acne may occur 2 to 3 weeks after beginning a topical retinoid.
b. Hyperpigmentation: In persons of color, retinoid-induced inflammation may cause hypo- or hyperpigmentation. This is an important reason to begin treatment with a low-potency agent, gradually increase application frequency, and use an emollient.
c. Teratogenicity: Because tretinoin is structurally similar to isotretinoin, concern exists about potential teratogenicity. However, there have been no reports of malformations occurring in infants exposed to tretinoin in utero.[1] Nevertheless, tretinoin and adapalene should be avoided during pregnancy and are classified category C (risk to the fetus cannot be ruled out). Tazarotene, in contrast, is category X (contraindicated in pregnancy) due to teratogenicity

concerns. This issue should be discussed if the drug is to be prescribed for a woman of childbearing potential.

Azelaic Acid (20%)

1. Mechanism of action: Antibacterial and comedolytic. As a result, it is most useful in the management of mild to moderate facial acne in those who cannot tolerate a topical retinoid.
2. Dosing: Applied twice daily
3. Adverse effects: Generally well tolerated but some patients experience pruritus, stinging, or erythema

Salicylic Acid

1. Mechanism of action: Promotes desquamation from follicles. May be beneficial for those who have comedonal acne but are unable to tolerate a topical retinoid.
2. Dosing: Applied once or twice daily. Available without a prescription as washes, scrubs, or pads.
3. Adverse effects: Drying, irritation

Oral Medications
Antibiotics

Oral antibiotics have greater efficacy than topical formulations and, for this reason, are used to treat those with more severe or extensive (i.e., chest and back) inflammatory acne. They should be used in conjunction with BPO (to reduce the likelihood of antibiotic resistance) and a topical retinoid. To avoid the development of antibiotic cross resistance, avoid the simultaneous use of different oral and topical antibiotics. Once the inflammatory component of the disease has been controlled and an appropriate topical treatment program is in place, discontinue the oral antibiotic. In the past, tetracycline and erythromycin were first-line therapies. However, the increasing prevalence of drug resistance among *P. acnes* limits their effectiveness. In addition, according to the Centers for Disease Control and Prevention, tetracycline is unavailable in the US at the time of this writing.[7] Doxycycline and minocycline often are preferred because they may be taken once daily, have better penetration into follicles, and have a lower prevalence of bacterial resistance.[2]

1. Doxycycline: Often a first choice, although shortages in the US at the time of this writing may limit use.[7]
a. Dosing: 50 mg to 100 mg once or twice daily
• To avoid gastrointestinal upset and pill esophagitis, take with food and a large glass of water, respectively.
• To prevent staining of dental enamel, use only in those ≥9 years of age.
• To prevent photosensitivity during sunny months, advise the use of a noncomedogenic broad-spectrum sunscreen (one with ultraviolet A and B protection).
b. Adverse effects (most common): Gastrointestinal upset, pill esophagitis, photosensitivity, headache (including that caused by benign intracranial hypertension)
2. Minocycline: May be a first choice (for severe acne) or a second choice (if doxycycline is ineffective).
a. Dosing: 50 mg to 100 mg once or twice daily
• To prevent gastrointestinal upset, take with food.
• To prevent staining of dental enamel, use only in those ≥9 years of age.
b. Adverse effects: Vertigo, dizziness, and headache (including that due to benign intracranial hypertension). Uncommon but important adverse effects include the following:
• Hyperpigmentation: Patients occasionally experience blue-black or gray discoloration in areas of acne scarring or normal skin (usually resolves with discontinuation of the drug) or generalized brown pigmentation (may persist).

- Lupus-like syndrome: Rare event that typically follows long-term minocycline use.[8] Symptoms and signs include malaise, arthralgias, arthritis, rash, or hepatitis. Generally resolves with drug withdrawal.
- Drug-induced hypersensitivity: Typically occurs during the first months of treatment. Characterized by diffuse erythema, respiratory symptoms, and facial swelling.
- Others: Stevens–Johnson syndrome, serum sickness-like eruption, autoimmune hepatitis.

3. Other antibiotics: A number of other antibiotics have been used to treat acne. Those most commonly employed include the following:
   a. Trimethoprim-sulfamethoxazole: An alternative for those who cannot tolerate or do not respond to other agents. It should be used with caution due to potentially severe adverse effects, including toxic epidermal necrolysis and Stevens–Johnson syndrome.
   b. Azithromycin: Efficacy has been demonstrated, although resistance among *P. acnes* may limit its use.

Hormonal Therapy

1. COCs improve acne by increasing sex hormone binding globulin and suppressing ovarian androgen production. Although three COCs have an FDA indication for the treatment of acne (Ortho Tri Cyclen, Estrostep, Yaz), others likely are beneficial.[1,2] COCs are not viewed as primary therapy for acne but as adjuncts to standard treatment in those who have resistant disease. The use of COCs and their possible adverse effects are discussed in Chapter 43.
2. Spironolactone has antiandrogenic properties and is used by some (off label) to treat young women who have recalcitrant severe acne and signs of androgen excess.[3]

Isotretinoin

Indicated for the treatment of severe, scarring acne recalcitrant to standard treatment. Those wishing to prescribe isotretinoin must register with iPLEDGE, a risk management system intended to prevent fetal exposure to the drug (https://www.ipledgeprogram.com/default.aspx). Recognizing that more than 90% of patients receive isotretinoin from a dermatologist, this section is intended to inform providers about the drug and possible adverse effects.

1. Mechanism of action: Reduces sebum production, normalizes follicular keratinization, decreases *P. acnes* colonization.
2. Dosing: 0.5 to 2.0 mg/kg/day divided twice daily for 16 to 20 weeks.[1] Most patients experience sustained clearing of acne.
3. Adverse effects: The most important of these include the following:
   a. Teratogenicity: Isotretinoin use during pregnancy is contraindicated due to the increased risk of spontaneous abortion and fetal malformations.[9] iPLEDGE requires that young women use two forms of effective contraception beginning 1 month before and extending to 1 month after the completion of treatment. Two negative pregnancy tests are required prior to receiving the initial prescription, and pregnancy tests are conducted monthly during treatment.
   b. Dermatologic: The most common adverse effect is cheilitis (erythema, fissuring, and peeling of the lips). Drying of nasal mucosae may lead to epistaxis. Dry skin and dry eyes (that may result in contact lens intolerance) are common.
   c. Musculoskeletal: Myalgias are common, and hyperostoses (bone spurs and calcification of tendons and ligaments) may occur, especially in those receiving long-term therapy.[9] Premature epiphyseal closure occurs rarely.[9]
   d. Gastrointestinal: Elevation of transaminases, triglycerides, and cholesterol may occur and, for this reason, regular monitoring is performed. Normalization generally occurs despite continued therapy. Concern has been raised about an association between isotretinoin use and the development of inflammatory bowel disease (IBD), although a recent well-designed case-control study found no increased risk.[10]
   e. Neuropsychiatric: A possible association between isotretinoin use and depression and suicidal ideation remains an issue of some concern. For most patients, successful acne treatment improves depressive symptoms and quality of life.[9] In addition, the majority of studies addressing the subject indicate no association with depression, and suicide rates are lower among those receiving isotretinoin than would be expected among the general population.[9] However, there are well-documented cases in which depressive symptoms appeared after beginning isotretinoin, resolved when the drug was withdrawn, and returned with rechallenge.[9,11] In view of this and the possibility that idiosyncratic reactions might occur, those caring for persons receiving isotretinoin should remain alert for the development of depression and suicidality. Beyond depression, patients may develop fatigue, headaches, and benign intracranial hypertension.[9]

FOLLOW-UP

Patients should return 3 to 4 months after beginning treatment. However, they should be encouraged to contact their provider sooner with questions or concerns about medication use or adverse effects. At the return visit, one can assess adherence, adverse effects, and the effect of treatment. Based on this information, the treatment plan can be maintained or revised.

REFERENCES

1. Krowchuk DP, Gelmetti C, Lucky AW. Acne. In: Schachner LA, Hansen RC, eds. *Pediatric Dermatology*. 4th ed. Philadelphia, PA: Mosby-Elsevier, 2011;827–850.
2. Eichenfield LA, Krakowski AC, Piggott C, et al. Evidence-based recommendations for the diagnosis and treatment of pediatric acne. *Pediatrics* 2013;131:S163–S186.
3. Szczepaniak D, Treadwell PA. Acne therapy in primary care: comprehensive review of current evidence-based interventions and treatment. *Adolesc Med* 2011;22:77–96.
4. Burris J, Rietkerk W, Woolf K. Acne: the role of medical nutrition therapy. *J Acad Nutr Diet* 2013;113:416–430.
5. Basak SA, Zaenglein AL. Acne and its management. *Pediatr Rev* 2013;34:479–497.
6. Yentzer BA, Ade RA, Fountain JM, et al. Simplifying regimens promotes greater adherence and outcomes with topical acne medications: a randomized controlled trial. *Cutis* 2010;86:103–108.
7. Centers for Disease Control and Prevention. Doxycycline shortage. Available at http://www.cdc.gov/std/treatment/doxycyclineShortage.htm. Accessed November 25, 2013.
8. Garner SE, Eady A, Bennett C, et al. Minocycline for acne vulgaris: efficacy and safety. *Cochrane Database Syst Rev* 2012;8:CD002086.
9. Lowenstein EB, Lowenstein EL. Isotretinoin systemic therapy and the shadow cast upon dermatology's downtrodden hero. *Clin Dermatol* 2011;29:652–661.
10. Etminan M, Bird ST, Delaney JA, et al. Isotretinoin and risk for inflammatory bowel disease: a nested case-control study and meta-analysis of published and unpublished data. *JAMA Dermatol* 2013;149:216–220.
11. Prevost N, English JC. Isotretinoin: update on controversial issues. *J Pediatr Adolesc Gynecol* 2013;26:290–293.

ADDITIONAL RESOURCES AND WEBSITES ONLINE

Miscellaneous Skin Conditions

Daniel P. Krowchuk

The identification and management of skin disorders is an important component of adolescent and young adult (AYA) health care. According to the National Ambulatory Medical Care Survey, an ongoing survey of office-based physician practice, in 2010, there were an estimated 47.9 million visits made by persons 13 to 26 years of age to general or family physicians, pediatricians, or internal medicine physicians.[1] In 17.8% of visits, a diagnosis of a dermatologic disorder was made.[1] This chapter reviews the identification and management of dermatologic diseases that affect AYAs, addressing the conditions most likely to be encountered by clinicians. For additional information, readers should consult a standard dermatology text or atlas. Of note, infestations (scabies and pediculosis) and molluscum contagiosum are discussed in Chapter 62.

DERMATITIS

The term dermatitis (or eczema) refers to inflammation of the epidermis and superficial dermis. Common forms of dermatitis that affect AYAs include atopic, allergic contact, and seborrheic.

Atopic Dermatitis

Atopic dermatitis (AD) is a chronic disease that is likely the result of multiple factors, including genetics, epidermal barrier dysfunction, immune dysregulation, and an immune response to *Staphylococcus aureus*. Among the more than 20% of children who develop AD, most have a resolution of symptoms by adolescence or adulthood.[2] However, 10% to 30% do not and a smaller number experience the onset of disease as an adult.[2]

Clinical Manifestations

1. In AYAs, AD is characterized by erythematous patches located in flexural areas, such as the antecubital and popliteal fossae. The face (including the eyelids), neck, and hands also may be involved (Fig. 22.1). A variant of hand dermatitis is dyshidrotic eczema in which deep-seated, intensely pruritic vesicles involve the lateral aspects of the digits or palms (e-Fig. 22.1). In persons of color, AD lesions are less erythematous and may be papular rather than flat. In addition, there may be areas of postinflammatory hypo- or hyperpigmentation.

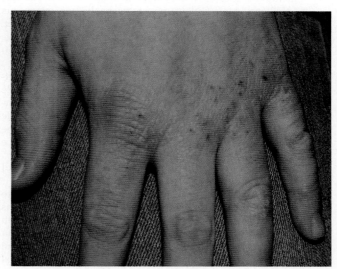

FIGURE 22.1 Atopic dermatitis involving the hand. Note the lichenfication (over the metacarpophalangeal joint of the index finger) and small crusted erosions.

2. Individuals who have AD also commonly exhibit:
   a. Xerosis
   b. Hyperlinear palms
   c. Keratosis pilaris: keratotic papules centered around follicles; typically located on the upper outer arms, thighs, and face (e-Fig. 22.2)
   d. Dennie–Morgan lines: prominent skin folds located beneath the eyes
   e. Ichthyosis vulgaris: polygonal scales located on the anterior and lateral legs
   f. Lichenification: thickening of the skin with accentuated skin creases (due to chronic scratching)
   g. Pityriasis alba: hypopigmented macules often located on the face; the borders are not sharply demarcated, rather there is a gradual transition from normal to abnormal color (e-Fig. 22.3)

Complications

Individuals who have AD are often colonized with *S. aureus*, likely because of increased bacterial adherence and failure to produce antimicrobial peptides. Defects in antimicrobial peptide production and T cell function increase susceptibility to viral infections, including molluscum contagiosum, warts, and eczema herpeticum.

Treatment

1. Daily measures:
   a. Avoid irritants: use fragrance-free skin-care products; a non-soap cleanser for bathing (e.g., a synthetic detergent like Cetaphil or Dove bar or a lipid-free cleanser like Cetaphil, CeraVe, or Aquanil); use an additive-free laundry detergent (e.g., All Free Clear, Tide Free, and others); wear cotton clothing.
   b. Hydrate the skin: apply a fragrance-free emollient immediately after a bath or shower. Lotions work well for many individuals but preservatives in some products may cause stinging. Creams or ointments are more effective emollients, although they may leave a greasy feel that some individuals find unpleasant.
2. Management of exacerbations:
   a. Topical corticosteroid: Apply twice daily if needed. Ointments offer greater efficacy and tolerability; however, as with emollients, some patients prefer creams because ointments have a greasy feel. Prescribe a sufficient amount of product. Recall that 3 g is required to cover an entire adult arm once.
      • Face: use a low-potency preparation (e.g., hydrocortisone 1% or 2.5%).
      • Extremities or trunk: use a mid-potency agent (e.g., triamcinolone acetonide 0.1% or fluocinolone acetonide 0.025%). For resistant or lichenified areas or when treating the hands, a higher-potency agent (e.g., fluocinonide 0.05% or mometasone furoate ointment 0.1%) may be needed. These agents should be used with caution since prolonged application may cause skin atrophy.
   b. Topical calcineurin inhibitors (e.g., tacrolimus [Protopic] and pimecrolimus [Elidel]):
      • Most useful for the management of AD in areas where potent corticosteroids cannot be used due to concerns about skin atrophy (e.g., the face, groin, axillae) or in areas of resistant disease (where they are often used in conjunction with topical corticosteroids [e.g., a topical corticosteroid is applied in the morning and the topical calcineurin inhibitor in the evening]).
      • Tacrolimus is indicated for the treatment of moderate-to-severe AD (the 0.03% concentration is approved for those 2 to 15 years of age and the 0.1% concentration for those ≥16 years of age); pimecrolimus is indicated for the treatment of mild-to-moderate AD in those ≥2 years of age.
   c. Antihistamine: A first-generation (sedating) antihistamine, like diphenhydramine or hydroxyzine, may be used at bedtime to provide relief from pruritus.
   d. Antibiotic: If signs of secondary bacterial infection are present (e.g., oozing, crusting), an anti-staphylococcal antibiotic may be administered orally for 7 to 10 days. For those who have severe or resistant AD, consider attempting to reduce *S. aureus* colonization by recommending: (1) twice-weekly bleach baths (1/4 cup of household bleach in a half-full bathtub) and (2) intranasal mupirocin twice daily for 5 days.

Allergic Contact Dermatitis

Allergic contact dermatitis (ACD) is a common problem; the prevalence of contact allergy to at least one antigen is 20%.[3] ACD occurs when an antigen penetrates the epidermis and sensitizes T lymphocytes. Within 12 to 24 hours of re-exposure to the antigen, an eruption appears at the site of contact. Often the offending agent can be identified based on the appearance of lesions and their distribution. In a minority of cases, dermatologic referral for patch testing may be necessary.

1. **Plant** (e.g., poison ivy, oak, or sumac):
   a. Clinical manifestations: ACD due to plants results in an acute dermatitis with erythematous papules, vesicles, or bullae. Lesions are present on exposed areas (e.g., face, extremities) and may be arranged in a linear distribution (at the site of contact with resin emanating from a damaged plant) (Fig. 22.2). If the exposure is indirect (e.g., you hug a dog that has run through poison ivy), a linear distribution of lesions is absent and one sees fine erythematous papules, not vesicles.
   b. Treatment: If the eruption is mild and limited in extent (e.g., <10% to 15% of the body surface), therapy may include a mid-potency topical corticosteroid (e.g., triamcinolone acetonide 0.1%), topical nonsensitizing anesthetic (e.g., pramoxine), and an oral first-generation antihistamine. When the eruption is extensive, severe, or involves critical areas (e.g., face, perineum), systemic corticosteroid therapy (e.g., prednisone orally for 12 to 21 days in a tapering dose) is indicated.
2. **Metal**: Nickel is among the most common contact allergens with a median prevalence of 8.6%.[3] Allergy to nickel is more common in those who have piercings and higher rates of allergy are associated with an increased number of piercings.[4] Nickel allergy produces a chronic dermatitis characterized by minimal erythema, scaling, and thickening of the skin. Commonly affected sites include the lobules of the ears (earrings), area below the umbilicus (belt buckle or clothing snap), umbilicus (piercing jewelry), neck (necklace), or wrist (bracelet or watch) (Fig. 22.3). Treatment is with an appropriate topical corticosteroid and nickel avoidance. Patients may be advised to:
   a. Choose nickel-free jewelry and eyeglass frames (i.e., items made of surgical-grade stainless steel, solid yellow gold, titanium, or pure sterling silver).
   b. Purchase clothing with snaps, buttons, and fasteners that are plastic or metal that is plastic coated or painted.
   c. Wear watchbands made of plastic, leather, or cloth.
3. **Preservatives, fragrances**: These products cause erythema and tiny papules. Commonly affected sites include the face or eyelids (cosmetics), axillae (deodorant), or neck (perfume). Treatment is avoidance of the offending agent (once identified) and the application of an appropriate topical corticosteroid.

Seborrheic Dermatitis

Seborrheic dermatitis is a chronic and relapsing inflammatory disorder that occurs in areas with numerous sebaceous glands. It affects 1% to 3% of adults and is especially common in AYAs in whom

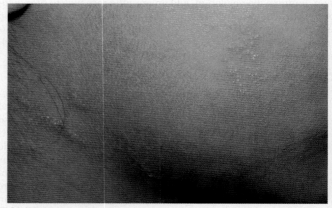

FIGURE 22.2 In contact dermatitis due to poison ivy, small erythematous papules are present, often in a linear arrangement as seen on the neck and the angle of the mandible.

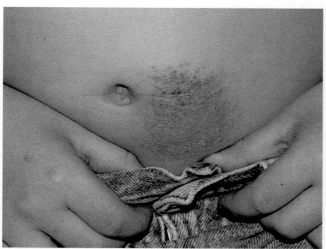

FIGURE 22.3 Contact dermatitis due to nickel in a clothing snap. There is an erythematous patch near the umbilicus. (From Goodheart HP. *Goodheart's photoguide of common skin disorders.* 2nd ed. Philadelphia, PA: Lippincott Williams & Wilkins, 2003.)

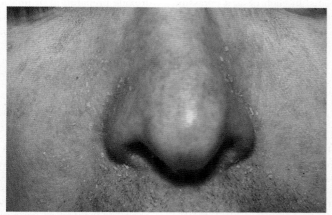

FIGURE 22.4 In adolescents and young adults, seborrheic dermatitis often involves the nasolabial folds with erythema and scaling. (From Goodheart HP. *Goodheart's same-site differential diagnosis: a rapid method of diagnosing and treating common skin disorders.* Philadelphia, PA: Lippincott Williams & Wilkins, 2010.)

sebaceous glands are most active.[5] Although the cause is not clearly understood, it may involve an inflammatory response to the yeasts of the genus *Malassezia* (formerly *Pityrosporum*).

Clinical Manifestations
Typical findings are scaling of the scalp (i.e., dandruff), or scaling and erythema of the eyebrows, eyelids, glabella, nasolabial or retroauricular creases, beard or sideburn areas, or ear canals (Fig. 22.4).

Treatment
1. Scalp: Advise the use of an antiseborrheic shampoo containing pyrithione zinc (e.g., Head and Shoulders, DHS Zinc, and others), selenium sulfide (e.g., Selsun, Exsel, and others), or ketoconazole (e.g., Nizoral). If facial skin is involved, allow some of the shampoo to contact these areas and then rinse (this is a useful adjunct to the topical therapies discussed below). If signs of inflammation are present (e.g., erythema or erosions), a topical corticosteroid solution (e.g., fluocinolone acetonide 0.1%) may be applied at bedtime if needed.

2. Skin: Control can be achieved using a low-potency topical corticosteroid (e.g., hydrocortisone 1%) and/or an agent active against yeast (e.g., clotrimazole, miconazole nitrate, or ketoconazole) applied twice daily if needed.

FUNGAL INFECTIONS

Tinea Versicolor
Tinea (pityriasis) versicolor is a common superficial infection with yeasts of the genus *Malassezia* (formerly *Pityrosporum*). The prevalence among adults in temperate climates is 1% to 4%, but it is particularly common among AYAs in whom sebaceous glands are highly active.[6] The sebum-rich environment appears to support lipophilic *Malassezia* spp. Although these organisms are part of the normal skin flora, hot and humid weather, sweating, and use of oils on the skin may trigger a change from the yeast form to the hyphal form, resulting in the appearance of rash.

Clinical Manifestations
Most patients have no symptoms but some report pruritus. The eruption is composed of well-defined round macules that may coalesce into large patches; scale may be present. Although lesions may be hypo- or hyperpigmented, most often, in more deeply pigmented individuals, they are hypopigmented (Fig. 22.5). The trunk is the primary site of involvement but the proximal extremities and sides of the neck may be affected. Tinea versicolor is usually diagnosed clinically. If uncertainty exists, a potassium hydroxide preparation performed on scale from a lesion will demonstrate short hyphae and spores (i.e., "spaghetti and meatballs") and a Wood's lamp examination will reveal a yellow-gold fluorescence of affected areas.

Differential Diagnosis
Eruptions that may be concentrated on the trunk and, therefore, mimic tinea versicolor include:

1. Pityriasis rosea (PR): Lesions are erythematous, oval thin plaques (not macules) with long axes oriented parallel to lines of skin stress.
2. Vitiligo: Lesions are depigmented (not hypopigmented) and lack scale.
3. Secondary syphilis: The eruption is composed of erythematous to violaceous to red-brown scaling papules. Lesions are widespread (not limited to the trunk) and often involve the

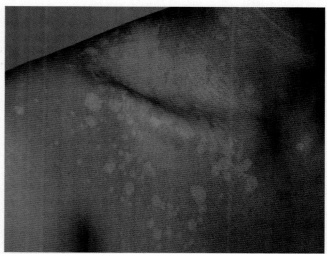

FIGURE 22.5 Tinea versicolor: there are numerous round hypopigmented macules. In the supraclavicular area, macules have coalesced to form a hypopigmented patch.

palms and soles. Affected individuals have systemic symptoms, including fever, malaise, and lymphadenopathy.

4. Confluent and reticulated papillomatosis of Gougerot and Carteaud: This uncommon disorder is often confused with tinea versicolor. Reticulated areas of hyperpigmentation that are hyperkeratotic (and, therefore, have a rough texture) are present on the central chest or back. Well-defined round or oval macules are not seen (e-Fig. 22.4).

Treatment

Several options exist for treatment. Because the recurrence rate may be as high as 60% in the first year, following any of the treatments listed below, prophylaxis once monthly for 3 months is warranted.[6] This may be accomplished using a single 8- to 12-hour application of selenium sulfide. It is important to counsel patients that even with effective treatment, several months will be required for normalization of pigmentation.

1. Topical agents:
   a. Selenium sulfide lotion 1% (available without a prescription) or 2.5% (requires prescription): Apply a thin coat to affected and adjacent areas for 10 minutes then shower. Repeat daily for a total of 7 days.
   b. Ketoconazole shampoo: Apply for 5 minutes once daily for 1 to 3 days.
   c. Terbinafine spray: Apply twice daily for 2 to 3 weeks.
   d. Imidazole creams (e.g., clotrimazole, miconazole nitrate, ketoconazole, and others): Effective for very localized infection (not practical in the treatment of large areas).
2. Oral agents: These are usually reserved for those who have resistant infections or cannot tolerate or effectively use a topical agent. Off-label options include the following:
   a. Itraconazole: 400 mg once or 200 mg/day for 7 days
   b. Fluconazole: 400 mg once

Tinea Pedis (Athlete's Foot)

Tinea pedis is the most prevalent dermatophyte infection in AYAs.

Clinical Manifestations

1. Interdigital form (caused by *Trichophyton [T.] rubrum* or *Epidermophyton [E.] floccosum*): Pruritus, fissuring, scaling, and maceration between the toes (Fig. 22.6)
2. Moccasin form (caused by *T. rubrum*): Widespread scaling that involves much or all of the sole and sides of the foot
3. Inflammatory form (caused by *T. mentagrophytes*): Vesicles or bullae located on the instep of the foot (Fig. 22.7).

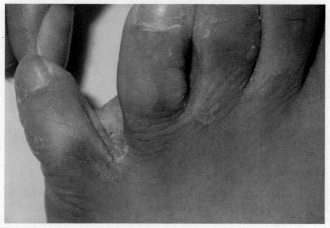

FIGURE 22.6 In the most common form of tinea pedis, scaling and maceration are present in the interdigital spaces.

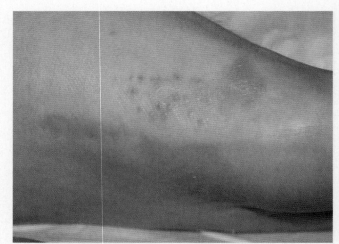

FIGURE 22.7 The inflammatory form of tinea pedis produces papules and vesicles near the instep of the foot.

Differential Diagnosis

Several disorders involve the feet and, therefore, may mimic tinea pedis. In each case, a potassium hydroxide preparation or fungal culture would be negative.

1. Contact dermatitis due to shoes: Involves the dorsum of the feet, not the interdigital spaces or plantar surfaces
2. AD (juvenile plantar dermatosis): Typically occurs in older children and less often in adolescents. Causes erythema, dryness, lichenification, and fissuring primarily of the plantar surfaces of the forefeet
3. Psoriasis: Causes erythema and thick (not fine) scale of the feet. Individuals often have lesions of psoriasis elsewhere.

Treatment

For most infections a fungistatic topical imidazole (e.g., miconazole nitrate, clotrimazole, econazole, etc.) applied twice daily until clearing occurs (typically 2 to 4 weeks) is effective. If this treatment fails, consider a topical agent that is fungicidal (e.g., terbinafine, naftifine). For widespread or resistant infection, an oral agent (e.g., griseofulvin, terbinafine, itraconazole, or fluconazole) may be required. If there is concomitant nail involvement (i.e., onychomycosis), oral terbinafine or itraconazole will be required.

Onychomycosis

The terms onychomycosis (nail infection by any fungus) and tinea unguium (infection by fungi called dermatophytes) are often used interchangeably. The vast majority of fungal nail infections are caused by dermatophytes (usually *T. rubrum*, *T. mentagrophytes*, and *E. floccosum*). The prevalence of onychomycosis is estimated to be as high as 12%.[7] Infection is uncommon before puberty and highest in those >65 years of age.[7]

Clinical Manifestations

Two forms of infection are recognized.

1. Subungual onychomycosis: The most prevalent form of infection that causes thickening of the nail and a yellow discoloration distally or laterally (the result of separation of the nail from the underlying nail bed) (Fig. 22.8)
2. Superficial white onychomycosis: Produces a white discoloration of the surface of the nail with powdery scale.

Differential Diagnosis

The clinical features of the disorders listed below often permit their differentiation from onychomycosis. However, if uncertainty exists, a fungal culture of a nail scraping or clipping can be helpful.

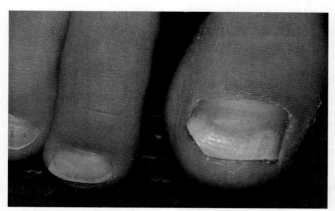

FIGURE 22.8 In onychomycosis, the nail becomes thick and yellow.

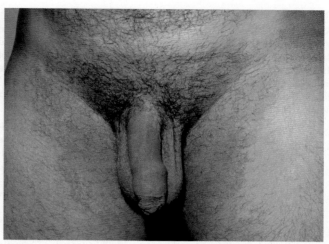

FIGURE 22.9 Tinea cruris is characterized by an erythematous patch that involves the proximal thigh and crural fold. Involvement may be bilateral as shown here or unilateral. (From Craft N, Taylor E, Tumeh PC, et al. *VisualDx: essential adult dermatology.* Philadelphia, PA: Lippincott Williams & Wilkins, 2010.)

1. Candidiasis: Uncommon in adolescents and usually involves the fingernails. Causes a chronic paronychia characterized by erythema and swelling of the proximal nail fold, loss of the cuticle, and nail dystrophy (that lacks yellow discoloration).
2. Psoriasis: Usually causes pitting of the nails; lesions of psoriasis are present elsewhere.
3. Pachyonychia congenita: Results in thickening and discoloration of the nails that may be difficult to differentiate clinically from onychomycosis. The condition usually has its onset in early childhood but may be delayed until adolescence.
4. Lichen planus: Causes longitudinal ridging or splitting of nails. Typical skin lesions (purple polygonal papules and plaques) are present elsewhere.

Treatment

Superficial white onychomycosis may respond to topical antifungal therapy. However, subungual onychomycosis requires oral therapy and options are listed below. One should consider potential drug interactions, adverse effects, and the need for laboratory monitoring.

1. Terbinafine 250 mg daily for 12 weeks
2. Itraconazole 200 mg daily for 12 weeks
3. Fluconazole is preferred by some but is not US Food and Drug Administration (FDA) approved for the treatment of onychomycosis.

Cure rates with oral therapy are as high as 80%; however, recurrences are common. To reduce the chance of recurrence, advise patients to dry carefully after bathing or showering and to apply an absorbent powder containing an antifungal agent (e.g., tolnaftate [e.g., Tinactin and others], or miconazole nitrate [Micatin, Desenex, Zeasorb AF, Lotrimin AF, and others]).

Tinea Cruris

Tinea cruris represents infection of the inguinal folds with the dermatophytes *T. mentagrophytes* or *E. floccosum*. It affects men more often than women and is uncommon before puberty.

Clinical Manifestations

Appears as a well-demarcated erythematous patch involving the proximal thigh and crural fold (may be unilateral or bilateral). The border of the lesion is elevated and scaling, and is typically more erythematous than the center. The scrotum and penis are spared (Fig. 22.9).

Differential Diagnosis

The clinical features usually permit diagnosis. If uncertainty exists, a potassium hydroxide preparation or fungal culture can be helpful. These would be negative in uncomplicated intertrigo and erythrasma, and would demonstrate pseudohyphae and spores in candidiasis.

1. Candidiasis: Bright red patch in the crural fold that also involves the scrotum and penis; satellite papules may be present.
2. Intertrigo: Maceration resulting from rubbing of moist skin surfaces creates a superficial erosion that is not as well defined as tinea cruris and lacks border elevation.
3. Erythrasma: Superficial infection caused by *Corynebacterium minitissiumum* that produces erythematous to brown patches in intertriginous areas (groin, axillae, gluteal cleft). Scale may be present but the borders of lesions are not elevated. Wood's lamp examination reveals a "coral-red" color fluorescence.

Treatment

Apply a topical imidazole cream twice daily as described in the section on tinea pedis. Tinea cruris may be a recurrent problem. Counsel patients to dry carefully after bathing or showering, avoid tight-fitting or occlusive clothing, and apply an absorbent powder to reduce moisture and friction.

⬤ VIRAL INFECTIONS

Warts

Warts are epidermal growths caused by various types of human papillomavirus (HPV). HPV types are often related to the clinical presentation; for example, types 1, 2, and 4 cause common warts on the hands and plantar warts, while types 2 and 10 cause flat warts. Warts are spread by direct contact, autoinoculation, or fomites (like showers or pool decking in the case of plantar warts).

Clinical Manifestations

1. Common warts: Skin-colored, often dome-shaped papules with a rough (i.e., verrucous) surface (e-Fig. 22.5). Occasionally, they exhibit a finger-shaped (i.e., filiform) appearance. Black specks that represent thrombosed capillaries may be seen on the surface of the wart.
2. Plantar warts: Skin-colored papules, nodules, or plaques that have a rough surface that are located on the plantar surface of the foot (e-Fig. 22.6). Because of the pressure exerted by walking, plantar warts are less elevated than common warts.
3. Flat warts: Skin-colored or pink, small (1 to 3 mm), smooth, flat-topped papules often located on the face or legs (e-Fig. 22.7).
4. Anogenital warts: Condylomata acuminata are skin-colored papules or plaques that involve the genitalia or perianal region (see Chapter 61).

Treatment

Warts often regress spontaneously and, therefore, observation without intervention is reasonable. However, many patients find the lesions unsightly and will request treatment. A number of therapeutic options exist but those most commonly employed are salicylic acid and cryotherapy (which have comparable efficacy).[8] Patients should be counseled that HPV may remain in the skin after successful treatment and, as a result, recurrence is possible.

1. Salicylic acid: Application of salicylic acid 17% liquid (available without a prescription) is a safe and effective first-line treatment, especially for common and plantar warts. Depending on the size of the wart, several weeks to 3 months may be required for resolution. A typical treatment plan is as follows:
   a. In the evening, shower, bathe, or otherwise moisten the wart and then dry with a towel.
   b. Rub the wart with an emery board or nail file (to debride the wart).
   c. Apply salicylic acid to the wart and allow it to dry. To avoid irritation, avoid applying salicylic acid to normal skin.
   d. Occlude the wart with tape.
   e. In the morning, remove the tape (which facilitates debridement).
   f. Repeat the above steps daily.
2. Cryotherapy: Destruction of a wart by freezing is effective but painful. Although a number of cryogens are available for in-office or home use, liquid nitrogen is most effective due to its lower temperature. The goal of treatment is to create a blister within the epidermis.
   a. Liquid nitrogen is applied using a spray device or a cotton-tipped applicator reinforced with additional cotton (to hold liquid nitrogen).
   b. It is applied until the wart and a 1-mm rim of normal skin turn white (typically 10 to 15 seconds).
   c. When the wart thaws, a second treatment may be performed.
   d. Counsel the patient that a blister may form and provide wound-care instructions.
   e. If no blister forms or if wart tissue remains after a blister heals, begin salicylic acid treatment as described above.
   f. Repeat cryotherapy in 4 weeks if necessary.
3. Cimetidine: Oral cimetidine has immunomodulatory effects, enhancing T cell function and cytokine production. Although data are conflicting, it may be of benefit, particularly in those who have numerous or resistant warts. A typical dose in AYAs is 400 mg twice daily for 6 to 8 weeks. Cimetidine is not FDA approved for the treatment of warts. If it is used, some recommend concomitant salicylic acid treatment as described previously.
4. Tretinoin: Topical tretinoin has been used off label to treat flat warts. The mechanism of action is not fully understood but it may be the result of the inflammatory response created in the skin. Tretinoin is applied to lesions nightly as tolerated.
5. Other treatment options include (a) intralesional injection of skin test antigens (e.g., *Candida*, *Trichophyton*); measles, mumps, and rubella vaccine; or bleomycin; or (b) the application of squaric acid. None of these are FDA approved for the treatment of warts. Referral for laser treatment or electrodessication and curettage may be considered for recalcitrant warts.

🔴 BACTERIAL INFECTIONS

Crusted (Nonbullous) Impetigo

Infection with *S. aureus* that produces erosions with a "honey-colored" crust often located near the nares. The differential diagnosis includes nummular eczema (often located on the extremities or trunk) or herpes simplex virus infection (typically produces clustered vesicles on an erythematous base). If infection is localized, a topical agent (e.g., mupirocin, retapamulin) may be used. For widespread or multifocal infection, an oral agent active against *S. aureus* is indicated.

Bullous Impetigo

Infection with specific phage types of *S. aureus* that elaborate an epidermolytic toxin. The toxin damages intercellular adherence resulting in the formation of fragile bullae that easily rupture leaving round, crusted erosions. The differential diagnosis includes thermal burns, insect bite reactions, or immunobullous diseases. Treatment with an oral anti-staphylococcal agent is indicated.

Folliculitis

Folliculitis represents inflammation centered around follicles. The most common form is caused by *S. aureus*. Hot tub folliculitis is caused by *Pseudomonas aeruginosa* acquired from hot tubs, swimming pools, or water parks.

Clinical Manifestations

Follicular-centered pustules with surrounding erythema (Fig. 22.10). Common sites of involvement are the thighs or buttocks, or areas exposed to pressure or friction applied by clothing. In those who have hot tub folliculitis, lesions are often concentrated in areas covered by bathing garments.

Treatment

Treatment options for staphylococcal folliculitis are presented below. Hot tub folliculitis requires no specific therapy as lesions resolve spontaneously over several days. Occasional patients experience a complication (e.g., conjunctivitis, otitis externa, cystitis) that requires appropriate antibiotic therapy.

1. Localized disease: Topical antibiotic (e.g., clindamycin, mupirocin, retapamulin)
2. Widespread disease: Oral anti-staphylococcal antibiotic for 7 to 10 days
3. Prevention:
   a. Use an antibacterial cleanser containing chlorhexidine or triclosan daily.
   b. Avoid tight-fitting clothing.
   c. If folliculitis is linked to shaving, change the razor blade frequently and use an antibacterial cleanser after shaving.

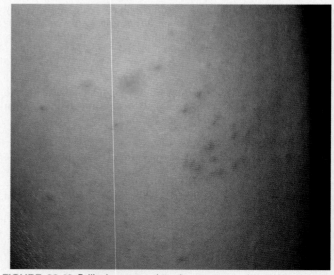

FIGURE 22.10 Follicular-centered erythematous papules and pustules are observed in folliculitis. This patient acquired infection from a hot tub.

d. If the above strategies fail, consider twice-weekly bleach baths (1/4 cup of household bleach in a half-full bathtub) and/or intranasal mupirocin twice daily for 5 days.

PAPULOSQUAMOUS DISEASES

These diseases are characterized by elevated lesions (papulo) that have scale (squamous). The two most common of these affecting AYAs, pityriasis rosea (PR) and psoriasis, will be discussed here.

Pityriasis Rosea

PR is a condition of unknown cause that may be the result of a viral infection. The prevalence of PR has been reported to be 1.3% but this likely represents an underestimate due to the failure to diagnose those who have atypical presentations.[9] PR occurs most often in those 10 to 35 years of age.[9]

Clinical Manifestations

1. Patients are usually well, although a minority experience a brief prodrome of malaise, headache, lymphadenopathy, or pharyngitis 1 to 2 weeks before the onset of the rash.
2. In 50% to 80% of patients, the rash begins with a herald patch, a scaling round or oval patch measuring 2 to 10 cm in diameter. The herald patch is usually located on the trunk, but may appear elsewhere.
3. Two to 21 days after the appearance of the herald patch, a generalized eruption begins that may be associated with pruritus. It is composed of oval thin plaques with scale that is located on the trailing edge of lesions (i.e., toward the center of lesions). This is unlike the scale of tinea corporis that is located at the leading edge of lesions (i.e., peripherally). Lesions are distributed symmetrically on the trunk with relative sparing of the face and extremities (Fig. 22.11). The long axes of lesions are arranged parallel to lines of skin stress, so that on the back, the arrangement of lesions suggests the appearance

of the branches of a fir tree. In persons of color, lesions may be papular and distributed "inversely" (i.e., concentrated on the extremities or in the groin with relative sparing of the trunk).

Differential Diagnosis

1. Tinea corporis or nummular eczema: May mimic the herald patch of PR. A lesion of nummular eczema usually exhibits crust not scale.
2. Viral exanthems or morbilliform drug eruptions: Lesions do not have scale or the unique orientation of those of PR.
3. Secondary syphilis: Unlike patients who have PR, those who have secondary syphilis are ill with fever and lymphadenopathy and often have lesions on the palms or soles.

Treatment

There is no specific treatment; resolution typically occurs in 6 to 8 weeks (range 2 to 12 weeks). Pruritus may be managed with a topical corticosteroid, an emollient containing menthol or phenol (agents that act as counterirritants distracting the body from the sensation of pruritus), or an oral first-generation (sedating) antihistamine. Judicious sun exposure may reduce pruritus or cause the eruption to resolve more rapidly.

Psoriasis

Psoriasis is an immune-mediated inflammatory skin disorder that affects an estimated 1% of the population.[10] In approximately one-third of patients, the disease first appears during childhood or adolescence.[10]

Clinical Manifestations

The lesions of psoriasis are well-defined erythematous papules and plaques that possess a thick, adherent scale. If scale is removed, punctate areas of bleeding appear (Auspitz sign). The eyebrows, ears, extensor surfaces of the elbows and knees, umbilicus, and gluteal cleft are commonly affected (Fig. 22.12). Lesions may appear at sites of trauma (the Koebner phenomenon), likely explaining involvement of the extensor elbows and knees. Many individuals have scalp disease with erythema and scale. Pitting, yellowing, or thickening of the nails occurs in a minority of patients. Although psoriasis may be associated with an oligoarthritis involving the metacarpophalangeal or proximal interphalangeal joints or axial skeleton, this occurs rarely in adolescents.

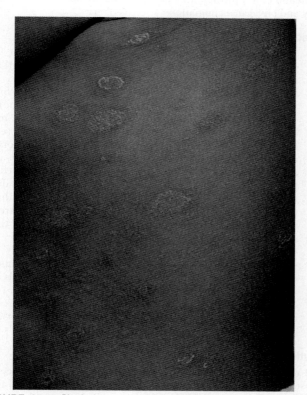

FIGURE 22.11 Pityriasis rosea: on the lateral trunk are oval scaling thin plaques. The long axes of lesions are arranged parallel to lines of skin stress.

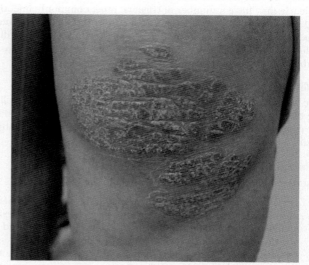

FIGURE 22.12 The lesions of psoriasis are erythematous scaling papules and plaques. Lesions are often located on the extensor surfaces of the extremities. (From Werner R. *Massage therapist's guide to pathology.* 5th ed. Philadelphia, PA: Lippincott Williams & Wilkins, 2012.)

Treatment

Typical topical treatment options are listed below. They are most useful for those who have a limited number and extent of lesions. Patients who have more widespread disease or those who fail to respond to topical treatment should be referred to a dermatologist for consideration of other topical or systemic agents.

1. Topical corticosteroid: For lesions on the trunk or extremities, a mid-potency agent like triamcinolone acetonide 0.1% may be applied twice daily. Those who fail to respond (or whose lesions are thick) may require a higher-potency product (like fluocinonide 0.05% [class 2]). However, when using potent preparations, caution should be exercised to avoid prolonged application that might result in skin atrophy. One way to avoid this is to apply the medication twice a day for 2 weeks and then twice daily Saturday and Sunday. This "pulsed" treatment maintains the steroid effect but reduces the likelihood of skin atrophy. Scalp involvement requires a solution (like fluocinolone acetonide oil 0.01% [class 6] or clobetasol propionate 0.05% [class 1]) or foam (like clobetasol propionate 0.05%).

2. Topical calcipotriene 0.005%: For those who do not respond adequately to a topical corticosteroid, calcipotriene may be valuable. It is a vitamin D_3 analog that normalizes epidermal proliferation. It is used in conjunction with a topical corticosteroid (each drug applied once daily). Although expensive, the most convenient formulation contains a class 1 corticosteroid and calcipotriene; it is applied once daily as needed.

3. Other treatments: Although effective, tars and anthralin are cosmetically displeasing and are generally considered second-line therapies. Tazarotene is a topical retinoid occasionally used in conjunction with a topical corticosteroid. A shampoo containing salicylic acid or tar can help remove thick scale from the scalp.

HYPERSENSITIVITY REACTIONS

Urticaria

Urticaria is a form of cutaneous hypersensitivity reaction in which there is vasodilation (causing erythema) and fluid leak from vessels (causing swelling). It affects 15% to 20% of individuals at some time during their lives.[11] Urticaria may be separated into acute (lasting <6 weeks) and chronic (lasting ≥6 weeks) forms. Acute urticaria may have a number of triggers, most commonly infection (e.g., viral, streptococcal, parasitic), foods (e.g., shellfish, peanuts, eggs, strawberries), medications (e.g., antibiotics [e.g., penicillin, sulfonamides], nonsteroidal anti-inflammatory agents, others [e.g., barbiturates, codeine]), or insect stings.

Clinical Manifestations

The lesions are wheals (hives) that may take many shapes, including rings, arcs, plaques, or papules (Fig. 22.13). Individual lesions are evanescent, typically lasting less than 3 hours and never longer than 24 hours.

Differential Diagnosis

Disorders that may mimic urticaria include the following:

1. Erythema multiforme (EM): Lesions are fixed in location (not evanescent); have a uniform morphology (not multiple lesion shapes); exhibit a central duskiness, vesicle, or crust; and favor the extremities with relative sparing of the trunk.

2. Urticarial vasculitis: Lesions last longer than 24 hours and have central duskiness or purpura.

3. Serum sickness-like eruption: Lesions are large, often purple rings or plaques associated with periarticular swelling; fever and arthralgias are often present.

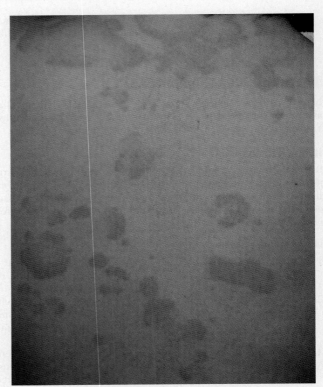

FIGURE 22.13 In urticaria, lesions take many shapes. In this patient there are erythematous papules, circles, incomplete circles, and plaques with polycyclic borders.

Evaluation

Evaluation for a precipitating factor should be dictated by the history and physical examination.

Treatment

1. Treat or remove any identified precipitant and avoid the use of nonsteroidal anti-inflammatory agents that may exacerbate urticaria.

2. H1 antihistamines are first-line therapy. Although a first-generation agent (e.g., diphenhydramine or hydroxyzine) is often used, sedation may be a problem. As a result, it may be prudent to begin therapy with a second-generation (e.g., loratadine, cetirizine) or third-generation (e.g., desloratidine, fexofenadine, levocetirazine) agent. If a response is not achieved, a first-generation antihistamine could be added at bedtime or the dose of the second- or third-generation drug increased (some advocate increasing the dose to two to three times that recommended).[11] Once lesions have resolved, treatment may be continued for several additional days and then discontinued.

3. Oral corticosteroids are second-line therapies generally reserved for severe disease. It is not uncommon for patients to experience a reappearance of lesions when corticosteroids are withdrawn.

4. Most episodes of urticaria resolve in about 2 weeks. If the condition persists or is recurrent, or if accompanied by an episode of anaphylaxis, allergy consultation is indicated.

Erythema Multiforme

EM represents a cutaneous hypersensitivity reaction that occurs most commonly in young adults. Traditionally, it is separated into two forms, EM minor and EM major. For convenience, both entities will be discussed here.

1. **EM** (formerly called EM minor)
   a. *Clinical manifestations:* Most cases (90%) are caused by infections, especially herpes simplex virus (prior herpes labialis is reported in 50% of patients with EM). Prodromal symptoms are absent and the rash begins as erythematous papules that have a predilection for acral surfaces, including the palms, soles, and face, with relative sparing of the trunk. Lesions remain fixed in location for up to 2 to 3 weeks before resolving. Over several days, a central violaceous discoloration or, occasionally, a vesicle or crust develops (Fig. 22.14). One-half of those who have EM have oral erosions that are few in number.
   b. *Treatment:* EM is self-limited, resolving in 2 to 3 weeks. No specific therapy is indicated. If EM is recurrent and thought to be the result of herpes simplex virus infection, consider daily oral antiviral prophylaxis.
2. **Stevens–Johnson syndrome (SJS) (formerly called EM major) and toxic epidermal necrolysis (TEN):** SJS and TEN represent more severe and potentially life-threatening hypersensitivity reactions to drugs (e.g., antibiotics [trimethoprim-sulfamethoxazole], anticonvulsants [lamotrigine, carbamazepine, phenytoin, phenobarbital], nonsteroidal anti-inflammatory agents) or, less commonly, infectious agents (e.g., *Mycoplasma pneumoniae*). SJS and TEN may represent the same disease process, differing only in extent of cutaneous involvement. The incidence (annually, worldwide, per million people) of SJS is 1.2 to 6 and of TEN 0.4 to 1.9.[12]
   a. *Clinical manifestations:* SJS/TEN typically begins 6 days to 2 weeks after initiating a drug.[4]
      • Patients experience prodromal symptoms, including fever, sore throat, rhinitis, cough, headache, vomiting, or diarrhea.
      • Within 14 days, erythematous or purpuric macules and patches appear on the trunk and extremities. Blisters form rapidly and rupture leaving large areas of denuded skin (e-Fig. 22.8). In SJS there is epidermal loss of <10% of the body surface, while TEN is diagnosed when patients lose >30% of the epidermal surface; those with involvement of 10% to 30% are said to have SJS/TEN overlap. In SJS and TEN, target lesions are absent or few in number.
      • Mucosal involvement is prominent with hemorrhagic crusting of the lips (e-Fig. 22.9), oral ulcers, and purulent conjunctivitis. The trachea, bronchi, and gastrointestinal tract may be involved.
   b. *Treatment:* Early discontinuation of the offending drug is essential. The use of systemic corticosteroids is controversial. Intravenous immunoglobulin may be beneficial. Plasmapheresis, tumor necrosis factor-alfa inhibitors, granulocyte colony-stimulating factor, *N*-acetylcysteine, and cyclosporine also have been used.[13] Supportive care (with careful attention to skin, eye, and fluid and electrolyte status) in a burn unit or intensive care unit is imperative. Monitoring for secondary bacterial infection is important since sepsis leading to multiorgan failure is the leading cause of death.[13]
   c. *Prognosis:* The mortality rate of SJS is 1% to 5%, and that of TEN is 25% to 30%.[13] Long-term complications involve the eye (impaired tear production and drainage, aberrant lashes), skin (altered pigmentation), and nails (dystrophy).

Erythema Nodosum

Erythema nodosum (EN) is a hypersensitivity reaction that results in inflammation of fat (panniculitis). Precipitants include infection (e.g., *Streptococcus pyogenes* [the most common infectious cause], tuberculosis, Epstein–Barr virus, *Yersinia enterocolitica*, histoplasmosis, coccidioidomycosis, leptospirosis), medications (e.g., estrogen in oral contraceptives, sulfonamides), inflammatory bowel disease, or collagen vascular disease. However, in most cases no precipitating factor is identified.

Clinical Manifestations

Patients develop tender erythematous nodules that are typically located on the extensor surfaces of both legs. Over several days, the nodules evolve from red to brown-red or purple and later to yellow-green (Fig. 22.15).

Evaluation

The evaluation is guided by the history and physical examination findings. In patients who have no known precipitants and appear healthy, some advise limited screening studies, including measurement of antistreptolysin-O and/or anti-DNase B titers, chest radiography, and screening for tuberculosis (PPD skin test or interferon gamma receptor assay).

Treatment

If identified, a precipitating factor should be treated or removed. EN generally resolves within several days to a few weeks. First-line treatment includes a nonsteroidal anti-inflammatory agent and relative rest. For those who fail to respond, consultation with a

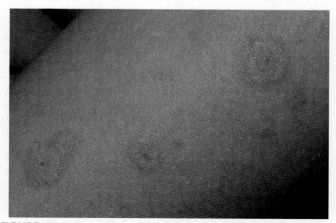

FIGURE 22.14 In erythema multiforme, target lesions are observed. These are erythematous papules that develop a central violaceous discoloration, vesicle, or crust.

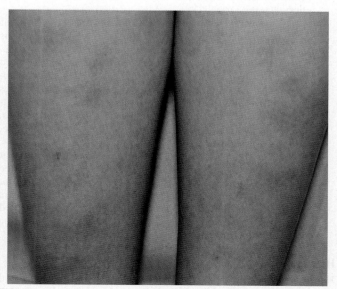

FIGURE 22.15 Erythema nodosum is characterized by violaceous nodules often located on the extensor surfaces of the legs.

dermatologist is appropriate to consider treatment with saturated solution of potassium iodide, colchicine, or prednisone.

Drug Eruptions

Drug eruptions represent a distinct form of hypersensitivity reaction. The major forms are discussed here (urticarial drug eruptions, SJS, and TEN were addressed previously).

1. **Exanthematous:** The most common form of drug eruption is one that mimics the appearance of a viral exanthem. Erythematous macules that may become slightly elevated begin on the trunk and spread to the face and extremities. The eruption appears 7 to 14 days after beginning a medication but may occur earlier if there has been prior drug exposure. Aminopenicillins, cephalosporins, sulfonamides, and anticonvulsants are most often responsible. Treatment involves removing the offending drug and administering an antihistamine. If the suspected drug is essential and no alternative exists, some advocate continuing the agent despite the eruption ("treating through"). In such cases, the eruption usually resolves but occasional patients experience worsening.

2. **Drug-induced hypersensitivity syndrome** (DIHS, also known as drug reaction with eosinophilia and systemic symptoms): DIHS is a severe reaction that likely results from defects in the metabolism of certain drugs. The agents most commonly implicated are anticonvulsants (e.g., phenobarbital, phenytoin, carbamazepine, and lamotrigine), antibiotics (e.g., sulfonamides, minocycline), and allopurinol. DIHS begins 2 to 6 weeks after initiating a drug. Patients develop fever and erythematous macules and papules (i.e., a morbilliform eruption); facial edema is often present. Hepatitis (possibly fulminant), pneumonitis, myocarditis, and nephritis may occur. Early withdrawal of the suspected drug is essential; systemic corticosteroids are employed in severe cases.

3. **Fixed drug eruption:** This unique eruption is characterized by an erythematous or dusky oval patch or plaque that occurs at the same body location each time the offending drug is administered (usually within 24 hours of restarting the agent). Lesions may blister and heal with hyperpigmentation (e-Fig. 22.10). Common sites of involvement are the distal extremities and the penis. Many drugs may cause a fixed drug eruption, including antibiotics (e.g., sulfonamides, tetracyclines), anticonvulsants (e.g., barbiturates, carbamazepine), and nonsteroidal anti-inflammatory agents.

4. **Photosensitivity eruptions:** May be classified as phototoxic or photoallergic.
   a. Phototoxic reactions: Occur when ultraviolet (UV) light (typically UVA) activates a drug. Phototoxic eruptions are mediated by nonimmunologic mechanisms (e.g., free radical damage to cells). Clinically, an exaggerated sunburn-like erythema appears 2 to 6 hours after exposure. Drugs commonly responsible include tetracyclines (doxycycline and other tetracycline), nonsteroidal anti-inflammatory agents, sulfonamides, fluoroquinolones, phenothiazines, and diuretics (e.g., furosemide, thiazide, hydrochlorothiazide).
   b. Photoallergic: Photoallergy is an uncommon disorder that is thought to be the result of delayed hypersensitivity. Once sensitized, within 24 hours of re-exposure to the drug an eczematous eruption (e.g., papules and vesicles) appears on sun-exposed areas. Extension of the rash to protected areas may occur. Sunscreens, particularly those containing benzophenones, are usually responsible.

Hair Loss

Hair loss without associated scarring of the scalp may be separated into generalized and localized forms. The most common causes will be discussed here.

1. Generalized hair loss:
   a. Telogen effluvium: Normally, approximately 90% of hairs are in a growing (anagen) state and 10% in a resting (telogen) state; 50 to 100 are lost each day. A stressful event such as a significant febrile illness, delivering an infant, or being born may shift the majority of hairs to a telogen state. Two to 4 months following the event, resting hairs are lost and replaced by growing hairs. Since hair regrowth occurs spontaneously, no treatment is necessary. Other causes of telogen effluvium include endocrine diseases (e.g., hypothyroidism, hypopituitarism) and medications (e.g., certain anticonvulsants, isotretinoin, cimetidine, terbinafine). Discontinuing an oral contraceptive also may be responsible.[14]
   b. Androgenetic alopecia (AGA): In men, AGA is believed to result from the effects of androgens on genetically susceptible hair follicles. Under the influence of dihydrotestosterone, genes are activated that reduce the length of the hair growth cycle and size of the follicles. As a result, shorter and finer hairs are produced. The role of androgens in women is less clear. In men, AGA usually begins in the 20s or 30s but may have its onset earlier (the prevalence in boys 15 to 17 years has been estimated to be 14%).[14] It is characterized by temporal and eventually frontal hairline recession. An estimated 3% of women aged 20 to 29 years develop AGA.[14] They experience diffuse hair loss that is most noticeable at the vertex. For women who have marked temporal recession or other signs of androgen excess, hormonal evaluation is indicated. The initial treatment of AGA in men is minoxidil 5% topically or finasteride orally; in women, minoxidil 2% topically or spironolactone orally may be employed.

2. Localized hair loss:
   a. Alopecia areata: Alopecia areata is an autoimmune disorder that results in one or more round or oval patches of complete hair loss; scaling and inflammation of the scalp are absent. At the periphery of lesions, one may see exclamation point hairs, short hairs that are broader distally than proximally. A minority of patients experience loss of all scalp hair (alopecia totalis) or body hair (alopecia universalis). For those who have one or two small patches of hair loss, no intervention is an option since there is a high rate of spontaneous remission within one year. Initial treatment generally involves a potent topical corticosteroid (like clobetasol foam) or intradermal corticosteroid injections performed every 4 to 6 weeks. One regimen for topical therapy is to apply the steroid at bedtime five consecutive nights followed by two nights without treatment (to avoid cutaneous atrophy). Minoxidil is often used in conjunction with a corticosteroid, especially if some hair regrowth is observed. If involvement is extensive, consultation with a dermatologist is indicated. The National Alopecia Areata Foundation is a source of support and resources for patients and families (www.naaf.org/site/PageServer).
   b. Traction alopecia: Thinning of the hair may result from constant, excessive traction as might result from tight braiding or ponytails. The hair loss is incomplete, symmetrically distributed, and located at sites where the hair is parted. Reducing traction on the hair generally results in regrowth.
   c. Trichotillomania (TTM) (hair-pulling disorder): Repetitive twirling, twisting, rubbing, or pulling hair may cause it to break, a disorder termed TTM. TTM is considered an impulse-control disorder that affects as many as 3.4% of AYAs.[14] Affected individuals often feel anxiety or tension before pulling and relief afterward. Most often the scalp is involved and affected individuals have well-defined patches of relative alopecia; within the patches are hairs of differing

lengths. Scaling is absent but petechiae or erosions may be present, particularly if hair is pulled. Other sites of involvement include the eyebrows, eyelashes, or extremities. For those with significant disease, consultation with a mental health provider may be helpful to consider cognitive behavioral therapy (e.g., relaxation training or habit reversal therapy).[14] No FDA-approved medications exist for the treatment of TTM. Selective serotonin reuptake inhibitors are frequently prescribed but no studies have demonstrated their efficacy.[15] In single trials, clomipramine, N-acetylcysteine, and olanzapine proved beneficial.[15] The Trichotillomania Learning Center provides information and resources for patients and families (www.trich.org).

OTHER CONDITIONS

Acanthosis Nigricans

Most often, acanthosis nigricans (AN) occurs in association with obesity and reflects insulin resistance. AN also may occur in certain syndromes (e.g., the HAIR-AN syndrome [*hyperandrognemia, insulin resistance, acanthosis nigricans*]) and in older adults may be associated with malignancy (in such cases, AN is of abrupt onset and widespread).

Clinical Manifestations

AN is a hyperpigmented "velvety" thickening of the skin typically observed at the nape and sides of the neck and in the axillae.

Treatment

If weight reduction can be achieved, the appearance of AN will improve. A topical retinoid applied daily or a keratolyic (like ammonium lactate or urea) applied twice daily may benefit some individuals.

Hidradenitis Suppurativa

Hidradenitis suppurativa is a chronic inflammatory disease of apocrine glands. It begins during the second or third decade of life and occurs more commonly in women. The prevalence is often stated to be 1%, although a recent study suggests that it may be as low as 0.053%.[16]

Clinical Manifestations

Involvement of the axillae or groin is typical; patients develop recurrent, tender nodules that rupture and drain. Over time, sinus tracts or hypertrophic scars may form (e-Fig. 22.11).

Treatment

Initial treatment includes long-term oral antibiotic therapy (with doxycycline or minocycline), twice-daily application of a topical antibiotic (like clindamycin), and regular use of an antibacterial soap (e.g., one containing triclosan or chlorhexidine). For those who have severe recalcitrant disease, surgical excision of the affected areas may be curative.

Hyperhidrosis

Hyperhidrosis, excessive sweating, affects 3% of the US population.[17] It may be primary (idiopathic) or secondary (resulting from an underlying disorder or medication). Primary hyperhidrosis typically has its onset between 14 and 25 years of age.[17]

Clinical Manifestations

Most often, primary hyperhidrosis involves the axillae, palms, and soles. Severe forms can adversely impact quality of life, compromising social or occupational activities.

Treatment

For axillary hyperhidrosis, one can recommend an over-the-counter antiperspirant containing aluminum chloride. If this fails, consider one of the following strategies:

1. Recommend a product containing a higher concentration of aluminum chloride (like Certain Dri [12%]) or prescribe a product containing aluminum chloride hexahydrate (like Xerac AC [6.25%] or DrySol [20%]). Ideally, these are applied at bedtime under occlusion with plastic wrap. If sweating is controlled (requires several days), occlusion can be discontinued and the frequency of application decreased (to every few days as needed).
2. For some individuals, tap-water iontophoresis may be beneficial. Devices are available to treat the underarms, hands, and feet. Information may be obtained at www.drionic.com.
3. An oral anticholinergic like glycopyrrolate is often effective but may cause dry mouth, dry eyes, or bladder or bowel dysfunction.
4. For those with recalcitrant axillary hyperhidrosis, intradermal injection of botulinum toxin or treatment with a device that employs electromagnetic energy may be useful. In those who have severe or widespread symptoms, thoracic sympathectomy may be considered.

Sun Exposure

Sun exposure is linked to the development of skin cancer and skin aging (i.e., wrinkling and laxity of the skin, mottled pigmentation, blackheads). The majority of skin cancers are nonmelanoma skin cancers (NMSCs, e.g., basal cell carcinoma and squamous cell carcinoma) that are associated with cumulative lifetime sun exposure. Approximately 2 million individuals in the US develop a NMSC each year and the incidence is rising, including among those <40 years of age. Rates of malignant melanoma also have been increasing. It was estimated that in 2014, 76,100 persons in the US would be diagnosed with malignant melanoma and 9,710 would die of this disease.[18] Among new cases, 0.5% are diagnosed in those <20 years of age and 6.2% in those 20 to 34 years of age.[19] Malignant melanoma is associated with intermittent intense UV exposure. Of note, both NMSC and malignant melanoma have been linked to tanning bed use; young age of use and UV dose appear to be important risk factors. Essential elements of sun protection for those at risk include:

- Use a broad-spectrum sunscreen (one that provides UVA and UVB protection). In the US, UVA protection is graded using a 4-star scale (1 star [low protection] to 4 stars [highest protection]). The sun protection factor (SPF) is primarily a measure of UVB protection; it is the ratio of the minimum dose of UV radiation needed to produce sunburn in sunscreen-protected skin to that of unprotected skin. In principle, therefore, application of an SPF 8 product would protect against sunburn eight times longer than using no sunscreen.[20]
  - Apply the sunscreen liberally—one ounce is required to cover the entire adult body once. Most people apply one-quarter to one-half this amount, a factor that diminishes the effective SPF (by the fourth or square root, respectively).[20,21] To provide a margin of error if too little is applied, choose a product with an SPF of 30 or more.
- Reapply the sunscreen frequently if sweating or swimming.
- Consider an alcohol-free product (to prevent stinging of the eyes) and one that is labeled "nonacnegenic," "noncomedogenic," or "won't block pores" (to avoid worsening acne).
- Wear sun-protective clothing (like a hat with a brim or shirts having an UV protective factor).
- Wear sunglasses that provide UV protection (labeled as blocking 99% to 100% of the full UV spectrum).
- Avoid tanning beds—consider sunless tanning products that can be applied at home or in a tanning facility.

Vitiligo

Vitiligo represents an acquired loss of pigment. It is likely an autoimmune phenomenon that occurs in genetically predisposed individuals. In the US and Europe, the prevalence is approximately 1%.[22]

Clinical Manifestations

Lesions are well-defined macules or patches that lack any pigment (i.e., are depigmented). Vitiligo may be separated into two forms: generalized (i.e., lesions are symmetrically distributed on the extremities, trunk, face, and neck) and segmental (i.e., involves only one area of the body and does not cross the midline). Occasionally, vitiligo is associated with other autoimmune disorders, including thyroiditis, adrenal insufficiency, pernicious anemia, and gonadal dysfunction. However, in the adolescent who is clinically well, routine screening for these disorders is generally not recommended.

Differential Diagnosis

The complete loss of pigment in vitiligo distinguishes it from other disorders characterized by a reduction in pigment (i.e., hypopigmentation), including tinea versicolor, pityriasis alba and other forms of postinflammatory hypopigmentation, and nevus depigmentosus. In addition, the lesions of tinea versicolor and pityriasis alba often have scale, and the lesions of pityriasis alba have indistinct borders.

Treatment

The treatment of localized vitiligo is with a potent topical corticosteroid or calcineurin inhibitor (the latter is especially useful in the treatment of facial lesions where the use of a potent topical corticosteroid may cause skin atrophy). Often the two drugs are used in combination (e.g., the calcineurin inhibitor is applied twice daily Monday–Friday and the corticosteroid twice daily Saturday and Sunday [to reduce the possibility of steroid-induced atrophy]). For those who have extensive disease, referral to a dermatologist is prudent (for consideration of UV light or laser therapy). Information and support can be found at the following sites: American Vitiligo Research Foundation (www.avrf.org), National Vitiligo Foundation (www.nvfi.org), and Vitiligo Support International (www.vitiligosupport.org).

REFERENCES

1. National Ambulatory Medical Care Survey. Available at http://www.cdc.gov/nchs/ahcd.htm. Accessed October 7, 2013.
2. Eichenfield LF, Tom WL, Chamlin SL, et al. Guidelines of care for the management of atopic dermatitis: section 1. Diagnosis and assessment of atopic dermatitis. *J Am Acad Dermatol* 2014;70:338–351.
3. Thyssen JP, Linneberg A, Menné T, et al. The epidemiology of contact allergy in the general population—prevalence and main findings. *Contact Dermatitis* 2007;57:287–299.
4. Warshaw EM, Kingsley-Loso JL, DeKowven JG, et al. Body piercing and metal contact sensitivity: North American contact dermatitis group data from 2007 to 2010. *Dermatitis* 2014;25:255–264.
5. Dessinioti C, Katsambas A. Seborrheic dermatitis: etiology, risk factors, and treatments: facts and controversies. *Clin Dermatol* 2013;31:343–351.
6. Hu SW, Bigby M. Pityriasis versicolor: a systematic review of interventions. *Arch Dermatol* 2010;146:1132–1140.
7. Scher RK, Rich P, Pariser D, et al. The epidemiology, etiology, and pathophysiology of onychomycosis. *Semin Cutan Med Surg* 2013;32(2, Suppl 1):S2–S4.
8. Kwok CS, Gibbs S, Bennett C, et al. Topical treatments for cutaneous warts. *Cochrane Database Syst Rev* 2012;(9):CD001781.
9. Drago F, Broccolo F, Rebora A. Pityriasis rosea: an update with a critical appraisal of its possible viral etiology. *J Am Acad Dermatol* 2009;61:303–318.
10. Shah KN. Diagnosis and treatment of pediatric psoriasis: current and future. *Am J Clin Dermatol* 2013;14:195–213.
11. Nichols KM, Cook-Bolden FE. Allergic skin disease: major highlights and recent advances. *Med Clin North Am* 2009;93:1211–1224.
12. Schwartz RA, McDonough PH, Lee BW. Toxic epidermal necrolysis, Part I: introduction, history, classification, clinical features, systemic manifestations, etiology, and immunogenesis. *J Am Acad Dermatol* 2013;69:173.e1–e13.
13. Schwartz RA, McDonough PH, Lee BW. Toxic epidermal necrolysis, Part II: prognosis, sequelae, diagnosis, differential diagnosis, prevention, and treatment. *J Am Acad Dermatol* 2013;69:187.e1–e16.
14. Tackett BN, Hrismalos EN. Alopecia in adolescents. *Adolesc Med* 2011;22:16–34.
15. Rothbart R, Amos T, Siegfried N, et al. Pharmacotherapy for trichotillomania. *Cochrane Database Syst Rev* 2013;(11):CD007662.
16. Cosmatos I, Matcho A, Weinstein R, et al. Analysis of patient claims data to determine the prevalence of hidradenitis suppurativa in the United States. *J Am Acad Dermatol* 2013;68:412–419.
17. Gordon JS, Hill SE. Update on pediatric hyperhidrosis. *Dermatol Ther* 2013;26:452–461.
18. Skin Cancer Foundation. Available at http://skincancer.org/skin-cancer-information/skin-cancer-facts#melanoma. Accessed November 20, 2014.
19. National Cancer Institute Surveillance, Epidemiology, and End Results Program. Available at http://seer.cancer.gov/statistics/html/melan.html. Accessed November 20, 2014.
20. Sambandan DR, Ratner D. Sunscreens: an overview and update. *J Am Acad Dermatol* 2011;64:748–758.
21. Faurschou A, Wulf HC. The relation between sun protection factor and amount of sunscreen applied in vivo. *Br J Dermatol* 2007;156:716–719.
22. Alikhan A, Felsten LM, Daly M, et al. Vitiligo: a comprehensive review, Part I: introduction, epidemiology, quality of life, diagnosis, differential diagnosis, associations, histopathology, etiology, and work-up. *J Am Acad Dermatol* 2011; 65:473–491.

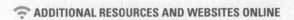

ADDITIONAL RESOURCES AND WEBSITES ONLINE

PART VI

Neurological and Sleep Disorders

23

Epilepsy

Gregory N. Barnes
S. Todd Callahan

Epilepsy is the most common chronic neurological condition, affecting 1% of the adolescent and young adult (AYA) populations. Seizures—the main symptoms of epilepsy—are defined as recurrent electroclinical episodes of disturbed central nervous system (CNS) function. Two-thirds of AYAs with epilepsy have the potential for excellent seizure control with medication.[1] Most patients have a likelihood of eventual remission of their epilepsy but this outcome is dependent on the epileptic syndrome. Advances in basic science, neurogenetics, and clinical research have contributed to a greater understanding of the mechanisms of epilepsies as a cause of neurological disease. New medications and surgical techniques have improved the outcome of intractable epilepsy and reduced the morbidity for all epilepsy patients.[2]

For the adolescent or young adult who is also navigating the stresses of peer relationships, independence, and body image, epilepsy can be particularly trying. Fear, prejudice, and stigma of epilepsy are common in society, creating even more challenges for AYAs with this disease. The goals of health care of the adolescent or young adult with epilepsy include making an accurate diagnosis of the epileptic syndrome; evaluation of seizure triggers; treatment of underlying etiologies where possible; appropriate use of anticonvulsant drugs; and recognition and treatment of neurocognitive and/or comorbid psychosocial problems.

ETIOLOGY

Seizures are caused by an excessive discharge of a population of cortical neurons. The location and pattern of spread of activity determine the clinical expression. Recurrent, *unprovoked* seizures are the hallmark of epilepsy. The etiology of epilepsy may be due to genetics or secondary to remote insult to the nervous system. Infection, trauma, metabolic disturbances, drugs, drug withdrawal, or fever may also provoke seizures acutely. Seizures that occur *only* in the setting of an acute provocation are not generally classified as epilepsy. In some AYAs with epilepsy, situations or specific stimuli such as strobe lights may provoke seizures (reflex seizures).

EPIDEMIOLOGY

The prevalence of epilepsy in the general population is 2 per 250 with a higher prevalence in children. The incidence is 0.7 to 1 per 1,000 in the general population.[3] The peak periods for the onset of idiopathic and age-related primary epilepsies are early childhood and adolescence. Epilepsy occurs slightly more often in males than in females (relative risk for males, 1.1 to 2.4 in various studies). In the US and Western Europe, epilepsy is slightly more common among lower socioeconomic groups. Epilepsy is more common in Mexico, South America, and Central America, and in immigrants from these areas in the US, at least partially due to the high incidence of cerebral cysticercosis. Mental retardation, cerebral palsy, and autism are associated with higher rates of epilepsy and lower rates of remission of childhood-onset epilepsy. Epilepsy is associated with an increased risk of death including sudden unexplained death.

CLINICAL MANIFESTATIONS

Table 23.1 lists classifications of seizures, based on the new international classifications.[4]

Seizure Components

The progression of a seizure is characterized by several temporal components:

1. An infrequent prodrome, which consists of altered behavior or mood occurring hours to days before the actual seizure. The individual may have an altered sensation or psychic symptom occurring just before other ictal manifestations.
2. The aura is actually part of the seizure, representing a simple partial seizure, usually with sensory, special sensory, or psychic symptoms.
3. The seizure event may include motor activity.
4. A postictal phase may include altered neurological function ranging from coma to mild lethargy, hemiplegia to minimal focal motor dysfunction, lasting minutes to 24 hours.

Grand Mal Seizures (Generalized Tonic–Clonic Seizures)

A generalized tonic–clonic seizure may have a brief, nondescript aura followed by the main seizure semiology. The main tonic phase involves forceful, postural contractions in flexion or extension. Usually, the early phase includes the following: early head deviation, a cry at the onset, loss of consciousness, fall to the ground, and biting the tongue or cheeks. In the clonic phase, the individual has bilateral, generally symmetrical, brisk jerking movements. Clonic movements have a discernible fast–slow component, as distinguished from other types of movement (writhing, sustained posturing, random bilateral nonsynchronous movements), which are less likely a part of a convulsion. After the tonic–clonic phase, the patient usually becomes flaccid, with or without incontinence of urine or stool, as the seizure stops. In the postictal state, the

TABLE 23.1
Classifications of Seizures

Generalized seizures: Bilaterally symmetrical, both in clinical and electroencephalographical manifestations, without focal features
1. Tonic–clonic, generalized convulsive, grand mal
2. Tonic seizures
3. Clonic seizures
4. Absence seizures
    a. Simple (impaired consciousness only): Classic petit mal
    b. Atypical: Disturbed consciousness plus myoclonic component, automatisms, autonomic component, or abnormality of postural tone
5. Akinetic (atonic) seizures
6. Myoclonic seizures

Partial seizures: Clinical and electroencephalographical onset is localized to one part of the brain (focal)
Simple partial seizures: No impairment of consciousness
1. Motor symptoms
2. Sensory symptoms
3. Autonomic symptoms
4. Special sensory (visual, auditory, olfactory, gustatory)
5. Psychic symptoms (fear, déjà vu, jamais vu, euphoria)

Complex partial seizures: Partial seizure with impairment of consciousness, includes most seizures described as "*psychomotor.*" Seizure may begin with impairment of consciousness or as a simple partial seizure and progress to impaired consciousness

Partial with secondary generalization: Either partial simple or complex partial seizures may secondarily generalize, producing a tonic–clonic or clonic convulsion similar to a primary generalized convulsion. A partial simple seizure may progress through a complex partial seizure or directly to a secondarily generalized seizure
1. Simple partial seizures progressing to generalized seizures
2. Complex partial seizures progressing to generalized seizures
3. Simple partial seizures progressing to complex partial seizures, progressing to generalized seizures

patient is initially unconscious with decreased tone and reflexes. Patients may have fixed pupils. During recovery, a sleeplike state is observed but the patient is responsive to arousal. After recovery, confusion or headaches may be present.

Typical Childhood Absence Epilepsy and Other Absence Seizures

Typical absence seizures in AYAs have no prodrome but often cluster after arousal from sleep. With abrupt onset and no aura, absence seizures are brief (3 seconds to 30 seconds) and are characterized by blank staring and loss of consciousness, usually without falling. In typical absence seizures, minor automatisms may be observed including blinking of eyes and movement of fingers. The seizure onset is abrupt and ends with near-immediate return to normal. In *atypical* absence seizures, the seizures may be (1) associated with automatisms, myoclonic movements, or loss of tone; (2) longer than 30 seconds; and/or (3) characterized by more gradual onset and less-immediate return to normal. After atypical absence seizures, there is no postictal confusion, but amnesia of the seizure is usual. One-third of absence seizures remit during adolescence (more likely in childhood absence epilepsy; less likely in adolescent-onset/juvenile absence epilepsy). The electroencephalogram (EEG) of typical absence seizures shows characteristic 3-Hz spike and wave activity. Other absence syndromes have generalized polyspike wave discharges, slow spike wave (Lennox–Gastaut syndrome), or faster 4- to 5-Hz spike wave (juvenile myoclonic epilepsy [JME] of Janz). Specific epileptic syndromes like JME with onset in adolescence combine absence with myoclonic seizures and occasional grand mal seizures, most prominent on arising in the morning.[5] Early morning myoclonus may be viewed

as "normal" by the patient and not reported without specific questioning. Patients with absence or absence plus myoclonic seizures are more likely to be photosensitive than those with other seizure types. While rare, "Video game"–related seizures are generally limited to these patients.

Myoclonic Seizures

Myoclonic jerks are brisk and irregular and may involve the trunk or extremities, in symmetric or asymmetrical fashion. The amplitude of myoclonic jerks may be small or large enough to cause the patient to fall. Patients are generally aware of the jerks if they are isolated. They may be unaware if myoclonic jerks are part of absence seizures. The differential diagnosis of myoclonic seizures includes tics, nonepileptic myoclonus, and other movement disorders. Myoclonus, usually occurring on rising in the morning, is a characteristic part of JME. Absence or generalized tonic–clonic seizures often occur in these patients. There is no prodrome, aura, or postictal period. The EEG usually shows bursts of spike wave or polyspike and wave in a generalized distribution. Photosensitivity may be demonstrated on EEG using strobe. Myoclonic seizures may be part of an epileptic encephalopathy, such as Lennox–Gastaut syndrome, beginning in early childhood and continuing in adolescence and young adulthood. Photomyoclonus occurs with exposure to a strobe or to strobe-like conditions in AYAs with photosensitive epilepsy. Other generalized seizures may also be present. Various degenerative conditions, including progressive myoclonic epilepsies and subacute sclerosing panencephalitis, may present during adolescence and young adulthood and may be characterized by myoclonic seizures.

Partial Simple Seizures

Benign focal epilepsy of childhood (also known as *benign Rolandic epilepsy (BRE)*) is the most common cause of focal motor seizures in childhood and early adolescence. Seizures in BRE are partial simple seizures usually involving the face or arm; seizures may secondarily generalize. Episodes are most likely to occur during drowsiness or sleep onset, or upon awakening. Seizures usually resolve by middle adolescence (14 to 16 years of age). Magnetic resonance imaging (MRI) of the brain in BRE is normal. In contrast, the onset of partial simple seizures during adolescence or young adulthood is more commonly associated with structural pathology (e.g., tumor, arteriovenous malformation, head injury, malformation, and stroke).

Sensory phenomena (aura) may be the only manifestation of a brief limited seizure. Most partial simple seizures are focal motor seizures in which consciousness is retained. Speech arrest and drooling may occur with ictal focus in the dominant hemisphere (left brain in the right-handed person). Focal clonic activity may "march" up an extremity or spread from arm to face or arm to leg, or vice versa. After the seizure, headache or postictal hemiparesis (Todd paralysis) may be present. BRE is associated with central temporal spikes, which are more commonly seen in sleep. The central temporal spikes are commonly bilateral, even if all observed seizures were on the same side. Other partial seizures may be associated with spikes or slowing in a unilateral distribution.

Partial Seizures with Complex Symptomatology

Partial seizures with complex symptomatology are seizures of focal onset accompanied by altered consciousness. These seizures may begin at any age. Although still unusual, structural pathology is more common than in generalized epilepsies or benign focal epilepsy of childhood. For instance, mesial temporal sclerosis may cause seizures of temporal lobe origin with onset during adolescence. Patients may report that "they know a seizure is coming," which may occur hours or days before a partial complex seizure. Headaches and changes in mood and/or appetite may also be reported.

Typical partial complex seizures consist of the following sequence (any of these symptoms may be absent other than the altered state of consciousness):

1. Initial sensory, autonomic, or psychic symptoms lasting seconds to minutes; common phenomena include fear, déjà vu, "rising feeling" in abdomen, tingling, and visual, auditory, olfactory, or gustatory hallucination. Flushing or pallor may be observed. Consciousness is generally retained, and patient remembers this part of the seizure.
2. A blank stare combined with impairment of responsiveness and consciousness. The patient is motionless and does not remember events clearly during this phase, if at all.
3. Automatisms such as hand wringing, picking, lip smacking, walking aimlessly, grunting, gagging, or swallowing. Although destructive or injurious behavior may occur, directed deliberate violence does not. Consciousness is impaired or lost during this phase, and the patient is amnestic of events during this phase.
4. Complex partial seizures from the frontal lobe may produce thrashing, agitated movements, bicycling leg movements, or pelvic thrusting, which are difficult to distinguish from nonepileptic seizures. After the seizure, confusion, stupor, headache, and lethargy may last seconds to hours.

Seizure triggers include sleep deprivation, alcohol, or drug ingestion. The EEG may demonstrate focal spikes in temporal, frontal, or parietal areas (usually unilateral), but may also be normal. Features that help differentiate various seizures reported as "little seizures" or "staring spells" (partial complex, typical, and atypical absence) are listed in Table 23.2.

ETIOLOGY/DIFFERENTIAL DIAGNOSIS OF SEIZURES

Etiology of Seizures

Symptomatic Seizures (due to Acute Systemic Disturbance or Trauma)
a. Acute metabolic disturbance (e.g., hypoglycemia, hyponatremia, and hypocalcemia)
b. Acute CNS infection (e.g., encephalitis and meningitis) or acute stroke
c. Intoxication (e.g., cocaine, alcohol, "ecstasy," phencyclidine, ketamine, and inhalants)
d. Drug or alcohol withdrawal (e.g., prolonged barbiturates, sedatives, and benzodiazepines use)
e. Acute head trauma (impact seizure and seizure in first few days after significant head trauma)
f. Convulsive syncope: Brief tonic or clonic movements occurring after primary syncope

Acquired (Symptomatic or Secondary) Epilepsies due to Remote History of CNS Insult
a. Cerebral malformations: Macroscopic or microscopic (cortical dysgenesis)
b. Intrauterine infections (e.g., cytomegalovirus and toxoplasmosis), perinatal insult, or postneonatal infections (e.g., meningitis, encephalitis, and brain abscess)
c. Posttraumatic epilepsy
d. Tuberous sclerosis, brain tumors, and other mass lesions
e. Vascular malformations and infarctions or cysticercosis
f. Genetic changes due to progressive or degenerative conditions
g. Unknown but presumed symptomatic: Epileptic encephalopathies such as Lennox–Gastaut syndrome, and Dravet syndrome

Idiopathic Epilepsy (Also Called Age-Related Epilepsies)
a. Primary generalized epilepsies (also called genetic generalized epilepsies)
b. Benign focal epilepsy of childhood

Differential Diagnosis of Paroxysmal Events That May Mimic Seizure Activity
1. Vasovagal syncope, migraine, or orthostatic hypotension
2. Cardiac disease: arrhythmias, low-output states, and mitral valve prolapse
3. Hyperventilation and anxiety states
4. Sleep disturbances:
   a. Narcolepsy: Catalepsy, sleep attacks, sleep paralysis, and hypnagogic hallucinations
   b. Drowsiness or sleep attacks in patients with obstructive sleep apnea or sleep deprivation
   c. Sleepwalking, rapid eye movement sleep disturbance, and other parasomnias
   d. Night terrors
   e. Periodic leg movements in sleep[6]
5. Movement disorders:
   a. Tics
   b. Paroxysmal kinesiogenic choreoathetosis
   c. Stiff-man syndrome and other syndromes of continuous muscle fiber activity
   d. Dystonias (paroxysmal torticollis, activity-related dystonias, dystonia musculorum deformans, and drug-related)
   e. Pseudohypoparathyroidism: AYAs with hypocalcemia secondary to pseudohypoparathyroidism may present with seizure-like episodes that are primarily dystonic
   f. Restless leg syndrome

TABLE 23.2

Features of Absence and Complex Partial Seizures

Type	Aura	Loss of Consciousness	Duration	Automatisms	Postictal State	Memory of Event	Electroencephalogram	Associated Abnormalities
Typical absence (Petit Mal)	None	Immediate	5–20 sec	Occasional simple automatisms	None	None	3-Hz spike wave	20% have grand mal seizures as well; mentally normal
Absence atypical	None	Immediate	5–45 sec	Occasional automatisms	None	None	Slow spike wave or polyspike	Myoclonus, drop attacks, grand mal; mental retardation more common
Complex partial	Often	Gradual or partial in some patients	5 sec–5 min	Frequent, more complicated	Frequent	Partial in some patients	Focal spikes	May have secondary generalization; structural lesions may underlie disorder

6. Pseudoseizures (nonepileptic seizures)
7. Episodic "staring" and inattention:
   a. Attention deficit disorder and
   b. Disorders of arousal.

Differentiating Grand Mal Seizures from Syncopal Episode

Table 23.3 compares grand mal seizures with syncopal episodes.

Differentiating Nonepileptic Seizures (Pseudoseizures) Versus Epilepsy

Table 23.4 compares pseudoseizures with epilepsy.

⬤ EVALUATION

History

Epilepsy is primarily a clinical diagnosis based on the history. The clinician should review the following with the observers of the event:

1. What was the adolescent or young adult doing before the episode began—sleeping, quiet, watching television, exercising, reading, or anxious? Where and when did the event occur?

TABLE 23.3

Grand Mal Seizures versus Syncopal Episodes

Component	Grand Mal	Syncope
Preictal	May have prodrome; aura may occur at time of loss of consciousness	Variable—may experience faint or dizzy feeling
Ictal	Violent body spasms; often cries out; sweaty appearance; may have incontinence after tonic–clonic component; coma after seizure	No stereotype; no abrupt onset; slowly falls to floor; cold and clammy May have mild twitching
Postictal	Gradual return to consciousness; confusion	Rarely; confusion

TABLE 23.4

Nonepileptic Seizures versus Epilepsy

Nonepileptic Seizures	Epileptic Seizures
Observers nearby	Observed or unobserved
Bizarre motor activity, back arching, pelvic thrusting	Usually stereotypic for a particular patient; automatisms of complex partial seizures may vary with activity and environment; generalized convulsions, usually tonic–clonic
No incontinence	May be incontinent of urine and stool
During ictus: Active pupillary reflex, normal corneal reflex	May have dilated unreactive pupils and lose corneal reflex during event
May occur in patients with epilepsy; may have abnormal EEG interictally, but no change during episode	Rhythmic spikes, slowing or electrodecremental EEG during episode, but may be normal
	Two- or threefold increase above baseline serum prolactin after convulsion or partial complex seizure is nearly invariable

2. Did the seizure occur just as the adolescent or young adult was falling asleep, just after awakening, or during deep sleep?
3. What was the first abnormality noted? What happened during the seizure? Did the adolescent or young adult seem to be aware that something was wrong?
4. Could observers get the adolescent or young adult's attention during the episode? Respond to commands? At what point did unresponsiveness start? How long did unconsciousness last?
5. Was there incontinence of urine or stool? What happened after the seizure?

Often, a review of the following points with the adolescent or young adult patient can be helpful:

1. What was the last event he or she remembers before the seizure?
2. Could the patient hear or understand people talking during the seizure? Could he or she respond?
3. What happened after the seizure? What is the first thing recalled after the event?
4. Were there any precipitating event such as sensory stimulation, activity, drugs, meals, medications, sleep pattern, stress, and menses? Have earlier seizures or similar events occurred?
5. Is there a family history of epilepsy, neurocutaneous syndromes, and other neurological conditions?
6. Was there any pertinent perinatal history, particularly birth injury, prematurity, and maternal infections?
7. Is there any history of CNS infections or trauma or drug history, including prescribed, over-the-counter, and "street" drugs and alcohol?
8. Is there any other recent changes in cognition, motor function, or other neurological function to suggest onset of neurological disease other than the seizures?
9. Has the adolescent or young adult traveled to and/or been around people from areas with endemic cysticercosis/Taenia solium?

Physical Examination

A general physical examination is recommended to evaluate for evidence of systemic disease. The clinician should look for signs of a neurocutaneous syndrome such as café au lait spots, depigmented macules, adenoma sebaceum (Fig. 23.1), shagreen patch, or subungual fibromas. Fundoscopic examination for optic disc edema (papilledema), focal abnormalities on neurologic exam and abnormalities in gait, or movements at rest and with activity (movement disorder) may suggest alternative explanations of symptoms. Episodes due to arrhythmia and/or syncope may be accompanied by abnormalities in blood pressure and pulse (arrhythmia), evidence of mitral valve prolapse, heart failure, or other abnormalities on cardiac examination. If absence (petit mal) seizures are suspected,

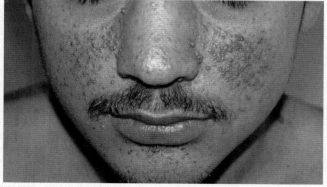

FIGURE 23.1 Adenoma sebaceum. (From Goodheart HP. *Goodheart's photoguide of common skin disorders.* 2nd ed. Philadelphia, PA: Lippincott Williams & Wilkins, 2003.)

the patient should be observed while hyperventilating for 2 to 3 minutes to determine if an episode can be induced.

Laboratory Evaluation

Complete blood cell count and routine chemistries including liver function tests are indicated before initiating anticonvulsant therapy (as baseline). Platelet count should be included if valproic acid will be used because thrombocytopenia is a potential side effect. In an apparently well adolescent or young adult without underlying medical problems, electrolytes, phosphorus, or magnesium have a very low yield for identifying a cause of seizures.

Rarely, an adolescent or young adult presenting with seizure-like episodes may be found to have very low blood calcium concentration because of pseudohypoparathyroidism. Because this condition is congenital, the calcium concentration is low from infancy and has usually already been identified. Measurement of blood glucose may be helpful if hypoglycemia is suspected, but only if the blood sample is obtained while the patient is symptomatic. These tests are not indicated on a routine basis in most AYAs with seizures.

A routine EEG study should be obtained during states of waking, hyperventilation, photic stimulation, drowsiness, and sleep. Hyperventilation is particularly useful if absence (petit mal) seizures are suspected. Photic stimulation is helpful if the patient reports that seizures occur when exposed to video games, television, rapid flashing lights, or in the car. An EEG while sleep-deprived increases the yield in patients with complex partial seizures, benign focal epilepsy of childhood, and some generalized epilepsies. MRI is indicated for focal seizures (except clear-cut BRE of childhood), seizures associated with neurological abnormalities, papilledema, neurocutaneous stigmata, or suspected degenerative conditions. Lumbar puncture is only indicated if infection or hemorrhage is suspected.

THERAPY

Anticonvulsant Therapy

After the diagnosis of epilepsy is made, two major components of therapy exist: drug therapy to control the seizures and counseling regarding psychosocial issues.

Drug Therapy
General Guidelines

- The clinician should start with a single anticonvulsant medication and consider the side effect profile because these factors will influence both safety and adherence.[7–10] For example, sodium valproate is effective for many seizure types; however, the side effects—including increased appetite, weight gain, transient hair loss, and menstrual irregularities—may be unacceptable to many AYAs.
- Medications should be adjusted slowly. Increase the dosage no more frequently than time increments equal to five times the drug's half-life until seizures are controlled or toxicity occurs except when control is urgent (frequent seizures or status epilepticus).
- Serum drug levels may be useful, but clinical response is more important.[11] Serum levels should not be frequently evaluated. Before changing to a second anticonvulsant medication due to poor response, serum levels can be helpful to detect fast metabolizers, which have been reported with most medications.
- Daily dosing should be based on the half-life of the drug. If seizures are refractory, more frequent dosing may be necessary, but increases the risk for drug toxicity and side effects. At least five half-lives are necessary for medication level to reach steady state after starting a medication or changing the dose. Most medications can be given twice a day (b.i.d.); adherence is better with b.i.d. than thrice-a-day (t.i.d.) schedules.[12,13]

- AYAs should have close follow-up, including monitoring of seizure frequency, physical examination, and evaluation for drug toxicity. Close follow-up also allows for early detection of nonmedical side effects (social, academic, independence, and vocational) and progression of the epilepsy itself.
- Unless allergic or serious idiosyncratic effects are evident, substitution with a second drug should only be considered when the dose of the first drug has been pushed to tolerance without controlling the seizures. When the second drug is at adequate serum levels, wean the first. Polytherapy is reserved for AYAs with refractory seizures unresponsive to trials of monotherapy with at least two to three different anticonvulsants at maximum tolerated levels. These individuals should be referred to a level 4 epilepsy center for further evaluation. AYAs with refractory focal epilepsy should also be referred to a level 4 epilepsy center because epilepsy surgery may be a therapeutic consideration.[14]
- Discontinuation of medication: In the adolescent or young adult who is seizure-free on medication, the clinician must assess the risks and benefits of continued therapy with anticonvulsants. Medications may be tapered and discontinued after the patient is seizure free for two to four years.[15,16] The estimated risk for recurrence of seizures after tapering is 30% to 40%, with the greatest risk occurring during the tapering period or in the first six months after discontinuation of the medication. Risk factors for recurrence are debated but include the following in at least some studies:
  1. Mental retardation or neurological abnormalities
  2. Long duration of seizures or many seizures before full control with medication
  3. Partial seizures (other than the benign focal epilepsies of childhood such as BRE), especially with a postictal Todd's paresis
  4. Abnormal EEG findings despite seizure-free period (highest risk: combination of focal slowing and focal epileptiform spikes)
  5. Nocturnal seizures
  6. History of febrile seizures
  7. Adolescent-onset seizures are less likely to remit than seizures with onset in earlier childhood.

Medication should be tapered one drug at a time (generally sedating drugs first), tapering each drug over six weeks to three months.

Drugs for Specific Seizure Types
Generalized Tonic–Clonic Seizures, Either Primarily or Secondarily Generalized

Older Generation: These medications are often accompanied by more side effects.[17,18]

a. Phenobarbital: Least expensive, can be given once a day. In developing countries, it is often the only drug available. In the US, it is less often used as first-line therapy due to concerns about cognitive slowing.
b. Phenytoin (Dilantin): Brand-name capsules can be used once a day. Using most generic capsules, liquid or chewable tablets, dose must be divided b.i.d. or t.i.d.
c. Valproic acid (Depakene or Depakote): Depakote is preferred. An extended-release form (Depakote ER) is available that is appropriate for once-a-day use in selected patients.
d. Primidone (Mysoline): Reserved for patients with refractory seizures.

Newer Generation: These medications are preferred due to their more favorable side effect profile

a. Lamotrigine (Lamictal): Useful for partial and generalized seizures, including AYAs with JME. Generally reserved for AYAs who are intolerant to valproic acid. Lamotrigine is recommended as first-line monotherapy for idiopathic generalized epilepsy among women of reproductive age (including those who are pregnant or breast-feeding).

b. Topiramate (Topamax): Effective but often significantly sedating and/or cognitively impairing, at least upon initiation. Tendency to cause mild anorexia and weight loss is viewed by some AYAs as an advantage over other anticonvulsants, which tend to promote weight gain. When used, dosage should be titrated slowly (weekly) to avoid cognitive dulling.

c. Felbamate (Felbatol): Effective for several seizure types, including generalized convulsive (tonic–clonic) seizures, drop attacks, and atypical absence seizures. It is only approved for children with Lennox–Gastaut syndrome (mixed generalized epilepsy). An initial alarming incidence of aplastic anemia has limited the use of felbamate to patients with refractory seizures who are able to give informed consent to its risks and comply with the requirement for frequent laboratory monitoring. The actual risk of aplastic anemia is probably very low, except in patients with other autoimmune conditions such as systemic lupus erythematosus.

d. Other newer anticonvulsants, occasionally useful for generalized convulsions, particularly those thought to be partial with secondary generalization, include levitiracetam (Keppra) and Zonisamide (Zonegran).[19,20]

In patients with mixed generalized seizures (i.e., generalized tonic–clonic plus myoclonic or absence seizures) or idiopathic generalized epilepsies, carbamazepine, phenytoin, oxcarbazepine (Trileptal), or tiagabine (Gabitril) occasionally may induce or exacerbate myoclonic, drop attacks or generalized tonic–clonic seizures. Valproic acid, preferably in the long-acting capsules (Depakote) or extended-release capsules (Depakote ER), is the drug of choice in mixed generalized epilepsies (grand mal plus myoclonic or absence) except Lennox–Gastaut syndrome. Rufinamide (Banzel) or clobazem (Onfi) is a drug of choice for AYAs with Lennox–Gastaut syndrome.

Childhood Absence Epilepsy

a. Ethosuximide (Zarontin): Standard first-line therapy, which is usually well tolerated for typical childhood absence epilepy (3-Hz spike wave EEG pattern) and the most effective drug in the recent childhood absence epilepsy clinical trial[21]

b. Valproic acid (Depakote): First choice if absence and generalized tonic–clonic seizures coexist, for atypical absence, or for JME

c. Lamotrigine (Lamictal): Second choice if generalized seizures coexist or for JME

d. Levetiracetam (Keppra): Third treatment choice if generalized seizures coexist or for JME

e. Felbamate (Felbatol): This is effective as monotherapy or adjunctive therapy for several seizure types in adults (not first line, see Drug section above), but is approved only for children and adolescents with Lennox–Gastaut syndrome (mixed generalized epilepsy).

Simple Partial Seizures (Focal Motor, Focal Sensory) and Complex Partial Seizures with or without Automatisms

a. Carbamazepine (Tegretol, Carbatrol): Generics are acceptable if same generic is consistently available; avoid switching brands. Two extended-release carbamazepine preparations allow b.i.d. dosing but are more expensive (Tegretol-XR and Carbatrol).

b. Oxcarbazepine (Trileptal): An alternative to carbamazepine for patients who have had an adverse behavioral reaction to carbamazepine at the therapeutic dose. Patients who are allergic to carbamazepine may also react to oxcarbazepine. Oxcarbazepine does not have an active metabolite. Pharmacokinetic interactions are less problematic than with

carbamazepine, making it appropriate for patients on other medications that are affected by or affect the cytochrome P-450 system—an important consideration for AYAs with multisystem disease needing many other medications (e.g., during chemotherapy or patients with acquired immunodeficiency syndrome).

c. Phenobarbital: See earlier discussion. Primidone (Mysoline): Reserve for patients with refractory epilepsy.

d. Phenytoin (Dilantin): See earlier discussion regarding generic forms.

e. Gabapentin (Neurontin): Approved for monotherapy and adjunctive treatment of partial-onset seizures. Gabapentin is not metabolized and does not change the metabolism of other medications. Consider use in multisystem disease when avoidance of alteration of drug metabolism of other agents is important (i.e., patients with organ transplant or those on chemotherapy, etc).

f. Lamotrigine (Lamictal): See earlier discussion. First-line or adjunctive treatment of partial seizures.

g. Topiramate (Topamax): See earlier discussion. First-line or adjunctive treatment for partial seizures

h. Tiagabine (Gabitril): Adjunctive treatment for partial seizures

i. Levetiracetam (Keppra): First-line or adjunctive treatment for partial seizures. Often used as first-line therapy in patients with hepatic dysfunction or during chemotherapy because it is excreted by kidneys and is not dependent on the P-450 system for its metabolism. The major concern is the relatively higher risk of behavior disturbance, particularly in AYAs who already have a history of agitated or aggressive behavior.

j. Clonazepam, clorazepate, or other benzodiazepines: Occasionally effective as monotherapy, but rapid development of tolerance and sedation are significant problems. May increase salivation and respiratory difficulties

k. Zonisamide (Zonegran): First-line or adjunctive therapy for partial seizures. Risks are similar to those of topiramate (sedation, renal stones, acidosis, anorexia, rash, oligohydrosis). Very long half-life makes it appropriate for once-daily dosing.

l. Felbamate (Felbatol): See earlier discussion. Reserve for patients with refractory epilepsy.

Side Effects of Anticonvulsant Drugs

Adverse effects of anticonvulsants can be divided into two major groups: 1) dose-related reactions; and 2) idiosyncratic reactions unrelated to drug level. Mild sedation is common with initiation of any anticonvulsant. For some, sedation and ataxia may be significant; therefore, initiation of treatment should generally start at low doses with slow increases over several weeks. Potential reproductive effects are also important to consider in females of childbearing potential.[18,22–26]

Dose-Related Effects

Toxic CNS effects are similar among most anticonvulsants. Excessive levels (or deliberate overdoses) produce ataxia, nystagmus, and sedation progressing to coma, with respiratory and cardiac depression at extremely high doses. Movement disorders (chorea) and tremor may be seen at toxic drug levels, primarily with phenytoin or carbamazepine.

Non-CNS dose-related effects are common. Alterations in vitamin D metabolism produce "chemical rickets," generally without clinically symptomatic abnormalities. Clinical rickets is occasionally seen in AYAs with multiple disabilities receiving anticonvulsants but having limited sun exposure and lacking vitamin D supplementation. Osteopenia is frequently found in studies of patients of all ages taking anticonvulsants chronically. If dietary intake of calcium is low, the health care provider should consider supplementation with oral calcium and vitamin D. Some anticonvulsants (phenytoin and carbamazepine) may have adverse effects on bone density by directly interfering with osteoblast proliferation.[27,28] Folate metabolism may also be altered, producing megaloblastic changes, usually without anemia.

For most AYAs taking anticonvulsants, health care providers should consider routinely supplementing with a multivitamin containing at least 400 µg of folic acid. AYA females taking anticonvulsants, particularly those with a potential for future childbearing, should take 1 to 4 mg of supplemental folic acid daily, depending upon which anticonvulsant they are taking (AYAs taking valproic acid are particularly at risk for deficiency).

Thyroid studies are commonly affected by anticonvulsant drugs, but usually without clinical evidence of hypothyroidism. In contrast, gastric distress is common with valproic acid, ethosuximide, banzel, and felbamate. These side effects may be minimized if the dose is divided or given with food.

Drug interactions are also common. Virtually all first-generation anticonvulsants induce hepatic microsomal enzymes, increasing clearance of themselves (autoinduction), each other, and various other medications including steroids, estrogens, and anticoagulants. Exceptions are the second-generation anticonvulsants, gabapentin (Neurontin), and levetiracetam (Keppra), which are excreted unchanged in the urine and do not affect other drug metabolisms. Conversely, several drugs significantly inhibit the metabolism of carbamazepine and to a lesser extent, of phenytoin. The most commonly encountered problematic interaction is with erythromycin (and the newer macrolides), which competitively inhibits carbamazepine metabolism to an extent that patients on previously stable doses may develop significant toxicity less than 24 hours after the addition of the antibiotic. A similar effect is seen with propoxyphene (Darvon) and with grapefruit juice. AYAs taking carbamazepine should be advised to avoid these drugs and grapefruit juice. Isoniazid (INH) inhibits both carbamazepine and phenytoin metabolism. Because INH is generally used on a long-term basis, the anticonvulsant drug can be adjusted to account for the decreased clearance.

Idiosyncratic (Non–Dose-Related) Side Effects
The following side effects may occur with any anticonvulsant.

- Allergic reactions such as skin rash, Stevens–Johnson syndrome, lupus-like syndromes, and even death can occur with any anticonvulsant, although most reported cases are associated with phenobarbital, phenytoin, carbamazepine, or lamotrigine.
- Bone marrow toxicity, usually reversible, has been reported with several anticonvulsants. Fatal aplastic anemia has been reported with carbamazepine and felbamate, primarily in older adults. High serum levels of valproic acid are associated with reversible bone marrow suppression, most commonly thrombocytopenia.
- Hepatic or pancreatic toxicity and metabolic abnormalities are seen in patients receiving valproic acid, primarily in infants, but can rarely occur with any anticonvulsant, at any age. These toxicities may include hyperammonemia, lactic acidosis, and Reye-like syndrome. Carnitine depletion, usually asymptomatic, may occur with valproic acid, particularly with long-term use in patients with poor muscle bulk. It is advisable to follow carnitine levels and supplement as needed. Valproic acid or topiramate can rarely cause serious pancreatitis. In a patient taking valproic acid or topiramate with abdominal pain or vomiting, serum lipase should be assessed.
- Adenopathy, "mononucleosis syndrome," and pseudolymphoma are primarily associated with hydantoin.
- Moderate hair thinning is relatively common with valproic acid. Frank alopecia does not occur. Other anticonvulsants may produce hair loss as part of allergic reactions.
- Weight changes: Weight gain is most frequently problematic with valproic acid but has been reported with many

anticonvulsants. Weight loss is common with felbamate, particularly at higher doses, and with valproic acid in young children. Topiramate and zonisamide often produce short-term anorexia and weight loss.

Reproductive Side Effects
There is a moderately increased risk of abnormal pregnancy outcome in women with epilepsy, regardless of specific drug treatment.[18,22–27,29] Facial malformations, particularly cleft palate, microcephaly, congenital heart disease, and minor malformations such as hypoplastic nails have been associated with the use of phenytoin and other anticonvulsants. These nonspecific malformations are more frequent in offspring of epileptic mothers, regardless of treatment. Open neural tube defects may be more frequent in fetuses exposed to valproic acid and carbamazepine.

All AYA females who are taking these anticonvulsants should also take a multivitamin containing at least 400 µg of folic acid. Female patients on anticonvulsants who are anticipating pregnancy should take 1 to 4 mg/day of folic acid. Unfortunately, a few case reports suggest that even higher doses of periconceptional folic acid may not be protective against the development of malformations. It is difficult to choose an anticonvulsant that is "completely safe." Risks to the developing fetus must be balanced against the risk of recurrent convulsions if medications are withdrawn. There is no reason to withhold oral contraceptives from a woman receiving anticonvulsants, but higher estrogen doses may be needed due to more rapid metabolism of the component hormones via induction of the cytochrome P-450 system.

Other Problems with Anticonvulsant Therapy
Because AYAs in whom epilepsy is well controlled often have no symptoms except for the drug side effects, it is tempting for them to take their medications only intermittently. These and other adherence problems are common. Suggestions for improving adherence include the following:

1. Provide clear explanations of prescribed medications and their expected side effects. Use medications with side effects that are most acceptable to the adolescent or young adult.
2. Foster the patient's growing responsibility for taking their medications. "Day-of-the-week" pillboxes, filled and checked weekly, with parental supervision, may help an adolescent or young adult patient to manage his or her own medications.
3. Discuss possible consequences of nonadherence with the adolescent or young adult, such as recurrent seizures and inability to get or keep a driver's license.

Alternative Treatments of Refractory Epilepsy
Vagus Nerve Stimulation
Vagus nerve stimulation (VNS) is a therapeutic option used as an adjunctive treatment for adolescents and adults with medically refractory epilepsy. The VNS device consists of a programmable, battery-operated generator and a silastic-coated lead, which are implanted subcutaneously in the chest, with the lead attached to the left vagus nerve. Multicenter trials evaluating the efficacy of VNS devices demonstrated a 50% or more reduction in seizures in approximately 40% of patients with refractory partial seizures. Newer data suggest that VNS may be effective for idiopathic and symptomatic generalized epilepsies. Common side effects include hoarseness of voice, local pain, paresthesias, dyspnea, and dysphagia. Uncommon complications include vocal cord paralysis and lower facial muscle weakness.

The Ketogenic Diet
The ketogenic diet is a tightly controlled, high-fat, low-carbohydrate diet used in the treatment of intractable epilepsy. Alternative seizure diets such as the modified Adkins diet or low-glycemic index diet are better tolerated by AYAs and have efficacy comparable

to the ketogenic diet. These diets are designed to place the body in a state simulating starvation, which results in the production of high levels of ketone bodies. Undertaking and adhering to this diet require strong commitments from both the patient and caregivers as well as the expertise of a dietitian and clinician familiar with diets. Expense may be substantial, including dietitian visits and special foods, which may not be covered by health insurance.

Epilepsy Surgery

Cortical resection or hemispherectomy may result in cessation or dramatic reduction of seizures for selected AYAs with intractable localization-related epilepsy. Key elements of surgical candidacy include intractability, a localized epileptic zone; and a low risk for new postoperative neurological deficits. Surgical options include temporal lobectomy, extratemporal and multilobar resections, functional or anatomic hemispherectomy, and corpus callosotomy. AYAs with uncontrolled or complicated epilepsy warrant referral to specialized centers with extensive pediatric epilepsy surgery experience that can offer comprehensive risk–benefit evaluation for each patient. There is evidence that early temporal lobectomy in AYAs with intractable complex partial seizures and mesial temporal sclerosis may improve long-term quality of life and overall outcome.

Other Important Treatment Issues
Educating and Dispelling Myths

Many myths about epilepsy can be dispelled by reassuring AYAs and their families and providing education about their condition. First, make sure that the adolescent or young adult understands that epilepsy is not contagious. Most seizure disorders can improve or resolve with age and can be prevented with medication. Epilepsy does not generally lower the patient's intelligence. He or she can participate in almost all activities. Epilepsy is generally not a "mental illness."

Many parents should also be given these reassurances, in addition to the following:

- There is no need to feel guilty. It is unlikely that anything the parent did (or did not do) caused the epilepsy.
- For AYAs, there is no need for special schooling solely because of epilepsy.
- Epilepsy does not *cause* learning disabilities. The prevalence of learning disabilities is higher in patients with epilepsy as a group. Some AYAs with epilepsy and learning disabilities may need neuropsychological testing and an individualized education plan. For instance, 30% of adolescents with idiopathic generalized epilepsies have attentional disorders that should be evaluated.

The adolescent or young adult and family should be educated about the following:

1. Diagnosis
2. Importance of careful observation and record keeping in a seizure diary
3. Avoidance of precipitating factors such as poor sleep
4. Side effects of medication
5. Prognosis and follow-up
6. Precautions and restrictions until seizure control is achieved, particularly regarding driving, swimming, and bicycle and motorcycle riding. Specific geographic requirements regarding reports to the Department of Motor Vehicles/Ministry of Transportation should be explained. Restrictions may need to be imposed regarding use of hazardous equipment such as power tools.
7. The need for effective contraception among sexually active AYA females who are taking anticonvulsant drugs. Supplementation with folic acid should be discussed with all AYA females with epilepsy who are of childbearing potential.

Family members, roommates, and caregivers should be aware of first aid for seizure episodes:

1. Help the person into a lying position if there is adequate warning.
2. Do not try to restrain the person.
3. Clear the area of dangerous objects.
4. Remove glasses and loosen tight clothing.
5. Turn the head to one side (or roll the person onto his or her side) to allow saliva to drain out and do not put anything into the person's mouth.
6. Report what you observe and try to time the episode with a watch.
7. Family members should be given specific criteria to call for paramedic help. For instance, if the seizure lasts longer than 5 to 10 minutes, or if seizures cluster without recovery, call for emergency medical help. Specific advice should be individualized, on the basis of the patient's seizure history.
8. In AYAs who have clusters of seizures or prolonged breakthrough seizures that require emergency care, family members can be taught to use a rectal dose of diazepam. In the US, a rectal gel form of diazepam is available in premeasured syringes as Diastat. The dose for AYAs is 0.2 mg/kg, rounded up to the next available size, with a maximum of 20 mg/dose. Intranasal or buccal midazolam has also been used to abort prolonged seizures or interrupt seizure clusters, but is "off-label" usage.

Miscellaneous Issues

In general, there is no need for restriction of activities once seizures are controlled, except for solo swimming, scuba diving, mountain climbing, or bicycling in areas with traffic. AYAs should generally be restricted from contact sports until seizures are controlled. The patient with epilepsy should wear a medical identification bracelet or necklace. This may reduce unnecessary trips to emergency facilities or unneeded testing if a seizure occurs away from home. Health care professionals should be aware of local driving laws that are relevant to AYAs with epilepsy. These should be explained to the patient along with the rationale for the laws. AYAs may be more adherent to medication in order to be seizure-free so that they can be licensed to drive. Laws regarding mandatory reporting to state Department of Motor Vehicles/Ministry of Transportation vary among the states. The patient's school should be informed if seizures are a recurring problem. If the adolescent or young adult has been seizure-free for an extended time, there is often no need to inform the teachers of the diagnosis, because this may cause unnecessary restrictions and lowered expectations. Abstinence from alcohol is usually desirable; more than a couple of drinks of alcohol a day may increase the risk of seizures in AYAs with epilepsy by lowering of the seizure threshold. Clinicians should anticipate other concerns which are specific to the AYA population. Because of their unpredictable and abrupt onset, threat of injury, and embarrassment, seizures can have significant impact on developing AYAs. Younger adolescents may be concerned about whether their body is normal. Middle adolescents may have concerns about their peers, driving, and sports restrictions. Older AYAs may be more concerned regarding vocational planning and perhaps future health insurance. Depression may occur among AYAs with epilepsy; thus, routine assessments for depression and suicidality are warranted.[30]

SPECIAL CONSIDERATIONS FOR FEMALES WITH EPILEPSY

Effect of Puberty on Epilepsy

Some AYA females with epilepsy experience changes in seizure activity that relate to changes in pubertal status, menstrual cycle, or pregnancy. In general, estrogen increases neuronal excitation and reduces inhibition, whereas progesterone has the opposite effect. Seizures may have their onset or change in frequency during puberty. Both JME and photosensitive seizures often present during puberty. In contrast, childhood absence epilepsy and BRE often remit during puberty.

With the rise of estrogen at ovulation and with the fall in progesterone during menses, seizures are more common during these times of the menstrual cycle. Foldvary-Schaefer and Falcone provide a comprehensive review of catamenial epilepsy.[31]

Reproductive Dysfunction and Contraception

Fertility in women with epilepsy is approximately one-third that of nonepileptic siblings.[26] This may reflect either a fear of consequences of pregnancy, social pressure not to become a parent, or physiological disruption to reproductive cycles. Anovulation is more common in females with epilepsy. Women with epilepsy appear to have a higher frequency of reproductive endocrine abnormalities including alterations of daily basal and pulsatile release of luteinizing hormone. Women with epilepsy may also have hormonal abnormalities because of anticonvulsant medication. Valproic acid in particular is associated with a syndrome similar to polycystic ovary syndrome as well as an isolated rise in circulating androgens. These hormonal abnormalities appear to be reversible with cessation of anticonvulsant medication.[29]

As discussed previously, there is an increased risk of abnormal pregnancy outcomes in women with epilepsy regardless of the specific drug treatment. The major issues with the use of contraception in AYAs with epilepsy are the interactions between certain anticonvulsants and their effect on the metabolism of hormonal contraceptives. The most significant problems are with those hormonal contraceptives with low doses of hormones used in combination with anticonvulsants that induce the cytochrome P-450 system (e.g., phenobarbital, primidone, phenytoin, carbamazepine, felbamate, topiramate, and vigabatrin). See Chapter 43 for a full discussion on these interactions and Figure 43.1 for the Center for Disease Control and Prevention's Criteria for Contraceptive Use.

REFERENCES

1. Camfield PR, Camfield CS. The prognosis of childhood epilepsy. *Semin Pediatr Neurol* 1994;1:102.
2. French JA, Gazzola DM. Antiepileptic drug treatment: new drugs and new strategies. *Continuum (Minneap Minn)* 2013;19(3 Epilepsy):643–655.
3. Kobau R, Zahran H, Thurman DJ, et al. Epilepsy surveillance among adults—19 States, Behavioral Risk Factor Surveillance System, 2005. *MMWR Surveill Summ* 2008;57(6):1–20.
4. Wheless JW, Kim HL. Adolescent seizures and epilepsy syndromes. *Epilepsia* 2002;43 (suppl 3):33.
5. Zifkin B, Andermann E, Andermann F. Mechanisms, genetics, and pathogenesis of juvenile myoclonic epilepsy. *Curr Opin Neurol* 2005;18(2):147–153.
6. Restless legs syndrome: detection and management in primary care. National Heart, Lung, and Blood Institute Working Group on Restless Legs Syndrome. *Am Fam Physician* 2000;62(1):108–114.
7. Buck D, Jacoby A, Baker GA. Factors influencing compliance with antiepileptic drug regimes. *Seizure* 1997;6:87.
8. French JA, Kanner AM, Bautista J, et al. Efficacy and tolerability of the new antiepileptic drugs I: treatment of new onset epilepsy. *Neurology* 2004;62:1252.
9. French JA, Kanner AM, Bautista J, et al. Efficacy and tolerability of the new antiepileptic drugs II: treatment of refractory epilepsy. *Neurology* 2004;62:1261.
10. Guerrini R, Zaccara G, la Marca G, et al. Safety and tolerability of antiepileptic drug treatment in children with epilepsy. *Drug Saf* 2012;35(7):519–533.
11. Browne TR. Pharmacokinetics of antiepileptic drugs. *Neurology* 1998;51(suppl 4):S2.
12. Chigier E. Compliance in adolescents with epilepsy or diabetes. *J Adolesc Health* 1992;13;375.
13. Mitchell WG, Scheier LM, Baker SA. Adherence to treatment in children with epilepsy: who follows "doctor's orders?" *Epilepsia* 2000;41:1616.
14. Jadhav T, Cross JH. Surgical approaches to treating epilepsy in children. *Curr Treat Options Neurol* 2012;14(6):620–629.
15. Sander JW. The use of antiepileptic drugs–principles and practice. *Epilepsia* 2004;45 (suppl 6):28.
16. Tennison M, Greenwood R, Lewis D, et al. Discontinuing antiepileptic drugs in children with epilepsy. *N Engl J Med* 1994;330:1407.
17. Mattson RH, Cramer JA, Colline JF, et al. Comparison of carbamazepine, phenobarbital, phenytoin, and primidone in partial and secondary generalized tonic-clonic seizures. *N Engl J Med* 1985;313:145.
18. Consensus statement: medical management of epilepsy. *Neurology* 1999;51 (suppl 4):S39–S44.
19. Goldberg-Stern H, Feldman L, Eidlitz-Markus T, et al. Levetiracetam in children, adolescents and young adults with intractable epilepsy: efficacy, tolerability and effect on electroencephalogram—a pilot study. *Eur J Neurol* 2013;17(3):248–253.
20. Glauser TA, Pellock JM. Zonisamide in pediatric epilepsy: review of the Japanese experience. *J Child Neurol* 2002;17:87.
21. Glauser TA, Cnaan A, Shinnar S; Childhood Absence Epilepsy Study Group. Ethosuximide, valproic acid, and lamotrigine in childhood absence epilepsy. *N Engl J Med* 2010;362(9):790–799.
22. Hiilesmaa VK. Pregnancy and birth in women with epilepsy. *Neurology* 1992;42:8.
23. Kaplan PW. Reproductive health effects and teratogenicity of antiepileptic drugs. *Neurology* 2004;63(10, suppl 4):S13.
24. Mikkonen K, Vainionpaa LK, Pakarinen AJ, et al. Long-term reproductive endocrine health in young women with epilepsy during puberty. *Neurology* 2004;62:445.
25. Morrell MJ. Guidelines for the care of women with epilepsy [Review]. *Neurology* 1998;51 (suppl 4):S21.
26. Morrell MJ. Epilepsy in women: the science of why it is special. *Neurology* 1999;53 (suppl 1):S42.
27. O'Connor SE, Zupanc ML. Women and epilepsy. *J Pediatr Pharmacol Ther* 2009;14(4):212–220.
28. Farhat G, Yamout B, Mikati MA, et al. Effect of antiepileptic drugs on bone density in ambulatory patients. *Neurology* 2002;58:1348.
29. Isojarvi JI, Laatikainen TJ, Knip M, et al. Obesity and endocrine disorders in women taking valproate for epilepsy. *Ann Neurol* 1996;39:579.
30. Baker GA. Depression and suicide in adolescents with epilepsy. *Neurology* 2006;66(6, suppl 3):S5.
31. Foldvary-Schaefer N, Falcone T. Catamenial epilepsy: pathophysiology, diagnosis, and management. *Neurology* 2003;61(suppl 2):S2.

📶 **ADDITIONAL RESOURCES AND WEBSITES ONLINE**

24

Headaches

Lilia C. Lovera
Walter M. Jay
M. Susan Jay

KEY WORDS

- Cluster headache
- Migraine headaches
- Primary headaches
- Secondary headaches
- Tension-type headache

Recurrent headaches are a frequent problem in adolescents and young adults (AYAs), accounting for numerous physician visits and lost days at school and work. By age 15, over 50% of adolescents have experienced at least one headache episode.[1] Most recurrent headaches are not associated with severe organic pathology. In contrast, the single, severe acute headache may be due to significant central nervous system (CNS) or systemic disease, particularly when it occurs in a patient without prior headache history.

EPIDEMIOLOGY

The prevalence of headaches by age 15 is 57% to 82%.[1,2] Most are infrequent and not disabling.

Migraine headaches have a prevalence of 8% to 23% among individuals 11 to 15 years old.[3,4] Half of those with migraine headaches develop symptoms before age 25.[5] In a large US-based population sample, the prevalence of chronic migraine among AYAs is 5% to 9%, with increasing prevalence throughout adolescence.[6] In general, headaches are more common in prepubertal males. After puberty, they are more common in females.[1,2]

HEADACHE TYPES

Headaches may be due to a primary headache disorder or secondary to another condition. The vast majority of headaches in AYAs are primary headache disorders including migraine (with or without aura), tension-type headache (TTH), and chronic daily headache. Primary headaches present with multiple acute attacks and complete remission between attacks. Commonly, secondary headaches may be due to systemic disease such as a viral illness or sinusitis.

CHARACTERISTICS

See **Table 24.1** for characteristics of common primary and secondary headaches.

Primary Headache Disorders

These include (A) migraine, (B) TTH, (C) trigeminal autonomic cephalgias (TACs), and some forms of (D) chronic daily headache.

TABLE 24.1

Common Headache Presentations

Type of Headache	Onset	Location	Pain Quality
Migraine without aura	Gradual	Unilateral or bilateral (especially in those <18 years old)	Throbbing, pulsating
Migraine with aura	Gradual	Unilateral	Throbbing, pulsating
Tension-type	Variable, usually afternoon	Bilateral, band-like	Steady pressure, dull
Cluster	2–3 a.m., abrupt	Unilateral, orbital, or temporal	Burning, boring, excruciating
Intracranial mass lesions	Gradual or sudden, but usually recent	Focal or general	Varied, often dull ache
Idiopathic intracranial hypertension	Variable	Vertex or diffuse	Dull

Migraine

1. **Migraine without aura, formerly "common migraine"**
   These are the most common, accounting for 60% to 85% of migraine headache cases.[7] See **Table 24.2** for criteria according to the International Headache Society (IHS). Common features include:
   - Symptoms that are often relieved by sleep or rest
   - Family history of migraines
   - Childhood history of motion sickness or cyclic vomiting
   - History of relief with triptans or ergot compounds is supportive of the diagnosis.
   - Pattern of headaches that varies over time, with exacerbations or onset that may be precipitated by puberty, college, or other life stressors
   - In some, episodes may be triggered by certain foods, including chocolate, tyramine-containing cheeses, red wines, and foods containing monosodium glutamate (MSG), nitrates, or nitrites.[8]

TABLE 24.2

IHS Criteria for Migraine without Aura

A. At least five attacks that fulfill criteria in B to D
B. Headache attacks that last 4 to 72 h (untreated or unsuccessfully treated)[a]
C. Headache has at least two of the following characteristics:
   1. Unilateral site[b]
   2. Pulsating quality
   3. Moderate to severe intensity
   4. Aggravation by or causing avoidance of routine physical activity (e.g., climbing stairs)
D. During headache, at least one of the following symptoms:
   1. Nausea or vomiting (or both)
   2. Photophobia and phonophobia
E. Not attributed to another disorder

[a]In patients aged under 18 y, duration may be 2–72 h.
[b]In patients aged under 18 y, headaches are more often bilateral.
From the Headache Classification Committee of the International Headache Society. The International Classification of Headache Disorders, 3rd edition (beta version). *Cephalalgia* 2013;33(9):629–808.

- Migraine headaches in children and adolescents under 18 years of age tend to be more often bilateral and become unilateral in late adolescence and young adulthood.[9]
2. **Migraine with aura, formerly "classic migraine"**
   An aura is a unilateral, fully reversible, visual, sensory, or other focal neurologic symptom that develops gradually and is followed by a headache and associated migraine symptoms. Given the paroxysmal neurologic symptoms, further evaluation and imaging may be required to rule out a transient ischemic attack especially at initial presentation.
   a. *Migraine with typical aura* occurs in 15% to 30% of patients with migraine with aura.[7]
      See Table 24.3 for diagnostic criteria according to IHS.
      - Visual auras occur in 90% of migraines with aura, followed by sensory auras, and less frequently, speech manifestations.[9]
      - Visual manifestations include blurred vision, zigzag lines, field defects, scintillations, or distortions.
   b. *Migraine with brainstem aura*, formerly "basilar migraine"
      - Represents 3% to 19% of childhood migraine with auras and are more common in female AYAs.[7,10]
      - Symptoms are characterized by vertigo, ataxia, dysarthria, diplopia, and decreased level of consciousness that are fully reversible.

TABLE 24.3

IHS Criteria for Migraine with Typical Aura

A. At least two attacks that fulfill criteria B and C
B. Migraine aura is fully reversible and consists of visual, sensory, and/or speech/language symptoms. There are no motor, retinal, or brainstem symptoms
C. At least two of the following four features:
   1. At least one aura symptom develops gradually over 5 min, and/or two or more different aura symptoms occur in succession
   2. Each aura symptom lasts 5–60 min
   3. At least one aura symptom is unilateral
   4. There is headache either with the aura or within 60 min of the aura
D. Not attributed to another disorder, and transient ischemic attack has been ruled out

From the Headache Classification Committee of the International Headache Society. The International Classification of Headache Disorders, 3rd edition (beta version). *Cephalalgia* 2013;33(9):629–808.

c. *Hemiplegic migraine*
   - Aura consists of fully reversible motor weakness with visual, sensory, or speech manifestations, followed by a migrainous headache.
d. *Retinal migraine*
   - Repeated attacks of a monocular visual disturbance; however, these are rare and other causes of monocular blindness should first be excluded.[9]
3. **Migraines and Menses**
   The IHS, in its Appendix to the third edition, defines two clinical entities—the pure menstrual migraine (PMM) and the menstrually related migraine (MRM). PMM is a migraine without aura with attacks occurring only 2 days before to 3 days after the onset of bleeding and at no other times of the menstrual cycle. In contrast, MRM may occur perimenstrually, like PMM, and at other times during the menstrual cycle. For the diagnosis to be made, headaches have to occur in two out of three consecutive cycles.[9] The perimenstrual migraine attack appears to be more closely linked with variations of sex hormones. Treatment options are discussed later in this chapter.[11,12]

TTH, Formerly "Tension" Headache

THHs are band-like and bilateral, with nonpulsating pain, and last 30 minutes to 7 days. There is no nausea or vomiting, but either photophobia *or* phonophobia may be present. They are not worsened by physical activity. The onset is usually gradual and may be related to stress and fatigue. There may be associated pericranial tenderness to palpation.[9,13,14]

Trigeminal Autonomic Cephalgias

This group of primary headache disorders includes headaches that are usually lateralized, with associated prominent cranial parasympathetic autonomic features (lacrimation, rhinorrhea, conjunctival injection) ipsilateral to the headache. TACs include cluster headaches, paroxysmal hemicranias, hemicrania continua (HC), and short lasting unilateral neuralgiform headaches with conjunctival injection and tearing. Cluster headaches are the most common.[9,15]

Cluster Headaches:
   - Found in <5% of AYAs
   - Male predominance and usually starting in late adolescence or adulthood, typical age at presentation is between 30 and 50 years.
   - Pain is steady boring or burning, usually localized behind one eye. Pain onset is sudden and severe, but brief, lasting from 15 to 180 minutes.
   - Rhinorrhea, lacrimation, conjunctival injection, and Horner syndrome ipsilateral to the pain are common during an attack. During clusters, multiple daily episodes occur, often in early morning hours, awakening patient from sleep.

Chronic Daily Headache

Chronic daily headache in AYAs includes chronic migraine, chronic TTH, new daily persistent headaches (NDPHs), and HC.

   - Chronic migraine and chronic TTH usually evolve from intermittent migraine or TTH, and are defined as headaches occurring on more than 15 days a month for over 3 months.
   - NDPH is an acute onset of daily headache in a patient with no history of headache, which persists for many weeks to months.[9,16]
   - HC, a chronic form of a TAC, is rare in AYAs. These usually respond well to treatment with indomethacin.[16]

Importantly, about half of patients with chronic daily headache also have a component of medication overuse.[9]

Secondary Headache

Although a new-onset headache may be the first attack of an episodic primary headache disorder, an acute, "first or worst" headache needs evaluation to rule out serious underlying pathology. Potential life-threatening causes for headaches include CNS infections (meningitis, brain abscess, epidural empyema), subarachnoid hemorrhage, intracranial hemorrhage, cerebral venous sinus thrombosis (CVST), severe hypertension, and cerebral ischemia. These patients will generally be referred to an emergency department for further evaluation. **Table 24.4** lists "Red flags" in the assessment of patients with headache that should prompt urgent evaluation. Important considerations for the use of hormonal contraceptives and intrauterine devices in AYA females with headaches are outlined in Chapters 43 and 44, respectively.

Other causes of secondary headache include sinusitis, non-specific headache due to fever, headache following seizure, acute dental disease, or eye or orbit pathology. The following are some common causes of secondary headaches that can be encountered among AYAs in the outpatient setting.[9,17]

Medication Overuse Headache, Formerly "Rebound" Headache

- Usually presents as a new type of headache or marked worsening of the preexisting headache in the setting of medication overuse in a patient with migraine or TTH
- Chronic headache occurring on more than 15 days/month for 3 months
- Associated with excessive use of analgesics on more than 10 to 15 days/month
- Frequency of use considered "overuse" depends on the type of analgesic.
- Education about overuse is important for prevention.[18]

Posttraumatic Headache

These headaches usually have a mixed migrainous and "tension" quality, with onset up to 7 days after head trauma. They may continue for weeks to months, but diminish gradually over time.[9,16]

Idiopathic Intracranial Hypertension, Formerly "Pseudotumor Cerebri"

- More common in young, obese females
- Pain is usually dull and vertex.
- Papilledema is common and visual fields may be abnormal, including enlarged blind spot or constricted peripheral fields. Visual obscuration (transient dimming or loss of vision with straining or position change) may be present.
- Double vision from cranial nerve VI palsy may occur.
- May be associated with oral contraceptive use, excessive vitamin A or D intake, rapid steroid taper, certain immunosuppressants (i.e., cyclosporine), tetracycline or minocycline intake (for acne or other indications), or isotretinoin (Accutane).
- A patient with headache and papilledema should be treated as an emergency as there is a significant risk of permanent visual loss if untreated.
- A postimaging lumbar puncture with careful measurement of opening pressure may be diagnostic and may even be therapeutic in the short term.[19]

TABLE 24.4
Common "Red Flags" in the Evaluation of Headaches

New, different, or "worst headache" of a person's life
Immunocompromised state
Exacerbation by head position
Alteration of consciousness
Seizure
Fever with nuchal rigidity
Nuchal rigidity
Papilledema
Abnormal neurologic exam: abnormal eye movements, ataxia, hemiparesis, abnormal reflexes, or hemisensory deficit

---

Headache Due to CVST

These headaches are often dull and accompanied by nausea and vomiting. Focal neurologic signs may or may not be present. Stroke due to CVST is rare, but women of childbearing age account for 75% of these cases.[20] Risk factors for CVST include thrombophilia (Factor V Leiden, prothrombin gene mutations) and oral contraceptive pill use.[9,20,21]

Headaches Due to Intracranial Mass Lesions

Headaches that are increasing in severity and frequency, or that occur nocturnally, should raise suspicion for intracranial mass lesions. These headaches are usually accompanied by other neurologic signs and symptoms, and neurologic and funduscopic exams are often abnormal.[9]

Headaches Due to Hydrocephalus (with or without Mass Lesion)

Headaches due to hydrocephalus are relatively constant and worse in the morning. The pain is dull, vertex, and increased by Valsalva maneuvers. Congenital aqueductal stenosis may cause symptom onset during adolescence.[16]

Headaches Due to Substance or Drug Abuse

Both drug use and withdrawal may cause headaches. These headaches are frequently associated with alcohol, cocaine, excessive use of over-the-counter (OTC) stimulants (ephedrine, pseudoephedrine, caffeine), inhalants, and other stimulants like "ecstasy" (also known as 3,4-methylenedioxymethamphetamine).[16]

Headaches Due to Other Medical Conditions

AYAs with chronic conditions like cystic fibrosis, chronic pulmonary disease, renal failure, sickle cell anemia, cancer, organ transplantations, or cyanotic congenital heart disease often also have headaches related to these conditions. Treatment targets the underlying condition and symptomatic relief of pain.[16]

DIAGNOSIS

In the evaluation of the AYAs with headache, the history and physical examination are crucial.

History

The history should include the following:

1. Onset: Age at first episode; events or illnesses surrounding onset; temporal pattern of headaches (time of day, day of week, and season)
2. Pattern and chronology of pain: Headache prodrome, location, quality (pounding, dull, sharp, stabbing), frequency, radiation, change in quality during episode, duration, severity, limitation of activities, and alleviating factors
3. Preceding and associated symptoms: Aura, photophobia, phonophobia, nausea, or vomiting
4. Headache triggers: Including stressors, illnesses, foods/diet/eating pattern (food additives, MSG, chocolate, nuts, cheeses, specific suspect foods; skipping meals), medications, exertion and orgasm, caffeine intake or withdrawal, alcohol intake, toxic exposures, and physical exposures (bright/flashing lights, temperature changes, strong odors).[16,22,23]
5. Other associated illnesses or symptoms: Including HIV risks. Changes in menstrual pattern or galactorrhea suggest pituitary lesion or pregnancy.
6. Medications (prescribed and OTC): Including analgesics, oral contraceptive pills, other medications used for headaches (acute or prophylactic), medications used for acne (tetracycline, minocycline, Accutane), vitamins and supplements
7. Substance abuse
8. Depression or mood disorders
9. School phobia or school avoidance and other secondary gains

10. Behavior between attacks: recent personality change or change in school performance
11. Family history of migraines or other headaches, epilepsy, affective disorders, or other neurologic conditions[16]

Physical Examination

A thorough physical examination should include careful neurological examination and a funduscopic exam. Pertinent physical findings include:

1. Vital signs: Elevated blood pressure or fever
2. Eyes, ears, nose, and throat: Papilledema, narrowing of vessels, optic atrophy, visual fields and visual acuity, sinus tenderness, acute or chronic otitis, poor dentition, and refractive error, TMJ pain, or dysfunction
3. Neck: Nuchal rigidity, spasm or tenderness of cervical neck muscles, or "trigger points"
4. General physical examination
5. Neurological examination: Head circumference, mental status, cranial nerves, motor and sensory examination, gait, reflexes, and coordination.[16,17]

Laboratory and Neuroimaging

When physical examination is normal, laboratory and radiological studies are seldom indicated in the evaluation of patients with recurrent headaches separated by periods of complete recovery. In contrast, an acute severe headache in a patient with no prior headache history should prompt further evaluation, because underlying systemic or CNS pathology is more likely and may be life threatening.

Neuroimaging and lumbar puncture should be considered to aid in the diagnosis and may be necessary on an emergency basis in the following: (1) an acute severe headache or a headache with increasing intensity; (2) headache with abnormal neurologic examination; (3) papilledema; and (4) headaches with co-occurring seizures.[16,24]

THERAPY

General Principles:

- Preventing a headache is better than having to get rid of it once it occurs.
- Look for precipitants and triggers, especially avoidable ones, as this is preferred over daily medications.
- Take the preferred abortive medication at the onset of the headache, the earlier the better.
- Do not underestimate the role of reassurance. Once the AYA is reassured, treatment beyond simple analgesics may be neither necessary nor desired by the patient.

Nonpharmacologic Measures

General strategies for headache management include patient education, maintaining a headache diary, adopting lifestyle changes, and behavioral interventions.

1. Headache diary: Patients should be encouraged to maintain a *detailed* record of headaches, medication intake (and results), as well as activities, foods, stresses, sleep pattern, and physical environment. This can help establish severity and frequency of headache while pointing out avoidable triggers. It is important to record medications used to determine if there may be a component of medication overuse. See Additional Resources for a list of common food triggers in migraineurs.
2. Lifestyle changes: Encourage patients to avoid skipping meals, maintain good hydration, adequate sleep (at least 8 hours nightly), and exercise 3 to 5 days weekly. Caffeine intake

should be stabilized (same amount every day) or weaned off completely. Alcohol intake and cigarette smoking should be stopped. Excessive gum chewing should also be discouraged.[25]
3. Behavioral interventions: Psychotherapy and counseling may be helpful. Relaxation techniques, deep breathing or imaging, may also help and can be learned from books or other aids.[26] Cognitive behavioral therapy may be helpful in the treatment of chronic migraine.[16,27]

Pharmacologic Measures
Treatment of Intermittent TTHs

Adopt the general strategies discussed above and encourage brief periods of relaxation or naps. Simple analgesics (e.g., acetaminophen and nonsteroidal anti-inflammatory drugs [NSAIDs]) are often effective, but patients should be counseled to avoid excessive use. If TTH evolve to chronic daily headache, prophylaxis with amitriptyline may be considered.[28]

Treatment of Cluster Headache

Cluster headaches are uncommon in AYAs, but are generally treated as in adults. Subcutaneous sumatriptan is the most effective abortive treatment and inhaled high-flow oxygen may relieve cluster headaches rapidly. Prednisone bursts have also been used in the acute phase. Verapamil is the most used prophylactic medication.[15,16]

Treatment of Medication Overuse Headache

Treatment requires weaning of overused analgesic medications. This can be done gradually or even abruptly while bridging on a steroid taper. Some require hospitalization for detoxification.

Treatment of Migraine Headaches: Abortive and Preventive Medication

Abortive Medications to Treat the Acute Episodic Migraine: These medications should all be taken soon after onset of symptoms. If headaches are occurring more than twice a week, beware of medication overuse as this may convert intermittent migraines to chronic migraines.

1. *Simple analgesics:* Ibuprofen, acetaminophen, or other NSAIDs. Avoid overuse by limiting to 3 to 4 days a week. Caffeine (as a tablet combined with analgesic or as a beverage) may potentiate the effect of the analgesic.
2. *Antiemetics:* IV, IM, and PR prochlorperazine, IM/IV metoclopramide, IV chlorpromazine, and PO/IV ondansetron. An antiemetic combined with or followed by an analgesic is very helpful if nausea or vomiting is prominent.[16]
3. *5-Hydroxytryptamine receptor agonists, "Triptans":* Oral almotriptan and rizatriptan, and nasal sumatriptan and zolmitriptan, are approved for use in adolescents. In addition, naratriptan and frovatriptan are approved for use in adults over 18. Triptans should not be taken more than 3 days/week and should not be mixed with ergot preparations. They are contraindicated in hemiplegic migraines, migraines with brainstem aura, and in patients with cardiovascular risk factors.
4. *Dihydroergotamine (DHE):* DHE nasal spray (migranal) may be used at home or school and is sometimes effective in AYAs who do not tolerate or respond to triptans. Side effects include nausea. DHE is contraindicated in patients with vascular disease, hemiplegic migraines, and in pregnancy.
5. *Sedative–analgesic combinations:* Barbiturate with acetaminophen or aspirin (Fiorinal, Fioricet) may be used sparingly given the high risk of dependence and development of medication overuse headaches.[29–31]

Migraine Preventive Therapy: Preventative therapy should be considered in patients when episodes occur more than four times a month and attacks interfere with daily functioning. The goals of preventive therapy are to reduce attack frequency and severity, improve response to abortive medications, and improve quality of life. Treatment should be continued until the headache pattern has markedly improved for about 6 months, then consider a trial of tapering-off medication.[30]

There are several therapeutic options that are recommended by the American Academy of Neurology for migraine prevention in adults (including young adults). These include several anticonvulsants, β-blockers, antidepressants, and, in the case of MRM, triptans.[32] Topiramate is the only Food and Drug Administration-approved medication for migraine prophylaxis in adolescents. Still, adolescents anecdotally benefit from many of the treatments used in adults.

- *Anticonvulsants:* Topiramate effectively decreases migraine frequency, with 100 mg/day demonstrating the best benefit-to-risk ratio. Side effects include paresthesias, fatigue, weight loss, cognitive disturbances, and acute closed angle glaucoma.[33] Changes in vision while on topiramate should prompt immediate evaluation.[34] Valproic acid and levetiracetam have also been reported to prevent migraines in adolescents. Recommendations for adults do not include levetiracetam. The dose required is often lower than that used for seizure control. Care should be taken when prescribing valproic acid to women of childbearing age given teratogenicity.[31–33]
- *β-Blockers:* Propranolol and timolol have shown some benefit in treating adolescents in a few studies. In young adults, metoprolol, propranolol, and timolol are effective. Side effects include fatigue, depression, and decreased exercise tolerance. Severe asthma, insulin-dependent diabetes, and depression are contraindications.[16,31,32]
- *Antidepressants:* Amitriptyline is useful for prophylaxis of migraines or mixed TTH and migraine headache in AYAs. Side effects include sedation, dry mouth, and arrhythmias.[28] Nortriptyline and desipramine can also be used. In young adults, venlafaxine may also be used.[32]
- *NSAIDs* (e.g., ibuprofen or naproxen): May be used in low doses for up to 2 months[16,35]
- *Cyproheptadine* (Periactin): May be useful in AYAs dosed at 2 to 4 mg three times a day. Side effects include sedation and weight gain.[16,31,35]
- *Calcium-channel blockers:* Flunarizine (not available in the US) has demonstrated significant headache reduction in adolescents. Other calcium-channel blockers have not been shown to be useful in AYAs.[32]
- *Supplements:* High-dose riboflavin (vitamin B_2), magnesium, and butterbur may prevent migraine in some patients.[16,35]

Treatment of Migraine Associated with Menses

PMM and MRM should initially be treated with preventive and abortive measures as any migraine headache. If ineffective, perimenstrual prophylaxis with NSAIDs or triptans can be used. Naproxen 550 mg once or twice daily started 1 to 2 days before the expected symptomatic period is effective. Triptans have some efficacy but are costly. For women taking hormonal contraception, there is anecdotal evidence that extended-cycle strategies (omitting placebo or reminder pills) may improve migraine symptoms.[11,36]

Treatment of Status Migrainosus

Status migrainosus is a severe, disabling migraine lasting more than 72 hours that is refractory to medications. These patients may require IV medications and may need to be referred to the emergency department for possible hospitalization. Status migrainosus may be treated with IV DHE dosed every 8 hours for 2 to 4 days. Sometimes, short courses of high-dose corticosteroids may end the episode.

Treatment of Chronic Daily Headache

Chronic daily headaches are sometimes mixed TTH and migraine headache. If they are frequent and disabling, they may be treated on a prophylactic basis with low-dose tricyclic antidepressants, usually amitriptyline.[28] In young adults with chronic migraine headache, onabotulinumtoxin A has also been shown to be effective.[37]

ACKNOWLEDGMENTS

The authors wish to acknowledge Dr. Wendy G. Mitchell, Dr. Kiaresh Sadrieh, and Dr. Lawrence S. Neinstein for their contributions to previous versions of this chapter.

REFERENCES

1. Linet MS, Stewart WF, Celentano DD, et al. An epidemiologic study of headache among adolescents and young adults. *JAMA* 1989;261(15):2211–2216.
2. Deubner DC. An epidemiologic study of migraine and headache in 10–20 year olds. *Headache* 1977;17(4):173–180.
3. Stewart WF, Linet MS, Celentano DD, et al. Age- and sex-specific incidence rates of migraine with and without visual aura. *Am J Epidemiol* 1991;134(10):1111–1120.
4. Lipton RB, Silberstein SD, Stewart WF. An update on the epidemiology of migraine. *Headache* 1994;34(6):319–328.
5. Stewart WF, Wood C, Reed ML, et al. Cumulative lifetime migraine incidence in women and men. *Cephalalgia* 2008;28(11):1170–1178.
6. Buse DC, Manack AN, Fanning KM, et al. Chronic migraine prevalence, disability, and sociodemographic factors: results from the American Migraine Prevalence and Prevention Study. *Headache* 2012;52(10):1456–1470.
7. Lewis DW. Pediatric migraine. *Neurol Clin* 2009;27(2):481–501.
8. Alpay K, Ertas M, Orhan EK, et al. Diet restriction in migraine, based on IgG against foods: a clinical double-blind, randomised, cross-over trial. *Cephalalgia* 2010;30(7):829–837.
9. Headache Classification Committee of the International Headache Society. The International Classification of Headache Disorders, 3rd edition (beta version). *Cephalalgia* 2013;33(9):629–808.
10. Dafer RM, Jay WM. Headache and the eye. *Curr Opin Ophthalmol* 2009;20(6):520–524.
11. Mathew PG, Dun EC, Luo JJ. A cyclic pain: the pathophysiology and treatment of menstrual migraine. *Obstet Gynecol Sur* 2013;68(2):130–140.
12. Casolla B, Lionetto L, Candela S, et al. Treatment of perimenstrual migraine with triptans: an update. *Curr Pain Headache Rep* 2012;16(5):445–451.
13. Pacheva I, Milanov I, Ivanov I, et al. Evaluation of diagnostic and prognostic value of clinical characteristics of migraine and tension type headache included in the diagnostic criteria for children and adolescents in International Classification of Headache Disorders—second edition. *Int J Clin Prac* 2012;66(12):1168–1177.
14. Lewis DW. Headaches in children and adolescents. *Am Fam Physician* 2002;65(4):625–632.
15. Lambru G, Matharu M. Management of trigeminal autonomic cephalalgias in children and adolescents. *Curr Pain Headache Rep* 2013;17(4):323.
16. Lewis DW. Headaches in children and adolescents. *Curr Probl Pediatr Adolesc Health Care* 2007;37(6):207–246.
17. Gunner KB, Smith HD. Practice guideline for diagnosis and management of migraine headaches in children and adolescents: part one. *J Pediatr Health Care* 2007;21(5):327–332.
18. Tepper SJ, Tepper DE. Breaking the cycle of medication overuse headache. *Cleveland Clin J Med* 2010;77(4):236–242.
19. Wall M. Idiopathic intracranial hypertension (pseudotumor cerebri). *Curr Neurol Neurosci Rep* 2008;8(2):87–93.
20. Paner A, Jay WM, Nand S, et al. Cerebral vein and dural venous sinus thrombosis: risk factors, prognosis and treatment—a modern approach. *Neuroophthalmology* 2009;33(5):237–247.
21. Ferro JM, Canhao P, Stam J, et al. Prognosis of cerebral vein and dural sinus thrombosis: results of the International Study on Cerebral Vein and Dural Sinus Thrombosis (ISCVT). *Stroke* 2004;35(3):664–670.
22. Kelman L. The triggers or precipitants of the acute migraine attack. *Cephalalgia* 2007;27(5):394–402.
23. Millichap JG, Yee MM. The diet factor in pediatric and adolescent migraine. *Pediatr Neurol* 2003;28(1):9–15.
24. Lewis DW, Ashwal S, Dahl G, et al. Practice parameter: evaluation of children and adolescents with recurrent headaches: report of the Quality Standards Subcommittee of the American Academy of Neurology and the Practice Committee of the Child Neurology Society. *Neurology* 2002;59(4):490–498.
25. Watemberg N, Matar M, Har-Gil M, et al. The influence of excessive chewing gum use on headache frequency and severity among adolescents. *Pediatr Neurol* 2014;50(1):69–72.
26. Powers SW, Andrasik F. Biobehavioral treatment, disability, and psychological effects of pediatric headache. *Pediatr Ann* 2005;34(6):461–465.
27. Powers SW, Kashikar-Zuck SM, Allen JR, et al. Cognitive behavioral therapy plus amitriptyline for chronic migraine in children and adolescents: a randomized clinical trial. *JAMA* 2013;310(24):2622–2630.
28. Couch JR; Amitriptyline Versus Placebo Study Group. Amitriptyline in the prophylactic treatment of migraine and chronic daily headache. *Headache* 2011;51(1):33–51.
29. Lewis D, Ashwal S, Hershey A, et al. Practice parameter: pharmacological treatment of migraine headache in children and adolescents: report of the American Academy of Neurology Quality Standards Subcommittee and the Practice Committee of the Child Neurology Society. *Neurology* 2004;63(12):2215–2224.

30. Brenner M, Lewis D. The treatment of migraine headaches in children and adolescents. *J Pediatr Pharmacol Ther* 2008;13(1):17–24.
31. Papetti L, Spalice A, Nicita F, et al. Migraine treatment in developmental age: guidelines update. *J Headache Pain* 2010;11(3):267–276.
32. Silberstein SD, Holland S, Freitag F, et al. Evidence-based guideline update: pharmacologic treatment for episodic migraine prevention in adults: report of the Quality Standards Subcommittee of the American Academy of Neurology and the American Headache Society. *Neurology* 2012;78(17):1337–1345.
33. Deaton TL, Mauro LS. Topiramate for migraine prophylaxis in pediatric patients. *Ann Pharmacother* 2014;48(5):638–643.
34. Alore PL, Jay WM, Macken MP. Topiramate, pseudotumor cerebri, weight-loss and glaucoma: an ophthalmologic perspective. *Semin Ophthalmol* 2006;21(1):15–17.
35. Holland S, Silberstein SD, Freitag F, et al. Evidence-based guideline update: NSAIDs and other complementary treatments for episodic migraine prevention in adults: report of the Quality Standards Subcommittee of the American Academy of Neurology and the American Headache Society. *Neurology* 2012;78(17):1346–1353.
36. Macgregor EA. Menstrual migraine: therapeutic approaches. *Ther Adv Neurol Disord* 2009;2(5):327–336.
37. Gerwin R. Treatment of chronic migraine headache with onabotulinumtoxinA. *Curr Pain Headache Rep* 2011;15(5):336–338.

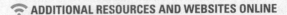

ADDITIONAL RESOURCES AND WEBSITES ONLINE

CHAPTER 25

Sleep Disorders

J. Aimée Coulombe
Shelly K. Weiss

KEY WORDS

- Apnea
- Excessive sleepiness
- Insomnia
- Parasomnias
- Prevention
- Screening
- Sleep
- Sleep disorders
- Sleep habits
- Treatment

Sleep is one of our basic needs. It is important for our physical, intellectual, and emotional health. Lack of sleep makes us tired and irritable, decreases short-term memory, and can result in decreased productivity at work and/or school, as well as sleep-related accidents. Sleep disturbances are common in adolescents and young adults (AYAs). Many young people acknowledge difficulties with sleep (often not obtaining adequate sleep) when specifically asked, although it may not be their chief complaint.

Given variation in classification systems (*Diagnostic and Statistical Manual of Mental Disorders-5, International Classification of Diseases-10, International Classification of Sleep Disorders-3*), rather than taking a purely diagnostic approach, this chapter focuses on common sleep problems experienced by AYAs, as they may be addressed by health care providers working in non-sleep specialty settings. These include sleep deprivation and excessive daytime sleepiness and the various sleep-related behaviors and disorders that are associated with them (e.g., insomnia, delayed sleep phase, sleep-disordered breathing (SDB) and apnea, and narcolepsy). Although less common in adolescence and young adulthood than in childhood, we also briefly describe parasomnias—undesirable physical (motor or autonomic) phenomena that occur exclusively or predominantly during sleep.

As in younger children and older adults, sleep disturbances in AYAs are multifactorial in etiology. They may arise from physiological and physical processes and symptoms (e.g., changes in chronobiology, difficulties in the transition from sleep to wakefulness, hormonal changes throughout the menstrual cycle, related to obstructive sleep apnea, pain, gastrointestinal reflux); symptoms related to mental health issues (e.g., anxiety, depression, stressors, and trauma); environmental and lifestyle factors (e.g., use of technology before bedtime and through the night, busy academic, social, or work schedules); parenting demands; and substance use and abuse (e.g., stimulants, barbiturates, or use of caffeine, nicotine, alcohol, hallucinogens, or other nonprescription substances).

SLEEP PHYSIOLOGY

Sleep is divided into rapid eye movement (REM) sleep and nonrapid eye movement (NREM) sleep. Studies of sleep physiology are carried out using polysomnography, which usually includes electroencephalogram (EEG), electrooculogram, electromyogram, and measures of respiratory function such as airflow, oxygen saturation, and end-tidal P_{CO_2} levels.

REM Sleep

REM sleep occupies about 25% of sleep time in AYAs and is characterized by a high autonomic arousal state including increased cardiovascular and respiratory activity, very low voluntary muscle tone, and rapid synchronous nonpatterned eye movements. The EEG pattern shows a low-voltage variable frequency resembling the awake state. Most dreams occur during REM sleep.

NREM Sleep

NREM sleep occupies 70% to 80% of sleep time in AYAs and is divided into three stages:

1. N1: Very light or transitional sleep, characterized on EEG by less than 50% alpha rhythm, and low-amplitude mixed-frequency activity
2. N2: Medium-deep sleep, characterized on EEG by the presence of sleep spindles, K-complexes, occupies about 50% of sleep
3. N3: Progressively deeper sleep, characterized on EEG by a general slowing of frequency and an increase in amplitude (delta waves). Muscular and cardiovascular activities are decreased and little dreaming occurs.

SLEEP PATTERN AND CHANGES DURING ADOLESCENCE AND YOUNG ADULTHOOD

Normal sleep usually consists of a brief period of N1 and N2, followed by a lengthier interval of N3 (slow-wave sleep). After approximately 70 to 100 minutes of NREM sleep, a 10- to 25-minute REM period occurs. This cycle is repeated four to six times throughout the night. The REM periods usually increase by 5 to 30 minutes each cycle, increasing the amount of REM sleep occurring in the second half of the night. The percentage of slow-wave sleep decreases and N2 increases between infancy and adolescence, a pattern that continues into adulthood.[1]

Another documented change in sleep, emerging in adolescence, is a delay in the circadian timing system.[2] With progressive pubertal development (documented by increasing sexual maturity ratings), there is a tendency toward a lengthening of the internal day and greater eveningness (a preference for later bedtimes and rise times). This tendency persists into young adulthood, before beginning to shift back to earlier bed and rise times in the early

20s.[3] Combined with lifestyle factors that further reinforce later bedtimes (e.g., social activities, electronic media use) and require early rising (e.g., academic and vocational schedules), sleep duration in AYAs is often truncated and insufficient. Although most adolescents require 8.5 to 9 hours of sleep per night, only 15% report sleeping at least 8.5 hours on school nights.[4] Similarly, although young adults require approximately 8 hours of sleep, the average sleep durations for these individuals are likely substantially less,[5] particularly when weeknight (versus weekend) sleep is considered. Only 35% of 18- to 29-year-olds report getting 8 or more hours of sleep on weeknights, whereas 60% report this amount of sleep on weekends.[6] It should be noted that attempts to catch up on sleep during the weekend are counterproductive, contributing to irregular sleep schedules and making sufficient weekday sleep more difficult to achieve.

COMMON SLEEP DISTURBANCES AND DISORDERS

Sleep Deprivation and Excessive Daytime Sleepiness Due to Insufficient Sleep

Excessive daytime sleepiness is common among AYAs. In a recent report of the American College Health Association (2013), 17.5% of college undergraduates endorsed that daytime sleepiness is a big or very big problem.[7] In the same publication, it was noted that 10.8% of undergraduate college students reported that they had no days in the past week where they had enough sleep to feel rested, and a further 30.4% that they only had enough sleep in 1 to 2 days of the past week. Although excessive daytime sleepiness may be caused by any factor that disrupts sleep (e.g., obstructive sleep apnea) or can be a symptom of narcolepsy, the most common cause of excessive daytime sleepiness is related to insufficient sleep ("inadequate sleep"). Inadequate sleep may be due to poor sleeping habits or late bedtimes. Demanding schedules that include academic, employment, and extracurricular activities, combined with circadian delays and early weekday wake times, can leave insufficient time for sleep. Electronic devices and social media, commonly used by AYAs, may further disrupt sleep during the night.[8] Additionally, young adults who are parents face additional sleep disruption associated with caring for young children who may themselves have difficulty sleeping.[9] This chronic sleep deprivation can cause complaints of fatigue or difficulty staying awake during school or work, adversely affecting performance. Mood, physical health, and safety may be compromised, with drowsy driving presenting a notable risk to the 16- to 25-year-old driver.[10] There are a wide variety of medications prescribed for AYAs (both for mental or physical health disorders) that can interfere with sleep, leading to insomnia or excessive daytime sleepiness. Compensatory behaviors, such as stimulant use, napping, sleeping in on weekends, poor food choices (e.g., excessive caffeinated foods or beverages), and reductions in activity, can be iatrogenic, maintaining inadequate sleep and precipitating other sleep disturbances (e.g., insomnia, phase delays, SDB/apnea).

Insomnia

Insomnia is characterized by dissatisfaction about sleep quality or duration. Subjective complaints include difficulty falling asleep at bedtime, waking up at night and having difficulty going back to sleep, waking up too early in the morning with an inability to return to sleep, or a complaint of nonrestorative sleep. The nocturnal difficulties lead to daytime symptoms including fatigue, decreased energy and/or problems with cognitive functions and mood disturbance.[11–13] AYAs most typically have insomnia that manifests as difficulties initiating sleep at bedtime or returning to sleep during the night following a typical period of arousal. Mechanisms underlying insomnia include maladaptive sleep-related cognitions (e.g., concerns about the effects of not getting enough sleep, doubt about

one's own ability to change sleep patterns) and behaviors (e.g., leaving inadequate time to relax and unwind before attempting to initiate sleep; use of technology before bed; using the bed and bedroom for activities other than sleep, thereby reducing the association between sleep and bed). Stress, anxiety, mood disorders, and substance abuse may all be bidirectionally associated with insomnia, and a growing body of literature suggests that insomnia predicts the development of psychological disorders over time.[14] Other less common causes of insomnia include physical illnesses associated with pain or discomfort, increased time in bed, or significant disruptions to sleep and daytime routines. Medications, such as selective serotonin reuptake inhibitors, stimulants, sympathomimetics, and corticosteroids, may also precipitate or perpetuate symptoms of insomnia.

Delayed Sleep Phase

A delayed sleep phase syndrome (DSPS) is a circadian phase disorder in which the timing of sleep is delayed. AYAs are particularly prone to this problem because of their busy evening schedules and an intrinsic biological preference for a later bedtime. When allowed to sleep for a normal length of time (e.g., weekends, vacations), the delayed sleep onset time will result in delayed waking time. Upon awakening, the individual will be refreshed. However, given the demands of early school and work start times, most individuals with DSPS will not be able to achieve sufficient sleep. They will have difficulty arising, experience daytime sleepiness, and be at risk of the myriad negative outcomes associated with inadequate sleep. When asked to fall asleep at a normal bedtime, well before physiologically ready, they will be at increased risk of engaging the maladaptive cognitions and behaviors associated with insomnia (described above). Difficulties with academic and occupational functioning, conflict with parents or significant others, and compensatory behaviors may further increase risk of developing a comorbid insomnia or other disorder. Based in part on normative data, Auger and Crowley[15] have proposed a weekday bedtime later than 12 a.m. as a potential indicator of DSPS in adolescents over age 14 years. Using a similar approach, Robillard et al.[16] have used a 1:30 a.m. or later sleep onset time and a 10:00 a.m. or later waking time as indicators of sleep phase delay in young adults, aged 19 to 24 years. It is important to note that these times are guidelines only.

SDB/Obstructive Sleep Apnea Syndrome

The main cause of SDB is obstructive sleep apnea syndrome (OSAS). This is the presence of complete or partial obstruction of the upper airway during sleep and is associated with the following history: frequent snoring (>3 nights/week), labored breathing during sleep, gasps/snorting noises, observer episodes of apnea, daytime sleepiness, and/or daytime neurobehavioral abnormalities plus others.[17] SDB/OSAS, either alone or in combination with other sleep disturbances, places AYAs at significant risk of inadequate sleep and its negative correlates including, but not limited to, excessive daytime sleepiness.[18]

Narcolepsy

Narcolepsy is a chronic neurological disorder characterized by two major abnormalities—excessive and overwhelming daytime sleepiness and intrusion of REM sleep phenomenon into wakefulness. The age at onset is usually between 10 and 25 years; however, the diagnosis is often delayed.[19] The first and primary manifestation of narcolepsy is excessive daytime sleepiness. The disorder is characterized by four classic symptoms: sleep attacks, cataplexy, sleep paralysis, and hypnagogic and hypnopompic hallucinations.

Sleep attacks are intrusive and debilitating periods of sleep during the day that may last anywhere from a few seconds to 30 minutes. These periods are often precipitated by sedentary, monotonous activity, and are more frequent after meals and later in the day.

Sleepiness is transiently relieved after short naps, but will gradually increase again within the 2 to 3 hours following the nap.

Cataplexy refers to abrupt, brief periods (seconds to minutes), bilateral loss or reduction of postural muscle tone while conscious, precipitated by intense emotions (e.g., anger, fright, surprise, excitement, or laughter). This is the most valuable symptom in the diagnosis of narcolepsy.

Sleep paralysis refers to the temporary loss of muscle tone occurring with the onset of sleep or upon awakening.

Hypnagogic hallucinations occur with the onset of sleep, while hypnopompic hallucinations occur upon awakening; hallucinations can be visual, auditory, tactile, or kinetic (with sensation of movement).

People without narcolepsy may have occasional sleep paralysis and/or hypnagogic hallucinations. In addition, people with narcolepsy may have automatic activity during periods of altered consciousness. Sleep attacks occur in 100% of individuals with narcolepsy, sleep attacks and cataplexy occur in 70%, sleep paralysis occurs in 50%, and hallucinations occur in 25%. Approximately 10% of individuals will experience all four classic symptoms.

Narcolepsy is a complex disorder caused by the loss of hypocretin (orexin)-producing neurons in the hypothalamus region of the brain.[20] The close association between narcolepsy–cataplexy and the human leukocyte antigen allele DQB1*0602 suggests an autoimmune etiology. There has also been recent interest in the association of narcolepsy with seasonal streptococcus, H1N1 infections and following a specific H1N1 influenza vaccine in Northern Europe.[20] Narcolepsy is diagnosed by clinical history and documentation of objective findings using both overnight polysomnography and daytime multiple sleep latency test (MSLT) and supported by genetic evaluation. The overnight polysomnography will exclude other sleep disorders, such as sleep apnea. The MSLT is a useful investigation in the diagnosis of narcolepsy. It will show a shortened time to sleep onset (sleep latency) and early onset of REM sleep.

Parasomnias

Parasomnias are undesirable phenomena that occur exclusively or predominantly during sleep. In general, the prevalence of parasomnias decreases with age.[21] Compared to the disturbances and disorders described above, the parasomnias described next, in and of themselves, are less frequently targeted for clinical intervention. Intervention is recommended when the parasomnia is severe enough to cause distress or dysfunction (e.g., nightmares significantly disrupt sleep or precipitate insomnia) or the individual is at risk of injury or harm (e.g., sleepwalking resulting in falls or leaving the house). Parasomnias may also be addressed during the course of intervention in an associated mental health disorder (e.g., anxiety- or trauma-related disorders). In this section, we focus on the more common parasomnias: nightmares, sleepwalking, and sleep terrors.

Nightmares

Nightmares occur during REM sleep, usually occurring in the last one-third to one-half of the sleep episode. They are the most common type of REM-related parasomnia (**Table 25.1**), with frequent nightmares affecting approximately 5% of the population and are more common in children than adults. Onset is usually before age 10 years; later onset is more suggestive of psychological causes, such as anxiety, distress, and trauma. Drug withdrawal, particularly from benzodiazepines, barbiturates, or alcohol, can also lead to nightmares. Nightmare content is often reflective of developmental milestones and stages, with AYAs expressing more social, academic, occupational, and safety-related concerns.[21] Nightmares may contribute to insomnia by increasing anxiety and therefore sleep onset latency (which is the time it takes to fall asleep after lights are turned off at bedtime).

TABLE 25.1

Characteristics of Sleep Terrors versus Nightmares

Characteristic	Sleep Terrors	Nightmares
Vocalization	Intense	Limited
Timing	In first 1/3 of night	Usually in second half of night
Autonomic activity	Marked increase	Slight increase
Arousal	Difficult	Easy
Motility	Marked	Limited
Recall	Minimal	Vivid
Sleep stage	NREM sleep	REM sleep

NREM, nonrapid eye movement; REM, rapid eye movement.

Sleepwalking and Sleep Terrors

Sleepwalking (somnambulism) and sleep terrors (pavor nocturnus) are disorders of impaired and partial arousal from deep slow-wave sleep. Both conditions occur in the first third of the sleep episode, during the rapid transition from N3 (slow-wave sleep) to lighter stages (N1/N2) of sleep. They are infrequently seen beyond adolescence. Characterized by a low level of awareness, clumsiness, a blank expression, and indifference to the environment, sleepwalking episodes usually last from 1 to 30 minutes. Sleep terrors, which are easily confused with, but distinct from nightmares (**Table 25.1**), are characterized by the outward expression of intense anxiety, fear, and vocalizations in the form of screams, moans, or gasps. Autonomic features include tachycardia, tachypnea, and sweating. As with sleepwalking, the individual experiencing a sleep terror appears to be relatively nonresponsive to the external environment or efforts to arouse him or her. Upon awakening, there is usually no recall of the experience. Psychological disturbances are thought to be a more likely cause of sleep terrors or sleepwalking if the onset is after age 12 years, the condition has persisted for several years, there is a negative family history, and there is maladaptive daytime behavior.

PREVENTION, IDENTIFICATION, AND TREATMENT

Although specific disturbances and disorders require unique assessments and interventions, comorbidity among disorders, shared risk and maintenance factors, and overlap in intervention strategies permit a staged approach to prevention, identification, and treatment. This approach may be particularly helpful in non-sleep specialty settings.

Prevention and Screening

Like diet and exercise, conversations about the promotion of healthy sleep habits should start early. Ideally, these conversations would be part of universal preventative health measures occurring across multiple systems and settings (e.g., home, school, media, health professionals' offices) and start early in children's lives. As independence and autonomy increase into adolescence and young adulthood, so can the individual's responsibility for maintaining healthy sleep habits. Some degree of monitoring by parents, while in the family home, and health professionals can be helpful. Although the transition out of the family home and into independent, peer, or romantic shared living arrangements can be a time when healthy sleep habits are vulnerable to disruption, a solid sleep foundation may help young adults maintain, or at least return to, healthier patterns following this transitional period.

TABLE 25.2
Side Bar

ABCs of SLEEPING
Developed by Bessey and colleagues[22], the ABCs of SLEEPING can be used to screen for and target sleep hygiene-related difficulties:

- *A*ge-appropriate *B*edtimes and waketimes with *C*onsistency: Ensure enough time for sleep, maintain regular sleep and rise times
- *S*chedules and routines: Reduce presleep arousal ("unwind" before bed), work with circadian rhythms
- *L*ocation: Minimize disturbances, reinforce associations between the bedroom and sleep
- No *E*lectronics in the bedroom or before bed
- *E*xercise and diet: Increase daytime activity, especially outdoors; reduce alcohol, energy drinks, caffeine, etc.
- *P*ositivity and relaxation: Address stress, anxiety, worries during the day; focus on relaxation, calm before bed
- *I*ndependence when falling asleep: Avoid becoming dependent on external stimuli (e.g., television, radio) to initiate sleep
- *N*eeds met during the day: Make time for socialization and entertainment earlier in the day rather than at night
- All of the above equals *G*reat sleep

To learn more about this tool, see "Additional Resources" (online ancillary content)

In addition to fostering healthy sleep, preventive counseling and screening can preclude the development of certain sleep disorders that are secondary to poor sleep habits. Prevention should include sleep education, monitoring of sleep and sleep habits, and building motivation to engage in healthy sleep behaviors. The ABCs of SLEEPING,[22] designed to organize sleep hygiene recommendations, can be used to structure screening and counseling efforts (**Table 25.2**). Other helpful screening and educational resources include the BEARS[23] screener, which provides a broad method of querying for many of the sleep disturbances described in this chapter (Bedtimes, Excessive sleepiness, Awakenings, Restlessness, and Snoring) and the sleep-smart tips for teens (which are also applicable to young adults) from the National Sleep Foundation (www.sleepfoundation.org).

History Taking, Sleep Diary, and Physical Examination
History
Following positive screening, the presenting sleep complaint(s) should be described and a history of other sleep problems in the individual and family should be taken. Information collected should include age at onset, timing during sleep, and the duration, frequency, and intermittent or continuous nature of the complaint. Daytime symptoms and effects should also be queried, including sleepiness, fatigue, and energy levels, mood and anxiety, cognitive difficulties (e.g., attention, memory, learning), and occupational and academic functioning. Symptoms of SDB/OSA should be elicited if possible from a parent, sibling, roommate, or partner. Compensatory behaviors (e.g., napping, substance use) and any treatment previously tried (description, length of trial, and result) should also be assessed. An academic and psychosocial history may further elucidate daytime factors that can be both consequences of, and contributors to, sleep disturbances. Corroborative history from parent(s) may be useful to determine if the perception of the complaint differs between people in the family. Thacher[5] provides an interesting discussion of the role of parents in diagnosing and treating sleep problems in young adults. If there is a bed partner or roommate, the significant other may also be asked to provide information. This can be particularly helpful for parasomnias, restlessness, and SDB.

Sleep History Tool
If not previously assessed using a tool like the ABCs of SLEEPING[22], a description of the bedroom environment; bedtime (weekdays

and weekends) and bedtime routines (what is done before sleep): sleep onset location; and the presence of light, noise, television, computer, or other electronics in bedroom should be requested, as should a description of sleep generally (i.e., time to fall asleep, amount of sleep, regularity of sleep and wake schedules). Additional information about what occurs after sleep onset (e.g., frequency, timing, and duration of arousals; behavior during arousals; presence of amnesia for event; response to intervention at time of arousal) can assist with the differential diagnoses of sleep disturbances such as difficulty returning to sleep related to insomnia, nightmares, sleep terrors, and other parasomnias.

Sleep Diary
A 1- to 2-week sleep diary, listing bedtimes, nighttime symptoms, time on awakening, daytime fatigue or sleepiness, and daytime naps, can be a very helpful tool in evaluating a sleep disturbance. Other assessment tools can include questionnaires and objective measures, such as home videos of nocturnal behaviors (e.g., for parasomnias) and actigraphy (a device that resembles a wrist-watch and is a computerized motion detector that measures activity as a proxy for sleep and waking). Medical, psychiatric, and surgical history (including history of tonsillectomy and adenoidectomy) should also be collected or considered, including prescription and over-the-counter medications, herbal products, dietary supplements, weight-loss products, performance-enhancing substances, stimulants as well as alcohol, cannabis, and other nonprescription drugs.

Physical Examination
Depending on the particular sleep complaint, health care providers may also wish to conduct a targeted physical examination. For example, a physical examination related to SBD/OSAS may reveal evidence of tonsillar hypertrophy, adenoidal facies, micrognathia/retrognathia, high-arched palate, failure to thrive, hypertension, and growth abnormalities (either underweight or overweight)[17]. It is important to note, however, that even if obstructive sleep apnea is present, there may be no abnormalities seen on physical examination.

Referral for Further Assessment
A referral for further assessment should be made in certain circumstances. It is often of benefit to refer to a sleep consultant about the need for a sleep study (overnight polysomnography), rather than ordering a sleep study right away. Sleep studies are used to evaluate a variety of conditions including SDB, some parasomnias, and disorders of hypersomnolence (combined with a daytime MSLT), but are often not necessary in the evaluation of other sleep disorders (e.g., insomnia).

Treatment
A staged approach to treatment is presented next. The treatment of all sleep disorders is beyond the scope of this chapter. The following strategies are foundational and will apply across most disturbances and disorders when there is an element of behavioral insomnia or inadequate sleep duration:

Identify sleep hygiene factors using data provided during screening and history taking, which may be contributing to or maintaining sleep disturbances (e.g., insufficient time for sleep, use of electronics in bedroom, variable sleep schedules).

Identify and encourage sleep-promoting behaviors (e.g., regular exercise; regularizing bedtime and wake time, including on weekends; reducing use of substances such as caffeine, alcohol, nicotine, and illicit substances; practicing wind down routines; increasing exposure to bright natural light in the morning, darkness at night).

Provide (or refer for) counseling related to existing situational stressors.

Use motivational interviewing (MI) techniques to assist with treatment planning and engagement. Although treatment will result in improved sleep and additional benefits, the changes required (e.g., earlier bedtimes, turning off electronics) will come at a cost (e.g., loss of social opportunities). MI can prevent these costs from becoming treatment barriers.

Relaxation techniques: Provide instruction or resources to facilitate the use of relaxation techniques.

Once these strategies are in place, more disorder-specific treatments can be applied, focusing on the more unique causes and characteristics of each disorder. These strategies are described in books and Web sites listed in the Additional Resources.

Sleep Disorder Clinics

For severe sleep disorders or diagnostic dilemmas, referral to a sleep disorder clinic or sleep consultant can be helpful. The National Sleep Foundation keeps an updated state-wise list of accredited sleep disorder centers (www.sleepfoundation.org). In addition, clinics in the US accredited by the American Academy of Sleep Medicine (listed by state) are available at www.aasmnet.org. Clinics in Canada (listed by province) are available at www.canadiansleepsociety.ca.

REFERENCES

1. Ohayon MM, Carskadon MA, Guilleminault C, et al. Meta-analysis of quantitative sleep parameters from childhood to old age in healthy individuals: developing normative sleep values across the human lifespan. *Sleep* 2004;27:1255–1273.
2. Carskadon MA, Tarokh L. Developmental changes in circadian timing and sleep: adolescence and emerging adulthood. In: Wolfson AR, Montgomery-Downs HE, eds. *The Oxford handbook of infant, child, and adolescent sleep and behavior.* New York, NY: Oxford University Press, 2013:70–77.
3. Roenneberg T, Kuehnle T, Pramstaller PP, et al. A marker for the end of adolescence. *Curr Biol* 2004;14(24):R1038–R1039.
4. National Sleep Foundation Sleep and Teens Task Force. *Adolescent sleep needs and patterns: research report and resource guide.* 2000. Available at http://sleepfoundation.org/sites/default/files/sleep_and_teens_report1.pdf.
5. Thacher PV. Late adolescence and emerging adulthood: a new lens for sleep professionals. In: Wolfson AR, Montgomery-Downs HE, eds. *The Oxford handbook of infant, child, and adolescent sleep and behavior.* New York, NY: Oxford University Press, 2013:586–602.
6. National Sleep Foundation 2002 Sleep in America Poll Task Force. *2002 "Sleep in America Poll."* 2002. Available at http://sleepfoundation.org/sites/default/files/2002SleepInAmericaPoll.pdf.
7. American College Health Association. *National College Health Assessment II, Reference Group Data Report Undergraduate Students Spring 2013.* Hanover, MD: American College Health Association, 2013.
8. Grandisar M, Short MA. Sleep hygiene and environment: role of technology. In: Wolfson AR, Montgomery-Downs HE, eds. *The Oxford handbook of infant, child, and adolescent sleep and behavior.* New York, NY: Oxford University Press, 2013:113–126.
9. Stremler R. Postpartum sleep: impact of infant sleep on parents. In: Wolfson AR, Montgomery-Downs HE, eds. *The Oxford handbook of infant, child, and adolescent sleep and behavior.* New York, NY: Oxford University Press, 2013:58–69.
10. Hershner S. Impact of sleep on the challenges of safe driving in young adults. In: Wolfson AR, Montgomery-Downs HE, eds. *The Oxford handbook of infant, child, and adolescent sleep and behavior.* New York, NY: Oxford University Press, 2013:441–454.
11. Morin C. Insomnia rounds (non-peer reviewed). 2012. Available at www.insomniarounds.ca.
12. American Psychiatric Association. *Diagnostic and Statistical Manual of mental disorders.* 5th ed. Arlington, VA: American Psychiatric Publishing, 2013.
13. American Academy of Sleep Medicine. International classification of sleep disorders: diagnostic & coding manual. 2nd ed. Westchester, IL: American Academy of Sleep Medicine, 2005.
14. Harvey AG, Alfano CA, Clarke G. Mood disorders. In: Wolfson AR, Montgomery-Downs HE, eds. *The Oxford handbook of infant, child, and adolescent sleep and behavior.* New York, NY: Oxford University Press, 2013:515–531.
15. Auger RR, Crowley SJ. Circadian timing: delayed sleep phase disorder. In: Wolfson AR, Montgomery-Downs HE, eds. *The Oxford handbook of infant, child, and adolescent sleep and behavior.* New York, NY: Oxford University Press, 2013:327–346.
16. Robillard R, Naismith SL, Rogers NL, et al. Delayed sleep phase in young people with unipolar or bipolar affective disorders. *J Affect Disord* 2013;145(2):260–263.
17. Marcus CL, Brooks LJ, Draper KA, et al. Diagnosis and management of childhood obstructive sleep apnea syndrome. *Pediatrics* 2012;130:576–584.
18. Archbold KH. Pediatric sleep apnea and adherence to positive airway pressure (PAP) therapy. In: Wolfson AR, Montgomery-Downs HE, eds. *The Oxford handbook of infant, child, and adolescents sleep and behavior.* New York, NY: Oxford University Press, 2013:362–369.
19. Sullivan SS. Narcolepsy in adolescents. *Adolesc Med State Art Rev* 2010;21(3):542–555, x–xi.
20. Singh AK, Mahlios J, Mignot E. Genetic association, seasonal infections and autoimmune basis of narcolepsy. *J Autoimmun* 2013;43:26–31.
21. Ivanenko A, Larson, K. Nighttime distractions: fears, nightmares, and parasomnias. In: Wolfson AR, Montgomery-Downs HE, eds. *The Oxford handbook of infant, child, and adolescent sleep and behavior.* New York, NY: Oxford University Press, 2013:347–361.
22. Bessey M, Coulombe A, Corkum P. Sleep hygiene in children with ADHD: findings and recommendations. *ADHD Rep* 2013;21(3):1–7.
23. Owens JA, Dalzell V. Use of the "BEARS" sleep screening tool in a pediatric residents' continuity clinic: a pilot study. *Sleep Med* 2005;6:63–69.

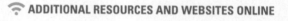 **ADDITIONAL RESOURCES AND WEBSITES ONLINE**

PART VII

Genitourinary Disorders

26 Renal and Genitourinary Tract Infections in Adolescents and Young Adults

Lawrence J. D'Angelo
Shamir Tuchman

Genitourinary tract infections are common in adolescents and young adults (AYAs). Those most often diagnosed include cystitis, pyelonephritis, urethritis, and asymptomatic bacteriuria.

 CYSTITIS

Epidemiology

1. Over the course of a lifetime, urinary tract infections (UTIs) occur three to five times more commonly in women than in men. For adolescents, this difference may be as great as 50-fold.
2. One in three females will have at least one episode of acute cystitis during adolescence or young adulthood.[1] Hooton et al.[2] defined the annual incidence of a lower UTI in a cohort of sexually active female university students to be 0.7 infections/person-year. One infection appears to predispose an individual to more, with Foxman[3] finding that 27% of young women had at least one recurrence within 6 months of the first infection and 2.7% had a second recurrence in this same period.
3. Risk factors for infection
   a. Females: Females are at greater risk than males because of a short urethra, which has close proximity to vaginal and rectal microorganisms. Other risk factors for UTIs include the following (although many of these risk factors are not well substantiated in the literature):
   - Coitus and coital behaviors (diaphragm use, coital frequency, use of spermicide-coated condoms, and having a new sexual partner)
   - Pregnancy
   - Previous UTIs
   - Nonsecretor of ABO blood group antigens (bind bacteria to vaginal epithelial cells)[4]
   - Catheterization or instrumentation of the urethra[5]
   - Anatomical abnormalities (e.g., urethral stenosis, neurogenic bladder, and nephrolithiasis)
   - Obesity[6]
   - Having a first-degree relative with a history of UTIs[7]
   b. Males: Because UTIs in general and cystitis in particular are so much less frequent in males, risk factors and pathophysiology are less well understood. In nonsexually active male adolescents, bladder and renal infections are more likely to result from structural or functional abnormalities

of the perineum and/or urinary tract. Additional factors may include the following:
- Blood group B or AB nonsecretor; P1 blood group phenotype
- Insertive anal intercourse[8]
- Sexual partner with vaginal colonization by uropathogens
- Uncircumcised[9]

Microbiology
Females

The most common organism causing acute cystitis is *Escherichia coli* (75% to 90%). Older literature suggested the importance of *Staphylococcus saprophyticus* in AYAs, but it now appears that other gram-negative organisms cause most of the remainder of the infections.[10] Organisms such as *Klebsiella* species, *Pseudomonas aeruginosa, Enterobacter* and *Proteus* species, *Staphylococcus aureus, Streptococcus faecalis,* and *Serratia marcescens* may play a greater role in recurrent or chronic, rather than in acute, infections. Gram-positive organisms such as *Staphylococcus saprophyticus,* enterococci, and group B streptococcus are less frequent pathogens; recent studies have shown that in women with symptoms suggestive of UTI, positive midstream cultures for the latter two organisms have a very low positive predictive value when compared to catheterized specimens,[11] implying that these are likely colonizers of the external periurethral area. In addition, emerging evidence suggests that *Mycoplasma genitalium* is associated with urethritis in women (see Chapter 56).[12]

Males

Approximately three-fourths of UTIs in male AYAs are due to gram-negative bacilli, but *E. coli* infections are not nearly as common as in women. Gram-positive organisms, particularly enterococci and coagulase-negative staphylococci, account for approximately one-fifth of infections. Sexually transmitted pathogens such as *Trichomonas vaginalis, Neisseria gonorrhoeae, Chlamydia trachomatis, Mycoplasma hominis,* and *Gardnerella vaginalis* can cause urethral, epididymal, and prostate infections that can be confused with UTIs in AYAs.[13] Furthermore, *M. genitalium* has been shown to cause nongonococcal urethritis (NGU) in men, with the highest prevalence in men who are *C. trachomatis* negative (see Chapter 56).[12]

Symptoms and Signs
Females

In women, the most common symptoms of UTIs are dysuria, frequency, hesitancy, suprapubic pain or pressure, overt pyuria and hematuria. These symptoms are often difficult to localize. For example, in female patients, dysuria can be related to infections in the bladder, urethra, vulva, or vaginal tract. In this case, the location and timing of the dysuria are occasionally helpful. Dysuria

Differential Diagnosis of Acute Dysuria in Women

Condition	Pathogen	Pyuria	Hematuria	Bacteriuria	Urine Culture[a]	Signs and Symptoms
Cystitis	*E. coli, S. saprophyticus, Proteus, Klebsiella* sp	Usually	Sometimes	Usually	$10^2->10^5$	Acute onset, severe symptoms, dysuria, frequency, urgency, suprapubic or low back pain, suprapubic tenderness, internal dysuria
Urethritis	*C. trachomatis, N. gonorrhoeae,* herpes simplex virus	Usually	Rarely	Rarely	$<10^2$	Gradual onset, mild symptoms, vaginal discharge or bleeding, lower abdominal pain, new sexual partner, cervical or vaginal lesions on examination
Vaginitis	*Candida* sp, *T. vaginalis*	Rarely	Rarely	Rarely	$<10^2$	Vaginal discharge or odor, pruritis, dyspareunia, external dysuria, no frequency or urgency, vulvovaginitis on examination

[a]Colony forming units (CFU)/mL

associated with cystitis or urethritis is often described as internal pain and is usually worse when a patient initiates micturition. External pain or "terminal pain" (at the end of micturition) is more often associated with other conditions such as a vulvar inflammation, upper genital tract infection, or a herpes simplex infection.

Table 26.1 lists the pathogens, incidence of pyuria and hematuria, urine culture findings, and signs and symptoms of acute dysuria in women.

Males

Apart from the preceding symptoms, male patients may also have symptoms associated with infections in the prostate (perineal or rectal pain), epididymis (scrotal discomfort or tender epididymis), or testicles (testicular pain and swelling).

Differential Diagnosis of Acute Dysuria

The most common complaint arousing suspicion of a UTI is dysuria. However, dysuria may be a symptom of infection elsewhere in the urinary tract or genital tract, particularly in AYAs.[14,15] The differential diagnosis of dysuria includes the following:

Females

1. Acute vaginitis and possible associated Skene glands infection secondary to sexually transmitted pathogens
2. Vulvovaginitis
3. Local dermatitis from chemicals and other agents such as soaps, contraceptive agents and foams, and feminine hygiene products
4. Subclinical pyelonephritis: Some females with only dysuria have an upper UTI. These infections may be more difficult to eradicate. There are no reliable and simple methods to distinguish them from lower UTIs.
5. Acute urethral syndrome: Symptomatic women with pyuria but no growth of urinary pathogens on culture are likely infected with one or more sexually transmitted pathogens and should be evaluated for these.[14]

Males

The differential diagnosis of cystitis and dysuria includes the following:

1. Urethritis (secondary to sexually transmitted organisms, including *N. gonorrhoeae, C. trachomatis, T. vaginalis, M. genitalium,* and others)
2. Prostatitis/epididymitis
3. Irritation from agents such as spermicidal foam
4. Trauma (usually associated with masturbation)

Diagnosis

1. History
   a. In females, it is important to elicit symptoms suggestive of vulvovaginitis, such as an abnormal vaginal discharge

or vaginal itching; with a vaginal infection, symptoms of frequency and urgency are less common. In males, a history of sexual exposure, type of sexual activity, past urinary tract problems, or trauma is important.
   b. Similarly in females, it is helpful to know if the patient uses any medications or irritants such as douches, feminine hygiene products, strong soaps, bubble bath, or contraceptive products that could cause a local dermatitis. In males, a history of mechanical irritation including frequent masturbation is important.
   c. For both males and females, inquiring about specific sexual practices is important.
   d. Determining whether there are signs of upper genitourinary tract disease is important. Fever and flank pain suggest acute pyelonephritis. Also important are factors suggestive of subclinical pyelonephritis, such as underlying urinary tract abnormalities, diabetes mellitus, UTIs in childhood, three or more previous UTIs, or acute pyelonephritis in the past.
2. Physical examination
   a. In both sexes, an examination of the abdomen and flank for tenderness should be performed.
   b. In females, an external genital or pelvic examination should be considered if the patient is sexually active or if there is history of a vaginal discharge.
   c. In males, examination should include inspection and palpation of the genitals to check for urethral discharge, meatal erythema, inflammation of the glans penis, penile lesions, an enlarged or tender epididymis or testis, or inguinal lymphadenopathy. A rectal examination is necessary if a diagnosis of prostatitis is under consideration.
3. Laboratory studies[16]
   a. Nonculture examination of urine
      • Either direct examination of *uncentrifuged* urine or Gram stain of a similar specimen are insensitive diagnostic tests, unless the culture has a bacteria colony count of at least 10^5 organisms/mL.
      • Several other chemical tests that use nitrate glucose oxidase or catalase to detect the presence of nitrites are commonly used diagnostic tests. Available by "dipstick," they are unfortunately dependent on the conversion of nitrate to nitrite, which is usually associated with infections caused by members of the Enterobacteriaceae bacterial family including *E. coli.* When the infection is caused by other organisms such as *S. saprophyticus* or *Enterococcus,* this test is most often negative.
      • Microscopic detection of pyuria on unspun urine necessitates counting cells in a hemocytometer (with ≥ 8 cells/mm^3 correlating with positive urine cultures) and

is rarely performed. Examination of centrifuged urine sediment, while possible, is not reliably standardized and may be positive with any cause of pyuria. Chemical testing for the presence of leukocyte esterase has limitations as well, although it may be conveniently combined on a dipstick for testing for urinary nitrites. When combined, these tests still have relatively low sensitivity but high specificity if both are positive. If nonculture testing is utilized, urine should be examined within 2 hours of collection.

b. Urine culture

• Urine cultures are usually not a routine part of the evaluation of every patient with symptoms consistent with a UTI. They are, however, necessary for those individuals who have recurrent or complicated infections (pyelonephritis) or in whom initial treatment has failed. Older criteria of a colony count of >100,000 CFU/mL of a typical urinary pathogen have been replaced by colony counts as low as $\geq 10^2$ CFU/mL or more commonly a count of 10^4 in a voided midstream specimen. However, while true for Enterobacteriaceae, this technique of sampling and diagnostic standard does not apply if other bacterial species (such as enterococci or group B strep) are isolated.[11]

4. Other tests

a. Females: In prepubertal women, those with three infections within 1 to 2 years should receive a more complete urinary tract evaluation, which may include a renal ultrasound and a voiding cystourethrogram. In postpubertal females with uncomplicated cystitis, evaluation even after recurrent episodes is unlikely to reveal significant abnormalities that would change either therapy or prognosis.

b. Males: Although some authorities recommend a full investigation after the first infection, this is probably of greater importance in the young child or infant. In AYAs, there is less evidence for such studies unless there is a suspected renal abnormality or if there is no response to therapy.

Recurrent Infections in Female AYAs

Approximately 20% to 25% of young women will have recurrent UTIs, defined as 2 infections in 6 months or 3 in 1 year.[17] Most of these AYA women do not have anatomical or functional abnormalities of the urinary tract. However, recurrent cystitis within 3 months of the original infection should call for a urine culture. Those female patients with a relapse of symptoms within 2 weeks of completion of therapy should also have their urine cultured, be treated with the selected antibiotic regimen for at least 7 days, and should have careful follow-up including a "test-of-cure" culture. Repeated infections not related to coitus, associated with persistent hematuria or recurrent pyelonephritis, or linked to renal insufficiency should result in an evaluation for an occult source of infection or urologic abnormality.

Evidence-based techniques for preventing recurrent infections include daily or every other day antimicrobial prophylaxis, postcoital prophylaxis, patient "self-diagnosis" combined with patient-initiated treatment (best for patients with one to two episodes annually), daily lactobacilli product administration, and methenamine salts. More controversial and still unsubstantiated approaches include daily ascorbic acid treatment, frequent use of cranberry products, the use of oral "immunostimulants," and a vaginal "vaccine" made of heat-killed uropathogenic bacteria.[18]

PYELONEPHRITIS

Pyelonephritis is an infection of the renal pelvis and medulla. Risk factors for pyelonephritis are similar to those for UTI (with the strongest factors being recent intercourse, a new sexual partner, and spermicide use), but also include maternal history of UTI and diabetes.[19] Most infections occur from bacterial ascent through the urethra and bladder.

The clinical and laboratory manifestations usually include the following: symptoms of acute cystitis, fever, costovertebral tenderness, elevated leukocyte count and erythrocyte sedimentation rate, urinalysis revealing leukocytes and bacterial casts, and/or a positive urine culture result.

The range of symptoms varies from mild flank pain to those of septicemia. Most cases of acute pyelonephritis in young women are caused by E. coli infection (>80%). Pyuria and gram-negative bacteria are usually present on examination of the urine. Urine culture specimens should always be obtained. Blood cultures should also be obtained from those whose diagnosis is uncertain, from immunosuppressed patients, from those in whom a hematogenous source is suspected, or from those who are ill enough to be hospitalized. If fever and flank pain persist after 72 hours of treatment, then cultures should be repeated and ultrasonography or computed tomography should be considered to evaluate for an abscess. Additional indications for imaging studies include recurrent pyelonephritis and persistent hematuria. Indications for hospitalization include persistent vomiting, suspected sepsis, uncertain diagnosis, and urinary tract obstruction. Other relative indications include anatomical urinary tract abnormalities, immunocompromised status, and inadequate access to follow-up care.

ASYMPTOMATIC BACTERIURIA

The prevalence of asymptomatic bacteriuria (reproducible growth of >10^5 CFU/mL) ranges from approximately 1% to 7%. There is a tendency toward spontaneous cure. However, women with this condition are at increased risk of an overt UTI (8% in the week after documented bacteria in the urine),[20] and, in individuals whose infection begins in childhood, there is a suggestion that their infection can lead to renal impairment. Asymptomatic bacteriuria during pregnancy is a risk factor for the development of acute pyelonephritis, for lower fetal birth weight, and for a higher incidence of prematurity. Treatment is mainly indicated for individuals who are (1) pregnant; (2) male; (3) individuals with renal tract abnormality or immunocompromised (diabetes, sickle cell disease, HIV infection, etc.); or (4) females with a history of UTI recurrence and concomitant pyuria.[21] Treatment should be with appropriate antibiotics selected on the basis of culture and subsequent sensitivities.

EPIDIDYMITIS/PROSTATITIS

Etiology

Epididymitis and prostatitis are inflammatory reactions of the male "upper" sexual/urinary tract. Epididymitis is the considerably more common of the two, but both are relatively infrequent and when they do occur in this age-group, they are usually secondary to sexually transmitted infections such as N. gonorrhoeae or C. trachomatis. Coliform bacteria, S. saprophyticus, M. hominis, U. urealyticum, and T. vaginalis have also been implicated as causative agents. Retrograde spread of pathogens is the usual mechanism of infection.[22]

Risk factors for both infections include sexual activity, strenuous physical activity, and prolonged periods of sitting such as that associated with long trips or sedentary jobs. Anatomical factors such as posterior urethral valves or urethral or meatal stenosis can also be a predisposing factor.

Diagnosis

Epididymitis usually presents with acute to subacute scrotal pain. Pain can affect one or both testes. Symptoms of lower UTI may be present (dysuria, frequency, hematuria) as can systemic symptoms such as fever, nausea, and vomiting.

If epididymitis is suspected, nucleic acid antibody testing for N. gonorrhoeae and C. trachomatis should be initiated from either

TABLE 26.2

Treatment of Genitourinary Tract Infections in AYAs

Cystitis/Lower UTI
- Nitrofurantoin monohydrate/macrocrystals (100 mg every 12 h for 5 d)
- Trimethoprim-sulfamethoxazole (160/800 mg every 12 h for 3 d)
- Fosfomycin (3 g IM in single dose)
- Cefpodoxime proxetil (200 mg every 12 h for 3 to 7 d)

In older adolescents (older than 16 y), the following quinolones are also acceptable:
- Ciprofloxacin (250 mg every 12 h for 3 d)
- Ofloxacin (200 mg every 12 h for 3 d)
- Levofloxacin (500 mg once daily for 3 d)

Patients with potentially complicating problems (diabetes, sickle cell disease, a history of a previous UTI, or symptoms for >1 wk): use a 7-d regimen of the above medications

In pregnancy, a 7-d regimen of the following is preferred:
- *Nitrofurantoin* (100 mg orally every 12 h for 5 d)

Postcoital or continuous prophylaxis to prevent recurrent infections in high-risk patients with asymptomatic bacteriuria, or those with recurrent infections:
- Trimethoprim (100 mg postcoital or daily)
- Trimethoprim-sulfamethoxazole (40/200 mg postcoital or daily)
- Nitrofurantoin (50–100 mg postcoital or daily)
- Norfloxacin (200 mg postcoital or daily)

Pyelonephritis/Upper UTIs
Oral Outpatient Therapy[a]:
- Trimethoprim-sulfamethoxazole (160/800 mg every 12 h for 14 d)
- Cefpodoxime proxetil (200 mg every 12 h for 14 d)
In older adolescents (older than 16 y), the following quinolones are also acceptable:
- Ciprofloxacin (500 mg every 12 h for 7–10 d)
- Levofloxacin (750 mg once daily for 5–7 d)
[a]All of the above regimens may be initiated with a one time dose of the following intravenous medications:
- Ceftriaxone, 1 g IV
- Ciprofloxacin, 400 mg IV
- Gentamicin, 5 mg/kg IV

Intravenous inpatient therapy:
- Ceftriaxone (1 g every 12 to 24 h)
- Ciprofloxacin (400 mg every 12 h)
- Gentamicin (5 mg/kg total, divided either every 8, 12, or 24 h [with or without ampicillin])
- Ticarcillin/clavulanate (3.1 g every 6 h)
- Imipenem/cilastatin (500 mg every 6 h)
These regimens should be maintained for 48–72 h or until the patient is afebrile and able to tolerate one of the oral medication regimens listed above. They should then complete 14 total days of antibiotic therapy.

Epididymitis/Prostatitis
Likely sexually transmitted organism:
- Ceftriaxone (250 mg IM in single dose) PLUS
- Doxycycline (100 mg PO b.i.d. for 10–14 d)

Likely enteric organism (anatomical defect or history of insertive anal intercourse)
- Levofloxacin (500 mg po every 24 h for 14 d [epididymitis]–28 d [prostatitis]) or
- Ofloxacin (300 mg every 12 h for 14 d [epididymitis]–28 d [prostatitis])

a urethral swab or urine. Urine dipsticks positive for leukocyte esterase or nitrates help to support the diagnosis in combination with clinical signs and symptoms. Physical findings may include scrotal swelling, tenderness of the epididymis, and associated tenderness of the testicle.

When testicular pain is the main presenting symptom and physical examination cannot distinguish between epididymal and testicular tenderness, the differential diagnosis must include testicular torsion and diagnostic testing with scrotal ultrasound with blood flow studies to assess perfusion and anatomy should be performed.

In prostatitis, symptoms and signs usually include penile/scrotal, suprapubic, perineal, groin, or back pain or pain that occurs during ejaculation. There may also be frequency, dysuria, and hesitation as well as systemic symptoms such as chills, fever, and malaise. Other symptoms may include hematospermia and hematuria. Physical examination usually reveals tenderness on rectal examination when the prostate is palpated.

In either condition, urinalysis may reveal bacteriuria or pyuria and urine cultures may be positive. However, absence of these laboratory findings does not eliminate either diagnosis if history and physical examination suggest infection.

TREATMENT OF RENAL AND URINARY INFECTIONS

In the face of a significant increase in the number of urinary pathogens demonstrating resistance to the agents, particularly trimethoprim-sulfamethoxazole (Tmp/Smx) and amoxicillin, historically used to treat UTIs,[23] the guidelines for treating acute uncomplicated UTIs have been updated. For this reason, local resistance patterns should be consulted before prescribing any antibiotic as first-line treatment of UTIs. Tmp/Smx should only be used if the local resistance rates of uropathogens do not exceed 20%. Ampicillin or amoxicillin should never be used as empirical treatment of UTIs; they should only be used if culture results show that the isolated bacteria are sensitive to these agents.[24] Table 26.2 summarizes the current recommendations for treating both lower and upper tract infections.

Oral antibiotic treatment remains appropriate for patients with pyelonephritis with mild to moderate illness and no associated nausea or vomiting (Table 26.2). Any of these regimens may be initiated with an initial dose of a one-time intravenous agent such as 1 g of ceftriaxone, 400 mg of ciprofloxacin, or 5 mg/kg of gentamicin, depending on local community resistance patterns.

Patients with severe illness, those who are unable to tolerate oral regimens, or those with significant underlying health issues (patients with diabetes, sickle cell disease, or immunodeficiency) should be admitted to the hospital and treated with one of the intravenous regimens listed in Table 26.2.

Patients with recurrent infections who elect either postcoital or daily prophylaxis should follow one of the regimens listed in Table 26.2, as determined by their urine culture and sensitivity results.

In epididymitis and prostatitis, treatment should be empirically initiated if either diagnosis is strongly considered, in accordance with the regimens listed in Table 26.2. Although antibiotics have good penetration into an acutely inflamed prostate gland or epididymis, epididymitis should be treated for 10 to 14 days while prostatitis should ideally be treated for 14 to 28 days.

REFERENCES

1. Foxman B. Urinary tract infection syndromes: occurrence, recurrence, bacteriology, risk factors, and disease burden. *Infect Dis Clin North Am* 2014;28(1):1–13. doi:10.1016/j.idc.2013.09.003.
2. Hooton TM, Scholes D, Hughes JP, et al. A prospective study of risk factors for symptomatic urinary tract infection in young women. *N Engl J Med* 1996;335:468–474.
3. Foxman B, Gillespie B, Koopman J, et al. Risk factors for second urinary tract infection among college women. *Am J Epidemiol* 2000;151(12):1194–1205.

4. Hooton TM. Recurrent urinary tract infection in women. *Int J Antimicrob Agents* 2001;17(4):259–268.
5. Uçkay I, Sax H, Gayet-Ageron A, et al. High proportion of healthcare-associated urinary tract infection in the absence of prior exposure to urinary catheter: a cross-sectional study. *Antimicrob Resist Infect Control* 2013;2:1–10. doi:10.1186/2047-2994-2-5.
6. Semins MJ, Shore AD, Makary MA, et al. The impact of obesity on urinary tract infection risk. *Urology* 2012;79(2):266–269. doi:10.1016/j.urology.2011.09.040.
7. Scholes D, Hawn TR, Roberts PL, et al. Family history and risk of recurrent cystitis and pyelonephritis in women. *J Urol* 2010;184(2):564–569. doi:10.1016/j.juro.2010.03.139.
8. Breyer BN, Vittinghoff E, Van Den Eeden SK, et al. Effect of sexually transmitted infections, lifetime sexual partner count, and recreational drug use on lower urinary tract symptoms in men who have sex with men. *Urology* 2012;79:188–193. doi:10.1016/j.urology.2011.07.1412.
9. Morris BJ, Wiswell TE. Circumcision and lifetime risk of urinary tract infection: a systematic review and meta-analysis. *J Urol* 2013;189:2118–2124. doi:10.1016/j.juro.2012.11.114.
10. Ronald, A. The etiology of urinary tract infection: traditional and emerging pathogens. *Dis Mon* 2003;49:71–82.
11. Hooton TM, Roberts PL, Cox ME, et al. Voided midstream urine culture and acute cystitis in premenopausal women. *N Engl J Med* 2013;369:1883–1891. doi:10.1056/NEJMoa1302186. PMID:24224622
12. Workowski KA, Bolan GA. Sexually Transmitted Diseases Treatment Guidelines, 2015. *MMWR Recomm Rep* 2015;64(3):1–135.
13. den Heijer CD, van Dongen MC, Donker GA, et al. Diagnostic approach to urinary tract infections in male general practice patients: a national surveillance study. *Br J Gen Pract* 2012;62:e780–e786. doi:10.3399/bjgp12X658313.
14. Huppert JS, Biro F, Lan D, et al. Urinary symptoms in adolescent females: STI or UTI? *J Adolesc Health* 2007;40:418–424.
15. Prentiss KA, Newby PK, Vinci RJ. Adolescent female with urinary symptoms: a diagnostic challenge for the pediatrician. *Pediatr Emerg Care* 2011;27:789–794. doi:10.1097/PEC.0b013e31822c10f6.
16. Wilson ML, Gaido L. Laboratory diagnosis of urinary tract infections in adult patients. *Clin Infect Dis* 2004;38:1150–1158.
17. Ikäheimo R, Siitonen A, Heiskanen T, et al. Recurrence of urinary tract infection in a primary care setting: analysis of a 1-year follow-up of 179 women. *Clin Infect Dis* 1996;22:91–99.
18. Geerlings SE, Beerepoot MA, Prins JM. Prevention of recurrent urinary tract infections in women: antimicrobial and nonantimicrobial strategies. *Infect Dis Clin North Am* 2014;28:135–147. doi:10.1016/j.idc.2013.10.001
19. Scholes D, Hooton TM, Roberts PL, et al. Risk factors associated with acute pyelonephritis in healthy women. *Ann Intern Med* 2005;142:20–27.
20. Hooton TM, Scholes D, Stapleton AE, et al. A prospective study of asymptomatic bacteriuria in sexually active young women. *N Engl J Med* 2000;343:992–997.
21. Cai T, Mazzoli S, Mondaini N, et al. The role of asymptomatic bacteriuria in young women with recurrent urinary tract infections: to treat or not to treat? *Clin Infect Dis* 2012;55:771–777. doi:10.1093/cid/cis534.
22. Trojian TH, Lishnak TS, Heiman D. Epididymitis and orchitis: an overview. *Am Fam Physician* 2009;79:583–587.
23. Swami SK, Liesinger JT, Shah N, et al. Incidence of antibiotic-resistant *Escherichia coli* bacteriuria according to age and location of onset: a population-based study from Olmsted County, Minnesota. *Mayo Clin Proc* 2012;87(8):753–759. doi:10.1016/j.mayocp.2012.02.025.
24. Gupta K, Hooton TM, Naber KG, et al. International clinical practice guidelines for the treatment of acute uncomplicated cystitis and pyelonephritis in women: a 2010 update by the Infectious Diseases Society of America and the European Society for Microbiology and Infectious Diseases. *Clin Infect Dis* 2011;52:e103–120. doi:10.1093/cid/ciq257.

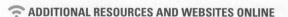 **ADDITIONAL RESOURCES AND WEBSITES ONLINE**

27

Enuresis

Diane Tanaka

KEY WORDS

- Daytime incontinence
- Desmopressin
- Detrusor overactivity
- Disturbed sleep
- Enuresis alarms
- Monosymptomatic enuresis
- Nocturnal polyuria
- Nonmonosymptomatic enuresis
- Primary enuresis
- Secondary enuresis
- Simple behavioral interventions

Enuresis is typically considered a childhood problem, but it affects 2% to 3% of teens and 0.5% to 2% of adults. Boys are affected more than girls by a ratio of 2:1. Even though enuresis spontaneously resolves by 15% per year, the longer enuresis persists, the lower the likelihood it will resolve spontaneously. The more severe the childhood enuresis, the more likely it will persist into adolescence and adulthood. About 53% to 82% of adolescents and young adults (AYAs) with enuresis have the moderate to severe form,[1,2] defined as >3 wet nights/week. Bladder dysfunction occurs more frequently in AYAs with enuresis.[1-3] As enuresis negatively impacts self-esteem and emotional well-being, it is reasonable to evaluate and treat enuresis in AYAs. Certain populations of AYAs have an increased incidence of nocturnal enuresis, including those with sickle cell anemia or anorexia nervosa[4,5] and those taking certain psychotropic medications. While there is reasonable evidence on effective treatments for nocturnal enuresis in children, there is a lack of evidence on treatments for AYAs.

STANDARDIZING TERMINOLOGY

The International Children's Continence Society has standardized enuresis terminology for children and adolescents[6]:

Enuresis: Discrete episodes of urinary incontinence occurring during sleep beyond the age of 5 years, which is the age at which bladder control is achieved.

Monosymptomatic nocturnal enuresis (MNE): Enuresis occurring in AYAs without other lower urinary tract symptoms and no history of bladder dysfunction.

Primary enuresis: never achieved dryness.

Secondary nocturnal enuresis: Nighttime wetting that occurs in AYAs who have a history of 6 months of dryness. This often occurs during stressful events or a vulnerable time in the teen's or young adult's life. The exact cause is often unknown.

Nonmonosymptomatic Enuresis (NME): Enuresis associated with other lower urinary tract symptoms, including urgency, increased or decreased urinary frequency, straining, hesitancy, or a weak or intermittent urinary stream.

Daytime incontinence: Incontinence during the day. Among AYAs who experience nocturnal enuresis, 18% to 29% also have significant daytime symptoms.[1,2,7] Females often have more daytime symptoms than males and may be associated with urinary tract infections (UTIs) and obstipation.

Evidence suggests that a significant proportion, if not most, of AYAs—especially older AYAs, and those with daytime wetness or other lower urinary tract symptoms—have NME and should be referred to a specialist.[3,8] Hence, this chapter will focus primarily on the management of AYAs with MNE, as they usually can be managed by primary care providers and adolescent medicine specialists.

ETIOLOGY OF MNE

Bladder maturation plays a key role in achieving urinary continence. The child must gain awareness of bladder filling, develop the ability to voluntarily suppress bladder contractions, and learn to coordinate sphincter and detrusor function. Daytime continence is usually achieved by 4 years of age. By age 5, most children have achieved nighttime bladder control.[4]

Major Contributors to MNE

Nocturnal Polyuria

Characterized by increased nighttime urine output. Increased fluid intake before bedtime, reduced response to antidiuretic hormone (ADH), and decreased secretion of ADH may be the mechanisms behind nocturnal polyuria.

Detrusor Overactivity

There may be a defect in the circadian rhythm of detrusor inhibition in teens with MNE. There is no clear pattern of urodynamic abnormality in MNE, unlike in AYAs with daytime incontinence. An increased rate of bladder contractions is seen during enuretic episodes, which has been confirmed with urodynamic studies. If the adolescent or young adult has MNE refractory to treatment, consider bladder dysfunction.[4]

Disturbed Sleep

Excessively deep sleep seems to contribute to MNE. Sleep studies have found that teens with MNE are more difficult to arouse than controls; may have frequent cortical arousals associated with unstable bladder contractions, but are unable to awaken completely; and that enuretic episodes may occur during any sleep stage, but can primarily occur during non-REM sleep.[4,9,10] Insomnia is found more often in AYAs with severe enuresis.[10]

Other Contributors to MNE

Maturational Delay

Spontaneous resolution of enuresis provides support for the role of maturational delay. An increased incidence of minor neurologic dysfunctions, including minor motor dysfunctions, has been found in studies of enuretic children.[11] However, studies have not investigated whether neurologic dysfunctions play a role in enuresis in AYAs.

Genetics

There is a 68% concordance between monozygotic twins and a 36% concordance between dizygotic twins. When both parents have a history of enuresis, 77% of their children are affected; in contrast, if neither parent has a history of enuresis, only 15% of their children are affected. An autosomal dominant form of primary nocturnal enuresis has been linked to chromosome 13q13-q14.3 in Danish families. Other genetic loci for enuresis have been found on chromosomes 12q13-q21 and 22q11.[4,11–13] Thirty percent of enuresis cases are sporadic, 50% appear to be autosomal dominant, and the remaining cases show autosomal recessive inheritance or polygenic inheritance.[13,14]

Abnormal Secretion of ADH

Studies indicate that decreased nocturnal secretion of ADH is a factor in the etiology of MNE.[15] There is evidence that the response to ADH secretion is subject to maturational development.

Small Bladder Capacity

The expected bladder capacity (in mL) for age can be calculated by multiplying the adolescent's age in years by 30 and then adding 30; after age 12, the estimated bladder capacity levels off at 390 mL.[6] Enuretic children have smaller bladder capacities than age-matched children without enuresis.[4,16–18] Early studies in children provided evidence that smaller bladder capacity is actually due to a functional decrease in capacity.[4] It is unclear to what extent this plays a role in AYAs.

Psychological Factors

Psychological stressors do not seem to cause enuresis. It is important to remember that the AYAs are not deliberately wetting the bed. An increased prevalence of emotional difficulties, including poor self-esteem, family stress, and family isolation, has been described in affected adolescents. However, this may be secondary to the enuresis rather than the cause. In many cultures, enuresis is psychosocially stigmatizing. Enuresis has been described in AYAs with anorexia nervosa.[5] It has also been described to occur early in treatment with second-generation antipsychotic medication, in particular clozapine.[18] ADHD and nocturnal enuresis have been noted to co-occur in children,[19] but persistence of this co-occurrence into AYAs has not been described.

● DIAGNOSIS

A thorough history, a focused physical exam, and a urinalysis are all that are needed to evaluate enuresis. Significant organic lesions are infrequent with MNE. A good voiding history is essential. The prevalence of an organic or psychological cause is more prevalent in secondary enuresis and daytime incontinence.

History

The history is the cornerstone of the evaluation of AYAs with enuresis:

1. Severity of enuresis: How many dry nights per month, most consecutive dry nights, frequency of urination, urgency of urination, evening fluid intake, and whether the bladder is emptied at bedtime.
2. Evaluate for NME or daytime incontinence: ask specifically about daytime incontinence, urgency, holding maneuvers, interrupted stream, weak stream, and straining.
3. History of UTIs
4. Symptoms of organic disease: Dysuria, intermittent daytime wetness, polydipsia, central nervous system trauma, constipation, or encopresis can indicate organic disease. AYAs with ectopic ureter will complain of constant wetness or dampness. Spinal tumors cause a change in gait, constipation, or encopresis. AYAs with neuromuscular disabilities may also suffer from enuresis.
5. Family history of enuresis or small bladders
6. Nocturia
7. Information regarding the AYAs' fluid intake and drinking habits is essential; however, the utility of a frequency/volume chart or "bladder diary" in AYAs has not been established.
8. Prior therapeutic modalities and results
9. The adolescent or young adult and their family's adjustment to the problem
10. Family member responsible for changing sheets and laundry
11. History of sleep disorders, such as night terrors or unusually deep sleep, as well as snoring, obstructive sleep apnea and difficulty arousing from sleep
12. General psychosocial review of family, peers, and school
13. Urgency of urination: The common causes of urgency of urination are UTIs, bacteria without dysuria, or constipation. Rare causes include a bladder calculus, a bladder foreign body, and hypercalciuria.
14. Bowel habits and constipation: If constipation is not treated, then it may be difficult to treat the enuresis. Ask about experiences of soiling or fecal incontinence.
15. AYAs' level of motivation to treat the enuresis: How concerned is the young person about their enuresis and do they want to do something about it?

Physical Examination

The physical examination in an adolescent or young adult with MNE is usually completely normal. However, the clinician should consider the following physical exam:

1. Check blood pressure.
2. Abdomen: Check for masses and palpate for stool.
3. If the history is consistent with constipation, consider performing a rectal exam to evaluate for hard stool.
4. Genitourinary tract: Check the urethral meatus for evidence of stenosis or abnormal location. Observe the urinary stream to see whether it is full and forceful or narrow and dribbling. Palpate the testes to confirm that they are descended and inspect the scrotum (an underdeveloped scrotum can be indicative of urologic abnormalities).
5. Look for midline defects in the lumbosacral area, abnormalities of the gluteal fold, or abnormal tufts of hair.
6. Perform a neurologic examination including:
   a. Gait
   b. Lower extremity: Motor and sensory
   c. Deep tendon reflexes
   d. Perineal sensation
   e. Rectal sphincter tone
   f. Bulbocavernosus reflex

Laboratory Tests

1. Urinalysis: Every AYA should have a urinalysis to screen for UTIs, diabetes mellitus, and diabetes insipidus. Look for the presence of glucose, protein, or white blood cells, and measure specific gravity. Urethral obstruction can be associated with hematuria.
2. Urine culture: Obtain a urine culture if the urinalysis suggests a UTI.
3. Uroflowmetry: A noninvasive measure of urine flow rate used to evaluate patients who are suspected of having NME, such as neurogenic bladder, urethral obstruction, overactive bladder, sphincter overactivity, or needing to use external pressure to void.

4. Imaging studies: Radiological studies are not needed routinely. If a urethral obstruction or a neurogenic bladder is suspected, then a voiding cystourethrogram is indicated (the neurogenic bladder will appear as a trabeculated "Christmas tree" or "pine cone" configuration). If a neurogenic bladder is suspected, consider a spinal magnetic resonance image to look for spinal cord abnormalities. Ultrasonography is indicated for patients with persistent daytime wetness or for patients with failure to empty the bladder. A prevoiding and postvoiding bladder ultrasonography can be obtained to rule out partial emptying (normal residual bladder volume is <10 mL). Ultrasound can also estimate bladder capacity and determine bladder wall thickness.

THERAPY

For therapy to be successful, both the family and the adolescent or young adult must be highly motivated to engage in treatment and be aware that successful treatment can take months. The approach to treatment is guided by the etiology of the enuresis if known, as well as the level of participation the adolescent or young adult and family want in the treatment process. It is important to inform the adolescent or young adult and family that enuresis is a common condition and it is not the fault of the AYA or the family. It should also be emphasized that punishment is not effective. Motivational interviewing can be effective, but its efficacy has mostly been shown in younger children.

Simple Behavioral Treatments

Simple behavioral treatments have been shown to be more effective than no treatment[20,21] in children. The advantage of these treatments is that the family and AYAs can initiate them with little input from a medical professional. As enuresis in AYAs is often more severe,[1,2] its response to simple behavioral treatments is less likely.

Evening Fluid Restriction

Daily fluid intake should be concentrated in the morning and early afternoon. Fluid intake and high-sugar beverages should be minimized in the evening. One recommended regimen is for the AYAs to drink 40% of their total daily fluid before noon, 40% in the afternoon, and only 20% after 5 p.m.

Parent-Awakening Programs

This intervention has been shown to be effective with children. The parent awakens the child, but the child finds the bathroom alone. Parents need to awaken their child at the parent's bedtime each night until the child or adolescent awakens quickly to sound for seven consecutive nights. This intervention is not effective for AYAs due to low rates of adherence, as well as the fact that they often have more severe enuresis.

Active Therapy

Enuresis alarms and medications are components of active therapy. Both are more effective than simple behavioral treatments, but require the involvement of medical professionals. If nocturnal polyuria has been identified as the cause of the AYAs' enuresis, then starting with a medication is advisable as first-line treatment.

Alarm Systems

Enuresis alarms have the highest cure rate of any available treatment for enuresis in children and AYAs.[20,21] While several studies have shown comparable cure rates between medications and alarms in the short term, these same studies showed persistent effectiveness only with the alarm.[22–26] The adolescent or young adult has the choice of wearing either an audio or tactile alarm. Alarms are comfortable, convenient, and inexpensive. Their disadvantages are that they are time intensive and the adolescent or young adult and parent must be motivated to use them properly. Alarms are first-line treatment for AYAs whose enuresis has not responded to simple behavioral interventions and who have wetting episodes at least twice a week. By learning to awaken as quickly as possible to the alarm, the AYAs eventually learn to awaken or to inhibit bladder contraction to the internal stimulus of a full bladder. It is recommended to test whether an adolescent or young adult can respond to parent awakening or alarm clock awakening before initiating alarm systems, as they need to awaken to sound or touch in order for the alarm to be effective. The adolescent or young adult should be seen for follow-up by the medical practitioner within 1 to 2 weeks of initiating alarm therapy. Alarm treatment should be continued until the adolescent or young adult has a minimum of 14 consecutive dry nights. This typically takes between 12 and 16 weeks (range 5 to 24 weeks). If the adolescent or young adult relapses, alarm therapy can be instituted again, with a rapid secondary response due to preconditioning from initial use of the alarm.

Types: Newer alarms are lightweight, easy to use, and relatively inexpensive ($54 to $150). They consist of two clips attached to the teen's underwear and connected to a wrist alarm or pajama collar alarm. The alarm buzzes if a small amount of wetness occurs on the underwear.

If the adolescent or young adult cannot afford to buy an enuresis alarm, then a clock radio, alarm clock, or wristwatch alarm set for 3 hours after going to sleep can be used. Recent studies on enuresis in AYAs find that adherence to alarm therapy is low.[21,26]

Results: Long-term cure rates average 70% in children and AYAs. Common reasons for alarm failure include the following:

- Parents discontinue the alarm too soon.
- The adolescent or young adult fails to awaken to the alarm.
- The adolescent or young adult refuses to use the alarm.
- The adolescent or young adult refuses to try any technique.
- The adolescent or young adult suffers from NME (may need oxybutynin in addition to an alarm).
- The adolescent or young adult wets during deep sleep when it is difficult to awaken him (combined treatment with drugs may be necessary; once the adolescent or young adult is dry on medications, the alarm can be restarted and the medications tapered).

Medications

Medications have been found to be more effective than simple behavioral interventions used to treat enuresis.[21–23] Medications allow focused treatment of enuresis in certain cases. If nocturnal polyuria plays a significant role in an adolescent or young adult's enuresis, then desmopressin (DDAVP) should be used as first-line treatment, as it decreases overnight urine production.[21,22,27–29] If bladder overactivity is identified, oxybutynin should be used.[22] Intermittent use of drugs is also appropriate for AYAs when needed for camping trips, school trips, vacations, or sleepovers. The major drugs available include the following:

DDAVP: First-line treatment of enuresis for AYAs who have not responded to fluid restriction or reward systems, and are not willing to use an alarm, as well as those in whom nocturnal polyuria is identified.

- Action: DDAVP is a synthetic analog of vasopressin. The mechanism of action is reduction of urine production by increasing water retention and urine concentration in the distal tubules. Treatment of enuresis using DDAVP is based on the hypothesis that ADH secretion at night is insufficient.
- Dose: DDAVP is tasteless and odorless and administered orally. It is given in the late evening to reduce urine production during sleep. The initial dose is 0.2 mg (one tablet) given 1 hour before bedtime. If there is a suboptimal result after 10 to 14 days on this dose, then increase to 0.4 mg (maximum dose). Due to the risk of hyponatremic seizures with the use of intranasal DDAVP, the US Food and Drug Administration no longer recommends its use for the treatment of nocturnal enuresis.[22,30]

- Assess the response to DDAVP 1 to 2 weeks after starting the medication. If there is a response, then treat for 3 months. The AYAs and family can decide whether to use the medication daily or just use it for certain events (e.g., overnight camp, sleepovers). If DDAVP is going to be used for these events, it is recommended that the medication be started 6 weeks before the event, so that there is adequate time to titrate to the appropriate effective dose.
- Results: The response to DDAVP improves with increasing age in patients with nocturnal enuresis. Best results are seen in patients older than 10 years. A family history of nocturnal enuresis after age 10 years and a normal bladder capacity also predicts a positive response to DDAVP. Seventy percent of AYAs with nocturnal enuresis who receive DDAVP stop their bed-wetting completely or reduce it significantly (30% are complete responders to DDAVP and 40% are partial responders). A positive effect of the medication is seen within a few days and is maintained as long as the drug is administered. Most patients have a relapse after drug withdrawal, particularly if the drug is stopped abruptly (relapse rates can be as high as 50% to 95%). Therefore, the drug should be tapered slowly. Long-term treatment lasting at least 1 year has become more routine. Several long-term studies indicate that 50% to 85% of AYAs on long-term treatment halved the number of wet nights and 40% to 70% became almost completely dry during treatment. Tolerance to DDAVP has not been found. During long-term therapy, treatment-free windows of 1 week every 3 months are essential to avoid treating AYAs who have become dry.[22]
- Side effects: Side effects are infrequent but can include symptomatic hyponatremia (limit fluid intake to 8 ounces 1 hour before to 8 hours after DDAVP administration), headache, abdominal discomfort, nausea, nasal congestion, rhinitis, nosebleeds, abdominal cramps, and sore throats. These symptoms usually disappear with a reduction in the dose.

Imipramine (Tofranil)
- Action: This drug combines an anticholinergic effect that increases bladder capacity with a noradrenergic effect that decreases bladder detrusor excitability. Imipramine is also thought to increase excretion of ADH from the posterior portion of the pituitary gland and it decreases the amount of time spent in REM sleep. It is considered a third-line treatment option (behind alarm therapy and DDAVP therapy) and is recommended only for use in AYAs who do not respond to alarm therapy or for whom DDAVP therapy is too expensive.
- Dose: Imipramine is taken 1 hour before bedtime. The duration of action is 8 to 12 hours. Start the patient at 50 mg/day and increase the dose weekly, as needed, to a maximum of 75 mg/day. A sustained-release form of imipramine, Tofranil-PM, is also available.
- Results: This medication is not well studied in AYAs. The relapse rate is higher when the drug is stopped abruptly or prematurely. The maximal effect of imipramine usually occurs in the first week of therapy. However, one should continue therapy for 1 month before deciding on efficacy and whether to adjust the dose. If there is no response after 3 months of treatment, gradually discontinue the medication.[22] The current recommendation is to treat for 3 to 9 months and then taper the drug by decreasing the dose by 25 mg decrements over 3 to 4 weeks.[22] If the patient has a relapse, one can repeat a course of therapy. The drug is most beneficial for occasional use when dryness is necessary (e.g., trips, vacations, sleepover parties). An advantage of imipramine over DDAVP is that it is less expensive ($5 a month for generic formulas versus $150 to $250 per month for DDAVP). Tolerance rates to imipramine are high and it is advised that the AYAs take 2-week medication holidays every 3 months in order to decrease the risk of developing tolerance.

- Side effects: Nervousness, gastrointestinal distress, syncope, and anxiety can occur. Because of imipramine's lethality when taken in overdose, both parents and AYAs need to be aware of its toxicity. Given the potential risk of fatal cardiac arrhythmias, a baseline electrocardiograph is recommended in AYAs who have a history of heart palpitations or syncope and/or a family history of sudden cardiac death or unstable arrhythmia.

Oxybutynin (Ditropan)
- **Action**: Oxybutynin provides an anticholinergic, antispasmodic effect that reduces uninhibited detrusor muscle contractions and increases bladder capacity. It is most beneficial for AYAs with small capacity bladders and who also have daytime frequency or enuresis associated with uninhibited bladder contractions. Therefore, it is not a recommended treatment for AYAs with MNE.[27,31]
- Dosage: A sustained-release formulation of oxybutynin is available (10 mg/day), as well as a conventional formulation (5 mg twice daily).
- Results: A success rate of 90% was reported in one study of individuals with daytime enuresis, bladder instability, or both. The drug is rarely helpful in patients with MNE. It is to be used in AYAs with NME, urge syndrome, or neurogenic bladder. However, emerging research shows that using DDAVP plus an anticholinergic medication in the treatment of MNE results in a quicker and more effective response than DDAVP alone.[32]
- Side effects: Dry mouth, flushing, drowsiness, and constipation.
- Combined drug therapy with enuresis alarms: Combining DDAVP with an alarm can be an effective treatment in AYAs with frequent enuresis. The drug can both prevent the necessity of awakening to use the bathroom and delay the filling of the bladder until early morning. The enuresis alarm is the backup system. After the AYAs are dry for 3 weeks, the drug is tapered gradually. However, studies have shown that the positive effects of the combined therapy are due to the impact of DDAVP, as once the medication is discontinued, relapses were seen. Long-term effects were due to successful use of alarm therapy.[22–26]

Treatment Relapses and Failures

Treatment relapse is defined as the recurrence of enuresis after having been dry for at least 1 month. The remedy is to reinstitute the treatment that was effective previously. Treatment failure occurs when the patient cannot remain dry despite using the alarm or combined therapy. For AYAs, the best approach is to put the young person in charge of solving the problem and emphasize that they will become dry once they learn to self-awaken.

When to Refer to a Specialist

If a urologic lesion is discovered, referral to an urologist is recommended. If an occult spinal dysraphism is detected, then neurosurgical referral is warranted. If the adolescent or young adult is having nightly nocturnal enuresis, or previous interventions have not worked, referral to an urologist or a physician who specializes in enuresis is indicated. Young people with NME should be referred to a specialist.

REFERENCES

1. Yeung CK, Sreedhar B, Sihoe JDY, et al. Differences in characteristics of nocturnal enuresis between children and adolescents: a critical appraisal from a large epidemiologic study. *BJU Int* 2006;97(5):1069–1073.
2. Yeung CK, Sreihoe JDY, Sit FKY, et al. Characteristics of primary nocturnal enuresis in adults: an epidemiologic study. *BJU Int* 2004;93(3):341–345.
3. Yeung CK, Sihoe JDY, Sit FKY, et al. Urodynamic findings in adults with primary nocturnal enuresis. *J Urol* 2004;171:2595–2598.
4. Tu ND, Baskin LS, Arnhym AM. Etiology and evaluation of nocturnal enuresis in children. In: Basow DS, ed. *UpToDate*. Waltham, MA: UpToDate, 2014.
5. Kanbur N, Pinhas L, Lorenzo A, et al. Nocturnal enuresis in adolescents with anorexia nervosa: prevalence, potential causes, and pathophysiology. *Int J Eat Disord* 2011;44:349–355.
6. Neveus T, Von Gontard A, Hoebeke P, et al. The standardization of terminology of lower urinary tract function in children and adolescents: report from the

standardization committee of the International Children's Continence Society. *J Urol* 2006;176:314–324.

7. Nappo S, Del Gado R, Chiozza ML, et al. Nocturnal enuresis in the adolescent: a neglected problem *BJU Int* 2002;90:912–917.

8. Walle JV, Rittig S, Bauer S, et al. Practical consensus guidelines for the management of enuresis. *Eur J Pediatr* 2012;171:971–983.

9. Esposito M, Gallai B, Parisi L, et al. Primary nocturnal enuresis as a risk factor for sleep disorders: an observational questionnaire-based multicenter study. *Neuropsychiatr Dis Treat* 2013;9:437–443.

10. Cohen-Zrubavel V, Kushnir B, Kushnir J, et al. Sleep and sleepiness in children with nocturnal enuresis. *Sleep* 2011;34(2):191–194.

11. Von Gontard A, Freitag CM, Seifen S, et al. Neuromotor development in nocturnal enuresis. *Dev Med Child Neurol* 2006;48:744–750.

12. Von Gontard A, Heron J, Joinson C. Family history of nocturnal enuresis and urinary incontinence: results from a large epidemiological study. *J Urol* 2011;185:2303–2307.

13. Arnell H, Hjalmas K, Jägervall M, et al. The genetics of primary nocturnal enuresis: inheritance and suggestion of a second major gene on chromosome 12q. *J Med Genet* 1997;34:360–365.

14. Von Gontard A, Schaumburg H, Hollmann E, et al. The genetics of enuresis: a review. *J Urol* 2001;166:2438–2443.

15. Rittig S, Schaumburg HL, Siggaard FS, et al The circadian defect in plasma vasopressin and urine output is related to desmopressin response and enuresis status in children with nocturnal enuresis. *J Urol* 2007;179:2389–2395.

16. Kawauchi A, Tanaka Y, Naito Y, et al. Bladder capacity at the time of enuresis. *Urol* 2003;61:1016–1018.

17. Hagstroem S, Kamperis K, Rittig S, et al. Bladder reservoir function in children with mononsymptomatic nocturnal enuresis and healthy controls. *J Urol* 2006;176:759–763.

18. Barnes TRE, Drake MJ, Paton C. Nocturnal enuresis with antipsychotic medication. *Br J Psychiatry* 2012;200:7–9.

19. Von Gontard A, Equit M. Comorbidity of ADHD and incontinence in children. *Eur Child Adolesc Psychiatry* 2015;24(2):127–140.

20. Caldwell PHY, Nankivell G, Sureshkumar P. Simple behavioral interventions for nocturnal enuresis in children. *Cochrane Database Syst Rev* 2013;19(7):CD003637.

21. Kalyanakrishnan R. Evaluation and treatment of enuresis. *Am Fam Phys* 2008;78(4):489–496.

22. Tu ND, Baskin LS. Management of nocturnal enuresis in children. In: Basow DS, ed. *UpToDate*. Waltham, MA: UpToDate, 2014.

23. Ozden C, Ozdal OL, Aktas BK, et al. The efficacy of the addition of short-term desmopressin to alarm therapy in the treatment of primary nocturnal enuresis. *Int Urol Nephrol* 2008;40:583–586.

24. Ahmed AF, Amin MM, Ali MM, et al. Efficacy of an enuresis alarm, desmopressin, and combination therapy in the treatment of Saudi children with primary monosymptomatic nocturnal enuresis. *Korean J Urol* 2013;54(11):783–790.

25. Robson WLM. Evaluation and management of enuresis. *N Engl J Med* 2009;360:1429–36.

26. Perrin N, Sayer L, While A. The efficacy of alarm therapy versus desmopressin therapy in the treatment of mono-symptomatic nocturnal enuresis: a systematic review. *Prim Health Care Res Dev* 2013;19:1–11.

27. Brown ML, Pope AW, Brown EJ. Treatment of primary nocturnal enuresis in children: a review. *Child Care Health Dev* 2011;37(2):153–160.

28. Lottmann HB, Alova I. Primary monosymptomatic nocturnal enuresis in children and adolescents. *Int J Clin Pract Suppl* 2007;155:8–16.

29. Shapiro E. Pediatric urology. Publications from the International Children's Continence Society. *Rev Urol* 2010;12(4):e202–e204.

30. Robson WLM, Leung AKC, Norgaard JP. The comparative safety of oral versus intranasal desmopressin for the treatment of children with nocturnal enuresis. *J Urol* 2007;178(1):24–30.

31. Neveus T, Eggert P, Evans J, et al. Evaluation of and treatment for monosymptomatic enuresis: a standardization document from the International Children's Continence Society. *J Urol* 2010;183(2):441–447.

32. Park SJ, Park JM, Pai KS, et al. Desmopressin alone versus desmopressin plus an anticholinergic in the first line treatment of primary monosymptomatic nocturnal enuresis: a multicenter study. *Pediatr Nephrol* 2014;29:1195–1200.

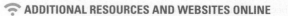 **ADDITIONAL RESOURCES AND WEBSITES ONLINE**

28 Asymptomatic Proteinuria and Hematuria

Shamir Tuchman
Lawrence J. D'Angelo

ASYMPTOMATIC PROTEINURIA

Asymptomatic proteinuria is defined as proteinuria not associated with hematuria, hypertension, or other symptoms of renal insufficiency. Proteinuria is a common finding during adolescence and young adulthood; however, it is most often transient and benign. Persistent asymptomatic proteinuria may be an early marker of chronic kidney disease (CKD). Routine urinary screening for proteinuria in adolescents and young adults (AYAs) is not recommended by either the American Academy of Pediatrics or the United States Preventative Service Task Force because 10% to 20% of AYAs will have proteinuria on routine urinalysis, but only 0.1% will have persistent proteinuria. Still, urinalyses are commonly performed during adolescence and young adulthood. The challenge for the clinician is to establish the significance of the proteinuria, exclude underlying treatable conditions, and identify the few individuals who need more extensive evaluation.

Pathophysiology

Indexed to body surface area, normal urine protein excretion in AYAs is less than 100 mg/m^2/day (approximately 4 mg/m^2/hour). Levels of proteinuria up to 250 mg/day may be normal in larger AYAs. Nephrotic range proteinuria is defined as protein excretion of ≥2,000 mg/m^2/day. Proteinuria may be quantified in two ways: (1) via a 24-hour sample (a cumbersome approach requiring the collection of all urine for 24 hours); or (2) by obtaining a spot urine protein-to-creatinine (Up/c) ratio (mg protein per mg creatinine). The latter provides a good approximation of the 24-hour excretion of protein in grams per day. The "second voided urine" is the most ideal specimen for this approach. It correlates well with the 24-hour urine protein excretion.[1,2] Proteinuria may occur as the results of four different mechanisms (**Table 28.1**), including:

1. *Increased permeability of the glomerular filtration membrane for mid- to high-molecular-weight proteins.* Larger and more negatively charged plasma proteins (e.g., albumin) are not appreciably filtered. However, proteinuria can occur when the permeability of the membrane changes.

2. *Changes in tubular reabsorption of low-molecular-weight (LMW) proteins.* Due to their smaller size, LMW proteins <25,000 Da are freely filtered at the glomerulus and almost completely reabsorbed in the proximal tubule. Any condition, whether acquired or congenital, that causes proximal tubular dysfunction can lead to LMW proteinuria.

3. *Increased production of plasma proteins (e.g., overflow proteinuria).* Patients with monoclonal gammopathies (e.g., multiple myeloma) may develop proteinuria due to the excessive production of immunoglobulins, which may overwhelm

TABLE 28.1

Mechanisms of Proteinuria

Category	Example
Factitious proteinuria	Highly concentrated urine Gross hematuria Contamination with antiseptic (chlorhexidine or benzalkonium) Highly alkaline urine Radiographic contrast media (affects specific gravity) High levels of cephalosporin/penicillin analogs Sulfonamide metabolites
Transient proteinuria	Benign positional proteinuria Transient proteinuria associated with exercise, stress, fever Urinary tract infection

Fixed proteinuria	Glomerular
	  Hyperfiltration
	    Diabetic nephropathy
	    Renal dysplasia, hypoplasia
	    Reflux nephropathy
	  Primary glomerulopathies
	    FSGS
	    Nail–patella syndrome
	    Fabry disease
	    Systemic disease(s): SLE
	Tubulopathies
	  Acquired
	    Nephrotoxic medications (antibiotics, nonsteroidal anti-inflammatory drugs)
	    Heavy metal poisonings (lead, mercury)
	  Inherited/genetic
	    Dent disease
	    Wilson disease
	    Genetic disorders associated with Fanconi syndrome

Overflow proteinuria	Monoclonal gammopathies (multiple myeloma)

the glomerular filtration membrane. These may not be detected by urine dipstick but can be diagnosed by urine protein electrophoresis.

4. *Functional proteinuria (e.g., fever, exercise, congestive heart failure) and orthostatic proteinuria due to changes in glomerular pressure and filtration.*

Epidemiology

Up to 10% to 20% of healthy AYAs may have proteinuria detected on a random urine sample.[2,3] The prevalence falls significantly with repeated testing, so a diagnosis of persistent proteinuria should be based on three separate urine specimens. In a study of 20-year old men, the prevalence of persistent proteinuria was 0.13%.[4]

Causes of Asymptomatic Proteinuria

The causes of asymptomatic proteinuria range from those that are known to be benign to those associated with significant renal disease. Significant renal disease is often suggested by the degree of proteinuria and the presence of associated findings like hypertension, hematuria, and/or elevated creatinine. Causes of asymptomatic proteinuria include the following:

Transient Proteinuria

Low-level proteinuria (<500 mg/m^2/day) may occur in the setting of recent exercise, stress, fever, dehydration, and urinary tract infection. Transient proteinuria has been reported in up to 12% of AYAs.[3] It is not associated with long-term renal morbidity.

Postural Proteinuria (Orthostatic or Benign Positional Proteinuria)

Postural proteinuria is a condition in which low- to moderate-level proteinuria develops in the standing or upright position and disappears in the recumbent position. It is found in up to 20% of school-age children, occurring more commonly in the second decade of life. Postural proteinuria is slightly more common in males.[2] It often resolves by young adulthood and is rarely associated with long-term renal disease. The diagnosis of postural proteinuria is confirmed when a random urine specimen is positive for protein and a first morning urine specimen is negative to trace for proteinuria. Patients with postural proteinuria may have up to 1,000 mg of protein in a 24-hour sample. Although a benign condition, postural proteinuria can rarely become fixed proteinuria signaling the presence of true renal disease; therefore, AYAs with postural proteinuria should have first morning urinalyses checked at regular intervals (i.e., well-child visits) to evaluate for the presence of fixed proteinuria.

Fixed Isolated Proteinuria

Persistent proteinuria that occurs in the absence of microscopic or gross hematuria may be due to glomerular and nonglomerular causes.

Glomerular Causes

Hyperfiltration Renal Injury: An important risk factor for progressive CKD, hyperfiltration occurs with excessive filtration through remaining functioning nephrons to maintain the glomerular filtration rate (GFR). This mechanism is important in *diabetic* and *reflux nephropathies* and *renal dysplasia.*

Glomerulopathies: Isolated fixed proteinuria may be due to primary glomerular diseases. An important example of this is focal segmental glomerulosclerosis (FSGS). FSGS can occur as a primary or secondary disease. Primary FSGS can be further subdivided into idiopathic disease or familial (monogenetic) forms. FSGS may present with a spectrum of disease ranging from asymptomatic moderate-level (500 to 2,000 mg/day) proteinuria to symptomatic disease with frank nephrosis. It carries a worrisome long-term prognosis with a significant proportion of patients progressing to end-stage renal disease (ESRD). Glomerulopathies that classically present with nephrosis such as minimal change disease (MCNS) or membranous nephropathy are rarely asymptomatic.

Systemic Disease: Proteinuria manifesting as albuminuria may be a renal manifestation of systemic disorders. Renal involvement occurs in about two-thirds of patients with systemic lupus erythematosus (SLE).[5] In those with isolated low-level proteinuria, this may be a sign of mild glomerular disease. However, in patients with nephrotic range proteinuria, this likely represents membranous disease. There is growing evidence that onset of SLE during adolescence and young adulthood is associated with more severe renal disease at presentation.[6]

Monogenetic Disorders: There are a group of rare genetic disorders associated with the occurrence of moderate to nephrotic range proteinuria that present in adolescence. One example is Fabry disease, which is associated with low- to moderate-level proteinuria in addition to other diverse manifestations of the disease.

Tubular Causes

Tubulointerstitial renal disease: Freely filtered LMW proteins are exclusively reabsorbed in the proximal tubule. As such, diseases causing generalized proximal tubular dysfunction may lead to low- to moderate-grade proteinuria called renal Fanconi syndrome. Fanconi syndrome may manifest secondary to (1) monogenetic disorders such as cystinosis, tyrisonemia, Wilson disease, Dent disease, or other inborn errors of metabolism or (2) an acquired condition due to reaction to penicillamine, aminoglycosides, heavy metals (mercury or lead), tenofovir, or other medication.

Overflow Causes

Conditions causing overflow proteinuria include myoglobinuria, hemoglobinuria, and multiple myeloma. These conditions are associated with overproduction of LMW proteins that can either overwhelm the reabsorptive capacity of the proximal tubule or cause damage to the filtration membrane or renal tubules directly. Myoglobinuria and hemoglobinuria are usually transient and multiple myeloma is rare.

Diagnostic Approach

The urine dipstick test is the most common qualitative test for protein in the urine. Urine dipsticks contain tetrabromophenol blue, which undergoes a colorimetric reaction in the presence of proteins with abundant amino acid groups (most commonly, albumin). The result is different shades of color corresponding to the concentration of the reacting proteins. The qualitative urine dipstick does not detect the presence of globulins, Bence Jones proteins, or LMW proteins.

When the urine dipstick test is positive for protein (1+ to 4+), the following diagnostic approach may be used to isolate the etiology.

1. Rule out a false-positive test—A false-positive test is more likely when any of these conditions are present: Alkaline urine (pH > 7.5), high urine specific gravity (≥ 1.025), exposure to iodinated contrast, or use of chlorhexadine antiseptic. If any are present, the test should be repeated.
2. Confirm true proteinuria by adding sulfosalicylic acid to urine or quantifying the Up/c ratio.
3. Repeat test on a second urine sample within one week to evaluate for persistence of proteinuria.
4. Compare a first morning Up/c ratio with that from a random urine specimen to evaluate for postural proteinuria.
5. If proteinuria is persistent, obtain a renal function panel (serum creatinine, sodium, potassium, chloride, bicarbonate, and phosphorus) to evaluate for abnormalities.
6. If proteinuria is persistent, obtain a renal ultrasound to evaluate for structural renal disease.
7. If a renal ultrasound fails to reveal structural renal disease, obtain tests to help diagnose systemic illness such as SLE as suggested by history and physical examination.

8. If the Up/c ratio is >2, obtain a serum albumin and total cholesterol to confirm the presence of hypoalbuminemia and hypercholesterolemia, consistent with nephrotic syndrome.

9. If signs of renal tubulopathy are present such as glucosuria, acidosis, and/or hypophosphatemia, obtain a urinary retinol binding protein (a marker of LMW proteinuria).

10. Consider a renal biopsy. While indications for performing a renal biopsy in asymptomatic proteinuria are not standardized, most pediatric nephrologists recommend obtaining a renal biopsy in asymptomatic adolescent patients with fixed proteinuria exceeding 1,000 mg/day (e.g., Up/c **ratio ≥ 1.0**). In general, the prognosis for asymptomatic orthostatic or persistent proteinuria of <500/day is good[7] and the yield of finding significant disease on renal biopsy is negligible. In patients with abnormal renal function and/or hypertension, lower levels of proteinuria should prompt consideration of renal biopsy.

In AYAs with nephrotic range proteinuria, the decision to proceed with a renal biopsy prior to a trial of corticosteroids hinges on the pre-biopsy probability of diagnosing FSGS versus MCNS. FSGS is likely to be resistant to treatment with corticosteroids. In adolescents between the ages of 12 and 18 years, FSGS has been found in approximately 23% of patients undergoing renal biopsy.[8] FSGS is also more likely to be the cause of nephrotic syndrome in Black adolescents. Therefore, a renal biopsy should be considered early in the evaluation of older adolescents or younger Black adolescents.

Prognosis

In general, isolated low-grade proteinuria (<500 mg/m²) is not associated with severe glomerular pathology. For proteinuria associated with clinical symptom or other urinary/laboratory findings, the prognosis depends on the underlying pathology. Even low-level microalbuminuria is a risk factor for renal complications in youth with hypertension, glomerulopathies associated with hematuria, and diabetes mellitus.[9]

HEMATURIA

Hematuria is defined as the presence of red blood cells (RBCs) in the urine. Screening for hematuria can be done with conventional urine dipsticks. The urine dipstick is able to detect one to five RBCs per high-powered field in urine, making this test very sensitive (>90%). Similarly, a negative urine dipstick test effectively excludes hematuria with a specificity approaching 99%. False-negative results for hematuria are rare but may occur in the presence of oxalates, pH < 5.1, or ascorbic acid (vitamin C). False-positive results may occur in the presence of hemoglobin, myoglobin, or semen.[10] Hemoglobinuria may develop from lysis of RBCs in the urine or from hemoglobin filtered due to intravascular hemolysis. As a result, true hematuria can only be confirmed by the presence of RBCs in spun urine sediment.

Epidemiology

In AYAs, the prevalence of hematuria is approximately 4.6%.[11] On a repeated urinalysis, the prevalence decreases to 1%.

Pathophysiology

Hematuria may be of glomerular or nonglomerular origin. Symptoms, laboratory tests, and direct urine microscopy often help the clinician determine the cause. Glomerular hematuria may be due to active glomerular inflammation (e.g., glomerulonephritis) or inherited abnormalities of the glomerular filtration membrane. The characteristic finding of glomerular hematuria on urine microscopy is the presence of dysmorphic RBCs with or without RBC casts. RBC casts form when RBCs are allowed to pass through the glomerulus and become obstructed in the tubular lumen, creating a mold of the lumen that is eventually flushed into the bladder.

Glomerular hematuria is often accompanied by proteinuria, hypertension, and/or abnormal renal function.

When hematuria is nonglomerular, the presence of symptoms may suggest the source of bleeding. Processes that cause distention of the renal capsule or irritation of the urothelium (lining of the urinary collecting system) may cause back, flank, abdominal, or pelvic pain depending on the site of injury. In contrast, bleeding within the renal parenchyma may be asymptomatic. In addition to pain, lower urinary tract bleeding may be suggested by the presence of dysuria, nausea, urinary frequency and/or urgency, or the presence of clots in the urine.

Differential Diagnosis

A systematic approach to evaluate hematuria includes determining whether the bleeding is glomerular or nonglomerular. If glomerular hematuria is thought to be present, the differential diagnosis may include both primary structural abnormalities and acquired inflammatory diseases. Table 28.2 summarizes the most commonly encountered diagnoses.

Diagnostic Approach

The initial approach to the adolescent or young adult with gross hematuria is summarized below:

1. Ensure that the urine is not being discolored by other pigments by microscopic exam for RBCs. Causes of pigmenturia may be endogenous (porphyrinuria, hemoglobinuria, myoglobinuria) or exogenous (foods and drugs).

2. Confirm that the hematuria is from the kidneys or urinary tract and not from other sources. False hematuria can be caused by vaginal bleeding or factitious hematuria.

3. If a glomerular source of hematuria is confirmed (by the presence of dysmorphic RBCs and/or RBC casts), obtain a renal function panel to assess the GFR and electrolytes, as well as serum complement levels C3 and C4 to narrow the differential.

4. If possible, obtain a urinalysis of parents and siblings to screen for a familial glomerulopathy.

5. In cases of significant proteinuria, a Up/c ratio and serum albumin will determine whether a nephritic/nephrotic syndrome is present.

6. If nonglomerular hematuria is present, further evaluation of potential etiologies is directed by the history, symptoms, associated comorbid conditions, and findings on microscopy.

7. Renal ultrasound is of limited diagnostic utility when a glomerular origin is suspected. Patients with active glomerulonephritis may have increased cortical echogenicity labeled as "medical renal disease." In contrast, a renal ultrasound should be obtained in the evaluation of nonglomerular gross hematuria to identify renal/bladder tumors, renal cysts, renal calculi, or hydronephrosis. Additional imaging, like computed tomography, should be reserved for evaluating renal trauma, nephrolithiasis, or to further delineate renal lesions seen on ultrasound.

8. In nonglomerular hematuria without an identified cause, a urine calcium-to-creatinine ratio should be obtained to evaluate for hypercalciuria (ratio ≥ 0.22). Hypercalciuria is one of the most common risk factors for the development of kidney stones. It is the most common metabolic abnormality identified in AYAs with kidney stones, being present in up to 42% of patients.[12]

9. In AYAs with African ancestry who present with gross hematuria of unclear etiology, consider screening for the presence of sickle cell trait with hemoglobin electrophoresis.

10. A kidney biopsy is usually not indicated for AYAs with asymptomatic hematuria. Renal biopsy may be indicated, when suspected glomerular hematuria occurs with hypertension, abnormal GFR, and/or proteinuria >1,000 mg/day, as these signs/symptoms are suggestive of more severe glomerular disease.

TABLE 28.2
Causes of Hematuria

Category	Example
Glomerular hematuria	
• Primary Glomerulopathies:	Alport syndrome Thin Basement Membrane (TBM) disease
• Acquired Glomerulopathies:	
Hypocomplementemic Glomerulonephritis	Post-infections glomerulonephritis (PIGN) Membranoproliferative glomerulonephritis (MPGN) Lupus Nephritis (SLE) Glomerulonephritis associated with chronic bacteremia Typical or atypical hemolytic uremic syndrome (HUS)
Normocomplementemic Glomerulonephritis	IgA Nephropathy Henoch-Schönlein purpura (HSP) Mesangioproliferative glomerulonephritis Anti-neutrophil cytoplasmic antibody-positive vasculitis Anti-glomerular basement membrane disease (anti-GBM)
Nonglomerular hematuria	
• Structural parenchymal disease	
Cystic renal disease	Isolated renal cysts Autosomal-dominant polycystic kidney disease (ADPKD) Cystic renal disease in Tuberous sclerosis (TS)
Noncystic renal disease	Medullary-sponge kidney with nephrocalcinosis/nephrolithiasis
• Renal parenchymal tumors	Renal cell carcinoma Renal medullary carcinoma (esp. sickle cell disease/trait) Angiomyolipomas in the context of Tuberous sclerosis (TS)
• Renal tubular hematuria	Acute papillary necrosis (sickle cell, diabetes, analgesic abuse) Sickle cell trait associated hematuria
• Renal trauma	Contusion, lacerations, disruption (inc. risk in enlarged kidneys)
• Vascular disease	Malignant hypertension AV malformations Renal arterial thrombi/Renal vein thrombosis
• Urothelial bleeding	
Structural/functional	Ureteropelvic junction (UPJ) obstruction Urethragia (predominantly males) Athlete's (runner's) hematuria Loin-pain hematuria syndrome
Inflammatory/ infectious	Acute cystitis/pyelonephritis BK-virus associated nephropathy (immunocompromised) Urethritis Prostatitis
Irritative	Nephrolithiasis Hypercalciuria Bladder tumors Hemorrhagic cystitis (cyclophosphamide exposure)
Coagulopathic (rare presentation)	Thrombocytopenia Congenital (hemophilia) or acquired (meds) coagulation defects

Specific Conditions
Marathon Runner's (Athlete's) Hematuria

Gross or microscopic hematuria is associated with many forms of vigorous exercise.[13] The typical history is one of normal urine prior to exercise and hematuria on the first specimen voided after exercise. This may last 24 to 48 hours, possibly in association with dysuria and suprapubic discomfort. The hematuria may be caused by a decrease in renal plasma flow, local bladder trauma, or leakage of blood from spiral vessels in the adventitia of minor calyces. The prognosis is benign.

Loin Pain-Hematuria Syndrome

This rare, poorly understood condition is characterized by recurrent bouts of gross or microscopic hematuria associated with unilateral or bilateral flank/abdominal pain. The pain may radiate to the pelvis and groin and can be severe and chronic. Examination of the urine reveals what appears to be glomerular hematuria with dysmorphic RBCs and/or RBC casts.[14] Loin pain-hematuria syndrome occurs primarily in women (70% of the diagnoses). Blood pressure and renal function are normal. The associated pain may be difficult to control, requiring consultation with specialists in pain medicine.

IgA Nephropathy (Berger Disease)

IgA nephropathy is a relatively common cause of gross hematuria in young adults. Eighty percent of patients are between 16 and 35 years old. The male-to-female ratio is 2:1 in North America. IgA nephropathy occurs more commonly in Asian and White youth.[15] The disease is commonly characterized by recurrent bouts of hematuria (usually gross) occurring shortly after infections. Urinary protein excretion varies from normal to nephrotic range. The decision to proceed with renal biopsy often hinges on the level of proteinuria. Renal function is usually normal at presentation, but up to 50% of individuals will progress to renal insufficiency.[16] Poor prognostic signs include hypertension, renal insufficiency, and persistent proteinuria (protein excretion >1 g/day). The diagnosis can only be made by renal biopsy. Henoch–Schönlein purpura can cause renal glomerular lesions that are indistinguishable from IgA nephropathy.

Hereditary Nephritis (Alport Syndrome)

Alport syndrome can be inherited as an X-linked (typically), autosomal-dominant, or autosomal-recessive condition. It is caused by mutations in the alpha-5 chain on type IV collagen, which explains both its renal and extrarenal manifestations. Alport syndrome is usually more severe in males and may present with a spectrum of clinical disease. Alport syndrome leads to ESRD in most males by the third to fourth decades of life.[17] In addition to hematuria, up to 85% of males have associated sensineuronal hearing loss.[18] Ocular manifestations, including anterior lenticonus and retinal abnormalities, occur in 20% to 30% of affected males.

Thin Basement Membrane Disease

Thin basement membrane disease (TBM) is characterized by glomerular hematuria (RBC casts) and normal renal function. TBM is inherited as an autosomal-dominant disease due to mutations in either the alpha-3 or alpha-4 chains of type IV collagen. Renal biopsy reveals diffuse thinning of the glomerular basement membrane. TBM affects approximately 1% of the population.[19] TBM is now known to lead to progressive CKD in a minority of patients, necessitating regular screening for the development of proteinuria, hypertension, and abnormal GFR.

REFERENCES

1. Leung YY, Szeto CC, Tam LS, et al. Urine protein-to-creatinine ratio in an untimed urine collection is a reliable measure of proteinuria in lupus nephritis. *Rheumatology* 2007;46(4):649–652.
2. Brandt JR, Jacoby A, Raissy HH, et al. Orthostatic proteinuria and the spectrum of diurnal variability of urinary protein excretion in healthy children. *Pediatr Nephrol* 2010;25(6):1131–1137.

3. Park YH, Choi JY, Chung HS, et al. Hematuria and proteinuria in a mass school urine screening test. *Pediatr Nephrol* 2005;20:1126–1130.

4. von Bonsdorff M, Koskenvuo K, Salmi HA, et al. Prevalence and causes of proteinuria in 20-year-old Finnish men. *Scand J Urol Nephrol* 1981;15(3):285–290.

5. Barsalou J, Levy DM, Silverman ED. An update on childhood-onset systemic lupus erythematosus. *Curr Opin Rheumatol* 2013;25(5):616–622.

6. Amaral B, Murphy G, Ioannou Y, et al. A comparison of the outcome of adolescent and adult-onset systemic lupus erythematosus. *Rheumatology (Oxford)* 2014;53(6):1130–1135.

7. Baskin AM, Freedman LR, Davis JS, et al. Proteinuria in Yale students and 30-year mortality experience. *J Urol* 1972;108:617.

8. Requião-Moura LR, Veras de S Freitas T, Franco MF, et al. Should adolescents with glomerulopathies be treated as children or adults? *Nephron Clin Pract* 2008;109(3):c161–c167.

9. Assadi FK. Value of urinary excretion of microalbumin in predicting glomerular lesions in children with isolated microscopic hematuria. *Pediatr Nephrol* 2005;20:1131.

10. Rao PK, Jones JS. How to evaluate 'dipstick hematuria': what to do before you refer. *Cleve Clin J Med* 2008;75(3):227–233.

11. Ferris M, Hogan SL, Chin H, et al. Obesity, albuminuria, and urinalysis findings in US young adults from the Add Health Wave III study. *Clin J Am Soc Nephrol* 2007;2(6):1207–1214.

12. Spivacow FR, Negri AL, del Valle EE, et al. Clinical and metabolic risk factor evaluation in young adults with kidney stones. *Int Urol Nephrol* 2010;42(2):471–475.

13. Van Biervliet S, Van Biervliet JP, Watteyne K, et al. Pseudonephritis is associated with high urinary osmolality and high specific gravity in adolescent soccer players. *Pediatr Exerc Sci* 2013;25(3):360–369.

14. Spetie DN, Nadasdy T, Nadasdy G, et al. Proposed pathogenesis of idiopathic loin pain-hematuria syndrome. *Am J Kidney Dis* 2006;47(3):419–427.

15. Hogg RJ. Idiopathic immunoglobulin A nephropathy in children and adolescents. *Pediatr Nephrol* 2010;25(5):823–829.

16. Berthoux FC, Mohey H, Afiani A. Natural history of primary IgA nephropathy. *Semin Nephrol* 2008;28(1):4–9.

17. Bekheirnia MR, Reed B, Gregory MC, et al. Genotype-phenotype correlation in X-linked Alport syndrome. *J Am Soc Nephrol* 2010;21(5):876–883.

18. Izzedine H, Tankere F, Launay-Vacher V, et al. Ear and kidney syndromes: molecular versus clinical approach. *Kidney Int* 2004;65(2):369–385.

19. Tryggvason K, Patrakka J. Thin basement membrane nephropathy. *J Am Soc Nephrol* 2006;17(3):813–822.

🛜 **ADDITIONAL RESOURCES AND WEBSITES ONLINE**

PART VIII

Infectious Diseases

29 Mononucleosis and Other Infectious Respiratory Illnesses

Terrill D. Bravender

INFECTIOUS MONONUCLEOSIS

Infectious mononucleosis (IM) is common in adolescents and young adults (AYAs). Usually, IM is an acute, self-limited, and benign lymphoproliferative disease caused by the Epstein–Barr virus (EBV). Although EBV is responsible for approximately 90% of cases, IM may also be caused by other infectious agents such as cytomegalovirus (CMV), toxoplasmosis, human herpes virus 6, and adenovirus.[1]

Etiology and Pathophysiology

EBV is a fragile, enveloped DNA herpes virus that cannot survive long outside of a host. Transmission occurs primarily through exposure to oropharyngeal secretions (hence its reputation as "the kissing disease"). EBV initially infects oral epithelial cells, then B lymphocytes, which spread the infection throughout the lymphoreticular system. There is a polyclonal B-cell proliferation with a significant T-cell response. The atypical white blood cells (WBCs) that are frequently seen on peripheral blood smears are mainly CD8 cytotoxic or suppressor cells. The immune response accounts for many of the clinical manifestations of IM such as lymphadenopathy and hepatosplenomegaly. Although a large number of B lymphocytes are infected, these are initially resting memory cells, which do not proliferate and thus have no oncogenic potential. For 3 to 4 months following acute infection, the number of infected cells decreases, but some infected cells continue to circulate indefinitely. Individuals remain infected for life, and 60% to 100% of seropositive, asymptomatic individuals intermittently shed EBV in an unpredictable fashion. EBV is present in the oropharyngeal secretions of up to 20% of asymptomatic adults. Over time, EBV infection of B cells may lead to cell transformation and establishment of lymphoblastoid cell lines. Such transformation occurs rapidly in vitro; in vivo, host immunity plays a critical role in containing the latent infection. Although multiple strains of EBV exist, it appears that a single episode of IM confers lifelong immunity, likely because the majority of patients are infected with multiple strains at the same time.

Epidemiology

Over 90% of adults have serologic evidence of past EBV infection. The highest rates of acute infection in the US are in older AYAs, particularly those living in close proximity to one another, such as in college or the military.

Age

Between 30% and 40% of AYAs who contract EBV will develop the symptoms of IM. About half of children have contracted EBV prior to age 5, when the infection is usually asymptomatic. Over 90% of adults have evidence of past infection. In the US, the annual incidence of IM for those between age 15 and 19 is 345 to 671 cases per 100,000 person-years. In contrast, the incidence for individuals aged 35 and older is only 2 to 4 cases per 100,000 person-years.

Gender

There are no gender differences in prevalence.

Race

In the US, IM is more prevalent among Whites than Blacks, likely reflecting earlier acquisition of EBV in Black children.

Season

There is no seasonal variation.

Household Contacts

An infected individual will transmit EBV to about half of susceptible household contacts. Exposure to an individual with acute infection may induce increased asymptomatic viral shedding in seropositive contacts.

Clinical Manifestations

The majority of EBV infections are either asymptomatic or associated with mild, nonspecific symptoms such as malaise, fever and chills, and anorexia. In those who develop IM, there is an incubation period of 4 to 7 weeks, after which there may be a 3- to 5-day prodrome of malaise, fatigue, headaches, anorexia, and myalgias. The traditional triad of IM includes the following:

1. Fever, lymphadenopathy, and pharyngitis
2. Lymphocytosis with atypical lymphocytes
3. Antibody response demonstrated by the presence of heterophile or EBV-specific antibodies

Signs and Symptoms

The common presentation includes fever, which may persist for several weeks, and sore throat, which can be severe and is associated with an exudative pharyngitis in up to 50% of individuals. Adenopathy is usually significant and is usually symmetrical, with posterior cervical lymph nodes more prominent than anterior. Splenomegaly and hepatomegaly may occur by the second week of the illness. Approximately 10% of individuals have a rash that may take on a number of different appearances—erythematous, maculopapular, morbilliform, urticarial, or erythema multiforme. Signs and symptoms are summarized in **Table 29.1**. Approximately

TABLE 29.1

Symptoms and Signs of Infectious Mononucleosis

Symptoms	Prevalence (%)
Sore throat	70–80
Malaise	50–90
Anorexia	50–80
Nausea	50–70
Headache	40–70
Myalgia	12–30
Cough	5–15
Abdominal pain	2–14
Arthralgia	5–10
Photophobia	5–10

Signs	Prevalence (%)
Lymphadenopathy	93–100
Fever	80–100
Tonsillopharyngitis	69–91
Palpable splenomegaly	11–60
Hepatomegaly	10–25
Palatal petechiae	25–35
Periorbital edema	25–35
Liver or splenic tenderness	15–30
Jaundice	5–10
Rash (usually maculopapular)	3–15[a]
Pneumonitis	<3

[a]Risk of rash is higher if exposed to ampicillin or amoxicillin.

TABLE 29.2

Potential Complications of Infectious Mononucleosis

Complication	Prevalence
Neurological:	<1%
Seizures	
Facial or peripheral nerve palsies	
Meningoencephalitis	
Aseptic meningitis	
Optic neuritis	
Reye syndrome	
Coma	
Brachial plexus neuropathy	
Transverse myelitis	
Guillain–Barré syndrome	
Acute psychosis	
Acute cerebellar ataxia	
"Alice in Wonderland" syndrome	
Hematological:	
Autoimmune hemolytic anemia (mild)	0.5%–3%
Thrombocytopenia purpura	Rare
Coagulopathy	Rare
Aplastic anemia	Rare
Hemolytic-uremic syndrome	Rare
Eosinophilia	Rare
Profound thrombocytopenia	Rare (Mild thrombocytopenia is common.)
Cardiac:	1.7%–6%
Pericarditis	
Myocarditis	
Electrocardiogram changes (nonspecific ST and T-wave abnormalities)	
Splenic rupture	0.1%–0.2%
Pulmonary:	
Airway obstruction	Rare (more common in young children)
Pneumonitis	Rare
Pleural effusions	Rare
Pulmonary hemorrhage	Rare
Gastrointestinal:	
Mild elevation of hepatocellular enzymes	80%–90%
Pancreatitis	Rare
Hepatitis with liver necrosis	Rare
Malabsorption	Rare
Dermatological:	3%–10%
Dermatitis	
Urticarial rash (may be cold-induced)	
Erythema multiforme	
Renal:	
Glomerulonephritis	Rare
Nephrotic syndrome	Rare
Mild hematuria or proteinuria	Up to 13%
Ophthalmological:	Rare
Conjunctivitis	
Episcleritis	
uveitis	
Other:	Uncommon
Bullous myringitis	
Orchitis	
Genital ulcerations	
Parotitis	
Monoarticular arthritis	

90% of patients who receive ampicillin or amoxicillin will develop an erythematous, maculopapular rash that typically appears about one week after starting antibiotics. Although the exact mechanism for the development of this rash is unknown, it appears that a true drug sensitization does occur in these patients. Whether this sensitization persists following resolution of IM is unknown.

Complications

Complications of IM are summarized in **Table 29.2**. Overall, the complication rate of IM is approximately 1% to 2%. Occasionally, patients will present with a major complication as their only manifestation of the disease. The typical clinical symptoms may not appear until later in the course of the illness.

Specific Complications

Splenic Rupture: Splenic rupture is seen in approximately 0.1% to 0.2% of cases of IM. At least half of cases are spontaneous without any history of trauma or unusual physical exertion. Typically, there is abrupt abdominal pain in the left upper quadrant that radiates to the top of the left shoulder, known as *Kehr sign*. This is followed by generalized abdominal pain, pleuritic chest pain, and signs and symptoms of hypovolemia. However, the onset may be insidious. Splenic rupture occurs between days 4 and 21 of the illness, with approximately half of cases occurring during the peak of the acute illness. Only about half of cases of splenic rupture have clinically significant splenomegaly noted before the rupture. All patients with IM should be considered at risk for splenic rupture, because clinical severity, laboratory results, and physical examination are not reliable predictors of risk.[2]

Airway Obstruction: Airway obstruction is an uncommon but life-threatening complication of IM related to massive lymphoid hyperplasia and mucosal edema. It is more common in younger adolescents and typically occurs approximately 1 week after the initial symptoms begin. Corticosteroids have been used to reduce the edema and hypertrophy of the lymphoid tissue. In more severe cases, acute tonsillectomy may be indicated. In emergency situations, intubation or tracheostomy may be necessary.

Streptococcal Pharyngitis: It was previously thought that EBV infection could potentiate adherence of β-hemolytic streptococci to epithelial cells membranes, with older reports identifying co-infection rates as high as 33%. More recent studies report a co-infection rate of 4%, which is the same as the general population.

Laboratory Evaluation

Antibody Testing

The standard rapid test for EBV-associated IM is the presence of heterophile antibodies. These immunoglobulin M (IgM) antibodies are induced by EBV infection and cross-react with unrelated antigens, typically horse, sheep, or bovine erythrocytes. These rapid test kits have sensitivities of 78% to 84% and specificities of 89% to 100% when compared to EBV-specific serologies, but sensitivity is lower (<50%) in children under 12 years of age. Sensitivity is also lower during the first week of symptoms; heterophile antibody levels peak between weeks two and five of the illness. About 10% of AYAs with EBV will remain heterophile antibody negative, but may be diagnosed by detection of EBV viral capsid antigen (VCA) IgM. Both IgM and immunoglobulin G (IgG) VCA antibodies peak 3 to 4 weeks after symptom onset. IgM levels then decline rapidly

and are undetectable by 3 months. Although VCA-IgG levels also decline, they are usually detectable for life. EBV early antigen (EA) antibodies develop early in the infection and usually persist for 1 to 2 months, although as many as 30% of infected individuals will have persistently high levels. Finally, about 2 to 3 months after symptom onset, antibodies against EBV nuclear antigen (EBNA) develop and persist indefinitely.[4] **Figure 29.1** shows the characteristic EBV antibody responses to various EBV antigens. **Table 29.3** shows the pattern of serologic results in various EBV stages.

Complete Blood Count

The WBC differential provides the traditional diagnostic criteria for IM >50% lymphocytes and at least 10% of the differential composed of atypical lymphocytes. The total WBC count is often elevated in the range of 10,000 to 20,000/mm³. Other common hematological abnormalities include a mild granulocytopenia and thrombocytopenia (usually in the range of 100,000 to 140,000/mm³) in approximately half of individuals with IM. Anemia is uncommon, although a mild hemolytic anemia may occur in up to 3% of cases.

Hepatic Transaminases

Transaminase levels are elevated in at least 90% of individuals, peaking during the second or third week of symptoms. Mild hepatitis is so common that entirely normal hepatic transaminases should lead the clinician to consider a diagnosis other than EBV infection.

Epstein–Barr Viral Detection

Serum-based EBV DNA nucleic acid amplification tests have been developed, and the magnitude of the viral load has been correlated with severity of illness. However, EBV viral load tests are not readily available for clinical use, and the primary use of these tests has been in immunocompromised patients at risk for EBV-associated malignancy.

Differential Diagnosis

In addition to other causes of EBV-negative mononucleosis such as CMV, toxoplasma gondii, rubella, adenovirus, and acute human immunodeficiency virus (HIV) infection, the differential diagnosis includes group A β-hemolytic streptococcal pharyngitis, nonspecific viral tonsillitis, mycoplasma pneumonia, Vincent angina (necrotizing

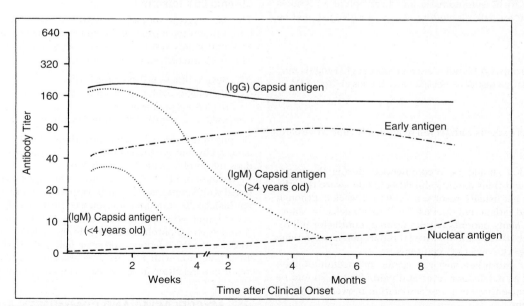

FIGURE 29.1 The evolution of antibodies to various EBV antigens in patients with IM is shown in the figure. The titers are geometric mean values expressed as reciprocals of the serum dilution. IgM and IgG antibody responses to EBV capsid antigen develop during the acute phase, as does an IgG response to EBV EA in most cases. The IgG response lasts for life, but the IgM response is transient and is shortest in very young children. Antibody response to nuclear antigen lasts for life and is typically quite late in onset. (From Sumaya CV. Epstein–Barr serologic testing: diagnostic indications and interpretations. *Pediatr Infect Dis* 1986;5:337.)

TABLE 29.3

Patterns of EBV Serology

| Types of Infection | Heterophile Antibody | VCA-IgG | VCA-IgM | Early Antigen | | EBNA |
				D-EA	R-EA	
Susceptible (nonimmune)	–	–	–	–	–	–
Acute primary infection	+	++	+	+	–	–
Remote past infection	–	+	–	–	–	+
Reactivated infection	+/–	+++	–	+	++	+/–

D-EA, diffuse early antigen; EBNA, Epstein–Barr nuclear antigen; Ig, immunoglobulin; R-EA, restricted early antigen; VCA, viral capsid antigen.

ulcerative gingivitis), diphtheria, viral hepatitis, and lymphoproliferative disorder or leukemia.

Diagnosis

The diagnosis is based on the following considerations:

Clinical Symptoms

IM should be suspected in an adolescent or young adult with fatigue, fever, splenomegaly, adenopathy, and pharyngitis.

Abnormal WBC *Count*

Patients will usually have the following:

 a. Relative lymphocytosis >50%.
 b. Absolute lymphocytosis >4,000/mm^3.
 c. Relative atypical lymphocytosis >10%.

Positive *Serology*

Almost all AYAs with IM have positive heterophile antibodies. If a patient continues to be symptomatic and heterophile antibodies are negative, titers for EBV (including VCA and EBNA) should be evaluated.

Other Tests

While testing for group A β-hemolytic streptococcal pharyngitis may be indicated, a positive test does not exclude the possibility of IM.

Management

The vast majority of patients with IM will require only supportive care.

Symptomatic Care

 a. Rest as needed should be recommended during the acute phase. AYAs and their parents should be made aware that the acute symptoms usually resolve over 1 to 2 weeks, although the associated fatigue may persist for 2 to 4 weeks, or sometimes longer. Many patients require up to 2 months for full recovery. About 10% of patients with IM report persistent fatigue 6 months after the onset of symptoms.
 b. Nonsteroidal anti-inflammatory agents or acetaminophen may be used as needed for fever and pain. Aspirin should be avoided, because there is a rare association between EBV and Reye syndrome.

Antimicrobials

In the absence of a bacterial co-infection, antibiotics should not be used. Acyclovir is not indicated; although it may reduce viral shedding, it does not impact the clinical course.[5]

Corticosteroids

Corticosteroids are not indicated. Despite their ineffectiveness and abundant recommendations discouraging their use, corticosteroids continue to be frequently prescribed for IM. The use of prednisone (40 to 60 mg daily, tapered over 1 to 2 weeks) is indicated only in patients with significant pharyngeal edema that threatens or causes respiratory compromise.[6]

Recommendations Regarding Physical Activity

AYAs with IM should refrain from vigorous physical activity for at least 1 month after the onset of symptoms.[3] In the past, it has been recommended that some athletes refrain from participation for a longer period; however, there is no evidence to support activity restriction for any time period greater than 4 weeks. The likelihood of splenic rupture decreases over time, and decisions about returning to play should be made on a case-by-case basis. Radiologic imaging of the spleen is not recommended. There is significant variability in splenic size, and such assessments have not been shown to predict splenic rupture risk.

Chronic EBV Infection

The vast majority of patients with EBV-associated IM develop lifelong immunity. Rarely, individuals may have very high titers of EBV antibodies and have chronic persistent active EBV infection. This is characterized by the following:

 1. Severe illness lasting >6 months
 2. Histologic evidence of end-organ disease, such as hepatitis, uveitis, or pneumonitis
 3. Evidence of EBV antigen or DNA in tissue

Despite some clinical similarities, there is little evidence that EBV causes chronic fatigue syndrome, and a positive IgG test for EBV does not imply a causal relationship.

Because of EBV's ability to alter cellular gene transcription combined with latent infection in B lymphocytes and, to a lesser degree, epithelial cells, immunocompromised hosts may be at risk for a variety of lymphoid and epithelial cancers.[7] In the rare genetic disorder X-linked lymphoproliferative syndrome, affected males are unable to control EBV infection and over half will die of IM. Rarely, host T-cell infection with EBV may be associated with hemophagocytic syndrome, resulting in severe pancytopenia and hepatitis.[8]

● MYCOPLASMA AND COMMUNITY-ACQUIRED PNEUMONIA

Community-acquired pneumonia (CAP) is the most common infectious cause of death in the world.[9] Although the vast majority of these deaths are in the elderly, CAP is a serious cause of illness in children, resulting in more than 150,000 hospitalizations each year in the US. However, in the absence of severe asthma or cardiac disease, AYAs (in contrast to infants and young children) are unlikely to develop severe illness; in a recent review of CAP hospitalization, only 10 of 492 admissions for CAP were adolescents and similar low rates were seen in young adults.[10]

The diagnosis of CAP is often straightforward (1) evidence of infection such as fever and/or leukocytosis, (2) lower respiratory tract signs and symptoms such as cough, sputum production, chest pain, or abnormal chest examination, and (3) an infiltrate on chest x-ray. Widespread vaccination of the pediatric population with conjugate pneumococcal vaccine has significantly reduced the rates of pneumococcal pneumonia; thus, atypical bacteria, such as *Mycoplasma pneumoniae*, have become more prominent. Clinicians should consider this as they choose antibiotic coverage for AYAs with CAP.[11] This section will focus on *M. pneumoniae*, a common cause of pneumonia in AYAs that may be asymptomatic but is often associated with pharyngitis, tracheobronchitis, and otitis media.

Etiology and Pathophysiology

Mycoplasma spp are about the same size as large viruses (approximately 150 to 250 nm). They are prokaryotes that do not have cell walls. Instead, they are bound by cell membranes containing sterols. Because they lack cell walls, they are resistant to β-lactam antimicrobials but are sensitive to antibiotics that interfere with protein synthesis, such as macrolides and tetracyclines.

By means of attachment proteins, *M. pneumoniae* adheres to ciliated and nonciliated respiratory epithelium, causing cellular damage to the trachea, bronchi, and bronchioles. The organism also causes ciliostasis, which may lead to prolonged cough. Transmission to the respiratory tract is through aerosolized inhalation. There is a high rate of transmission to family members and other close contacts, with an incubation period of 3 to 4 weeks. Many of the nonpulmonary findings are related to the immune response to infection.

Epidemiology

Because laboratory testing for *M. pneumoniae* is infrequently performed except in seriously ill hospitalized patients, prevalence data are scarce. Infection is endemic in many areas and may result in cyclical epidemic outbreaks every few years. Localized outbreaks often occur in schools, military bases, summer camps, college dormitories, and prisons. *M. pneumoniae* has been found to be the causative agent of CAP in more than 50% of children over age 5, and has been identified in up to 50% of adults with cough and upper respiratory symptoms.[12]

Clinical Manifestations

Symptoms are often insidious in onset, heralded by malaise, headache, and low-grade fever. Cough develops after 3 to 5 days. Though initially nonproductive, cough may progress to production of frothy white sputum.[13] Sputum production is not as copious as in typical bacterial pneumonia. The cough may become paroxysmal, and occasionally chest pain and hemoptysis occur. In patients with no prior history of asthma, dyspnea is uncommon. Patients may also have nasal congestion and rhinorrhea.

Individuals do not usually appear very ill, and physical findings are often minimal. When present, individuals may have mild pharyngitis, conjunctivitis, or lymphadenopathy. Bilateral bullous myringitis is suggestive of mycoplasma infection, but this is rare and the previously reported association has been questioned.[14] Chest examination is usually benign. If pneumonia is present, there may be isolated crackles or areas of wheezing over one or both of the lower lobes. Signs of pleural effusion are occasionally present.

Complications

Nonrespiratory infections and complications may occur 1 to 21 days after initial respiratory symptoms. Because evidence of past infection is so common, one must use caution when using serologic testing for diagnosis of an *M. pneumoniae* infection in individuals with extrapulmonary manifestations and no respiratory tract symptoms. In the past, the failure to isolate *M. pneumoniae* from nonrespiratory clinical specimens led to the conclusion that extrapulmonary complications were due to cross-reacting antibodies or by an unidentified toxin. However, through the use of polymerase chain reaction (PCR) testing, *M. pneumoniae* has been identified in cerebrospinal fluid and serum, both of which are indicative of dissemination.[15] Cross-reacting antibodies may still be the cause for hemolysis and cutaneous manifestations. Reported complications include almost every organ system, including the development of arthralgias and arthritis, severe rash including Stevens–Johnson syndrome, hemolytic anemia, Guillain–Barré syndrome, conjunctivitis, and uveitis.

Laboratory Evaluation

Traditionally, cold agglutinins have also been used for bedside diagnosis; however, PCR testing on nasopharyngeal swab is increasingly available and affords the most utility.[16] Serology may be helpful in the evaluation of more severely ill patients, but acute and convalescent titers are required. The WBC count is usually normal. Radiographic findings often appear worse than the clinical observations. Chest x-ray often has a peribronchial interstitial pattern, frequently in the lower lobes. Hilar adenopathy (34%) and pleural effusions (20%) are also seen.

Differential Diagnosis

The differential diagnosis includes streptococcal pneumonia, viral pneumonia (such as adenovirus, parainfluenza, and influenza), and pneumonia caused by *Chlamydia* or *Legionella*. In at-risk individuals, one should also consider tuberculosis, Q fever (*Coxiella*), rickettsial infections, and fungal infections.

Diagnosis

The diagnosis of *Mycoplasma* infections is usually based on clinical suspicion. In rare instances, a more precise diagnosis may be required. See laboratory evaluation described earlier.

Management

Although most infections with *M. pneumoniae* are self-limited and resolve without treatment, antibiotic therapy has been shown to decrease the length and severity of illness. Since the early 2000s, there have been increasing reports of macrolide-resistant *M. pneumoniae*, particularly in Asia. As many as 90% of isolates in China are now macrolide resistant, and there have been case reports of resistance in the US.[17] If symptoms persist and there is concern about resistance, the use of fluoroquinolones may be considered. Otherwise, any of the following is an appropriate choice:

a. Azithromycin: 500 mg on day 1, then 250 mg daily on days 2 through 5
b. Clarithromycin: 500 mg twice a day for 7 days
c. Erythromycin: 500 mg four times a day for 7 days
d. Tetracycline: 500 mg four times a day for 7 days
e. Doxycycline: 100 mg twice a day for 7 days

PERTUSSIS

Pertussis, meaning "intense cough," is frequently unrecognized and underdiagnosed in AYAs. The term "pertussis" is more appropriate than "whooping cough," because many patients, particularly AYAs, do not "whoop." Pertussis infection continues to cause fatal illness in vulnerable neonates and incompletely immunized infants. AYAs are a major source of infection for these vulnerable populations.

Etiology

Bordetella spp are small gram-negative coccobacilli. *Bordetella pertussis* is the sole cause of epidemic pertussis and the usual cause of sporadic pertussis. Only *B. pertussis* produces pertussis toxin (PT), which plays a major role in the virulence of the infection. *B. parapertussis* may occasionally cause pertussis, but accounts for fewer than 5% of *Bordetella* isolates in the US.

Transmission is through close contact with respiratory secretions. Intrafamilial spread is quite common in both immunized and unimmunized individuals.[18] The incubation period is commonly 5 to 10 days but may be as long as 21 days. Pertussis is primarily a mucosal disease; although the organism may invade alveolar macrophages, there is neither a systemic invasion nor a bacteremic phase of the illness.

Epidemiology

Despite widespread vaccination, there are approximately 30 to 50 million annual cases of pertussis worldwide, resulting in about 300,000 deaths. More than 90% of cases are in parts of the world where vaccination rates remain very low. The incidence of pertussis demonstrates a cyclic pattern, with peaks occurring every 2 to 5 years—this was true in the prevaccine era as well as today. Before widespread vaccine use, pertussis was the leading cause of death due to infectious disease in children under 14 years old. Routine childhood vaccination led to a significant decrease in disease burden, and the rate of pertussis infection reached its lowest level in 1976. Since then, rates of infection have increased significantly, even in highly immunized populations. There have been several epidemic outbreaks in the US, and even the interepidemic rates have not returned to the low levels of 1976. The number of reported cases in the US increased from 4,570 in 1990, 9,971 in 2001, to 27,550 cases in 2010. While there were only18,719 cases reported in 2011, the number of cases skyrocketed to 48,277 in 2012.[19] Most of the recent increase in pertussis illness has been attributed to disease in AYAs, who now account for half of all cases in the US. The increased infection burden is thought to be a combination of waning immunity, vaccine refusal, and improved recognition and diagnosis of the illness. In AYAs with prolonged cough illness, 13% to 20% are caused by *B. pertussis* infection.

Clinical Manifestations

The clinical severity of pertussis varies widely and may be influenced by age, immunization history, degree of exposure, past antibiotic administration, and concomitant infections. Classic pertussis is divided into three stages:

Catarrhal

This begins after the incubation period with nasal congestion and rhinorrhea, sometimes accompanied by low-grade fever, sneezing, and watery eyes. Patients are most contagious at this time, but the symptoms are indistinguishable from a routine upper respiratory tract infection. These symptoms begin to wane after 1 to 2 weeks, as the paroxysmal stage begins.

Paroxysmal

The onset of cough marks the beginning of the paroxysmal stage. Initially dry and intermittent, the cough progresses to the paroxysms that are characteristic of pertussis. An otherwise well-appearing patient may have episodic coughing fits with choking, gasping, and feelings of strangulation and suffocation. A forceful inspiratory gasp sounding like a "whoop" is most frequently heard in young infants. Post-tussive emesis is common. At its peak, these episodes may occur hourly.

Convalescent

During this stage, the number, severity, and duration of the coughing paroxysms diminish.

The duration of classic pertussis is 6 to 10 weeks. AYAs, particularly those who have been immunized, are unlikely to show distinct stages of illness. AYAs may complain only of coughing episodes, without fever or congestion, but the illness often leads to days or weeks of interrupted sleep and time away from school. The physical examination between coughing episodes may be completely normal.

Pertussis is most contagious from approximately 1 to 2 weeks before the onset of cough and for 2 to 3 weeks after coughing begins. Complications are primarily seen in infants and young children and include seizures, pneumonia, apnea, encephalopathy, and death. AYAs rarely develop serious complications, but secondary bacterial pneumonia and adult respiratory distress syndrome have been reported.

Laboratory Evaluation

Profound Leukocytosis

Profound leukocytosis with WBC counts from 15,000 to as high as 100,000/mm^3 due to an absolute lymphocytosis may be seen, particularly in the catarrhal phase.

DNA Amplification

PCR for the diagnosis of pertussis is rapid and accurate, having a sensitivity of 97% and specificity of 93%.

Culture

The incubation period is 10 to 14 days; so culture rarely guides treatment decisions. False-negative cultures may occur after the second week of illness or if antibiotics have been administered.

Serology

IgM and IgG antibodies to pertussis toxin are the most commonly used. Serologic testing may be difficult to interpret, particularly in AYAs who have been immunized in the past year. Acute and convalescent samples are no longer used clinically because of the high number of immunized individuals and their typical presentation late in the course of illness.

Differential Diagnosis

The differential diagnosis includes adenoviral infection, mycoplasma pneumonia, chlamydia pneumonia, and influenza.

Diagnosis

Based on recommendations developed at the 2011 Global Pertussis Initiate Conference, pertussis should be suspected in patients over 10 years old who present with paroxysms of cough without fever plus one of the following: whoop, apnea, sweating episodes between paroxysms, post-tussive emesis, or worsening symptoms at night.[20]

When clinical suspicion warrants, confirmatory testing should be performed. Specimens for PCR testing must be obtained from the posterior nasopharynx and not the anterior nasopharynx or throat. Alternatively, nasopharyngeal aspiration with saline may yield better diagnostic results, but is not always practical in the clinical setting. The proper test is based on symptom duration:

1. Cough <2 weeks: PCR and culture
2. Cough for 2 to 4 weeks: PCR and serology
3. Cough >4 weeks: serology

Management

All individuals with suspected or confirmed pertussis should receive appropriate antibiotic therapy. Treatment administered early in the illness may provide some clinical benefit and also decreases the spread of infection. Any of the following oral antibiotics may be used:

1. Azithromycin 500 mg on day 1 and 250 mg on days 2 to 5.
2. Clarithromycin 500 mg twice daily for 7 days.
3. Erythromycin 500 mg 4 times daily for 14 days.
4. Trimethoprim-sulfamethoxazole 1 double-strength tablet twice daily for 14 days may be used for those who are unable to tolerate macrolides.

Symptomatic treatment of cough with various agents, including corticosteroids, albuterol, montelukast, and antihistamines have minimal impact and are not recommended.[21]

Control Measures

1. Treatment with a full course of antibiotics is indicated for all household contacts of an infected patient within 3 weeks of symptom onset in the index patient regardless of immunization status. The dose and duration of prophylactic antibiotics are the same as used for treatment. Prompt antibiotic administration can limit secondary transmission, because pertussis immunity is not absolute and even those with subclinical disease may be able to transmit the illness to others. Treatment is particularly important for those who have close contact with infants or young children.
2. Nonhousehold contacts of the infected individual should be monitored for symptoms for 21 days after the most recent contact.
3. Students with pertussis should be excluded from school. Individuals are considered noninfectious after 5 days of antibiotic therapy and may return to school then. If unable to take antibiotics, individuals are considered infectious for 21 days after the onset of cough.

Immunization

Universal pertussis immunization is recommended for children starting at 2 months of age and has been widely used in combination with diphtheria and tetanus toxoids (diphtheria, tetanus, pertussis [DTP]) since the 1940s. Less reactogenic, acellular pertussis vaccines (DTaP), containing purified inactivated components of the *B. pertussis* organism, are highly effective and have replaced the use of the whole cell vaccine in the US.

Natural and vaccine-induced immunity to pertussis wanes over time, leaving adolescents and adults susceptible to infection. Two acellular pertussis vaccines are licensed for use in adolescents (Tdap). Adolescents (aged 11 to 18 years) who have completed the recommended childhood DTaP series should receive a Tdap booster, preferably at their 11 or 12 year annual visit. Adults (aged 19 to 64 years) should receive a single Tdap booster in lieu of a Td booster.[22]

⬤ INFLUENZA

Influenza is an acute respiratory illness that is highly contagious, affects all age-groups, and has caused epidemics for hundreds of years. Although most influenza infections in AYAs are self-limited, those with chronic illnesses such as asthma or cardiac disease may develop a serious life-threatening infection. Additionally, AYAs often serve as the reservoir for influenza, and those who are unvaccinated may be responsible for infecting high-risk individuals such as infants.[23]

Etiology

Influenza viruses are orthomyxoviruses that are enveloped with two important surface glycoproteins: hemagglutinin (HA) and neuraminidase (NA). Influenza viruses are classified as A, B, or C. Influenza A and B viruses are responsible for seasonal epidemics, whereas C virus is responsible for mild, common cold-like illnesses. Influenza A viruses are further categorized into subtypes on the basis of HA and NA. Since 1977, there have been two predominant circulating subtypes, influenza A (H1N1) and influenza A (H3N2). Influenza B is not subtyped. Influenza A and B are indistinguishable clinically, but influenza A (H3N2) viruses are generally associated with the most severe epidemics.

Influenza viruses are negative-sense RNA viruses that contain eight separate gene segments. During virus replication, point mutations in the gene segments can lead to minor antigenic virus variants. Minor antigenic changes occur frequently and lead to yearly epidemics of influenza illness. Transmission is person to person through respiratory droplets or by direct contact with articles recently contaminated by nasopharyngeal secretions. The incubation period is only 1 to 4 days, and a single infected person may transmit the virus to a large number of susceptible individuals. Individuals are most infectious during the 24 hours before and through the peak of symptoms. Viral shedding continues for approximately 7 days after the onset of symptoms. Seasonal epidemics typically occur during the winter. Local outbreaks can peak within 2 weeks of onset and last 4 to 8 weeks.

Epidemiology

Although influenza may be sporadically identified through the year, epidemics typically occur annually during the winter months. Influenza A generally occurs annually, whereas influenza B recurs every 3 or 4 years. Local epidemics are maintained by high infection rates in young children. During these outbreaks, infection rates may be as high as 40% for school-aged and preschool children, as opposed to infection rates in young adults of 10% to 20%. For most adolescents, influenza results in nothing more than a "bad cold"; however, it is a cause of morbidity, particularly among young children and those with underlying medical conditions. During the past four influenza seasons, hospitalization rates have ranged from 16 to 77 hospitalizations per 100,000 population for those ages 0 to 4 years, 4 to 27 for those 5 to 17 years, and 4 to 23 for those 18 to 49 years.[24] Hospitalization rates for those with high-risk conditions such as asthma or heart disease may be as high as 200 per 100,000 population.

Clinical Manifestations

Patients typically develop sudden onset fever and chills associated with a nonproductive cough, myalgias, sore throat, malaise, and headache. The fever, often as high as 40°C, peaks within 24 hours of the onset of symptoms, and may last 5 days. The dry, hacking cough may persist for 1 week after other symptoms have resolved. Nausea, vomiting, and diarrhea, seen in younger children, are infrequent in AYAs. Patients appear unwell, with injected conjunctiva, hyperemic mucous membranes, and clear rhinorrhea.

Complications

Influenza has been associated with primary viral pneumonia, encephalitis, encephalopathy, Guillain–Barré syndrome, Reye syndrome, and myositis.

Laboratory Evaluation

During influenza season or in the setting of a known influenza outbreak, diagnostic testing using a nasopharyngeal swab or wash should be considered in any patient who presents within 5 days of the onset of acute febrile respiratory symptoms. Immunocompromised or hospitalized patients with such symptoms should be tested regardless of the timing of symptom onset. Rapid influenza diagnostic tests (RIDTs) are immunochromatographic lateral flow and membrane-based immunoassays that can provide results in less than 30 minutes. These are now the tests of choice for confirmatory influenza testing and have supplanted immunofluorescence, PCR, and viral cultures at most centers.[25]

Differential Diagnosis

The differential diagnosis includes bacterial infections such as streptococcal pneumonia, chlamydia pneumonia, and mycoplasma pneumonia and viral infections such as adenovirus, parainfluenza, respiratory syncytial virus, and rhinovirus.

Diagnosis

Even during peak influenza activity, the clinical diagnosis of influenza can be difficult because many other circulating respiratory viruses cause similar symptoms. During episodes of peak disease activity, it is impractical to test every patient with signs and symptoms of influenza. Therefore, the diagnosis is often made based on the clinical presentation informed by the clinician's assessment of the prior probability of influenza based on local rates of influenza activity. There are few data examining the validity of the clinical diagnosis of influenza in adolescents. The reported positive predictive value of the clinical diagnosis in adults varies widely, from 18% to 87% compared to laboratory-confirmed influenza. During a seasonal outbreak, the diagnosis should be considered in any adolescent or young adult with sudden onset of fever and dry, nonproductive cough.

Management

Most AYAs who contract influenza will require supportive care only. Ibuprofen or acetaminophen may be used for fever, headache, and myalgia. Patients should be advised not to use aspirin because of the potential for the development of Reye syndrome. Antiviral medications should be prescribed for patients with underlying illness (regardless of timing) and otherwise healthy patients who present for treatment within 48 hours of the onset of symptoms. These medications have been shown to decrease the time to symptom resolution by 1 to 2 days and to decrease viral shedding. Due to resistance, amantadine and rimantadine are no longer recommended. NA inhibitors that block the release of virions from infected cells continue to be effective. Two are currently available, one oral and one an inhaled powder: (1) oseltamivir, 75 mg by mouth twice daily for 5 days and (2) zanamivir two inhalations (5 mg each inhalation) twice daily for 5 days. Zanamivir may induce bronchospasm and should not be used in individuals with asthma or other respiratory disease.

Immunization

Annual universal immunization is strongly recommended.[26] Current options include (1) an inactivated trivalent influenza vaccine (IIV3) containing two A antigens (representing both the H1N1 and H3N2 subtypes) and a B antigen, (2) an inactivated quadrivalent vaccine (IIV4) containing an additional B antigen, or (3) a live attenuated quadrivalent vaccine (LAIV4). Vaccine viruses for IIV and LAIV are grown in chicken eggs. IIV3 and IIV4 are killed virus products administered by intramuscular injection, whereas LAIV4 is a live attenuated virus product administered using an intranasal sprayer. Neither IIV nor LAIV should be given to those with a history of an anaphylactic hypersensitivity to eggs or to other specific vaccine components. IIV3 and IIV4 can be used for both healthy AYAs as well as those with high-risk medical conditions. Use of LAIV4 should be restricted to healthy AYAs only and should not be administered to those with high-risk medical conditions or individuals who are pregnant. When vaccine is limited, priority should be given to individuals who are immunosuppressed or those with underlying chronic disease such as asthma, diabetes, hemoglobinopathies, and renal dysfunction. Additionally, all health care personnel and individuals who plan to be pregnant during the influenza season should make special efforts to be vaccinated.

REFERENCES

1. Bravender T. Epstein-Barr virus, cytomegalovirus, and infectious mononucleosis. *Adolesc Med State Art Rev* 2010;21(2):251–264.
2. Foreman BH, Mackler L. Can we prevent splenic rupture for patients with infectious mononucleosis? *J Fam Pract* 2005;54(6):547.
3. Burroughs KE. Athletes resuming activity after infectious mononucleosis. *Arch Fam Med* 2000;9(10):1122.
4. Ruf S, Wagner HJ. Determining EBV load: current best practice and future requirements. *Expert Rev Clin Immunol* 2013;9(2):139–151.
5. Candy B, Chalder T, Cleare AJ, et al. Recovery from infectious mononucleosis: a case for more than symptomatic therapy? A systematic review. *Br J Gen Pract* 2002;52:844.
6. Chan SC, Dawes PJ. The management of severe infectious mononucleosis tonsillitis and upper airway obstruction. *J Laryngol Otol* 2001;115(12):973.
7. Ambinder RF. Epstein-Barr virus-associated lymphoproliferative disorders. *Rev Clin Exp Hematol* 2003;7(4):362.
8. Chen CJ, Huang YC, Jaing TH, et al. Hemophagocytic syndrome: a review of 18 pediatric cases. *J Microbiol Immunol Infect* 2004;37(3):157.
9. Wunderink RG, Waterer GW. Community-acquired pneumonia. *N Engl J Med* 2014;370(6):543–551.
10. Griffin MR, Zhu Y, Moore MR, et al. U.S. hospitalizations for pneumonia after a decade of pneumococcal vaccinations. *N Engl J Med* 2013;369:155–163.
11. Queen MA, Myers AL, Hall M, et al. Comparative effectiveness of empiric antibiotics for community-acquired pneumonia. *Pediatrics* 2014;133(1):e23–e29.
12. Korppi M, Neiskanen-Kosma T, Kleemola M. Incidence of community-acquired pneumonia in children cause by *Mycoplasma pneumoniae*: serological results of a prospective, population-based study in primary health care. *Respirology* 2004;9(1):109–114.
13. Atkinson TP, Balish MF, Waites KB. Epidemiology, clinical manifestations, pathogensis and laboratory detection of *Mycoplasma pneumoniae* infections. *FEMS Microbiol Rev* 2008;32(6):956–973.
14. Mellick LB, Verma N. The *Mycoplasma pneumoniae* and bullous myringitis myth. *Pediatr Emerg Care* 2010;26(12):966–968.
15. Waites KB. What's new in diagnostic testing and treatment approaches for *Mycoplasma pneumoniae* infections in children? *Adv Exp Med Biol* 2011;19:47–57.
16. Loens K, Goossens H, Ieven M. Acute respiratory infection due to *Mycoplasma pneumoniae*: current status of diagnostic methods. *Eur J Clin Microbiol Infect Dis* 2010;16(3):162–169.
17. Principi N, Esposito S. Macrolide-resistant Mycoplasma pneumoniae: its role in respiratory infection. *J Antimicrob Chemother* 2013;68(3):506–511.
18. Bisgard KM, Pascual FB, Ehresmann KR, et al. Infant pertussis: who was the source? *Pediatr Infect Dis J* 2004;23:985.
19. Bettiol S, Wang K, Thompson MJ, et al. Symptomatic treatment of the cough in whooping cough. *Cochrane Database Syst Rev* 2012;(5):CD003257.
20. Spector TB, Maziarz EK. Pertussis. *Med Clin North Am* 2013;97:537–552.
21. Cherry JD, Tan T, Wirsing von Konig CH, et al. Clinical definitions of pertussis: summary of a global pertussis initiative roundtable meeting, February 2011. *Clin Infect Dis* 2012;54:1762.
22. Centers for Disease Control and Prevention. Updated recommendations for use of tetanus toxoid, reduced diphtheria toxoid and acellular pertussis (Tdap) vaccine form the Advisory Committee on Immunization Practices, 2010. *MMWR* 2011;60(1):13–15.
23. Dharan NJ, Sokolow LZ, Cheng PY, et al. Child, household, and caregiver characteristics associated with hospitalization for influenza among children 6–59 months of age. *Pediatr Infect Dis J* 2014;33:e141–e150.
24. Epperson S, Blanton L, Kniss K, et al. Influenza activity—United States, 2013–14 season and composition of the 2014–15 influenza vaccines. *MMWR* 2014;63:483–490.
25. Labella AM, Merel SE. Influenza. *Med Clin North Am* 2013;97:621–645.
26. Committee on Infectious Diseases. Recommendations for prevention and control of influenza in children, 2013–2014. *Pediatrics* 2013;132(4):e1089–e1104.

🛜 **ADDITIONAL RESOURCES AND WEBSITES ONLINE**

CHAPTER 30

Viral Hepatitis

Mary E. Romano
Lynette A. Gillis

KEY WORDS

- Hepatitis A
- Hepatitis B
- Hepatitis C
- Hepatitis vaccine
- Viral hepatitis

ETIOLOGY

Hepatitis refers to inflammation of the liver due to infectious or noninfectious causes. Infectious causes include hepatitis viruses (HAV, HBV, HCV, HDV, and HEV), Epstein–Barr virus, and Cytomegalovirus. This chapter will specifically discuss types A, B, C, D, and E. The majority of viral hepatitis in the US is caused by hepatitis A, B, and C.

1. HAV is an RNA virus in the *Picornaviridae* family.
2. HBV is a DNA virus in the *Hepadnaviridae* family. The virion, also referred to as a Dane particle, is 42 nm in diameter. The circular DNA virus is contained in a 28 nm core surrounded by a 7 nm lipid envelope (Fig. 30.1).
   a. Hepatitis B surface antigen (HBsAg) is contained within a lipid envelope.
   b. Hepatitis B core antigen (HBcAg) surrounds the circular DNA virus.
   c. Spherical and tubular particles (20 to 22 nm) may be found circulating in the blood. These particles are excess virus coat material and contain HBsAg.
3. HCV is an RNA virus in the *Flaviviridae* family. There are seven major genotypes, more than 80 subtypes, and minor variants referred to as quasispecies. Genotype 1 is most common in the US. Treatment and anticipated response vary by HCV genotype.
4. HDV can only co-infect or superinfect in the presence of HBV. HDV is referred to as a subviral satellite due to its inability to cause infection on its own.
5. HEV is an RNA virus.

EPIDEMIOLOGY

Hepatitis A

1. HAV is transmitted primarily through the fecal–oral route in contaminated food or water. HAV can be transmitted through close personal contact in group settings (household, day care, residential facility).
2. HAV does not cause chronic disease. Viral shedding is highest in the 2 weeks prior to onset of symptoms and is minimal approximately 1 week after the onset of jaundice. Infected children shed the virus longer than adults and are often asymptomatic, making them an important source of infection.
3. Overall, rates of hepatitis A have decreased by 90% in the last 10 years due to the expanded recommendations for vaccination of all children and adolescents.[1] Rates were once higher for males, but are now similar for both genders.
4. Rates of hepatitis A are highest among young adults aged 20 to 29 years.[2] Serologic evidence of hepatitis A increases with age as a result of natural infection and more widespread uptake of hepatitis A vaccine.

Hepatitis B

1. HBV is transmitted through percutaneous or permucosal exposure to infected bodily fluids and/or blood. This can occur through perinatal exposure, sexual contact, contaminated needles, or close personal contact with an infected individual (i.e., sharing personal items, contact with open sores or secretions). Among adults with HBV, about 60% report "no risk factors" for HBV infection.[3] However, according to Centers for Disease Control and Prevention (CDC) data, when queried about selected behaviors, the most frequently reported risk factors among adults with HBV are ≥2 sexual partners (33%), men who have sex with men (MSM) (19%), and shared needles (18%).[3]
2. HBV may be found in the blood and *all* bodily secretions (saliva, breast milk, tears, stool, urine, semen, vaginal secretions, and respiratory droplets).
3. The estimated prevalence of hepatitis B is 0.4% in the US.[4] Foreign-born persons have significantly higher rates of infection, particularly chronic HBV infection.
4. Incidence rates of acute HBV have continued to decline in all age-groups.[2] In 2011, the highest incidence rates of acute HBV were seen in adults aged 30 to 39 years and the lowest in children <19 years. The greatest decline in acute incidence rates was in young adults aged 20 to 29 years. The acute incidence rates are higher in males than females, but this gap has narrowed in the last decade. The decline in infection rates is mostly attributed to HBV vaccination and a national strategy to eliminate HBV infection.

Hepatitis C

1. HCV is a blood-borne pathogen. The primary route of transmission is maternal-fetal in children and intravenous (IV) drug use in adolescents and young adults (AYAs).[2] Sexual exposure, particularly MSM, is the next highest risk factor. Screening procedures have essentially eliminated HCV infection related to transplantation or receipt of blood products.
2. Rates of acute HCV infection have increased 45% from 2007 to 2011.[2] The largest rate of increase was seen in those 0 to 19 years (0.05 to 0.1/100,000) and 20 to 29 years of age (0.75 to 1.18/100,000).

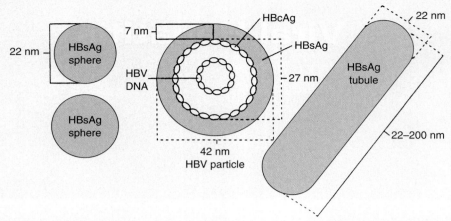

FIGURE 30.1 Hepatitis B virion (Dane particle) and spherical and tubular HBsAg particles found in serum of infected persons. HBcAg and HBsAg: hepatitis B core and surface antigens, respectively. (Adapted from Kalser MH, Howard RB. Hepatic and pancreatic disorders. *Postgrad Med* 1986;79:199.)

3. An estimated 75% to 85% of newly infected individuals will develop chronic HCV infection.[5] There are an estimated 3.2 million people in the US with chronic HCV, making it the most common blood-borne infection. Although prevalence rates are highest in adults aged 45 to 68 years, isolated reports have shown increasing rates among AYAs (15 to 24 years).[2] AYAs with reported IV drug use are at highest risk.

4. There have been significant increases in screening efforts for pregnant women, blood donors, and individuals at risk for HCV infection. In 2010, the Food and Drug Administration (FDA) approved point-of-care testing for HCV in order to expedite notification of results and referral to care.[5]

Hepatitis D

HDV is transmitted primarily through blood and sexual contact and only in those already infected with HBV. It is uncommon in children, but can be acquired by AYAs with preexisting HBV infection. Risk factors include IV drug use and high-risk sexual activity, particularly MSM. The risk from contaminated blood and clotting products has been reduced in recent years due to improved screening techniques.

Hepatitis E

1. HEV is transmitted though the fecal–oral route and is largely the result of contaminated water. Animals are thought to be a reservoir for this virus.

2. Hepatitis E is a significant problem in developing countries and is endemic in Asia, Africa, and the Middle East. Seroprevalence rates in North America and Europe are between 1% and 3%.[6] Cases of HEV in North America and Europe were previously thought to be due to travel; however, recent studies have identified strains that are distinctly different from those found in endemic developing countries.[7]

3. Hepatitis E is typically self-limited but can be a serious disease. The infection is particularly serious for pregnant women—up to 20% develop fulminant hepatitis.[6] There are case reports of HEV causing chronic liver disease in immunocompromised patients.[7]

⬤ CLINICAL MANIFESTATIONS

Symptoms

It is impossible to determine the cause of hepatitis based on the initial clinical presentation. If the date of exposure is known, the incubation period may suggest the diagnosis. The approximate incubation period for these diseases are as follows[2]:

- Hepatitis A: 2 to 6 weeks
- Hepatitis B: 2 to 6 months

- Hepatitis C: 2 weeks to 6 months
- Hepatitis D co-infection: 2 to 3 months
- Hepatitis D superinfection: 2 to 8 weeks
- Hepatitis E: 2 weeks to 3 months

Early viral hepatitis is often characterized by right upper quadrant pain and flu-like symptoms, including fatigue, low-grade fever, malaise, myalgias, and arthralgias. Cholestasis may also be present, resulting in acholic stools, dark urine, and jaundice.[8]

1. About 20% of individuals with hepatitis A will present with diarrhea.[8]

2. Hepatitis B is associated with arthritis, arthralgias, and rash due to circulating immune complexes.[8] The arthritis is usually symmetric, affects smaller joints and typically spares the feet. Rash is present in patients with HBV up to 50% of the time and is typically urticarial although maculopapular and petechial rashes have been reported.

Laboratory Findings

1. Laboratory findings include relative lymphocytosis, elevated transaminases, elevated total/conjugated bilirubin, and mild elevation of alkaline phosphatase.[8,9] Only 20% of patients with HCV infection develop symptoms with acute illness.[9]

2. The CDC case definition for acute hepatitis requires the discrete onset of symptoms and either jaundice or elevated serum transaminase levels. Serum alanine aminotransferase (ALT) is often more significantly elevated than aspartate aminotransferase (AST) unless cirrhosis is already present.[8,9] In more serious disease, decreased albumin and increased prothrombin time are present. Decreased serum complement is found in patients with HBV arthritis. Joint fluid contains white blood cells ranging from 2,000 to 90,000 cells/mL.

⬤ VIRAL ANTIGENS AND ANTIBODIES

Laboratory evaluation for viral antigens/antibodies can help to differentiate the causative agent. CDC laboratory criteria for diagnosis of acute hepatitis are as follows[10]:

1. **Hepatitis A—CDC criteria for acute hepatitis A[10]:**
   a. Immunoglobulin M (IgM) antibody to HAV (anti-HAV).
   - HAV in stool is the first marker. It is shed in stool 2 weeks before and 1 week after the onset of jaundice and corresponds to the period of greatest infectivity. Children can shed HAV for months, much longer than adults infected with HAV. A carrier state does not occur. IgM anti-HAV antibodies are present 5 to 10 days prior to the onset of

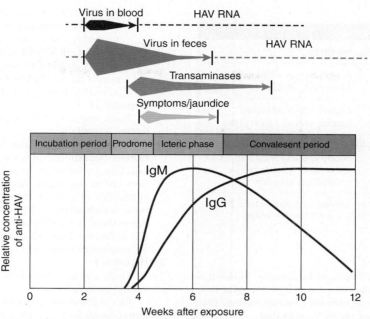

FIGURE 30.2 Immunologic and biologic course for HAV infection divided into four clinical stages. HAV RNA genomic material can be detected over a finite period of time (dotted lines) in some individuals in the absence of documented infectivity. An HAV carrier state does not occur. (From Knipe DM, Howley PM. *Fields virology.* Vol 2. 6th ed. Philadelphia, PA: Lippincott Williams & Wilkins, 2015.)

symptoms and remain positive for up to 6 months. IgG anti-HAV antibodies rise much more slowly and remain positive conferring lifelong protection (Fig. 30.2).

2. **Hepatitis B—CDC criteria for acute hepatitis B[10]:**

   a. HBsAg positive *and*
   b. IgM antibody to HBV core antigen (anti-HBc) positive
   c. Figure 30.3 details the course of hepatitis b serology.
      - HBsAg becomes positive about 1 month after acute exposure and is usually undetectable by 15 weeks, although some individuals have persistence of this antigen for life. The presence of HBsAg indicates either acute HBV infection or a carrier state and the ability to transmit HBV.
      - Anti-HBsAg antibodies develop during convalescence or as a result of immunization and indicate immunity to disease.
      - Anti-HBcAg antibodies (HBcAb) appear in the window between the disappearance of HBsAg and the appearance of anti-HBsAg antibodies. Anti-HBcAg IgM and IgG appear simultaneously, but IgM disappears by 8 months. The presence of IgG antibodies alone indicates infection of >6 months duration.
      - HBeAg appears during the incubation period, and its presence indicates active viral replication and high infectivity. Persistence of HBeAg positivity beyond 12 weeks indicates likely progression to a chronic carrier state. The appearance of anti-HBeAg antibodies coincides with the disappearance of HBeAg and serves as a marker of decreased viral activity and infectivity. **Table 30.1** summarizes the infectivity risk of HBV. Reactivation of disease can occur, particularly in immunosuppressed states. When reactivation occurs, there is reemergence of HBeAg and disappearance of anti-HBeAg antibodies.
      - HBV DNA can be measured and quantified, but it is not routinely used for diagnosis. It may be used to help monitor response to therapy.

3. **Hepatitis C: CDC criteria for acute hepatitis C[10]:**

   a. Antibody to HCV (anti-HCV) screening-test-positive. (Criteria for positive values for specific lab assays as per CDC

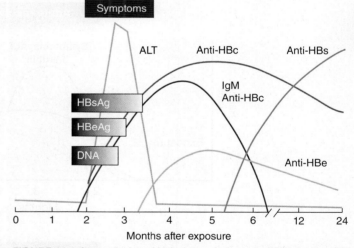

FIGURE 30.3 Immunologic and biologic course for acute HBV infection. ALT, alanine aminotransferase; anti-HBc, antibody to HBcAg; anti-HBe, antibody to hepatitis B e-antigen; anti-HBs, antibody to HBsAg. (From Perrillo RP, Regenstein FG. Viral and immune hepatitis. In Kelley WN, ed. *Textbook of internal medicine.* 3rd ed. Philadelphia, PA: J.B. Lippincott, 1996.)

can be found at http://www.cdc.gov/hepatitis/HCV/LabTesting.htm) *or*

   b. HCV recombinant immunoblot assay (HVC RIBA) positive *or*
   c. HCV RNA nucleic acid test (NAT) positive (including qualitative, quantitative or genotype testing)

And, if done, meets the following two criteria:

   d. Absence of IgM antibody to hepatitis A virus (IgM anti-HAV) *and*
   e. Absence of IgM antibody to HBcAg (IgM anti-HBc)
      - HCV antibodies are detectable about 7 weeks after exposure and are positive for life.
      - HCV RNA may be detected as early as 2 weeks after exposure to the virus.

TABLE 30.1
Infectivity for Acute Hepatitis B Virus

HBsAg	Anti-HBc	HBeAg	Anti-HBe	Infectivity
+	+	+	−	Acute infection or chronic carrier; very infectious
+	+	−	−	Acute or recent infection; possible chronic carrier state; moderately infectious
+	+	−	+	Recent infection or chronic carrier state; good prognosis; probably low infectivity

Anti-HBc, antibody to hepatitis B core antigen; anti-HBe, antibody to hepatitis B e-antigen; HBeAg, hepatitis B e-antigen; HBsAg, hepatitis B surface antigen.

- Antibodies against HCV may not be detected in infected patients who are immunocompromised or receiving dialysis. In contrast, patients with autoimmune disease may have a false positive test for HCV antibodies.
- Chronic HCV disease is characterized by persistence of HCV antibodies and HCV RNA. A single negative test

for HCV RNA using currently available NAT testing is considered sufficient to rule out chronic infection in an antibody-positive individual with no ongoing exposure. However, HCV RNA testing may be transiently negative as HCV antibodies are rising and so the CDC recommends repeat RNA testing ≥6 months after exposure for definitive diagnosis (Fig. 30.4).

4. **Hepatitis D**

There are no US FDA-approved tests for HDV. Commercial testing is available.

Infection with HDV can occur only with or after HBV infection. Superinfection is more likely to result in chronic disease than co-infection. Anti-HDV antibodies (IgM and IgG) are detected in acute and chronic infections, with persistence of antibodies in chronic infection. Delta antigen (HDVAg) has been documented in 20% of patients with acute infection.[10] Since there is no FDA-approved test for delta antigen in the US, definitive diagnosis of chronic HDV is made by immunohistochemical analysis of liver tissue for HDV.[10]

5. **Hepatitis E**

There are no FDA-approved tests for HEV. Commercial testing is available.

HEV is detectable in stool 1 week prior and 1 week after symptoms appear. Total and IgM anti-HEV antibodies are detectable at 3 weeks.[10] IgM antibodies decline by 13 weeks, but total antibodies remain positive for life, conferring lifelong protection.[10]

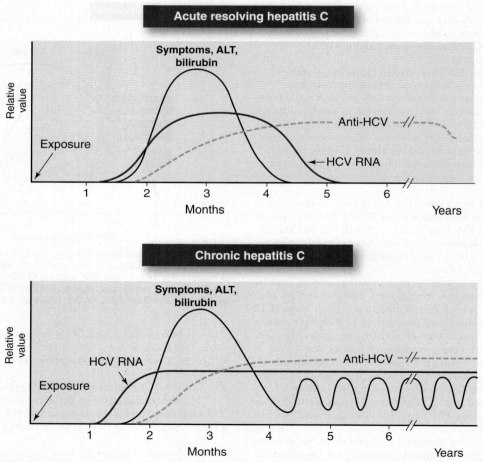

FIGURE 30.4 Immunologic and biologic course for HCV infection. **A:** Acute resolving hepatitis C. Self-limited infection with disappearance of HCV RNA and persistence of anti-HCV. **B:** Chronic hepatitis C. Chronic illness with exacerbation and remission of clinical symptoms. Persistence of HCV RNA. Development of anti-HCV does not affect clinical outcome in individuals with chronic HCV infection. (From Rubin R, Strayer DS. *Rubin's pathology: clinicopathologic foundations of medicine.* 5th ed. Philadelphia, PA: Lippincott Williams & Wilkins, 2008.)

CLINICAL COURSE

1. Hepatitis A: Acute hepatitis A has an abrupt onset. Symptoms generally vary by age. Approximately 70% of older children, adolescents, and adults have symptomatic infection. Clinical infection does not usually last longer than 2 months; however, 10% to 15% of individuals have relapsing signs and symptoms of illness. HAV can cause fulminant hepatitis or autoimmune hepatitis.[11]

2. Hepatitis B: Clinical signs and symptoms of acute hepatitis occur more often in AYAs. While perinatal HBV acquisition is almost always asymptomatic, up to 50% of AYAs will present with acute clinical signs and symptoms after HBV exposure.[11] When symptomatic, prodromal symptoms last about 10 days prior to onset of jaundice. Jaundice lasts 1 to 3 weeks although malaise and fatigue may last for months following initial infection. Pregnant women with acute HBV infection are at significantly higher risk of acute liver failure and death. The risk of progression to chronic disease decreases with age. Only 2% to 6% of adults progress to chronic infection compared to 90% of infected infants and 30% of children <5 years.[12]

   The majority of individuals who develop chronic HBV infection are asymptomatic but capable of transmitting the infection. A minority of individuals with chronic HBV are not only infectious but also have active liver disease with abnormal serum transaminases. The risk of premature death from cirrhosis or hepatocellular carcinoma (HCC) is 15% to 25% in chronic carriers.[11] Adults who have had a chronic HBV infection since childhood develop HCC at a rate of 5% per decade. Up to 25% of infants and older children who acquire HBV infection eventually develop HCC or cirrhosis.[11]

3. Hepatitis C: Seventy percent of individuals with acute HCV infections are asymptomatic, while only 25% develop jaundice.[13] Chronic disease develops in 75% to 85% of infected individuals. Co-infection with HBV and/or HIV, alcohol or IV drug use, male sex, and acquisition of infection >40 years of age are risk factors for disease progression.[13] Within 20 years of acquiring HCV infection, approximately 20% of individuals with chronic disease will go on to develop cirrhosis and 5% will die of complications of liver disease and/or carcinoma.[13]

4. Hepatitis D: Infection with HDV can occur only in the presence of HBV.
   - Co-infection occurs when both HDV and HBV are simultaneously contracted and is typically a self-limited condition. Less than 5% of co-infected individuals develop chronic infection; however, co-infection usually results in a more severe acute hepatitis than is caused by HBV infection alone.[2]
   - Superinfection occurs when an individual with chronic HBV acquires HDV. Superinfection results in a severe acute hepatitis and is more likely to result in fulminant hepatitis than in other hepatitis types.
   - Chronic infection with both HDV and HBV is associated with more rapid disease progression although progression to carcinoma is similar to HBV infection alone. Mortality rates for chronic HDV/HBV infection are about 10 times higher than with chronic HBV infection.[2]

5. Hepatitis E: The clinical course of HEV is similar to HAV, with asymptomatic shedding of virus prior to and after clinical infection. Symptomatic infection is most likely to occur in those 15 to 44 years of age.[14] Although typically self-limited, the mortality rate is about 1% in the general population. Pregnant women are more likely to experience severe illness and death. Mortality rates for women in their third trimester are between 10% and 30%.[15] Acute HEV does not progress to chronic infection, but HEV infection can lead to chronic liver disease and cirrhosis in individuals who are receiving chemotherapy or who have undergone organ transplant.[2]

TABLE 30.2
Differential Diagnosis of Hepatitis

Infectious	Noninfectious
Hepatitis A through E	Drug induced
Cytomegalovirus	Toxin induced
Epstein–Barr virus	Alcohol induced
Varicella	Nonalcoholic steatohepatitis (NASH)
Enterovirus	Genetic
Coxsackie B	α-1 Antitrypsin deficiency
ECHO virus	Wilson disease
Rubella	
Adenovirus	Autoimmune hepatitis

DIFFERENTIAL DIAGNOSIS

The differential diagnosis of hepatitis includes both infectious and noninfectious causes (**Table 30.2**).[8,9]

- A thorough risk assessment is important to evaluate for exposure to drugs or toxins, alcohol use, or risk factors for viral hepatitis.
- Specific testing should include anti-HAV IgM, HBsAg, anti-HBcAg IgM, anti-HCV enzyme immunoassay, and a mononucleosis spot test.[8,9]
- RNA for HCV should be obtained if hepatitis C is suspected.[8,9]
- Liver tests including ALT, AST, albumin, PT/PTT, -glutamyl transferase (GGT), and conjugated bilirubin should be considered to assess for hepatocellular necrosis, liver failure, and cholestasis.[8,9]
- Hepatic ultrasound can detect inflammation, cirrhosis, or HCC and can determine the optimal location for percutaneous liver biopsy.[8,9]
- Percutaneous liver biopsy is considered the gold standard to assess the degree of inflammation and fibrosis in chronic infection; however, biopsy is rarely needed as part of the diagnostic evaluation of acute infection.[8,9]

TREATMENT

Acute Hepatitis

Treatment of acute hepatitis is typically supportive and includes monitoring for progression or resolution of clinical or laboratory abnormalities. In rare cases, patients may require hospitalization for IV hydration or closer monitoring. Activity should be modified as clinically indicated. There is no evidence that diet affects course or outcome of acute disease.

- The adolescent or young adult should be advised to avoid any alcohol or drug use as well as any hepatotoxic drugs (acetaminophen, oral contraceptives, steroids).
- Serum transaminases and bilirubin should be checked weekly during the acute phase of illness and then every 2 to 3 weeks until they return to baseline.
- Severe disease is indicated by elevated prothrombin time, albumin <2.5 g/dL, and evidence of ascites, edema, or encephalopathy.
- In the setting of clinical (encephalopathy, ascites, edema) or laboratory (elevated PT/PTT, low albumin) findings of liver disease, closer monitoring is warranted.

Chronic Infection

In general, chronic infection should be managed by a liver specialist.

1. Chronic hepatitis B: There are two classes of medication used to treat chronic HBV.
   - Interferon α/pegylated interferon α is an immunomodulator that improves host response to HBV. Pegylated interferon α has a longer half-life. Pegylated interferon α is approved for individuals >3 years of age.[13,16]
   - There are five nucleos(t)ide analogs used to reduce viral replication. Three are approved for use in adolescents: lamivudine (approved for use in youth ≥3 years); adefovir (≥12 years); entecavir (≥16 years). Telbivudine and tenofovir are also approved for use in adults. Resistance to nucleos(t)ide inhibitors can develop over the course of treatment. Treatment is recommended for those with evidence of active hepatic necrosis (ALT > 1.5 times normal) and viral replication (HBV ≥ 2,000 IU/mL) in conjunction with liver biopsy histopathology.[13,16]
2. Chronic hepatitis C: Treatment includes combination therapy with pegylated interferon α and ribavirin. Ribavirin suppresses viral replication and is approved for individuals over 3 years of age. Ribavirin is teratogenic, and this should be discussed with female patients of childbearing age. Treatment duration is dependent on HCV genotype. Genotype 1 generally requires a longer duration of treatment, while genotypes 2 and 3 generally have a more rapid response. Treatment is recommended only for those with active disease and viral replication since treatment without active liver disease has not been shown to alter the course of illness.[12,13]

● COMPLICATIONS

1. Acute hepatitis
   a. Myocarditis
   b. Pancreatitis
   c. Atypical pneumonia
   d. Aplastic anemia
   e. Transverse myelitis
   f. Glomerulonephritis
   g. Arthritis
2. Fulminant hepatitis
3. Chronic carrier state
4. Chronic hepatitis
5. Cirrhosis
   a. Chronic liver failure
   b. HCC

● PREVENTION

General Disinfection

1. Heat sterilization
   a. Boiling in water at 100° C for 10 minutes
   b. Steam autoclaving at 121° C and 15 lb/in³ for 15 minutes
   c. Dry heat of 160° for 2 hours
2. Other methods
   a. Sodium hypochlorite 2.5% for 30 minutes
   b. Formalin 40% for 12 hours
   c. Glutaraldehyde 2% for 10 hours

Hygiene

Recommended guidelines for contacts of infected patients include the following:

1. Avoid sharing razors, toothbrushes, food utensils, or towels.
2. Careful personal hygiene including proper hand washing after contact.
3. Avoid (or handle carefully) secretions, including saliva and urine.

4. Needle precautions.
5. Hepatitis A/E: Isolate patients until jaundice peaks; use stool precautions.

● PROPHYLAXIS

Hepatitis A

Adequate hand hygiene, water sanitation, and food hygiene are essential to prevent the spread of hepatitis A. Two agents are available for HAV prophylaxis—hepatitis A vaccine and human immune serum globulin (HISG). Only HISG is approved for postexposure prophylaxis.[11,17]

HAV Vaccine

Based on the success of vaccination programs in high incidence areas, in 2005, the ACIP recommended that all children between 12 and 23 months of age receive immunization against HAV. Children and adolescents who were not immunized by 2 years of age should receive the vaccine at subsequent visits. Adults at high risk for HAV exposure or who are likely to have severe complications from disease should also be vaccinated, as soon as risk is identified (Table 30.3). If the potential exposure can be anticipated (i.e., travel), vaccine should be given at least 2 weeks before that exposure.[11,17]

Two Vaccines are Available: HAVRIX (GlaxoSmithKline) for those >2 years and VAQTA (Merck) for those >12 months. Both are inactivated vaccines with adult and pediatric formulations (Table 30.4). Both vaccines are highly immunogenic. Greater than 97% of children and adolescents will become seropositive within 1 month of receiving the first dose, and 100% will become seropositive after 2 doses. Protection is afforded within 4 weeks of the initial dose, and the 2nd dose is required for long-term protection. There are currently no data on the need for reimmunization in immunocompetent AYAs. It is estimated that protective levels of HAV antibodies are sustained for at least 20 years. The vaccine can be given at the same time as other vaccines and HISG. In both instances, the injections should be administered at separate injection sites.

Single-antigen HAV vaccine is also recommended for postexposure prophylaxis in certain individuals. In healthy individuals 1 to 40 years of age, single-antigen vaccine at the age-appropriate dose may be used as postexposure prophylaxis within 2 weeks of exposure. These individuals should then complete the vaccine series at the recommended interval. Vaccine can also be used when HISG cannot be obtained.

A combination HAV and HBV vaccine was approved in 2001 called Twinrix (GlaxoSmithKline). It is approved for in adults (>18 years old) and is given at 0, 1, and 6 months. Twinrix is approved for active immunization only.

TABLE 30.3

Persons at Increased Risk of Hepatitis A Infection

Travelers to countries of high/intermediate risk (*all* except Canada, Western Europe, Scandinavia, Japan, New Zealand, and Australia)

Those in close contact with an international adoptee from a country of high/intermediate risk

Men who have sex with men

IV and illicit drug users

Persons with clotting factor disorders

Persons with occupational risk (direct exposure to person with HAV or actual virus)

Persons with chronic liver disease

TABLE 30.4

Hepatitis A Vaccine Dose/Schedule

Age (y)	HAVRIX				VAQTUA			
	Dose (Elisa Units)	Volume (mL)	Number of Doses	Schedule (mo)	Dose (Units)	Volume (mL)	Number of Doses	Schedule (mo)
1–18	720	0.5	2	0, 6–12	25	0.5	2	0, 6–18
>19	1,440	1	2	0, 6–12	50	1	2	0, 6–12

Human Immune Serum Globulin

HISG provides passive, and therefore temporary, protection against HAV. HISG is indicated in the following situations:

a. HISG should be used as postexposure prophylaxis for exposed, susceptible/unvaccinated persons aged 40 years or older as there is inadequate evidence regarding the efficacy of vaccine for postexposure prophylaxis in this age-group.

b. HISG should also be used for postexposure prophylaxis in children less than 12 months of age, immunocompromised persons, persons with chronic liver disease, and those with a vaccine allergy.

Prophylactic HISG should be used in individuals who will receive the HAV vaccine ≤2 weeks prior to anticipated exposure/travel, those who refuse vaccine, or those who cannot receive the vaccine due to age (<12 months) or allergy. A dose of 0.02 mL/kg provides protection for 3 months. A dose of 0.06 mL/kg should be given if travel/exposure is anticipated to be ≥5 months.

Susceptible persons should receive HISG as soon as exposure is determined. Efficacy of HISG has not been established >2 weeks after exposure. Postexposure HISG is given intramuscularly at a dose of 0.02 mL/kg. When this dose is given within 14 days of exposure, efficacy is 80% to 90%. Unless contraindicated, HAV vaccine should be given simultaneously at a separate injection site. Because HISG decreases their efficacy, live viral vaccines should be delayed after HISG administration (>3 months for measles, mumps, rubella; >5 months for varicella). Individuals who have received at least 1 dose of HAV vaccine ≥1 month prior to exposure/travel do not need HISG.

Hepatitis B

Two agents are available for HBV prophylaxis—hepatitis B vaccines and hepatitis B immunoglobulin (HBIG). Hepatitis B vaccines provide active immunization against HBV infection and are recommended for both preexposure and postexposure prophylaxis. HBIG provides passive and temporary protection and is indicated for postexposure prophylaxis but only in certain exposure settings. The CDC's strategy to eliminate transmission of HBV infection in the US includes the following[3,11]:

• Universal vaccination of infants beginning at birth
• Prevention of perinatal infection by routine screening of all pregnant women for HBsAg and the provision of immunoprophylaxis to infants born to HBsAg-positive women (and to infants born to women in whom HBsAg status is unknown)
• Vaccination of previously unvaccinated children and adolescents
• Vaccination of previously unvaccinated adults at increased risk for infection (**Table 30.5**)

Because high-risk behavior is common and may not be identified during young adulthood, some have advocated for universal immunization for young adults not previously vaccinated.

HBV Vaccine

Two HBV vaccines are available: Recombivax HB and Energix-B (GlaxoSmithKline).[3,11] Both are available in pediatric and adult

TABLE 30.5

Persons at Increased Risk of Hepatitis B Infection

Sexual exposure
• Men who have sex with men
• Sexual contact of HBsAg-positive person
• Multiple sexual partners
• Person receiving STI treatment

Percutaneous/mucosal exposure
• Current or previous IV drug use
• Household contacts of HBsAg-positive person
• Residents/staff of facilities for developmentally disabled
• Persons with diabetes mellitus or end stage renal disease
• Health care workers with exposure to blood or blood contaminated bodily fluids.

Persons with HIV

Travel to a country with high/intermediate risk

TABLE 30.6

Hepatitis B Vaccine Dosing

Age	Recombivax HB		Energix-B	
	Dose (μg)	Volume (mL)	Dose (μg)	Volume (mL)
Adolescents				
11–15 y	10[a]	1	N/A	N/A
11–19 y	5	0.5	10	0.5
Adults (>20 y)	10	1.0	20	1.0
Dialysis/immunocompromised persons				
<20 y[b]	5	0.5	10	0.5
>20 y	40[c]	1.0	40[d]	2.0

[a]Adult formulation on 2 dose schedule.
[b]No specific recommendations have been made for higher doses.
[c]Special formulation at standard 3 dose schedule.
[d]Two 1.0 mL doses given at same site at 0, 1, 2 and 6 months.
Modified Centers for Disease Control and Prevention. Hepatitis A. In: Atkinson W, Wolfe S, Hamborsky J, eds. *Epidemiology and prevention of vaccine-preventable diseases.* 12th ed. Washington, DC: Public Health Foundation, 2012:Ch 9 (115–138).

formulations. Recombivax HB and Energix-B can be used interchangeably within the vaccine series. Adult/pediatric formulations of Recombivax HB can be used interchangeably; however, pediatric and adult formulations of Energix-B cannot be used interchangeably. Pediatric Energix-B is only approved for individuals under age 20 years, while the adult formulation of Energix-B can be used for individuals aged 11 years and older. The appropriate dose for age should be used (**Table 30.6**). Recombivax HB is approved for 2 dose scheduling in adolescents aged 11 to 15 years.

TABLE 30.7

Recommendations for Hepatitis B prophylaxis after Percutaneous or Permucosal Exposure

Exposed Person	HBsAg Positive	Treatment When Source Is	
		HBsAg Negative	Status Unknown
Unvaccinated	HBIG 1 dose[a] HBV vaccine series	HBV vaccine series	HBV vaccine series
Previously vaccinated			
Known responder	No treatment	No treatment	No treatment
Known nonresponder			
After 3 doses	HBIG 1 dose 2nd HBV vaccine series	No treatment	If source high risk, treat as if HBsAg+
After 6 doses	HBIG 2 doses[b]	No treatment	If source high risk, treat as if HBsAg+
Response unknown	Test exposed person for HBsAg Ab - Ab positive (>10ml): no treatment - Ab negative: HBIG 1 dose and HBV vaccine booster dose[c]	No treatment	Test exposed person for HBsAg Ab - Ab positive (>10ml): no treatment - Ab negative: HBV vaccine booster dose[c]

HBsAg: Hepatitis B surface Antigen; HBIG: Hepatitis B immune globulin
[a]Dose of HBIG 0.06ml/kg given intramuscularly
[b]HBIG doses should be 1 month apart
[c]Test antibody response after booster vaccine. Check at 1-2 months if no HBIG given; 4-6 months if HBIG given. If antibody response is inadequate (< 10ml) give 2 additional doses to complete 3 vaccine series.
Modified Centers for Disease Control and Prevention. Epidemiology and Prevention of Vaccine-Preventable Diseases. Atkinson W, Wolfe S, Hamborsky J, eds. 12th ed., Washington DC: Public Health Foundation, 2012. Ch 9 (115–138)

- Vaccine schedule: The vaccine schedule for children and AYAs is 3 doses given preferably at 0, 1, and 6 months. The minimal interval between dose 1 and 2 is 4 weeks and between dose 2 and 3 is 8 weeks. There should be no less than a 16-week interval between the first and third doses.
- Recombivax HB may be given on a 2 dosing schedule. Two 1 mL (10 µg) doses may be given 4 to 6 months apart. This is only approved for use in adolescents 11 to 15 years of age, and the series must be completed by 16 years of age.
- For adults over 18 years, Twinrix, a combination HBV and HAV vaccine, may be administered in a 3-dose series.

Efficacy: After receiving 3 doses of HBV vaccine, >95% of adolescents and >90% of adults will develop an adequate antibody response.[11] The vaccine is 80% effective in preventing infection in those who complete the vaccine series. Individuals who are immunocompromised or on hemodialysis require higher doses of vaccine to ensure adequate antibody response. In AYAs, HBV vaccine must be given in the deltoid muscle because the vaccine is less effective when other sites are used. Antibody levels wane over time. Up to 60% of vaccinated individuals lose detectable antibodies within 9 to 15 years after vaccination. However, protection against HBV infection and disease seems to persist. Booster doses are not needed in immunocompetent individuals.

Pre-/Postvaccine Testing
- Routine screening of AYAs prior to initiation of vaccine series is not recommended. Prevaccine screening is only recommended for those at high risk of HBV infection. Anti-HBsAg or anti-HBcAg can be used for screening purposes. Anti-HBs will not identify individuals who are carriers and therefore antibody negative. Anti-HBc will detect all previously infected persons.[11]
- Postvaccination testing for immunity is also not recommended routinely. Postvaccine serology testing is advisable only for individuals who are expected to have a poor response to vaccine or for whom HBV immune status will affect subsequent management. Risk factors for poor vaccine response include age >40 years at vaccine receipt, administration of the vaccine in a location other than the deltoid, and immunocompromised state. Postvaccination testing should be done 1 to 6 months after completion of vaccine series, since lack of antibodies many

years postvaccination may be part of the normal antibody waning seen in all persons. Individuals found to be nonresponders to vaccine should have the vaccine administered a second time on the usual 0, 1, and 6 month schedule in the deltoid muscle.[11]
- Revaccination produces adequate antibody response in 15% to 25% of nonresponders after one additional dose and 30% to 50% after 3 additional doses if given in the deltoid.[3,11] Revaccination after primary vaccine was given in the buttocks induces an adequate antibody response in >75% of people. Individuals who fail to respond to a second vaccine series should be screened for chronic HBV infection by checking HBsAg. If negative, these individuals should be considered HBV susceptible and treated appropriately if future HBV exposure occurs.

Hepatitis B Immunoglobulin

HBIG provides passive protection against HBV and is indicated after HBV exposure in susceptible persons.[3,11] Susceptible persons include infants born to mothers with known HBV, unimmunized individuals with HBV exposure, or known vaccine nonresponders. Exposure may occur at birth, through contaminated blood or through sexual contact. HBIG dose is 0.06 mL/kg given intramuscularly. The dose for newborns is 0.5 mL. Since HBV vaccine is typically administered at the same time, postexposure, HBIG should be given at a different injection site.

Hepatitis B Postexposure Prophylaxis

Prophylactic treatment to prevent HBV is recommended in certain situations—perinatal exposure, exposure to contaminated blood, and sexual contact.[3,11] Testing of pregnant women for blood and sexual contacts is recommended as soon as possible after exposure but should not delay treatment within the recommended treatment window.

a. *Perinatal exposure*: Infants born to HBsAg-positive mothers should receive HBV vaccine and HBIG as soon as possible after birth (ideally within 12 hours) at separate injection sites.[3,11] If HBV and HBIG are not given within 12 hours of delivery, they should be administered as soon as possible within 1 week after delivery. Subsequent vaccine doses should be given at 1 to 2 months and 6 months. Administration of vaccine and HBIG shortly after birth is 85% to 95% effective in preventing transmission. When HBV status is unknown, infants should receive vaccine within 12 hours of birth and subsequently be given HBIG if indicated based on mother's screening results (see "Considerations during Pregnancy" section below).

b. *Exposure to blood*: Passive prophylaxis with HBIG and/or HBV vaccine is indicated in certain situations (**Table 30.7**).[3,11] Decisions about prophylaxis depend on whether the source of exposure can be tested for HBsAg or is known to be HBsAg positive. When postexposure prophylaxis is indicated, it should be given as soon as possible. Efficacy of postexposure prophylaxis beyond 7 days has not been determined. CDC Recommendations for HBV postexposure prophylaxis can be found at http://www.cdc.gov/mmwr/preview/mmwrhtml/rr6210a1.htm

c. *Sexual Contacts of HBsAg-positive persons*: Treatment of sexual contacts should occur within 14 days of exposure.[3,11] Sexual contacts should be screened for hepatitis antibodies (anti-HBcAg and anti-HBsAg), but this screening should not delay treatment beyond 14 days. Treatment consists of HBIG (0.06 mL/kg), followed by the HBV vaccine series. Vaccine series may be started simultaneously at a different injection site. HBIG is 75% effective at preventing HBV infection.

d. *Household contacts of persons with acute HBV*: HBIG is not routinely given to household contacts of individuals with HBV unless there is known exposure to blood or the contact is younger than 12 months and there is an acute infection in the primary caregiver. *All* household contacts should receive HBV vaccine.[3,11]

Hepatitis C

There is no vaccine or immunoglobulin available for hepatitis C. If percutaneous exposure occurs, the source of exposure should be tested for HVC RNA as soon as possible. Exposed individuals should be tested immediately for HCV RNA as this is the first antigen to appear in the bloodstream. Exposed individuals should be tested again 2 to 8 weeks later for HCV RNA plus HCV antibodies and ALT.[2]

Hepatitis D

HDV infection occurs only in the presence of HBV; therefore, prevention of HBV will prevent HDV infection. Persons with exposure to HBV and HDV should be treated in the same manner as those exposed to HBV alone.

CONSIDERATIONS DURING PREGNANCY

1. Hepatitis A: There is no maternal to fetal HAV transmission during pregnancy although transmission can occur during delivery. Infants born to mother with active HAV can be screened by checking HAV IgM antibodies. The safety of HAV vaccine during pregnancy has not been determined. The theoretical risk is assumed to be low as the vaccine is made with inactivated virus.[11,18]

2. Hepatitis B: Transmission of HBV from mother to infant during the perinatal period is significant. Infants born to mother who are HBeAg and HBsAg positive have a 70% to 90% risk for chronic HBV by age 6 months without appropriate postexposure prophylaxis. The risk for chronic infection is only 10% when the mother is HBsAg positive but HBeAg negative. Unless appropriately vaccinated, children who are not infected at birth remain at risk due to long-term close personal contact. Appropriate postexposure prophylaxis prevents the development of chronic HBV in 90% to 95% of treated infants.[3,11] Therefore, the CDC recommends the following:

a. All pregnant women should be tested for HBsAg early in pregnancy even if they have a history of HBV vaccination.

b. Pregnant women without prenatal screening who engage in high-risk behaviors for HBV or with clinical hepatitis should be tested at time of delivery.

c. If testing of the mother is not possible, the infant should be given HBV vaccine within 12 hours of birth and should complete series according to schedule for infants born to HBsAg-positive mothers.

d. If mother is found to be HBsAg positive, the infant should receive HBIG and HBV vaccine within 12 hours of birth and no later than 7 days after birth. HBIG dose is 0.5 mL. HBV vaccine should be given again at 1 to 2 months and 6 months. Testing for protective antibodies should be done 3 to 9 months after completion of vaccine series. Special vaccine recommendations exist for preterm infants weighing <2,000 g.

e. Infants of HBsAg-positive mothers may begin breast-feeding at birth, even before HBV vaccine and HBIG are administered. Careful attention should be paid to avoid any nipple trauma or bleeding.

3. Hepatitis C: Pregnant women should be screened for HCV only if significant risk factors are present (IV drug use, high-risk sexual activity, HIV infection). Approximately 4% of infants born to HCV-infected mothers will become infected with HCV.[5] Transmission occurs at the time of birth, and no prophylaxis is available. Interferon and ribavirin are not approved for use in pregnancy. Transmission risk is increased in the presence of maternal HCV viremia at delivery and if the mother is co-infected with HIV. There has been no proven benefit to delivery by cesarean section; however, attention should be paid to avoid prolonged rupture of membranes or use of a scalp monitor. If HCV viral load is low, there is no contraindication to breast-feeding unless the mother's nipples are bleeding or traumatized. Infants born to HCV-positive mothers should be tested for HCV between 2 and 6 months and again between 18 to 24 months.[5,12] Screening for HCV RNA should only be done at 2 to 6 months since HCV antibodies from the mother may persist until the infant is 18 months of age. Testing for HCV RNA and HCV antibodies should be done at 18 to 24 months.

4. Hepatitis E: While typically self-limiting, HEV infection results in a higher rate of fulminant hepatitis and even death during pregnancy. This has been thought to be secondary to the effect of hormonal changes on the immune system. Mortality rates among pregnant women are higher in certain geographical regions, particularly India. In areas where HEV is endemic, it is the most common cause of hepatitis during pregnancy.[6,15]

ACKNOWLEDGMENT

The authors wish to acknowledge Praveen S. Goday for contributions to previous versions of this chapter.

REFERENCES

1. Centers for Disease Control and Prevention. Surveillance for acute viral hepatitis—United States, 2007. *MMWR Surveill Summ* 2009;58(3):1–27.
2. Centers for Disease Control and Prevention; National Division for HIV/AIDS, STD & TB Prevention, Division of Viral Hepatitis. *Viral hepatitis surveillance, United States, 2011*. Available at http://www.cdc.gov/hepatitis/Statistics/2011Surveillance/. Accessed January 10, 2014.
3. Centers for Disease Control and Prevention. A comprehensive immunization strategy to eliminate transmission of hepatitis B virus infection in the United States. Recommendations of the Advisory Committee on Immunization Practices (ACIP), Part 1: immunization of infants, children, and adolescents. *MMWR* 2005;54(RR-16):1–23.
4. Kim WR. Epidemiology of hepatitis B in the United States. *Hepatology* 2009;49 (suppl 5):S28–S34.
5. Mack L, Gonzalez-Peralta RP, Gupta N, et al. NASPGHAN practice guidelines: diagnosis and management of hepatitis C infection in infants, children, and adolescents. *J Pediatr Gastroenterol Nutr* 2012;54(6):838–855.
6. Clemente-Casares P, Pina S, et al. Hepatitis E virus epidemiology in industrialized countries. *Emerg Infect Dis* 2003;9(4):448–454.
7. Halac U, Béland K, Lapierre P, et al. Cirrhosis due to chronic hepatitis E infection in a child post-bone marrow transplant. *J Pediatr* 2012;160(5):871–874.
8. Clemente M, Schwarz K. Hepatitis: general principles. *Pediatr Rev* 2011;32(8):333–340.

9. Hochman JA, Balistreri WF. Chronic viral hepatitis: always be current. *Pediatr Rev* 2003;24(12):399–410.

10. Centers for Disease Control and Prevention: Division of Viral Hepatitis; National Center for HIV/AIDS, Viral Hepatitis, STD, and TB Prevention, Division of Viral Hepatitis. *Viral Hepatitis-Resource Center*. Available at http://www.cdc.gov/hepatitis/Resources/Professionals/Training/Serology/training.htm. Accessed January 5, 2014.

11. Centers for Disease Control and Prevention. *Epidemiology and prevention of vaccine-preventable diseases.* 12th ed. Washington, DC: Public Health Foundation, 2012.

12. Ghany M, Strader D, Thomas D, et al. Diagnosis, management, and treatment of hepatitis C: an update. *Hepatology* 2009;49(4):1335–1374.

13. Murray K, Shah U, Mohan N, et al; Chronic Hepatitis Working Group. Chronic hepatitis. *J Pediatr Gastroenterol Nutr* 2008;47(2):225–233.

14. Hughes J, Wilson M, Teshale E, et al. The two faces of hepatitis E virus. *Clin Infect Dis* 2010;51(3):328–334.

15. Navaneethan U, Al Mohajer M, Shata MT. Hepatitis E and pregnancy: understanding pathogenesis. *Liver Int* 2008;28(9):1190–1199.

16. Jonas M, Block J, Haber B, et al. Treatment of children with chronic hepatitis B virus infection in the United States: patient selection and therapeutic options. *Hepatology* 2010;52(6):2192–2205.

17. Centers for Disease Control and Prevention. Prevention of hepatitis A through active or passive immunization. Recommendations of the Advisory Committee on Immunization Practices (ACIP). *MMWR* 2006;55 (RR-7):1–23.

18. Spradling PR, Rupp L, Moorman AC, et al. Hepatitis B and C virus infection among 1.2 million persons with access to care: Factors associated with testing and infection prevalence. *Clin Infectious Dis* 2012;55(8):1047–55.

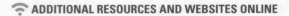 **ADDITIONAL RESOURCES AND WEBSITES ONLINE**

31

Human Immunodeficiency Virus Infections and Acquired Immunodeficiency Syndrome

Lisa K. Simons
Marvin E. Belzer

Human Immunodeficiency Virus Infections and Acquired Immunodeficiency Syndrome

KEY WORDS

- Acquired immunodeficiency syndrome (AIDS)
- Antiretroviral therapy (ART)
- Exposure
- Human immunodeficiency virus (HIV)
- Prevention
- Preexposure prophylaxis (PrEP)
- Testing
- Transmission
- Treatment
- Virus

TABLE 31.1

Clinical Manifestations of Acute HIV-1 Infection

Features	Overall % (n = 378)
Fever	75
Fatigue	68
Myalgia	49
Skin rash	48
Headache	45
Pharyngitis	40
Cervical adenopathy	39
Arthralgia	30
Night sweats	28
Diarrhea	27

Adapted from Daar ES, Pilcher CD, Hecht FM. Clinical presentation and diagnosis of primary HIV-1 infection. *Curr Opin HIV AIDS* 2008;3(1):10–15.

As of December 2012, over 35 million people worldwide were living with human immunodeficiency virus (HIV), the virus responsible for the advanced immunocompromised condition known as acquired immunodeficiency syndrome (AIDS). The number of people living with HIV continues to rise with the combined effects of improving therapies and high rates of new infections, particularly among adolescents and young adults (AYAs). While antiretroviral therapy (ART) allows most adherent youth to live healthy lives with simple once-a-day regimens, existing challenges for care providers involve identifying HIV-positive youth, engaging them in care, and assisting them with long-term adherence to medications.

In July 2013, 3 years after the establishment of the National HIV/AIDS Strategy, the nation's first comprehensive federal plan addressing the domestic epidemic, President Barack Obama released an Executive Order instituting the HIV Care Continuum Initiative.[1] Also referred to as the HIV treatment cascade, the "HIV care continuum" provides a framework for understanding engagement in care as a spectrum, ranging from "not in care" (either aware or unaware of HIV status) to "fully engaged in HIV primary care." For individuals to fully benefit from treatment, they need to be aware of their infection, engage and remain in medical care, and obtain and adhere to ART. Accordingly, HIV service delivery in the US has shifted toward a public health model with strategies simultaneously aimed at improving testing and early diagnosis, enhancing linkage and retention in care, and supporting access and adherence to ART.

ETIOLOGY, PATHOGENESIS, AND NATURAL HISTORY

The causative agent of AIDS is HIV, a single-stranded RNA retrovirus that infects and leads to the destruction of CD4$^+$ T lymphocytes. HIV-1 is the cause of most cases of AIDS in the world. HIV-2, a retrovirus related to HIV-1, is found primarily in Central Africa and generally has a slower progression (20 years versus 5 to 10 years with HIV-1) but a similar spectrum of disease.

Acute HIV infection presents as a mononucleosis-like illness in many but not all patients, 2 to 6 weeks after infection. The illness typically lasts 1 to 2 weeks and causes nonspecific constitutional symptoms as well as myalgias, lymphadenopathy, and sore throat (Table 31.1). Without a high index of suspicion, the diagnosis may be unrecognized by clinicians.

While the phase of illness following acute infection is one of clinical latency, it is now clear that viral production is steady at an estimated 10 billion virions daily. During this time, T cell production and destruction remain precariously balanced.

A slow but steady depletion of CD4$^+$ T cells occurs in all but a small percentage of untreated patients, who are referred to as long-term nonprogressors. Without treatment, the average rate of decline of CD4$^+$ T cells is about 50/mm^3/year and most patients develop AIDS (severe immune deficiency) over a period of 8 to 10 years. Approximately 10% of newly infected individuals will rapidly progress to an AIDS diagnosis within 4 years. Numerous studies indicate that ART can suppress the viral load to undetectable levels in most patients. Viral suppression is associated with a steady immune reconstitution in most patients. Even patients with severe depletion of their immune systems can often return to excellent health after successful treatment.

AYAs identified with HIV early, who successfully initiate ART, should have a near-normal life span if good adherence persists and risks, such as drug use, are avoided.[2] There is growing evidence that chronic HIV infection elicits systemic inflammation that accelerates risk for cardiovascular illness. Even with effective antiretroviral treatment, HIV-positive individuals have higher cardiovascular risk, and cardiovascular disease has emerged as an important cause of death in patients with HIV.[3] Research is in progress to determine if therapy with medications like statins can reduce inflammation and cardiovascular risk.[4]

Another area of emerging research is neurocognitive function in HIV-positive adolescents. In one study of 220 recently diagnosed youth (mean age 21) naive to ART, 67% of participants demonstrated neuropsychological testing consistent with asymptomatic HIV-associated neurocognitive disorder.[5] There were high rates of impairment in learning and memory as well as executive functioning that clearly impact clinicians' approach to patient management. Research examining the impact of ART on neurocognitive changes is ongoing.

EPIDEMIOLOGY

Prevalence

At the end of 2009, the Centers for Disease Control and Prevention (CDC) estimated that 1,148,200 persons aged 13 and older were living with HIV infection in the US, including 207,600 (18.1%) persons unaware of their infection. *Youth aged 13 to 24 made up 7% of the 1.1 million living with HIV.*[6]

Incidence

From 2008 through 2011, the number of new HIV infections in the US remained stable, at approximately 50,000 new cases each year. *In 2010, one in four new infections occurred in AYAs aged 13 to 24.*[6]

Age

AYAs are particularly impacted by HIV. In 2010, the CDC reported an estimated 12,000 new HIV infections in youth aged 13 to 24. Although young people in this age group represented 16% of the US population in 2010, they accounted for 26% of all new diagnoses made that year. Young adults aged 20 to 24 have the highest number of new cases of HIV compared with other age groups. The CDC estimates that approximately 60% of all youth living with HIV in the US are unaware of their infection.[6]

Ethnicity

Communities of color continue to be disproportionately impacted by HIV infection. Among youth in the US aged 13 to 24, 60% of new infections occurred in Blacks and 20% in Hispanic in 2010.[6]

Gender

At the end of 2010, 75% of adolescents and adults aged 13 years or over living with HIV were men and 25% were women. Figure 31.1 shows that the number of young males living with HIV is higher than females, and this difference increases with age. It is important to note that while transgender individuals are at highest risk for HIV, data for these communities are lacking as a result of the absence of uniform data collection approaches.

Transmission

Figures 31.2 and 31.3 show the common routes of transmission for males and females diagnosed with HIV/AIDS in 2011. Most new cases in males occur in men who have sex with men (MSM), while the majority of new infections among females are transmitted through heterosexual contact and intravenous (IV) drug use.[6] Young men who have sex with men (YMSM), especially Black and Hispanic YMSM, are at especially high risk of acquiring HIV.

TRANSMISSION

HIV can be transmitted only by the exchange of body fluids. Blood, semen, vaginal secretions, and breast milk are the only fluids documented to be associated with HIV infection. Although HIV is found in saliva, tears, urine, and sweat, no case has been documented that implicates these fluids as agents of infection.

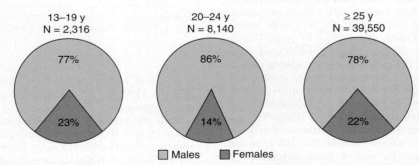

FIGURE 31.1 Diagnosis of HIV infection among persons aged 13 years and older, by sex and age group, 2011—United States and 6 dependent areas. (From Centers for Disease Control and Prevention. *HIV surveillance in adolescents and young adults.* Slide set available at http://www.cdc.gov/hiv/pdf/statistics_surveillance_Adolescents.pdf. Accessed 2014.)

Transmission category	13–19 y No.	13–19 y %	20–24 y No.	20–24 y %
Male-to-male sexual contact	1,664	92.8	6,354	90.8
Injection drug use (IDU)	23	1.4	117	1.7
Male-to-male sexual contact and IDU	37	2.1	232	3.3
Heterosexual contact[a]	67	3.7	294	4.2
Other[b]	0	0.0	0	0.0
Total	**1,794**	**100**	**6,998**	**100**

FIGURE 31.2 Diagnosis of HIV infection among adolescent and young adult males, by age group and transmission category 2011—United States and 6 dependent areas. (From Centers for Disease Control and Prevention. *HIV surveillance in adolescents and young adults.* Slide set at available at http://www.cdc.gov/hiv/pdf/statistics_surveillance_Adolescents.pdf. Accessed 2014.)
[a]Heterosexual contact with a person known to have, or to be at high risk for, HIV infection.
[b]Includes hemophilia, blood transfusion, perinatal exposure, and risk factor not reported or identified.

Transmission category	13–19 y		20–24 y	
	No.	%	No.	%
Injection drug use	37	7.0	101	8.8
Heterosexual contact[a]	485	92.7	1,041	91.2
Other[b]	0	0.3	0	0.0
Total	**523**	**100**	**1,142**	**100**

FIGURE 31.3 Diagnosis of HIV infection among adolescent and young adult females, by age group and transmission category 2011—United States and 6 dependent areas. (From Centers for Disease Control and Prevention. *HIV surveillance in adolescents and young adults*. Slide set at available at http://www.cdc.gov/hiv/pdf/ statistics_surveillance_Adolescents.pdf. Accessed 2014.)
[a]Heterosexual contact with a person known to have, or to be at high risk for, HIV infection.
[b]Includes hemophilia, blood transfusion, perinatal exposure, and risk factor not reported or identified.

IV Drug Use

HIV is easily transmitted by needle sharing. Because of the unreliability and frequent unacceptance of needle bleaching and unacceptance or inaccessibility of drug treatment, almost all public health organizations support needle exchange programs. In these programs, injection drug users can exchange dirty needles for clean ones while at the same time gaining access to condoms, bleach, and referral resources. Many programs across the US have shown that injection drug use does not increase in the community or in an individual user when needle exchange is available. Moreover, HIV and other blood-borne disease transmissions (e.g., hepatitis) are markedly reduced with the availability of needle exchange programs.[7]

Sex

Sexual transmission of HIV is thought to have a hierarchy of relative risk. Receptive anal intercourse without condoms is riskiest, followed by insertive anal intercourse and vaginal intercourse. Oral sex is categorized as less risky but has been shown to transmit HIV. Studies have shown that the proper and consistent use of latex condoms or dental dams can markedly reduce the risk for HIV transmission during sex.[8]

Vertical Transmission

Universal opt-out HIV screening of pregnant women, antiretroviral treatment and prophylaxis, use of cesarean delivery when appropriate, and avoidance of breast-feeding have greatly reduced perinatal HIV transmission in the US. With early diagnosis, appropriate treatment, and avoidance of breast-feeding, transmission risk is reduced to 2% or less.[9] According to the CDC, in 2011, an estimated 192 children younger than 13 years were infected with HIV, 127 of these being perinatally infected.[6]

⬤ HIV PREVENTION

The HIV prevention paradigm has shifted significantly in recent years. Primary prevention efforts to reduce the HIV risks of uninfected persons have expanded beyond behavioral interventions to include biomedical interventions like preexposure prophylaxis (PrEP), public health strategies like HIV counseling and testing, and structural interventions that address community partnerships and collaboration, including increasing access to condoms. The White House and other public health leaders have increasingly emphasized secondary prevention (reducing transmission risks from persons living with HIV) through "Treatment as Prevention."

Primary Prevention
Preexposure Prophylaxis

PrEP is an HIV prevention method that uses a daily antiretroviral pill to reduce transmission to HIV-negative individuals at high risk of infection. In a multinational study of 2,470 sero-negative MSM and 29 transgender women, participants were randomly assigned to emtricitabine/tenofovir (Truvada®), a two-drug combination

antiretroviral pill, or a placebo. All received HIV testing, condoms, and risk reduction counseling. PrEP was found to reduce the risk of transmission by 44% among all participants and by 92% in those with detectable drug levels. No differences were detected in high-risk sexual practices or sexually transmitted infections (STIs) between the two groups.[10] Two large trials conducted in Africa, Partners-PrEP and TDF2, demonstrated the efficacy of PrEP with antiretrovirals in heterosexual individuals at high risk of HIV acquisition.[11,12] Based on these results, the US Food and Drug Administration (FDA) approved the use of daily emtricitabine/tenofovir in 2012 for uninfected adults (including adolescents aged 18 and older) at high risk of acquiring HIV, to be used in combination with safe sex practices. Recommendations include the integration of behavioral interventions with ongoing HIV testing for those choosing to utilize PrEP.

While initial studies suggest that PrEP may be a promising strategy for HIV prevention, research studies focusing specifically on adolescents are needed prior to development of recommendations for the use of PrEP in adolescents under 18 years. Questions remain as to whether the use of PrEP in youth is cost effective, whether youth engaging in high-risk behaviors can adhere to daily use of PrEP, and whether or not high-risk youth will continue to use condoms at the same rate as they did prior to the introduction of PrEP. Current studies are examining the efficacy, safety, and tolerability of PrEP in adolescents (under 18 years). Research is also investigating whether topical PrEP or intermittent use of oral PrEP is effective.

Nonoccupational Postexposure Prophylaxis

Nonoccupational postexposure prophylaxis (nPEP) after injection drug use, sexual, or other nonoccupational exposure to HIV may be recommended to prevent HIV infection for persons seeking care within 72 hours of exposure to blood, genital secretions, or other potentially infectious body fluids. Expert consultation is available through the National HIV/AIDS Clinician's Consultation PEPline at 1-888-448-4911 (see Additional Resources at the end of this chapter) to help clinicians determine if the exposure represents substantial risk and which antiretroviral regimen is most appropriate. Sexual assault survivors should always be offered nPEP. When PEP is recommended, it should be initiated as early as possible after exposure (ideally within 72 hours). nPEP typically consists of a 28-day two- or three-drug antiretroviral regimen. Sequential follow-up HIV testing should be organized by the clinician. It is unknown if treatment for exposures initiated after 72 hours provides any reduction in HIV infection risk.

HIV Prevention Education

AYAs frequently receive general HIV education in school settings. More targeted approaches with high-risk populations like YMSM, transgender women, or women of color are best employed utilizing evidence-based interventions that are strongly connected to HIV and STI screening, such as those published by the CDC (http://www.effectiveinterventions.org/en/HighImpactPrevention/Interventions.aspx). The CDC has also increased focus on community-level structural changes involving changing policy, laws, access to services, and so on.

VIII

Appropriate educational interventional goals for HIV-negative AYAs include the following:

1. Reducing misinformation about and prejudice against HIV-positive persons
2. Helping to reduce high-risk behavior, including recommendations to decrease unprotected sexual activity, numbers of sexual partners, and experimentation with drugs
3. Supporting AYAs who choose abstinence
4. Increasing use of condoms and other barrier methods by AYAs who are sexually active
5. Encouraging young people in sexual relationships to get HIV tested along with their partners
6. Referral and/or linkage to behavioral and biomedical interventions (e.g., nPEP and PrEP) as appropriate.

HIV/AIDS prevention education should be conducted at schools, religious organizations, youth organizations, medical facilities, and meetings with parents. Media (Internet, television, radio, magazines) are powerful methods to impart information that may change AYAs' attitudes. Outreach to youth where they congregate can be an especially effective method of reaching high-risk populations such as homeless, gang involved, or out-of-school youth. Involving peers in the education process can also be helpful.

It is important to offer HIV/AIDS education in a language and format that the adolescent or young adult can understand. The information must be simple, accurate, and direct. Previously, the federal government allocated many resources to *abstinence-only* prevention education, despite a lack of evidence that this approach was effective. *Abstinence-based* education, which promotes abstinence but also provides information on how to reduce risk if sexually active, has been shown to delay the onset of sexual activity in some studies. Information on peer-reviewed programs that have been shown to be effective can be found at http://www.effectiveinterventions.org/en/Home.aspx.

Secondary Prevention

Since the onset of the HIV epidemic, prevention strategies in the US have largely targeted persons at risk for acquiring HIV and have been aimed at reducing sexual and drug-using risk behaviors. While these continue, new efforts have been initiated that place a greater emphasis on targeting HIV transmission by those living with HIV. These efforts include peer navigation programs (where AYAs diagnosed with HIV are supported by peers who are living with HIV or have experience with HIV), medication adherence interventions, and behavioral interventions that focus on reducing STIs. Data indicate that less than half of youth infected with HIV are aware of their status and of those in care, less than half have adequately suppressed their HIV.

The most significant change in the landscape for HIV prevention is the emphasis on the role of HIV treatment as a method of HIV prevention, a shift resulting from mounting evidence suggesting that treating HIV-positive individuals reduces HIV transmission to uninfected partners. In 2011, a landmark study conducted by the HIV Prevention Trials Network (HPTN 052) was stopped three years earlier than planned when it became clear that treating HIV-positive individuals with ART regardless of their T cell count significantly reduced the risk of heterosexual transmission and that it would be unethical to continue recruiting for the study. The randomized study showed that by suppressing detectable viremia, ART produced a 96% reduction risk in sexual transmission of HIV to uninfected partners.[13] "Treatment as prevention," which refers to the personal and public health benefits of treating HIV-positive individuals with ART, has driven treatment guidelines to recommend that HIV-positive individuals consider taking antiretroviral medications as soon as they are prepared to be adherent.

⬤ HIV TESTING

Early diagnosis and entry into care are critical steps in addressing the HIV epidemic, yet many HIV-positive individuals, especially youth, remain unaware of their status. The importance of HIV testing cannot be overstated. A number of factors, including consent, confidentiality, and appropriate counseling, should be considered when screening for HIV in AYAs.

Consent and Confidentiality

Health care practitioners must balance the protection of AYAs' rights against the amount of information needed to deliver proper care. Laws governing an individual's ability to consent for HIV testing and receive confidential care vary within the US and from country to country. Current US regulations are described here:

Individuals older than 18 years who are competent: The CDC recommends that patients in all health care settings receive HIV testing as part of routine primary medical care. Separate informed consent (from the general medical consent) need not be done and prevention counseling should not be required for HIV diagnostic testing or as part of HIV screening programs.

Individuals between 12 and 17 years: The laws vary widely from state to state. According to the Guttmacher Institute, all 50 states and the District of Columbia allow minors to consent to STI services, although some states specify a minimum age (generally 12 or 14 but 16 in South Carolina) one must reach before they can provide consent.[14] Thirty-one states explicitly include HIV testing and treatment as part of STI services for which minors can consent.[14] Many states allow (but do not require) physicians to notify a minor's parents that their child is seeking STI services.

Individuals younger than 12 years and incompetent adolescents: For these individuals, a third party (parent or guardian) authorizes testing. However, this authorization may be restricted by state laws.

An increasing number of states have statutes governing HIV testing. Without such a statute, general laws regarding minors apply. It is not clear whether HIV testing would fall under the category of consent for STI services in states that do not declare HIV to be an STI. Clinicians worldwide need to be familiar with local laws regarding the following:

1. Consent for testing: Who can consent? What is the required informed consent? Are pretest and posttest counseling available?
2. Who can receive the results of these tests and under what circumstances?
3. Where can test results be recorded?
4. What can be written in the chart regarding testing and test results?

To Whom Should HIV Testing Be Offered?

In 2006, the CDC modified its recommendations to advise that HIV testing be routine for all sexually active adolescents and adults between the ages of 13 and 64 years when they access health care. Youth should be advised that they will be tested and given the option to decline. Following initial testing, persons at high risk should be screened at minimum once annually. Prevention counseling is not required but does continue to offer benefit for health care systems that have the ability to provide this service. At the time of this publication, laws in all but two states (Nebraska and New York) were consistent with these CDC recommendations.[15] Clinicians in the US can access more information regarding state-specific laws at http://www.cdc.gov/hiv/policies/law/states/index.html. Clinicians practicing outside of the US should be familiar with local laws governing HIV testing.

The following groups are at high risk and should have repeat testing at least annually:

1. MSM regardless of sexual orientation (note that many youth in this group may not self-identify as gay or bisexual)
2. Transgender women (MTF) who have sex with men

3. Youth who share needles (e.g., steroid injections and recreational drugs)
4. Youth with partners from the above three groups
5. Youth who have had intercourse or shared needles with HIV-positive persons
6. Youth with other STIs
7. Sexually active youth from economically disadvantaged areas or areas of known high seroprevalence
8. Youth with multiple sexual partners

Who Should Have HIV Testing Deferred?

Expert opinion suggests testing be deferred in the following situations:

1. Suicidal teens and those who indicate they would seriously consider suicide if HIV positive
2. Intoxicated and drug-withdrawing youth
3. Severely mentally ill youth who cannot provide consent for testing

When Should Testing Be Repeated for Youth with Positive Confirmatory HIV Test Results?

Testing should be repeated for the following persons:

1. Any youth who desires a second test
2. Any youth who is claiming to be HIV positive but has unreliable documentation
3. Youth who are at extremely low risk and have a single positive test result
4. Youth with normal CD4$^+$ T cells and undetectable viral load, who are not taking antiretroviral medications and have had only a single positive test result in the past

Youth-Specific Testing

Testing can occur in a number of settings. Many testing sites now have counselors (including peers) who are specifically trained to work with AYAs and may therefore be perceived as youth friendly. Counselors should have specialized training to address identified risks and knowledge of effective interventions and resources for youth. Often, these sites are colocated where other services or activities are available for youth (e.g., homeless shelters, free clinics, schools, recreational centers, mobile testing vans). Youth-specific testing should be recommended whenever possible, because it can be an effective component of prevention education. In particular, testing that is targeted to subpopulations of youth highly impacted by HIV can support National HIV/AIDS Strategy goals for identification of the large percentage of youth who are unaware of their HIV status. However, this approach should not deter from routine testing in all clinical settings, which is a strategy critical to identification of the 60% of youth who are infected but unaware aware of their status.

🔵 HIV COUNSELING AND TESTING

The primary goals of HIV testing are detection of HIV-positive patients and linkage to appropriate health care and supportive services. The CDC has moved in a direction of increasing access and removing barriers to HIV testing through new testing technologies and approaches, including the option of not requiring prevention counseling. While HIV prevention counseling is no longer required for HIV testing, for many adolescents, pretest counseling is a highly "teachable" moment.

HIV Tests

The technology for HIV testing continues to evolve at a rapid pace. Available assays rely on various methods, including detection of (1) HIV antibodies, (2) the viral p24 antigen, and (3) viral nucleic acid. Standard and rapid HIV tests are now available with sensitivities and specificities exceeding 99%.

Standard Testing

Standard testing uses an enzyme immunoassay (EIA) to detect HIV antibodies. To exclude false-positive results, positive EIA results should be followed by a confirmatory Western blot analysis, which detects antibodies to specific viral proteins and has nearly 100% specificity. An isolated positive EIA test should never be reported to a patient as a positive test result for HIV (see below). Western blot tests can be indeterminate, most commonly for patients in the window phase between acute infection and seroconversion. The time delay from HIV infection to positive Western blot averages 21 days with newer test reagents, although rare cases of prolonged seroconversion (6 months or longer) have been reported. However, many patients with indeterminate tests will later test HIV negative by EIA or Western blot. It is recommended that testing be repeated until a definitive positive or negative result occurs, typically at 1, 3, and 6 months following an indeterminate Western blot. In confusing cases, including indeterminate results, false reporting, and patients who are potentially in the window period, HIV RNA determination by polymerase chain reaction (PCR) may be helpful in clarifying serostatus.

Rapid HIV Antibody Tests

Rapid HIV antibody tests offer preliminary test results within 1 to 40 minutes, providing a critical opportunity for counseling and linkage to care while eliminating the need for return visits. Easy administration allows for rapid, low-cost screening in high-volume settings such as emergency departments. For these reasons, rapid tests have become the screening of choice in the US and many parts of the world. One recent study has shown that youth accept and prefer point-of-care testing over traditional tests.[16]

Since 2002, the FDA has approved a number of rapid HIV tests for use on serum, whole blood (fingerstick samples), and oral secretions. Rapid tests have excellent diagnostic accuracy, with sensitivities and specificities over 99%. The CDC Web site (http://www.cdc.gov/hiv/testing/laboratorytests.html) has extensive information on the use of rapid HIV testing, including specific recommendations for providers regarding the Clinical Laboratory Improvement Amendments Program, counseling, and quality assurance guidelines. In 2010 and 2013, respectively, the FDA approved the INSTI HIV-1 antibody test, which provides results in as little as 60 seconds, and the OraQuick In-home HIV Test, the first rapid over-the-counter home-use oral secretion testing kit.

Rapid HIV tests report results as positive, negative, or indeterminate. As with standard EIA tests, positive results should be followed by confirmatory testing. If a Western blot is used for confirmation, patients must be educated that the preliminary test is positive but there is no definitive diagnosis until confirmation tests return. Indeterminate results also require further testing, either with a repeat antibody test, Western blot or, if acute HIV infection is suspected, with viral RNA test and fourth-generation tests (described below). A negative test result does not need to be confirmed.

New testing algorithms have been adopted in many organizations that include the use of a second rapid test kit (different than initial) to confirm positive test results during the same visit. If a second rapid HIV test is used for confirmation, the patient is given a presumptive positive result and connected to services for further diagnostic evaluation (e.g., viral load). Use of a two-test rapid HIV testing algorithm rather than traditional confirmatory testing with a Western blot may improve linkage to care in some settings.[17]

Fourth-generation HIV Tests

New fourth-generation HIV tests have the advantage of detecting the viral p24 antigen as well as HIV antibodies. Combination antibody–antigen tests may allow HIV detection during acute infection before HIV antibodies are formed, effectively shortening the window period. These tests can be used for screening and are particularly helpful for use in acute settings such as delivery rooms and occupational exposures. While not yet widely available, a rapid combination antibody–antigen test was approved by the FDA in August 2013.

Viral Nucleic Acid Tests

Viral nucleic acid tests remain the test of choice for detection of early or acute HIV infection. PCR-based tests are frequently used to detect HIV RNA. Time to positivity is determined by the sensitivity of the individual test, and ultrasensitive assays are now capable of detecting very low levels of viremia as early as five days following infection.

Posttest Counseling for Positive Test Results

Posttest counseling should be given in-person and should include the following:

1. Provide the results of the test: This should be done in a direct manner at the beginning of the posttest session. If a screening antibody test was reactive and a two-test rapid HIV testing algorithm is not standard care, then a Western blot is ordered. It is imperative to explain that the screening was positive and that a definitive diagnosis cannot be made until confirmatory results return.
2. Allow the adolescent or young adult time to express feelings and reactions: It is important to give the adolescent or young adult hope by reiterating the advances in medical treatment discussed during the pretest session.
3. Assess the adolescent or young adult's understanding of the result: This is best assessed by asking the adolescent or young adult directly what the test result means to him or her. The youth should be supported in identifying behavior change goals to reduce their risk of transmitting the virus to others. The youth should also understand that although the virus is probably present for life, a positive antibody test does not mean one has AIDS. Antibody-positive youth should be advised as follows:
   a. Do not donate blood, semen, or body organs.
   b. Employ safer sex practices.
   c. Inform physicians and dentists of HIV status.
   d. Encourage sexual partners, children, and needle contacts to seek evaluation and testing (many counties in the US and other countries have anonymous partner notification programs).
   e. No evidence exists that HIV is transmitted to family household members or to close contacts by routes other than sexual intercourse, exposure to infected blood, and perinatal transmission.
   f. Household items may be shared by HIV-positive individuals and household members. Personal hygiene items (i.e., razors and toothbrushes) should not be shared.
   g. Bathroom facilities may be used by all household members.
4. Refer the patient to an HIV specialist, preferentially one who is experienced with AYAs. Ideally, the clinic will have a multidisciplinary team that includes a clinician, social worker, nurse, and other caregivers to assist the patient with managing their disease. It is highly advisable to get multiple contact methods (phone, email, Facebook, other social media, etc.) from the patient so that they can be reached in subsequent weeks to ensure they have been linked to care.

● MANAGEMENT OF HIV INFECTION IN AYAs

Initial Assessment

History and Physical Examination

The history and physical examination should evaluate the following:

1. Prior exposure to diseases that are likely to reactivate, including tuberculosis (TB), syphilis, herpes genitalis, herpes zoster, and cytomegalovirus (CMV) infections
2. Number of children, their ages, and their health status
3. Injection drug-use history and history of alcohol and other drug use

4. Sexual history, past history of STIs
5. History of mental health problems, such as depression and anxiety
6. Prior immunizations
7. A review of systems, focusing particularly on the following:
   a. Systemic: Anorexia, weight loss, fevers, night sweats
   b. Skin: Pruritis, rashes, pigmented lesions
   c. Lymphatic: Increased size of lymph nodes
   d. Eyes, ears, nose, and throat: Change in vision, sinus congestion
   e. Cardiopulmonary: Cough, dyspnea
   f. Gastrointestinal: Dysphagia, abdominal pain, and diarrhea
   g. Musculoskeletal: Myalgias, arthralgias
   h. Neurological: Memory loss, neuralgias, motor weakness, and headache
   i. Genitourinary: Bumps, ulcers, dysuria, or discharge
8. Careful measurement of weight, height, body mass index, and vital signs
9. Careful physical examination assessing the following:
   a. Skin: Seborrhea, folliculitis, Kaposi sarcoma (KS) lesions, psoriasis, tinea, herpetic lesions, genital lesions, and molluscum contagiosum
   b. Eye: Visual acuity and fields, cotton-wool spots, and hemorrhagic exudates on fundoscopic examination
   c. Mouth: Periodontal disease (gingivitis), oral hairy leukoplakia (white plaques along lateral aspect of tongue), thrush, oral ulcers, and KS lesions
   d. Lymphatic: Asymmetrical, tender, enlarged nodes, particularly posterior cervical, axillary, and epitrochlear nodes
   e. Cardiopulmonary: Rales, murmurs (in injection drug users)
   f. Gastrointestinal: Hepatosplenomegaly
   g. Genitourinary: Herpetic lesions, warts; penile discharge in males; cervical discharge or vaginal discharge in females
   h. Anal: Perianal ulcers, fissures, and condyloma
   i. Neurological: Focal findings, altered mental status

Laboratory Evaluation

Initial assessment should include the following:

1. Complete blood count (anemia, leukopenia, or thrombocytopenia)
2. Chemistry panel (hypergammaglobulinemia, hypoalbuminemia, hypocholesterolemia, elevated liver enzymes, or decreased renal function)
3. Urinalysis
4. $CD4^+$ T cell count and percentage
5. Viral load (HIV RNA PCR)
6. HIV-resistance testing in patients with acute or recent seroconversion
7. TB screening with either purified protein derivative (PPD, tuberculin skin test) or interferon-gamma release assays (IGRA)
8. Serology for hepatitis A, B, and C, toxoplasmosis, and varicella if previous infection or immunization status is not known
9. Chest radiograph (CXR) is recommended by the CDC for detection of asymptomatic TB and to serve as a baseline study; however, due to low yield of CXR abnormalities, it is not universally obtained in patients with a negative TB screen
10. Tests for syphilis, gonorrhea, and chlamydia infections if sexually experienced
11. Papanicolaou test (Pap smear) in women who have ever been sexually active, regardless of age. If normal, the Pap smear should be repeated in 6 months.

Vaccinations

For more detailed information, refer to the Advisory Committee on Immunization Practices (ACIP) general recommendations on immunization.[18]

1. Hepatitis A: Recommended for all previously unvaccinated individuals at risk for infection. Specific indications include but are not limited to MSM, persons who use injection or

non-injection illicit drugs, persons with chronic liver disease, and persons traveling to or working in countries with high or intermediate endemicity of hepatitis A.

2. Hepatitis B: Recommended for all patients without evidence of hepatitis B immunity or chronic infection. Retrospective studies demonstrate that many AYAs with HIV do not develop antibodies to hepatitis B after three immunizations. Physicians can consider a fourth immunization or repeating the series after the patient begins ART.

3. Human papillomavirus (HPV): Recommended for both males and females living with HIV through the age of 26 years if they did not receive or complete the series. Given the high HPV burden in those infected with HIV, vaccination has the potential to be very beneficial. While immunogenicity and safety of HPV vaccination have been studied in adult men with HIV, investigations with HIV-positive adolescents are ongoing.

4. Influenza: While intranasal vaccination is contraindicated, the inactivated vaccine should be offered annually.

5. Measles, mumps, rubella (MMR): MMR is generally considered safe in most patients with HIV but is contraindicated in individuals with severe immunosuppression (defined as CD4$^+$ count below 200 cells/μL or CD4$^+$ less than or equal to 15%).

6. Meningococcal vaccination: HIV-positive individuals are likely at increased risk for meningococcal disease. Their response rates to the vaccine may be suboptimal, however, and ACIP recommends a two-dose primary series with conjugated vaccine (given at least eight weeks apart) for HIV-positive adolescents receiving their first vaccine between ages 11 and 18.

7. Tetanus, diptheria, and acellular pertussis (Tdap): HIV is not a contraindication to Tdap vaccination; follow general AYA vaccination schedules. However, the immune response in those who are immunosuppressed might be suboptimal.

8. Pneumococcal: If neither pneumococcal conjugate vaccine (PCV13) nor pneumococcal polysaccharide vaccine (PPSV23) has been received previously, administer one dose of PCV13 as soon as possible after diagnosis and one dose of PPSV23 8 weeks later. If PCV13 has been received previously, administer one dose of PPSV23 at least 8 weeks after the most recent dose of PCV13. A single revaccination of PPSV23 five years after the first dose is recommended for individuals with HIV.

9. Polio: Patients requiring primary or booster immunizations should only receive the inactive form.

10. Varicella (chickenpox): The ACIP recommends that HIV-infected patients without a history of clinical varicella infection (i.e., chickenpox or shingles) and lacking varicella antibody should be considered for primary varicella vaccination as long as the patient's CD4$^+$ count is >200 cells/μL.

Follow-up

Patients should have their medical and psychosocial needs assessed at least every 3 months. Most patients on ART should be seen monthly, because adherence issues frequently arise. These appointments should focus on identifying signs and symptoms of disease progression, assessing coping skills, and reinforcing secondary prevention education. Antiretroviral management is reviewed below. Secondary prevention focuses on preventing the spread of HIV to others but also in preventing unplanned pregnancy and STIs that are commonly seen in youth. Follow-up should include the following:

1. Complete blood count and CD4$^+$ T cell count every 3 to 6 months
2. HIV RNA by PCR every 3 months
3. PPD or IGRA yearly
4. Venereal Disease Research Laboratory (VDRL) or a rapid plasma reagin test for syphilis yearly. These tests should be conducted more frequently for YMSM in high-prevalence regions.
5. Pap smear—regardless of age—annually (after two normal Pap smears at 6-month intervals in the first year after HIV diagnosis) in sexually experienced women. While there are no specific guidelines on obtaining anal Pap smears in MSM, some clinicians screen annually.

6. Regular discussion of safer sex and family planning
7. Discussion of disclosure including options for partner notification
8. Discussion of nutrition, exercise, disease progression, medication options, and potential clinical trials
9. Regular evaluation of mental health status
10. Ongoing referral and linkage to identified resources (e.g., housing, transportation, employment, education)

Manifestations of HIV Infection

Early manifestations of HIV are listed in **Table 31.2**.

Opportunistic diseases, including infections and neoplasms, typically occur after immune suppression reaches a certain level. **Table 31.3** lists some common diseases and the corresponding CD4$^+$ T cell count associated with these illnesses.

The management of conditions associated with HIV is beyond the scope of this chapter and is frequently left to HIV specialists. Updated treatment information is available on several Web sites listed at the end of this chapter.

TABLE 31.2

Early Manifestations of HIV Infection

Chronic lymphadenopathy	Pruritic papular eruptions
Unexplained weight loss	Oral hairy leukoplakia
Xerosis	Recurrent tinea infections
Severe molluscum contagiosum	Leukopenia
Seborrheic dermatitis	Exacerbations of psoriasis
Isolated thrombocytopenia	Fatigue and malaise

TABLE 31.3

Opportunistic Diseases

CD4$^+$ T cell count (per mm^3)	Condition
200–500	Thrush KS Tuberculosis reactivation Herpes zoster Bacterial sinusitis/pneumonia Herpes simplex
100–200	Pneumocystis carinii pneumonia All of the above
50–100	Systemic fungal infections Primary tuberculosis Cryptosporidiosis Cerebral toxoplasmosis Progressive multifocal leukoencephalopathy Peripheral neuropathy Cervical carcinoma
0–50	Cytomegalovirus disease Disseminated MAC Non-Hodgkin lymphoma Central nervous system lymphoma AIDS dementia complex

MAC, Mycobacterium avium complex; AIDS, acquired immunodeficiency syndrome. From Phari JP, Murphy RL. *Contemporary diagnosis and management of HIV/AIDS infections.* Newton, PA: Handbooks in Health Care, 1999 with permission.

Management of STIs

1. Uncomplicated chlamydia, gonorrhea, trichomonas, and syphilis are generally treated in the same manner as in AYAs without HIV.
2. Pelvic inflammatory disease can be more difficult to treat in women with HIV, especially in those with significant immune dysfunction (low CD4$^+$ T cell count). In general, the CDC treatment guidelines (http://www.cdc.gov/STD/treatment/) are followed but the threshold for hospitalization for administration of IV antibiotics is lowered.
3. Cervical dysplasia has been shown to be very prevalent in women with HIV, who are at significantly higher risk for invasive cervical cancer than women who are not infected with HIV. High-risk serotypes such as HPV-16 seem to be more common, and spontaneous regression appears to be less common. Abnormal Pap smears in women with HIV should be managed following recommendations for the general population. Whenever possible, refer adolescents with HIV and abnormal Pap smear results to care providers with HIV experience.

Management of Family Planning

Risk of Mother–Child Transmission

With the marked improvements in prevention of mother–child transmission of HIV, family planning has changed. Many HIV-positive women acknowledge their interest in having children. Physicians should be honest about the risks of mother–child transmission. Transmission risk is linearly correlated with maternal viral load. Without treatment, the risk of mother–child transmission of HIV is approximately 23%. This risk is reduced to <2% for those achieving viral suppression with ART. The current standard of care is to treat HIV-positive women who desire pregnancy with a minimum of three antiretrovirals. The CDC has developed specific guidelines on the prevention of mother–child transmission.[19]

There are also concerns about HIV transmission between serodiscordant partners when unprotected vaginal intercourse is the method of conception. For these couples, chance of transmission is reduced (but not eliminated) when the positive partner's viral load is suppressed on ART. While not yet widely available, PrEP for the HIV-negative partner in addition to timed intercourse (limiting unprotected intercourse to times of peak fertility) may also reduce risk of transmission. When both partners are HIV positive, there is a chance of superinfection (infection with a second HIV strain); however, that exact risk is unknown.

Contraception

As with any AYAs, it is important to discuss birth control with HIV-positive youth. Unplanned pregnancies can disrupt an already complex situation for youth with HIV. As condom use frequently drops when young women use hormonal contraceptives, contraceptive counseling in these youth is complicated by the competing desires of preventing transmission of HIV to sexual partners (using condoms) and preventing unplanned pregnancy (usually with a more effective hormonal method). Data from a cohort of HIV-positive adolescents indicated that most adolescents reported condoms as their main method of contraception.[20] Unfortunately, the rate of conception was >20% during the first year of the study, and it was high in those reporting other contraceptive use as well, highlighting the need to discuss contraception and adherence frequently. Long-acting reversible contraception (LARC), which offers the advantage of not requiring ongoing effort on the part of the user, is safe to use in AYA women with HIV and may be a more effective method of contraception. Condom use to prevent HIV transmission is highly recommended for AYA women using all methods of contraception, including LARC.

Drug interactions in women on ART are important to consider. Contraceptives utilizing estrogen may be less effective in patients using medications that increase estrogen metabolism, such as protease inhibitors (including antiretroviral boosting medications

like norvir), specific non-nucleoside reverse transcription inhibitors (efavirenz and nevirapine), and the combination ART pill elvitegravir/cobicistat/emtricitabine/tenofovir disoproxil fumarate (Stribild). For young women at high risk for pregnancy, the use of estrogen-containing contraception may be better paired with ART regimens that do not include these medications. Contraceptive pill use also adds to the pill burden in patients taking other medications. As mentioned above, LARC (implantable and intrauterine devices) are effective options in women living with HIV and offer the additional benefits of avoiding drug interactions with estrogen and not increasing pill burden. Interactions between etonogestrel (implant) and the antiretroviral drug efavirenz are possible.[21]

Sports Participation

When Ervin "Magic" Johnson announced that he was HIV positive, many questions surrounding the advisability of vigorous exercise occurred. To date, there have been no studies documenting a positive or negative impact of exercise on HIV. Currently, we recommend using common sense in guiding HIV-positive youth on sports participation.

Evaluation of Specific Syndromes

The clinician's index of suspicion for opportunistic infections (OI) should correlate with the state of the patient's immune system, best approximated by the CD4$^+$ T cell count. Clinicians should have a low threshold for seeking consultation with an HIV or infectious disease specialist for patients experiencing severe or persistent symptoms.

Pulmonary (Cough or Shortness of Breath)

1. If the CD4$^+$ T cell count is 200/µL or less or the percentage of CD4$^+$ T cells is 14% or less, *Pneumocystis pneumonia* (PCP) should be considered. Workup for PCP should include CXR and pulse oximetry, induced sputum, and bronchoscopy.
2. In patients with a CD4$^+$ T cell count higher than 200/µL and a percentage higher than 14%, it is unlikely to be PCP. Evaluate for bronchitis, sinusitis, TB, and viral or bacterial pneumonia and consider CXR and sinus films. Sinus problems are frequent and often severe in individuals with HIV, especially those with advanced immune deficiency.

Fever

1. Diagnostic evaluation for those with severe immunosuppression (CD4$^+$ T cell count <200/µL) and without specific organ system signs or symptoms should include workup for PCP, *Mycobacterium avium* complex (MAC), and CMV.
   a. CXR: Interstitial infiltrates are consistent with PCP or infection with MAC or CMV; focal infiltrates are consistent with TB or bacterial pneumonia.
   b. Labs: Anemia and elevated alkaline phosphatase are common with MAC; elevated lactate dehydrogenase is common in PCP.
   c. Blood cultures for bacteria, virus (CMV), fungus, and acid-fast bacillus
   d. Consider serum cryptococcal antigen.
      If fever persists and above tests are inconclusive, consider the following:
   e. Lumbar puncture: May detect cryptococcal infection
   f. Bone marrow biopsy: May identify disseminated MAC, CMV, or fungus
   g. Ophthalmology consultation: May detect evidence of CMV
   h. Sinus films
   i. Body computed tomography (CT): May detect lymphoma
2. In patients with mild immunosuppression (CD4$^+$ T cell count 200 to 500/µL), look for common illnesses (viral or bacterial) and consider TB, sinusitis, and pneumonia.
3. In patients with minimal immune suppression (CD4$^+$ T cell count >500/µL), avoid costly workups unless conservative evaluation fails.

Diarrhea

Always assess whether symptoms could be medication related.

1. In patients with severe immunodeficiency (CD4+ T cell count <200/μL):
   a. If diarrhea is mild, consider empiric treatment with diphenoxylate (Lomotil) or loperamide (Imodium).
   b. If diarrhea is severe, check stool for ova and parasites and enteric pathogens including *Cryptosporidium, Cyclospora,* and *Isospora.*
   c. If these tests are inconclusive, consider colonoscopy looking for CMV, MAC, *Microsporidia,* and *Isospora.*
2. In patients without severe immunodeficiency, diarrhea is usually self-limited, and costly evaluations should be avoided. Consider evaluation for parasites, *Clostridium difficile,* and bacteria if the patient is sexually active, is homeless, or has traveled abroad recently.

Neurological (New or Worsening Headaches, Seizures, Focal Neurological Symptoms or Signs)

In patients with severe immunodeficiency (CD4+ T cell count <200/μL):

a. Emergency CT or magnetic resonance imaging of head: Multiple enhancing ring lesions are usually indicative of toxoplasmosis; primary central nervous system lymphoma is also common.
b. Lumbar puncture for cell count, protein, glucose, cryptococcal antigen, Gram stain, bacterial and fungal cultures, routine acid-fast bacillus, and VDRL.

Dysphagia

In patients with severe immunodeficiency (CD4+ T cell count <200/μL), if oral thrush is present, consider empiric treatment for *Candida* with fluconazole. In the absence of oral thrush or if empiric treatment fails, consider endoscopy to look for fungus, CMV, and herpes simplex virus.

Prophylaxis

Prophylaxis is one of the most important ways that patients with severe immunosuppression can maintain their health. Patients who have severe immune suppression but are not ready for ART should still be encouraged to use prophylaxis to prevent OI. The CDC frequently publishes updated guidelines for primary prophylaxis that can be found on their Web site (http://aidsinfo.nih.gov/guidelines).

1. *Pneumocystis:* Initiate when the CD4+ T cell count is 200/μL or less. Patients who start ART and in whom the CD4+ T cell count rises above 200/μL for 3 to 6 months may safely discontinue prophylaxis.
   a. Drug of choice: Trimethoprim-sulfamethoxazole (TMP-SMX) one double-strength (DS) tablet daily (for those patients with allergies to sulfa who either anticipate requiring a prolonged course or for whom using alternative medications is impractical, desensitization can be performed).
   b. Alternatives: Dapsone 100 mg/day orally (check for glucose-6-phosphate dehydrogenase deficiency before using); nebulized pentamidine 300 mg every 4 weeks through Respirgard II nebulizer (may be the method of choice in nonadherent youth); Atovaquone 1,500 mg orally a day with meals
2. *Tuberculosis:* Initiate in AYAs who are PPD positive (>5 mm) or who have a positive IGRA without evidence of active TB and with no prior history of treatment for active or latent TB. Treat AYAs who are close contacts of a person with infectious TB, regardless of screening result. More information is available on the CDC Web site (http://www.cdc.gov/tb/publications/LTBI/treatment.htm#1).
   a. Drug of choice: Isoniazid 300 mg plus pyridoxine 25 mg daily OR Isoniazid 900 mg biweekly (via direct observed therapy) plus pyridoxine 25 mg daily for 9 months. While

6-month isoniazid regimens may be considered for some HIV-negative individuals, a 9-month regimen is still recommended for patients living with HIV due to greater efficacy.
   b. Alternative: Rifampin 600 mg daily for 4 months (rifampin is contraindicated in patients taking protease inhibitors). In cases when rifampin is contraindicated, rifabutin may be substituted. A directly observed 12-dose once-weekly regimen of isoniazid and rifapentine may be considered for HIV-positive individuals who are not on ART.
3. *MAC:* Initiate when the CD4+ T cell count is 50/μL or less. Prophylaxis can probably be discontinued if the cell count rises above 100/μL for 3 to 6 months after initiation of ART.
   a. Drug of choice: Clarithromycin 500 mg twice daily or azithromycin 1,200 mg orally once a week
   b. Alternative: Rifabutin 300 mg orally once a day.
4. *Toxoplasma gondii:* Initiate when the CD4+ T cell count is <100/μL or if serology results are positive for *T. gondii* immunoglobulin G.
   a. Drug of choice: TMP-SMX one DS tablet once a day
   b. Alternative: TMP-SMX one DS tablet three times weekly; TMP-SMX one single-strength tablet daily; Dapsone 50 mg orally once daily plus pyrimethamine 50 mg/week plus leucovorin 25 mg weekly.

Antiretroviral Therapy

The CDC regularly updates guidelines on the use of antiretrovirals for adolescents and adults (http://aidsinfo.nih.gov/guidelines) and should be consulted with the assistance of an HIV specialist in determining whether a patient should be treated with ART. Although a full discussion of the use of antiretrovirals is beyond the scope of this chapter, some basic principles pertaining to youth are important.

Initiating ART

In March 2012, the US Department of Health and Human Services released new guidelines recommending ART for all people living with HIV, regardless of immune status (CD4+ T cell count), to reduce the risk of disease progression and for prevention of HIV transmission. As noted in the section on secondary prevention, "treatment as prevention" was driven largely by the results of HPTN 052, a multisite randomized controlled study, which demonstrated that effective ART reduces sexual transmission of HIV in HIV-serodiscordant couples by over 96%.

While guidelines have changed, there is considerable attention to the issue of a patient's ability to adhere strictly to a regimen for many years and perhaps for the rest of the patient's life. Decisions to initiate therapy must be made jointly by a well-informed patient and their health care providers. Empowering patients through education on their ability to control HIV through the proper use of medications, while at the same time helping them develop a realistic time frame and plan for initiating therapy, is the key to eventual adherence and the reaching of mutual agreement on treatment.

There are currently over 30 FDA-approved antiretroviral drugs that belong to one of six classes based on their mode of preventing HIV replication. There are an increasing number of medication formulations that allow two to three different medications to be placed into one single pill or fewer pills per medication. These have allowed for considerable simplification of antiretroviral regimens. While the advent of one pill once-daily regimens may impact youth's desire to start early, the risk of nonadherence must always be considered. Nonadherence with some medications has high risks for quick development of HIV resistance, while other combinations have much higher barriers to resistance. HIV specialists must consider these factors and review them with the HIV-positive patient.

The general principles of ART are listed in **Table 31.4**. The primary aim is to initiate a regimen containing a minimum of three antiretroviral medications with the goal of reducing the patient's viral load to an undetectable level on a highly sensitive assay for HIV RNA. Incomplete suppression, through either inadequate

TABLE 31.4
Summary of the Principles of Therapy of HIV Infection

1. HIV replication results in immune system damage and progression to AIDS if untreated. Regular, periodic measurement of HIV RNA levels (viral load measurements)
   a. Determines the risk for HIV disease progression
   b. Guides decisions to initiate and change antiretroviral treatment regimens (ART)
   c. In addition, measurement of $CD4^+$ T cell counts monitors the extent of immune dysfunction
2. The goal of ART is suppression of HIV replication to below the levels of detection by sensitive viral load assays. The most effective means of suppression of HIV replication is through treatment with simultaneous combinations of antiretroviral drugs to which the virus is susceptible
3. Each antiretroviral drug used in combination therapy should always be used according to optimum schedules and dosages
4. The decision to start ART should be made only after a conversation between the patient and physician has taken place. Adolescents with HIV should be encouraged to initiate ART as soon as they and their physicians feel confident that they are ready to begin
5. Women should receive optimal ART regardless of pregnancy status
6. These principles apply to HIV-positive children, adolescents, and adults, although the treatment of HIV-positive children involves unique pharmacological, virologic, and immunological considerations
7. HIV-positive persons should be considered infectious even with an undetectable viral load; however, the risk of transmission is markedly reduced in patients with undetectable viral loads. Adolescents should be counseled to avoid sexual or drug-use behaviors that would transmit HIV or other infectious pathogens

AIDS, acquired immunodeficiency syndrome; ART, antiretroviral therapy.
Adapted from US Department of Health and Human Services. Report of the NIH panel to define principles of therapy of HIV infection. *MMWR* 1998;47(R-55):1.

TABLE 31.5
Barriers to Adherence

Barriers for the general population	1. Complexity of the medical regimen 2. Lack of social support 3. Adverse effects of treatment 4. Distrust of health providers 5. Lack of understanding about the medication 6. Difficulty coming to terms with a life-threatening illness

Additional barriers for adolescents	Developmental capacities of adolescence can create barriers to adherence
	1. Early adolescence
	  a. Concrete, not yet abstract, thinking (undeveloped problem-solving skills)
	  b. Preoccupation with self and questions about pubertal changes
	2. Middle adolescence
	  a. Need for acceptance from peers (desire not to appear different)
	  b. Present orientation (decreased ability to plan for future doses and grasp future implications of disease)
	  c. Busy, unstructured lives (difficulty remembering to take pills)
	3. Late adolescence
	  a. Establishment of independence (the need to challenge authority figures and restructure regimens)
	  b. Feelings of immortality (disbelief that HIV can hurt them)

Additional barriers for adolescents living with HIV	1. For most, fear of disclosure of their HIV status to family and friends 2. For many, lack of adult or peer support to reinforce their adherence 3. For youth establishing independence, the conflict between needing to challenge authority figures and needing to depend on adult providers for support in taking ART 4. For asymptomatic adolescents, difficulty accepting the implications of a serious illness when they still feel well 5. For some who still think concretely, difficulty grasping the concept that there is a connection between strict adherence to ART and prevention of disease progression 6. For homeless and transient youth, lack of refrigeration or a place to store medicines and lack of a daily routine

HIV, human immunodeficiency virus; ART, antiretroviral therapy.

medication or nonadherence, may lead to the development of HIV strains that are resistant to the antiretrovirals.

The patient's ability to adhere to the drug regimen must be considered. Research has indicated that physicians are notoriously poor at predicting how likely a patient is to take medication. **Table 31.5** reviews some basic concepts about AYAs and adherence to ART. Predictors of poor adherence include psychosocial problems such as poor support, mental health problems, substance abuse, and homelessness. Factors such as patients' trust in their health care providers or concerns that taking medication might inadvertently disclose their HIV status to family, friends, roommates, or coworkers must be considered. Also, critical are medication-inherent factors such as the number of pills, the frequency of dosing, the size or taste of pills, potential side effects (many youth fear rashes that might disclose their HIV status), and food and timing requirements. Forgetting, not feeling like taking medication, and not wanting to be reminded of HIV infection were the most common barriers reported by participants in one sample of nearly 500 adolescents living with perinatally and behaviorally acquired HIV.[22]

In general, one should try to keep regimens as simple and tolerable as possible. Because studies have demonstrated that AYA adherence to ART is often poor, it is important to choose regimens such that, if resistance develops, options can still be maintained for the future. Close monitoring for nonadherence by multiple providers including psychosocial support staff is critical and monthly follow-up appointments are needed for most patients. The use of pill boxes, cell phone alarms, and mobile applications can help youth stay organized although these methods have yet to be studied in randomized trials.

In summary, viral load suppression with ART in HIV-positive adolescents not only impacts the individual's disease progression but also reduces HIV transmission in the population. Medication has been demonstrated in many cases to produce immune reconstitution in even the most damaged immune systems as long as the virus is sensitive to the medication and the patient has not developed a terminal or untreatable complication. Initiation and selection of a treatment regimen should occur only after a thoughtful conversation between the patient and clinician with expertise in HIV care, after taking into consideration the patient's ability to adhere and numerous psychosocial factors. Helping patients prepare for ART and maintain treatment once begun is a challenging task best undertaken by a multidisciplinary team.

RECOMMENDATIONS FOR HEALTH-CARE PROVIDERS

Primary care practitioners should:

1. Be aware of the disproportionate burden of HIV infection in youth, especially in high-risk populations such as YMSM, and especially in AYAs of color.

2. Obtain thorough histories and counsel regularly on risk reduction behaviors.
3. Understand HIV testing and counseling.
4. Comanage HIV-positive individuals with HIV specialists.
5. Initiate the evaluation of common symptoms such as fever, cough, headache, and diarrhea.
6. Be familiar with community resources available for AYAs in need of more intensive HIV prevention interventions.

REFERENCES

1. White House Press Office. *Executive Order—HIV Care Continuum Initiative.* Available at http://www.whitehouse.gov/the-press-office/2013/07/15/executive-order-hiv-care-continuum-initiative. Accessed February 12, 2014.
2. Samji H, Cescon A, Hogg RS, et al. Closing the gap: increases in life expectancy among treated HIV-infected individuals in the United States and Canada. *PLoS One* 2013;8(12):e81355.
3. Lo J, Abbara S, Shturman L, et al. Increased prevalence of subclinical coronary atherosclerosis detected by coronary computed tomography angiography in HIV-infected men. *AIDS* 2010;24(2):243–253.
4. Moore R, Bartlett J, Gallant J. Association between use of HMG CoA reductase inhibitors and mortality in HIV-infected patients. *PLoS One* 2011;6(7):e21843.
5. Nichols SL, Bethel J, Garvie PA et al. Neurocognitive functioning in antiretroviral therapy-naïve youth with behaviorally acquired human immunodeficiency virus. *J Adolesc Health* 2013;53(6):763–771.
6. Centers for Disease Control and Prevention. *Monitoring selected national HIV prevention and care objectives by using HIV surveillance data—United States and 6 U.S. dependent areas—2010.* HIV Surveillance Supplemental report 2012;17(3, Pt A). Available at http://www.cdc.gov/hiv/library/reports/surveillance/index.html. Accessed June 22, 2015.
7. Centers for Disease Control and Prevention. Syringe exchange programs—United States 2008. *MMWR* 2010;59(45):1488–1491.
8. Centers for Disease Control and Prevention. *Male latex condoms and sexually transmitted diseases.* http://www.cdc.gov/condomeffectiveness/docs/Condoms_and_STDS.pdf. Accessed June 22, 2015.
9. Centers for Disease Control and Prevention. *HIV among pregnant women, infants and children.* Available at http://www.cdc.gov/hiv/risk/gender/pregnantwomen/facts/index.html. Accessed February 12, 2014.
10. Grant RM, Lama JR, Anderson PL, et al. Preexposure chemoprophylaxis for HIV prevention in men who have sex with men. *N Engl J Med* 2010;363(27):2587–2599.
11. Baetem JM, Donnel D, Ndase P, et al. Antiretroviral prophylaxis for HIV prevention in heterosexual men and women. *N Engl J Med* 2012;367(5):399–410.
12. Thigpen MC, Kebaabetswe PM, Paxton LA, et al. Antiretroviral preexposure prophylaxis for heterosexual HIV transmission in Botswana. *N Engl J Med* 2012;367(5):423–434.
13. Cohen MS, Chen YQ, McCauley M, et al. Prevention of HIV-1 infection with early antiretroviral therapy. *N Engl J Med* 2011;365:493–505.
14. Guttmacher Institute. *State policies in brief: minors access to STI services.* Available at http://www.guttmacher.org/statecenter/spibs/spib_MASS.pdf. Accessed February 12, 2014.
15. Centers for Disease Control and Prevention. *State HIV testing laws: consent and counseling.* Available at http://www.cdc.gov/hiv/policies/law/states/testing.html. Accessed February 12, 2014.
16. Turner SD, Anderson K, Slater M, et al. Rapid point-of-care HIV testing in youth: a systematic review. *J Adolesc Health* 2013;53(6):683–691.
17. Martin EG, Salaru G, Paul SM, et al. Use of a rapid HIV testing algorithm to improve linkage to care. *J Clin Virol* 2011;52 (suppl 1):S11–S15.
18. Centers for Disease Control and Prevention. General recommendations on immunization—recommendations of the Advisory Committee on Immunization Practices (ACIP). *MMWR* 2011;60(2):1–64.
19. Centers for Disease Control and Prevention. *Recommendations for use of antiretroviral drugs in pregnant HIV-infected women for maternal health and interventions to reduce perinatal HIV transmission in the United States.* Available at http://aidsinfo.nih.gov/contentfiles/lvguidelines/perinatalgl.pdf. Accessed February 12, 2014.
20. Belzer ME, Rogers AS, Camarca M, et al. Adolescent medicine HIV/AIDS research network. Contraceptive choices in HIV-infected and HIV at-risk adolescent females. *J Adolesc Health* 2001;29 (suppl):93.
21. Panel on Antiretroviral Guidelines for Adults and Adolescents. *Guidelines for the use of antiretroviral agents in HIV-1-infected adults and adolescents.* Department of Health and Human Services [Table 18b]. Available at http://aidsinfo.nih.gov/contentfiles/lvguidelines/AdultandAdolescentGL.pdf. Accessed June 22, 2014.
22. MacDonell K, Naar-King S, Huszti H, et al. Barriers to medication adherence in behaviorally and perinatally infected youth living with HIV. *AIDS Behav* 2013;17(1):86–93.

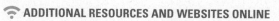 **ADDITIONAL RESOURCES AND WEBSITES ONLINE**

VIII

PART IX

Conditions Affecting Nutrition and Weight

32

Obesity

Nancy A. Crimmins
Stavra A. Xanthakos

Over the past 30 years, rising rates of obesity have occurred not only in the US, but also worldwide. Globally, obesity has nearly doubled since 1980, with nearly 11% of adults aged 20 and over estimated to be obese in 2008. Overweight and obesity are the fifth leading cause for global deaths, causing an estimated 2.8 million annual deaths in adults. Within the US, more than one-third of adults (age-adjusted 34.9%) are now obese based on the most recent national health surveys in 2011 to 2012.[1] Although the rate of obesity is slightly lower in younger adults aged 20 to 39, it remains strikingly high at 30.3%.[2] In adolescents, rates of obesity quadrupled from 5.0% in 1980 to 20.5% in 2011 to 2012.[3] The prevalence in emerging young adults aged 20 to 24 has gone up from 24.1% to 28.7% from 2001–2002 to 2007–2008 with significant worsening in this population and rates significantly worse than adolescents.[4] Health care providers who care for adolescents and young adults (AYAs) will encounter a substantial number of affected young people with obesity. As such, they need to be prepared to accurately diagnose obesity and the related health problems and counsel on appropriate prevention and treatment options for this age group.

DEFINING OVERWEIGHT AND OBESITY IN AYAS

Body mass index (BMI), a simple index of weight-for-height (kg/m²), is the most commonly used and recommended tool to screen for excess adiposity at all ages. Adult overweight is defined as a BMI of ≥25 kg/m² and adult obesity as a BMI of ≥30 kg/m². However, using a set BMI cut-point in adolescents is not feasible due to growth-related changes in weight and height. Therefore, age- and gender-specific BMI percentile distributions in the Centers for Disease Control and Prevention (CDC) growth charts are the preferred reference (www.cdc.gov/growthcharts/).

Adolescent Obesity

The recommended definition for adolescent obesity is a BMI threshold of ≥95th percentile for age and gender or BMI of >30 kg/m² (whichever is lower).[5,6]

Overweight

Overweight is defined as a BMI of ≥85th percentile for age and gender, but less than the 95th percentile or 30 kg/m² (whichever is lower).

Severely Obese

Approximately 4% to 6% of all youth in the US have been recognized as "severely obese." These youth carry a much higher burden of cardio-metabolic risk factors and have a propensity to remain severely obese into adulthood. In the Bogalusa Heart Study, severely obese youth (defined as ≥99th percentile for age and gender) had a nearly five-fold increase (33% versus 7%) of having three or more cardiovascular risk factors compared to those at the 95th percentile.[7] In addition, 100% of these youth remained obese as adults, with 88% still severely obese as adults (BMI ≥ 35 kg/m²).[7] The current recommended definition for extreme pediatric obesity is a BMI of 120% or 1.2 × the 95th percentile BMI or a BMI of ≥35 kg/m² (whichever is lower).[8] Of note, a BMI of 35 kg/m² is higher for most youth, except for boys approximately18 years of age and girls ≥16 years.

BMI

BMI is a very useful screening tool but has limitations. A high BMI may reflect a larger fat-free mass in very athletic AYAs with high muscle mass.[9] There are also racial and ethnic differences in percentages of body fat at the same BMI, with Mexican American and South Asian children having higher percentages and African-American children lower percentages of body fat than children of White European heritage.[10] However, at this time, the same BMI reference percentiles are currently recommended for all US youth. Skin-fold thickness and waist circumference have also been used to measure and track excess adiposity using percentile cutoffs.[11] These methods are not currently recommended for routine clinical use, as they require specific training to perform accurately and consistently.[5]

EPIDEMIOLOGY OF OBESITY IN AYAS

Data from national health surveys performed between 1976 and 2012 show that the prevalence of obesity in 12- to 19-year-olds of both genders has essentially quadrupled from 1997–1980 to the present 2011–2012 survey[12,13] (Table 32.1). Data from 2011 to 2012 show a 20.5% prevalence of obesity among adolescents 12 to 19 years of age, with a prevalence of 20.3% in males and 20.7% in females.[3] The prevalence of obesity among young adults aged 20 to 24 is even higher at 28.7%.[4] There has been a relative plateau in obesity prevalence among all children and adolescents since 2003 to 2004.[3] However, disparities in obesity rates remain among ethnic and racial groups, with Hispanic youth and non-Hispanic Black youth having the highest prevalence rates, followed closely by non-Hispanic White youth, while non-Hispanic Asian youth have the lowest rates (Table 32.1).

Despite an overall plateau in pediatric obesity, there has been a continued rise in severe obesity regardless of the definition used (see above).[8] This may portend a substantial rise in morbidity and

TABLE 32.1

Obesity Prevalence in Adolescents Aged 12 to 19 Years (US National Health and Nutrition Examination Surveys)

	NHANES II 1976–1980	NHANES III 1988–1994	NHANES 1999–2002	NHANES 2009–2010	NHANES 2011–2012
Females 12–19 (%)	5.3	9.7	15.4	17.1	20.7
Males 12–19 (%)	4.8	11.3	16.7	19.6	20.3
Both sexes 12–19 (%)	5.0	10.5	16.1	18.4	20.5
Obesity Prevalence by Race/Ethnicity, Both Sexes, Aged 12–19 y					
Non-Hispanic White (%)	–	–	13.7	16.1	19.6
Non-Hispanic Black (%)	–	–	21.1	23.7	22.1
Non-Hispanic Asian (%)	–	–	–	–	11.1
Hispanic youth (%)[a]	–	–	22.5	23.9	22.6

Obesity Prevalence has Risen Steeply among Adolescents, Ages 12–19) in Serial United States National Health and Nutrition Examination Surveys (NHANES).
[a]NHANES 1999–2002 and 2009–2010 surveys described obesity rates in Mexican American youth, while NHANES 2011–2012 described obesity rates in Hispanic youth.
Adapted from data presented in Fryar CD, Carroll MD, Ogden CL. Prevalence of obesity among children and adolescents: Unites States, Trends 1963 to 1965 through 2009 to 2010. Health E-Stat. September 2012. Available from http://www.cdc.gov/nchs/data/hestat/obesity_child_09_10/obesity_child_09_10.htm. Accessed March 21, 2014; Hedley AA, Ogden CL, Johnson CL, et al. Prevalence of overweight and obesity among US children, adolescents, and adults, 1999–2002. *JAMA* 2004;291:2847; Ogden CL, Carroll MD, Kit BK, et al. Prevalence of obesity and trends in body mass index among us children and adolescents, 1999–2010. *JAMA* 2012;307:483; and Ogden CL, Carroll MD, Kit BK et al. Prevalence of childhood and adult obesity in the United States, 2011–2012. *JAMA* 2014;311:806.

mortality in our next generation of young adults, given the higher number of cardiovascular risk factors and likelihood to remain severely obese as adults.[7] Severe obesity at age 18 years is associated with a significant increased risk of premature death in adulthood with a hazard ratio for death from all causes of 2.46 (95% confidence interval (CI), 1.91, 3.16) for severely obese and 1.41 (95% CI, 1.15, 1.73) for those obese at age 18 compared to those of normal weight.[14]

CAUSES OF OBESITY

Obesity is a complex condition influenced by multiple intrinsic and extrinsic risk factors, ultimately contributing to a fundamental imbalance between calories consumed and calories expended.

Environmental and Behavioral Risk Factors

Major societal changes over the past century have likely played the greatest role in our current epidemic of obesity. These include:

1. Improvements in food production and government subsidies resulting in greater availability of cheaper energy-dense (and frequently nutrient-poor) foods high in sugar and fat.
2. Decrease in home-cooked family meals and greater reliance on commercially prepared foods, in part due to more dual wage-earner families. Processed food products are often specifically designed by manufacturers to be intensely appealing to natural human taste preferences for sweet, salty, and fatty foods.
3. Concurrent technological advances that have dramatically reduced energy expenditure in both work and leisure-time activities. Television and computer gaming devices are ubiquitous in the homes and bedrooms of many AYAs. This not only contributes to increased sedentary behavior, but may result in reduced sleep duration, which has been linked to increased food intake.[15,16]

Familial or Genetic Risk Factors

Weight is a heritable trait. The concordance of fat mass in monozygotic twins ranges from 70% to 90% compared to 35% to 45% in dizygotic twins.[17] Furthermore, adoption studies have shown a much stronger correlation of BMI with the adoptee's biological parents compared to their adoptive parents.[17] However, the specific genes involved have proven difficult to isolate and replicate in genome-wide association studies.

1. Monogenic mutations: Monogenic mutations are a rare cause of obesity. The most common is a mutation in melanocortin-4

receptor (MC4R), which leads to alterations in leptin-melanocortin signaling and loss of satiety. The prevalence of MC4R mutations in obese children ranges from 0.5% to 5.8%,[18] with clinical onset of obesity by age 2 years. Mutations in the LEP and LEPR can also lead to early-onset obesity, as well as hyperphagia, delayed puberty, and immune dysfunction. Although true leptin deficiency is rare, mutations in LEPR were found to have a prevalence of 3% in a cohort of early-onset obesity and hyperphagia.[19] Leptin levels in individuals with leptin receptor mutations are elevated; however, levels can also be elevated due to the leptin resistance frequently seen in patients with obesity and insulin resistance. Therefore, measuring leptin concentrations alone cannot diagnose mutations in the receptor and genetic analysis must be performed to diagnose mutations.

2. Other genes: Other genes implicated in the development of obesity include genes in the melanocortin-leptin signaling system (proopiomelanocortin, melanocortin 2-receptor); brain-derived neurotropic factor (BDNF) and its receptor tyrosine receptor kinase B; and the fat mass and obesity-associated (FTO) gene. Genetic syndromes associated with obesity include Prader–Willi, Bardet–Biedl, and Alstrom syndromes. AYAs with developmental delay, dysmorphic features, or organ dysfunction should be referred to a genetics specialist for evaluation to rule out syndromes with obesity as a component.

Hormonal Causes of Obesity

Hormonal causes of obesity should be suspected in cases where there is poor linear growth and/or symptoms of endocrine disease. Although thyroid disease is often suspected as a cause of obesity, it is rarely the cause of significant weight gain unless severe thyroid hormone deficiency exists. Further complicating the picture, mild elevation of thyroid-stimulating hormone with normal free thyroxine (T_4), consistent with subclinical hypothyroidism, is often seen in obesity and does not require thyroid hormone replacement. Growth hormone (GH) deficiency should be suspected if insulin-like growth factor (IGF-1) and IGF-binding protein-3 are low and can be confirmed on GH-stimulation testing. Cushing syndrome is very uncommon in adolescents. The first signs of Cushing syndrome are weight gain and growth arrest. Later in the course, the classic signs and symptoms develop, including central obesity, thick striae, acne, facial flushing, virilization, and psychological disturbances. Diagnosis of Cushing syndrome is difficult as no one single test confirms the diagnosis and interpreting results require

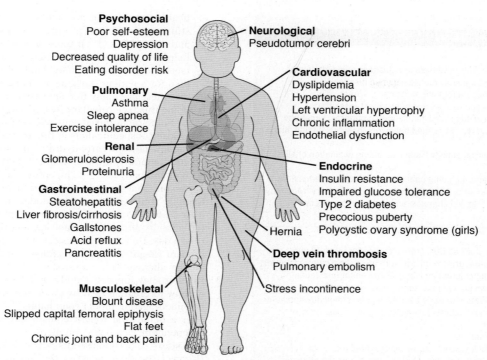

FIGURE 32.1 Health risks of obesity in AYAs. (Adapted from Figure 1 in Xanthakos, SA, Daniels SR, Inge TH. Bariatric surgery in adolescents: an update. *Adolesc Med Clin* 2006;17(3):589–612).

input from an endocrinologist. Furthermore, it must be determined if the cause of excess cortisol is ACTH dependent (pituitary adenoma or ectopic production of ACTH such as by carcinoid tumor) or ACTH independent (adrenal overproduction of cortisol).

Medications, Chronic Illness, and Obesity

Although relatively uncommon, certain medications including systemic high-dose steroids and some atypical antipsychotics are known to promote excess and rapid weight gain.[20,21] Insatiable appetite leading to very rapid and severe obesity can also result from damage to or tumors affecting the hypothalamic area.[22]

HEALTH EFFECTS AND MEDICAL EVALUATION OF OBESITY

Regardless of the cause of obesity, associated health problems are well described in AYAs, particularly those suffering from severe obesity. Complications due to obesity include a wide number of problems previously considered "adult" conditions (Fig. 32.1). Because obesity affects a wide range of organ systems, AYAs with obesity should undergo a thorough review of systems and comprehensive medical evaluation (Table 32.2).

Among adolescents, the onset of puberty can also affect the risk of metabolic disease. A transient state of insulin resistance develops during puberty and peaks at sexual maturity rating 3 in both sexes.[23] The exact mechanisms are not known, but increased insulin resistance is likely due to the concurrent spike in GH secretion. Glucose tolerance is usually maintained by an increase in insulin production from β cells in the pancreas. However, the increase in insulin resistance seen in puberty can cause metabolic disease to manifest in peripubertal obese children who already have baseline insulin resistance and genetic predisposition to disease. Obesity can in turn impact the timing and characteristics of puberty. Obese adolescents tend to be taller than expected for genetic potential and it is common to see some advancement in skeletal maturation. Obese females may undergo earlier sexual maturation, possibly due to higher levels of leptin, an adipokine that indicates adequate fat mass for reproduction and is thought to be

permissive for puberty to occur. Conversion of adrenal androgens to estrogens in adipose tissue may also play a role. Despite earlier sexual maturation, obese females often exhibit menstrual irregularities. Obesity and insulin resistance are risk factors for polycystic ovarian syndrome (PCOS) (see Chapter 49), characterized by chronic anovulation and hyperandrogenism. However, obesity can also lead to suppression of gonadotropins independent of hyperandrogenism with blunting of luteinizing hormone during sleep.[24]

TREATMENT OPTIONS FOR OBESE AYAs

Prevention

Prevention is the best cure when it comes to obesity. Efforts need to be made to control and/or reverse weight gain as soon as it is recognized that a healthy-weight adolescent is crossing percentiles for weight or a young adult is increasing their BMI above 25 kg/m². Anticipatory guidance to promote a healthy-weight status for AYAs includes the following:

1. Encourage healthy nutritional practices in early puberty when there is programmed propensity to increase fat cells.
2. Identify unhealthy eating attitudes and harmful eating behaviors including dieting, overeating, and binging, all of which are associated with overweight.
3. Encourage a lifestyle of activity and participation rather than one of inactivity and observation.
4. Discourage or limit television viewing, video games, computer-based and other sedentary pastimes.
5. Encourage family time including meals and activities.

Treatment in the Primary Care Setting

Once overweight or obesity is present, the mainstay of treatment remains behavioral interventions to promote optimal nutritional balance and increased physical activity. Surveying the patient to determine what has been tried, successful or failed in the past is critical to avoid repeating recommendations that have not met with success in the past.

TABLE 32.2
Medical Evaluation of Obesity

History

1. Family history of obesity, cardiovascular disease, hyperlipidemia, hypertension, type 2 diabetes mellitus, thyroid disease
2. Onset of obesity, triggers for weight gain (e.g., illness, injury, depression, medication usage), and past weight-loss efforts
3. Diet history including diet recall, family-eating patterns, unhealthy eating attitudes, and weight-related behaviors including dieting, binge eating, purging
4. Sedentary and physical activity history, including evaluation of all screen time
5. Full review of systems including headaches, orthopedic complaints, snoring, daytime sleeping, abdominal pain, hip pain, urinary frequency, polydipsia, polyuria, bowel changes, and irregular menses or amenorrhea

Physical Examination

1. Plot weight, height, BMI on CDC growth curves for those 18 and younger. Short stature, growth failure, or relative short stature (shorter than expected genetic potential) may indicate endocrine cause
2. Measure blood pressure with the appropriate sized cuff
3. Pubertal staging. Watch for early puberty in girls (breast development before age 8). Delayed puberty in females suggests possibility of endocrine disorder
4. Skin, hair, and extremities:
   a. Acanthosis nigricans suggests insulin resistance
   b. Striae that are thick, violet in color, and located on the abdomen, buttocks, and thighs are suggestive of Cushing syndrome
   c. Hirsutism is suggestive of polycystic ovarian syndrome
   d. Polydactyly may indicate Bardet–Biedl syndrome
5. Papilledema suggests pseudotumor cerebri
6. Thyromegaly suggests hypothyroidism

Laboratory Tests and Diagnostic Evaluations, as Indicated

1. Basic screening: Thyroid-stimulating hormone, fasting blood glucose, hemoglobin A1C, fasting lipid profile, and liver function tests
2. For evaluation of type 2 diabetes, a fasting plasma glucose (FPG): FPG of 100–125 mg/dL represents impaired fasting glucose and FPG ≥ 126 mg/dL or above represents diabetes
   Alternative tests include a 2-h glucose tolerance test or a casual glucose
   a. Impaired glucose tolerance defined as blood glucose ≥140 mg/dL at 2 h and diabetes as blood glucose ≥200 mg/dL. Patient should be in usual state of health and not taking oral steroids or medications that can affect blood glucose for ≥2 wk
   b. A casual glucose >200 mg/dL plus polyuria, polydipsia, and weight loss
3. For diagnosis of polycystic ovarian syndrome: (1) clinical or biochemical evidence of androgen excess including acne, hirsutism, elevated testosterone or free testosterone; and (2) oligomenorrhea. Luteinizing hormone:follicle-stimulating hormone ratio of >2.0 supportive but not diagnostic alone. A 17-hydroxyprogesterone and dehydroepiandrosterone-sulfate level can rule out late-onset congenital adrenal hyperplasia and adrenal tumors, respectively.
4. If symptoms of obstructive sleep apnea are present, a polysomnography study is warranted

1. Dietary interventions: Specific dietary interventions that are recommended include[25,26]:
   - Avoid consumption of sugar-sweetened beverages.
   - Increase intake of fruits and vegetables with a goal of ≥5 servings a day.
   - Eat regular meals, including breakfast, and avoid "grazing" throughout the day, especially after school.
   - Limit fast food to no more than once a week.

   It is, however, important to note that some of these recommendations are widely accepted presumptions that are not necessarily supported by randomized controlled clinical trials.[27,28] Nonetheless, because they are likely to confer health benefits and are unlikely to cause harm, they are still considered first-line recommendations for overweight and obese AYAs.[25,26] If these simple interventions fail, it is helpful to involve a dietitian to identify specific dietary risk factors and tailor an individualized and balanced dietary plan for a patient. Logging of intake and activity is helpful and there are many free apps that can assist the patient in doing this (see Ancillary Resources).

   Some randomized controlled studies have examined the efficacy of specific diets in the treatment of obesity, including low-fat, low-carbohydrate, and low-glycemic index diets. Generally, these diets are equally effective in reducing BMI and body fat.[29–32] The optimal dietary plan is therefore the one that the patient is most likely to follow.

2. Exercise and activity recommendations: AYAs should get at least 1 hour of moderate to vigorous activity a day.[25,26] Sedentary activity should be reduced to less than 2 hours of screen time a day. However, exercise changes alone rarely lead to significant weight loss; patients must also be counseled to make dietary changes to be successful.

3. Psychosocial support: Family members need to be educated on how to create a healthy environment at home and should be encouraged to model good habits.[25,26] Parental BMI change after a behavioral weight control intervention was the only independent significant predictor of adolescent BMI change in a study of 86 adolescents between 13 and 16 years old.[33] However, the older the AYAs, the less likely parental influences will lead to changed behaviors in the patient. Contrary to intuition, setting realistic goals or readiness to change do not appear to predict amount of weight loss or treatment adherence in those seeking weight-loss treatments.[27] Therefore, basic screening for depression, low self-esteem, and substance use should be considered as they could potentially impair motivation and the AYAs' ability to carry out lifestyle changes.

Tertiary Interventions When Lifestyle and Dietary Counseling Fail

1. Comprehensive weight management programs: These multidisciplinary interventions typically involve more frequent visits of every 1 to 2 weeks, with psychological support, physician supervision, and intensive dietitian and exercise support.[25] Comprehensive interventions of medium (26 to 75 contact hours) to high intensity (>75 contact hours) are the most effective approach with a 1.9 to 3.3 kg/m^2 unit difference favoring intervention at 12 months.[34] However, such programs are resource intensive and therefore expensive. Since these programs are not always covered by third-party payers, they may not be accessible to all patients. Further, the frequency of visits required for optimal success is sometimes incompatible with employment or school commitments or prohibitive if distance or transportation issues exist.

2. Medications: Adjunctive weight-loss medications may be attempted when intensive lifestyle modifications have failed to prevent weight gain or to achieve weight loss and in cases where significant obesity-related comorbidities exist. Orlistat (Xenical, Alli) is the only US Food and Drug Administration (FDA)-approved medication for weight loss in patients 12 to 18 years old. It prevents the absorption of dietary fat by inhibiting gastrointestinal lipases. In a randomized controlled study in adolescents, 120 mg orally three times daily achieved a 0.55 unit decrease in BMI compared to a 0.31 increase with placebo ($p = 0.001$).[35] However, it can cause stomach pain, gas, diarrhea, and leakage of oily stool.

   Metformin is often used to treat impaired glucose tolerance or diabetes in AYAs. Increasingly, there has also been interest in the impact of metformin on weight loss. Although it has not been FDA-approved for weight loss, evidence suggests that

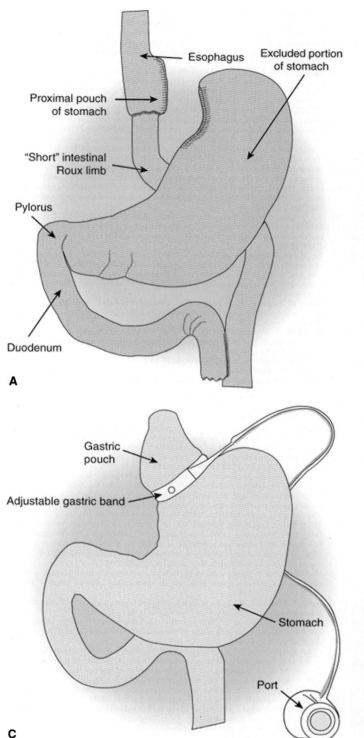

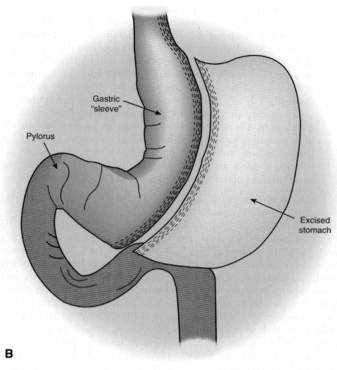

FIGURE 32.2 Types of weight-loss surgeries performed in AYAs. **A:** Roux-en-Y gastric bypass (RYGB) creates a small gastric pouch by stapling off the body of the stomach. A Roux limb of jejunum is anastomosed to the gastric pouch, while the excluded stomach and bypassed duodenum are connected distally to the jejunum. **B:** The sleeve gastrectomy (SG) is created by stapling off and removing the body of the stomach, leaving a narrow gastric "sleeve" that remains in continuity with the bowel. **C:** Adjustable gastric band (AGB) is an inflatable silicone band placed around the neck of the stomach, which slows and decreases food consumption. A catheter connects the band to a subcutaneous port so that the band can be inflated or deflated by injecting or removing saline. (From Nettina SM. *Lippincott manual of nursing practice.* 10th ed. Philadelphia, PA: Lippincott Williams & Wilkins, 2013.)

it may be modestly helpful in reducing BMI in obese adolescents compared to placebo and that it may temper weight gain caused by atypical antipsychotic use in youth.[36–38]

For those 18 and older, a new once-daily, controlled-release combination of phentermine/topiramate (Qysmia) has recently been FDA-approved for management of obesity. This drug results in statistically significant weight loss compared to placebo with an approximate 9% to 10% reduction in weight over 2 years. Although generally well tolerated,[39] there is potential for significant birth defects (cleft lip/palate) if the fetus (primarily

first trimester) is exposed to topiramate. As such, AYA females of reproductive potential should have effective contraception and pregnancy monitoring during Qysmia therapy.

3. Bariatric Surgery: Unfortunately, comprehensive lifestyle interventions are often least successful for the severely obese who are also often excluded from clinical trials of obesity medications. Given the paucity of effective treatments, there has been increasing application of weight-loss surgery (WLS), particularly in adolescents.[40] Current recommendations for adolescents have lowered the threshold to 35 kg/m² for those

with severe comorbidities including type 2 diabetes, pseudo-tumor cerebri, severe nonalcoholic steatohepatitis, and severe obstructive sleep apnea, which is aligned with recommendations in adults.[41] Adolescents should be evaluated in a program that is able to assess and support the unique developmental and medical needs of adolescents. Young adults are generally considered to be appropriate for an adult bariatric program. Typically a 3- to 6-month period of preparation is required for an adolescent or young adult to become adequately prepared for surgery. Absolute contraindications for surgery include inability to understand or provide informed assent/consent for the procedure, active psychiatric illness, or substance abuse, a medical cause for obesity that can be treated (i.e., Cushing syndrome) or planned pregnancy within 12 months of surgery.

WLS techniques that have been used in AYAs include the roux-en-y gastric bypass (RYGB) (Fig. 32.2A), the sleeve gastrectomy (SG) (Fig. 32.2B), and the adjustable gastric band (AGB) (Fig. 32.2C). Perioperative risk appears to be lower for both SG and the AGB, compared to RYGB.[42] However, the AGB is not approved for adolescents <18 years of age, in part due to concerns about a higher rate of long-term device-related complications and reoperations in adults with longer-term follow-up. Some programs will offer the AGB "off-label" but it is generally declining in use even among adults, while the use of SG is increasing. All types of WLS can result in micronutrient deficiencies, and lifelong supplementation and monitoring for nutrient deficiencies are critical.

On average, BMI declines 28% to 37% postoperatively in adolescents depending on the type of WLS, with RYGB > SG > AGB.[42,43] Baseline BMI is the strongest predictor of postoperative BMI; an adolescent with very high BMI (>60 kg/m^2) is likely to still have a high postoperative BMI (BMI > 40 kg/m^2) despite substantial weight loss.[44] Nonetheless, significant improvements in cardiovascular risk factors and comorbidities occur. A minority of AYAs (10% to 15%) can also experience significant weight regain but there are no specific predictors for those who are at risk for suboptimal weight loss or significant weight regain.

SUMMARY

Obesity remains a significant problem for youth in the US, affecting one in five adolescents and nearly one in three young adults. Comprehensive screening for key health complications is recommended and the burden is particularly high in the severely obese. Lifestyle and dietary counseling in the primary care setting remains the recommended first-line treatment for most patients, but if these measures fail, more intensive lifestyle interventions, adjunctive medications, and bariatric surgery (for appropriate candidates) may be considered.

ACKNOWLEDGMENTS

The authors wish to acknowledge Marcie B. Schneider for her contributions to the previous versions of this chapter.

REFERENCES

1. World Health Organization. *Obesity and overweight, fact sheet No. 311*. Available at http://www.who.int/mediacentre/factsheets/fs311/en/. Accessed February 26, 2014.
2. Ogden CL, Carroll MD, Kit BK, et al. *Prevalence of obesity among adults: United States, 2011–2012*. NCHS Data Brief. 2013; no. 131. Hyattsville, MD: National Center for Health Statistics, 2013.
3. Ogden CL, Carroll MD, Kit BK, et al. Prevalence of childhood and adult obesity in the United States, 2011–2012. *JAMA* 2014;311(8):806–814.
4. Park MJ, Scott JT, Adams SH, et al. Adolescent and young adult health in the United States in the past decade: little improvement and young adults remain worse off than adolescents. *J Adolesc Health* 2014;55:3–16.
5. Krebs NF, Himes JH, Jacobson D, et al. Assessment of child and adolescent overweight and obesity. *Pediatrics* 2007;120 (suppl 4):S193–S228.
6. Koplan JP, Liverman CT, Kraak VI. Preventing childhood obesity: health in the balance: executive summary. *J Am Diet Assoc* 2005;105(1):131–138.
7. Freedman DS, Mei Z, Srinivasan SR, et al. Cardiovascular risk factors and excess adiposity among overweight children and adolescents: the Bogalusa Heart Study. *J Pediatr* 2007;150(1):12–17.
8. Kelly AS, Barlow SE, Rao G, et al. Severe obesity in children and adolescents: identification, associated health risks, and treatment approaches: a scientific statement from the American Heart Association. *Circulation* 2013;128(15):1689–1712.
9. Demerath EW, Schubert CM, Maynard LM, et al. Do changes in body mass index percentile reflect changes in body composition in children? Data from the Fels Longitudinal Study. *Pediatrics* 2006;117(3):e487–e495.
10. Ehtisham S, Crabtree N, Clark P, et al. Ethnic differences in insulin resistance and body composition in United Kingdom adolescents. *J Clin Endocrinol Metab* 2005;90(7):3963–3969.
11. Fernandez JR, Redden DT, Pietrobelli A, et al. Waist circumference percentiles in nationally representative samples of African-American, European-American, and Mexican-American children and adolescents. *J Pediatr* 2004;145(4):439–444.
12. Ogden CL, Flegal KM, Carroll MD, et al. Prevalence and trends in overweight among US children and adolescents, 1999–2000. *JAMA* 2002;288(14):1728–1732.
13. Hedley AA, Ogden CL, Johnson CL, et al. Prevalence of overweight and obesity among US children, adolescents, and adults, 1999–2002. *JAMA* 2004;291(23):2847–2850.
14. Ma J, Flanders WD, Ward EM, et al. Body mass index in young adulthood and premature death: analyses of the US National Health Interview Survey linked mortality files. *Am J Epidemiol* 2011;174(8):934–944.
15. Allison KR, Adlaf EM, Dwyer JJ, et al. The decline in physical activity among adolescent students: a cross-national comparison. *Can J Public Health* 2007;98(2):97–100.
16. Burt J, Dube L, Thibault L, et al. Sleep and eating in childhood: a potential behavioral mechanism underlying the relationship between poor sleep and obesity. *Sleep Med* 2014;15(1):71–75.
17. Xia Q, Grant SF. The genetics of human obesity. *Ann N Y Acad Sci* 2013;1281:178–190.
18. Valette M, Bellisle F, Carette C, et al. Eating behaviour in obese patients with melanocortin-4 receptor mutations: a literature review. *Int J Obes* 2013;37(8):1027–1035.
19. Farooqi IS, Wangensteen T, Collins S, et al. Clinical and molecular genetic spectrum of congenital deficiency of the leptin receptor. *N Engl J Med* 2007;356(3):237–247.
20. Correll CU, Manu P, Olshanskiy V, et al. Cardiometabolic risk of second-generation antipsychotic medications during first-time use in children and adolescents. *JAMA* 2009;302(16):1765–1773.
21. Zhang FF, Rodday AM, Kelly MJ, et al. Predictors of being overweight or obese in survivors of pediatric acute lymphoblastic leukemia (ALL). *Pediatr Blood Cancer* 2014; 61(7):1263–1269.
22. Rosenfeld A, Arrington D, Miller J, et al. A review of childhood and adolescent craniopharyngiomas with particular attention to hypothalamic obesity. *Pediatr Neurol* 2014;50(1):4–10.
23. Goran MI, Gower BA. Longitudinal study on pubertal insulin resistance. *Diabetes* 2001;50(11):2444–2450.
24. Rosenfield RL. Clinical review: adolescent anovulation: maturational mechanisms and implications. *J Clin Endocrinol Metab* 2013;98(9):3572–3583.
25. Barlow SE. Expert committee recommendations regarding the prevention, assessment, and treatment of child and adolescent overweight and obesity: summary report. *Pediatrics* 2007;120 (suppl 4):S164–S192.
26. August GP, Caprio S, Fennoy I, et al. Prevention and treatment of pediatric obesity: an endocrine society clinical practice guideline based on expert opinion. *J Clin Endocrinol Metab* 2008;93(12):4576–4599.
27. Casazza K, Fontaine KR, Astrup A, et al. Myths, presumptions, and facts about obesity. *N Engl J Med* 2013;368(5):446–454.
28. Spear BA, Barlow SE, Ervin C, et al. Recommendations for treatment of child and adolescent overweight and obesity. *Pediatrics* 2007;120 (suppl 4):S254–S288.
29. Mirza NM, Palmer MG, Sinclair KB, et al. Effects of a low glycemic load or a low-fat dietary intervention on body weight in obese Hispanic American children and adolescents: a randomized controlled trial. *Am J Clin Nutr* 2013;97(2):276–285.
30. Ebbeling CB, Leidig MM, Feldman HA, et al. Effects of a low-glycemic load vs low-fat diet in obese young adults: a randomized trial. *JAMA* 2007;297(19):2092–2102.
31. Nordmann AJ, Nordmann A, Briel M, et al. Effects of low-carbohydrate vs low-fat diets on weight loss and cardiovascular risk factors: a meta-analysis of randomized controlled trials. *Arch Intern Med* 2006;166(3):285–293.
32. Kirk S, Brehm B, Saelens BE, et al. Role of carbohydrate modification in weight management among obese children: a randomized clinical trial. *J Pediatr* 2012;161(2):320–327.
33. Sato AF, Jelalian E, Hart CN, et al. Associations between parent behavior and adolescent weight control. *J Pediatr Psychol* 2011;36(4):451–460.
34. Whitlock EP, O'Connor EA, Williams SB, et al. Effectiveness of weight management interventions in children: a targeted systematic review for the USPSTF. *Pediatrics* 2010;125(2):e396–e418.
35. Chanoine JP, Hampl S, Jensen C, et al. Effect of orlistat on weight and body composition in obese adolescents: a randomized controlled trial. *JAMA* 2005;293(23):2873–2883.
36. Kendall D, Vail A, Amin R, et al. Metformin in obese children and adolescents: the MOCA trial. *J Clin Endocrinol Metab* 2013;98(1):322–329.
37. Wu RR, Zhao JP, Jin H, et al. Lifestyle intervention and metformin for treatment of antipsychotic-induced weight gain: a randomized controlled trial. *JAMA* 2008;299(2):185–193.
38. Klein DJ, Cottingham EM, Sorter M, et al. A randomized, double-blind, placebo-controlled trial of metformin treatment of weight gain associated with initiation of atypical antipsychotic therapy in children and adolescents. *Am J Psych* 2006;163(12):2072–2079.
39. Smith SM, Meyer M, Trinkley KE. Phentermine/topiramate for the treatment of obesity. *Ann Pharmacother* 2013;47(3):340–349.
40. Tsai WS, Inge TH, Burd RS. Bariatric surgery in adolescents: recent national trends in use and in-hospital outcome. *Arch Pediatr Adolesc Med* 2007;161(3):217–221.
41. Pratt JS, Lenders CM, Dionne EA, et al. Best practice updates for pediatric/adolescent weight loss surgery. *Obesity (Silver Spring)* 2009;17(5):901–910.
42. Inge TH, Zeller MH, Jenkins TM, et al. Perioperative outcomes of adolescents undergoing bariatric surgery: the Teen-Longitudinal Assessment of Bariatric Surgery (Teen-LABS) study. *JAMA Pediatr* 2014;168(1):47–53.
43. O'Brien PE, Sawyer SM, Laurie C, et al. Laparoscopic adjustable gastric banding in severely obese adolescents: a randomized trial. *JAMA* 2010;303(6):519–526.
44. Inge TH, Jenkins TM, Zeller M, et al. Baseline BMI is a strong predictor of nadir BMI after adolescent gastric bypass. *J Pediatr* 2010;156(1):103–108.

CHAPTER 33

Feeding and Eating Disorders

Debra K. Katzman
Neville H. Golden

KEY WORDS

- Anorexia nervosa
- Avoidant/restrictive food intake disorder
- Binge-eating disorder
- Bulimia nervosa
- Eating disorders
- Family-based treatment
- Medical complications
- Multidisciplinary

The focus of this chapter is on feeding and eating disorders in adolescents and young adults (AYAs). Feeding and Eating Disorders in the 5th edition of the *Diagnostic and Statistical Manual of Mental Disorders* (DSM-5) include several changes to better represent the disturbances in eating throughout the lifespan.[1] In the DSM-5, feeding disorders of early infancy and childhood, pica, and rumination have been combined with eating disorders in a new section called Feeding and Eating Disorders. The diagnostic classifications in this section include (1) anorexia nervosa (AN), (2) bulimia nervosa (BN), (3) binge-eating disorder (BED), (4) avoidant/restrictive food intake disorder (ARFID), (5) pica, (6) rumination disorder, (7) other specified feeding or eating disorder, and (8) unspecified feeding or eating disorder. This chapter focuses on feeding and eating disorders most commonly seen in AYAs: AN, BN, BED, and ARFID. These feeding and eating disorders are characterized by weight-control behaviors and eating attitudes and behaviors that commonly result in medical complications. Individuals with feeding and eating disorders benefit from prompt diagnosis and aggressive multidisciplinary, developmentally appropriate treatment.

The epidemiologic and treatment data included in this chapter predate the changes in the DSM-5 and these changes are likely to affect the results of future epidemiologic and treatment studies.

ANOREXIA NERVOSA

The core features of AN include significantly low weight, fear of gaining weight, and a disturbance in the way body weight, shape, or size is experienced. There are two separate subtypes, the restricting type, AN-R (those who control their weight through dieting, fasting, or exercising) and a binge-eating/purging subtype, AN-B/P (those who purge calories to control weight and/or routinely binge-eat) (**Table 33.1**).[1]

Etiology

The etiology of AN is multifactorial with biological, psychological, and sociocultural factors all contributing to the development of the disorder. Over the last decade, research has focused on the contributions of genetics to biological vulnerability, the personality type associated with AN, and the potential role of neurotransmitters in the etiology of the disorder.

TABLE 33.1	
DSM-5 Diagnostic Criteria for Anorexia Nervosa[1]	
A	Restriction of energy intake relative to requirements, leading to a significantly low body weight in the context of age, sex, development trajectory, and physical health. Significantly low weight is defined as a weight that is less than minimally normal or, for children and adolescents, less than that minimally expected
B	Intense fear of gaining weight or of becoming fat, or persistent behavior that interferes with weight gain, even though at a significantly low weight
C	Disturbance in the way in which one's body weight or shape is experienced, undue influence of body weight or shape on self-evaluation, or persistent lack of recognition of the seriousness of the current low body weight
Restricting type	During the last three months, the individual has not engaged in recurrent episodes of binge-eating or purging behavior (i.e., self-induced vomiting or the misuse laxatives, diuretics, or enemas). This subtype describes presentations in which weight loss is accomplished primarily through dieting, fasting, and/or excessive exercise
Binge-eating/ purging type	During the last three months, the individual has engaged in recurrent episodes of binge-eating or purging behavior (i.e., self-induced vomiting or the misuse of laxatives, diuretics, or enemas)

There is a familial predisposition to eating disorders, with female relatives most often affected. There is a higher rate of AN among identical twins compared to fraternal twins. In addition, relatives of individuals with an eating disorder are at higher risk of developing an eating disorder. These findings suggest that genetic factors may predispose some people to eating disorders. To date, no single gene or combination of genes has been identified. Studies suggest that certain areas of the human genome may harbor susceptibility genes for AN on chromosome 1.[2]

Researchers have discovered disturbances in a number of different neurotransmitters including serotonin, norepinephrine, and dopamine in those with AN. There is evidence that starvation, binging, and excessive exercising can lead to changes in neurotransmitters, and conversely, there is evidence that neurotransmitter abnormalities can lead to these behaviors. The role of disturbances in transmission of serotonin, a neurotransmitter known to play a role in modulating appetite, obsessional behavior, and impulsivity, has received particular interest.

Weight concerns and societal emphasis on thinness are pervasive in westernized societies, and adolescent girls tend to be more vulnerable to these influences. The slim body ideal is thought to be the key contributor to the gender differences seen in both AN and BN. In a biologically predisposed individual, feelings of ineffectiveness and loss of control during adolescence, compounded by societal pressures to be thin, can lead to dieting to obtain a sense of control. Dieting itself leads to further preoccupation with shape and weight, perpetuating the cycle. Many of the behaviors, physical signs, and symptoms seen in AN can be attributed to malnutrition.

Epidemiology

1. Prevalence and incidence:
   a. Estimated prevalence in young women is 0.3% to 0.5%.[3]
   b. Estimated incidence rate is 8 cases per 100,000 population per year.
   c. Incidence rates are highest in 15- to 19-year-old girls.
   d. Rates for partial syndrome are typically higher.
   e. College students: 5.2% (6.2% females and 3.4% males) have a body mass index (BMI) less than 18.5; 1.4% of undergraduates state that an eating disorder disrupted their academics; 34.7% state that they are very or slightly overweight; and 52% state they are trying to lose weight.[4]
2. Age:
   a. Commonly begins during adolescence; >90% of individuals with eating disorders are diagnosed before age 25 years.
   b. Peak age at onset is mid-adolescence (13 to 15 years) with a range of 10 to 25 years.
   c. Increasing prevalence in children and younger adolescents
3. Gender:
   a. 85% to 90% of AYAs with AN are female.
   b. 16.7% of adolescents under age 14 with AN are male.[5]
4. Comorbidity:
   a. May coexist with other psychiatric conditions (e.g., anxiety disorders, depression, obsessive-compulsive disorder (OCD), and substance abuse disorders)
   b. May coexist with medical conditions (e.g., diabetes mellitus, cystic fibrosis, and celiac disease).

Risk Factors[6]

1. Age and gender:
   a. Adolescence
   b. Female
2. Early childhood eating problems:
   a. Picky eating, digestive and early eating-related problems
   b. Struggles concerning meals
3. Weight concerns/negative body image/dieting:
   a. Adolescent girls who diet are more likely to develop an eating disorder than girls who do not diet.
4. Perinatal events:
   a. Prematurity, small for gestational age, and cephalohematoma
   b. Young women with a history of AN may also be at increased risk for adverse perinatal events.
5. Personality traits:
   a. Perfectionism
   b. Anxiety
   c. Low self-esteem
   d. Harm avoidance
   e. Obsessionality
6. Early puberty
7. Chronic illness:
   a. Increased risk in teenagers with diabetes mellitus
8. Physical and sexual abuse:
   a. Individuals who have been sexually abused have the same or only slightly higher incidence of AN as those not abused.
9. Family history/family psychopathology:
   a. Elevated rates of psychiatric disorders (anxiety disorders and mood affective disorders) in first-degree relatives of patients with AN
10. Competitive athletics:
    a. Participation in sports that place a high emphasis on body weight and appearance (e.g., ballet and gymnastics).

Clinical Manifestations
Behaviors

1. Dieting: May follow comments about body weight, shape, or size
2. Relentless pursuit of thinness:
   a. Initially, weight loss reinforced by positive comments from others
   b. Later, preoccupation with food, shape, and weight progresses and patient loses control over eating.
3. Distorted body image: Results in continued weight loss, leading to a state of emaciation
4. Unusual eating attitudes and behaviors:
   a. Denial of hunger
   b. Consumes low-calorie and/or low-fat foods
   c. Avoids previously enjoyed foods
   d. Eats the same foods at the same time each day
   e. Breaks food into small portions, eats foods of the same color, hides food, or secretly throws food away
   f. May consume large amounts of water or diet sodas with caffeine to satisfy hunger or cause diuresis
   g. Enjoys reading cookbooks, collecting recipes, watching cooking shows on television, cooking, and preparing food for others, although will not eat
5. Increased physical activity:
   a. May stand constantly, move arms and legs, run up and down stairs, jog, do floor exercises or calisthenics in an effort to expend energy
   b. As weight loss continues, activity level often increases
6. Purging behaviors: May include vomiting, use of diuretics, fasting, excessive exercise, or herbal remedies or complementary and alternative medicines (CAM)
7. Frequent weighing:
   a. Weighing oneself daily or multiple times a day
   b. Weight on the scale determines how the individual feels about him/herself
8. Wears baggy or layered clothing: Conceals weight loss or to keep warm
9. Poor self-esteem
10. Isolation:
    a. Withdrawal from friends and family
    b. Minimizes contact with criticizing or teasing peers
    c. Avoids social situations associated with food
11. Inflexibility: Difficulties with "set-shifting" (ability to flexibly shift a cognitive response) that may result in a strong sense of "right and wrong"
12. Irritability and mood changes:
    a. Starvation can cause mood changes
    b. Comorbid mental illness can contribute to mood disturbance.

Signs and Symptoms

Signs and symptoms may be minimal but can include the following:

1. Signs:
   a. Weight loss:
      - Restriction of energy intake leading to a significantly low body weight (a weight that is less than minimally normal, or for children and adolescents, less than minimally expected) in the context of age, sex growth and developmental trajectory, and physical health.

- Any significant or unexpected weight loss or failure to make expected weight gain during a period of growth is cause for concern.
- Physical signs of malnutrition including loss of subcutaneous tissue, temporal wasting, loss of muscle mass, and prominence of bony protuberances
  b. Amenorrhea:
  - Amenorrhea is no longer a criterion for the diagnosis of AN, but
  - 20% to 30% develop amenorrhea before significant weight loss; 50% develop it at the same time as the weight loss; and 25% develop it following weight loss.
  - Resumption of menses usually occurs within 3 to 6 months of achieving a weight approximately 95% of median BMI.[7]
  c. Pubertal delay: AN can delay the start or progression of puberty.
  d. Growth: There is no general agreement on the impact of AN on growth. Some studies have shown that adolescents who develop AN before growth is complete may develop growth retardation, whereas others have shown that preservation of height potential can occur because of a prolonged growth period secondary to delayed bone age. Regardless, it is important to review the growth chart to determine whether the patient has crossed growth percentiles.
  e. Skin and body hair:
  - Dry skin with hyperkeratotic areas
  - Yellow or orange discoloration, most noticeable on the palms and soles
  - Pitting and ridging of the nails
  - Lanugo hair—fine downy hair commonly seen on the back, stomach, or face
  - Hair loss or thinning
  f. Recurrent fractures
  g. Hypothermia: Oral body temperature may be 35°C or lower
  h. Bradycardia: One of the most common cardiac findings
  i. Hypotension: Hypotension associated with significant postural changes
  j. Acrocyanosis
  k. Edema, usually dependent
  l. Systolic murmur sometimes associated with mitral valve prolapse
2. Symptoms:
  a. Cold intolerance
  b. Postural dizziness and fainting
  c. Early satiety, abdominal bloating, discomfort, and pain
  d. Constipation
  e. Fatigue, muscle weakness, and cramps
  f. Poor concentration

Laboratory Features

1. Hematological:
  a. Leukopenia: May be a relative lymphocytosis
  b. Anemia: Not common, usually a late finding
  c. Thrombocytopenia
  d. Decreased serum complement C3 levels (normal C4 levels); no evidence for increased susceptibility to bacterial infection
  e. Decreased erythrocyte sedimentation rate (ESR); if the ESR is elevated, consider another diagnosis.
2. Chemistry:
  a. Hypokalemia: Hypokalemia with an increased serum bicarbonate level may indicate frequent vomiting or use of diuretics, whereas nonanion gap acidosis is common with laxative abuse. Caloric restriction alone does not usually cause hypokalemia.
  b. Hyponatremia: Secondary to excess water intake
  c. Hypophosphatemia

  d. Hypomagnesemia
  e. Hypocalcemia
  f. Increased blood urea nitrogen (BUN)
  g. Mildly increased serum transaminases
  h. Increased cholesterol
  i. Increased serum carotene level (15% to 40% of patients)
  j. Decreased vitamin A level
  k. Decreased serum zinc and copper levels
3. Endocrine:
  a. Thyroid:
  - Thyrotropin (TSH): Usually normal
  - Thyroxine (T_4): Usually normal or slightly low
  - 3,5,3′-Triiodothyronine (T_3): Often low, probably representing increased conversion of T_4 to reverse T_3
  - Thyroid changes represent adaptation to starvation, do not require thyroid hormone replacement, and will reverse with weight restoration.
  b. Growth hormone (GH):
  - Decreased insulin-like growth factor 1 levels
  - GH levels normal or elevated
  c. Prolactin: Usually normal
  d. Gonadotropins:
  - Basal levels of luteinizing hormone (LH) and follicle-stimulating hormone (FSH): Usually low
  - Twenty-four-hour LH secretory pattern: Prepubertal with low LH levels and no spikes or occasional nocturnal spikes
  - Blunted response of FSH and LH to gonadotropin-releasing hormone stimulation
  e. Sex steroids:
  - Estradiol: Low in females (<30 pg/mL)
  - Testosterone: Low in males
  f. Cortisol:
  - Basal levels normal or slightly high
  - Decreased response of adrenocorticotropic hormone (ACTH) to corticotropin-releasing hormone
  - Normal cortisol response to ACTH stimulation
4. Cardiac:
  a. Electrocardiogram (ECG): Bradycardia, low-voltage changes, prolonged QTc interval, T-wave inversions, and occasional ST-segment depression
  b. Echocardiogram: Decreased cardiac size and left ventricular wall thickness, pericardial effusion, and increased prevalence of mitral valve prolapse
5. Gastrointestinal (GI):
  a. Upper GI tract series: Usually normal findings; with occasional decreased gastric motility. May demonstrate features of the superior mesenteric artery syndrome
  b. Barium enema: Normal findings
6. Renal and metabolic:
  a. Decreased glomerular filtration rate
  b. Elevated BUN concentration
  c. Decreased maximum concentration ability (nephrogenic diabetes insipidus)
  d. Metabolic alkalosis
  e. Alkaline urine
7. Low bone mineral density (BMD):
  a. Females with AN have low BMD and are at increased fracture risk.
  b. Oral estrogen–progesterone combination pills have not been proven to be effective in increasing BMD.[8,9]
  c. Bisphosphonates (alendronate and risedronate) have shown no significant effect on spine BMD in adolescents[10] but positive effect in adults.[11]
  d. 17β-estradiol transdermal patch to older girls with AN (bone age ≥ 15 years) and small but increasing doses of ethinyl estradiol to younger girls (bone age < 15 years, in whom growth is not complete) showed increased spine and hip BMD.[12] However, complete catch-up did not occur.

TABLE 33.2

Medical Complications of Eating Disorders

System	Anorexia Nervosa	Bulimia Nervosa
Fluid and electrolytes	• Dehydration, elevated BUN/creatinine • Hypokalemia • Hyponatremia • Hypochloremic alkalosis • Hypophosphatemia • Hypomagnesemia • Hypoglycemia • Ketonuria • Edema	• Dehydration, elevated BUN/creatinine • Hypokalemia (from vomiting or from laxative or diuretic use) • Hypophosphatemia (especially when binging occurs after a prolonged period of dietary restriction) • Hypomagnesemia • Edema
Head, eyes, ears, nose and throat	• Dry, cracked lips and tongue	• Dry lips and tongue • Palatal scratches • Erosion of dental enamel • Dental caries
Cardiovascular	• Bradycardia • Orthostatic hypotension • Orthostatic blood pressure or heart rate changes • Cardiac arrhythmias • Electrocardiographic abnormalities (prolonged QT interval, low voltage, T-wave abnormalities) • Reduced myocardial contractility • Mitral valve prolapse • Pericardial effusion • Congestive heart failure	• Dizziness • Orthostatic blood pressure or heart rate changes • Cardiac arrhythmias • Ipecac cardiomyopathy
Gastrointestinal	• Delayed gastric emptying • Constipation • Elevated transaminases • Superior mesenteric artery syndrome • Rectal prolapse • Gallstones	• Parotid swelling • Esophagitis • Mallory–Weiss tears • Rupture of the esophagus or stomach • Acute pancreatitis • Paralytic ileus secondary to laxative abuse • Cathartic colon • Barrett esophagus
Pulmonary		• Aspiration pneumonia • Pneumomediastinum

System	Anorexia Nervosa	Bulimia Nervosa
Renal	• Elevated BUN/creatinine • Decreased glomerular filtration rate • Renal calculi • Edema • Renal concentrating defect • Enuresis (most commonly nocturnal)	• Elevated BUN/creatinine • Massive edema (after withdrawal of laxatives)
Endocrine	• Primary or secondary amenorrhea • Pubertal delay • Growth retardation and short stature • Low T3 syndrome • Hypercortisolism • Partial diabetes insipidus	• Irregular menses
Hematological	• Anemia • Leukopenia • Thrombocytopenia • Low ESR	
Musculoskeletal	• Muscle wasting and generalized muscle weakness • Reduced BMD • Increased fracture risk	• Fatigue, muscle weakness, and cramps • Reduced BMD (if previously at a low weight or amenorrheic)
Dermatologic	• Acrocyanosis • Dry, yellow skin (hypercarotenemia) • Lanugo • Brittle nails • Thin, dry hair • Hair loss	• Calluses on the dorsum of hand (Russell's sign)
Neurological	• Syncope • Seizures • Peripheral neuropathies • Structural brain changes (enlarged lateral ventricles and deficits in both gray and white matter volumes) • Decreased concentration, memory, and thinking ability	• Syncope • Seizures

e. Current recommendations for low BMD in AN include sustainable weight restoration through optimizing nutritional intake, resumption of spontaneous menses, and optimal calcium (1,300 mg/day of elemental calcium) and vitamin D (600 to 1,000 IU units/day) intake. Despite intervention, BMD may not return to normal.

Medical Complications

Table 33.2 outlines the medical complications seen in AYAs with AN.

Diagnosis and Differential Diagnosis

The diagnosis of AN should be suspected in any AYAs with unexplained weight loss and food avoidance.

1. Medical conditions:
   a. Inflammatory bowel disease
   b. Malabsorption—cystic fibrosis, celiac disease
   c. Endocrine conditions—hyperthyroidism, Addison's disease, diabetes mellitus

d. Collagen vascular disease
e. Central nervous system (CNS) lesions—hypothalamic or pituitary tumors
f. Malignancies
g. Chronic infections—tuberculosis, human immunodeficiency virus
h. Immunodeficiency
2. Psychiatric conditions:
a. Mood disorders
b. Anxiety disorders
c. Somatization disorder
d. Substance abuse disorder
e. Psychosis

Evaluation

History

Helpful questions regarding eating, weight-control behavior, and other issues include:

1. Why has individual and/or family come for assessment?
2. How does she/he feel about her/his appearance?
3. Is she/he trying to change her/his appearance?
4. Any change in weight? If yes, what methods were used?
5. How much does the patient want to weigh?
6. Does the patient binge? Describe a "binge?" Frequency of binges?
7. What methods of purging are used (vomiting, laxative abuse, diuretics, ipecac, diet pills, herbal medications, or other CAM)?
8. Highest and lowest weight and when?
9. Feeling that one's body affects her/his mood?
10. Is there a part of the patient's body that she/he is uncomfortable with and why?
11. Does the disordered eating interfere with the individual's life? How much time does he or she spend preparing food, exercising, and weighing him/herself?
12. How much does the patient worry about eating or her/his weight?
13. Previous treatment, including hospitalizations? Where? What type and for how long?
14. Exercise history? Type, amount, and frequency?
15. Twenty-four-hour dietary recall?
16. Menstrual history including age of menarche, last normal menstrual period, frequency of menses, changes in menses, medications including hormonal contraceptives?
17. Family medical and psychiatric history (family members with an eating disorder, mental illness, or substance abuse disorder)
18. Prior or current history of sexual, physical, or emotional abuse?
19. Family's understanding of patient's eating problem? What have parent(s)/caregiver/family members done to support the individual?

Instruments

Several instruments have been developed to aid in the diagnosis of eating disorders and the differentiation of AN from BN. These include the following:

1. *Eating Attitudes Test (EAT-26)*: This screening test is a 26-item self-report questionnaire that examines attitudes and behaviors regarding food, weight, and body image. A score >21 is suggestive of an eating disorder and warrants further evaluation.[13] The EAT-26 has been validated for use in adolescents.
2. *Eating Disorders Inventory*: A 91-item questionnaire that can be used both for screening and monitoring the emergence of an eating disorder in a high-risk group but not for diagnosis. It assesses drive for thinness, body dissatisfaction, bulimic behaviors as well as other dimensions associated with eating disorders including ineffectiveness, perfectionism, interpersonal distrust, interoceptive awareness, and maturity fears. Scores reflect percentiles for normal populations.[14]
3. *Eating Disorders Examination Questionnaire (EDE-Q)*: The EDE-Q[15] is a 38-item self-report version of the Eating Disorders Examination administered to assess eating disorder pathology. The questionnaire assesses restraint and concerns about eating, body weight, and shape.
4. *Kids' Eating Disorders Survey (KEDS)*: The KEDS[16] is a 14-item self-report instrument requiring a second-grade reading level. It includes a three-point scale and eight figure drawings for assessing body shape concerns. Normal values are available.

Nutritional Assessment

1. Twenty-four-hour dietary recall:
a. Types of foods and beverages
b. Portion sizes
c. Specific foods or food groups that are intentionally avoided (e.g., fats, carbohydrates, or protein)
d. Excessive amount of fluid intake including caffeinated products (coffee, tea, iced tea, or soda) to reduce hunger and alter body weight
2. Diet products or CAM
3. Dietary calcium intake:
a. Adolescents require 1300 mg of elemental calcium/day
b. May require oral supplementation
4. Anthropometric measurements: Height, weight, BMI, and skinfold measures

Physical Examination

1. Measure weight and height and calculate BMI and plot on Centers for Disease Control and Prevention growth charts:
a. Weight—measure in hospital gown after patient has emptied her/his bladder
b. Calculate BMI = weight (kg)/height (m^2).
c. Calculate percentage median BMI = patient's BMI/ median BMI for age and sex × 100.
d. Obtain previous growth charts—may indicate falling off percentiles for weight, height, or BMI
2. Sexual Maturity Rating: Assure that puberty is proceeding in a normal manner.
3. Focus on signs of malnutrition described above.

Recommended Laboratory Tests

1. Complete blood cell (CBC) and platelet count and ESR
2. Serum chemistry including BUN, creatinine, electrolytes (including calcium, magnesium, and phosphorus) and liver function tests
3. Serum albumin level
4. T_3, T_4, and TSH levels
5. LH, FSH, estradiol, and prolactin level if amenorrheic
6. ECG
7. BMD
a. In females who have been amenorrheic for >6 months
b. No definitive recommendations for males

Optional laboratory tests include:

1. Upper GI tract series and small bowel series
2. Barium enema
3. Celiac screen
4. Computed tomography or magnetic resonance imaging of the head.

Treatment

1. Team approach: Treatment is best conducted by an interdisciplinary team of individuals who are skilled and knowledgeable in working with AYAs with eating disorders. The treatment team typically consists of a physician, therapist, and nutritionist. Excellent communication among team members is paramount.

2. Diagnosis: Early diagnosis and intervention is important.
3. Medical and nutritional intervention: Goals include nutritional rehabilitation, weight restoration, and reversal of the acute medical complications.
4. Psychological intervention: Empiric research supports that family-based treatment (FBT) is an effective first-line treatment for adolescents with AN.[17] FBT is based on the importance of empowering parents/caregivers as the principal resource in effectively changing the eating disorder behaviors. Coexisting mental illness such as an anxiety disorder or depression should also be considered in making treatment recommendations.
5. Pharmacological treatment: Some individuals with eating disorders may benefit from the use of psychotropic medications. Fluoxetine does not augment the inpatient treatment of AN.[18,19] One study reported that fluoxetine prevented relapse in AYAs with AN who have attained 85% expected body weight (EBW),[18] whereas another study failed to demonstrate any benefit from fluoxetine in weight-restored patients with AN.[20] The most common medications used include the following selective serotonin reuptake inhibitors: fluoxetine, sertraline, paroxetine, fluvoxamine, and citalopram. These medications are also useful in treating comorbid depression or OCD. The US Food and Drug Administration has required manufacturers of these medications to include a "black box" warning label alerting health care providers and consumers to an increased risk of suicidal thinking and behavior in those being treated with the medications. The atypical antipsychotic medications such as risperidone, olanzapine, and quetiapine may be effective in reducing anxiety and obsessional thinking in AN, but do not appear to increase rate of weight gain over and above standard treatment. While psychopharmacology may have a role in treating comorbid symptoms in patients, it should not be the first line of treatment.[21]
6. Treatment setting:
   a. Inpatient, outpatient, partial hospitalization, or residential settings
   b. Indications for hospitalization outlined in **Table 33.3**.[22]
   c. Goals of hospitalization include weight gain and reversal of the acute medical complications.
   d. Nutritional rehabilitation
      • Essential for underweight or those who are medically compromised
      • Weight restoration via oral route, whenever possible
      • Short-term nasogastric feeding may be necessary.
      • Studies show that 1,400 to 2,000 kcal/day with regular nutritional advancements[23–26] results in consistent and safe weight gain with negligible adverse effects.
      • Inpatient weight gain of 2 to 3 pounds a week is optimal.
      • Refeeding syndrome—a constellation of cardiac, hematological, and neurological symptoms is associated with refeeding a malnourished patient.
      • Most serious feature of refeeding is sudden unexpected death associated with hypophosphatemia and cardiac arrhythmias.
      • Refeeding hypophosphatemia has been associated with the degree of malnutrition on admission and the rate of weight loss prior to admission.[24]
   e. Some medical complications may not be completely reversible (growth retardation, reduced bone mass, and structural brain changes)with nutritional rehabilitation (Fig. 33.1).[27]

Clinical and Laboratory Findings Associated with Sudden Death

1. Prolonged QTc interval
2. Hypophosphatemia
3. Ipecac cardiomyopathy
4. Severe emaciation (<70% of EBW)

TABLE 33.3

Indications for Hospitalization in an Adolescent with an Eating Disorder

One or more of the following justify hospitalization:
1. Severe malnutrition (weight ≤75% median body mass index for age and sex)
2. Dehydration
3. Electrolyte disturbances (hypokalemia, hyponatremia, hypophosphatemia)
4. ECG abnormalities (e.g. prolonged QTc or severe bradycardia)
5. Physiological instability
   Severe bradycardia (heart rate <50 beats/min daytime; <45 beats/min at night)
   Hypotension (<90/45 mm Hg)
   Hypothermia (body temperature <96°F)
   Orthostatic changes in pulse (>20 beats/min) or blood pressure (>20 mm Hg systolic and >10 mm Hg diastolic)
6. Arrested growth and development
7. Failure of outpatient treatment
8. Acute food refusal
9. Uncontrollable binging and purging
10. Acute medical complications of malnutrition (e.g., syncope, seizures, cardiac failure, pancreatitis)
11. Acute psychiatric emergencies (e.g., suicidal ideation, acute psychosis)
12. Comorbid diagnosis that interferes with the treatment of the eating disorder (e.g., severe depression, obsessive-compulsive disorder, severe family dysfunction)

Adapted with permission from Golden NH, Katzman DK, Sawyer SM, et al. Position paper of the Society for Adolescent Health and Medicine: medical management of restrictive eating disorders in adolescents and young adults. *J Adolesc Health* 2015;56:121–125.

Outcome

More than 100 studies have been conducted on the outcome of AN over the last 50 years with wide variability in the results. Comparisons among studies are limited by differences in definitions of recovery cases, length of follow-up, and type of data collected. General consensus is that the prognosis for young people with AN is better than that for adults, due in part to the shorter duration of symptoms in this population. Between 40% and 70% of adolescents with AN recover, 20% to 30% improve but continue to have persistent symptoms, and 20% develop a chronic form of the illness.[6]

In a well-designed prospective study, 95 adolescents with AN (aged 12 to 17) were followed up at 6- to 12-month intervals for 10 to 15 years.[28] There was full recovery in 75.8%, partial recovery in an additional 10.5%, and chronicity or no recovery in 13.7%. However, the time to full recovery was prolonged and ranged from 57 to 79 months. Readmission to the hospital within the first year of treatment occurred in 30% of patients but did not portend a poor prognosis. Adolescents with AN can fully recover, but the time to recover may take many years. Findings pertaining to recovery include:

1. Weight restoration: 40% to 63% of adolescents achieve a weight >90% EBW at one-year follow-up.[29]
2. Menses: 68% of adolescents with AN followed for 1 year and 95% of those followed for 2 years were menstruating at follow-up.[7]
3. Eating difficulties:
   a. Eating difficulties take longer to resolve.
   b. One-third of patients were eating normally at follow-up and half were still purposefully avoiding high-calorie foods.
4. Psychological disturbances:
   a. Psychiatric comorbidity common in follow-up
   b. Lifetime incidence of depression in 50% to 68%; anxiety disorders (especially OCD and social phobia) in 30% to 65%; substance abuse in 12% to 21%; and comorbid personality disorders in 20% to 80%

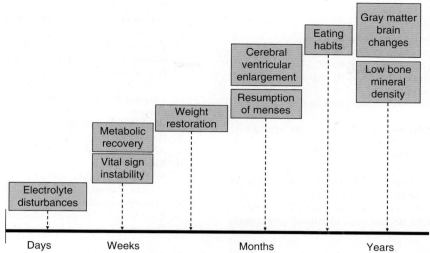

FIGURE 33.1 Timeline for resolution of the medical complications of anorexia nervosa. (Reprinted with permission from Golden NH, Meyer W. Nutritional rehabilitation of anorexia nervosa. Goals and dangers. *Int J Adolesc Med Health* 2004;16(2):131. Freund Publishing House Ltd.)

  c. Good or satisfactory psychosocial functioning ranged from 22% to 73%.
  d. One-third of patients with AN "cross over" to BN at some time in their illness.
5. Psychosocial: Most patients were engaged in full-time employment, with good work attendance.
6. Mortality:
  a. Mortality rate ranges from 2% to 8% with a standardized mortality ratio of 4.4 to 6.2.[30]
  b. Causes of death are suicide and the medical complications of starvation.
  c. Greatest risk for mortality occurs in the first 10 years of follow-up.
7. Factors associated with a good prognosis:
  a. Short duration of illness
  b. Early identification and intervention
  c. Early onset (<14 years old)
  d. No associated comorbid psychological diagnoses
  e. No binging and purging
  f. Supportive family
8. Factors associated with a poor prognosis:
  a. Longer duration of illness
  b. Binging and purging
  c. Comorbid mental illness (mood disorders, substance abuse)
  d. Lower body weight at presentation

AN appears to have lower recovery rates than BN.

BULIMIA NERVOSA

BN is an eating disorder characterized by recurrent binge-eating accompanied by inappropriate compensatory behaviors including self-induced vomiting, laxative abuse, enemas, diuretics, excessive exercise, prolonged fasting, abuse of stimulants (including methylphenidate, cocaine, over the counter 'natural' supplements, caffeine), and underdosing of insulin (for those with diabetes mellitus) to control weight or to purge calories consumed during a binge eating. These behaviors must occur, on average, at least once a week for 3 months (**Table 33.4**).[1]

Epidemiology

1. Prevalence:
  a. Up to 15% of individuals report binge-eating or purging behaviors. The numbers are even higher for college students with

TABLE 33.4
DSM-5 Diagnostic Criteria for Bulimia Nervosa[1]

A. Recurrent episodes of binge eating. An episode of binge eating is characterized by both of the following:
  1. Eating, in a discrete period of time (e.g., within any 2-hour period), an amount of food that is definitely larger than what most individuals would eat in a similar period of time under similar circumstances
  2. A sense of lack of control over eating during the episode (e.g., a feeling that one cannot stop eating or control what or how much one is eating)
B. Recurrent inappropriate compensatory behaviors in order to prevent weight gain, such as self-induced vomiting; misuse of laxatives, diuretics, or other medications; fasting; or excessive exercise
C. The binge-eating and inappropriate compensatory behaviors both occur, on average, at least once a week for 3 months
D. Self-evaluation is unduly influenced by body shape and weight
E. The disturbance does not occur exclusively during episodes of anorexia nervosa

23% of college women and 14% of college men reporting binging at least once each week, and 23% of the females and 9% of the males using vomiting, laxatives, or diuretics for weight control.
  b. Lifetime prevalence of BN in young females living in western industrialized countries is estimated to be 1% to 4%.
2. Age:
  a. Onset during late adolescence or early adulthood
  b. Modal age at onset of 18 to 19 years
  c. Rare in those less than 14 years old.
3. Gender:
  a. 90% to 95% are female.
  b. Recently, increased prevalence in males, particularly those who participate in sports with weight classes/restrictions (e.g., wrestlers)
4. Comorbidity:
  a. 80% of patients with BN report a lifetime prevalence of another psychiatric condition.
  b. Major comorbid conditions are affective disorders (50% to 80%), anxiety disorders (13% to 65%), personality disorders (20% to 80%), and substance abuse disorders (25%).[6]
  c. Patients tend to be more impulsive than those with AN.
  d. May engage in shoplifting, stealing, self-destructive acts, and sexual acting out.

Risk Factors

1. Age and gender:
   a. More likely to develop during adolescence
   b. Females affected more than males
2. Early childhood eating and health problems:
   a. Childhood eating problems (pica, early digestive problems, and weight reduction efforts)
3. Weight concerns, negative body image, and dieting
4. Personality traits:
   a. Negative affect, impulsivity, stressful life events, and family conflict
5. Early puberty/early menarche
6. Family history:
   a. Increased risk of developing BN if a family member has an eating disorder; concordance rates are higher for monozygotic than for dizygotic twins and range from 27% to 83%.
   b. Susceptibility locus for BN has been identified on chromosome 10p.[31]
7. Childhood sexual abuse.

Clinical Manifestations

Behaviors

1. Binging and purging
   a. Binging:
      - Rapid consumption of a large amount of high-calorie food (as high as 3,000 to 5,000 kcal) in a short period of time
      - Self-perceived loss of control over eating
      - Triggers—negative mood, interpersonal stress, hunger due to dietary restriction, and negative feelings related to body image. Typically occur in afternoon after skipping breakfast or lunch, or late in the evening.
   b. Purging (specific behaviors outlined above)
   c. Binge–purge cycles:
      - After a binge, feelings of guilt and shame together with fear of weight gain result in purging.
      - Purging may have a calming effect and relieve guilt after a binge episode leading to recurrent cycles of binging and purging in an attempt to manage feelings of depression and anxiety.
      - Binging and purging are usually done secretly.
      - Patients distressed by abnormal eating behaviors.
         Initially, the binge–purge activity may be infrequent, but with time, it may increase to daily or even several times a day. Some individuals with BN will purge even after ingesting normal or small amounts of any food that might be considered high in calories or fat. Therefore, over time, what began as a diet or weight-control measure turns into a means of mood regulation with the binging and purging behaviors becoming a source of coping.
2. Evidence of purging:
   a. Frequent trips to the bathroom, particularly after eating.
   b. Signs and/or smells of vomit, presence of empty food containers, or packages of laxatives or diuretics
3. Evidence of binge eating:
   a. Disappearance of food or the presence of empty wrappers and containers indicating the consumption of large amounts of food
   b. Stealing, hoarding, hiding food, or eating in secret
4. Frequently weighing
5. Preoccupation with food
6. Overly concerned with food, body weight, shape, and size
7. Self-evaluation is unduly influenced by body shape and weight.

Signs and Symptoms

1. Signs
   a. Body weight is usually normal or above normal.
   b. Marked weight fluctuations

   c. Skin changes: Calluses on the dorsum of the hand secondary to abrasions from the central incisors when the fingers are used to induce vomiting (Russell's sign)
   d. Enlargement of the salivary glands: Commonly parotid glands; usually bilateral and painless
   e. Dental enamel erosion (perimolysis): Usually occurs in the lingual, palatal, and posterior occlusal surfaces of the teeth
   f. Edema (fluid retention)
2. Symptoms
   a. Weakness and fatigue
   b. Headaches
   c. Abdominal fullness and bloating
   d. Nausea
   e. Normal or irregular menses
   f. Muscle cramps
   g. Chest pain and heartburn
   h. Easy bruising (from hypokalemia/platelet dysfunction)
   i. Bloody diarrhea (in laxative abusers).

Medical Complications

Table 33.2 outlines the medical complications seen in AYAs with BN.

Diagnosis and Differential Diagnosis

1. Medical conditions:
   a. Chronic cholecystitis
   b. Cholelithiasis
   c. Peptic ulcer disease
   d. Gastroesophageal reflux disease
   e. Superior mesenteric artery syndrome
   f. Malignancies (including CNS tumors)
   g. Infections—acute bacterial and viral GI infections, parasitic infections, and hepatitis
   h. Pregnancy
   i. Oral contraceptives: Nausea can be a side effect of oral contraceptives/hormone replacement therapy
   j. Medications—some have side effects that include nausea and vomiting, or food cravings.
2. Psychiatric conditions:
   a. AN-binge/purge subtype
   b. BED
   c. Major depressive disorder, with atypical features
   d. Borderline personality disorder
   e. Kleine–Levin syndrome

Evaluation

Evaluation includes a complete history and physical examination. Laboratory screening includes:

1. CBC count
2. BUN and creatinine, electrolytes, glucose, calcium, phosphorus, magnesium
3. Serum amylase
4. ECG with rhythm strip
5. Urinalysis—specific gravity

Treatment

The treatment requires an interdisciplinary team approach. The first step is to make a diagnosis and address the eating disorder as soon as possible. The principles of treatment include the following:

1. Medical and nutritional intervention: The goals of medical intervention include careful medical monitoring and the correction of any medical complication, in particular electrolyte abnormalities. A structured meal plan including three normal meals a day will reduce the physiological drive to binge. Individuals should be encouraged and supported to avoid foods that trigger a binge (e.g., ice cream or baked goods). Moderate exercise can also be helpful. Patients should have routine

dental care and consultation should be sought for those with dental damage secondary to vomiting.

2. Psychological intervention: In adults, cognitive-behavioral therapy (CBT) is the first-line therapy for BN.[32] Treatment with CBT reduces binge eating and purging activity in 30% to 50% of patients and improves attitudes about body shape and weight. CBT focuses on strategies to cope with the emotional triggers that lead to binge eating and purging and addresses ways to modify abnormal attitudes to eating, body shape, and weight. In adolescents with BN, 39% of those treated with FBT were no longer binging or purging compared with 18% receiving supportive psychotherapy.[33]

3. Pharmacologic treatment: Multiple studies have demonstrated a positive effect of a number of different antidepressants for treating BN. Fluoxetine is the only medication approved by the FDA for the treatment of BN and is most effective at a dose of 60 mg daily.[34] Treatment with fluoxetine results in a decrease in binge-eating and purging episodes in 55% to 65% of subjects. A combination of antidepressant medication and CBT appears to be superior to either modality alone.

4. Treatment settings: The treatment settings for individuals with BN are similar to those outlined for AN. The majority of patients with BN can be treated as outpatients.

Outcome

Most individuals with BN recover over time with recovery rates ranging from 35% to 75% at 5 years of follow-up. BN tends to be a chronic relapsing condition and approximately one-third of patients relapse in 1 to 2 years. Comorbidity is frequent but mortality is low.

Full recovery rates in women with BN tend to be higher than that in women with AN. No predictors of recovery have consistently been reported across studies but a poor outcome has been associated with poor self-esteem, long duration of illness prior to presentation, high frequency of binging and purging, and a history of substance abuse.[6]

BINGE-EATING DISORDER

BED became formally recognized as an eating disorder in the DSM-5 (**Table 33.5**).[1] BED is characterized by recurrent and persistent binge-eating that occurs at least weekly, for more than 3 months. BED is not associated with recurrent inappropriate compensatory behaviors. Patients with BED may eat rapidly, eat irrespective of hunger or satiety, eat alone because of embarrassment, and experience negative feelings after a binge. Individuals with BED are commonly overweight or obese and may not present with associated physical findings.

BED typically begins in adolescence or young adulthood and is common in adolescent and college-age samples. Community-based surveys suggest that BED occurs in 1% to 2% of young people between the ages of 10 and 19 years. The lifetime prevalence of BED is 2.8%. BED affects women slightly more often than men. BED is as common among females from racial or ethnic minority groups as for White females. The disorder is more prevalent among those in weight-loss treatment than in the general population.

The causes of BED are still unknown although it appears to run in families. The disorder is associated with increased medical morbidity and mortality and increased health care utilization. Treatment approaches currently being studied include CBT, interpersonal psychotherapy, and psychotropic medications such as antidepressants. Although the course for BED is comparable to that of BN, remission rates are higher for BED.

AVOIDANT RESTRICTIVE FOOD INTAKE DISORDER

Avoidant restrictive food intake disorder (ARFID) replaces and expands the DSM-IV diagnosis of feeding disorder of infancy or early childhood (**Table 33.6**).[1] The signature feature of ARFID is a

TABLE 33.5

DSM-5 Diagnostic Criteria for Binge-Eating Disorder[1]

A. Recurrent episodes of binge eating. An episode of binge eating is characterized by both of the following:
1. Eating, in a discrete period of time (e.g., within any 2-hour period), an amount of food that is definitely larger than what most people would eat in a similar period of time under similar circumstances
2. A sense of lack of control over eating during the episode (e.g., a feeling that one cannot stop eating or control what or how much one is eating)
B. The binge-eating episodes are associated with three (or more) of the following:
1. Eating much more rapidly than normal
2. Eating until feeling uncomfortably full
3. Eating large amounts of food when not feeling physically hungry
4. Eating alone because of feeling embarrassed by how much one is eating
5. Feeling disgusted with oneself, depressed, or very guilty afterward
C. Marked distress regarding binge eating in present
D. The binge eating occurs, on average, at least once a week for three months
E. The binge eating is not associated with the recurrent use of inappropriate compensatory behavior as in bulimia nervosa and does not occur exclusively during the course of bulimia nervosa or anorexia nervosa

TABLE 33.6

DSM-5 Diagnostic Criteria for Avoidant Restrictive Food Intake Disorder[1]

A. An eating or feeding disturbance (e.g., apparent lack of interest in eating or food; avoidance based on the sensory characteristics of food; concern about aversive consequences of eating) as manifested by persistent failure to meet appropriate nutritional and/or energy needs associated with one (or more) of the following:
1. Significant weight loss (or failure to achieve expected weight gain or faltering growth in children)
2. Significant nutritional deficiency
3. Dependence on enteral feeding or oral nutritional supplements
4. Marked interference with psychosocial functioning
B. The disturbance is not better explained by lack of available food or by an associated culturally sanctioned practice
C. The eating disturbance does not occur exclusively during the course of anorexia nervosa or bulimia nervosa, and there is no evidence of a disturbance in the way in which one's body weight or shape is experienced
D. The eating disturbance is not attributable to a concurrent medical condition or not better explained by another mental disorder. When the eating disturbance occurs in the context of another condition or disorder, the severity of the eating disturbance exceeds that routinely associated with the condition or disorder and warrants additional clinical attention

disturbance in eating or feeding as exhibited by persistent failure to meet appropriate nutritional and/or energy needs leading to significant clinical consequences, such as weight loss, failure to achieve expected weight gain, or faltering growth in children; nutritional deficiency; dependence on enteral feeding or oral nutritional supplements; or marked interference with psychosocial functioning. ARFID can occur in children, adolescents, and adults. The disturbance cannot be attributed to AN or to a medical condition. Recent studies suggest that the incidence of ARFID is approximately 14% but can vary between sites.[35] ARFID is more common among males compared to those with AN or BN. Patients with ARFID have a low body weight, but not as low as that found in patients with AN. In addition, patients with ARFID are younger and have a longer duration of illness compared with children and adolescents with AN and BN. Although treatment interventions have not yet been studied, it is currently recommended that treatment include medical monitoring, nutritional interventions and advice, and psychological interventions.

MALES AND EATING DISORDERS

Approximately 10% of AYAs suffering from eating disorders are male. The percentage of males with eating disorders is higher in young adolescent males than in adult males. The reasons for the growing prevalence of eating disorders in younger adolescent males remain unclear. Research indicates that eating disorders in adolescent males are clinically similar to eating disorders in females. Body image concerns appear to be one of the strongest variables in predicting eating disorders in males. Adolescent males at increased risk for developing an eating disorder include:

1. Participation in athletic activities where there is a focus on body weight and body image—body builders, wrestlers, dancers, swimmers, runners, rowers, gymnasts, and jockeys
2. Struggles with sexual identity conflict
3. Comorbid mental disorders
4. Family history of an eating disorder.

Although males of all types of sexual orientation develop eating disorders, several studies report that there is an increased incidence of homosexuality among males with eating disorders.

FEMALE ATHLETE TRIAD

The female athlete triad is a syndrome consisting of low energy availability, menstrual dysfunction, and reduced BMD in female athletes.[36] The key feature is that in these athletes, caloric intake is insufficient for energy expenditure. The resulting "energy deficit" causes hypothalamic amenorrhea (primary or secondary) and a low estrogen state. The low estrogen state is associated with osteoporosis and increased fracture risk (see Chapter 19).

Females at greatest risk are those participating in sports that emphasize a lean physique (e.g., figure skating, gymnastics, ballet, long distance running, and swimming). The triad is not restricted to elite athletes but is also seen with increasing frequency in recreational athletes. Frequent weigh-ins, consequences for weight gain, and pressure from parents or athletic coaches may also increase an athlete's risk.

Many female athletes with the triad do not meet strict DSM-5 criteria for AN or BN,[1] but engage in similar disordered eating behaviors such as dietary restriction, prolonged fasting, self-induced vomiting, or the use of laxatives, diuretics, or diet pills to lose weight or maintain a thin physique. Body weight can be low, but often is in the normal range and usually there is no body image distortion.

This disorder often goes unrecognized because of the subtlety of the symptoms, the secretive nature of the disorder, and the belief that amenorrhea is a common consequence of athletic training. Although the triad is more prevalent in elite athletes, one or more components of the triad can occur in up to 1/4 of high school athletes. Early recognition of the female athlete triad is important and therefore requires careful screening and assessment. Every female athlete with amenorrhea should have a complete history and physical examination to evaluate for an underlying eating disorder and to rule out other treatable causes of amenorrhea. Principles of treatment include increasing caloric intake, calcium and vitamin D supplementation, restricting the intensity of training (if necessary), and monitoring for resumption of menses. Adolescent athletes, their parents, and coaches should be educated about this disorder and the associated health risks.

REFERENCES

1. American Psychiatric Association. *Diagnostic and Statistical Manual of mental disorders.* 5th ed. Arlington, VA: American Psychiatric Publishing, 2013.
2. Grice DE, Halmi KA, Fichter MM, et al. Evidence for a susceptibility gene for anorexia nervosa on chromosome 1. *Am J Human Genet* 2002;70(3):787–792.
3. Hoek HW, van Hoeken D. Review of the prevalence and incidence of eating disorders. *Int J Eat Disord* 2003;34(4):383–396.
4. American College Health Association. *American College Health Association–National College Health Assessment II: Reference Group Undergraduates Executive Summary.* Hanover, MD: American College Health Association, 2013.
5. Pinhas L, Morris A, Crosby RD, et al. Incidence and age-specific presentation of restrictive eating disorders in children: a Canadian Paediatric Surveillance Program study. *Arch Pediatr Adolesc Med* 2011;165(10):895–899.
6. Walsh BT, Bulik CM, Attia E, et al. Defining eating disorders. In: Evans DL, Foa EB, Gur RE, et al., eds. *Treating and preventing adolescent mental health disorders: what we know and what we don' know.* 2nd ed. New York, NY: Oxford University Press, The Annenberg Foundation Trust and Sunnylands, and the Annenberg public Policy Center of the University of Pennsylvania, 2005.
7. Golden NH, Jacobson MS, Schebendach J, et al. Resumption of menses in anorexia nervosa. *Arch Pediatr Adolesc Med* 1997;151(1):16–21.
8. Golden NH, Lanzkowsky L, Schebendach J, et al. The effect of estrogen-progestin treatment on bone mineral density in anorexia nervosa. *J Pediatr Adolesc Gynecol* 2002;15(3):135–143.
9. Strokosch GR, Friedman AJ, Wu SC, et al. Effects of an oral contraceptive (norgestimate/ethinyl estradiol) on bone mineral density in adolescent females with anorexia nervosa: a double-blind, placebo-controlled study. *J Adolesc Health* 2006;39(6):819–827.
10. Golden NH, Iglesias EA, Jacobson MS, et al. Alendronate for the treatment of osteopenia in anorexia nervosa: a randomized, double-blind, placebo-controlled trial. *J Clin Endocrinol Metab* 2005;90(6):3179–3185.
11. Miller KK, Meenaghan E, Lawson EA, et al. Effects of risedronate and low-dose transdermal testosterone on bone mineral density in women with anorexia nervosa: a randomized, placebo-controlled study. *J Clin Endocrinol Metab* 2011;96(7):2081–2088.
12. Misra M, Katzman D, Miller KK, et al. Physiologic estrogen replacement increases bone density in adolescent girls with anorexia nervosa. *J Bone Min Res* 2011;26(10):2430–2438.
13. Garner DM, Garfinkel PE. The eating attitudes test: an index of the symptoms of anorexia nervosa. *Psychol Med* 1979;9(2):273–279.
14. Garner DM, Olmsted MP. More on the eating disorder inventory. *Am J Psychiatry* 1986;143(6):805–806.
15. Fairburn CG, Beglin SJ. Assessment of eating disorders: interview or self-report questionnaire? *Int J Eat Disord* 1994;16(4):363–370.
16. Childress AC, Brewerton TD, Hodges EL, et al. The Kids' Eating Disorders Survey (KEDS): a study of middle school students. *J Am Acad Child Adolesc Psychiatry* 1993;32(4):843–850.
17. Lock J, Le Grange D, Agras WS, et al. Randomized clinical trial comparing family-based treatment with adolescent-focused individual therapy for adolescents with anorexia nervosa. *Arch Gen Psychiatry* 2010;67(10):1025–1032.
18. Kaye WH, Nagata T, Weltzin TE, et al. Double-blind placebo-controlled administration of fluoxetine in restricting- and restricting-purging-type anorexia nervosa. *Biol Psychiatry* 2001;49(7):644–652.
19. Attia E, Haiman C, Walsh BT, et al. Does fluoxetine augment the inpatient treatment of anorexia nervosa? *Am J Psychiatry* 1998;155(4):548–551.
20. Walsh BT, Kaplan AS, Attia E, et al. Fluoxetine after weight restoration in anorexia nervosa: a randomized controlled trial. *JAMA* 2006;295(22):2605–2612.
21. Golden NH, Attia E. Psychopharmacology of eating disorders in children and adolescents. *Pediatr Clin N Am* 2011;58(1):121–138, xi.
22. Golden NH, Katzman DK, Sawyer SM, Ornstein RM, Rome ES, Garber AK, Kohn M, Kreipe RE. Medical management of restrictive eating disorders in adolescents and young adults. Position Paper of the Society for Adolescent Health and Medicine. *J Adolesc Health* 2015; 56:121–125.
23. Garber AK, Mauldin K, Michihata N, et al. Higher calorie diets increase rate of weight gain and shorten hospital stay in hospitalized adolescents with anorexia nervosa. *J Adolesc Health* 2013;53(5):579–584.
24. Golden NH, Keane-Miller C, Sainani KL, et al. Higher caloric intake in hospitalized adolescents with anorexia nervosa is associated with reduced length of stay and no increased rate of refeeding syndrome. *J Adolesc Health* 2013;53(5):573–578.
25. Leclerc A, Turrini T, Sherwood K, et al. Evaluation of a nutrition rehabilitation protocol in hospitalized adolescents with restrictive eating disorders. *J Adolesc Health* 2013;53(5):585–589.
26. Whitelaw M, Gilbertson H, Lam PY, et al. Does aggressive refeeding in hospitalized adolescents with anorexia nervosa result in increased hypophosphatemia? *J Adolesc Health* 2010;46(6):577–582.
27. Katzman DK. Medical complications in adolescents with anorexia nervosa: a review of the literature. *Int J Eat Disord* 2005;37 (suppl):S52–S59; discussion S87–S59.
28. Strober M, Freeman R, Morrell W. The long-term course of severe anorexia nervosa in adolescents: survival analysis of recovery, relapse, and outcome predictors over 10–15 years in a prospective study. *Int J Eat Disord* 1997;22(4):339–360.
29. Forman SF, Grodin LF, Graham DA, et al. An eleven site national quality improvement evaluation of adolescent medicine-based eating disorder programs: predictors of weight outcomes at one year and risk adjustment analyses. *J Adolesc Health* 2011;49(6):594–600.
30. Franko DL, Keshaviah A, Eddy KT, et al. A longitudinal investigation of mortality in anorexia nervosa and bulimia nervosa. *Am J Psychiatry* 2013;170(8):917–925.
31. Bulik CM, Devlin B, Bacanu SA, et al. Significant linkage on chromosome 10p in families with bulimia nervosa. *Am J Human Genet* 2003;72(1):200–207.
32. Hay P. A systematic review of evidence for psychological treatments in eating disorders: 2005–2012. *Int J Eat Disord* 2013;46(5):462–469.
33. Le Grange D, Crosby RD, Rathouz PJ, et al. A randomized controlled comparison of family-based treatment and supportive psychotherapy for adolescent bulimia nervosa. *Arch Gen Psychiatry* 2007;64(9):1049–1056.
34. Fluoxetine in the treatment of bulimia nervosa. A multicenter, placebo-controlled, double-blind trial. Fluoxetine Bulimia Nervosa Collaborative Study Group. *Arch Gen Psychiatry* 1992;49(2):139–147.
35. Ornstein RM, Rosen DS, Mammel KA, et al. Distribution of eating disorders in children and adolescents using the proposed DSM-5 criteria for feeding and eating disorders. *J Adolesc Health* 2013;53(2):303–305.
36. Nattiv A, Loucks AB, Manore MM, et al. American College of Sports Medicine position stand. The female athlete triad. *Med Sci Sports Exerc* 2007;39(10):1867–1882.

 ADDITIONAL RESOURCES AND WEBSITES ONLINE

PART X

Functional and Other Unexplained Medical Conditions

34

Disorders of Somatic and Musculoskeletal Pain

Bethany A. Marston
David M. Siegel

Adolescent and young adult (AYA) patients who present with somatic illnesses as well as those who present with complaints of physical pain who lack clear or sufficient physical findings to explain their symptoms are a challenge to the physician. There are many potential explanations for such symptoms, but these can be difficult to accurately diagnose or manage, and some remain incompletely understood.

PSYCHOSOMATIC DISORDERS

Adjustment Disorder

Adjustment disorder is an excessive or exaggerated reaction to an identifiable life stressor. It is more than would be expected and can manifest as physical, psychological, and/or cognitive symptoms and impairment.

Potential stressors for AYAs that can lead to excessive and abnormal reactions include the following somatic symptoms:

- Physical changes of puberty
- The cognitive developmental progression from concrete to formal operational thinking
- Changing demands and expectations in the family, and social, academic, and vocational realms

Milder and more time-limited psychological disequilibrium can also precipitate bodily discomfort and lead to physical complaints such as light-headedness, nausea, headache, palpitations, and so on. All of these are commonly associated with emotional distress and may serve in the patient's mind as "legitimate" reasons to see the clinician; more acceptable to the patient and family than overtly expressed psychological problems.

Psychophysiological Disorders

In psychophysiological disorders, physical symptoms are observable and often fall into biological processes that are understood by the clinician and the disease course is clearly influenced by psychological function. For example, the patient with asthma experiences increased bronchospasm when under stress, leading to increased episodes of coughing, wheezing, and shortness of breath.

Although managing and optimally preventing these exacerbations is not necessarily easy or rapidly accomplished, the connection between the psychological and the physical, once shared with and understood by the patient and family, is not typically rejected or denied. The "medical legitimacy" of the primary physiological disorder (i.e., asthma) represents a common ground of acceptance between clinician and patient/family and also provides the clinician with a familiar and well-understood template for medical treatment. Beyond the strictly medical treatment, however, the clinician must attempt to facilitate the AYAs and parent(s) successfully identifying sources of stress and anxiety that contribute to inadequate control of the primary disease and its symptoms. This exploration may very well be enigmatic and may require open-ended questions, thoughtful probing, and multiple visits. Sometimes, referral to a health psychologist or medical family therapist is productive.

Somatic and Related Disorders

Complaints of significant somatic symptoms without identifiable biomedical etiology are frequent in AYA patient encounters and had previously been classified as somatoform somatization disorder. However, the *Diagnostic and Statistical Manual of the American Psychiatric Association*, 5th edition (DSM–5) articulates a new categorization template. This new template is clearer and provides a useful set of diagnostic labels and descriptions, recognizing that the majority of these patients present to medical as opposed to mental health settings. This group of conditions is now referred to as somatic symptom and related disorders, they all share the "prominence of somatic symptoms associated with significant distress and impairment."[1] Beginning with the most common, these include:

1. *Somatic symptom disorder*: Persistent (>6 months) somatic symptom(s) that cause psychosocial impairment, with persistent thoughts about the seriousness of symptoms, anxiety about symptoms or general health, or excessive time and energy devoted to symptoms or health concerns. Incorporation of affective, cognitive, and behavioral components rather than just somatic symptoms alone is central in making the diagnosis.

   The newer criteria for somatic symptom disorder require the presence of a symptom or symptoms with associated excessive or disproportionate thoughts, feelings, or behaviors that surround these, and the emphasis is on this disruptive or maladaptive response.[2] The symptom may be medically "explained" or not. This category encompasses most of those previously diagnosed with somatization disorder, undifferentiated somatoform disorder, and some of those with hypochondriasis, and DSM-5 further posits that the revised labels may be less stigmatizing, particularly in the case of hypochondriasis. The prior category of somatization disorder was also cumbersome and restrictive, requiring a complex tally of symptoms in different categories, while undifferentiated somatoform disorder was so broad as to be of questionable clinical usefulness. Some in the field have concerns that the current definitions may lead to overdiagnosis of somatic symptom disorder in those with medical illness.[3]

2. *Illness anxiety disorder*: Persistent (>6 months) preoccupation with having a serious undiagnosed illness, anxiety about health, or excessive health behaviors or maladaptive avoidance of situations perceived as health threats, accompanied by minimal somatic symptoms and not better explained by another disorder

3. *Conversion disorder*: Neurologic symptoms that are found, after appropriate neurological assessment, to be incompatible with neurological pathophysiology

4. *Psychological factors affecting other medical disorders*: Presence of one or more clinically significant psychological or behavioral factors that adversely affect a medical condition by increasing the risk for suffering, death, or disability

5. *Factitious disorder*: The falsification of medical or psychological signs and symptoms in oneself or others that are associated with the individual taking surreptitious actions to misrepresent, simulate, or cause signs or symptoms of illness or injury in the absence of obvious external rewards.

In contrast to somatoform disorders, in which symptoms are associated with unconscious conflict, factitious disorders are those of conscious falsification of symptoms and signs to create a sick role, thought to be motivated by the need to be cared for. Factitious disorders, especially those that are chronic, such as Munchausen syndrome and particularly Munchausen syndrome by proxy,[4] are serious and in some instances difficult to distinguish from somatoform conditions. These also need to be distinguished from malingering, which is not considered a psychiatric condition, in which there is conscious and intentional exaggeration or falsification of symptoms for an obvious secondary gain.

There are some general principles that can apply to how the clinician approaches AYAs when the above clinical entities are under consideration.

1. Biopsychosocial assessment: Biomedical and psychosocial factors must be evaluated at the onset. This will allow the clinician to understand the psychological stressors and conflicts, as well as the biomedical elements that together serve to limit the differential diagnosis. It also makes the eventual diagnosis of a psychosomatic disorder more acceptable to families in that this conclusion does not arise late in the evaluation process, that is, diagnosis of exclusion. Elements of the assessment include:
   a. Detailed history focused on the presenting symptoms: It is important not to neglect the symptoms that brought the patient and family to the provider. Focusing on the symptoms can give the AYAs the message that the provider is taking their concerns seriously, and does not need to reinforce the perception of medical illness.
   b. Physical examination focused on symptoms
   c. Laboratory and imaging studies: These should be chosen on the basis of the history and physical examination and should be limited to the least number of minimally invasive tests required to clarify the diagnosis or rule out important alternate possibilities.

2. Evaluation for psychiatric disease: Mood disorders (especially major depression, anxiety disorders), and even schizophrenia can all manifest with somatization, and sometimes physical symptoms may be the only complaints with which the AYAs initially present. When further questioning and interaction with the patient and family support the presence of significant psychiatric illness, formal mental health consultation is warranted. A less severe mood or anxiety disorder uncovered during the evaluation of somatic complaints may be managed by the adolescent/young adult care provider.

3. Evaluation for personality disorders: Beyond Axis I psychiatric diagnoses, somatic symptoms/somatic symptom disorder can also be associated with certain personality (Axis II) disorders. Those patients with enduring attitudes and habitual patterns of response that characterize obsessive-compulsive personality disorder or histrionic personality disorder are at higher risk for developing somatic symptom disorder. Adolescents with personality traits of dependency or neurotic preoccupation with self also have a greater tendency to experience and describe unexplained physical symptoms. The diagnosis of personality disorders per se, however, is generally not applicable to those under 18 years of age.

4. Evaluation of environmental factors: In addition to personality disorders, environmental factors can also underlie the emergence and perpetuation of various chronic pain syndromes. Somatic complaints in parents, family members, or peer contacts should be examined as possible models for, and contributors to, the patient's own symptoms and behaviors. Cultural norms and expectations might also reinforce a form of illness and an expression of distress that emphasizes and serves to support physical pain. An awareness on the part of providers as to the patient's cultural milieu is critical in placing preoccupation with somatic symptoms (as well as many other behaviors) in appropriate context.

Other aspects of a teen or young adult's present or past experience might also bear on somatic symptoms and provide insights for the provider into the possible meaning for the behavior. For example, a patient whose early life experience did not include consistent parental support and caretaking (or were exposed to overt trauma and/or abuse) might develop physical symptoms as a means to meet dependency needs. When these patients become increasingly demanding about diagnostic evaluations, and angry and hostile with the clinician about the lack of a physical diagnosis or the inadequacy of treatment, these emotions may actually be expressions of deeper and unconscious feelings about early caretakers that are now displaced onto the clinician.

In summary, important areas to help the practitioner understand somatic symptoms without biomedical explanation include the following:

- Symptoms of mental illness or psychiatric diagnosis
- Association with personality traits or disorder
- Modeling or reinforcement of somatic symptom behavior by the family, peer, or cultural environment
- Placement of somatic symptoms in the context of the patient's present or past experiences, circumstances, and culture

FUNCTIONAL PAIN DISORDERS

Fibromyalgia

Fibromyalgia and juvenile fibromyalgia are conditions of chronic widespread musculoskeletal pain. This disorder sometimes goes by other names, and precise definitions vary.

Epidemiology

1. Estimates of prevalence vary, but US-based hospital-based pediatric rheumatology clinics report that 7.65% of new patients seen were diagnosed with fibromyalgia[5] and in the community a 1% to 6% prevalence has been reported.[6,7]

2. The clinical characteristics of the condition are similar regardless of age, though the developmental and psychosocial differences between adolescence and adulthood bear on the disease's impact and some aspects of treatment.

Clinical Presentation

1. The predominant complaint is chronic widespread musculoskeletal pain defined as affecting the upper and lower as well as left and right sides of the body.

2. Most patients describe poor sleep quality, fatigue, mood disruption, and difficulty concentrating.

3. Many will have other somatic manifestations including headache, irritable bowel or other abdominal symptoms, dysmenorrhea, subjective swelling or color changes, dizziness, or multiple chemical sensitivities[8]
4. Symptoms may develop additively over time, and may not be recognized early due to relatively normal physical exam findings, but can have profound effects on function. Because of this, many patients present with concerns about arthritis, lupus, or other underlying rheumatologic conditions, and patients and families are often frustrated when no ready explanation for these symptoms is found on routine testing.

Pathophysiology

A biopsychosocial model, considering both biologic and environmental factors, is useful for understanding the effects of fibromyalgia on function and approaches to management. Although the factors that cause juvenile fibromyalgia are incompletely understood, pain processing appears to be altered in several ways in adult fibromyalgia and related conditions, and much of this research probably applies equally to younger patients.

1. The concept of central sensitization may be important in understanding this disorder; pain results from abnormal pain processing in the brain, resulting in a perception of pain at much lower levels of noxious stimulus (e.g., pressure or heat). As compared to normal controls:
   a. Functional magnetic resonance imaging has demonstrated increased cortical activity in pain-processing regions in fibromyalgia patients in response to pressure stimuli.[9]
   b. Patients with fibromyalgia demonstrate increased levels of pain neurotransmitters such as substance P and glutamate, and decreased levels of inhibitory substances such as dopamine, serotonin, and norepinephrine.[10]
2. Peripheral nerve abnormalities may also play a role. Small fiber neuropathy, including altered detection thresholds for temperature, mechanical, and pressure sensation, have recently been described.[11]
3. Genetic, environmental, and family influences are also important in the development of fibromyalgia. Juvenile and adult fibromyalgia are much more common in females than males, and are more common in those with affected relatives. There are some suggested HLA linkages and potential polymorphisms in some neurotransmitter genes that may be associated with increased susceptibility, but details and specificity remain unclear.[12]
4. Personality and family traits that may increase fibromyalgia symptoms or severity, including emotional sensitivity or anxiety, poor family functioning, poor coping responses such as pain catastrophization, and sedentary behaviors have also been described.

Diagnosis

Although these features may all influence a patient's symptoms and function, there are no absolutely confirmatory tests for the diagnosis of fibromyalgia. Classification criteria in both pediatric and adult populations depend on a thorough history and physical exam.

1. Self-reported symptoms of chronic widespread pain, fatigue, sleep disruption, cognitive changes, and other associated features (Table 34.1)[13] are well correlated with prior classification criteria that relied on clinical findings of tender points.
2. History and physical exam should focus on differentiating fibromyalgia from other conditions, and on excluding comorbid diagnoses, which may contribute to pain or functional difficulties.
   • Further evaluation with laboratory testing or imaging is appropriate when patients have atypical findings including the presence of asymmetric tenderness, primarily small joint tenderness, any joint swelling or limitation to passive range of motion, enthesitis, or objective systemic findings such as rash, fever, or weight loss.

TABLE 34.1

Fibromyalgia Diagnostic Criteria

Criteria
Patient satisfies diagnostic criteria for fibromyalgia if the following are met:
1. Widespread pain index (WPI) ≥7 and symptoms severity (SS) scale score ≥ 5 or WPI 3–6 and SS scale score ≥ 9
2. Symptoms have been present at a similar level for at least 3 mo
3. The patient does not have a disorder that would otherwise explain the pain

Ascertainment

1. WPI: note the number of areas in which the patient has had pain over the last week. In how many areas has the patient had pain? Score will be between 0 and 19

Should girdle, left	Hip (buttock, trochanter), left	Jaw, left	Upper back
Should girdle, right	Hip (buttock, trochanter), right	Jaw, right	Lower back
Upper arm, left	Upper leg, left	Chest	Neck
Upper arm, right	Upper leg, right	Abdomen	
Lower arm, left	Lower leg, left		
Lower arm, right	Lower leg, right		

2. SS scale score:
   Fatigue
   Waking unrefreshed
   Cognitive symptoms
   For each of the three symptoms above, indicate the level of severity over the past week using the following scale:

   0 = no problem
   1 = slight or mild problems, generally mild or intermittent
   2 = moderate, considerable problems, often present and/or at a moderate level
   3 = severe: pervasive, continuous, life-disturbing problems

   Consider somatic symptoms in general, indicate whether the patients has[a]:

   0 = no symptoms
   1 = few symptoms
   2 = a moderate number of symptoms
   3 = a great deal of symptoms

The SS scale score is the sum of severity of the three symptoms (fatigue, waking unrefreshed, cognitive symptoms) plus the extent (severity) of somatic symptoms in general. The final score is between 0 and 12

[a]Somatic symptoms that might be considered: muscle pain, irritable bowel symptoms, fatigue/tiredness, thinking or remembering problem, muscle weakness, headache, pain/cramps in the abdomen, numbness/tingling, dizziness, insomnia, depression, constipation, pain in in the upper abdomen, nausea, nervousness, chest pain, blurred vision, fever, diarrhea, dry mouth, itching, wheezing, Raynaud's phenomenon, hives/welts, ringing in the ears, vomiting, heartburn, oral ulcers, low or change in taste, seizures, dry eyes, shortness of breath, loss of appetite, rash, sun sensitivity, hearing difficulties, easy bruising, hair loss, frequent urination, painful urination, and bladder spasms.
Reprinted with permission from Wolfe F, Clauw DJ, Fitzcharles MA, et al. The American College of Rheumatology preliminary diagnostic criteria for fibromyalgia and measurement of symptom severity. *Arthritis Care Res (Hoboken)* 2010;62:600–610.

Management

Management of fibromyalgia is challenging, and placing a priority on nonpharmacologic treatment, especially in young people, is very important.

1. *Cognitive-behavioral therapy* is helpful to reduce pain catastrophization, improve coping and problem-solving skills, develop relaxation techniques, and minimizing associated depression and anxiety.

2. *Exercise therapy*, using aerobic and strength training approaches, can reduce pain, improve function, and ward off an increasingly sedentary activity pattern, which will otherwise lead to alterations in strength, balance, and posture, exacerbating pain and making exercise programs more likely to cause injuries and setbacks.

3. *Sleep Hygiene*: For adolescents in particular, stress the importance of adhering to good sleep hygiene, especially in the setting of emerging life challenges and demands that can precipitate flares in the disease.

4. *Medications* approved for fibromyalgia in adults have not been approved for pediatric patients, but clinical trials for some are underway. Categories of drugs used in fibromyalgia include:

   a. Serotonin-norepinephrine reuptake inhibitors
      • Duloxetine and milnacipran have been approved in adults, although venlafaxine may also be helpful.
   b. γ-aminobutyric acid analog antiepileptics
      • Pregabalin (approved in adult fibromyalgia) and gabapentin have indications for neuropathic pain and both are used clinically.
   c. Seratonin reuptake inhibitors may help with associated mood symptoms in some but have not been shown in adults to improve pain.
   d. Tricyclic antidepressants
      • Amitriptyline at low doses, and the muscle relaxant cyclobenzaprine that is chemically similar, are used off-label with benefit in some patients, particularly those in whom nonrestorative sleep is a prominent feature.

Prognosis

1. Early studies of juvenile fibromyalgia outcome were encouraging, with a long-term prognosis that appeared much better than that in adults; approximately 70% of children no longer met classification criteria after 2 years.[14] This was attributed at least in part to early diagnosis, which led to more timely patient awareness and acceptance, as well as initiation of therapy.[15]

2. More recent studies have shown that the majority of patients who seek treatment for juvenile fibromyalgia will still have increased pain and potentially reduced quality of life several years later.[16]

Complex Regional Pain Syndrome

Complex regional pain syndrome (CRPS) is a noninflammatory condition that includes regional pain, hyperesthesia/allodynia, vasomotor disturbances including swelling and color change, and eventually dystrophic changes. It has many other names, and is sometimes broken down into two types:

- Type I (also known as reflex sympathetic dystrophy), in which there is no definable nerve injury, is vastly more common.
- Type II (formerly known as causalgia), in which a nerve lesion is present.

Epidemiology

1. More common in girls
2. Average age at diagnosis in pediatric studies is about 13.[17,18]

Clinical Presentation

1. History and presenting symptoms include the following:
   • High-achieving, often under psychological stress
   • Same characteristics are prevalent in patient's family.
   • History of recent injury, which may be trivial
   • Pain is dramatically out of proportion to the mechanism or degree of injury.
   • Pain in one body region, usually a limb
   • Allodynia
   • Increased sensitivity to touch
   • Localized edema
   • Temperature changes (affected side is warmer or cooler than contralateral side)
   • Changes in color (may appear as pallor, cyanosis, or erythema)

2. Physical exam findings:
   • Extreme sensitivity to touch or pressure over the affected region, which does not follow a dermatomal pattern.
   • The affected limb is often cool to the touch and cyanotic; sometimes exhibits edema or hyperhidrosis, but less commonly is warm and ruddy.
   • Findings are typically limited to one limb. Lower extremities are more commonly affected in pediatric patients, unlike in adults. Occasionally, multiple sites may be affected.
   • Later findings may include thickened skin, muscle wasting, and eventually restriction of movement or contractures. These are seen less often in children than in adults.[18]

Diagnosis

Diagnosis on clinical presentation is sufficient and extensive investigative studies are not encouraged except in instances of clinical ambiguity.

1. If further testing is required to confirm the diagnosis of CRPS, objective markers of autonomic function such as resting sweat output, resting skin temperature, or quantitative sudomotor axon reflex testing can be pursued.

2. Imaging studies can be helpful, though findings may depend on duration of symptoms.
   • In early stages, scintigraphy (bone scan) may reveal increased uptake of technetium-99m on delayed bone imagings, though a normal scan does not rule out the diagnosis.
   • Plain X-rays are less helpful early in disease, but patchy demineralization within the affected area can be seen in some cases, particularly associated with chronicity of symptoms and signs. MRI can reveal skin thickening and edema or contrast enhancement of soft tissue in early stages, and changes in skin thickness and muscle atrophy are sometimes seen in later stages.

Differential Diagnosis

Alternate diagnoses can be distinguished using clinical, laboratory, or imaging features, and may include:

- Localized infection
- Atypical injury
- Vasculitis
- Raynaud's phenomenon
- Peripheral neuropathy
- Deep vein thrombosis or thrombophlebitis
- Arterial insufficiency
- Thoracic outlet syndrome (in the case of upper extremity involvement)
- Rheumatoid or juvenile arthritis
- Connective tissue disease including lupus or systemic sclerosis
- Conversion or factitious disorders

Management

As in fibromyalgia syndrome, optimal management is multifaceted. Prior to presentation, many patients have tried conservative treatment with rest, immobilization, and over-the-counter analgesics, which usually provide little relief. Lack of use of the involved limb actually contributes to disease progression and deterioration, so immobilization should be discouraged. A broad range of pharmacologic agents and interventions have been attempted in practice, but most remain poorly studied.

Early patient education is key for successful early functional improvement and outcome. This should include:

1. The nature of neuropathic pain, which does not indicate tissue damage.
2. The need for working to improve function of the affected area despite pain.
   • Most patients and families are initially quite resistant to therapeutic recommendations focused on aggressive use of the affected limb along with friction-mediated desensitization,

which is experienced as completely contrary to the person's intuitive sense that conscientious rest of the affected area and a minimum of physical contact are most comfortable and appropriate. As such, the health professional team must engage both education and consistent encouragement to support the patient in proceeding with therapy, including incorporation of pain management and coping strategies as early as possible.

3. Therapy
   - A recent review[19] summarizing trials in adults found strong evidence for physical therapy-based interventions to improve pain and function.
   - Aggressive and multidisciplinary (physical therapy, occupational therapy, psychologic) outpatient approaches are successful at both relieving pain and normalizing function in the majority of children, though for a small subset, progression to inpatient treatment is necessary.[20]
4. Medications
   A variety of medications have been studied in adults, but there is less evidence for the use of any pharmacologic agent or procedure for management of CRPS in young adolescents. Regardless, the use of invasive or painful procedures especially should be avoided.
   - There is fairly strong evidence that bisphosphonates improve pain in CRPS, though these should be used with caution in growing adolescents.
   - There is moderate evidence for transient benefit from low-dose intravenous ketamine, though there are significant concerns about safety and efficacy over time.
   - Reports of other interventions remain limited, though spinal cord stimulation, tadalafil, and intravenous immunoglobulin have been used.[19]
   - Many other agents have been tried with variable success in small or uncontrolled trials, and some experts advocate for the use of tricyclic antidepressants, and/or anticonvulsants such as gabapentin, as have been applied with other forms of chronic neuropathic pain.[21]
   - Results of treatment with systemic corticosteroids have been conflicting, though there may be utility in early stages, and nonsteroidal anti-inflammatory drugs consistently have little benefit.[22]
5. Procedures
   - Preliminary findings around the use of repetitive transcranial magnetic stimulation suggest benefit, but it is unclear if this is a feasible long-term approach.
   - Some forms of regional blockade have been described and may be helpful.
6. Psychological
   - Although CRPS is not a primarily psychological disorder, psychological and family interventions are important. Most patients with CRPS, and their families, experience significant personal and family stress as well as dysfunction.
   - Treatment approaches including early mobilization and aggressive physical therapy (PT) are painful for the patient and psychologic treatment can help promote adherance to PT.
7. Prognosis
   By maintaining a supportive structure and persistent adherence to a rehabilitative approach, a gradual and substantial recovery is a realistic treatment outcome for young patients with CRPS.

Other Functional Pain Syndromes

Many young people develop functional pain syndromes that are not primarily musculoskeletal. A detailed discussion of these is beyond the scope of this chapter, but they may frequently overlap with amplified musculoskeletal pain syndromes.

1. Functional abdominal pain and irritable bowel syndrome are quite common.
   - Similar to fibromyalgia, the approach consists of evaluating other potential biomedical causes of symptom and assessment for psychological stressors/triggers.
   - Management should focus on symptom-specific strategies, enhancement of coping, and identification of goals that are based on functional improvement as opposed to symptom eradication. As with other chronic pain syndromes, decrease in psychological and emotional distress is also an important target, and speaks to the central role of mental health professionals on the treatment team.
2. Other common pain syndromes include chronic daily headache, temporomandibular pain, interstitial cystitis or chronic pelvic pain, chronic back pain, and others. In our experience, though these can co-occur with fibromyalgia, they are generally less responsive than the latter to a rehabilitation approach that incorporates physical and occupational therapy modalities, along with mental health and behavioral strategies.

Chronic Fatigue Syndrome

While some patients with fibromyalgia syndrome may experience profound fatigue along with widespread pain, there are AYAs who do not manifest amplified pain and whose dominant symptom is persistent, overwhelming, and disabling fatigue leading to the diagnosis of chronic fatigue syndrome (see Chapter 35).

REFERENCES

1. American Psychiatric Association. *Diagnostic and Statistical Manual of mental disorders*. 5th ed. Arlington, VA: American Psychiatric Association; 2013.
2. Dimsdale JE, Creed F, Escobar J, et al. Somatic symptom disorder: an important change in DSM. *J Psychosom Res* 2013;75:223–228.
3. Frances A. DSM-5 somatic symptom disorder. *J Nerv Ment Dis* 2013;201:530–531.
4. von Hahn L, Harper G, McDaniel SH, et al. A case of factitious disorder by proxy: the role of the health-care system, diagnostic dilemmas, and family dynamics. *Harvard Rev Psychiatry* 2001;9:124–135.
5. Bowyer S, Roettcher P. Pediatric rheumatology clinic populations in the United States: results of a 3 year survey. Pediatric Rheumatology Database Research Group. *J Rheumatol* 1996;23:1968–1974.
6. Clark P, Burgos-Vargas R, Medina-Palma C, et al. Prevalence of fibromyalgia in children: a clinical study of Mexican children. *J Rheumatol* 1998; 25:2009–2014.
7. Weir PT, Harlan GA, Nkoy FL, et al. The incidence of fibromyalgia and its associated comorbidities: a population-based retrospective cohort study based on International Classification of Diseases, 9th Revision codes. *J Clin Rheumatol* 2006;12:124–128.
8. Aaron LA, Burke MM, Buchwald D. Overlapping conditions among patients with chronic fatigue syndrome, fibromyalgia, and temporomandibular disorder. *Arch Intern Med* 2000;160:221–227.
9. Gracely RH, Petzke F, Wolf JM, et al. Functional magnetic resonance imaging evidence of augmented pain processing in fibromyalgia. *Arthritis Rheum* 2002;46:1333–1343.
10. Kashikar-Zuck S, Ting TV. Juvenile fibromyalgia: current status of research and future developments. *Nat Rev Rheumatol* 2014;10:89–96.
11. Uceyler N, Zeller D, Kahn AK, et al. Small fibre pathology in patients with fibromyalgia syndrome. *Brain* 2013;136:1857–1867.
12. Arnold LM, Fan J, Russell IJ, et al. The fibromyalgia family study: a genome-wide linkage scan study. *Arthritis Rheum* 2013;65:1122–1128.
13. Wolfe F, Clauw DJ, Fitzcharles MA, et al. The American College of Rheumatology preliminary diagnostic criteria for fibromyalgia and measurement of symptom severity. *Arthritis Care Res (Hoboken)* 2010;62:600–610.
14. Yunus MB, Masi AT. Juvenile primary fibromyalgia syndrome. A clinical study of thirty-three patients and matched normal controls. *Arthritis Rheum* 1985;28:138–145.
15. Siegel DM, Janeway D, Baum J. Fibromyalgia syndrome in children and adolescents: clinical features at presentation and status at follow-up. *Pediatrics* 1998;101:377–382.
16. Kashikar-Zuck S, Cunningham N, Sil S, et al. Long-term outcomes of adolescents with juvenile-onset fibromyalgia in early adulthood. *Pediatrics* 2014;133:e592–e600.
17. Sherry DD, Wallace CA, Kelley C, et al. Short- and long-term outcomes of children with complex regional pain syndrome type I treated with exercise therapy. *Clin J Pain* 1999;15:218–223.
18. Tan EC, Zijlstra B, Essink ML, et al. Complex regional pain syndrome type I in children. *Acta Paediatr* 2008;97:875–879.
19. Cossins L, Okell RW, Cameron H, et al. Treatment of complex regional pain syndrome in adults: a systematic review of randomized controlled trials published from June 2000 to February 2012. *Eur J Pain* 2013;17:158–173.
20. Brooke V, Janselewitz S. Outcomes of children with complex regional pain syndrome after intensive inpatient rehabilitation. *PM R* 2012;4:349–354.
21. Stanton-Hicks MD, Burton AW, Bruehl SP, et al. An updated interdisciplinary clinical pathway for CRPS: report of an expert panel. *Pain Prac* 2002;2:1–16.
22. Kalita J, Vajpayee A, Misra UK. Comparison of prednisolone with piroxicam in complex regional pain syndrome following stroke: a randomized controlled trial. *QJM* 2006;99:89–95.

ADDITIONAL RESOURCES AND WEBSITES ONLINE

Fatigue and the Chronic Fatigue Syndrome

Peter C. Rowe

Fatigue is a private, subjective experience that, unlike muscle weakness, is difficult to quantify. It usually refers to an unpleasant, overwhelming sense of exhaustion that affects mental and physical activity, and differs from sleepiness or lack of motivation.[1] Acute fatigue is a common symptom in adolescents and young adults (AYAs); 20% to 35% report fatigue of at least moderate severity over the preceding month. Acute fatigue usually is readily explained by factors such as inadequate sleep, excessive work or physical training demands, psychosocial factors, iron deficiency, or self-limited medical conditions. Because it can be the initial sign of a life-threatening underlying medical or psychiatric condition—ranging from vasculitis to severe depression—or associated with more protracted and potentially disabling medical conditions such as chronic fatigue syndrome (CFS), the challenge is to differentiate the benign and self-limited from the disabling or dangerous conditions.

CAUSES OF FATIGUE

Fatigue can be associated with virtually any disease of any organ system.[2] Most causes of acute fatigue are readily apparent from the history, physical examination, and simple laboratory studies. Common causes include recent inadequate sleep or poor sleep hygiene, psychological distress, and infection.

Sleep requirements remain constant or increase through adolescence, averaging 9 hours per night, but many biologic, social, and scholastic pressures result in lower average amounts of sleep, closer to 7 hours nightly on weeknights.[3,4] In addition, most AYAs sleep more on weekends than they do during the week. Sleep disorders are increasingly being recognized as a cause of fatigue and/or daytime sleepiness in AYAs (see Chapter 25). These include the following:

1. *Insomnia* is defined as decreased sleep quality and/or quantity due to trouble falling asleep and/or maintaining sleep. Insomnia may be a symptom of an underlying medical or psychological disorder, part of a delayed sleep phase syndrome (DSPS), or unexplained. DSPS is a common disorder "in which an individual's internal circadian pacemaker is not in synchrony with internal or environmental time."[5]
2. *Obstructive sleep apnea* occurs in up to 1% to 3% of adolescents and may be caused by enlarged tonsils and adenoids, obesity, retrognathia, or nasal obstruction.

3. *Other sleep disorders* are uncommon; they include narcolepsy, idiopathic hypersomnia, Kleine–Levin syndrome, periodic leg movements during sleep, and restless leg syndrome.

Psychological disorders that can be associated with too little sleep and increased fatigue include depression, anxiety, stressful situations, or bipolar disorder. Generally, a thorough history from the patient and parent will illuminate symptoms of a mental health disorder that correspond to the onset of excessive fatigue.

Fatigue can also result from medications including antihistamines, sedatives, antidepressants, and other psychotropic medications, alcohol, or illicit drugs. In addition, infectious diseases such as mononucleosis, hepatitis, chronic infectious diseases such as HIV, tuberculosis, or Lyme disease, or bacterial endocarditis may also result in daytime sleepiness. Finally, endocrine disorders including thyroid disease, adrenal disease, or diabetes mellitus as well as other systemic illnesses (e.g., connective tissues diseases, anemia, neoplasms, congenital heart disease, asthma, inflammatory bowel disease, or kidney or liver failure) will also produce fatigue.

Red flags for more serious conditions include unexpected weight loss, fevers, abnormalities on the neurologic examination, generalized lymphadenopathy, adventitious sounds on the lung examination in someone without asthma, fatigue during exertion, clubbing, bronzing of the skin, and erythematous, swollen joints.

CHRONIC FATIGUE SYNDROME

CFS is a relatively common disorder affecting AYAs. It has a heterogeneous group of precipitating and perpetuating factors, and is characterized not only by fatigue but also by an inability to engage in cognitive and physical exertion without a marked exacerbation of symptoms. To maximize functioning of affected individuals, symptomatic treatment should begin before 6 months of fatigue have elapsed and prior to diagnostic confirmation of CFS.

Definition

The International CFS Study Group criteria outlined in Fukuda et al.[6] were developed to ensure a consistent research definition (**Table 35.1**) but have also served as the clinical definition.

Epidemiology

Population-based studies have shown that CFS affects previously healthy, active individuals from all socioeconomic strata and from all races.[7] Prevalence estimate varies depending on the CFS definition, but has been estimated at 1 to 3 per 1000 in AYAs.[8] While CFS is much more common after age 10, when present in younger children, the symptoms are similar to those who are older.[9] Females are more likely to develop CFS than males, in a ratio of 2-4:1. Across the globe, CFS is a common reason for home tutoring and prolonged inability

TABLE 35.1

International Consensus Committee Criteria for Chronic Fatigue Syndrome[a]

Fatigue criteria
The fatigue must be clinically evaluated, otherwise unexplained after evaluation, persistent or relapsing for more than 6 months, of new or definite onset (not lifelong), not the result of ongoing exertion, not substantially alleviated by rest, associated with a substantial reduction in previous levels of occupational, educational, social, or personal activities.

Symptom criteria
The fatigue must be accompanied by concurrent occurrence of four or more of the eight symptom criteria, all of which must have persisted or recurred during the 6 or more months of the illness:

- Self-reported impairment in short-term memory or concentration
- Sore throat
- Tender cervical or axillary lymph glands
- Unrefreshing sleep
- Muscle pain
- Multi-joint pain without joint swelling or redness
- Headaches of a new type, pattern, or severity
- Postexertional malaise lasting more than 24 hours

[a]Exclusionary criteria and conditions that can be comorbid with CFS, and ambiguities in the 1994 definition can be found in Fukuda K, Straus SE, Hickie I, et al. The chronic fatigue syndrome: a comprehensive approach to its definition and study. Ann Intern Med 1994;121:953–959.; Reeves WC, Lloyd A, Vernon S, et al. Identification of ambiguities in the 1994 chronic fatigue syndrome research case definition and recommendations for resolution. *BMC Health Serv Res* 2003;3:25.

TABLE 35.2

Prevalence of Fukuda Symptoms in AYAs with CFS

Symptom	Prevalence (Range) (%)
Unfreshing sleep	84–96
Postexertional malaise	80–96
Memory/concentration problems	79–84
Headaches	75–78
Muscle pain	59–73
Joint pain	48–67
Sore throat	43–57
Tender nodes	31–44

TABLE 35.3

Other Symptoms Reported with Moderate Severity in AYAs with CFS

Symptom	Prevalence (Range) (%)
Lightheadedness	70–100
Abdominal pain	50–70
Nausea	40–55
Temperature fluctuations	50
Heart racing	40–45
Shortness of breath	35–40
Chest pain	35–40

to attend regular school classes. The factor that most closely predicts school attendance is physical functioning as opposed to mental health and/or behavioral issues.[10]

Symptoms

See **Tables 35.2** and **35.3** for symptoms (Fukada and other common symptoms, respectively) in AYAs with CFS.

Etiology

Infection

The onset of CFS can be abrupt—associated with a flu-like or mono-like infection—but gradual onset of symptoms is also common.[11] However, no single pathogen has been identified as a cause for all CFS. Finally, evidence of persistent infection has not been detected in those with CFS.

- While fatigue affects virtually all patients at the onset of infectious mononucleosis, only 13% of these patients meet CFS criteria after a 6-month duration of this symptom.[12]
- After certain other acute infections, up to 10% of AYA patients can develop CFS; the severity of the initial infection appears to be a main risk factor, not the patient's premorbid behavioral state.[13]
- Immune abnormalities are variable, and autoimmune phenomena are occasionally present; there are no clear features consistent with a classical immunodeficiency disorder.[14]

Mental Health

Depressive and anxiety disorders must be evaluated carefully to disentangle the presence of these disorders and CFS. Depression shares some clinical features with CFS, including fatigue, nonrestorative sleep, and difficulty concentrating. However, AYAs with depression are distinguished from those with CFS by the dominance of low mood and loss of pleasure in activities.

For those AYAs with CFS, adjusting to a chronic, debilitating illness can sometimes lead to depression. As many as half of CFS patients develop depression at some time during the course of their illness. Such patients need to be assessed for the severity of depression and evaluated for treatment. Providers need to be aware that various classes of antidepressant drugs may worsen CFS symptoms. In addition, depression or other psychological disorder may warrant referral to a mental health profession.

- Studies in children and youth with CFS suggest a 40% to 50% prevalence of anxiety and 25% to 50% prevalence of depression.[15]
- When present in CFS patients, the severity of depression is usually mild; anhedonia and symptoms of self-reproach are uncommon.
- Among patients with depressive disorders, fatigue is less severe than those with CFS and often improves with exercise. In contrast, after a period of activity that exceeds their usual baseline, individuals with CFS often have a marked exacerbation of fatigue, cognitive dysfunction, pain, and other symptoms—often lasting more than a day.[16]
- CFS symptoms are present on weekends and summers, thus differentiating CFS from school phobia. While some AYAs improve during the summer months because they can rest and sleep duration can be increased, symptoms do not disappear.
- It is appropriate to provide medication to ameliorate symptoms of depression and anxiety if warranted, but these medication will not relieve or cure the major symptoms of CFS.

Autonomic Dysfunction

In AYAs, observations over the past two decades confirm that CFS symptoms (fatigue, lightheadedness, and cognitive problems) are usually made worse by prolonged upright posture.[17,18] This orthostatic intolerance is commonly accompanied by one or both of the following circulatory disorders:

- Neurally mediated (or vasovagal) hypotension during prolonged (40 to 45 minutes) head-up tilt, characterized by reproduction of fatigue and orthostatic symptoms, and associated with a 25 mm Hg reduction in systolic blood pressure[17-20]
- Postural tachycardia syndrome, defined as a greater than 40-beat increase in heart rate with standing for adolescents[21] or a 30-beat change in adults, together with reproduction of associated orthostatic symptoms (lightheadedness, headache, cognitive difficulties, nausea), in the first 10 minutes of quiet standing or head-up right tilt table testing[22]

Treatment of orthostatic intolerance can be associated with improvements in overall function, including energy and tolerance of activity in those with chronic fatigue and CFS.[17,18]

EVALUATION OF CFS

History

First, it is most helpful to ask a patient to list his or her current symptoms to get a sense of the possible areas that will require evaluation. In those with CFS, the symptoms tend to be predictably similar from one patient to another rather than a random collection of somatic complaints. After getting a sense of the onset of the illness and changes since it began, explore the details of each symptom on the list, asking about the frequency, severity, aggravating and relieving factors, and the timing of each in relation to other symptoms. A careful history includes the following:

- Past medical history
- Diet
- Sleep patterns
- Mood and anxiety
- School performance
- Relationships with family and friends
- Medication and drug use
- Family history

Critical historical items of importance to explore include the following:

- Orthostatic intolerance, which is indicated by:
  - increased fatigue or lightheadedness when standing still, or in a hot shower or bath, or in hot weather;
  - frequent adoption of postural counter-maneuvers (sitting with knees to chest, doing homework in a reclined position, legs crossed when standing, fidgeting);
  - avoidance of low-impact activities such as shopping; and
  - worsening of fatigue after long periods of sitting (such as at the end of a 90-minute class).
- Menstrual periods
  - Does fatigue worsen in the days before the onset of menses?
- Impact on daily life
  - What activities must the individual now limit or avoid?
  - Do they continue to participate in social activities or sports?
- Family history
  - Higher rate of CFS and other similar disorders (fibromyalgia, irritable bowel disease, temporomandibular joint dysfunction, anxiety, syncope, joint laxity, celiac disease, milk protein intolerance) in first-degree relatives of affected patients

Physical Examination

The physical examination should include a careful neurologic examination, measurement of joint hypermobility, and evaluation for postural dysfunctions. Patients with CFS usually have abnormal findings (see below). Orthostatic testing is warranted in most,

especially those reporting frequent lightheadedness and chronic fatigue. This can take two forms:

- In-office standing tests: 5 minutes supine, then 10 minutes of quiet standing, leaning against a wall. Record changes in heart rate and blood pressure each minute, as well as changes in orthostatic symptoms and fatigue on a 0 to 10 scale between supine and standing. The test must be observed due to the risk of syncope.
- Laboratory head-up tilt table test: Prolonged testing of 40 to 45 minutes is required to identify neurally mediated hypotension. Shorter 10-minute tests will only identify postural orthostatic tachycardia syndrome (POTS) or, less commonly, orthostatic hypotension. (Care should be taken in those with more severe impairment, as prolonged orthostatic testing can aggravate symptoms, often for several days; some centers administer 1 to 2 L of intravenous saline after the test to reduce the risk of an exacerbation).

Common abnormalities on physical examination include the following:

- Tachycardia or hypotension during prolonged upright posture, often associated with a purple discoloration in the dependent limbs, termed acrocyanosis[22]
- Joint hypermobility, which has been reported in 60% of those with CFS[23]; some CFS patients will also meet criteria for Ehlers–Danlos syndrome.[24]

Due to the joint laxity, the hypermobile CFS patient is at risk for postural dysfunctions (head-forward posture, thoracic kyphosis, lumbar lordosis) and accompanying areas of muscle guarding, tenderness, and limited range of motion[25] that may benefit from evaluation and treatment by a physical therapist.

Laboratory Studies

There is no single test to confirm a diagnosis of CFS. However, the clinician should perform the following to exclude other important causes of chronic fatigue:

- Complete blood count, with white blood count and differential and platelet count
- Serum chemistries including electrolytes, urea, creatinine, total protein, albumin, calcium, alanine aminotransferase (ALT), aspartate aminotransferase (AST), and alkaline phosphatase
- T_4 free, thyroid-stimulating hormone
- C-reactive protein or erythrocyte sedimentation rate
- Urinalysis

Other testing is dependent on the history and physical examination (e.g., antinuclear antibody testing in someone with a malar rash). The following should be considered:

- Ferritin or other measures of iron deficiency
- Vitamin B_{12}, especially in vegans or those on proton pump inhibitors
- Celiac disease screening
- Serology for certain infections, including Lyme disease in endemic areas. Serology for Epstein–Barr virus and Cytomegalovirus can help with categorizing whether the illness might have been initiated by these organisms, but usually does not change management.
- Magnetic resonance imaging of the brain and cervical spine is not routinely indicated, but important if there is occipital headache, nystagmus, worsening of symptoms on neck movement, or hyperreflexia (chronic fatigue can be a presenting feature of Chiari I malformation and cervical spine stenosis).[26]

MANAGEMENT OF CFS

The goal of treatment is to improve function and activity and to ameliorate specific symptoms. No single pharmacologic agent has been identified to be universally helpful in CFS. While data have demonstrated moderate efficacy for intravenous immunoglobulin (IVIG) in adolescents,[27] the results from adult studies are mixed.[28] Clinicians need to remember that some medications can cause harm, such as corticosteroids, which lead to adrenal insufficiency. Treating the adolescent or young adult with CFS requires careful attention by the patient and the practitioner to the factors that provoke and exacerbate symptoms. Treatment of this disease requires a willingness by the patient to try several medications before the best management of symptoms is achieved, and requires the understanding that medications often treat symptoms but will not cure the disorder. The clinician should use an iterative clinical treatment process that includes the following:

- Develop working hypotheses about the dominant influences on fatigue symptoms.
- Explain and demystify CFS and provide reassurance about the potential for improved functioning.
- Initiate nonpharmacologic therapies as listed below.
- Begin pharmacologic treatment as indicated, focusing on the dominant influences on symptoms first before proceeding with other symptoms (e.g., orthostatic intolerance, sleep dysfunction, pain, headache, food and environmental allergies, menstrual dysfunction, low mood, anxiety).
- Reassess at regular intervals (every 1 to 2 months depending on level of severity) and repeat steps 1 to 4

Nonpharmacologic Treatments
Behavioral Interventions
- Ascertain the level of depressed mood and anxiety, and treat accordingly.
- Coping skills training can be helpful for some, including relaxation and breathing techniques and distraction.
- Cognitive behavioral therapy (CBT)—emphasizing the importance of a daily routine, encouraging exercise—is also helpful,[28,29] as it has been for a wide range of medical conditions. However, improvements are not always sustained, and CBT has not been studied extensively with severely affected CFS patient populations.

Sleep
- Aim for a specified, regular bedtime, recognizing that this is not always possible in those with more challenging reversals of circadian rhythms.
- Eliminate use of electronic devices, that is, smartphones, iPads after "lights out," which aggravate fatigue.[30]
- Avoid sleeping more than 12 hours at a time. Longer periods of sleep promote low blood volume and can aggravate orthostatic intolerance.
- If insomnia is impressive and unresponsive to relaxation techniques and standard sleep hygiene measures (e.g., avoiding daytime naps, avoiding caffeine in the evening), pharmacologic treatment may be needed.[31]

Exercise
- Encourage gradual increases in daily activity.
- Manual physical therapy can be a bridge to tolerating exercise; recumbent exercise initiated slowly may help, especially in the early days of treatment.
- Emphasize gradual increases in exercise and activities, with specific rest cycles between activities to avoid the "push-crash" cycle of excessive activity on a good day followed by prolonged postexertional collapse.

Orthostatic Intolerance
- Avoid conditions that aggravate symptoms (prolonged standing, warm environments).
- Increase fluid intake (2 to 3 L daily in most AYAs)
- Increase sodium intake according to taste, supplemented by buffered salt tablets.

- Utilize the muscle pump function of the lower limbs with postural counter-maneuvers: crossing legs and shifting from one leg to the other while standing, sitting with knees higher than hips, leg muscle contraction exercises before standing.
- Recommend compression garments or support hose at 20 to 30 mm Hg compression (waist high > thigh high > knee high) and body shaper garments or abdominal binders.

Educational Accommodations
AYAs still in school who report orthostatic intolerance are likely to report feeling worse in the morning, when blood volume is lowest, and do somewhat better as the day progresses. Symptoms wax and wane, often unpredictably from day to day, are often worse after vigorous exercise, and persist longer after viral respiratory illnesses. Educational accommodations can include one or more of the following:

- A later start to the school day
- A reduction in course load
- An excuse from gym, or permission to self-modulate exercise
- Salty snacks and water bottle in classroom
- Permission to get up and move around in class
- Extended time for tests
- Flexibility with assignments and deadlines
- For those with moderate to severe CFS, consider these:
  - a skipped day midweek to rest/recover,
  - half day attendance, and
  - home and hospital teaching.

Pharmacologic Treatment
For orthostatic intolerance, medication options include agents that will

- Increase blood volume, including fludrocortisone, low-dose oral contraceptive pills (particularly helpful as a first-line agent in females with orthostatic intolerance and dysmenorrhea or worse fatigue with menses),[32] or desmopressin.
- Block the elevated catecholamine levels that are associated with orthostatic intolerance, using low-dose β-blockers, possibly selective serotonin reuptake inhibitors.
- Improve vasoconstriction using midodrine, stimulant medications, or serotonin norepinephrine reuptake inhibitors, or pyridostigmine bromide.[22,33]

For reports of headaches and chronic pain, the clinician should consider the following:

- Physical therapy if there is a biomechanical contributor, head-forward posture, slumped shoulders, kyphosis, neck tilt, or other postural dysfunctions.
- Over-the-counter medications that have been demonstrated to be effective for migraine headaches, such as riboflavin 400 mg daily and coenzyme Q10 300 mg daily
- For severe and chronic migraines, daily medication to prevent headaches may include atenolol, cyproheptadine, or topiramate.
- For those reporting chronic pain symptoms, tricyclic antidepressants in low doses can be used with caution, but can aggravate lightheadedness.
- Medications used for widespread fibromyalgia pain in adults include gabapentin, duloxetine, and pregabalin.[34]

Outcomes
Health outcomes for the adolescent or young adult with CFS are thought to be better than that for adults with this disorder. For some, it takes several years before recovery is noted, while a select few have persistent disability. While full recovery is possible, long-term data identify persistent limitations in quality of life even among some of those who report resolution of the illness.[35]

ACKNOWLEDGMENTS

The author wishes to acknowledge Martin Fisher, Marvin Belzer, and Lawrence Neinstein for their contributions to previous versions of this chapter.

REFERENCES

1. Jones JF, Kohl KS, Ahmadipour N, et al. Fatigue: case definition and guidelines for data collection, analysis, and presentation of immunization safety data. *Vaccine* 2007;25:5685–5696.
2. Cavanaugh RM. Evaluating adolescents with fatigue: ever get tired of it? *Pediatr Rev* 2002;23:337–347.
3. Caskadon MA. Sleep in adolescents: the perfect storm. *Pediatr Clin N Am* 2011;58:637–647.
4. Fisher M. Fatigue in adolescents. *J Pediatr Adolesc Gynecol* 2013;26:252–256.
5. Millman RP; Working Group on Sleepiness in Adolescents/Young Adults; American Academy of Pediatrics Committee on Adolescence. Excessive sleepiness in adolescents and young adults: causes, consequences, and treatment strategies. *Pediatrics* 2005;115:1774–1786.
6. Fukuda K, Straus SE, Hickie I, et al. The chronic fatigue syndrome: a comprehensive approach to its definition and study. *Ann Intern Med* 1994;121:953–959.
7. Jason LA, Richman JA, Rademaker AW, et al. A community-based study of chronic fatigue syndrome. *Arch Intern Med* 1999;159:2129–2137.
8. Rimes KA, Goodman R, Hotopf M, et al. Incidence, prognosis, and risk factors for fatigue and chronic fatigue syndrome in adolescents: a prospective community study. *Pediatrics* 2007;119:e603–e609.
9. Davies S, Crawley E. Chronic fatigue syndrome in children aged 11 years old and younger. *Arch Dis Child* 2008;93:419–422.
10. Crawley E, Sterne JAC. Association between school absence and physical function in paediatric chronic fatigue syndrome/myalgic encephalopathy. *Arch Dis Child* 2009;94:752–756.
11. Nijhoff SL, Maijer K, Bleijenberg G, et al. Adolescent chronic fatigue syndrome: prevalence, incidence, and morbidity. *Pediatrics* 2011;127:e1169–e1175.
12. Katz BZ, Shiraishi Y, Mears CJ, et al. Chronic fatigue syndrome after infectious mononucleosis in adolescents. *Pediatrics* 2009;124;189–193.
13. Hickie, I, Davenport T, Wakefield D, et al. Post-infective and chronic fatigue syndromes precipitated by viral and non-viral pathogens: prospective cohort study. *BMJ* 2006;333:575. doi:10.1136/bmj.38933.585764.AE.
14. Bansal AS, Bradley AS, Bishop KN, et al. Chronic fatigue syndrome, the immune system and viral infection. *Brain Behav Immun* 2012;26:24–31.
15. Bould H, Lewis G, Emond A, et al. Depression and anxiety in children with CFS/ME: cause or effect? *Arch Dis Child* 2011;96:211–214.
16. Hawk C, Jason LA, Torres-Harding S. Differential diagnosis of chronic fatigue syndrome and major depressive disorder. *Int J Behav Med* 2006;13:244–251.
17. Rowe PC, Bou-Holaigah I, Kan JS, et al. Is neurally mediated hypotension an unrecognised cause of chronic fatigue? *Lancet* 1995;345:623–624.
18. Bou-Holaigah I, Rowe PC, Kan J, et al. Relationship between neurally mediated hypotension and the chronic fatigue syndrome. *JAMA* 1995;274:961–967.
19. Stewart JM, Gewitz MH, Weldon A, et al. Orthostatic intolerance in adolescent chronic fatigue syndrome. *Pediatrics* 1999;103:116–121.
20. Wyller VB, Due R, Saul JP, et al. Usefulness of an abnormal cardiovascular response during low-grade head-up tilt-test for discriminating adolescents with chronic fatigue from healthy controls. *Am J Cardiol* 2007;99:997–1001.
21. Singer W, Sletten DM, Opfer-Gehrking TL, et al. Postural tachycardia in children and adolescents: what is abnormal? *J Pediatr* 2012;160:222–226.
22. Raj SR. Postural tachycardia syndrome. *Circulation* 2013;127:2336–2342.
23. Barron DF, Cohen BA, Geraghty MT, et al. Joint hypermobility is more common in children with chronic fatigue syndrome than in healthy controls. *J Pediatr* 2002;141:421–425.
24. Rowe PC, Barron DF, Calkins H, et al. Orthostatic intolerance and chronic fatigue syndrome associated with Ehlers-Danlos syndrome. *J Pediatr* 1999;135:494–499.
25. Rowe PC, Marden CL, Flaherty M, et al. Impaired range of motion of limbs and spine in chronic fatigue syndrome. *J Pediatr* 2014;165:360–366.
26. Heffez DS, Ross RE, Shade-Zeldow Y, et al. Clinical evidence for cervical myelopathy due to Chiari malformation and spinal stenosis in a non-randomized group of patients with the diagnosis of fibromyalgia. *Eur Spine J* 2004;13:516–523.
27. Rowe KS. Double-blind randomized controlled trial to assess the efficacy of intravenous immunoglobulin for the management of chronic fatigue syndrome in adolescents. *J Psychiat Res* 1997;31:133–147.
28. Chambers D, Bagnall A-M, Hempel S, et al. Interventions for the treatment, management and rehabilitation of patients with chronic fatigue syndrome/myalgic encephalomyelitis: an updated systematic review. *J R Soc Med* 2006;99:506–520.
29. Nijhof SL, Bleijenberg G, Uiterwaal CSPM, et al. Effectiveness of internet-based cognitive behavioral treatment for adolescents with chronic fatigue syndrome (FITNET): a randomised controlled trial. *Lancet* 2012;379:1412–1418.
30. Van den Bulck J. Adolescent use of mobile phones for calling and for sending text messages after lights out: results from a prospective cohort study with a one-year follow-up. *Sleep* 2007;30:1220–1223.
31. Friedberg F, ed. *ME/CFS: a primer for clinical practitioners, 2012*. Available at http://www.iacfsme.org/Portals/0/PDF/PrimerFinal3.pdf. Accessed March 4, 2014.
32. Boehm KE, Kip KT, Grubb BP, et al. Neurocardiogenic syncope: response to hormonal therapy. *Pediatrics* 1997;99:623–625.
33. Grubb BP. Neurocardiogenic syncope. *N Engl J Med* 2005;352:1004–1010.
34. Carville SF, Arendt-Nielsen S, Bliddal H, et al. EULAR evidence-based recommendations for the management of fibromyalgia syndrome. *Ann Rheum Dis* 2008;67(4):536–541.
35. Brown MM, Bell DS, Jason LA, et al. Understanding long-term outcomes of chronic fatigue syndrome. *J Clin Psychol* 2012;68:1028–1035.

ADDITIONAL RESOURCES AND WEBSITES ONLINE

Chronic Abdominal Pain

Paula K. Braverman

Chronic abdominal pain is a common complaint among adolescents and young adults (AYAs). The differential diagnosis of chronic abdominal pain includes functional gastrointestinal disorders (FGIDs) and organic disorders related to anatomic abnormalities, inflammation, or tissue damage. The Rome III criteria have been developed to characterize FGID among different age-groups. There is ongoing research into the pathophysiology of the brain–gut axis related to FGID as well as pharmacologic and dietary treatment options. Efforts to treat chronic abdominal pain can lead to intense frustration among patients, families, and health care providers alike. The approach to this problem is particularly challenging, and in most cases, there is no specific organic abnormality found. This chapter reviews the epidemiology, pathophysiology, differential diagnosis, clinical approach, and available treatment modalities for chronic abdominal pain with an emphasis on FGID.

DEFINITION

In the past, children with chronic abdominal pain were commonly diagnosed as having recurrent abdominal pain (RAP). In 2005, the Subcommittee on Chronic Abdominal Pain of the North American Society for Pediatric Gastroenterology, Hepatology, and Nutrition published a report recommending that the term "RAP" be eliminated and concluded that abdominal pain exceeding 1 or 2 months, whether long lasting, intermittent, or constant, should be considered chronic.[1,2] The differential diagnosis of chronic abdominal pain includes FGIDs and organic disorders related to anatomic abnormalities, inflammation, or tissue damage. The Rome criteria are a diagnostic system developed to characterize and standardize the diagnosis of FGIDs. FGIDs are disorders of the gastrointestinal (GI) system in which symptoms cannot be explained by organic abnormalities but are based on clinical symptoms in children, adolescents, and adults.[3] This chapter will focus on the diagnosis and treatment of chronic abdominal pain with an emphasis on FGID.

DIFFERENTIAL DIAGNOSIS AND CLINICAL MANIFESTATIONS OF CHRONIC ABDOMINAL PAIN

FGID

FGIDs, characterized by persistent and recurring GI symptoms, include a number of separate idiopathic disorders that can affect any part of the GI tract.

Epidemiology

The exact prevalence of FGIDs in AYAs is unknown for several reasons:

1. There may be overlapping symptoms, and individuals may have more than one FGID as defined by the Rome criteria.[4–6]
2. The prevalence of FGID differs depending on the version of Rome criteria applied and the population studied, including the geographic region or country, suggesting different perceptions and sociocultural interpretations of symptoms.[4,5,7]
3. Many prevalence studies in children/adolescents used the older RAP terminology or simply asked about abdominal pain symptoms rather than using the Rome criteria.
4. The Rome criteria may not accurately reflect the clinical presentation. This was specifically discussed in the 2012 Multinational Irritable Bowel Syndrome Initiative report indicating that the Rome criteria are not necessarily adequate or most relevant for the clinical diagnosis of irritable bowel syndrome (IBS).[8]

Despite these limitations, the following studies provide some estimates of the prevalence of chronic abdominal pain in children and AYAs:

1. Results from a systematic review on RAP found a prevalence of 0.3% to 19% in children and adolescents in the US and Europe.[9]
2. The National Longitudinal Study of Adolescent Health study of a nationally representative sample of 13- to 18-year-olds found 3.2% with daily abdominal pain and 15% with pain more than twice a week.[10]
3. A prospective Norwegian study on 4- to 15-year-olds referred for evaluation of RAP found that 87% met criteria for one or more FGID and 43% had IBS using the Rome III criteria.[11]
4. A study in Japan utilizing Rome III criteria in 3,976 students between 10 and 17 years of age found a prevalence of 13.9% for one or more FGID.[12]
5. A systematic review of the worldwide literature assessing IBS among individuals 15 years and older found prevalence rates from 7% to 21%, with a pooled prevalence of 11% for those less than age 30.[13]

Etiology of FGIDs

The etiology of FGID is still not well understood; however, recent studies indicate multidimensional causes. Current theories suggest that FGIDs are due to the following:

1. Dysregulation or impairment of the bidirectional communication in the "brain–gut axis" involving[14,15]:
   a. Neural systems (neurotransmitters, e.g., *serotonin, noradrenaline*) and the autonomic and enteric nervous systems, which affect motility and secretions
   b. Gut and peripheral immune systems (e.g., *cytokines, mast cell activation, T-cell activation*)
   c. Endocrine systems (hypothalamic–pituitary–adrenal axis)
2. Visceral hypersensitivity (hyperalgesia) with alteration in the neural processing of visceral stimuli, resulting in lower pain thresholds and/or alterations in pain perception. Possible disturbance in pain processing is evidenced by brain imaging studies demonstrating activation of certain areas of the brain and structural brain changes.[16]
3. Other factors influencing the brain–gut axis, including genetic predisposition psychological factors (stress, anxiety, trauma, pain, mood, cognitive function, expectation, conditioning), and physical factors (infection, mucosal inflammation, alteration in enteric microbiota).[15–17]

Diagnostic Criteria

The Rome III criteria include categories for infant/toddlers, children and adolescents aged 4 to 18 and for adults.[3] A key criterion in diagnosing FGIDs is that there is no evidence of structural disease to explain the symptoms. Different FGIDs can co-occur in the same AYAs.[6] The following are the relevant differences in the Rome III categories by age-group. The Full Rome III criteria are laid out at http://www.romecriteria.org/criteria/

1. The child/adolescent components are classified by symptom pattern or area of symptom location, whereas the adult components are divided into six domains (**Table 36.1**).
2. The Rome III criteria for adults define FGID as abdominal pain starting 6 months prior to diagnosis and meeting criteria for active symptoms for the previous 3 months. For children/adolescents, many of the categories require only active symptoms for 2 months and do not specify a time frame for onset of symptoms.
3. The criteria for the same diagnostic category of FGID differ by age-group.

Table 36.2 outlines the age-related Rome III criteria for several diagnostic entities common to both the child/adolescent and adult age-groups, including functional abdominal pain, IBS, and functional dyspepsia.

Organic Causes of Chronic Abdominal Pain

Causes of Chronic Pain Commonly Associated with Dyspepsia

Gastroesophageal reflux; peptic ulcer disease; biliary tract obstruction; gall bladder dyskinesia; chronic pancreatitis; gastroparesis

Causes of Chronic Pain Commonly Associated with Altered Bowel Pattern

Inflammatory bowel disease (IBD); celiac disease; lactose intolerance; colitis; complications of constipation (encopresis, megacolon); infection (parasites and bacteria)

1. IBD can be manifested by the following:
   a. Poor growth
   b. Anemia, elevated erythrocyte sedimentation rate (ESR), and elevated fecal calprotectin[18,19]
   c. Bloody stools—although stools may be positive for hemoccult without signs of diarrhea
   d. Systemic symptoms—arthritis, iritis, hepatitis, and erythema nodosum

---

TABLE 36.1

Rome III Classification for FGIDs

Adult Categories	Child/Adolescent Categories
Functional Esophageal Disorders	**Vomiting and Aerophagia**
Functional heartburn Functional chest pain of presumed Esophageal origin Functional dysphagia Globus	Adolescent rumination syndrome Cyclic vomiting syndrome Aerophagia
Functional Gastroduodenal Disorders	**Abdominal Pain-Related Functional GI Disorder**
Functional dyspepsia Belching disorders Nausea and vomiting disorders Rumination syndrome in adults	Functional dyspepsia IBS Abdominal migraine Childhood functional abdominal pain Childhood functional abdominal pain syndrome
Functional Bowel Disorders	**Constipation and Incontinence**
IBS Functional bloating Functional constipation Functional diarrhea Unspecified functional bowel disorder	Functional constipation Nonretentive fecal incontinence
Functional Abdominal Pain Syndrome	
Functional Gallbladder and Sphincter of Oddi Disorders	
Functional gallbladder disorder Functional biliary sphincter of Oddi disorder Functional pancreatic sphincter of Oddi disorder	
Functional Anorectal Disorder	
Functional fecal incontinence Functional anorectal pain Functional defecation disorders	

Adapted from *Rome Foundation* Available at http://www.romecriteria.org/. Accessed March 15, 2014.

---

2. Celiac disease is one of the most common genetic diseases (HLA class II haplotypes DQ2 and DQ8). There is evidence that the prevalence is increasing worldwide, with current estimates of 1% in the general population[20] and 10% to 15% in those with an affected first-degree relative.[21] This disease is often under recognized and under diagnosed by health care providers, with only 10% to 15% of those affected having been diagnosed and treated.[20] Celiac disease can be symptomatic or asymptomatic and may not be diagnosed until adulthood. Extraintestinal manifestations become more prevalent with increasing age.[20,22] Celiac disease can be manifested by the following signs and symptoms:
   a. GI symptoms include diarrhea, constipation, abdominal pain, anorexia, vomiting, weight loss, bloating, malabsorption, and malnutrition.[20,22]
   b. Extraintestinal manifestation include fatigue, dermatitis, osteopenia, short stature, delayed puberty, iron deficiency anemia resistant to oral iron, hepatitis, arthritis, aphthous stomatitis, dental enamel hypoplasia, seizures, recurring headache, unexplained infertility in females, and psychiatric disorders (anxiety, panic attacks, depression).[20,21]

TABLE 36.2

ROME III Criteria for Selected Diagnoses in Children/Adolescents and Adults

Functional Abdominal Pain

Children and Adolescents

Childhood Functional Abdominal Pain
Criteria at least once a week for at least 2 mo before diagnosis and include all of the following:
a. Episodic or continuous abdominal pain
b. Insufficient criteria for other FGIDs
c. No evidence of inflammatory, anatomic, metabolic, or neoplastic process that explains subject's symptoms.

Childhood Functional Abdominal Pain Syndrome
Must satisfy criteria for childhood functional abdominal pain and have at least 25% of the time one or more of the following:
a. Some loss of some daily functioning
b. Additional somatic symptoms such as headache, limb pain, or difficulty sleeping

Adults

Functional Abdominal Pain Syndrome
Criteria fulfilled for the last 3 mo with symptom onset at least 6 mo prior to diagnosis. Must include all of the following:
a. Continuous or nearly continuous abdominal pain
b. No or only occasional relationship of pain with physiological events (e.g., eating, defecation, or menses)
c. Some loss of daily functioning
d. The pain is not feigned (e.g., malingering)
e. Insufficient symptoms to meet criteria for another functional gastrointestinal disorder that would explain the pain

Irritable Bowel Syndrome

Children and Adolescents
Criteria fulfilled at least once per week for at least 2 mo prior to diagnosis and must include both of the following:
a. Abdominal pain/discomfort associated with two or more of the following at least 25% of the time:
   • Improvement with defecation
   • Onset associated with change in frequency of stool
   • Onset associated with change in form (appearance) of stool
b. No evidence of an inflammatory, anatomic, metabolic, or neoplastic process that explains the subject's symptoms.

Adults
Criterion fulfilled for the last 3 mo with symptom onset at least 6 mo prior to diagnosis
Recurrent abdominal pain or discomfort at least 3 d/mo in the last 3 mo associated with two or more of the following:
a. Improvement with defection
b. Onset associated with a change in frequency of stool
c. Onset associated with change in form (appearance) of stool

Functional Dyspepsia

Children and Adolescents
Criteria fulfilled at least once for week for at least 2 mo prior to diagnosis. Must include all of the following:
1. Persistent or recurrent pain or discomfort centered in the upper abdomen (above the umbilicus)
2. Not relieved by defecation or associated with the onset of a change in stool frequency or stool form (i.e., not IBS)
3. No evidence of an inflammatory, anatomic, metabolic, or neoplastic process that explains the subject's symptoms

Adults
Criteria fulfilled for the last 3 mo with symptom onset at least 6 mo prior to diagnosis
1. One or more of the following:
   a. Bothersome postprandial fullness
   b. Early satiety
   c. Epigastric pain
   d. Epigastric burning
AND
2. No evidence of structural disease (including at upper endoscopy) that is likely to explain the symptoms

Adapted from *Rome Foundation*. Available at http://www.romecriteria.org/. Accessed March 15, 2014.

c. Associated conditions include diabetes mellitus (10% prevalence), thyroiditis, IgA deficiency, Addison disease, Down syndrome, and Turner syndrome.[20,21]

d. Celiac disease is associated with an increased risk for malignancies, including small bowel adenocarcinoma, esophageal cancer, and non-Hodgkin lymphoma.[22]

Diagnosis is dependent on suspecting the disease, screening with serologic testing (anti-tTG IgA), and then small bowel biopsy for confirmation in those with positive serology.[20–22] Patients with celiac disease can also have FGIDs including IBS, which can contribute to challenges in deciding who to screen.[20,23,24]

Causes of Chronic Pain Commonly Associated with Paroxysmal Abdominal Pain

Musculoskeletal pain; bowel obstruction; ureteral obstruction

Other Causes of Chronic Abdominal Pain

The differential diagnosis includes gynecologic conditions, referred pain form the lungs or spine, systemic conditions such as diabetic ketoacidosis or sickle cell crisis.

⬤ DIAGNOSIS

Based on the current literature, the Subcommittee on Chronic Abdominal Pain in Children was unable to produce an evidence-based procedural algorithm for the diagnostic evaluation of chronic abdominal pain in children and adolescents. The conclusions drawn by the subcommittee[1,2] are detailed below:

History

1. Some patients have features of more than one FGID.
2. The pain frequency, severity, location, or impact on lifestyle cannot distinguish functional and organic disorders. Timing of the symptoms, including postprandial pain and nighttime awakening, were not found to be helpful.
3. "Alarm symptoms or signs" suggestive of organic disease requiring further diagnostic testing include, but are not limited to, (a) involuntary weight loss; (b) family history of IBD; (c) deceleration in linear growth; (d) unexplained fever; (e) GI blood loss; (f) significant vomiting—cyclical vomiting, bilious emesis; (g) chronic severe diarrhea; (h) persistent right upper or right lower quadrant pain.
4. Family history: (a) Parental history of anxiety, depression, and somatization is not helpful in distinguishing between functional and organic disorders. (b) Overall family functioning (e.g., cohesion, conflict, marital satisfaction) does not differ between those with FGIDs and healthy families or those with acute illness.
5. Issues regarding the relationship of pain to current stress and emotional and behavioral concerns include (a) a history of anxiety, depression, and more negative life event stress does not distinguish functional from organic abdominal pain; (b) a relationship that exists between daily stress and pain episodes as well as increased negative life events and persistent symptoms; (c) no evidence to support the concept of emotional/behavioral symptoms predicting the severity of pain, course of the pain episode, or response to treatment; and (d) evidence to support that adolescents with FGIDs are at risk for emotional problems and psychiatric disorders (e.g., anxiety and depression) later in life.

Physical Examination

FGIDs are usually associated with normal findings on physical examination or mild pressure tenderness without rebound commonly located in the upper abdomen.

Diagnostic Tests
Testing for Organic Disorders

The following tests can be considered in the evaluation of a possible organic disorder in children, adolescents, and adults.[23,25]

1. Primary screening tests
   a. Complete blood count with differential, ESR, C-reactive protein, chemistry profile with liver function tests
   b. Urinalysis with or without culture
   c. Stool samples obtained for evidence of occult blood, ova, and parasites (including stool for Giardia antigen).
2. If diarrhea is present, additional studies to be considered include the following:
   a. Stool for *Clostridium difficile* toxin, lactose breath test, celiac panel, fecal calprotectin. Because of undiagnosed celiac disease, there is discussion in the literature about increasing screening for this disease in adolescents and adults. The American College of Gastroenterology recommends screening in patients with IBS associated with diarrhea and mixed symptoms.[20–23]
3. If dyspepsia is present, additional studies to be considered include the following:
   a. Testing for *Helicobacter pylori* (stool antigen or urea breath test)
   b. Serum amylase and lipase
4. Radiologic studies (upper GI series with small bowel follow through; hepatobiliary scintigraphy with cholecystokinin infusion; abdominal, renal, or pelvic ultrasound) or referral to a gastroenterologist for possible endoscopy or colonoscopy can be considered to rule out organic disease in patients with alarm symptoms or specific symptoms such as dyspepsia unresponsive to treatment, right upper quadrant pain, dyspepsia with recurrent vomiting, or symptoms and/or physical examination suggestive of pelvic pathology or urinary tract abnormalities.

Diagnostic Tests—Additional Considerations

The Subcommittee on Chronic Abdominal Pain in Children found that[1,2]:

1. No studies have been done to specifically evaluate the use of laboratory tests to distinguish between functional and organic abdominal pain even in the face of alarm signals.
2. There is no evidence that ultrasonography of the abdomen or pelvis, endoscopy, biopsy, or pH monitoring in the absence of alarm signals significantly detects organic disease.
3. FGID can be diagnosed by a primary care clinician when there are no alarm symptoms, the physical examination is normal, and there is a negative stool sample for occult blood. Testing is sometimes necessary to reassure the patient and family, especially when the pain is significantly affecting the patient's quality of life.

Similarly, a position statement from the American College of Gastroenterology Task Force concluded that organic disease is unlikely in patients under 50 years old with typical IBS symptoms without alarm features, and therefore, routine diagnostic testing is not recommended (with the exception of conducting celiac serology in some patients). Rectal bleeding and nocturnal pain did not discriminate IBS from organic disease, but anemia, weight loss, and family history of colorectal cancer, IBD, or celiac disease were important alarm features that warrant further investigation.[23]

Although inconclusive, there is some evidence that short-chain poorly absorbed carbohydrates may trigger GI symptoms. Lactose intolerance may also mimic or coexist with FGIDs. Although the data are controversial, some individuals also appear to have gluten sensitivity with negative serology and intestinal biopsies.[21,23,25] Keeping a pain diary for 1 to 3 weeks may be helpful to document the pattern, timing, severity, association with food or beverage, and precipitating factors. In addition to helping the clinician work through the differential diagnosis, this type of diary provides a way for AYAs to be directly involved in their care plan.

Approach to the Evaluation of FGIDs

If after a careful history and physical examination there is no obvious organic source for the chronic abdominal pain, the practitioner should explain to the AYAs that the evaluation seems to indicate a FGID. Although a serious underlying disease is not suspected, AYAs should appreciate that the symptoms they are experiencing are real. It is also useful to explain the concepts of visceral hypersensitivity and disordered brain–gut communication in terms that the AYAs and family can understand. If further clarification of the history is needed, the adolescent or young adult should be asked to keep a pain diary with a follow-up appointment scheduled in 1 to 3 weeks. If there are alarm signals or further diagnostic tests are necessary for reassurance, selected screening utilizing laboratory tests and/or radiologic studies can be performed.

TREATMENT OR THERAPEUTIC APPROACH

FGIDs are best treated in the context of a biopsychosocial model, which may include psychological interventions, dietary changes, and some specific pharmacologic therapy to reduce the frequency and severity of the symptoms. Pharmacologic therapy should be used judiciously for specific symptomatology and specific functional GI conditions. Psychological and physical pain triggers should be identified so that they can be modified or reversed. The goal of treatment is to resume normal functioning and return to daily activities rather than focusing on the pain itself.

Treatment Options for FGIDs

The Subcommittee on Chronic Abdominal Pain in Children found a paucity of studies evaluating pharmacologic and dietary treatments in children and adolescents.[1,2] Many of the studies in adults have focused on IBS. Treatment options include the following[1,2,23,25–29]:

Pharmacologic Treatments

The following medications have some evidence of effectiveness from pediatric and adult studies:

1. Enteric-coated peppermint oil capsules—thought to have smooth muscle relaxing properties—may reduce abdominal pain in children and adults with IBS.
2. H_2 receptor antagonists or proton-pump inhibitors may relieve some symptoms of ulcer-like dyspepsia.
3. Pizotifen—a serotonin antagonist has been effective prophylactically for abdominal migraine. This drug has not yet been approved for use in the US. In some studies, propanolol and cyproheptadine have been shown to be effective.
4. 5-HT$_3$ antagonist (alosetron) has been helpful in adult women with severe diarrhea-predominant IBS. Because of potential side effects (severe constipation, ischemic colitis, bowel perforation), it is available only under a restricted prescribing program.
5. Tricyclic antidepressants used at low doses and selective serotonin reuptake inhibitors may improve symptoms of abdominal pain in adults with IBS and children with functional abdominal pain. Data in children and adolescents are conflicting. Tricyclic antidepressants appear particularly useful in cases of IBS with refractory diarrhea in adults.
6. The chloride channel-2 agonist (lubiprostone), a bicyclical fatty acid compound that activates chloride-rich fluid secretion in the intestine, is approved for treatment of chronic idiopathic constipation in adults and IBS with constipation in women at least 18 years old.
7. Guanylin cyclase-C receptor agonist (linaclotide), which increases release fluid with chloride and bicarbonate into the intestine and accelerates GI transit, is approved for treatment of adults with chronic idiopathic constipation and IBS with constipation.
8. Polyethylene glycol has been used for children with chronic constipation.

Other symptomatic treatment options:

1. Antispasmodic or anticholinergic agents (e.g., hyoscyamine, dicyclomine) may be used for symptomatic relief on short-term basis.
2. Antidiarrheals (loperamide) may reduce stool frequency in diarrhea-predominant IBS, but may not improve pain or bloating compared to placebo.
3. Probiotics may improve IBS symptoms in children, adolescents, and adults.
4. Short-term trials have shown that nonabsorbable antibiotics (rifaximin) are more effective than placebo for symptoms of bloating in adults with IBS.

Fiber and Dietary Modifications

1. High-fiber diet has been recommended in both constipation-predominant and diarrhea-predominant IBS, as well as functional abdominal pain. Soluble fiber (ispaghula/psyllium) is best supported by the evidence; insoluble fiber is not effective. Excessive fiber should be avoided because it may cause gas and distension as well as exacerbation of constipation and diarrhea. If foods high in fiber are unsuccessful, supplements are available over the counter.
2. Dietary carbohydrates—malabsorption may be a provocative stimulant. A diet low in fermentable oligosaccharides, disaccharides, monosaccharides, and polyols can provide symptom relief in some individuals. These include foods with lactose, sorbitol, mannitol, and fructose and include milk products, fruits, vegetables, some grains, chewing gum, and excessive carbonated beverages.
3. Gluten-free diet: Some individuals with nonceliac gluten sensitivity may have improvement on a gluten-free diet, but the data are controversial.

Psychological Interventions

Counseling consists of reassuring the adolescent or young adult and their family that the abdominal pain which accompanies FGID is real and that no specific organic disease has been found. The practitioner should stress that the pain is not "in the young person's head" but is a real manifestation, which can be exacerbated, by stress. It is important to reassure the adolescent or young adult that they are physically healthy and can continue with all activities. Often young people with FGID miss a lot of school or work. If this is the case, the family, teachers, school nurse, and employer should work together with the individual to keep him or her in school or at work. Significant changes in or atypical characteristics of the pain should prompt reevaluation.

If significant depression, anxiety, or family problems are uncovered, the adolescent or young adult and family can be referred for further psychological or family assessment. However, psychological intervention may be helpful even in less severe cases. Cognitive behavioral therapy and hypnotherapy have been demonstrated to be successful for treating functional disorders in children, adolescents, and adults. Guided imagery which leads to muscle relaxation has been shown to be beneficial in children. Ultimately, the goal is to reduce illness behavior. Prompt recognition and intervention are important. Long-term follow-up studies have shown that children with persistent abdominal pain are at increased risk for developing psychiatric disorders (including anxiety and depression) during adolescence and adulthood.[1,30]

REFERENCES

1. Di Lorenzo C, Colleti RB, Lehman HP, et al. Chronic abdominal pain in children, Subcommittee on Chronic Abdominal Pain, Technical Report. *Pediatrics* 2005;115:e370–e381.
2. Di Lorenzo C, Colleti RB, Lehman HP, et al. Chronic abdominal pain in children, Subcommittee on Chronic Abdominal Pain, Clinical Report. *Pediatrics* 2005;115:812–815.
3. *Rome Foundation*. Available at http://www.romecriteria.org/. Accessed March 15, 2014.
4. Choung RS, Locke GR. Epidemiology of IBS. *Gastroenterol Clin North Am* 2011;40(1):1–10.
5. Chang F-Y, Cehn P-H, Wu T-C, et al. Prevalence of functional gastrointestinal disorders in Taiwan: questionnaire-based survey for adults based on Rome III criteria. *Asia Pac J Clin Nutr* 2012;21:594–600.
6. Drossman DA. The functional gastrointestinal disorders and the Rome III process. *Gastroenterology* 2006;130:1377–1390.

7. Corazziari E. Definition and epidemiology of functional gastrointestinal disorders. *Best Prac Res Clin Gastroenterol* 2004;18:613–631.
8. Pimentel M, Talley NJ, Quigely E, et al. Report from the multinational irritable bowel syndrome initiative 2012. *Gastroenterology* 2013;144: e1–e5.
9. Chirkara DK, Rawat DJ, Talley NJ. The epidemiology of childhood recurrent abdominal pain in western countries: a systematic review. *Am J Gastroenterol* 2005;200:1868–1875.
10. Youssef NN, Atienza K, Langseder AL, et al. Chronic abdominal pain and depressive symptoms: analysis of the National Longitudinal Study of Adolescent Health. *Clin Gastroenterol Hepatol* 2008;6:329–332.
11. Helgeland H, Flagstad G, Grotta J, et al. Diagnosing pediatric functional abdominal pain in children (4–15 years old) according to the Rome III criteria: results from a Norwegian prospective study. *J Pediatr Gastroenterol Nutr* 2009;29:309–315.
12. Sagawa T, Okamura S, Kakiazaki, et al. Functional gastrointestinal disorders in adolescents and quality of school life. *J Gastroenterol Hepatol* 2013;28:285–290.
13. Lovell RM, Ford AC. Global prevalence of and risk factors for irritable bowel syndrome: a meta-analysis. *Clin Gastroenterol Hepatol* 2012;10:712–721.
14. Mayer EA, Tillisch K. The brain-gut axis in abdominal pain syndromes. *Annu Rev Med* 2011;62:381–396.
15. Kennedy PJ, Clarke G, Quigley EMM, et al. Gut memories: towards a cognitive neurobiology of irritable bowel syndrome. *Neurosci Biobehav Rev* 2012;36:310–340.
16. Elsenbruch S. Abdominal pain in irritable bowel syndrome: a review of putative psychological, neural and neuro-immune mechanisms. *Brain Behav Immun* 2011;25:386–394.
17. Simren M, Barbara G, Flint H, et al. Intestinal microbiotica in functional bowel disorders: a Rome foundation report. *Gut* 2013;62:159–176.
18. VanReheenen PF, Van de Vijer E, Fidler V. Faecal calprotectin for screening of patients with suspected inflammatory bowel disease: diagnostic meta-analysis. *BMJ* 2010;341:c3369. doi:10.1136/bmj.c3369.
19. Henderson P, Anderson NH, Wilson DC. The diagnostic accuracy of fecal calprotectin during the investigation of suspected pediatric inflammatory bowel disease: a systematic review and meta-analysis. *Am J Gastroenterol* 2014;109:637–645. doi:10.1038/aj g2013.131.
20. Guandalini S, Assiri A. Celiac disease a review. *JAMA Pediatr* 2014;168(3):272–278. doi:10.1001/jamapediatrics.2013.3858.
21. Fasano A, Catassi C. Celiac disease. *N Engl J Med* 2012;367:2419–2426.
22. Rubio-Tapia A, Hill ID, Keely CP, et al. ACG clinical guidelines: diagnosis and management of celiac disease. *Am J Gastroenterol* 2013;108:656–676.
23. American College of Gastroenterology Task Force on irritable bowel syndrome. An evidence-based systematic review on the management of irritable bowel syndrome. *Am J Gastroenterol* 2009;104 (suppl 1):S1–S35.
24. Saps M, Adams P, Bonilla S, et al. Abdominal pain and functional gastrointestinal disorders in children with celiac disease. *J Pediatr* 2013;162:505–509.
25. Rasquin A, Di Lorenzo C, Forbes D, et al. Childhood functional gastrointestinal disorders: child/adolescent. *Gastroenterol* 2006;130:1527–1537.
26. Gibson PR, Barrett JS, Muir JG. Functional bowel symptoms and diet. *Intern Med J* 2013;43:1067–1074.
27. Ford AC, Vandvik PO. Irritable bowel syndrome. *Clin Evid* 2012;01:410.
28. Camilleri M, DiLorenzo C. Brain-gut axis: from basic understanding to treatment of IBS and related disorders. *J Pediatr Gastroenterol Nutr* 2012;54:446–453.
29. Korternick JJ, Oekeloen L, Benninga MA, et al. Probiotics for childhood functional gastrointestinal disorders: a systematic review and meta-analysis. *Acta Paediatr* 2014;103(4):365–372. doi:10.1111/apa.12513.
30. Shelby GD, Shirkey KC, Sherman AL, et al. Functional abdominal pain in childhood and long-term vulnerability to anxiety disorders. *Pediatrics* 2013;132:475–482.

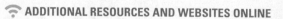 **ADDITIONAL RESOURCES AND WEBSITES ONLINE**

PART XI

Sexuality and Contraception

37 Adolescent and Young Adult Sexuality

Devon J. Hensel
Kimber L. Hendrix

KEY WORDS

- Romantic relationships
- Sexual behavior
- Sexual health
- Sexuality

Adolescence and young adulthood is recognized as an important period in the development of lifelong sexual health. Sexuality is a normal and primary developmental element of puberty and the several years that follow. Many key biologic, psychological, social, and behavioral aspects of adult sexuality begin to unfold during this period of time. Among many changes, adolescents and young adults (AYAs) develop new sexual feelings and interests, initiate close relationships, and explore a wide range of partnered and solo sexual behaviors.

Many AYAs can find it difficult to discuss sexuality in a direct and open manner. As a result, it is common for people to equate the emergence of sexuality with potential consequences of sexual behavior, such as sexually transmitted infections (STIs) or unintended pregnancy. Yet, it is important to remember that formative experiences with different aspects of sexuality provide AYAs with the skills they will need to be sexually independent and responsible adults.

Health care providers play an important role in the development of sexuality, as both AYAs and their parents value clinical guidance on a variety of sexuality-related topics. Clinicians are uniquely positioned to deliver AYA sexual and reproductive health services, such as taking a sexual history or prescribing contraception, and take a patient-centered approach to discussing the ancillary emotional or interpersonal issues associated with AYA sexuality, such as emerging readiness for sex or refusing any unwanted sex. Professionals need to be prepared to have informed, supportive, and nonjudgmental conversations with their adolescent and young adult patients and to facilitate similar conversation between them and their parents.

This chapter provides an overview of the key changes in heterosexual AYA sexuality (see Chapters 38 and 39 for additional information on sexuality issues for gay, lesbian, bisexual, and transgendered [GLBT] youth). Using data from several different nationally representative studies, we address the development of close relationships in adolescence and young adulthood and the association of these relationships to the emergence of partnered and nonpartnered sexual behaviors. This information is intended to improve physician's and other health care provider's ability to directly and regularly engage sexuality-related topics with their AYAs and families, to anticipate initiation of sexual health changes, and to proactively devise counseling strategies that may improve health outcomes.

CLOSE RELATIONSHIPS IN ADOLESCENCE AND YOUNG ADULTHOOD

Close relationships—both romantic and nonromantic—play an important role in the development of sexuality during adolescence and young adulthood. Each partnership's emotional and behavioral characteristics provide a context for young people's ongoing learning and organizing of sexuality. Different relationships can fulfill different needs, such as intimacy, companionship, or sexual behavior(s), at different points in time, with changes in these relationships helping AYAs transition from childhood to later adult sexuality.

Relationship Forms and Meaning

Several studies have articulated the trajectory of young men's and women's close relationships changes in industrialized countries from early adolescence to early adulthood.[1-5]

Between pre- and early adolescence:

- Relationship interests shift from same-gender friendship groups to mixed-gender friendship groups in early adolescence to opposite-gender dyadic friendships and some romantic interests.
- Initial romantic partnerships are typically short lived (e.g., "going together") and are usually arranged by intermediaries, such as peers or friends, rather than by the adolescent themselves.
- Early relationships are limited in physical and emotional investment, and typically consist of interaction occurring at school, on the phone, or in groups.

During middle adolescence:

- Young men and women become increasingly aware of their romantic feelings toward the specific members of the opposite gender.
- The relationships associated with these feelings increase in both the importance adolescents ascribe to them and in the time adolescents spend with partners.
- Interactions typically become "one-on-one," and can become the venue for the emergence of "lighter" partnered sexual behaviors, such as kissing or hand-holding.

By late adolescence:

- Most young people have had and/or are in a serious romantic relationship.
- These dyads are associated with the emergence of learning more adult-like emotional and communication qualities, such as expressing feelings for one's partner, negotiating conflict, or recognizing sexual satisfaction.

- Young men and women may also make decisions about more involved types of partnered sexual behavior (e.g., genital touching, oral sex, or vaginal sex).

During young adulthood:

- Relationships move into a period of increased degree of investment and confidence in the relationship.
- AYAs further hone the characteristics found in earlier relationships. These characteristics can include better communication with one's partner, greater comfort with one's own sexuality, and increased sexual activity.
- Young women may be more confident than young men in navigating these relationships, as the social dynamics contained in these relationships often mimic those in friendships.

    Increasing attention has also been paid to "friends with benefits" (FWB) and "hook up" relationship typologies in adolescence and young adulthood.[6,7] While sexual activity can occur in both, and these two forms are often used interchangeably in popular media, studies suggest important differences between the two.

FWB relationships typically:

- Combine traits of friendships and romantic relationships.
- Draw on psychological intimacy and trust afforded by a friendship with the sexual intimacy of a romantic relationship.
- Avoid expectations of commitment or exclusivity often present in romantic relationships.
- Often characterized in popular and medical literature as an early adult phenomenon (particularly among college students), but also endorsed by adolescents as distinctly different from romantic relationships and casual sex partners, but not different from friendship except for sexual activity.

"Hook Ups":

- Characterized as no-strings-attached sexual behaviors.
- Typically occurs once, usually between people who are strangers or acquaintances.
- Unlike traditional romantic relationships, they have no expectations.

Developmental Benefits in Relationships

Close partnerships in adolescence and young adulthood help individuals learn the emotional and behavioral skills they will need to manage sexual relationships during their lifetime.[1–5]

- *Emotional* skills include learning how to develop intimacy, building trust and fidelity, first expressing love and affection, how to negotiate conflict, how to resolve conflicting emotions, and how to successfully end relationships.
- *Behavioral* skills include learning about a wide range of "lighter" (e.g., hugging, hand-holding, and kissing) and more involved (e.g., oral sex and penile-vaginal intercourse) partnered sexual acts, understanding and advocating for sexual pleasure, communicating likes and dislikes, or balancing power in relationships.
- FWB and "hook up" relationships can also include opportunities for experiencing exploration, particularly because they are perceived to be low risk.

⬤ SEXUAL BEHAVIOR IN ADOLESCENCE AND YOUNG ADULTHOOD

Traditional discussions of AYA sexual behavior commonly center on three partnered behaviors: giving or receiving oral sex, penile-vaginal sex, and penile-anal sex. While these behaviors are important pieces in understanding AYA sexuality, it is also vital to consider the role of other intimate partnered contact (e.g., kissing, hugging, holding hands, genital touching), any nonpartnered behaviors (e.g., solo masturbation), and the absence of any "behavior" (e.g., sexual

abstinence). Understanding specifically what AYAs are (or are not) participating in when they say they are "having sex" is key to a health care provider being prepared to assess ongoing levels of sexual risk as well as contraceptive and condom use needs.[8–11]

Sexual "Abstinence"

Overview

- Many cultural terms (e.g., "abstinence," "virginity" or "celibacy") are used to describe AYAs' nonparticipation in sexual activity.
- These terms make it challenging to accurately know how and when AYAs may voluntarily opt out of specific types of sexual activity.
- A clinician should not assume no sexual contact is occurring if an adolescent or young adult says that he or she is "sexually abstinent."
  - Avoidance of any and all sexual activity that occurs by one's self, or with partners.
  - Avoiding a limited scope of behaviors, such as those that carry a risk of pregnancy or STIs, while still participating in other behaviors.

Prevalence

- The National Survey of Family Growth (NSFG)[12] suggests that about three-quarters of 15- to 17-year-olds (females: 73%; males: 74%) and about one-third of 18- and 19-year-olds (females: 37.3%; males: 36.1%) have never had sex.
- The Youth Risk Behavior Survey (YRBS)[13] demonstrates that about half of all young people in high school have never had sex (females: 54%; males: 52.5%), with a decrease in reported abstinence between grade 9 (females: 71.9%; males: 68%) and grade 12 (females: 37.2%; males: 34.6%).
- About one-third of college students (females: 30.0%; males: 34%) report not having any oral, vaginal, or anal sex in the past year.[14]
- Young people sometimes differentiate between "primary" sexual abstinence (an absence of any lifetime sexual intercourse experience, usually penile-vaginal sex) and "secondary" sexual abstinence (first time sexual experience followed by periods without sexual activity).
- Both "primary" and "secondary" abstainers participate in nonpenetrative partnered sexual behaviors (e.g., kissing, breast fondling, genital stimulation, and oral-genital sex), often because they believe these behaviors do not "count" as sexual experience.

Context

- Choosing "primary" and "secondary" sexual abstinence could occur for a variety of reasons.
  - Avoid perceived social or health risks
  - Uphold moral or religious commitments
  - Peer or parental pressure
  - Saving sexual experience for one's future spouse
- Age wise:
  - Younger AYAs typically see themselves as less "ready" for sex.
  - Older AYAs balance their moral (e.g., "doing the right thing") with their behavioral (e.g., avoiding specific activities) ideals in deciding.

Solo Masturbation

Overview

Solo masturbation is perhaps the most difficult of all sexual behaviors to study.[15,16]

- Historically, participation in solo masturbation has been stigmatized.
- Many social and gender norms still proscribe masturbation, particularly among women.
- Very few nationally representative studies ask questions about masturbation.

Prevalence

- The National Study of Sexual Health Behavior (NHSSB) suggests that:[17,18]
  - The majority of adolescent males (62.6% to 80.0%) and adolescent females (43.3% to 58.0%)[19] as well as among emerging adult men (e.g., over the age of 18) (86.1% to 94.3%) and women (66.0% to 84.6%) have ever masturbated in their lifetime.
  - About half of adolescent men (42.9% to 58.0%), a quarter of adolescent women (24.1% to 25.5%), about 60% of young adult men (61.1% to 62.8%), and between a quarter and a half of young women (26.0% to 43.7%) have masturbated in the past month.
  - About half of adolescent males (49.1%) and a fifth (22.1%) of adolescent women reported masturbating two or more times per week.

Context

- Solo masturbation serves important functions in developing sexuality.[15,16,20,21]
  - Learning about the geography of one's body
  - Learning about sexual response
  - Learning about one's own personal sexual likes and dislikes, and communicating these preferences to partners
- Solo masturbation may be used as a "safe sex" alternative to avoid STI or pregnancy.
- Solo masturbation can be used to experience sexual pleasure in the absence of a partner, when one does not desire to have sex with a partner, or as a follow-up to partnered sexual activities that were not sexually fulfilling.

Partnered Masturbation

Overview

- The term "partnered masturbation" can refer either to two individuals who self-masturbate in the presence of one another or to individuals stimulating the genitals of their partner.
- Similarly to solo masturbation, very few nationally representative studies ask questions about partnered masturbation.

Prevalence

- The NHSSB suggests that:[17,19]
  - *Lifetime* reports of partnered masturbation increase with age among adolescent men (3.2% to 21.1%) and adolescent women (7.2% to 26.0%),[19] as well as in young adult women (38.8% to 46.9%) and young adult men (49.3% to 54.5%).
  - More than half of adolescent males (57.8%) and about 10% of adolescent females reported partnered masturbation in the *past 90 days*, with increased reporting between 14 years and 17 years.
  - Less than a fifth of young adult women (16.1% to 18.4%) and young adult men (14.5% to 15.0%) have participated in partnered masturbation in the past month.

Context

Partnered masturbation may occur for a variety of reasons and in different contexts.[3,18,21,22]

- It can serve as an important source of partner-focused sexual learning:
  - Negotiating sexual needs and desires
  - Understanding shared intimacy and pleasure
- Partnered masturbation often precedes first vaginal sex.
- It can occur early in the early stages of a relationship, or when a sexual encounter or partner is more casual.
- Like solo masturbation, partnered masturbation may also serve as a "safer" behavior choice to avoid STI or pregnancy.
- Some individuals may choose partnered masturbation as one of multiple sexual behaviors enacted with a partner, such as part of "foreplay" prior to vaginal sex, or as the ending behaviors in a given sexual episode.

Oral Sex

Overview

- The term "oral sex" can refer to a number of different sexual practices, and can take on a variety of meanings in different contexts for AYAs.
  - The most common definition: stimulation of the vaginal or penile genital area by use of the mouth, tongue, or teeth, both received from a partner and/or given to a partner.
  - Other venues of stimulation (e.g., to the anus) are possible and are practiced.
- Variability in these definitions creates challenges for assessing the prevalence of oral sex.
- It is important that health care providers ask specific questions about oral sexual practices and the motivations surrounding those practices.

Prevalence

- Slightly under half of college women (46.0%) and men (42.0%) report having any oral sex in the past 30 days.[14]
- The NSFG demonstrates that[23]:
  - Under half of 15- to 19-year-old young women report ever giving (41%) and/or receiving oral sex (43%).
  - About half of 15- to 19-year-old men report receiving oral sex, and 35% in the same age-group have ever given oral sex.
  - The majority of 20- to 24-year-old men (82%) and women (85%) report ever participating in oral sex.
- The NHSSB suggests that[17]:
  - *Receiving* oral sex in one's lifetime varies among adolescent women (10.1% to 25.8%) and adolescent men (13.0% to 34.4%), as well as in young adult women (62.0% to 79.1%) and men (59.4% to 73.5%).
  - Lifetime reports of giving oral sex also vary in adolescence (females: 12.8% to 29.1%; males: 8.3% to 20.2%) and over the age of 18 (females: 61.2% to 77.6%; men: 60.9% to 70.9%).
  - Less than a fifth of adolescent males and females report giving or receiving oral sex in the last month, whereas nearly half of men and women over the age of 18 report giving and/or receiving oral sex in the past month.

Context

Oral sex occurs during adolescence and young adulthood for a variety of reasons.[24–27]

- Individuals may believe that participating in oral sex may bring social status or popularity.
- Oral sex may also occur if individuals perceive it is less risky than vaginal sex or anal sex.
- Some younger adolescents may participate in oral sex as a means of "preserving virginity," particularly if they believe it does not "count" as sex.
- Choosing a specific oral sex act (e.g., receiving versus giving, or a specific body site) may occur based on what a partner or a young person desires.
- Oral sex may also occur as one behavior in a larger sexual routine that a given couple has, such as part of "foreplay."
- Older AYAs may participate in oral sex specifically to enhance emotional intimacy or to effectively achieve sexual pleasure and orgasm.

Penile-Vaginal Sex

Overview

Penile-vaginal sex is perhaps the most culturally significant sexual behavior in Western societies.

- During adolescence, it is constructed as the traditional way that an individual "loses their virginity" or has their "first sex".
- It is the behavior most often referenced in association to the concept of "abstinence."
- The first experience of penile-vaginal sex often influences how people experience it in the future.

IX

Prevalence

- About half of college women (52.0%) and men (44.0%) report having penile-vaginal sex in the past 30 days.[14]
- The NSFG demonstrates that[23]:
  - Under half of 15- to 19-year-old young women (47%) and young men (49%) report ever having vaginal sex.
  - The majority of 20- to 24-year-old men (85%) and women (87%) report ever having vaginal sex.
- The NHSSB suggests that[17,19]:
  - About a fifth (males: 20.5%; females: 22.6%) of adolescents report lifetime experience with vaginal sex, with increased reporting between the ages of 14 and 17 years.
  - Similarly, a majority of both young adult women (64.0% to 85.6%) and men (62.5% to 70.3%) report lifetime experience with vaginal sex.
  - About 15% of all adolescent males and females report having had vaginal sex in the past three months, with an increase in reporting between the ages of 14 and 17 (females: 1.1% to 26.9%; males: 8.8% to 25.0%).
  - About half of young adult women (43.1% to 61.9%) and between a third and half of young adult men (31.0% to 52.0%) report participating in penile-vaginal sex in the past month.

Context

AYAs may choose penile-vaginal sex for a variety of reasons.[27–29]

- Individuals may choose vaginal sex for emotional reasons (e.g., to express love or intimacy), physical reasons (e.g., sexual interest or stress reduction) or social reasons (e.g., increased social status or popularity).
- The frequency of vaginal sex may increase over time in relationships as relationship quality and sexual satisfaction also grow.
- Vaginal sex is also more likely in a given sexual episode when it has recently occurred, or it becomes part of a person's usual sexual routine.

Penile-Anal Sex

Overview

- Penile-anal sex is typically a most difficult sexual behavior to discuss.
- People often feel social stigma associated with reporting their participation in anal sex.
- Both the difficulty discussing anal sex, and the social stigma associated with anal sex could make physicians falsely assume:
  - Young people do not participate in anal sex.
  - It occurs infrequently.
  - When it does happen, it is coerced, particularly for young women.

Prevalence

- Very few college women (4.0%) and men (7.0%) report having penile-anal sex in the past 30 days.[14]
- The NHSSB suggests that[17,19]:
  - Less than 5% of male and female adolescents report any lifetime experience with penile-anal sex and less than 2% of either group participated in anal sex in the past three months.
  - More young adult women (20.0% to 39.9%) than men (9.7% to 23.7%) report lifetime participation in penile-anal sex and less than 10% of either group chose anal sex in the past month.
  - Frequency of anal sex increases as AYAs become older.

Context

AYAs' participation in penile-anal sex can vary across different contexts.[27,30–34]

- Penile-anal sex occurs in both AYAs' main and casual relationships, as well as in monogamous and nonmonogamous relationships.

- Similar to their perceptions about oral sex, some AYAs may not consider penile-anal sex as "having sex," and may use it as a means to preserve virginity.
- Others may perceive penile-anal sex to be a "safer" alternative to vaginal sex, as it poses no risk of pregnancy.
- Anal sex may occur as an act of physical pleasure or emotional intimacy with one's partner, in deference to partner requests, or in response to imbalanced relationship power.
- Anal sex is more likely in a given sexual episode if a couple also has other sexual behaviors (particularly penile-vaginal sex), or if it has occurred recently (e.g., the past few days or week).

OUTCOMES ASSOCIATED WITH SEXUAL BEHAVIOR

While most AYAs participate in sexual behavior without issue, some young people do experience adverse sexual outcomes, including unintended pregnancy and STIs. More information associated with the prevalence and organization of these conditions can be found in Chapter 40 (pregnancy) and Chapters 56 to 60 (STIs).

CLINICIAN RECOMMENDATIONS

Health care providers play a direct and important role in assuring sexual and reproductive health care during adolescence and young adulthood. Sexuality continues to be a recommended dimension of preventative health across the life span, and it additionally intersects with several specific goals in Healthy People 2020.[35] Moreover, AYAs value medical professional guidance on a variety of sexual topics. Thus, health care providers should be prepared to address concerns and questions posed by both AYAs and their families. Outlined below are some points to support these interactions.

1. *All clinically associated visits, including preventative, immunization, acute care, follow-up, and otherwise, can and should be used as opportunities to (re)address adolescent or young adult sexual health issues*. The regularity of preventative health visits declines during adolescence, and a physician may not find enough time in the course of a preventative visit to completely discuss all sexual health concerns. Moreover, some AYAs may not have insurance or a usual source of care. Thus, expanding sexual health support to all provider–patient interactions may ensure a greater breadth, depth, and continuity of sexuality care during this critical time frame.

2. *Providers should remember that regular and complete sexual health assessments are necessary for both male and female AYAs*. Common sex/gender norms about sexuality, or statistics about disparities in STIs, may cause health care professionals to incorrectly assume their adolescent or young adult female patients are at greater sexual risk than their adolescent or young adult male patients. As a result, they may screen females more regularly or in more depth for sexual risk, or proactively offer sexual health counseling, as compared to males. Yet, since the long-term morbidity and mortality associated with adverse sexual outcomes affect young people regardless of gender, it is important for health care providers to be equally versed in understanding sexuality and sexual health in all their AYA patients.

3. *Solo masturbation may emerge earlier than other partnered sexual behaviors*, and/or may cause some adolescents or young adults' significant anxiety, guilt, or embarrassment. In early adolescence, providers may initiate a conversation with patients regarding emerging sexual feelings, using this as a lead in to normalizing solo masturbation: *Many young people express sexual feelings by masturbating, or exploring what feels good on their own bodies. This is a completely normal thing to do, and it can help you better learn about your own body. Have you heard anything about it from your parents, your friends, or other people that you might be confused about? Can I answer any questions for you about it?*

As AYAs become older, or enter into close relationships, the conversation can also be used to normalize both solo masturbation as a means of delaying sex or being able to communicate to a partner about how they liked to be touched.

4. *Beginning in early adolescence, health care providers should regularly (re)assess AYAs' close/intimate relationships.* Health care providers should expect participation in these relationships to emerge as adolescents enter middle school or junior high, and to begin asking about them as a means of establishing rapport on this topic.

    Questions to facilitate this early conversation may include the following:

    Is there anyone you like at school/church/etc.? What do you like about him or her? What kinds of things do you do together? How often do you see him or her?

5. *It is also important to revisit partnerships mentioned in prior conversation,* to gauge changes in the relationship's importance, as well as to get a sense for the types of emotional experiences the adolescent or young adult has in that relationship. These qualities, both positive and negative, offer important insight as to where the provider can help support the development of attributes an adolescent or young adult finds satisfying and where a provider might be able to support a solution for attributes in which the young person feels stuck, afraid, or otherwise unsafe.

    Questions or prompts might include:

    - *What's new with your love life? The last time you were here, you mentioned a person named X. Is she or he still important to you?*
    - *What kinds of things have changed since we last spoke? What about X makes you happy? What about X bothers you? Do you have anyone new you're spending time with? What does Y mean to you?*

6. *The emotional content in a relationship also provides cues as to when lighter or more involved partnered sexual behaviors may emerge.* In the context of every partnership, health care practitioners should ask specific questions about how and when the young person expresses sexual or physical affection for partners, and assess any risk associated with those activities.

    Questions may include the following:

    - *How do you and X express affection for each other? Do you hold hands? Hug? What other kinds of things do you do with X?*
    - *Did you know that some of the activities you mentioned could increase the likelihood that you could...? [get pregnant/catch a STI]. I'd like to talk about how we can make sure you protect yourself while you are with X.*
    - *You mentioned that sometimes X pressures you to... [touch genitals/have vaginal sex/have oral sex]. How does that make you feel? What can I do to help you stop that from happening again?*

    In the context of ongoing assessment, these questions can be amended: *Last time you were here, you mentioned that you and X liked to [hold hands and kiss]. Is that still how you prefer to spend time together? Are [condoms/birth control pills/abstinence] still working for you? How can I help you?*

7. *Providers also need to be vigilant about clarifying what an adolescent or young adult means when they say they are "sexually abstinent,"* including periods when they do and do not have relationships with partners. Such questions could include *When you say you (or you and X) are abstinent, what does that mean to you (or the two of you)?*

    It would be helpful for clinicians to be equipped to provide appropriate information around any misperceptions AYAs may have about sexual risk reduction in their behavior choices, as well as to support their motivations for remaining abstinent, or changing their approach to abstinence. It may be helpful to begin both these conversations with a question related to why they chose abstinence: *Why is abstinence important for you? What does it provide to you (or you and X)?*

In this manner, the health care provider gains a sense of any perceived moral, religious, or safety benefits an adolescent or young adult derives from his or her version of abstinence, and provides appropriate points of risk-reduction counseling. Questions or prompts could include: *You mentioned that [activities X, Y, and Z] are "safer" and that's why you (or you and X) do them together. Did you know that some of them could actually increase the likelihood that you could...? [get pregnant/catch a STI]. I'd like to talk about how we can make sure you protect yourself while you are with X.*

8. *Health professionals need to be aware of the ongoing presence of FWB or "hook up" relationships, even when an adolescent or young adult has been in, or is currently in, a more regular relationship.* When one of these relationships is noted, they can ask patients how well they know their partner's sexual history, what sexual risks they perceive, and what methods they are using to reduce adverse sexual outcomes. Providers should also be prepared to adjust their counseling around condom and contraceptive use, as well as sexual refusal strategies, in the context of these partnerships.

    Questions or prompts might include: *You mentioned you are/were [kissing/holding hands/having oral/vaginal/anal sex] with Y [the last time you were here], but that s/he wasn't your boy/girlfriend. What does that mean? How are you protecting yourself with this partner?*

9. *Clinicians need to be aware that the various motivations for and perceptions about different sexual behaviors change over time, and these motivations and perceptions can influence both participation and perception of risk.* Understanding and revisiting these elements, particularly in the context of new and ongoing relationships, will help providers tailor sexual health education around those specific motivations.

    Questions and prompts could include: *You mentioned that [activities X, Y, and Z] are what you and [A] do together. What is your favorite part of those activities? What benefits do you feel they bring to your partnership or to you as a person?*

    Similar to discussion about different versions of sexual abstinence, a follow-up sentence could be: *You said that [having sex without a condom...increases intimacy/increases sexual pleasure], but it also increases the likelihood that you could.... [get pregnant/catch a STI]. I'd like to talk to about ways to [increase intimacy/increase sexual pleasure] that won't increase your risk for [getting pregnant/getting s STI]...*

10. *Encourage open, honest, and direct sexual communication between AYAs and their parents.* It may be useful to remind parents that despite increasing independence, their children still need, and value, guidance from them. Reinforce the importance of knowing and asking questions about their child's close relationships, and empower parents to check in on the emotional and behavioral content in these relationships. It may be necessary to assure parents that asking about specific experiences will not "cause" their children to participate in them (e.g., vaginal sex), but it will provide parents an ongoing sense of the young person's readiness to manage them. Likewise, help AYAs initiate "tough" conversations with their parents, vetting any advanced concerns they may have about parents' being angry or upset regarding sexual issues. If necessary, provide a neutral space for AYAs and their parents to talk out specific issues, helping to guide the conversation to specific issues and validating emotions and concerns on both sides.

SEXUAL BEHAVIOR OUTCOMES

While the majority of AYAs transition into sexual relationships and sexual behavior without issue, some do experience adverse sexual outcomes, such as unintended pregnancy and STIs. More information on the prevalence and organization of these outcomes is provided in Chapter 40 (pregnancy) and Chapters 56 to 62 (STIs).

REFERENCES

1. Collins WA, Madsen SD. Relationships in adolescence and young adulthood. In: Perlman D, Vangelisti A, eds. *Handbook of personal relationships*. Cambridge: Cambridge University Press, 2006:191–209.
2. Connolly J, McIsaac C. Romantic relationships in adolescence. In: Underwood MK, Rosen LH, eds. *Social development: relationships in infancy, childhood, and adolescence*. New York, NY: Guilford Press, 2011:180–206.
3. O'Sullivan LF, Cheng MM, Harris KM, et al. I wanna hold your hand: the progression of social, romantic and sexual events in adolescent relationships. *Perspect Sex Reprod Health* 2007;39(2):100–107.
4. Giordano PC, Manning WD, Longmore MA. Affairs of the heart: qualities of adolescent romantic relationships and sexual behavior. *J Res Adolesc* 2010;20(4):983–1013. doi:10.1111/j.1532-7795.2010.00661.x.
5. Giordano PC, Manning WD, Longmore MA, et al. Developmental shifts in the character of romantic and sexual relationships from adolescence to young adulthood. Early Adulthood in a Family Context. In: Booth A, Brown SL, Landale NS, et al., eds. New York, NY: Springer, 2012:133–164.
6. Furman W, Shaffer L. Romantic partners, friends, friends with benefits, and casual acquaintances as sexual partners. *J Sex Res* 2011;48(6):554–564. doi:10.1080/00224499.2010.535623.
7. Garcia JR, Reiber C, Massey SG, et al. Sexual hookup culture: a review. *Rev Gen Psychol* 2012;16(2):161.
8. Loewenson PR, Ireland M, Resnick MD. Primary and secondary sexual abstinence in high school students. *J Adolesc Health* 2004;34(3):209–215. doi:10.1016/j.jadohealth.2003.05.002.
9. Ott MA, Pfeiffer EJ, Fortenberry JD. Perceptions of sexual abstinence among high-risk early and middle adolescents. *J Adolesc Health* 2006;39(2):192–198. doi:10.1016/j.jadohealth.2005.12.009.
10. Bersamin MM, Fisher DA, Walker S, et al. Defining virginity and abstinence: adolescents' interpretations of sexual behaviors. *J Adolesc Health* 2007;41(2):182–188. doi:10.1016/j.jadohealth.2007.03.011.
11. Abbott DA, Dalla RL. 'It's a choice, simple as that': youth reasoning for sexual abstinence or activity. *J Youth Stud* 2008;11(6):629–649. doi:10.1080/13676260802225751.
12. Martinez G, Copen CE, Abma JC. Teenagers in the United States: sexual activity, contraceptive use, and childbearing, 2006–2010 National Survey of Family Growth. *Vital Health Stat* 2011;23(31):1.
13. Kann L, Kinchen S, Shanklin SL, et al. Youth risk behavior surveillance—United States, 2013. *MMWR Surveill Summ* 2014;63 (suppl 4):1–168.
14. American College Health Association. *American College Health Association-National College Health Assessment II: Canadian Reference Group Data Report Spring 2013*. Bethesda, MD: American College Health Association, 2013.
15. Kaestle C, Allen K. The role of masturbation in healthy sexual development: perceptions of young adults. *Arch Sex Behav* 2011:1–12. doi:10.1007/s10508-010-9722-0.
16. Das A. Masturbation in the United States. *J Sex Marital Ther* 2007;33(4):301–317. doi:10.1080/00926230701385514.
17. Herbenick D, Reece M, Schick V, et al. Sexual behavior in the United States: results from a national probability sample of men and women ages 14–94. *J Sex Med* 2010;7:255–265. doi:10.1111/j.1743-6109.2010.02012.x.
18. Robbins CL, Schick V, Reece M, et al. Prevalence, frequency, and associations of masturbation with partnered sexual behaviors among US adolescents. *Arch Pediatr Adolesc Med* 2011;165(12):1087–1093. doi:10.1001/archpediatrics.2011.142.
19. Fortenberry JD, Schick V, Herbenick D, et al. Sexual behaviors and condom use at last vaginal intercourse: a national sample of adolescents ages 14 to 17 years. *J Sex Med* 2010;7:305–314. doi:10.1111/j.1743-6109.2010.02018.x.
20. Hogarth H, Ingham R. Masturbation among young women and associations with sexual health: an exploratory study. *J Sex Res* 2009;46(6):558–567. doi:10.1080/00224490902878993.
21. Coleman E. Masturbation as a means of achieving sexual health. *J Psychol Hum Sex* 2003;14(2/3):5–16. doi:10.1300/J056v14n02_02.
22. Fortenberry JD. *The science of adolescent sexual health. State of sexual freedom in the United States*. 2011:76.
23. Copen CE, Chandra A, Martinez G. *Prevalence and timing of oral sex with opposite-sex partners among females and males aged 15–24 years: United States, 2007–2010*. Hyattsville, MD: National Center for Health Statistics, 2012.
24. Cornell JL, Halpern-Felsher BL. Adolescents tell us why teens have oral sex. *J Adolesc Health* 2006;38(3):299–301. doi:10.1016/j.jadohealth.2005.04.015.
25. Bay-Cheng LY, Fava NM. Young women's experiences and perceptions of Cunnilingus during adolescence. *J Sex Res* 2011;48(6):531–542. doi:10.1080/00224499.2010.535221.
26. Chambers WC. Oral sex: varied behaviors and perceptions in a college population. *J Sex Res* 2007;48(1):28–42.
27. Hensel DJ, Fortenberry JD, Orr DP. Variations in coital and noncoital sexual repertoire among adolescent women. *J Adolesc Health* 2008;42(2):170–176.
28. Meston C, Buss D. Why humans have sex. *Arch Sex Behav* 2007;36(4):477–507. doi:10.1007/s10508-007-9175-2.
29. Sayegh MA, Fortenberry JD, Shew M, et al. The developmental association of relationship quality, hormonal contraceptive choice and condom non-use among adolescent women. *J Adolesc Health* 2006;39(3):388–395. doi:10.1016/j.jadohealth.2005.12.027.
30. Hensel DJ, Fortenberry JD, Orr DP. Factors associated with event level anal sex and condom use during anal sex among adolescent women. *J Adolesc Health* 2010;46(3):232–237.
31. Houston AM, Fang J, Husman C, et al. More than just vaginal intercourse: anal intercourse and condom use patterns in the context of "main" and "casual" sexual relationships among urban minority adolescent females. *J Pediatr Adolesc Gynecol* 2007;20(5):299–304.
32. Lescano CM, Houck CD, Brown LK, et al. Correlates of heterosexual anal intercourse among at-risk adolescents and young adults. *Am J Public Health* 2009;99(6):1131–1136.
33. Maynard E, Carballo-Diéguez A, Ventuneac A, et al. Women's experiences with anal sex: motivations and implications for STD prevention. *Perspect Sex Reprod Health* 2009;41(3):142–149. doi:10.1363/4114209.
34. Herbenick D, Reece M, Schick V, et al. An event-level analysis of the sexual characteristics and composition among adults ages 18 to 59: results from a National Probability Sample in the United States. *J Sex Med* 2010;7:346–361. doi:10.1111/j.1743-6109.2010.02020.x.
35. U.S. Department of Health Human Services. *Healthy People 2020*. Washington, DC: U.S. Government Printing Office, 2011.

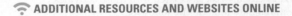

ADDITIONAL RESOURCES AND WEBSITES ONLINE

CHAPTER 38

Lesbian, Gay, and Bisexual Adolescents and Young Adults

Eric T. Meininger

KEY WORDS

- Bisexual
- Gay
- Homosexuality
- Lesbian
- LGB
- Queer
- Sexual minority
- Sexual orientation

HOMOSEXUALITY

Sexuality is an emotionally charged issue. It is a difficult topic to address, not only for adolescents and young adults (AYAs) but also for their family and health care provider, especially among those who identify as a sexual minority. The health care provider needs to be equipped to address the concerns of AYAs with a homosexual, bisexual, or questioning orientation and the fears of others, including parents, who are questioning their feelings. This chapter reviews minority sexual orientations in the context of AYAs' health, including features of counseling youth, young adults (YAs), and their parents.

General Considerations and Terminology

Sexual Orientation

Sexual orientation is a multidimensional personal framework composed of sexual identity (the self-assigned label), sexual behavior (the gender of partners), and sexual attraction (an individual's attractions to the same or opposite sex).[1,2] Sexual orientation is not discrete—individuals tend to fall along a continuum of sexual expression and desires rather than into distinct categories. These dimensions may not be in full concordance, reflecting the diversity of intimate human relationships. The phrase sexual preference implies choice and should not be used in reference to sexual orientation.

Gender Identity

Gender identity relates to an individual's innate sense of maleness or femaleness and should not be confused with or used interchangeably with sexual orientation. It usually develops at a much younger age (see Chapter 39).

Homosexuality

Although there is no absolute definition, *homosexuality* usually reflects "a persistent pattern of homosexual arousal accompanied by a persistent pattern of absent or weak heterosexual arousal."[3] Most homosexual individuals have a gender identity that is consistent with their biologic sex. Homosexuality is recognized as a nonpathologic variant of human sexuality.[4] Homosexual men are often informally referred to as "gay," while women may be referred to as "gay" or "lesbian."

Bisexuality

A *bisexual* person is erotically attracted to both men and women. This does not preclude long-term monogamous relationships, nor does it imply promiscuity.

Complicating all of the definitions above is the fact that the dimensions of sexual orientation (identity, behavior, and attraction) may occur in ways that seem contradictory to health care providers or others. Lesbian, gay, or even "queer" is a sexual identity label a person may or may not adopt. A person need not have had sex with a person of the same gender to identify as lesbian or gay, and a person who is sexually active with partners of the same gender may not identify as lesbian or gay. Young people who engage in sex with persons of the same gender may identify as homosexual or bisexual, but sometimes as heterosexual, curious, or questioning. Today, the term "sexual minority" or "queer" may be used to refer to the lesbian, gay, bisexual, and transgender populations collectively.

Prevalence

Homosexuality has existed in all societies and cultures. Prevalence estimates vary according to the time, place, and different measures of homosexuality used in research. Although sexual orientation is thought to be determined before adolescence, its expression may be postponed until early adulthood or indefinitely, making it difficult to determine the actual prevalence of homosexuality during adolescence.

Highly reliable prevalence, incidence, and acquisition patterns of homosexuality data are difficult to identify because:

- there is a lack of consistent clear definitions of homosexuality,
- the reluctance of some individuals to disclose sexual orientation information due to stigma, and
- the costliness of recruiting large enough samples that include a meaningful sample of homosexual individuals for analysis.

Many early studies used nonprobability samples as large population studies have historically not included questions to capture the dimensions of sexual orientation.[5]

Adolescents

In a large, population-based study of 35,000 junior and senior high school students in Minnesota,[6] greater than one-fourth of 12-year-old students were unsure about their sexual orientation. By 18 years of age, the figure dropped to 5% and uncertainty gave way to heterosexual or homosexual identification. Reported homosexual attractions (4.5%) exceeded fantasies, the latter being more common in girls (3.1%) than in boys (2.2%). Overall, 1.1% of students described themselves as predominantly homosexual or bisexual. The prevalence of reported homosexual experiences remained constant among girls (0.9%), but increased from 0.4% to 2.8% in boys between the ages of 12 and 18 years. Childhood and adolescent sexual behavior is not necessarily predictive of an adolescent's sexual orientation. Only about a third of teens who reported homosexual experience or fantasies identified themselves as homosexual or bisexual. Complicating the matter is that some children who have had involuntary or coercive same-gender sex may experience confusion about their sexual orientation as AYAs. A study by Garofalo et al.,[7] based on a question added to the Massachusetts Youth Risk Behavior Survey, found that 2.5% of youth self-identified as gay, lesbian, or bisexual. There is a growing recognition that youth who are "unsure" of their sexual orientation make up a sizeable number of youth[6] with unique stresses and morbidity.

Young Adults

The National Health and Social Life Survey (NHSLS) of 1992 used several dimensions of sexuality, including behavior, desire, and identification.[8] The prevalence of homosexual contact since puberty was approximately 10% of men and 5% of women, and 5% and 4%, respectively, had had homosexual contact since age 18 years. Because estimates in this study were based on small sample sizes, the numbers have been questioned in this sample. A more recent survey, the National Survey of Sexual Health and Behavior (2010),[9] estimates that 6.8% of men and 4.5% of women identify as homosexual, gay, lesbian, or bisexual, but did not ask questions on same-sex desire. The National College Health Assessment,[10] which surveys YAs who are college students, asked questions about multiple dimensions of sexuality, including attraction, behavior, and identity. The most recent survey data available suggest that almost 3.0% of YAs identify as lesbian or gay and almost 5.0% identify as bisexual.[10] A sizeable minority (2.5%) still identified as unsure.[10]

Etiology of Homosexuality

Significant evidence points to fundamental biologic differences between heterosexual and homosexual persons. These findings have included the following:

Genetic

The clustering of homosexuality within some families has long been recognized. As compared to dizygotic twins, the greater concordance of homosexuality in monozygotic twins highlights the role of genetic constitution. Among identical twins, concordance rates for homosexuality are reported in the range of 48% to 66%. A chromosomal location (Xq28) has been identified and is thought to be involved in male homosexuality; a specific gene has not yet been identified. No clear patterns of inheritance have been established.[11]

Neuroendocrine

Although heterosexual and homosexual adults have comparable levels of circulating sex steroids, it has been proposed that perinatal hormones organize and activate key areas of the brain early in life. This might contribute to the eventual development of neuroanatomical and neuropsychological functional differences related to sexual orientation.

Brain: Genetic, hormonal, and other biologic factors may influence behavior by their effect on the structure and functioning of the brain. In humans, brain regions correlated with homosexuality include the interstitial nuclei of the anterior hypothalamus (designated INAH1, INAH2, INAH3, and INAH4), the supraoptic nucleus, the anterior commissure, and the corpus callosum. The evidence is quite limited, and findings vary among studies.

Less well understood is the way that biology interacts with the environment and experience in shaping the expression of sexual orientation. Well-designed studies have not found differences in the familial and social backgrounds of homosexual and heterosexual men and women, nor any evidence that homosexuality is related to abnormal parenting, sexual abuse, or other traumatic events. Indeed, knowledge of other homosexual individuals is not

necessary for the development of a homosexual orientation,[12] nor do homosexual parents have an influence on the sexual orientation of their children.[13] However, environment can modulate the expression of fundamental biologic predisposition by influencing the social behavior and visibility of homosexual persons, complicating whether environmental factors are the result, rather than the cause.

Early descriptions of sexual orientation identified stages of acquisition of a homosexual identity (sensitization, identity confusion, identity assumption, commitment).[14,15] This appears to be an effect of a previous age cohort defined by events that were occurring. More recent research has identified that critical aspects of sexual orientation develop during preadolescence, typically as a period of sexual questioning which is relatively well adjusted, and not influenced by stigma.[16]

Prior research found that gay and lesbian adolescents generally reported first awareness of same-sex attractions by 10 or 11 years of age, self-identification as homosexual at age 13 to 15 years, and first same-sex experiences near the time of self-identification.[17] Self-identification usually precedes sexual debut with either male or female partners.[18] Girls appear to "come out" later, in the context of a relationship; whereas boys appear to come out at a younger age, in the context of sexual encounters.[18,19] With increasing visibility of sexual minority role models for adolescents, young people may be more likely to self-identify as a sexual minority before sexual debut.[20] As more population-based surveys are available, it is clear that self-identification likely varies by race, ethnicity, income level, or geographic location.[5]

Homophobia or Sexual Prejudice

While bias against sexual minorities is decreasing in many segments of society, it is still pervasive. The term "homophobia" was coined in 1967 to signify an irrationally negative attitude toward homosexuals.[21] Because a phobia is a fear, the term is somewhat of a misnomer. Prejudice, characterized by hostility, is a more accurate term, but homophobia or heterosexism is still commonly used.[4] Greenberg[22] found that two particularly prominent influences fostered homophobia in the US—religious fundamentalism and heterosexism, the belief that heterosexuality is inherently morally superior to homosexuality. In interviews with gay, lesbian, and bisexual adolescents, D'Augelli[23] found that 81% experienced verbal abuse, 38% had been threatened with physical harm, 15% reported a physical assault (6% with a weapon), and 16% reported a sexual assault. In the anonymous Minnesota school-based survey, gay, lesbian, and bisexual adolescents reported sexual abuse more than twice as often as the general adolescent population.[24]

Health Concerns

Lesbian, gay, and bisexual (LGB) AYAs, like their peers, may face adverse medical consequences related to lifestyle choices, low self-esteem, or unsafe sexual behaviors. The vast majority do not have negative health outcomes as a result of their sexuality; however, they do, as a group, experience a unique variety of stressors due to stigma, bias, rejection, and bullying. On average, perhaps as a consequence of these stressors, sexual minorities develop mental or physical health issues at rates higher than the general population of young people.

Early research on LGB AYAs classified risk factors associated with identifying as a sexual minority. Later researchers added protective factors, but still considered sexual orientation the independent variable. In the last decade, academics are increasingly adopting social stress theory to conceptualize the stigma and prejudice associated with a minority status.[2] Minority stress theory[25] expands on the social stress theory by distinguishing the excess stress that individuals from stigmatized categories are exposed to as a result of their minority social position. Meyer[25] conceptualized minority stress as three-fold: (1) distal (external objective stressful events both chronic and acute), (2) expectations of such events and the hypervigilance this requires, and (3) proximal (internalization of negative societal attitudes). Dual minority status (female and lesbian or Hispanic and gay) adds another layer of stressors that increase negative outcomes.

Thus, providers must be sensitive to a variety of these issues when providing care to homosexual or questioning (LGBQ) AYAs.

Cancer

The risk of breast cancer and its complications among lesbians may be heightened by nulliparity, delayed pregnancy, alcohol use, obesity, and nonuse of screening services. This is an area of ongoing research. Ovarian, lung, and colorectal cancers have been virtually unexplored in LGB communities.[26]

Eating Disorders

Gay males reported a significantly higher prevalence of poor body image, frequent dieting, binge eating, or purging than heterosexual males in a population-based survey of Minnesota schools.[27] YA college men surveyed in 2008 who identified as gay, unsure, or bisexual reported more clinical eating disorders and disordered eating behaviors compared to their heterosexual peers.[28] All sexual minority college students were significantly more likely to report dieting to lose weight compared to their heterosexual peers.[28]

Pregnancy and Parenthood

A survey of adolescents revealed that lesbian or bisexual women were equally likely to have had intercourse with men, but more likely than their heterosexual peers to report a pregnancy (12% versus 5%).[27] LGB YA college students were less likely to be involved in a pregnancy in the last 12 months (0.6% lesbians and gays, 4.5% bisexuals, 5.1% heterosexuals), but this was not necessarily planned. 43.9% of heterosexual YAs, 33.5% gays/lesbians, and 66.7% bisexuals said the pregnancy was unintentional.[29] Among sexually experienced adolescents, lesbian or bisexual women were also more likely to have engaged in prostitution during the previous year (9.7% versus 1.9%).[29] Similar data are not currently available in YAs.

Intimate Partner Violence

LGB YAs are often overlooked in discussions of violence against women and may therefore not have access to needed resources. Abuse of YAs within the LGB community has been invisible to health care workers, and has historically been unacknowledged by the LGB community as well. (see Chapter 73) College student YAs who identify as LGB report significantly higher lifetime rates of domestic violence (both men and women) compared to their heterosexual peers.[29] Rates reported by bisexual YA students are significantly higher (45.6%) compared to both lesbian/gay (35.7%) and heterosexual students (25.6%).[24]

Runaway and Homelessness

Parental rejection, abandonment, and violence contribute to the disproportionately high numbers of LGB teens in the homeless youth community. D'Augelli et al.[19] found that 10% of mothers and 26% of fathers of LGB adolescents in community centers rejected their children after they revealed their sexual orientation. With damaged self-esteem and few support networks, teens living on the streets may turn to prostitution, theft, or selling drugs as a means of survival. One in 10 LGB-identified YAs report having experienced at least one episode of homelessness, more than twice the rate of their heterosexual peers.[30]

School Problems

Adolescents facing a hostile school environment may exhibit declining school performance or school avoidance or dropout. Conversely, they may excel in schoolwork by concentrating on their studies in lieu of social and romantic relationships.[31] Russell et al.[32] found that middle and high school students who identified having attraction to same or both sexes were more likely to have been in a fight that resulted in a need for medical treatment and more likely to have witnessed violence than their peers. YA LGB college students report a significantly higher likelihood of being in a physical fight and sustaining an injury in the last 12 months than non-LGB-identified students.[33]

Substance Abuse

Statewide surveys have found that LGB adolescents are more likely to use tobacco than their heterosexual peers.[34] They are also significantly more likely to initiate tobacco use at a younger age (48% LGB youth versus 23% heterosexual Massachusetts youth used cigarettes before age 13 years). Higher use is also found when surveying LGB-identified college YAs (34.7% lesbian/gay YAs, 35.6% bisexuals, and 25.8% heterosexuals report current tobacco use).[33] Remafedi and Carol[35] reported that LGB youth and professionals who interact with them recommend culturally specific approaches to tobacco prevention and cessation programs.

Rosario et al.[36] reported that rates of illicit substance use were 6.4 times higher among lesbian or bisexual girls and 4.4 times higher among gay or bisexual boys than in national samples of heterosexual peers. Similarly, in a survey of college-attending YAs, LGB students are significantly more likely to have used alcohol, illicit substances, or another person's prescription drugs in the last year compared to heterosexual peers. Similarly, methamphetamine use has been increasing, and there is a strong correlation between methamphetamine use and human immunodeficiency virus (HIV).[37,38] Because adolescents are forced to cope with the stigma of their sexual orientation at a developmental point of limited skills and resources, they may turn to alcohol or other substances as a means to escape fear and to control emotional distress. Substance use may result in unsafe sexual practices, leading to sexually transmitted infections (STIs) or HIV infections (syndemic effect).

Suicide

Rates of attempted suicide among homosexual youths have been found to be consistently higher than expected in the general population of adolescents, ranging from 20% to 42%.[39] As compared to gender-matched heterosexual comparison groups, the risk of attempted and completed suicide appears to be especially accentuated in males. Suicide attempts often occur in proximity to "identity assumption" and may be associated with family conflict. Identified risk factors are young age at first awareness of homosexuality, experience of rejection based on sexual orientation, substance use, and perceived gender nonconformity. The severity of attempts is comparable with other adolescents. Suicide rates remain higher into young adulthood, with 1.4% of lesbian/gay and 5.0% of bisexual college students reporting a suicide attempt in the last year, compared to 0.8% of heterosexual college students.[33]

HIV and Other STIs

The most common and serious sexually related conditions arise from unprotected penile-anal intercourse. The epithelial surfaces of the fragile rectal mucosa are easily damaged during sex, facilitating the transmission of pathogens. Rectal intercourse has been shown to be the most efficient route of infection by hepatitis B virus, cytomegalovirus, and HIV.

Oral-anal or digital-anal contact can transmit enteric pathogens such as the hepatitis A virus. Unprotected oral sex can also lead to oropharyngeal disease and gonococcal and nongonococcal urethritis for the insertive partner. Certain STIs, particularly ulcerative diseases such as syphilis and herpes simplex virus infection, can facilitate the spread of HIV.

Concordance between female sexual partners suggests that bacterial vaginosis is sexually transmitted among lesbians.[40] Human papillomavirus (HPV) and trichomonas infections may also be transmitted between women. Though possible, female-to-female sexual transmission of HIV is inefficient, and women who only engage in same-sex behavior are less likely than other AYAs to acquire STIs in general.

IX

Men who have sex with other men (MSM) continue to be at great risk for HIV infection. In a study of HIV risk among 15- to 22-year-old MSM in seven US cities from 1994 to 1998, Valleroy et al.[41] interviewed and tested approximately 3,500 men who were recruited in public venues. Four out of ten (41%) reported unprotected anal intercourse (UAI) in the last 6 months (range 33% to 49% across cities), and the prevalence of HIV infection was 7.2% (range 2.2% to 12.1%). In a subsequent study of 23- to 29-year-old MSM in six US cities from 1998 to 2000, Valleroy et al.[42] found 46% of 2,401 men reported UAI in the last 6 months (range 41% to 53%), and HIV prevalence was 12.3% (range 4.7% to 18%). Altogether, 77% of the men found to be HIV seropositive from 1994 to 2000 did not know they were infected. In both of these studies, HIV prevalence was found to be higher in MSM of color than among White MSM.

Syphilis is also a concern. In the last decade, cases of primary and secondary syphilis have nearly doubled, with the largest increase occurring among MSM, particularly YAs.[43] The Centers for Disease Control and Prevention (CDC) recommends screening all sexually active MSM at least annually, with more frequent screening for MSM who have multiple or anonymous sex partners.[43]

Health Assessment

History

When evaluating an LGB adolescent or YA for medical problems, the practitioner must create an environment of trust. Begin by assuring the adolescent or YA patient that all information will be kept in confidence (unless the adolescent or YA poses a danger to self or others). Explain that you will ask personal questions and that an honest response will help you give the best possible care. Ask questions in a nonjudgmental manner that conveys an attitude of empathy, curiosity, and respect. This will maximize the likelihood of an honest response.

Ask about factors in an adolescent or young adult's environment that they may encounter, which raise their level of minority stress, whether it is bullying in a school setting, intimate partner violence, or hostility in the workplace. Explore also an adolescent or young adult's protective factors, which may help moderate distress – connection to caring adults, friends, and safety in the school or workplace. Psychological distress in LGB individuals tends to decrease during normal development over the period of adolescence and into young adulthood as AYAs develop improved coping skills.[44]

Inquiring about specific sexual practices will help determine the adolescent's or YA's risk for STIs and will direct laboratory studies. It also provides an opportunity to offer education regarding prevention of STIs and risk reduction. For those AYAs who are involved sexually, specific questions should include type of intercourse (penile-vaginal, orogenital, penile-anal, receptive or insertive, oral-anal, or vaginal-vaginal), number of lifetime and recent sexual partners, use of barrier methods, prior history of STIs, symptoms suggestive of STIs, and HIV status of the adolescents or YAs or their partner(s).

STI Screening

Not all sexual minority AYAs require a full STI evaluation. If the history indicates that the teen is either not sexually active or scrupulously avoids risk, a simple physical examination and routine recommended screening may suffice. The reliability of the young person's history should be considered. If a question of veracity exists, it may be wise to offer more frequent follow-up appointments to establish a rapport and create an honest dialogue. Practitioners might routinely offer STI and HIV testing to high-risk populations such as incarcerated individuals, persons involved in the sex industry, or institutionalized or homeless young people. Appropriate screening of the sexually active GLB adolescent or YA with risk factors identified during the sexual history might include a physical examination and laboratory testing for HIV, gonorrhea, chlamydia, syphilis, trichomonas, HPV infection, and other illnesses as indicated.

Specific STIs or Conditions

LGB AYAs are at risk of contracting the same STIs as their heterosexual counterparts. A few specific conditions related to sexual practices that are more common among gay AYAs, such as rectal HPV infection from penile-anal intercourse or pharyngeal gonorrhea from oral-genital intercourse, are elaborated later in this chapter. For more detailed information, refer to Chapters 56 to 62.

Enteric Illnesses: AYAs who engage in unprotected oral or anal sex are at higher risk of contracting various enteric pathogens. Male or female AYAs who engage in anal intercourse may experience local pain, bleeding, or skin lesions due to trauma, allergy to latex or lubricants, or STIs. Persistent gastrointestinal (GI) symptoms in AYAs who engage in anal intercourse should prompt a comprehensive history and physical examination. Pathogens include, but are not limited to, *Entamoeba histolytica, Giardia lamblia, Shigella, Neisseria gonorrhoeae, Treponema pallidum* (syphilis), *Chlamydia trachomatis*, HPV (warts), and herpes simplex virus.

Diagnostic evaluation may include stool cultures for invasive bacteria and microscopic evaluation for ova and parasites. Tests for gonorrhea, chlamydia, and herpes should be obtained when proctitis is suggested by rectal discharge, tenesmus, or pain. Also consider anoscopy, anal Papanicolaou smear, and screening for syphilis and HIV.

Chlamydia: Treatment for chlamydia is outlined in Chapter 57. However, clinicians should be aware of lymphogranuloma venereum (LGV), a systemic disease caused by *C. trachomatis* (serovars L1, L2, or L3) that occurs only rarely in the US. As of September 2004, the Netherlands saw a 19-fold increase in confirmed cases in MSM. Most cases were also coinfected with HIV. LGV should be considered in young MSM who have proctitis, proctocolitis, or painful inguinal lymphadenopathy as a presenting complaint.[45]

Gonorrhea: Gonococcal infections may be asymptomatic or associated with pharyngitis, urethritis, and proctitis. Treatment for gonorrhea is outlined in Chapter 57. Clinicians should be aware of increasing antibiotic resistance in *N. gonorrhoeae*, especially in MSM. As of 2012, the CDC no longer recommends fluoroquinolones or oral cephalosporins in treating any gonococcal infections.[46]

Syphilis: Since the mid-1990s, there has been growing concern about a resurgence of risky sexual behavior in MSM, possibly leading to an increase in HIV transmission. Reviews of sexual behavior data suggest that rates of UAI have been increasing among MSM. There have been outbreaks of syphilis[47] and gonorrhea among MSM in US cities and increases in newly diagnosed HIV infections in MSM from 1999 to 2002.[48]

Detecting the primary lesion of syphilis at the anus, where it may not be seen or felt, can be difficult. Although generally painless, rectal syphilis can cause discomfort or may appear as an atypical lesion with shaggy borders, resembling carcinoma. Regular syphilis screening is recommended for sexually active MSM. There is evidence that coinfection with HIV may alter the course of syphilis. Syphilis in HIV-seropositive individuals may not respond to traditional therapy or may have an accelerated course. Evaluation and treatment for syphilis is outlined in Chapter 59.

Hepatitis: Historically, there has been a higher prevalence of hepatitis B in the gay male community than in the general population. The Advisory Committee on Immunization Practices (ACIP) recommends universal hepatitis B vaccination for all ages. The fecal-oral route can transmit hepatitis A during orogenital and oral-anal sex. Because of this and the potential morbidity among infected adults, the hepatitis A vaccine series is recommended for all MSM.

Cytomegalovirus Infection: As many as 80% of homosexual males who engage in sex with multiple partners will acquire cytomegalovirus within a year.[49] This infection is largely asymptomatic but may lead to a severe mononucleosis-like illness, particularly in immunosuppressed HIV-seropositive AYAs.

HPV Infection: Condyloma acuminatum (genital warts) can be found on the penis, vagina, or rectal area. Management of internal warts is complicated and should be carried out in consultation with an expert. Treatment for condyloma is outlined in Chapter 61. HPV is the cause of cervical dysplasia, which can be a risk factor for cervical cancer. It can also cause dysplasia in the anal or rectal mucosa, increasing the risk for anal or rectal carcinoma. All sexually active YA females, whether they identify as heterosexual, bisexual, or lesbian, should be screened routinely with a Papanicolaou smear (guidelines can be found in Chapter 61). Anal Papanicolaou smears can also be used to screen for anal condyloma. The benefit of screening for anal carcinoma is an area of ongoing research. A quadrivalent vaccine for the prevention of HPV (types 6,11,16,18) is now recommended for females and males between the ages of 11 and 26.[50] A nine valent vaccine is also available and can be used in females 9 to 26 and for males at age 11 to 21. Males 22 to 26 may be vaccinated with the nine valent vaccine. Vaccination of females is recommended with 2vHPV, 4vHPV or 9vHPV. Vaccination of males is recommended with 4vHPV or 9vHPV (see Chapters 2 and 61) http://www.cdc.gov/mmwr/preview/mmwrhtml/mm6411a3.htm.

Herpes Simplex: Herpes simplex infections of the penis, vagina, mouth, or rectum can occur. Findings associated with herpes simplex proctitis include fever, difficulty with urination or defecation, sacral paresthesias, inguinal adenopathy, severe anorectal pain, tenesmus, constipation, perianal ulcerations, and the presence of diffuse ulcerations or vesicular or pustular lesions in the distal 5 cm of the rectum. Treatment of herpes simplex is outlined in Chapter 60.

HIV Infection: Acquired immunodeficiency syndrome (AIDS) and HIV are discussed in Chapter 31. Because of limited social networks, meeting sexual partners through the Internet or online social networks has become an increasingly popular and potentially risky behavior, especially for MSM. Benotsch et al.[51] found that one-third of MSM reported having met a sexual partner online. LGB and transgender AYAs may be at particular risk for HIV exposure because of their relative inexperience and weaker position of power in negotiating drug use and condoms. Drug use (e.g., methamphetamines, marijuana, ecstasy, and others) has been shown to increase the likelihood of UAI in MSM. Recommend a barrier method of protection for all sexually active AYAs. Discuss social media and substance use with the patient and recommend the following harm-reduction practices:

- Abstain from sex or risky sexual practices such as anal intercourse.
- Reduce number of sexual partners. Screen for social media use as a means of meeting new partners.
- Use condoms or barriers consistently during insertive and receptive oral, anal, and vaginal sex.
- Use latex—not natural lambskin—condoms, because the latter have been shown to be potentially porous. Polyurethane condoms are an acceptable, albeit more expensive, alternative for AYAs with a sensitivity to latex.
- Lubricants should be water or silicone-based products, rather than oil-based ones that can weaken latex and contribute to pruritus ani.
- Avoid substance use during sex. Brainstorm harm-reduction techniques to increase the likelihood of condom use during sex.
- Avoid sharing needles. If needles must be used, they should be clean, fresh from a sealed pack, or flushed with household bleach and then water.

Counseling Issues

The American Academy of Pediatrics (AAP) recognizes the physician's responsibility to provide health care and anticipatory guidance for all AYAs. The removal of homosexuality from the American Psychiatric Association's (APA's) *Diagnostic and Statistical Manual of Mental Disorders*[52] in 1973 signaled a change in our understanding and counseling of homosexual AYAs and their families.

Given the opportunity to grow up in a supportive environment, most gay and lesbian AYAs are no more likely to experience serious mental health problems than the general adolescent population.[53] Minority stress, whether experienced as direct violence, internalized prejudice or external events, engenders guilt, shame, and psychological problems. Practitioners must be prepared to counsel worried families in their attempt to understand their AYAs. If a health care provider is unable to accept homosexuality as a nonpathologic variant of the breadth of normal human sexuality, he or she should be prepared to refer the individual to an appropriate resource.

Counseling the Teen or YA

1. Create an open environment in which the young person feels comfortable discussing issues of sexuality.
2. Do not minimize an adolescent's concerns regarding sexual orientation. Stating, "it's just a phase" may actually intensify the young person's confusion.
3. Discussing homosexuality with an undecided AYA will not make them homosexual.
4. Assure the young person that homosexuality is a normal variation of sexual orientation and that sexual orientation is biologically driven.
5. Do not expect teens to define their sexual orientation prematurely. Sexual orientation unfolds during adolescence. Assuring them that questions about their sexual orientation will resolve over time may take some of the urgency out of the issue, "Am I, or am I not?" Remember, health care providers are not responsible for labeling, nor even identifying youth who are nonheterosexual.[54]
6. The position of the APA, the AAP, the American Medical Association, and the Pan American Health Organization is that conversion therapy (i.e., attempts to repair or "cure" them of homosexuality) is not useful and may be damaging. In a review of outcomes, Haldeman[55] found that attempts to replace homosexual fantasies with heterosexual ones were unsuccessful among men who had not experienced sexual attraction to women. Such attempts may contribute to guilt, low self-esteem, and psychological problems.
7. Regardless of whether AYAs have resolved uncertainty about their sexual orientation, helping to prevent STIs, unplanned pregnancies, and the spread of HIV/AIDS infection is of paramount importance. This is a prime reason to inquire about AYAs' sexual practices.
8. Not all sexual minority youth experience difficulties with their orientation. As with other healthy AYAs, well-adjusted sexual minority individuals need sensitive and informed health care services. Some individuals will appreciate the opportunity to discuss their unique experiences or concerns as an LGB individual.

Counseling Concerned Parents

The following are some suggestions for helping families:

1. Help parents explore and address their feelings of anger, fear, shame, guilt, or grief. Their child's sexual orientation is not a result of their parenting style.
2. Offer correct information about homosexuality.
3. Explain that not every emotional problem manifested by a young person is a result of his or her sexual orientation.
4. Challenge society's dichotomous belief that homosexuality is bad and that heterosexuality is good.
5. Explore religious beliefs and provide appropriate referrals. Affirming groups exist in most faiths and religious denominations.

XI

6. Discuss HIV/AIDS prevention with parents. Some parents automatically associate homosexuality with illness.

7. Supplement counseling with referrals to support groups. The addresses of a number of organizations can be found in the Resources section of this chapter.

8. Finally, help parents understand that AYAs who just "came out" are the same persons who sat in front of them before the disclosure. Their child's main need has been, is, and will always be love and acceptance.

ACKNOWLEDGMENT

The author would like to thank Gary Remafedi for his role in shaping and editing the previous editions of this chapter, and Dillon J. Etter for assistance in editing and updating references in the current chapter.

REFERENCES

1. Sell RL, Becker JB. Sexual orientation data collection and progress toward healthy people 2010. *Am J Public Health* 2001;91:876–882.
2. Brewster KL, Tillman KH. Sexual orientation and substance use among adolescents and young adults. *Am J Public Health* 2012;102:1168–1176.
3. Spitzer RL. The diagnostic status of homosexuality in DSM-III: a reformulation of the issues. *Am J Psychiatry* 1981;138:210.
4. Adelson SL; American Academy of Child and Adolescent Psychiatry (AACAP) Committee on Quality Issues (CQI). Practice parameter on gay, lesbian, or bisexual sexual orientation, gender nonconformity, and gender discordance in children and adolescents. *J Am Acad Child Adolesc Psychiatry* 2012;51:957–974.
5. Institute of Medicine (US) Committee on Lesbian, Gay, Bisexual, and Transgender Health Issues and Research Gaps and Opportunities. *The health of lesbian, gay, bisexual, and transgender people. Building a Foundation for Better Understanding*. Washington, DC: National Academy Press, 2011.
6. Remafedi G, Resnick M, Blum R, et al. Demography of sexual orientation in adolescents. *Pediatrics* 1992;89:714.
7. Garofalo R, Wolf RC, Kessel S, et al. The association between health risk behaviors and sexual orientation among a school-based sample of adolescents. *Pediatrics* 1998;101:895–902.
8. Laumann EO, Gagnon JH. *The social organization of sexuality: sexual practices in the United States*. Chicago, IL: University of Chicago Press, 1994.
9. Herbenick D, Reece M, Schick V, et al. Sexual behavior in the United States: results from a national probability sample of men and women ages 14–94. *J Sex Med* 2010;7 (suppl):255–265.
10. American College Health Association, (ACHA-NCHA-II). *Reference Group Data Report—Spring, 2014* Hanover, MD: American College Health Association, 2014. Available at http://www.acha-ncha.org/docs/ACHA-NCHA-II_ReferenceGroup_DataReport_Spring2014.pdf. Accessed January 11, 2015.
11. James WH. Biological and psychosocial determinants of male and female human sexual orientation. *J Biosoc Sci* 2005;37:555–567.
12. Friedman RC, Downey JI. Psychoanalysis and the model of homosexuality as psychopathology: a historical overview. *Am J Psychoanal* 1998;58:249–270.
13. Gartrell NK, Bos HM, Goldberg NG. Adolescents of the U.S. national longitudinal lesbian family study: sexual orientation, sexual behavior, and sexual risk exposure. *Arch Sex Behav* 2011;40:1199–1209.
14. Troiden RR. Becoming homosexual: a model of gay identity acquisition. *Psychiatry* 1979;42:288–299.
15. Troiden RR. Homosexual identity development. *J Adolesc Health Care* 1988;9:105–113.
16. Carver PR, Egan SK, Perry DG. Children who question their heterosexuality. *Dev Psychol* 2004;40:43–53.
17. Smith SD, Dermer SB, Astramovich RL. Working with nonheterosexual youth to understand sexual identity development, at-risk behaviors, and implications for health care professionals. *Psychol Rep* 2005;96:651–654.
18. Remafedi G. Predictors of unprotected intercourse among gay and bisexual youth: knowledge, beliefs, and behavior. *Pediatrics* 1994;94:163–168.
19. D'Augelli AR, Hershberger SL, Pilkington NW. Lesbian, gay, and bisexual youth and their families: disclosure of sexual orientation and its consequences. *Am J Orthopsychiatry* 1998;68(3):361–71.
20. Floyd FJ, Bakeman R. Coming-out across the life course: implications of age and historical context. *Arch Sex Behav* 2006;35:287–296.
21. Weinberg GH. *Society and the healthy homosexual*. New York, NY: St. Martin's Press, 1992.
22. Greenberg DE. *The construction of homosexuality*. Chicago, IL: University of Chicago Press, 1988.
23. D'Augelli AR. *Sexual orientation milestones and adjustment among lesbian, gay, and bisexual youths from 14 to 21 years of age*. Paper presented at the Seventh Biennial Conference of the European Association for Research on Adolescence. Jena, Germany, June 3, 2000.
24. Saewyc EM, Bearinger LH, Heinz PA, et al. Gender differences in health and risk behaviors among bisexual and homosexual adolescents. *J Adolesc Health* 1998;23:181–188.
25. Meyer IH. Prejudice, social stress, and mental health in lesbian, gay, and bisexual populations: conceptual issues and research evidence. *Psychol Bull* 2003;129:674–697.
26. Brown JP, Tracy JK. Lesbians and cancer: an overlooked health disparity. *Cancer Causes Control* 2008;19:1009–1020.
27. French SA, Story M, Remafedi G, et al. Sexual orientation and prevalence of body dissatisfaction and eating disordered behaviors: a population-based study of adolescents. *Int J Eat Disord* 1996;19:119–126.
28. Matthews-Ewald MR, Zullig KJ, Ward RM. Sexual orientation and disordered eating behaviors among self-identified male and female college students. *Eat Behav* 2014;15(3):441–444.
29. Saewyc E, Bearinger L, Blum R, et al. Sexual intercourse, abuse, and pregnancy among adolescent women: does sexual orientation make a difference? *Fam Plann Perspect* 1999;31:127.
30. McLaughlin KA, Hatzenbuehler ML, Xuan Z, et al. Disproportionate exposure to early-life adversity and sexual orientation disparities in psychiatric morbidity. *Child Abuse Negl* 2012;36(9):645–655.
31. Treadway L, Yoakam J. Creating a safer school environment for lesbian and gay students. *J Sch Health* 1992;62:352–357.
32. Russell ST, Franz BT, Driscoll AK. Same-sex romantic attraction and experiences of violence in adolescence. *Am J Public Health* 2001;91:903–906.
33. *College student health survey report 2007–2011*. 2013:1-1-59. Available at http://www.bhs.umn.edu/surveys/survey-results/2007-2011_LGB_CSHSReport.pdf. Accessed January 12, 2015.
34. Garofalo R, Wolf RC, Wissow LS, et al. Sexual orientation and risk of suicide attempts among a representative sample of youth. *Arch Pediatr Adolesc Med* 1999;153:487–493.
35. Remafedi G, Carol H. Preventing tobacco use among lesbian, gay, bisexual, and transgender youths. *Nicotine Tob Res* 2005;7:249–256.
36. Rosario M, Hunter J, Gwadz M. Exploration of substance use among lesbian, gay, and bisexual youth: prevalence and correlates. *J Adolesc Res* 1997;12:454–476.
37. Purcell DW, Moss S, Remien RH, et al. Illicit substance use, sexual risk, and HIV-positive gay and bisexual men: differences by serostatus of casual partners. *AIDS* 2005;19:S37–S47.
38. Colfax G, Coates TJ, Husnik MJ, et al. Longitudinal patterns of methamphetamine, popper (amyl nitrate), and cocaine use and high-risk sexual behavior among a cohort of San Francisco men who have sex with men. *J Urban Health* 2005;82 (1, suppl 1):i62–i70.
39. Remafedi G. Sexual orientation and youth suicide. *JAMA* 1999;282:1291–1292.
40. Berger BJ, Kolton S, Zenilman J, et al. Bacterial vaginosis in lesbians: a sexually transmitted disease. *Clin Infect Dis* 1995;21:1402–1405.
41. Valleroy L, MacKellar D, Karon J, et al. HIV prevalence and associated risks in young men who have sex with men. *JAMA* 2000;284:198–204.
42. Valleroy L, Secura G, MacKellar D, et al. *High HIV and risk behavior prevalence among 23- to 29- year-old men who have sex with men in 6 US cities*. 8th Conference on Retroviruses and Opportunistic Infections. Chicago, IL, 2001. Abstract 211.
43. Patton ME, Su JR, Nelson R, et al. Primary and secondary syphilis—United States, 2005–2013. *MMWR* 2014;63:402–406.
44. Birkett M, Newcomb ME, Mustanski B. Does it get better? A longitudinal analysis of psychological distress and victimization in lesbian, gay, bisexual, transgender, and questioning youth. *J Adolesc Health* 2015;56:280–285.
45. Centers for Disease Control and Prevention. Lymphogranuloma venereum among men who have sex with men—Netherlands, 2003–2004. *MMWR* 2004;53:985–988.
46. Centers for Disease Control and Prevention. Update to CDC's sexually transmitted diseases treatment guidelines, 2010: oral cephalosporins no longer a recommended treatment for gonococcal infections. *MMWR* 2012;61:590–594.
47. Centers for Disease Control and Prevention. Trends in reportable sexually transmitted diseases in the United States, 2003: national data on chlamydia, gonorrhea, and syphilis, 2005. Available at from http://www.cdc.gov/std/stats/trends2003.htm. Accessed August 7, 2014.
48. Guenther-Grey CA, Varnell S, Weiser JI, et al. Trends in sexual risk taking among urban young men who have sex with men (1999–2002). *J Natl Med Assoc* 2005;97:38S–43S.
49. Mintz L, Drew L, Miner RC, et al. Cytomegalovirus infections in homosexual men: an epidemiological study. *Ann Intern Med* 1983;99:326–329.
50. Markowitz LE, Dunne EF, Saraiya M, et al. Human Papillomavirus Vaccination: Recommendations of the Advisory Committee on Immunization Practices (ACIP). *MMWR* 2014;63(5):1–29.
51. Benotsch EG, Kalichman S, Cage M. Men who have met sex partners via the Internet: prevalence, predictors, and implications for HIV prevention. *Arch Sex Behav* 2002;31:177–183.
52. American Psychiatric Association. *Diagnostic and statistical manual of mental disorders*. 4th ed. Washington, DC: American Psychiatric Association, 1994.
53. Gonsiorek JC. Mental health issues of gay and lesbian adolescents. *J Adolesc Health Care* 1988;9:114–122.
54. Frankowski BL; American Academy of Pediatrics; The Committee on Adolescence. Sexual orientation and adolescents. *Pediatrics* 2004;113:1827–1832.
55. Haldeman DC. Sexual orientation conversion therapy for gay men and lesbians: a scientific examination. In: Gonsiorek JC, Weinrich JD, eds. *Homosexuality: research implications for public policy*. Newbury Park, CA: Sage Publications Inc, 1991:149.

📶 ADDITIONAL RESOURCES AND WEBSITES ONLINE

CHAPTER 39

Transgender Youth and Young Adults

Johanna Olson

GENERAL CONSIDERATIONS

"Transgender" is a broad term that is used to describe individuals who experience incongruence between their assigned gender at birth and their internal sense of "maleness" or "femaleness." For many transgender people, this incongruence causes gender dysphoria, the persistent distress about the misalignment of assigned gender and experienced gender. Many transgender people pursue a phenotypic gender transition utilizing hormones and/or surgery to more closely align their bodies with their internal gender identities. The last decade has seen a large increase in the number of transgender youth seeking medical intervention in the US, Canada, and Europe in early and middle adolescence.[1,2] Unfortunately, little formal education about the care of these extraordinary youth is incorporated into either medical school or residency curricula.

Historically, the experience of gender incongruence has been assigned clinical diagnostic codes that fall under the umbrella of psychopathological conditions. The diagnosis "Gender Identity Disorder" was removed from the *Diagnostic and Statistical Manual of Mental Illness* (DSM) and replaced by "Gender Dysphoria" in 2013.[3] The transgender experience should not be considered psychopathological, but the distress that results from the incongruence may often lead to functional problems that should be addressed by a team that includes both medical and mental health professionals.

Terminology

The elements that make up an individual's psychosexual identity include, but are not limited to, assigned sex at birth, gender identity, gender expression, and sexual attraction. Assigned sex at birth is generally determined by genital anatomy at the time of birth, and is recorded on the birth certificate accordingly. In many states across the US, this can be changed if someone identifies later as a different gender. There are still some states that do not allow this change. Gender identity is an individual's internal sense and experience of "maleness" or "femaleness." For transgender adolescents and young adults (AYAs), this is incongruent with their assigned sex at birth. Gender expression includes how an individual presents his or her gender with clothing, hair, name, pronouns, and mannerisms, as well as gender performance; how an individual acts with respect to the cultural constructs and expectations around gender. Sexual attraction refers to who an individual finds romantically and sexually attractive. Sexual attraction is often mistakenly conflated with gender identity. Transgender AYAs have a range of sexual attraction identity labels, and should not be assumed to have any particular sexual orientation labels based on their assigned sex at birth. For example, an individual assigned a male gender at birth, who has a transfeminine identity, might be sexually and romantically attracted to men, women, both, neither, or any-gendered people. From a health care perspective, risk for sexually transmitted infections (STIs) and necessary screening should rely on assessment of specific sexual behavior and presence of specific body parts. Gender identity, gender expression, and sexual attraction are not binary. There are an infinite number of places along the spectrum of male → female or masculine → feminine that all people might identify. Additionally, they may fluctuate over time, particularly gender expression. Transgender AYAs may make socioculturally strategic decisions about gender expression in different environments. For younger adolescents, realization that there is a spectrum of identities that are not limited to the male/female binary is important information for them to have in their gender exploration process.

While professionals, academics, families, and allies adopt language to define the gender identities of others, it is critical to recognize that individuals should, and do, self-identify their own gender. Mental and medical health providers should be cognizant that the lexicon is dynamic, particularly among transgender AYAs, and best approached by asking each individual how he or she identifies himself or herself before assigning a label. Some AYAs may prefer not to identify themselves as transgender in any way, and identify simply as "boy/man" or "girl/woman."

Increasingly common is the emergence of AYAs who identify as "nonbinary." These young people reject the traditional gender binary categories of male and female, and instead consider themselves both, neither, or something else entirely. The approach to non-binary–identified AYAs requires attention to each individual's needs. Gender nonconforming or transgender AYAs should be asked about their preferred name and pronoun at each office visit. Inquiring about each young person's identity, name, and pronoun preference can help to foster trust and develop rapport between provider and patient.

Prevalence

There continues to be a lack of information accurately or consistently describing the prevalence of transgender individuals, and studies from around the world report a broad range from 1:200

to 1:100,000.[4-6] While specific prevalence rates are unknown, it is the case that increasing numbers of transgender youth are seeking care in clinics around the world.[1,2] In the most recent data from the American College Health Association's National College Health Assessment, 0.2% of respondents reported their gender as transgender.[7]

Etiology

Many theories have attempted to explain the cause of gender incongruence, ranging from hormone imbalance in utero to parental psychopathology or history of trauma.[8,9] To date, no clear etiology has been identified that adequately provides a causal explanation for the transgender experience. The phenomenon of gender incongruence continues to be classified within the mental health domain, and transgender individuals are still in many cases required to complete a comprehensive psychiatric evaluation, as well as live for a certain amount of time in their authentic gender role in order to receive medical intervention for phenotypic transition. Additionally, attempts are still made to try and dissuade or change individual's experienced gender identity with "corrective" therapy. While this approach has been repudiated by most medical and mental health professional societies, there are still some institutions that practice this outdated and damaging intervention with transgender people.

Coming Out Process

Transgender AYAs experience initial awareness about their gender incongruence in many ways. Many recognize from very early childhood that their gender is different than the one they were assigned at birth. Some are able to articulate their experience to parents, family members, or others in early childhood, and some are not. Many AYAs describe a history of feeling "different" but not necessarily ascribing that difference to gender incongruence until later in adolescence. It is common for young people to acquire language around the transgender phenomenon from the popular media or the Internet. Limited data and clinical experience seem to indicate a bimodal distribution of transgender awareness in transgender boys/young men with one peak in early childhood and a second around or shortly after the experience of puberty. Among transgender girls/young women, there is more commonly awareness of gender incongruence during early childhood, although later discovery is also not uncommon. This may be due to the societal inability to tolerate "boys in girls' clothing," which might subsequently drive parents/caregivers to seek professional care earlier. For youth who discover their transgender identity in adolescence, disclosure often occurs first among close friends, followed by parents and extended family. Parent/caregiver response to the disclosure of transgender identity is critical to the well-being and future of these youth. Parents who are accepting, open, and supportive help mitigate the multitude of psychosocial challenges faced by transgender youth.[10]

Emotional and Behavioral Health
Mood Disorders and Anxiety

Transgender youth frequently have symptoms of mood disorders and anxiety that are intimately entangled with the experience of gender incongruence. Many AYAs presenting for gender transition are already engaged in mental health services, and are often prescribed psychotropic medications. However, a diagnosis of depression or other mood disorder should not preclude an adolescent or young adult from initiating puberty suppression or cross-sex hormone therapy. Anecdotal information suggests that individuals often are able to wean or discontinue psychotropic medications altogether after initiating gender transition. Close partnering with mental health professionals is strongly advised in cases where AYAs are experiencing significant mental health morbidities.

Homelessness

Transgender AYAs are disproportionately represented among the population of young people experiencing homelessness. While a broader understanding and greater tolerance of gender nonconformity is occurring in the US and other parts of the world, it is still common for gender and sexual minority youth to be rejected by their families of origin. Transgender youth in the foster system are much less likely to remain in foster families, and more often placed in group homes. Youth experiencing homelessness are at increased risk for violence, poverty, drug use, human immunodeficiency virus (HIV), survival sex, and exposure to environmental hazards.

Violence

Transgender youth commonly report being victims of violence, hate crimes, sexual assault (see Chapter 73), harassment, bullying, and physical assault in school, communities, places of employment, and, too often, in their own homes. Assessment for history of and exposure to potential violence is an important part of screening at each visit.

Suicide

Suicidal ideation and attempts are extraordinarily high among transgender people compared to the population at large.[11] A recent study reported that 77% of transgender people over the age of 16 had seriously considered suicide, with 43% reporting an attempted suicide. One-third of those who had attempted had done so before the age of 15.[12] Discussing suicidality with transgender youth is critical, and should be revisited frequently. Even youth who are undergoing hormone treatment should be frequently queried about suicidal thoughts, plans, and attempts because gender incongruence is a permanent state even if phenotypic gender transition is undertaken. Gender dysphoria and its subsequent sequelae are difficult to predict and fluctuate over time.

Health Concerns
Substance Use

Transgender AYAs use drugs and alcohol more than their cisgender (nontransgender) peers to cope with anxiety and distress related to gender dysphoria. Screening and referral for problematic drug use are important in these youth.

Eating Disorders

Clinical reports of eating disorders among transgender AYAs are common. Body dysphoria is pervasive and should be assessed at the initial visit with transgender patients seeking care. Again, the presence of an eating disorder should not preclude initiation of cross-sex hormones, but needs to be simultaneously addressed by an experienced mental health professional.

Obesity

Excessive weight gain in order to hide endogenous body shape is common among both transgender boys/young men and girls/young women. Both feminizing and masculinizing hormones can increase appetite; therefore, encouraging youth to have healthy eating habits and advising to engage in regular exercise should be incorporated into routine anticipatory guidance.

Pregnancy

Specific sexual behaviors and acts should not be assumed in transgender AYAs. Inquiry about specific sexual acts using thoughtful and appropriate language will give providers more accurate information about pregnancy risk. Additionally, all youth should be counseled that exogenous hormone use is not adequate birth control. Transgender young women can still impregnate other individuals, and transgender young men can become pregnant despite testosterone use. Transgender AYAs should be advised to use birth control if they are engaging in sexual behaviors with associated pregnancy risk.

Sexually Transmitted Infections

Transgender boys/young men who are taking testosterone are at increased risk for STIs due to thinning and drying of the vaginal walls. Youth should be reminded that if they are having receptive genital sex, adequate lubrication and care will help avoid tearing and undue exposure to infections. HIV infection rate is increased among transgender young women due to unprotected sex, survival sex, unmonitored hormone injections, and injection drug use. Transgender young men may also engage in sex work in order to survive; the concomitant use of needles for injecting hormones and drugs should not be overlooked by the provider as it represents a significant health risk.

Medical Intervention

The approach to care for transgender youth is dependent on the age and sexual development of youth at presentation, presence of a social support system, medical condition, and the individual desires of the youth.

Hormones

- Adolescents can be given gonadotropin-releasing hormone analogs (GnRHa) in early puberty (sexual maturity rating [SMR] 2 or 3) to suppress the development of undesired secondary sexual characteristics.[13]
- Older AYAs can be prescribed cross-sex hormones to induce secondary sexual characteristics that more closely match their internal gender identity.

Hormone scheduling doses and medical monitoring are outlined in the *Endocrine Society's Clinical Care Guidelines*. (https://www.endocrine.org/~/media/endosociety/Files/Publications/Clinical%20Practice%20Guidelines/Endocrine-Treatment-of-Transsexual-Persons.pdf)

Hormone Therapy Risk

- *GnRH analogs:* For youth who are starting GnRH analogs, the most concerning issue is slower accrual of bone mineral density (BMD). In the earliest studies of youth undergoing pubertal suppression for gender-related concerns, BMD did not diminish during a year of treatment, but was lower than age-matched peers, indicating that BMD accrued at a prepubertal rate during treatment. However, BMD recovered after cross-sex hormones were added.[14] Other clinical reports of emotional instability and weight gain have been reported in youth on GnRH analog treatment.
- *Cross-sex hormone use:* Very little information is available documenting the medical side effects of cross-sex hormone use in transgender adolescents. In older youth, little is known about the physiologic impact of cross-sex hormones. Potential side effects may be extrapolated with caution from dissimilar populations.
- *Estrogen and androgen blocker therapy:* In transgender females taking estradiol and androgen antagonists, side effects may include venous thromboembolic events liver damage, prolactinoma, gallstones, and hyperkalemia (from spironolactone use). Less dangerous side effects include nausea, mood swings, decreased libido, shrinking of the testicles (often desirable), and decreased muscle mass. Desired changes include breast development, softening of the skin, increased emotions, slowed growth of facial and body hair, and diminished erections. All youth should be counseled about likely loss of fertility, and if male pubertal development has progressed to the later SMRs, sperm banking should be discussed as an option for those young people interested in future biologic offspring.

- *Testosterone therapy:* In transgender males, the following side effects should be considered and discussed with patients undergoing testosterone therapy: liver damage, insulin resistance, changes in lipid profile, and polycythemia. Less dangerous side effects include acne, increased libido, and premature hair thinning/balding. Desired side effects include deepening of the voice, development of facial hair, male pattern body hair, clitoral enlargement, increased muscle mass and strength.

While there are transgender men who have discontinued testosterone use, resumed ovulation, and carried and birthed their own children, it is unclear when in the course of testosterone treatment fertility is no longer an option. Harvesting eggs is expensive and difficult, and is not commonly done, but should be discussed with patients interested in preserving reproductive tissue for future use. In youth who begin treatment in SMR 2 or 3, viable reproductive tissue will not have developed and will likely not be suitable for harvesting.

Surgery

- Males: Surgical interventions for transgender males may include male chest reconstruction for those who have undergone female breast development prior to intervention and genital surgery for gender confirmation. Male chest reconstruction is increasingly being performed on minors, but genital surgery is generally delayed until youth reach the age of majority.
- Females: For transgender females, breast augmentation may be required, as well as genital reconstruction for gender confirmation. Genital surgery in transgender young women is usually delayed until youth reach the age of majority.

Preintervention Assessment

The current standard of care recommends assessment of AYAs by mental health therapists skilled in gender-related care prior to initiation of medical intervention. There are varying opinions about the "gatekeeper" model of care for transgender people, but most agree it is prudent to involve competent mental health providers prior to, as well as during, the time youth are undergoing gender transition. Mental health therapists provide AYAs with a necessary "toolbox" of resiliency skills necessary to navigate gender transition in adolescence or early adulthood. Historically, the role of mental health professionals has been emphasized in the period of time leading up to hormone initiation, but recent data and clinical experience indicate that it is the period immediately following initiation of hormones that may be the most challenging and that patients may benefit more from mental health involvement in this time period.

Other Issues for Transgender AYAs

Sex-Segregated Facilities

Laws governing the use of appropriate sex-segregated facilities for transgender people vary across the US. Many college campuses are moving toward supporting transgender people utilizing the sex-segregated facilities that correspond to an individual's gender identity, but this is certainly not universally applied. Additionally, there have been a handful of states that have legislated appropriate access to sex-segregated locker rooms and restrooms in the K-12 school setting. These laws are still rare, and are not always enforced in every school.

Electronic Records

Most electronic record systems document a gender marker that corresponds to the gender on an individual's birth certificate. This applies to schools as well as health care facilities. There is no consensus, nor systematized approach as to how to address the issue of incongruence between an electronic gender marker and an individual's identity; it becomes the purview of each institution about how to manage this discrepancy. Additionally, prior to someone getting their name changed, a birth name of record is often what appears in an electronic documentation system. Transgender AYAs are often challenged with advocating for specific chart notations to be made that alert providers and administrators to use appropriate pronouns and names. This issue, if poorly managed, can lead to an individual's transgender status being inadvertently disclosed. In many states, birth certificates can be amended and reissued to accurately reflect name and gender with a physician's declaration document. Unfortunately, gender markers are limited to the binary choice of male or female, and leave no options for those with nonbinary identities.

Approach to the Transgender AYA and Family

Transgender AYAs should be treated with the same dignity and respect as any other youth or young adult. Preference for names, pronouns, and use of specific names for body parts that feels most comfortable should be solicited and subsequently honored. Medical and mental health professionals should model nonjudgmental and compassionate communication with youth in front of parents, caregivers, and other family members. The needs of youth with gender dysphoria should be taken seriously, as the sequelae of untreated gender dysphoria can be life-threatening. Because there is such a strong correlation between parental support and well-being of transgender youth, parents and caregivers who are struggling to understand and accept their transgender children should be referred to local support groups, family gender conferences, and appropriate literature.

⬤ ACKNOWLEDGMENTS

The author wishes to acknowledge Eric Meininger and Gary Remafedi for their contributions to previous versions of this chapter.

REFERENCES

1. de Vries ALC, Cohen-Kettenis PT. Clinical management of gender dysphoria in children and adolescents: the Dutch approach. *J Homosex* 2012;59:301–320.
2. Spack NP, Edwards-Leeper L, Feldman HA, et al. Children and adolescents with gender identity disorder referred to a pediatric medical center. *Pediatrics* 2012;129:418–425.
3. American Psychiatric Association. *Diagnostic and Statistical Manual Of mental disorders.* 5th ed. Arlington, VA: American Psychiatric Publishing, 2013.
4. De Cuypere G, Van Hemelrijck M, Michel A, et al. Prevalence and demography of transsexualism in Belgium. *Eur Psychiatry* 2007;22:137–41.
5. Veale J. Prevalence of transsexualism among New Zealand passport holders. *Aust N Z J Psychiatry* 2008;42:887–889.
6. Gates G. *How many people are LGBT?* Los Angeles, CA: UCLA School of Law, Williams Institute. Available at http://williamsinstitute.law.ucla.edu/wp-content/uploads/Gates-How-Many-People-LGBT-Apr-2011.pdf. Accessed February 25, 2014.
7. National College Health Assessment II, American College Health Association. *Reference Group Executive Summary, Spring 2012*:17. Available at http://www.acha-ncha.org/docs/ACHA-NCHA-II_ReferenceGroup_ExecutiveSummary_Spring2012.pdf. Accessed January 8, 2015.
8. Meyer-Bahlburg HF. From mental disorder to iatrogenic hypogonadism. *Arch Sex Behav* 2010;39:461–476.
9. Gooren L. The biology of human psychosexual differentiation. *Horm Behav* 2006;50:589–601.
10. Travers R, Bauer G, Pyne J, et al. *Impacts of strong parental support for trans youth: a report prepared for Children's Aid Society of Toronto and Delisle Youth Services, Trans PULSE Project.* Available at http://transpulseproject.ca/wp-content/uploads/2012/10/Impacts-of-Strong-Parental-Support-for-Trans-Youth-vFINAL.pdf. Accessed February 25, 2014.
11. Clements-Nolle K, Marx R, Katz M. Attempted suicide among transgender persons, *J Homosex* 2006;51:53–69.
12. Bauer GR, Pyne J, Francino MC, et al. Suicidality among trans people in Ontario: implications for social work and social justice. *Service Social* 2013;59:35–62.
13. Hembree WC, Cohen-Kettenis P, Delemarre-van de Waal HA, et al. Endocrine treatment of transsexual persons: an Endocrine Society clinical practice guideline. *J Clin Endocrine Metab* 2009;94:3132–3154.
14. Delemarre-van de Waal HA, Cohen-Kettenis PT. Clinical management of gender identity disorder in adolescents: a protocol on psychological and paediatric endocrinology aspects. *Eur J Endocrin* 2006;155 (suppl 1):S131–S137.

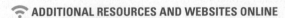 **ADDITIONAL RESOURCES AND WEBSITES ONLINE**

40

Adolescent and Young Adult Pregnancy and Parenting

Joanne E. Cox
Madeline Beauregard

Although adolescent and young adult (AYA) pregnancy rates have declined by more than 50% and 25% respectively since a peak year in 1991, many more young people experience unplanned pregnancy in the US than in other industrialized countries.[1,2] Over 80% of teen pregnancies and 70% of pregnancies to unmarried women aged 20 to 24 years are unplanned.[3] Unplanned pregnancies are prevalent especially in AYAs who are Black or Hispanic, low-income and in those who have not completed high school. In 2008, there were 620,000 unplanned pregnancies in teens 15 to 19 years old, whereas women aged 20 to 24 years experienced 1,080,000 unplanned pregnancies, resulting in considerable public cost.[3]

There are significant trends in comparing AYA pregnancy and birth rates (see Figs. 40.1–40.3).

- **Pregnancy rates**: Pregnancy rates increase with age up through age 29 (Figs. 40.1 and 40.2). The percentage of pregnancies that end in births also increases with age, while the percentage ending in abortions decreases and miscarriages remain fairly constant (Fig. 40.2).

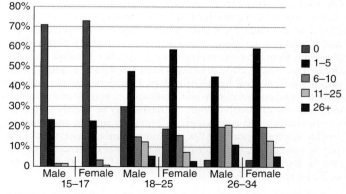

FIGURE 40.1 Lifetime number of opposite sex sexual partners by gender and age-group, in the United States, 2006 to 2010. (From Lepkowski JM, Mosher WD, Davis KE, et al. The 2006-2010 National Survey of Family Growth: sample design and analysis of a continuous survey. *Vital Health Stat* 2010;2:1-36. PMID: 20928970.)

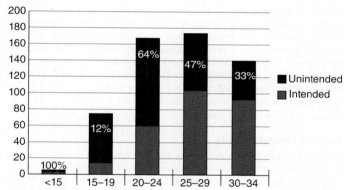

FIGURE 40.2 Pregnancy rates (per 1,000) by age of mother and intention, United States 2010. (From Finer LB, Zolna MR. Unintended pregnancy in the United States: Incidence and disparities, 2006. *Contraception* 2011;84(5): 478–485. doi:10.1016/j.contraception.2011.07.013.)

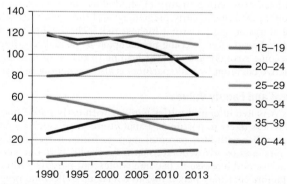

FIGURE 40.3 Trends in birth rates (per 1,000) by age-group of mother, in the United States, 1990 to 2013. (From Hamilton BE, Martin JA, Osterman MJK, et al. Births: preliminary data for 2013. *Natl Vital Stat Rep* 2014;63(2):1–20.)

- **Intention**: The percentage of total pregnancies that are unintended decreases with age (Fig. 40.1). Despite the rates of unintended pregnancies being highest in women aged 20 to 24, this comprises 64% of all pregnancies in comparison to 82% in the 15 to 19 age-group.
- **Birth rates trends**: In 2013, teen birth rates reached a nadir of 26.6 per 1,000 girls aged 15 to 19 years, compared to 81.2 per 1,000 women aged 20 to 24 years in 2013.[1] Trends show a decrease of birth rates in AYAs until age 29 years, with rates rising over time in those aged 30 years and over (Fig. 40.3).

Variables that affect AYA birth rates include ethnicity, socioeconomic status, and geographic location. Over the last 15 years, Hispanic teens have had the highest rate of teen births.[1] Teen birth rates also vary considerably by state. In 2012, New Mexico had the highest teenage birth rate at 47.5 per 1,000 females aged 15 to 19 years. This compares to New Hampshire, with the lowest teenage birth rate at 13.8 per 1,000 females aged 15 to 19 years. From another perspective, by 2012, the teen birth rate in California had decreased by 64% since 1991. Comparatively, the teen birth rate in West Virginia has seen the smallest decline since 1991, with a 24% change since 1991.[3]

- **College students:** Among college-age students who reported having vaginal intercourse, 1.4% of females had experienced unintended pregnancy in the last year and 1.5% of males reported impregnating their partner.[4]

FACTORS CONTRIBUTING TO AYA PREGNANCY

Poverty

Poverty is the strongest factor associated with unplanned AYA pregnancy. Recent evidence suggests that both long-term exposure to poverty and living in impoverished neighborhoods during adolescence independently increase the risk of adolescent and unplanned pregnancy.[5] For AYAs, living in poverty may be associated with lack of hope for the present and future that translates into overall risky behaviors and lack of attention for the consequences. A baby can represent success and hope for the future for AYAs faced with economic and educational obstacles.

Rates of Sexual Activity

While there has been a decline in lifetime report of sexual activity, 15- to 19-year-old prevalence rates are 60.6% for Blacks, 49.2% for Hispanics, and 43.7% for Whites.[6] Males are slightly more likely to be sexually experienced than females; and, sexual activity increases with grade, among ninth through twelfth graders.

Physical and Sexual Abuse

Abusive relationships are common features in the lives of AYA mothers. Adolescents with a history of child abuse or neglect are twice as likely to experience early pregnancy, and those with histories of sexual abuse or neglect are at highest risk.[7] Those who have been sexually abused often become preoccupied by sexualized thoughts and become sexually active early, leading to risk of pregnancy. Reproductive coercion by male partners is also a potential risk factor.

Cultural and Family Values

Many AYAs live in communities familiar with early parenthood; so they are less likely to postpone sexual intercourse. Adolescents living in families with little parental support, little restriction of risky behaviors, and poorly defined goals are more likely to become sexually active and likewise to become adolescent parents. Other cultural factors that may play a role in decisions to become pregnant include peer pressure, early dating, and lack of religious affiliation. Although more adolescents have delayed pregnancy, they often experience unplanned pregnancy as young adults.

Early initiation of sexual activity is not unusual if other family members have a prior history of becoming pregnant during adolescence. Adolescent parents may have mothers, sisters, or brothers who were teen parents. Pregnancy can result in both joy or excitement and increased stress, which potentially either increases or decreases a sibling's risk of pregnancy.[8]

Psychological

Mental health problems such as depression may influence a young woman's decision to become pregnant. Pregnant and parenting young people have high rates of depression, but they also often have poor social supports and conflicted relationships while living

in low-income, violence prone neighborhoods, all of which predispose them to mental health disorders.[9] Other risky behaviors are associated with concomitant sexual activity including alcohol and drug use.[6]

Early Puberty and Development

Since 1900, the average age at onset of menarche has significantly decreased. This earlier physical maturation has widened the gap between reproductive capacity and cognitive and emotional maturation and has increased the risk of unintended pregnancy in this age-group.

Many developmental characteristics of adolescents, particularly of younger teens, interfere with decision making regarding sexual activity and the successful use of contraceptives. These include a limited ability to plan for the future or to foresee the consequences of their actions and a sense of personal invulnerability.

Media

Exposure to highly sexualized media has long been considered a risk factor for AYA unplanned pregnancy. This was especially true in the US, where the sexualized medial culture seemed at odds with a national focus on abstinence education and restriction on contraceptive availability. However, the popular *16 and Pregnant* and *Teen Mom* shows may have reversed that association. Data have suggested that some of the pregnancy decline is the result of accurately reporting the reality of pregnancy and parenting at a young age.[10]

Access to and Adherence with Contraception

Obtaining and adhering to contraceptives remains critical to minimizing the number of unplanned AYA pregnancies. In 2011, about 11% of male high school students and 15% of female high school students did not use any method to prevent pregnancy during their most recent sexual intercourse. Among those who did use some method of contraception, the condom was most popular. About 67% of males and 54% of females used a condom during their most recent sexual intercourse. About 13% of males and 23% of females used a birth control pill during their most recent sexual intercourse.[6]

Although lack of negative attitudes toward pregnancy may be a factor in failure to use contraception, access to confidential counseling and prescriptions is also important. AYAs who feel that pregnancy will inhibit their career or educational goals are more likely to comply with contraception.[11] Yet, access remains problematic. In a recent study, half of adolescents reported not using contraception prior to an unplanned birth; and lack of access to contraception was associated with unplanned births.[11]

Many environmental, social, and psychological barriers interfere with decision making regarding sexual activity and contraception among AYAs. Significant obstacles to successful contraception include inaccurate information, accessibility, contraceptive acceptability, and partner issues (see Chapter 41). Some young women chose not to protect themselves from pregnancy because they desire to have a baby. AYAs may experience barriers to acquiring contraception from their health providers. Providers may not address sexuality and contraception use, and patients may be embarrassed to initiate the discussion. Some clinicians may be overtly judgmental of sexuality and contraception. Providers may be unwilling to provide contraception to AYAs without parent consent. Clinicians may be unnecessarily concerned about safety of contraceptives, especially long-acting reversible contraceptive (LARC) methods such as the intrauterine device (IUD) (see Chapter 44).[12]

REPEAT PREGNANCY

Repeat teen birth has decreased in number over the past 2 decades, but accounts for 18.3% of total births to teen mothers. Low-income, non-White adolescents experience a disproportionate number of repeat births.[13] Repeat pregnancy has adverse effects on parenting while increasing stress and reducing maternal economic and educational outcomes. Inconsistent contraceptive use and high-risk sexual activity are known predictors of repeat pregnancy. LARC has demonstrated efficacy in preventing repeat pregnancies.[14,15]

Multiple interventions have been tested to decrease repeat pregnancy. Teen-tot medical homes, motivational interviewing, and home-visiting show promise.[16,17] AYA mothers with strong sense of both control over their contraceptive decision making and intent to prevent pregnancy are most likely to avoid rapid repeat pregnancy.

ADOLESCENT PREGNANCY PREVENTION INTERVENTIONS

Many adolescent pregnancy prevention interventions have been implemented and studied over the last 2 decades. They generally fall into three categories: (1) clinic-based models with emphasis on counseling and access to contraception, (2) school-based abstinence-only and comprehensive educational programs, and (3) school-linked community programs.[18]

Program designs are varied and may be developed by parents, schools, physicians, religious groups, social agencies, and/or government departments. Successful programs include elements of abstinence promotion, contraceptive information/availability, sexual education, school completion strategies, job training, and other youth development strategies such as volunteerism, involvement in the arts or sports. Components of successful programs should be based on the age and developmental stage of the target group. A randomized controlled trial of abstinence-only education for 6th and 7th graders showed reduction in sexual initiation rates by 9th grade.[19] However, abstinence-only programs for high school students have been associated with increased unprotected sexual activity.[20]

Research strongly supports a two-pronged approach to primary prevention by using methods to delay sexual initiation and by providing contraceptive education and availability, if necessary. No research exists that links contraceptive education with increased sexual activity.

EVALUATION AND MANAGEMENT OF THE PREGNANT AYAs

When an adolescent or young adult presents to a health care facility for reproductive health services or advice, it is important to provide an environment that is welcoming, comfortable, and confidential.

Role of the Practitioner

Determining whether a pregnancy is intentional or unintentional is imperative in planning the management of the pregnancy. Both the age of the mother and her intentions behind the pregnancy may significantly affect the management of the pregnancy. Unplanned pregnancy can be a crisis for the young woman and her family. The provider is uniquely positioned to offer guidance and support.

Pregnancy requires that the provider gives balanced attention to the pregnant patient's medical issues and her counseling needs. The young woman should be granted confidentiality as they discuss choices and plans. It is vital that the practitioner be familiar with their local laws on adolescent confidentiality as they vary geographically. In ideal circumstances, the AYAs' family and her partner need to be considered as a plan is formulated to manage the pregnancy. However, the practitioner must ascertain whether there has been sexual coercion, history of physical abuse, as well as whether the potential for abuse exists. Opportunities for intervention include the following:

- Diagnosis of pregnancy and facilitated decision making
- Open, nonjudgmental service planning
- Screening for depression, substance use and domestic violence
- Management of pregnancy, if the adolescent or young adult chooses to continue the pregnancy
- Preparation for parenthood, if the adolescent or young adult chooses to raise the child
- Referrals for subspecialty services, as needed
- Support, if the adolescent or young adult chooses adoption
- Family planning and safe-sex education

Open, nonjudgmental service planning is critical. Despite a provider's personal preferences, the provider needs to counsel the patient about her options or refer to a provider who is comfortable about counseling pregnant AYAs. If they are not available within the provider's own health program, appropriate referrals for care should be made. Timeliness is important, because some of the choices are only available during the early weeks of the pregnancy.

Common Presentations of Pregnancy

AYAs may present with various complaints that may suggest early pregnancy. The most frequent objective concern is a missed or an abnormal menstrual period. Others may report abdominal pain, fatigue, breast tenderness, and vomiting or appetite changes. Patients with such concerns should be questioned about sexual activity, contraceptive use, and desire for a pregnancy test. Adolescents may need extra time to discuss the concerns and fears they have about a possible pregnancy. A flexible approach can allow patients to make healthy decisions for their particular situation.

Pregnancy Tests

The development of sensitive and specific pregnancy tests has significantly facilitated the early diagnosis of a pregnancy. Young women are often unsure of their last menstrual period (LMP). This is even more likely in adolescents who may not yet have regular menstrual cycles. Pregnancy tests measure levels of human chorionic gonadotropin (hCG), a glycoprotein that is secreted by invasive cytotrophoblast cells in early pregnancy and implantation. The most common is a radioimmunoassay (RIA) that detects serum levels of the β subunit of hCG as low as 7 mIU/mL. Most urine pregnancy tests will detect hCG when levels exceed 25 mIU/mL, thus giving a positive test result around the first missed menstrual period with an accuracy of 93%.[21]

1. hCG levels during pregnancy: It is important for the practitioner to remember that hCG levels change significantly during the course of pregnancy and that the results must be interpreted based on the particular test used (sensitivity and specificity). Serum hCG is detectable 8 days after conception in about 5% of women and by day 11 in more than 98% of women. At 4 weeks gestation, serum hCG doubling times are approximately 2.2 days, but only every 3.5 days by 9 weeks' gestation. Levels peak at 10 to 12 weeks' gestation and then decline rapidly until a slower rise begins at 22 weeks' gestation, which continues until term.[22]
   a. Abnormally elevated levels can indicate either a multiple-gestation pregnancy or a molar pregnancy. Anticonvulsants, phenothiazine, and promethazine may increase serum hCG levels.
   b. Abnormally low levels can indicate a spontaneous abortion or ectopic pregnancy. Low levels may also indicate delayed ovulation or implantation. Diuretics and promethazine can decrease hcG levels.
2. hCG levels after pregnancy: Levels gradually decrease after a delivery or abortion, and the initial decrease is quite rapid. After 2 weeks, the serum hCG level should be <1% of the level when the pregnancy was terminated.
   a. Term delivery: Levels should drop to <50 mIU/mL by 2 weeks—undetectable by 3 to 4 weeks.

b. First-trimester abortion: Initial hCG levels are much higher. If the abortion is at 8 to 10 weeks and initial hCG levels are more than 150,000 mIU, then levels at 2 weeks can be 1,500 mIU/mL and detectable for 8 to 9 weeks.

3. Types of pregnancy kits
   a. Immunometric tests: These tests are based on enzyme-linked immunosorbent assay (ELISA) techniques that identify two antibodies for hCG, making these tests specific for the β subunit of hCG. The urine test kits provide accurate qualitative response within 2 to 5 minutes and measures hCG levels as low as 5 to 50 mIU/mL. This provides positive test results as soon as 10 days after fertilization. These are the most common tests used in most family planning and young women's health clinics.
   b. Home pregnancy testing (HPT): HPTs are popular because they are convenient, quick, and confidential. HPTs are commonly used in the week after the missed menstrual period. During this period of pregnancy, urine hCG values are extremely variable. The problem with this technique is that the young person may not follow instructions and this causes an inaccurate result, that is, performing test too early.
   c. Quantitative β-hCG RAI: This expensive, highly sensitive test for specific levels of serum hCG takes 4 hours to complete and is positive 10 to 18 days post conception. However, it has no advantage over the immunometric urine tests for the regular clinical setting. The major use is in identifying an abnormal pregnancy such as ectopic pregnancy, or threatened miscarriage by checking either the doubling time or hCG disappearance over time.

4. False-positive and false-negative results
   a. False-negative hCG test results most often involve urine and are due to a misreading or interpretation of color changes. There may be a hCG concentration below the sensitivity threshold of the test being used, a miscalculation of LMP, delayed ovulation, or delayed menses from early pregnancy loss. Elevated lipids, immunoglobulin levels, and low serum protein levels can interfere with the serum test.
   b. False-positive test results with immunometric tests are rare but can also occur with laboratory error. Very rarely, pregnancy test results are positive from hCG production from a nonpregnancy source such as tumors of the ovaries, breast, and pancreas. For this reason, clinical correlation with the laboratory finding is essential. Should the laboratory result be inconsistent with the clinical presentation, it is imperative that the provider verifies the pregnancy test, using the more sensitive tests available.

5. Ultrasound estimated crown to rump length is an accurate method for estimating duration of pregnancy starting between 10 and 14 weeks. It has accuracy plus or minus 5 days.[23]

6. The physical examination is also an essential element of the initial evaluation. The pelvic examination will help determine the gestational age of the fetus and will identify any problems that may require immediate attention.

7. Uterine enlargement indicates the following:
   • 8 weeks of gestation: Uterine enlargement detected.
   • 12 weeks of gestation: Uterus palpated at symphysis pubis.
   • 20 weeks of gestation: Fundal height at umbilicus. At this point in the pregnancy, fetal movements should be detected, and fetal heart sounds should be audible by Doppler study.

8. Other signs
   • Softening of the cervix.
   • Discoloration of the cervix (it may appear purple or hyperemic).
   • Uterine softness.
   • Should vaginal bleeding be present or abdominal pain be elicited, it suggests pregnancy complications, such as a threatened abortion or an ectopic pregnancy.

Gestational Age

Most AYAs will want to know the gestational age of the fetus. Providers should carefully determine the LMP. Those having regular cycles lasting approximately 28 days are best able to predict the gestational age, which is calculated by counting the weeks since the LMP. A pregnancy wheel can be very helpful for calculating gestational age by dates.

The expected date of delivery (also called the expected date of confinement) can be obtained from the pregnancy wheel or is estimated using the Nägele rule: add 7 days to the first day of the LMP, subtract 3 months from the month of the LMP, and add 1 year to the calculated date. If the uterus is smaller than expected by menstrual dates, the providers should consider an error in pregnancy test, an ectopic pregnancy, an incomplete or missed spontaneous abortion, or fertilization occurred later than reported dates suggest. If the uterus is larger than expected, considerations include the following: twins, uterine fibroids, uterine anomaly, hydatidiform mole, or earlier fertilization.

⬤ PREGNANCY COUNSELING

Counseling the pregnant patient about her pregnancy options is perhaps the most important aspect of early pregnancy management. Providers who offer pregnancy tests should be prepared to provide such counseling and medical assessment, including pelvic examination for confirmation of gestational age of the fetus, sexually transmitted infection (STI) screening, and multivitamins prescription with folate supplementation.

Critical elements of counseling the pregnant adolescent or young adult include the following:

1. An assessment of the individual's expectations and desires regarding the possible pregnancy. Privacy and confidentiality are critical. A preliminary assessment of any stressors or safety concerns is useful while counseling the adolescent or young adult about her test results. A private discussion permits the provider to consider the adolescent or young adult independent of others who may become involved with the young person and the pregnancy.

2. Confidentiality: AYAs are entitled to confidentiality, although family members sometimes disagree. AYAs should be reminded that any discussions remain confidential, unless the adolescent wishes to inform or include others. This allows the adolescents or young adults to make their own choices regarding disclosure of the pregnancy. Occasionally, there are mental health concerns, such as the threat of suicide or homicide, or abuse that require involvement of others. The practitioners should familiarize themselves with the medical confidentiality laws of their geographic area particularly in regards to statutory rape, parental consent for termination, and guidelines for judicial bypass.

3. Support of the partner or concerned adult: The patient may be accompanied by a partner or adult. In such instances, a provider should offer the patient the choice of including this person in a portion of the pregnancy counseling session. If the pregnancy test result is positive, the patient should be encouraged to seek the support of adults (e.g., parents, grandparents, or other trusted adult). These adults could form a "core of support" for the adolescent or young adult should she elect to carry the pregnancy to term or decide to terminate the pregnancy. The patient's partner may also share in the decision-making process. It is vital, however, to screen AYAs for safety in both their relationship and family domains.

4. Nonjudgmental approach: The provider needs to provide the opportunity for open discussion when counseling AYAs about a positive pregnancy test result. The provider should allow the individual to express her wishes for this pregnancy, without imposing the provider's personal values on the youth.

5. Presenting options: The adolescent or young adult needs need to consider many options for this pregnancy, which include the following:
   • Carrying the pregnancy to term and assuming parental responsibility
   • Family-centered care for the adolescent and her new baby, thereby sharing childcare responsibility among the baby's extended family
   • Placing the baby with adoptive parents after the baby is born
   • Terminating the pregnancy (e.g., induced abortion)

TERMINATING THE PREGNANCY

Among girls 15 to 19 years old, the percentage of unintended pregnancies that result in abortion is 37%. This rate is increased in younger populations; almost 49% of unwanted pregnancies result in abortion in girls younger than 15 years. Among women aged 20 to 24, 23% of all pregnancies result in abortion. This number climbs to 41% when the pregnancy is unintended. The abortion rate for women aged 15 to 44 has reached a nadir of 16.9/1,000.[24] There are many possible explanations for this trend, such as a decline in the availability and accessibility of abortions nationwide. Abortions are a service that is frequently offered in free-standing clinics that are separate from the more traditional, primary health care programs. Thus, a referral to another facility is generally required for this procedure and some AYAs lack the skills to negotiate health services in a new health facility. In the US, mandatory waiting periods and Medicaid restrictions have also decreased access to abortion services.

Providers of patients who seek an abortion should be aware that careful follow-up and psychological support are needed while the adolescent or young adult explores this option. Health care providers should be aware of their local laws governing adolescents who seek abortion services. For instance, parental notification laws apply in the majority of US states. Careful attention to legal considerations, including the rights of parents, will be important as the provider advocates for the adolescent. Any financial barriers that may interfere with the adolescent's ability to obtain the abortion should also be reviewed.

Patients who are certain about their decision to terminate the pregnancy should be encouraged to do so in the early stages of the pregnancy. This will minimize both the complications and the costs of the procedure. Most induced abortions are performed within 8 weeks of conception.

After an adolescent or young adult has decided to end her pregnancy, she may need help in selecting the best method. There are more options for those who have earlier terminations, but adolescents may delay in making this decision until after 15 weeks. Methods in the first 12 weeks are safe and include vacuum aspiration, curettage, and medical terminations with either methotrexate-misoprostol or mifepristone-misoprostol.

Between 12 and 24 weeks, methods include dilation and evacuation, amnioinfusion, and uterotonic/hypertonic techniques. Most young women have a first-trimester abortion and decide between a medical or surgical method.

Choice of Medical versus Surgical Early Abortion Methods
Medical Method
Advantages of the medical method are that it avoids surgery and anesthesia, is less painful, may be easier emotionally, provides the patient with more control, is a more private process, and has less risk of infection. Medical methods are successful, with need for surgical intervention avoided in 84% to 98% of women.[25]

Disadvantages include bleeding, cramping and nausea, more waiting and uncertainty, extra clinic visit, limited to pregnancies up to 7 to 9 weeks, and risk of methotrexate-induced birth defects if abortion is incomplete.

Types of Medical Methods
First Trimester: Two methods in the US include mifepristone (RU-486) with misoprostol and methotrexate with misoprostol.

1. Mifepristone-misoprostol: Mifepristone is a progesterone antagonist that is an effective abortifacient. The efficacy increases with the addition of a prostaglandin analog such as misoprostol. The earlier in pregnancy that these are used, the higher the efficacy. In women with pregnancies <7 weeks, 97% have a complete abortion.[25] The technique involves at least three visits:
   a. First visit: Mifepristone 600 mg
   b. Two days later: Misoprostol dose. Some abortions are complete before this visit. If not, 400-μg are given orally. In those who have not aborted, two-thirds occur within 4 hours of the prostaglandin administration.
   c. Two weeks later: Checkup to ensure completed abortion.
2. Methotrexate and misoprostol: methotrexate is a cytotoxic drug that is lethal to trophoblastic tissue. When used with misoprostol, the combination is about 95% successful in terminating early pregnancies, but effect takes longer than mifepristone and misoprostol.[25]

Surgical Method
Advantages are as follows: quicker (one visit); more certain; AYAs can be less involved; can be done under general anesthesia; and continuation of pregnancy is rare.

Types of Surgical Methods
In the US, surgical methods are the most common method of termination of pregnancy.

1. Vacuum aspiration
   a. The most widely used and standard first-trimester surgical method
   b. Relatively simple technique requiring small cervical dilation
   c. May be performed with local anesthesia
   d. Can be done in an office through 14 weeks' gestation
2. Dilation and evacuation
   a. Most common second-trimester method of abortion
   b. Requires more dilation than the aspiration method. Laminaria or other osmotic dilators are often inserted before the procedure to gradually dilate the cervix. This may be a 1- to 2-day procedure.
   c. Is commonly used for procedures between 13 and 16 weeks, although many clinicians use this procedure up through 20-plus weeks
   d. Para cervical or general anesthesia is used before evacuating the uterus.

Second Trimester: Medical techniques for second-trimester abortions include hypertonic saline instillation, hypertonic urea instillation, and prostaglandin E_2 suppository insertion. These techniques account for less than 1% of all abortions in the US. Most have been replaced by dilation and evacuation procedures, which are faster, safer, and less expensive.

Abortion Risks and Complications
Short-term: Infection occurs in up to 3% of all women. This is minimized by prior diagnosis and treatment of gonorrhea and chlamydia, as well as by the use of prophylactic antibiotics. Infection from retained products requires antibiotics and an additional procedure. Intrauterine blood clots occur in <1% of procedures. Use of laminaria and skillful technique lowers the risk of cervical trauma. Young women have lower risks of trauma.

Other complications include bleeding (0.03% to 1%) and failed abortion (0.5% to 1%). The mortality rate is less than 1 per 100,000 abortions.

Long-term Post-Abortion Complications

Medical: There are no long-term complications of abortion from the most common methods. First-trimester abortion with vacuum aspiration does not appear to affect fertility rates or cause future spontaneous abortions.

Psychological: Although some studies report that adolescent and young women may consider abortion to be a stressful experience, these symptoms are often short lived and can be mitigated with support before, during, and after the procedure. A population-based longitudinal study showed no association between abortion and subsequent depression in women aged 15 to 27 years.[26] The young women obtaining an abortion were also less likely to experience a subsequent pregnancy than either of the other two groups. It is important to note that post-abortion stress may be higher in adolescents under age 18 years especially if they perceived high levels of conflict with parents.

MEDICAL MANAGEMENT OF THE PREGNANT ADOLESCENT

Prenatal care is a major factor predicting a positive outcome for an AYA birth. Factors associated with adequate prenatal care are increased age, a longer interpregnancy interval, partner/social support, and participation in a specialized pregnancy program. These programs often include a multidisciplinary team, including medicine, social work, nursing, and nutrition. The following is a brief guide on the important areas of prenatal care for the adolescent patient.

1. Initial evaluation: this should include a thorough history, including both a family history of chronic illness and a personal medical history. A drug history for tobacco, alcohol, and substance use is important. Risk for human immunodeficiency virus (HIV) infection should be assessed. Due to young people's reluctance to disclose sensitive information during an initial visit, practitioners should continue to assess risk status throughout the pregnancy. A complete physical examination and pelvic examination should be performed.

   Laboratory evaluation should include complete blood cell count, urinalysis, blood type and group, syphilis serology, sickle cell test in Black patients, test for Tay–Sachs disease for Mediterranean or Jewish heritage, rubella titer, Papanicolaou test if older than 21 years, Gonococcal and Chlamydia tests, hepatitis B serology, and HIV antibody counseling and testing.
2. Topics to be covered on successive visits include physiology of pregnancy, maternal nutrition, substance abuse, STIs and HIV infection, discussion and referral to a prepared childbirth class, childbirth, breast-feeding and infant nutrition, infant care and development, contraception, sexuality, and post-delivery care needs.
3. Nutrition: Ideal weight gain should be 25 to 40 pounds. The adolescent or young adult should be advised against dieting during pregnancy. A prenatal vitamin supplement, containing iron and folic acid, should be prescribed. Additional iron is required if iron deficiency is diagnosed. AYAs consuming <1,000 mg of calcium per day should be given a calcium and vitamin D supplement. Pregnant AYAs may become obese. Consumption of fruits and vegetables and avoidance of sugar-sweetened beverages and energy-dense foods should be encouraged.
4. Prenatal visits: AYAs should have visits every 2 to 4 weeks, through the 7th month. Visits are every 2 weeks in the 8th month, and weekly thereafter.
5. Psychosocial aspects: It is essential to consider that the pregnant AYAs' acceptance of the pregnancy and their relationship

with their parents or the father of the child may change during the course of the pregnancy. Depression is a common before, during, and after a teen pregnancy. Screenings at every prenatal visit are important.
6. Substance abuse: Due to the serious consequences of substance use for both mother and infant, a thorough assessment of past and present drug use is necessary at pregnancy diagnosis and throughout the prenatal period. The following is a list of common substances and their effects during pregnancy.
   a. Alcohol: Fetal alcohol syndrome including prenatal and postnatal growth retardation; facial dysmorphogenesis (microcephaly, short palpebral fissures, cleft palate, and micrognathia); abnormalities of the central nervous system (CNS); and increased risk of cardiac defects, joint abnormalities, hepatic fibrosis, mental retardation, and learning difficulties.
   b. Amphetamines: May cause malformations.
   c. Cocaine: Increased risk of spontaneous abortion and premature delivery; neurobehavioral deficits in the newborn; increased prevalence of abruptio placentae; increased risk of genital and urinary tract defects, including prune belly syndrome, hypospadias, and hydronephrosis.
   d. Heroin: Intrauterine growth retardation; neonatal abstinence syndrome (infant irritability, tremor, convulsions, or poor feeding due to heroin withdrawal); increased risk of hepatitis, HIV, and other infections in the mother.
   e. Lysergic acid diethylamide: Increased risk of congenital abnormalities, including hydrocephalus, spina bifida, and myelomeningocele.
   f. Marijuana: Questionable increased risk of birth defects.
   g. Nicotine: Impaired growth; increased risk of spontaneous abortion.
7. Medications and pregnancy: The US Food and Drug Administration classifies drug classes A through D in terms of whether benefits out way risks during pregnancy. Pregnant AYAs should be advised to avoid over-the-counter medications and herbal supplements. Up-to-date information regarding the risks of medications in pregnancy can be found at www.otispregnancy.org and http://toxnet.nlm.nih.gov.
8. The chronically ill AYAs: Pregnancy in chronically ill patients presents specific challenges and requires coordination with their specialty care providers. Each illness is associated with specific risks.
9. HIV disease: Practitioners should offer HIV counseling and testing to all pregnant patients. Education regarding the risks of perinatal transmission should also be provided. Pregnant women infected with HIV should be referred for appropriate treatment and supportive services. Some women found to be infected may choose to terminate their pregnancy once their HIV status is known. Due to the risks of HIV transmission through breast milk, breast-feeding is not recommended for HIV-infected mothers. Infants will require treatment after delivery.
10. Domestic violence: Several studies have demonstrated increased risk for domestic violence during and prior to teen pregnancy. Violence can be severe, leading to injuries and death.[27] Battering often starts or becomes worse during pregnancy. Prenatal risk assessment should include specific questions regarding family and partner violence. Practitioners must be knowledgeable about domestic violence reporting laws in their state and should be familiar with community resources.

MEDICAL COMPLICATIONS OF PREGNANCY

Adolescents are not at a higher risk of developing complications during early pregnancy. Potential complications for AYAs are as follows:

1. Spontaneous abortion: A spontaneous abortion may occur in 20% of all pregnancies. A spontaneous abortion occurring in the first 20 weeks of pregnancy usually results from abnormal chromosomal development in the fetus or abnormalities of the pelvic structure within the adolescent.

   Abdominal cramping and vaginal bleeding characterize the early stages of a miscarriage, or a spontaneous abortion. The term "threatened abortion" refers to pregnancies complicated by bleeding and cramping, but the cervix remains long and closed. Should the condition progress, the pregnancy is nonviable, and an abortion is considered "inevitable." Physical changes include a widening of the cervical os and an increase in the bleeding and cramping. A "complete abortion" occurs when all the products of conception have passed. A sonogram will confirm the absence of the fetus, and physical examination will show that cervical os is closed. If the miscarriage is considered an incomplete abortion, a dilation and evacuation procedure will be necessary to prevent blood loss and infection.

2. Ectopic pregnancy is more likely to occur in those with a history of prior STIs or in women who are 35 years or older. Ectopic pregnancies occur in 2% of this higher-risk population. Abdominal cramping and bleeding suggest an ectopic, or extrauterine, pregnancy.

3. Hydatidiform mole, or gestational trophoblastic disease, may occur in 1 of 1,000 pregnancies each year. Although AYAs commonly experience vaginal bleeding and abdominal cramping with a problem pregnancy, those with a hydatidiform mole usually have severe and profuse bleeding. The uterus is larger than expected given the estimated gestational age of the fetus, and the hCG levels are often >100,000 mIU/mL. Ultrasound of the uterus demonstrates the characteristic cluster of grapes appearance of the mass.

   An immediate procedure is needed to terminate a molar pregnancy. Treatment with dilation and suction is the treatment of choice, although the procedure is complicated because it places the patient at increased risk for severe hemorrhage. Close follow-up of the serum hCG level is required to ensure that the tumor has been adequately removed. The hCG level should remain <2 mIU/mL for 1 year. If the hCG level remains elevated, it suggests that the tumor has not been sufficiently removed; if the hCG level rises, the tumor may have recurred. The patient should use a reliable method of contraception for the year after the diagnosis of trophoblastic disease.

Adoption

While most AYAs who continue their pregnancy intend to raise their baby, some will express an interest in placing their child in a home with adoptive parents. Few consider this option at the time that the pregnancy test is obtained, although it is important that the pregnant adolescent or young adult be counseled about this option. In most states and the District of Columbia, mothers who are minors may legally place their child for adoption without parental involvement. Less than 10% of the babies born to unmarried teens are placed in adoptive homes. Unmarried teen mothers who place their children for adoption are more likely to be White, have higher socioeconomic status and educational aspirations, and be from suburban residences.

OTHER CONSEQUENCES OF ADOLESCENT PREGNANCY

Child Outcomes

For adolescents ≥15 years, pregnancies do not have increased risk of adverse outcomes if they receive adequate prenatal care. However, for teens <15 years, there are increased risks, independent of prenatal care, for prematurity, low birthweight, and mortality.

Factors associated with pregnancy outcome are variations in prenatal care, nutritional status, prepregnancy weight, STI exposure, smoking, and substance use.

Although there have been no recent long-term outcome studies, the children of teen mothers face significant challenges with risks of developmental delay, behavioral problems, school failure, mental health problems, and high-risk behaviors during adolescence.[14] Sons are at increased risk for incarceration and teen fatherhood, and daughters are at increased risk for pregnancy, thus continuing family cycles of teen pregnancy. Toxic stress associated with poverty, violence exposure experienced in childhood may contribute to poor child developmental and psychological outcomes.[28] Rapid repeat pregnancy is also associated with poorer child developmental outcomes.

Growth and Development

No definitive data suggest that adolescent pregnancy adversely affects growth and development although some recent studies have suggested small potential decreases in hip-bone mineralization and ultimate height in the very young pregnant adolescents. Young adolescents (e.g., <15 years) may not fully understand the long-term implications of childbirth, particularly in the early stages of the pregnancy.

Education and Socioeconomic Issues

Adolescent parenthood is associated with socioeconomic disadvantage. Mothers, who give birth prior to age 20, often delay school completion. Factors linked to higher educational attainment for adolescent mothers are race (Blacks do better than Whites), growing up in a smaller family, the presence of reading materials in the home, mother's employment, and higher parental educational level.[29] While 80% of young mothers receive governmental assistance at some point in time, most eventually do not receive public assistance.

Subsequent Childbirth

Repeat pregnancy is often targeted by adolescent parenting interventions because short interpregnancy intervals are associated with adverse pregnancy, neonatal, and child outcomes. The rate of second births to adolescent mothers has declined over the past decade. However, within 2 years, 10% to 40% of teen mothers become pregnant again. Protective factors against repeat adolescent pregnancy are older maternal age (>16 years), participation in a specialized adolescent parent program, use of effective contraception, school attendance, new sex partner, and avoidance of interpersonal violence.

MALE AYAs AS FATHERS

Young fathers rarely receive the same degree of attention and support that is offered to mothers, yet AYA men are at high risk for unplanned pregnancy. Fathers may not be included in decisions regarding pregnancy options, or establish a long-term supportive relationship with the mother of the child. However, child outcomes improve when fathers participate in the child's care.[14] Even if not romantically involved, AYA parents need to negotiate their family responsibilities and plan childcare together.

Whenever possible, the providers should attempt to discuss reproductive health issues with their male patients who are sexually active. This is easily done during health maintenance visits, but it should also be done during acute visits for STI evaluation. Asking the male patient about whether he has fathered a child is reasonable when he indicates that he is sexually active. Supportive counseling should be available to male adolescents who are actively involved with babies they have fathered and to male adolescents who have pregnant girlfriends.

CARE OF YOUNG PARENTS AND THEIR CHILDREN

Parenting is the most common outcome, yet it is, in many respects, the most difficult commitment to fulfill, because it requires the young woman, and ideally young man, to assume long-term responsibility for a baby. A comprehensive care program that is designed to address the health and social needs of pregnant AYAs is optimal. Essential elements for prenatal programs include a complement of medical, psychological, social, and educational services; and linkages to mother/infant programs.[16]

Family-centered Care for the Mother and Newborn

Because adolescents are rarely able to assume independence after the birth of a baby, the adolescent's family (or community) needs to offer help; yet, young mothers are often lonely with inadequate support systems. Living arrangements may be unpredictable. Providers who care for the young parents will need to be linked to community-based services for extended families. Home-visiting programs can benefit both AYAs.

Adolescent parents benefit from comprehensive postnatal programs that combine medical care for the teens and their children with parenting education and social support. Patient-centered medical home practices or teen-tot clinics provide pregnant and parenting adolescents with integrated primary care and social/mental health services.[29,30] They can improve infant immunization rates and parenting abilities and assist with the teen's return to school. Contraception, especially access to LARCs, should be readily available as well as immunizations and well-baby care. Young parents are at increased risk for depression, school failure, poor parenting, and domestic violence and should be screened at each visit. Home-visiting programs can also be effective as well as school-based programs.[15,16] Program staff should encourage enrollment of children in early education programs such as Head Start. Long-term continuous relationships with caring providers are essential to positive outcomes.

REFERENCES

1. Hamilton BE, Martin JA, Osterman JC, et al. *Births: preliminary data for 2013.* Natl Vital Stat Rep. Available at http://www.cdc.gov/nchs/data/nvsr/nvsr63/nvsr63_02.pdf. Accessed January 9, 2014.
2. Neinstein LS. *The new adolescents: an analysis of health conditions, behaviors, risks and access to services among emerging young adults 2013.* Available at http://www.usc.edu/studentaffairs/Health_Center/thenewadolescents. Accessed November 26, 2014.
3. The National Campaign to Prevent Teen and Unplanned Pregnancies. Available at http://thenationalcampaign.org. Accessed February 22, 2014.
4. American College Health Association. *College health assessment report: international and domestic UPC students.* University of Southern California. Available at https://engemannshc.usc.edu/files/2012/12/NCHA-Report-2014-University-Park-Campus-International-and-Domestic.pdf. Accessed November 26, 2014.
5. Wodtke GT. Duration and timing of exposure to neighborhood poverty and the risk of adolescent parenthood. *Demography* 2013;50:1765–1788.
6. Centers for Disease Control and Prevention. *Youth online: high school YRBS.* Available at http://nccd.cdc.gov/youthonline/App/Results.aspx?TT=&OUT=&SID=HS& QID=H59&LID=&YID=&LID2=&YID2=&COL=&ROW1=&ROW2=&HT=&LCT=& FS=&FR=&FG=&FSL=&FRL=&FGL=&PV=&TST=&C1=&C2=&QP=G&DP=&VA =CI&CS=Y&SYID=&EYID=&SC=&SO. Accessed June 16, 2014.
7. Noll JG, Shenk CE. Teen birth rates in sexually abused and neglected females. *Pediatrics* 2013;131:e1181–e1187.
8. East PL, Slonim A, Horn EJ, et al. Effects of adolescent childbearing on Latino siblings: changes in family dynamics and feelings toward the teen mother. *Hisp J Behav Sci* 2011;33(4). doi:10.1177/0739986311423368.
9. Hodkinson S, Beers L, Southammakosane C, et al. Addressing the mental health needs of pregnant and parenting adolescents. *Pediatrics* 2013;133:114–122.
10. Kearney MS, Levine PB. *Media influences on social outcomes : the impact of MTV's 16 and pregnant on teen childbearing.* NBER Working Paper No 19795 2014.
11. Santelli J, Orr M, Lindberg LD. Pregnancy intentions, contraceptive use at the time of conception, and pregnancy-related behaviors among adolescents. *J Adolesc Health* 2010;46:S53.
12. Rubin SE, Campos G, Marken S. Primary care physicians' concerns may affect adolescents' access to intrauterine contraception. *J Prim Care Community Health* 2013;4:216–219.
13. Centers for Disease Control and Prevention. Vital signs: repeat births among teens—United States, 2007–2010. *MMWR* 2013;62:249–255.
14. Savio Beers LA, Hollo RE. Approaching the adolescent-headed family: a review of teen parenting. *Curr Probl Pediatr Adolesc Health Care* 2009;39:216–233.
15. Tocce KM, Sheeder JL, Teal SB, et al. Rapid repeat pregnancy in adolescents: do immediate postpartum contraceptive implants make a difference? *Am J Obstet Gynecol* 2012;206:481.e1–e7.
16. Ruedinger E, Cox JE. Adolescent childbearing: consequences and interventions. *Curr Opin Pediatr* 2012;24:446–452.
17. Barnet B, Rapp T, DeVoe M, et al. Cost-effectiveness of a motivational intervention to reduce rapid repeated childbearing in high-risk adolescent mothers: a rebirth of economic and policy considerations. *Arch Pediatr Adolesc Med* 2010;164:370–376.
18. Lavin C, Cox JE. Teen pregnancy prevention: current perspectives. *Curr Opin Pediatr* 2012;24:462–469.
19. Jemmott JB III, Jemmott LS, Fong GT. Efficacy of a theory based abstinence only intervention over 24 months. *Arch Pediatr Adolesc Med* 2010;164:152–159.
20. Dailard C. Recent finds from the 'add health' survey: teens and sexual activity. *Guttmacher Report on Public Policy* 2001:4(4). Available at http://www.guttmacher.org/pubs/tgr/04/4/gr040401.html. Accessed November 30, 2014.
21. Johnson SR, Godbert S, Perry P, et al. Accuracy of a home-based device for giving an early estimate of pregnancy duration compared with reference methods. *Fertil Steril* 2013;100:1635–1641.e1.
22. Larsen J, Buchanan P, Johnson S, et al. Human chorionic gonadotropin as a measure of pregnancy duration. *Int J Gynaecol Obstet* 2013:123:189–195.
23. Whitworth M, Bricker L, Neilson JP, et al. Ultrasound for fetal assessment in early pregnancy [Review]. *Cochrane Database Syst Rev* 2010;4:CD007058.
24. Jones RK, Jerman J. Abortion incidence and service availability in the United States. *Perspect Sex Reprod Health* 2014;46(1):3–14. doi:10.1363/46e0414.
25. Raymond EG, Shannot C, Weaver MA, et al. First-trimester medical abortion with mifepristone 200 mg and misoprostol: a systematic review. *Contraception* 2013;98:264–269.
26. Pederson W. Abortion and depression: a population-based longitudinal study of young women. *Scand J Public Health* 2008;36:424–428.
27. Cheng D, Horon IL. Intimate-partner homicide among pregnant and postpartum women. *Obstet Gynecol* 2010;115:1181–1186.
28. Garner AS, Shonkoff JP; Committee on Psychosocial Aspects of Child and Family Health et al. Early childhood adversity, toxic stress, and the role of the pediatrician: translating developmental science into lifelong health. *Pediatrics* 2012;129(1):e233-e246.
29. Cox JE, Buman MP, Woods ER, et al. Evaluation of raising adolescent families together: a medical home for teen mothers and their children. *Am J Public Health* 2012;102:1879–1885.
30. Pinzon JK, Jones VF; Committee on adolescent; Committee on early childhood. Care of adolescent parents and their children. *Pediatrics* 2012;130:e1743–e1756.

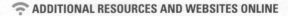 **ADDITIONAL RESOURCES AND WEBSITES ONLINE**

Contraception

Romina L. Barral
Melanie A. Gold

Currently, adolescence and young adulthood can last for over 15 years. Since puberty occurs earlier in life and with an extended period until adult roles, there is a prolonged time period for contraceptive needs. Sexual activity, abortion, and birth rates among adolescents and young adults (AYAs) increased in the 1960s and 1970s, but those rates started to decline early in the 1990s, partially in response to the acquired immunodeficiency syndrome (AIDS) epidemic and also better contraceptive methods. Despite this progress, significant risk-taking behaviors remain and the need for higher usage of effective contraception continues.

EPIDEMIOLOGY

Pregnancy Rates

In 2009, the national pregnancy rate was approximately 102.1 pregnancies per 1,000 women aged 15 to 44 years, about 11.8% below the peak in 1990 (115.8).[1] The highest rate was among 25- to 29-year-old women (162 per 1,000) followed by women aged 20 to 24 years (158.3 per 1,000). The pregnancy rate for teenagers fell 43.6% during 1990 to 2009 (65.3 per 1,000 in 15- to 19-year-olds), to the lowest reported since 1976.

- The pregnancy rate for 15- to 17-year-olds declined from 77.1 per 1,000 in 1990 to 36.4 per 1,000 in 2009.
- The rate for older teenagers 18 to 19 years of age declined by over one-third during this time period, from 167.7 per 1,000 in 1990 to 106.3 per 1,000 in 2009.
- Pregnancy rates for women in their early 20s declined by 22.5% from 1990 to 2009.
- Declines in pregnancy rates for women aged 25 to 29 years were less marked from 1990 to 2009 falling 9.5% during the same time period (179 to 162).

Birth and Terminations of Pregnancy

Rates for all three age-groups (15 to 19, 20 to 24, and 25 to 29) fell for births, induced abortions (largest percent declines), and fetal losses. Patterns were generally similar across race and Hispanic ethnicity. Despite these declines,[1] the teen birth rates in the US are significantly higher than other industrialized nations with marked racial and ethnic disparities.[2]

The Centers for Disease Control and Prevention (CDC) analyzed data from the National Survey of Family Growth (NSFG) collected in 1995, 2002, and 2006 to 2010 and found that the decline in teen birth rates since 1995 were attributed to significant increases in the proportion of female adolescents who were abstinent, and, among sexually experienced female adolescents, increases in the proportion who were using effective contraception.

Sexual Activity and Contraceptive Usage

The percentage of teenagers who reported having had recent sex (defined and measured within the last month, 3 and 12 months), and the percentage using a method of contraception at first and last intercourse, remained unchanged from 2002 through 2006 to 2010. At the same time, males' report of using condoms and of dual methods at *first* intercourse increased, as did males reporting that their female partners were using oral contraceptives and dual methods at *last* intercourse.[3] Of note, although they reported an increase in these behaviors, the percentage of 15- to 19-year-olds reporting dual method use at last intercourse remained low at 13.1% in 2002 and 14.8% in 2006 to 2010.[3] The 2006 to 2010 data showed that female adolescents are adopting newer contraceptive methods: a larger proportion reported using hormonal methods other than the pill at first intercourse, and a higher percentage had ever used emergency contraception (EC) (14%), the contraceptive patch (10%), and the contraceptive ring (5%). Reported oral and injectable contraceptive use did not change significantly since 2002 (20.7% in 2002 versus 20.3% in 2006 to 2010).[3] Overall, initial declines in sexual activity and increases in contraception use explain the declines in teen pregnancy and birth rates (1998 to 2002). The lack of change in these risk behaviors between 2002 and 2006 to 2010 is reflected in trends in teen pregnancy and birth rates, that "with the exception of small fluctuation, have failed to continue to drop."[3]

Despite increased availability of newer, more effective contraceptive methods, disparities in unintended pregnancies and birth rates across major sociodemographic groups persist due to variations in contraceptive use and access. More notably, there is a marked underutilization of the most effective methods across all ages and races.

CONTRACEPTIVE METHODS

The 2008 report on national pregnancy rates found that of the nearly 6.6 million pregnancies, 51% were unintended.[4] Women aged 15 to 19 years reported greater unintended pregnancy rates (82%) compared to those who were 20 to 24 years old (64%). Most of these pregnancies are the result of contraceptive failure or non-use. Both the effectiveness inherent to each method (perfect use) and how correctly and consistently each method is used (typical use) can affect overall effectiveness of each contraceptive method (Table 41.1). The gap between perfect use and typical use increases with methods that are more user-dependent. Adolescents represent a group with higher than usual failure rates for many user-dependent methods as well as higher discontinuation rates compared to adult women. The CHOICE study, conducted in St Louis, found that girls aged 14 to 19 years have higher rates of discontinuing reversible contraception compared to women aged 20 years and older, at the 24 months follow-up (adjusted hazard ratios for risk of discontinuation = 1.40, 95% CI 1.22, 1.60).[5] Estimates of contraceptive failure from the 2002 NSFG showed that women younger than 30 years of age have higher probability of contraceptive failure (specifically pills, condom, and withdrawal) compared to the relevant reference groups (older than 30-year-old women) for the first 12 months of use.[6] The most commonly used methods of contraception reported by sexually active teenagers are male condoms, followed by withdrawal and combination oral contraceptives (COCs). These methods have differing effectiveness: Typical-use failure rate is 15% for condoms, 27% for withdrawal, and 8% for COCs.[7] More importantly, adolescents often use these methods inconsistently (nearly half "take breaks") or discontinue them early (up to half discontinued COCs within the first 6 months of use).

Throughout this chapter we reference the United States Medical Eligibility Criteria for Contraceptive (US MEC),[8] an excellent resource that provides guidance on contraceptive method safety for women with specific medical conditions. In addition, although this chapter provides an overview on most contraceptive methods, we refer the reader to Chapters 42 to 44 for information on specific contraceptive methods.

LONG-ACTING REVERSIBLE CONTRACEPTIVE METHODS

Long-acting reversible contraceptives (LARCs), also called highly effective reversible contraceptives (or HERCs), include intrauterine contraception (IUC) and subdermal implants. These are top-tiered contraceptive methods based on effectiveness, with failure rates of less than 0.1% per year for both perfect and typical use (see Chapter 44). These methods have the highest rates of continuation and satisfaction of all reversible contraception.[9] The American College of Obstetricians and Gynecologists (ACOG), the American Academy of Pediatrics (AAP), the CDC, and the World Health Organization (WHO) all recognize the potential impact of LARCs to reduce unintended pregnancies.[10] In fact, the ACOG recommends that LARCs be "first-line" choice for most women, emphasizing they are safe and appropriate for most women and adolescents and that, given the high risk of unintended pregnancy, adolescents may benefit from increased access to LARCs.[9] This was supported by a policy statement released by the AAP (September 2014).[11]

An analysis of data from the 2002 and 2006 to 2010 NSFG report confirms that the proportion of all LARC users across the US increased significantly between 2007 (3.7%) and 2009 (8.5%) among almost every subgroup of 15- to 44-year-old women; women of all ages, races/ethnicities, marital and educational statuses, income levels, and religions reported significant increases. The highest levels of use were reported among women aged 25 to 39 years, married and cohabiting women, women covered by Medicaid, women with a religious affiliation other than Catholic or Protestant, and those with no religious affiliation.[12] Another analysis of

NSFG data compared use of LARCs from 2007 to 2009 and found that for adolescents aged 15 to 19 years, use of LARCs tripled from 1.5% to 4.5%, with most or all of this increase noted among women aged 18 to 19 years, and these percentages increased from 4% to 7% for women aged 20 to 24 years and 5% to 10% for those aged 25 to 29 years. "Discrepancies by race and ethnicity seen in 2002 continued through 2007 but were largely eliminated by 2009. The latest figures also show no real differences by income level. Women born in the US appear to be catching up to women born outside the US, who already had a higher level of use, likely due to a greater prevalence of these methods in Mexico".[12]

Despite the increases reported, LARC use in the US lags behind use in other developed countries around the world. The United Nations 2011 Report on World Contraceptive Use reported LARC use among 15% of 15- to 49-year-old women who are married or in union in most other developed countries, including 11% of British women, 23% of French women, 27% of Norwegian women, and 41% of Chinese women. The large majority of LARC use is the intrauterine device (IUD).[13]

In the US, multiple reasons have been identified for lack of LARC use, including, but not limited to:

- women's lack of knowledge about and nonaccepting attitudes toward the methods, restrictive counseling and practice patterns among providers, myths and misconceptions among both users and providers
- high initial up-front costs associated with initiating these methods (despite better cost-effectiveness over time)
- pervasive misconceptions about risks and benefits of use.[14]

LARCs may have another advantage. One cause of unintended pregnancy among teenagers and young adult women is the rate of sexual assault, which is higher for youth than among any other group. Dating violence among the adolescent population is also an increasing risk affecting this age-group, and strong associations of intimate partner violence (IPV) with unintended pregnancy have been observed in prior studies. Male partners may be manipulating condom use and contraceptive methods in an attempt to get their partners pregnant, such as flushing COCs down the toilet, removing vaginal rings, and poking holes in condoms. LARCs are ideal for women in these violent or coercive settings to prevent unwanted pregnancies resulting from sexual assault or IPV. In fact, the copper IUD allows for discrete contraception because it is less likely to affect menstrual cycle regularity. Although the removal of an IUD may be more challenging, the strings can be cut high up in the cervical os if there is a need to hide the presence of the IUD or concern that the partner may feel or pull on the strings.

Intrauterine Devices
Current Use

Data from National Health Statistics Report[15] found that ever use of an IUD among 15- to 44-year-old women in the US declined from 1982 (18%) through 2002 (5.8%), but increased between 2002 and 2006 to 2010 (7.7%). The type of IUD used (hormonal versus copper) was not assessed by the surveys used in this report. Adolescents continue to report using less effective contraceptive methods. Data that assessed IUD use per age-group, published in the NHSR in 2012, reported that in the period of 2006 to 2010, 2.7% of adolescents, aged 15 to 19 years, who used contraception reported using an IUD, compared to 5.6% in women aged 20 to 24 years, and an average of 5.9% of women aged 25 to 44 years. Although IUDs are extremely effective and safe methods with the lowest adverse side effect profiles, there are multiple myths and misconceptions about their use among both providers and users. The most frequent cited misconceptions among patients include fear of the IUD causing an abortion, previously overestimated risk of pelvic inflammatory disease (PID), secondary infertility after IUD removal, the IUD causing ectopic pregnancies, hair loss, as well as osteoporosis and cancer.

TABLE 41.1

Percentage of Women Experiencing an Unintended Pregnancy During the First Year of Typical Use and Perfect Use of Contraception and the Percentage Continuing Use at the End of the First Year—the United States

| Method | Women Experiencing an Unintended Pregnancy Within the First Year of Use | | Women Continuing Use at 1 y[c] (%) |
	Typical Use[a] (%)	Perfect Use[b] (%)	
No method[d]	85	85	
Spermicides[e]	29	18	42
Withdrawal	27	4	43
Fertility awareness-based methods	25		51
Standard days method[f]		5	
TwoDay method[f]		4	
Ovulation method[f]		3	
Sponge			
Parous women	32	20	46
Nulliparous women	16	9	57
Diaphragm[g]	16	6	57
Condom[h]			
Female (Reality)	21	5	49
Male	15	2	53
Combined pill and POP	8	0.3	68
Evra patch	8	0.3	68
NuvaRing	8	0.3	68
Depo-Provera	3	0.3	56
IUD			
ParaGard (Copper-T)	0.8	0.6	78
Mirena (LNG-IUS)	0.2	0.2	80
Implanon	0.05	0.05	84
Female sterilization	0.5	0.5	100
Male sterilization	0.15	0.10	100
Emergency contraceptive pills[i]	Not applicable	Not applicable	Not applicable
Lactational amenorrhea methods[j]	Not applicable	Not applicable	Not applicable

[a]Among typical couples who initiate use of a method (not necessarily for the first time), the percentage who experience an unintended pregnancy during the first year if they do not stop use for any other reason. Estimates of the probability of pregnancy during the first year of typical use for spermicides, withdrawal, fertility awareness-based methods, the diaphragm, the male condom, the pill, and Depo-Provera are taken from the 1995 NSFG corrected for underreporting of abortion; see the text for the derivation of estimates for the other methods.

[b]Among couples who initiate use of a method (not necessarily for the first time) and who use it *perfectly* (both consistently and correctly), the percentage who experience an unintended pregnancy during the first year if they do not stop use for any other reason. See the text for the derivation of the estimate for each method.

[c]Among couples attempting to avoid pregnancy, the percentage who continue to use a method for 1 year.

[d]The percentages becoming pregnant in the typical-use and perfect-use columns are based on data from populations where contraception is not used and from women who cease using contraception to become pregnant. Of these, approximately 89% become pregnant within 1 year. This estimate was lowered slightly (to 85%) to represent the percentage who would become pregnant within 1 year among women now relying on reversible methods of contraception if they abandoned contraception altogether.

[e]Foams, creams, gels, vaginal suppositories, and vaginal film.

[f]The TwoDay and Ovulation methods are based on evaluation of cervical mucus. The Standard Days method avoids intercourse on cycle days 8–19.

[g]With spermicidal cream or jelly.

[h]Without spermicides.

[i]Treatment initiated within 72 hours after unprotected intercourse reduces the risk for pregnancy by at least 75%. The treatment schedule is 1 dose within 120 hours after unprotected intercourse and a second dose 12 hours after the first dose. Both doses of Plan B can be taken at the same time. Plan B (1 dose is 1 white pill) is the only dedicated product specifically marketed for emergency contraception. The Food and Drug Administration has in addition declared the following 22 brands of oral contraceptives to be safe and effective for emergency contraception: Ogestrel or Ovral (1 dose is 2 white pills); Levlen or Nordette (1 dose is 4 light-orange pills); Cryselle, Levora, Low-Ogestrel, Lo/Ovral, or Quasence (1 dose is 4 white pills); Tri-Levlen or Triphasil (1 dose is 4 yellow pills); Jolessa, Portia, Seasonale, or Trivora (1 dose is 4 pink pills); Seasonique (1 dose is 4 light blue-green pills); Empresse (1 dose is 4 orange pills); Alesse, Lessina, or Levlite (1 dose is 5 pink pills); Aviane (1 dose is 5 orange pills); and Lutera (1 dose is 5 white pills).

[j]Lactational amenorrhea method is a highly effective *temporary* method of contraception. However, to maintain effective protection against pregnancy, another method of contraception must be used as soon as menstruation resumes, the frequency or duration of breast-feeding is reduced, bottle feeds are introduced, or the baby reaches 6 months of age.

Adapted from Trussell J. Contraceptive efficacy. In: Hatcher RA, Trussell J, Nelson AL, et al., eds. *Contraceptive technology.* 19th revised ed. New York, NY: Ardent Media, 2007.

IX

Patients are also concerned and confused about the amount of bleeding following IUD insertion, weight changes, and the amount of pain during insertion, as well as misperceiving that insertion must take place at a particular time during the menstrual cycle. In addition, providers have misconceptions regarding the need to obtain parental consent and safety for inserting IUDs in nulliparous women, the latter of which has been successful and preferable. The CHOICE study showed that teens prefer LARCs to other methods,[5] and the ACOG states that nulliparity is not a contraindication to IUD use (see Chapter 44).[9]

Advantages

Hormonal IUDs are not only effective for contraception, but also provide other noncontraceptive health benefits, such as decreasing dysmenorrhea, menorrhagia, and endometriosis. IUDs are among the most efficacious contraceptive methods, with the advantage of being estrogen free. The copper IUD is also not only the most effective EC method available, but also the only highly effective method of contraception available for patients with contraindication to any type of hormonal method, such as patients with autoimmune disorders and positive antiphospholipid antibodies.[8]

Current Availability in the US

Copper 10 Year IUD (Paragard)

Manufactured by Teva, it is the most effective EC method when used within 5 days of unprotected sexual intercourse.

Levonorgestrel-IUDs: 5 Year IUD (Mirena) and 3 Year IUD (Skyla)

Both are manufactured by Bayer. Skyla was approved by the Food and Drug Administration (FDA) on January 9, 2013.

Implants (Etonogestrel (ETG) Implant or Nexplanon)
Current Use

According to a secondary analysis of the 2002 and 2006 to 2010 NSFG, 0.4% of contraceptors aged 15 to 44 years in the US used the contraceptive implant in 2002, compared to 0.8% in 2009 ($p = 0.003$).[12] Several studies have confirmed its high efficacy, convenience, and cost-effectiveness. However, restricted availability of trained providers, limited marketing, and high initial cost has contributed to limited use in the US.

Advantages

ETG implants provide highly effective, discreet, easy to use, convenient, long-acting, estrogen-free contraception. Implants are a good choice for postpartum adolescents and young women whose risk for a blood clot is elevated and for whom estrogen is contraindicated. The ETG implant effectively inhibits ovulation by preventing LH surge and inhibits endometrial proliferation. These two effects explain its use as an option in the hormonal treatment of endometriosis. Funk et al.[16] reported an 81% improvement in dysmenorrhea among 18- to 40-year-old women who used the ETG implant and presented with a baseline history of dysmenorrhea. Despite the irregular vaginal bleeding reported with the ETG implant use, a Brazilian study showed a 0.6 g/dL *increase* in hemoglobin and 1.5% *increase* in hematocrit among 37 female adolescents, aged 16 to 19 years, during implant use compared to those not using contraception. The study concluded that the increase was probably due to amenorrhea and reduced bleeding volume or frequency of periods.[17]

Current Availability in the US

Nexplanon, manufactured by Merck & Co., is the only implant currently marketed in the US; it is a 40-mm × 2-mm single rod containing 68 mg of ETG, the biologically active metabolite of desogestrel, covered with a rate-controlling membrane of ethylene vinyl acetate that slowly releases the ETG.

INJECTABLES (DEPOT MEDROXYPROGESTERONE ACETATE: DEPO-PROVER OR DMPA)
Current Use

Depo-Provera or DMPA has become a popular contraceptive choice and is widely used among AYA women in the US. According to NSFG data (from 2006 to 2010), approximately 3.5% of all female adolescents, aged 15 to 19 years, use DMPA as their contraceptive method. For 20- to 24-year-olds and 25- to 29-year-olds, 3.3% to 3.4% reported DMPA use compared to 0.6% to 1.7% reported DMPA use among 30- to 44-year-old women (see Chapter 43).[18]

Advantages

Advantages of this intermediate-acting contraceptive include the following:

- High effectiveness including a 2-week grace period, which can be ideal for AYA women who have poor adherence to other user-dependent methods
- Estrogen-free contraceptive
- Convenience and low maintenance as well as intercourse and partner independent
- Initial cost of approximately $50 per injection for each 12-week interval of use
- Ideal method for breast-feeding women; given its lack of negative impact on lactation and infant's growth[19,20]
- For young women with sickle cell disease, DMPA is particularly beneficial because it reduces the incidence of sickle cell crises.[21]
- Likewise, for women with seizure disorders, DMPA raises the seizure threshold, resulting in a lowering of seizure episodes.[22] In addition, DMPA does not have drug interactions with common anticonvulsants that compromise the effectiveness of other oral and implantable contraceptive methods.
- Amenorrhea is common with longer-term use (50% after the first year of use, 75% after 2 years, and 80% by 5 years of use).[23] Amenorrhea is a side effect that is frequently desired by AYA women and can prevent anemia and iron deficiency.
- Other benefits include decreased incidence of primary dysmenorrhea, endometriosis, ovulation pain, improvement of menstrual symptoms (breast tenderness, mood swings, headaches, nausea, and cyclic menstrual cramps), and functional ovarian cysts.[24]
- DMPA also decreases risk of endometrial cancer by 80%, and decreases incidence of uterine fibroids and ectopic pregnancies.
- Because DMPA creates thick mucus and amenorrhea, there is a decreased incidence of PID in adolescents with cervicitis who use DMPA.

Availability in the US

DMPA is the only injectable preparation for contraception available in the US. It was FDA approved for contraception in October 1992. Its intramuscular (IM) formulation consists of 150 mg of medroxyprogesterone acetate (a pregnane 17α-hydroxyprogesterone-derivative) in an aqueous suspension of microcrystals in a lipid base, and is administered in the gluteal or deltoid area every 11 to 13 weeks. This preparation works as a long-acting delivery system due to the low solubility of the microcrystals. The FDA approved a micronized formulation of 104 mg DMPA in December 2004 that can be administered subcutaneously in either the abdomen or thigh (DMPA-SC).

COMBINATION METHODS: COCs, CONTRACEPTIVE PATCH, AND CONTRACEPTIVE RING

Combined methods include COCs, the combined hormonal patch (P), and the combined vaginal ring (R). The combined hormonal patch and vaginal ring are relatively newer contraceptive methods. Combination hormonal contraceptives do not protect against sexually transmitted infections (STIs) or HIV (see Chapter 43).

Combination Oral Contraceptive Pills

Current Use

COCs have been the most common contraceptive method used by women and their partners in the US, second to female sterilization. COC use has remained stable since 1995 (28%) until the last data collected in 2006 to 2010 (27%). Approximately 50% of women under age 25 years use COCs: 53% of those aged 15 to 19 and 47% of those aged 20 to 24 years according to the last data analyzed in the last National Health Statistics reports.

Advantages

COCs have many noncontraceptive benefits and are first-line off-label therapy for women who experience heavy or prolonged menstrual bleeding, infrequent or painful menses, recurrent luteal phase ovarian cysts, family history of ovarian cancer, personal risk factors for endometrial cancer, acne and hirsutism, and polycystic ovary syndrome (PCOS). COCs also regulate menstrual periods, improve premenstrual syndrome (PMS) and premenstrual dysphoric disorder (PMDD), and decrease anovulatory bleeding, pain caused by ovulation (Mittelschmerz disease syndrome), menstrual migraines, risk of benign breast conditions, episodes of sickle cell crises, catamenial seizures, iron deficiency anemia, symptoms of endometriosis, and risk of uterine fibroids. They have favorable impact on bone for high-risk women. In addition, extended use of COCs are an off-label for treatment of anemia due to heavy or prolonged menstrual bleeding and control of menses in developmentally delayed women who often struggle with menstrual hygiene.[14]

Availability

Different formulations are available: monophasic, multiphasic, and variable combinations, but they all have similar advantages and effectiveness.[24] Even though COC components and doses have changed over time with new hormone compounds being introduced, the two chief components remain the same: estrogen and progestin. The first estrogen was mestranol, currently replaced by ethinyl estradiol (EE) in most formulations, but in different doses (ranging from 50 μg down most recently to 10 μg). Ten different progestins have been used in COCs that are available in the US. There are different progestin classification systems, but the most commonly used categorizes progestins in generations: The first three generations of progestins are derived from 19-nortestosterone and the fourth generation is drospirenone. Newer progestins are hybrids.

Contraceptive Ring and Patch

Current Use

Ever use of the contraceptive ring among sexually experienced female adolescents aged 15 to 19 in the US has been reported as 5.2% in 2006 to 2010.[21] Contraceptive patch use increased from 1.5% in 2002 to 10.3% in 2006 to 2010[3] There are no data on use patterns among women aged 20 to 24 years of age.

Advantages

Ring and patch advantages are similar to COCs, with the benefit that neither method requires daily use nor oral administration and they are verifiable methods, which could facilitate consistent and correct use. Both methods have comparable cycle control to COCs. More specifically, the ring has excellent cycle control, especially in the first 6 months of use, and is less likely to produce irregular bleeding compared to COCs. Patch users experience more break through bleeding in the first 2 cycles of use compared to COC users.

Availability

The vaginal contraceptive ring (Nuvaring) was FDA approved in 2001. It is a soft, translucent, and flexible ethylene vinyl acetate copolymer ring with a 4 mm cross-sectional diameter. It releases 120 μg of etonogestrel and 15 μg of EE daily. The ring is designed to be placed vaginally and kept in for 3 weeks, then removed for 7 days to allow withdrawal bleed before insertion of a new ring.

In 2002, the FDA approved a transdermal contraceptive patch (Ortho Evra), a beige colored 20 cm² patch that releases 6 mg of norelgestromin and 0.75 mcg of EE daily. The patch is applied to upper arms or torso (excluding the breasts), lower abdomen or buttocks for 7 days, and replaced weekly for 3 weeks, allowing a patch-free week for withdrawal bleeding before starting the next cycle.

Progestin-Only Pills

Current Availability

The progestin dose is lower in progestin-only pills (POPs) compared to the dose in COCs (hence it is called the "mini-pill"). Worldwide, commercially available POPs contain low doses of levonorgestrel (LNG), norethindrone (norethisterone), ethynodiol diacetate, or desogestrel. In the US, the only available POPs contain 0.35 mg norethindrone (Micronor, Nor-QD, Jolivette, Camila, Heather, Nora-BE or Errin). Packs of POPs contain 28 active pills with no placebo pills or hormone-free week, and, for maximum efficacy, they must be taken within 3 hours of the same time every day.

Advantages

The pill-taking regimen for POPs is fixed: The same color pill is taken every day at the same time without a "placebo" week; there are no days without pill taking, and there are no placebo pills in the pack. Since POPs do not contain estrogen, there is no increase in risk of stroke, myocardial infarction, or venous thromboembolism.[25] POPs may be a good choice when an adolescent wants an oral contraceptive but cannot tolerate estrogen-related side effects. Due to the limited duration of action of POPs compared to COCs, adherence to the narrow time frame acceptable to maintain effective contraceptive coverage may be particularly difficult; nevertheless, POPs can be an acceptable alternative that should be offered to adolescents who want an oral progestin-only contraceptive method.

HELPING AN ADOLESCENT OR YOUNG ADULT WOMAN SELECT THE CONTRACEPTIVE METHOD THAT IS RIGHT FOR HER

When helping an adolescent or young adult woman choose a method of contraception, the characteristics of method, as well as patient needs, should be taken into account. On one side, the patient and clinician together should consider method convenience, effectiveness, STI and PID risk reduction, minimizing adverse effects, and maximizing noncontraceptive benefits of each method. On the other side, AYA women face challenges that include difficulty with access, cost, confidentiality, and age- and life-stage-appropriate medical services, as well as complexities inherent to different adolescent developmental stages (concrete thinking, incomplete understanding of direct consequences of risk-taking behaviors, importance of adherence to medication regimens, lack of independence in terms of financial costs/insurance and transportation issues, etc.). Patients with certain health conditions need particular consideration when selecting a suitable and safe contraceptive. Figure 41.1 summarizes medical eligibility criteria for contraceptive use. For example, estrogen-containing methods are contraindicated for those who have migraine headaches with aura, a history of thromboembolic events, etc. Also, some methods provide particular noncontraceptive benefits, such as DMPA for those with sickle cell disease or a seizure disorder, or those on concomitant medications that decrease the effectiveness of hormonal contraceptives that go through first-pass metabolism.

The CDC United States Selective Practice Recommendations for Contraceptive use 2013 (US SPR)[7] recommend that all women

Summary Chart of US Medical Eligibility Criteria for Contraceptive Use

Updated June 2012. This summary sheet only contains a subset of the recommendations from the US MEC. For complete guidance, see: http://www.cdc.gov/reproductivehealth/unintendedpregnancy/USMEC.htm

Most contraceptive methods do not protect against sexually transmitted infections (STIs). Consistent and correct use of the male latex condom reduces the risk of STIs and HIV.

Key:
1   No restriction (method can be used)
2   Advantages generally outweigh theoretical or proven risks
3   Theoretical or proven risks usually outweigh the advantages
4   Unacceptable health risk (method not to be used)

Condition	Sub-condition	Combined pill, patch, ring I	C	Progestin-only pill I	C	Injection I	C	Implant I	C	LNG–IUD I	C	Copper-IUD I	C
Age		Menarche to <40=1; ≥40=2		Menarche to <18=1; 18-45=1; >45=1		Menarche to <18=2; 18-45=1; >45=2		Menarche to <18=1; 18-45=1; >45=1		Menarche to <20=2; ≥20=1		Menarche to <20=2; ≥20=1	
Anatomic abnormalities	a) Distorted uterine cavity									4		4	
	b) Other abnormalities									2		2	
Anemias	a) Thalassemia	1		1		1		1		1		2	
	b) Sickle cell disease‡	2		1		1		1		1		2	
	c) Iron-deficiency anemia	1		1		1		1		1		2	
Benign ovarian tumors	(including cysts)	1		1		1		1		1		1	
Breast disease	a) Undiagnosed mass	2*		2*		2*		2*		2		1	
	b) Benign breast disease	1		1		1		1		1		1	
	c) Family history of cancer	1		1		1		1		1		1	
	d) Breast cancer‡												
	i) current	4		4		4		4		4		1	
	ii) past and no evidence of current disease for 5 years	3		3		3		3		3		1	
Breastfeeding (see also Postpartum)	a) < 1 month postpartum	3*		2*		2*		2*					
	b) 1 month or more postpartum	2*		1*		1*		1*					
Cervical cancer	Awaiting treatment	2		1		2		2		4	2	4	2
Cervical ectropion		1		1		1		1		1		1	
Cervical intraepithelial neoplasia		2		1		2		2		2		1	
Cirrhosis	a) Mild (compensated)	1		1		1		1		1		1	
	b) Severe‡ (decompensated)	4		3		3		3		3		1	
Deep venous thrombosis (DVT)/Pulmonary embolism (PE)	a) History of DVT/PE, not on anticoagulant therapy												
	i) higher risk for recurrent DVT/PE	4		2		2		2		2		1	
	ii) lower risk for recurrent DVT/PE	3		2		2		2		2		1	
	b) Acute DVT/PE	4		2		2		2		2		2	
	c) DVT/PE and established on anticoagulant therapy for at least 3 months												
	i) higher risk for recurrent DVT/PE	4*		2		2		2		2		2	
	ii) lower risk for recurrent DVT/PE	3*		2		2		2		2		2	
	d) Family history (first-degree relatives)	2		1		1		1		1		1	
	e) Major surgery												
	(i) with prolonged immobilization	4		2		2		2		2		1	
	(ii) without prolonged immobilization	2		1		1		1		1		1	
	f) Minor surgery without immobilization	1		1		1		1		1		1	

FIGURE 41.1 US Medical Eligibility Criteria that rates the safety of contraceptive methods for women with a variety of underlying medical conditions. (From Centers for Disease Control and Prevention (CDC), *Division of Reproductive Health, National Center for Chronic Disease Prevention and Health Promotion.* United States Medical Eligibility Criteria (USMEC) for Contraceptive Use, 2010: Summary Chart of US Medical Eligibility Criteria for Contraceptive Use. Updated June 2012. Available at: http://www.cdc.gov/reproductivehealth/unintendedpregnancy/USMEC.htm.)

Condition	Sub-condition	Combined pill, patch, ring I	C	Progestin-only pill I	C	Injection I	C	Implant I	C	LNG–IUD I	C	Copper-IUD I	C
Depressive disorders		1*		1*		1*		1*		1*		1*	
Diabetes mellitus (DM)	a) History of gestational DM only	1		1		1		1		1		1	
	b) Non-vascular disease												
	(i) non-insulin dependent	2		2		2		2		2		1	
	(ii) insulin dependent‡	2		2		2		2		2		1	
	c) Nephropathy/ retinopathy/ neuropathy‡	3/4*		2		3		2		2		1	
	d) Other vascular disease or diabetes of >20 years' duration‡	3/4*		2		3		2		2		1	
Endometrial cancer‡		1		1		1		1		4	2	4	2
Endometrial hyperplasia		1		1		1		1		1		1	
Endometriosis		1		1		1		1		1		2	
Epilepsy‡	(see also Drug Interactions)	1*		1*		1*		1*		1		1	
Gallbladder disease	a) Symptomatic												
	(i) treated by cholecystectomy	2		2		2		2		2		1	
	(ii) medically treated	3		2		2		2		2		1	
	(iii) current	3		2		2		2		2		1	
	b) Asymptomatic	2		2		2		2		2		1	
Gestational trophoblastic disease	a) Decreasing or undetectable ß-hCG levels	1		1		1		1		3		3	
	b) Persistently elevated ß-hCG levels or malignant disease‡	1		1		1		1		4		4	
Headaches	a) Non-migrainous	1*	2*	1*	1*	1*	1*	1*	1*	1*	1*	1*	
	b) Migraine												
	i) without aura, age <35	2*	3*	1*	2*	2*	2*	2*	2*	2*	2*	1*	
	ii) without aura, age ≥35	3*	4*	1*	2*	2*	2*	2*	2*	2*	2*	1*	
	iii) with aura, any age	4*	4*	2*	3*	2*	3*	2*	3*	2*	3*	1*	
History of bariatric surgery‡	a) Restrictive procedures	1		1		1		1		1		1	
	b) Malabsorptive procedures	COCs: 3 P/R: 1		3		1		1		1		1	
History of cholestasis	a) Pregnancy-related	2		1		1		1		1		1	
	b) Past COC-related	3		2		2		2		2		1	
History of high blood pressure during pregnancy		2		1		1		1		1		1	
History of pelvic surgery		1		1		1		1		1		1	
HIV	High risk	1		1		1*		1		2	2	2	2
	HIV infected (see also Drug Interactions)‡	1*		1*		1*		1*		2	2	2	2
	AIDS (see also Drug Interactions)‡	1*		1*		1*		1*		3	2*	3	2*
	Clinically well on therapy	If on treatment, see Drug Interactions								2	2	2	2
Hyperlipidemias		2/3*		2*		2*		2*		2*		1*	
Hypertension	a) Adequately controlled hypertension	3*		1*		2*		1*		1		1	
	b) Elevated blood pressure levels (properly taken measurements)												
	(i) systolic 140–159 or diastolic 90–99	3		1		2		1		1		1	
	(ii) systolic ≥160 or diastolic ≥100‡	4		2		3		2		2		1	
	c) Vascular disease	4		2		3		2		2		1	

FIGURE 41.1 (*Continued*) US Medical Eligibility Criteria that rates the safety of contraceptive methods for women with a variety of underlying medical conditions. (From Centers for Disease Control and Prevention (CDC), *Division of Reproductive Health, National Center for Chronic Disease Prevention and Health Promotion.* United States Medical Eligibility Criteria (USMEC) for Contraceptive Use, 2010: Summary Chart of US Medical Eligibility Criteria for Contraceptive Use. Updated June 2012. Available at: http://www.cdc.gov/reproductivehealth/unintendedpregnancy/USMEC.htm.)

Condition	Sub-condition	Combined pill, patch, ring I	C	Progestin-only pill I	C	Injection I	C	Implant I	C	LNG-IUD I	C	Copper-IUD I	C
Inflammatory bowel disease	(Ulcerative colitis, Crohn's disease)	2/3*		2		2		1		1		1	
Ischemic heart disease‡	Current and history of	4		2	3	3		2	3	2	3	1	
Liver tumors	a) Benign												
	i) Focal nodular hyperplasia	2		2		2		2		2		1	
	ii) Hepatocellular adenoma‡	4		3		3		3		3		1	
	b) Malignant‡	4		3		3		3		3		1	
Malaria		1		1		1		1		1		1	
Multiple risk factors for arterial cardiovascular disease	(such as older age, smoking, diabetes and hypertension)	3/4*		2*		3*		2*		2		1	
Obesity	a) ≥30 kg/m² body mass index (BMI)	2		1		1		1		1		1	
	b) Menarche to < 18 years and ≥ 30 kg/m² BMI	2		1		2		1		1		1	
Ovarian cancer‡		1		1		1		1		1		1	
Parity	a) Nulliparous	1		1		1		1		2		2	
	b) Parous	1		1		1		1		1		1	
Past ectopic pregnancy		1		2		1		1		1		1	
Pelvic inflammatory disease	a) Past, (assuming no current risk factors of STIs)												
	(i) with subsequent pregnancy	1		1		1		1		1	1	1	1
	(ii) without subsequent pregnancy	1		1		1		1		2	2	2	2
	b) Current	1		1		1		1		4	2*	4	2*
Peripartum cardiomyopathy‡	a) Normal or mildly impaired cardiac function												
	(i) < 6 months	4		1		1		1		2		2	
	(ii) ≥ 6 months	3		1		1		1		2		2	
	b) Moderately or severely impaired cardiac function	4		2		2		2		2		2	
Postabortion	a) First trimester	1*		1*		1*		1*		1*		1*	
	b) Second trimester	1*		1*		1*		1*		2		2	
	c) Immediately post-septic abortion	1*		1*		1*		1*		4		4	
Postpartum (see also Breastfeeding)	a) < 21 days	4		1		1		1					
	b) 21 days to 42 days												
	(i) with other risk factors for VTE	3*		1		1		1					
	(ii) without other risk factors for VTE	2		1		1		1					
	c) > 42 days	1		1		1		1					
Postpartum (in breastfeeding or non-breastfeeding women, including post-cesarean section)	a) < 10 minutes after delivery of the placenta									2		1	
	b) 10 minutes after delivery of the placenta to < 4 weeks									2		2	
	c) ≥ 4 weeks									1		1	
	d) Puerperal sepsis									4		4	
Pregnancy		NA*		NA*		NA*		NA*		4*		4*	
Rheumatoid arthritis	a) On immunosuppressive therapy	2		1		2/3*		1		2	1	2	1
	b) Not on immunosuppressive therapy	2		1		2		1		1		1	
Schistosomiasis	a) Uncomplicated	1		1		1		1		1		1	
	b) Fibrosis of the liver‡	1		1		1		1		1		1	
Severe dysmenorrhea		1		1		1		1		1		2	

FIGURE 41.1 (*Continued*) US Medical Eligibility Criteria that rates the safety of contraceptive methods for women with a variety of underlying medical conditions. (From Centers for Disease Control and Prevention (CDC), *Division of Reproductive Health, National Center for Chronic Disease Prevention and Health Promotion.* United States Medical Eligibility Criteria (USMEC) for Contraceptive Use, 2010: Summary Chart of US Medical Eligibility Criteria for Contraceptive Use. Updated June 2012. Available at: http://www.cdc.gov/reproductivehealth/unintendedpregnancy/USMEC.htm.)

Condition	Sub-condition	Combined pill, patch, ring I	C	Progestin-only pill I	C	Injection I	C	Implant I	C	LNG–IUD I	C	Copper-IUD I	C
Sexually transmitted infections (STIs)	a) Current purulent cervicitis or chlamydial infection or gonorrhea	1		1		1		1		4	2*	4	2*
	b) Other STIs (excluding HIV and hepatitis)	1		1		1		1		2	2	2	2
Sexually transmitted infections (cont.)	c) Vaginitis (including trichomonas vaginalis and bacterial vaginosis)	1		1		1		1		2	2	2	2
	d) Increased risk of STIs	1		1		1		1		2/3*	2	2/3*	2
Smoking	a) Age < 35	2		1		1		1		1		1	
	b) Age ≥ 35, < 15 cigarettes/day	3		1		1		1		1		1	
	c) Age ≥ 35, ≥15 cigarettes/day	4		1		1		1		1		1	
Solid organ transplantation‡	a) Complicated	4		2		2		2		3	2	3	2
	b) Uncomplicated	2*		2		2		2		2		2	
Stroke‡	History of cerebrovascular accident	4		2	3	3		2	3	2		1	
Superficial venous thrombosis	a) Varicose veins	1		1		1		1		1		1	
	b) Superficial thrombophlebitis	2		1		1		1		1		1	
Systemic lupus erythematosus‡	a) Positive (or unknown) antiphospholipid antibodies	4		3		3	3	3		3		1	1
	b) Severe thrombocytopenia	2		2		3	2	2		2*		3*	2*
	c) Immunosuppressive treatment	2		2		2	2	2		2		2	1
	d) None of the above	2		2		2	2	2		2		1	1
Thrombogenic mutations‡		4*		2*		2*		2*		2*		1*	
Thyroid disorders	Simple goiter/hyperthyroid/hypothyroid	1		1		1		1		1		1	
Tuberculosis‡ (see also Drug Interactions)	a) Non-pelvic	1*		1*		1*		1*		1		1	
	b) Pelvic	1*		1*		1*		1*		4	3	4	3
Unexplained vaginal bleeding	(suspicious for serious condition) before evaluation	2*		2*		3*		3*		4*	2*	4*	2*
Uterine fibroids		1		1		1		1		2		2	
Valvular heart disease	a) Uncomplicated	2		1		1		1		1		1	
	b) Complicated‡	4		1		1		1		1		1	
Vaginal bleeding patterns	a) Irregular pattern without heavy bleeding	1		2		2		2		1	1	1	
	b) Heavy or prolonged bleeding	1*		2*		2*		2*		1*	2*	2*	
Viral hepatitis	a) Acute or flare	3/4*	2	1		1		1		1		1	
	b) Carrier/Chronic	1	1	1		1		1		1		1	
Drug Interactions													
Antiretroviral therapy	a) Nucleoside reverse transcriptase inhibitors	1*		1		1		1		2/3*	2*	2/3*	2*
	b) Non-nucleoside reverse transcriptase inhibitors	2*		2*		1		2*		2/3*	2*	2/3*	2*
	c) Ritonavir-boosted protease inhibitors	3*		3*		1		2*		2/3*	2*	2/3*	2*
Anticonvulsant therapy	a) Certain anticonvulsants (phenytoin, carbamazepine, barbiturates, primidone, topiramate, oxcarbazepine)	3*		3*		1		2*		1		1	
	b) Lamotrigine	3*		1		1		1		1		1	
Antimicrobial therapy	a) Broad spectrum antibiotics	1		1		1		1		1		1	
	b) Antifungals	1		1		1		1		1		1	
	c) Antiparasitics	1		1		1		1		1		1	
	d) Rifampicin or rifabutin therapy	3*		3*		1		2*		1		1	

I = initiation of contraceptive method; C = continuation of contraceptive method; NA = Not applicable

* Please see the complete guidance for a clarification to this classification: www.cdc.gov/reproductivehealth/unintendedpregnancy/USMEC.htm

‡ Condition that exposes a woman to increased risk as a result of unintended pregnancy.

FIGURE 41.1 (*Continued*) US Medical Eligibility Criteria that rates the safety of contraceptive methods for women with a variety of underlying medical conditions. (From Centers for Disease Control and Prevention (CDC), *Division of Reproductive Health, National Center for Chronic Disease Prevention and Health Promotion.* United States Medical Eligibility Criteria (USMEC) for Contraceptive Use, 2010: Summary Chart of US Medical Eligibility Criteria for Contraceptive Use. Updated June 2012. Available at: http://www.cdc.gov/reproductivehealth/unintendedpregnancy/USMEC.htm.)

be counseled about the full range of effective contraceptive options for which they are medically eligible so that they can pick the optimal method for themselves (Fig. 41.1). Although there are highly effective, reversible methods available in offering hormonal contraceptive methods including IUDs and implants to AYA women, it is important to assess STI, HIV, and PID risk, and discuss with patients that LARCs and other moderately effective hormonal methods do not prevent STIs or HIV. Consistent and correct use of male latex condoms reduces the risk for HIV infection and other STIs, including chlamydial, gonorrhea, and trichomoniasis infections. In addition, it is important to discuss that certain infections, such as herpes simplex virus (HSV), human papillomavirus (HPV), molluscum contagiosum, and pubic lice, can be transmitted despite condom use.

SPECIAL ISSUES IN PROVIDING CONTRACEPTION TO AYAs WITH CHRONIC MEDICAL CONDITIONS

The recommendations for contraception use among young women who have varying medical conditions is well described in the US MEC for Contraceptive Use (Fig. 41.1).[7] This is an excellent resource with a chart that includes recommendations on each contraceptive method and for most chronic illness http://www.cdc.gov/reproductivehealth/unintendedpregnancy/usmec.htm.

Included on this Web site are the initial and updated recommendations, as well as charts in English and Spanish in both MS word and pdf format. The CDC has a new app that includes the US MEC[7] that is available for the iphone and ipad. The following section includes contraceptive recommendations and considerations in AYAs with psychiatric (depressive disorders are covered in the above outlined recommendations) and intellectual disabilities that are not covered in this chart.

Psychiatric Disease and Intellectual Disabilities

Adolescents with psychiatric conditions frequently have their family planning needs overlooked. Issues arising may include the following:

- Recognition of the contraceptive need
- Individuals capacity to give informed consent
- Ability to utilize some of the contraceptive methods

Some individuals with mental illness may have a dual diagnosis, including substance abuse or seizure disorder. Barrier methods provide needed reduction in the risk of acquiring an STI, but they may not be used consistently. LARC methods may be an excellent primary form of contraception, but potential interactions with medications (e.g., seizure medications) need to be considered in this recommendation, in particular with a contraceptive implant. AYAs with intellectual disabilities in an institutional setting may benefit from a LARC where compliance may be a problem with other methods. This population is potentially vulnerable for exploitation, so both sex education and an effective form of contraception is important. Oral contraceptives in this setting may have low compliance rates.

EMERGENCY CONTRACEPTION

EC is the only contraceptive method designed to prevent pregnancy after intercourse.

Prevention of Ovulation versus Implantation

Emergency contraceptive pills (ECPs) do not interrupt an established pregnancy, defined by medical authorities, including the FDA, National Institutes of Health (NIH), and the ACOG as beginning with implantation. Therefore, ECPs are not abortifacients. When advising women, it is important to clarify that ECPs, like any of the other hormonal contraceptives (including COPs, POPs,

DMPA, implant, ring, and patch), prevent pregnancy primarily by delaying or inhibiting ovulation and inhibiting fertilization, but it is not scientifically possible to rule out definitively that a method may inhibit implantation of a fertilized egg in the endometrium. However, the best available evidence shows that both the mechanism of action of LNG and ulipristal acetate (UPA) ECPs to prevent pregnancy can be fully accounted for by mechanisms that do not involve interference with post-fertilization events. Of note, the very high effectiveness of the copper IUD implies a possible post-fertilization effect.[26]

The National Centers for Health Statistics reported in February 2013 that during the 2006 to 2010 period, one in nine sexually experienced women aged 15 to 44 used EC at least once. EC use was most common among women aged 20 to 24 years, those who never married, Hispanic or non-Hispanic White women, and those who had attended college. This study also showed that most women who used EC had done so once or twice. The reasons for EC use were noted to differ by age, ethnic/racial, and educational level of the groups: around 50% of women reported having used it because of fear of method failure (often older women, non-Hispanic White women, and women with more education), and the other 50% cited the main reason as having had unprotected sex (more common among Non-Hispanic Black and Hispanic women and those with less education). Legal over-the-counter (OTC) access to EC for girls younger than 17 years old was restricted during the time the data for this report was collected.

Advance Prescription

Writing AYA women an advance prescription of EC, before it is needed, may facilitate access by reducing the cost of obtaining EC for those whose insurance covers EC by prescription. Studies have shown that adolescents are more likely to use EC if it has been prescribed in advance of need[27]; these studies also showed no increase in sexual activity or decrease in use of ongoing contraceptive use. However, a majority of practicing pediatricians and pediatric residents do not routinely counsel patients about EC and have not prescribed it. The AAP released a policy statement on EC in 2012 encouraging education of providers on available EC, routine counseling and advanced EC prescription as a public health strategy to reduce teen pregnancy.[28]

Relative Effectiveness

The exact effectiveness of ECPs is difficult to measure, and some researchers believe the effectiveness may be lower than that reported on package labels. Overall, the copper IUD is the most effective EC method, followed by UPA or Ella and then POPs containing LNG.[26,29,30] The use of COCs for EC (Yuzpe method) is no longer a standard of care. When used for EC, the Copper-T IUD is 99% effective in reducing pregnancy risk.[31] There is no mention of the effectiveness of Ella in the patient package insert or provider label. However, the observed and expected pregnancies reported in two Phase III clinical trials suggest effectiveness rates of 60% and 66%. The failure rate has been described as approximately 1.4%.[31] The effectiveness listed on the Plan B/Next Choice package is 89%. The failure rate has been described as approximately 2% to 3%.[31] UPA is at least as effective as LNG when used within the first 72 hours after unprotected intercourse. *However, UPA is more effective than LNG when used between 72 and 120 hours after unprotected intercourse, and, therefore, constitutes a better option for women who require EC on the 4th and 5th days after unprotected intercourse.*[32] Two trials comparing UPA 30-mg single dose to LNG 1.5-mg single dose in a meta-analysis found that UPA was more effective compared to LNG within 72 hours after unprotected intercourse (RR 0.63), which was significant at a marginal level ($p = 0.08$).[30,33] When the 72- to 120-hour data from the Glasier 2010 trial were included in meta-analysis, UPA was associated with lower risk of pregnancy than LNG and the difference was significant at the 0.05 level.[29]

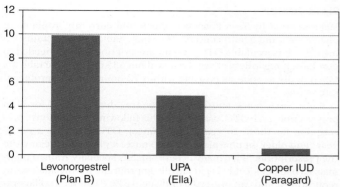

FIGURE 41.2 Pregnancies expected per 1,000 women who had unprotected sex in the past week.

The published literature on combined progestin-estrogen ECPs estimates a range of effectiveness between 56% and 89% in reducing pregnancy risk. Data clearly show that the progestin-only ECP regimen is more effective than the Yuzpe method. Five trials reviewed by Cochrane with data from 4,221 women[29] compared the Yuzpe regimen with LNG 0.75 mg given twice 12 hours apart. Data showed that LNG was more effective in preventing pregnancy than the Yuzpe regimen (RR 0.54; 95% CI 0.36 to 0.80).

The effectiveness rates listed on Figure 41.2 have known discrepancies. Also, as mentioned before, most published efficacy data for ECPs are probably overestimates.

COPPER IUD FOR EC (PARAGARD)

The copper IUD is manufactured by Teva. According to guidelines from ACOG, for EC the copper IUD should be inserted within 5 days of unprotected intercourse.[34] This method can be used beyond 5 days, as long as the time of ovulation can be reasonably determined and the insertion occurs no more than 5 days after ovulation.[7] This insertion timing would ensure insertion before implantation, if one is seeking a contraceptive action versus an early abortifacient.[31]

Mechanism of Action

A foreign body sterile inflammatory process, via production of cytotoxic peptides and activation of enzymes, leads to inhibition of sperm motility, reduced sperm capacitation and survival, and increased phagocytosis. Copper also causes an increase in copper ions, enzymes, prostaglandins and macrophages in uterine and tubal fluids, impairing sperm function and preventing fertilization.[24] The very high effectiveness of the copper-releasing IUD when used for EC implies that it may also act by preventing implantation of the blastocyst.[35]

Advantages

The copper IUD is the only EC that can also provide 10 to 12 years of ongoing highly effective contraception for women with no copper allergy. In addition to being one of the most cost-effective ongoing methods of contraception, it is the most effective EC and therefore the best choice when unprotected sexual intercourse occurs around the time of ovulation. Women who have intercourse around ovulation should ideally be offered a copper IUD. It is also the best option for women with elevated body mass index (BMI >24), since data show no clinical concern of lower effectiveness with increased BMI[30] as compared to UPA and LNG EC methods. The copper IUD should also be considered, as in the case of all IUDs, for patients who have privacy concerns or who have partners who sabotage their contraception.

Side Effects

Menstrual disturbances such as menorrhagia and dysmenorrhea are common with copper IUDs. Menses can have increased length, flow, and discomfort during the first several cycles after the copper IUD is inserted. Dysmenorrhea and heavy menses are the most frequent reasons for copper IUC removal.[24] Average blood loses may increase up to 55%, although rarely leading to anemia.[36] Because the copper device does not contain hormones, it does not cause progestin-related side effects seen with LNG-IUDs. Rates of expulsion, perforation, and risk of PID do not differ when a copper IUD is used for EC compared to regular, ongoing use of an IUD for contraception. A recent study comparing IUD use among nulliparous and parous women found similar rates of complications, discontinuation, and expulsion. This study found that copper IUD users had a rate of PID of 3.5 per 1,000 women-years, rates of (ectopic) pregnancy of 0.6% to 1.1% per year, and rates of expulsion of 0% to 1.2% per year. Nulliparous women did not show more complications compared to parous women. There was not a significantly higher IUD removal rate among nulliparous women compared to parous women. Main reasons for removal were "menstrual problems" and "contraception no longer necessary."[37]

The copper IUD is largely underused for EC. Harper et al.[38] recently conducted a survey among 1,246 clinicians (response rate 65%) in a California State family planning program, where US FDA-approved contraceptives are available at no cost to low-income women. The results showed that the large majority of clinicians (85%) never recommended the copper IUD for EC, and most (93%) required two or more visits for an IUD insertion. Recommendation of the copper IUD for EC is rare, despite its high efficacy and long-lasting contraceptive benefits. Although same day insertion of IUDs for EC and ongoing contraception use could greatly enhance access, especially to young women, and is ideal clinical practice, this service requires clinic flow and scheduling adjustments.

ULIPRISTAL ACETATE OR UPA (ELLA) FOR EC

Ulipristal acetate or UPA is a second-generation progesterone receptor (PR) modulator, which has been marketed in Europe since 2009 and was FDA approved in 2010 [http://www.rhtp.org/contraception/emergency/documents/FDAApprovedEmergencyContraceptiveChartDecember2011-PRINTABLE_000.pdf]. It is manufactured by Watson Pharmaceuticals. UPA is available in health clinics, and only by prescription in pharmacies in both Europe and the US, regardless of age. Pharmacy prices tend to be $5 to $10 more than Plan B OneStep. Since it is prescription only, it is covered by some private and public insurance. Ella may be ordered from online prescription service—https://www.ella-kwikmed.com. The pill is mailed the following day, and the cost of the product plus shipping is $42.

Mechanism of Action

UPA is a derivative of 19-norprogesterone that binds to PRs to produce an antiprogesterone contraceptive effect. Antiglucocorticoid and antiandrogen activities were observed at doses 50-fold greater than that necessary for an antiprogestin effect. One tablet of 30 mg of UPA is taken orally as soon as possible within 120 hours (5 days) of unprotected intercourse or a known or suspected contraceptive failure. UPA has different mechanism of action, depending on the time of the menstrual cycle when it is administered. When administered during the mid-follicular phase, UPA inhibits folliculogenesis, leading to delayed ovulation and decreased estradiol concentrations. When administered during the LH surge, follicular rupture is delayed by 5 to 9 days. Changes in endometrial thickness may affect luteal implantation.[39] Even on the day of the LH peak, UPA could delay ovulation for 24 to 48 hours after administration. These results suggest that UPA may have a direct inhibitory effect on follicular rupture that allows UPA to be effective, even when administered before ovulation when LH has already started to rise, a time when LNG is no longer effective. The effect of UPA on the endometrium has also been demonstrated to be dose-dependent. Treatment with 10 to 100 mg of UPA resulted in inhibition of downregulation of PRs, reduced endometrial thickness, and delayed histologic maturation with the highest dose, while the effect of lower doses equivalent to the 30 mg used for EC were similar to that of placebo.[26]

Advantages

Clinical trials show that UPA is a well-tolerated and effective method of EC when used within 120 hours of intercourse. Unlike LNG, UPA's effectiveness does not decline with delay in treatment. Therefore, UPA is an excellent option for women in need of EC who present "late" after unprotected intercourse.[30] Obese and overweight women also have a higher oral EC failure rate. Data from a meta-analysis of two randomized controlled trials comparing the efficacy of UPA showed that the risk of pregnancy was more than three-fold greater for obese women (BMI of 30 kg/m^2 or greater, OR = 3.60, CI 1.96–6.53; p < 0.0001) and more than 1.5 times higher for overweight women (BMI 25 to 30 kg/m^2) when compared with women with normal BMI, regardless of which EC regimen was taken.[40] For obese women, the risk of pregnancy was greater for those taking LNG compared to UPA users. LNG showed a rapid decrease in efficacy with increasing BMI, reaching the point where it appeared no different from pregnancy rates expected among women not taking LNG at a BMI of 26 kg/m^2 compared with 35 kg/m^2 for UPA. For both ECs, pregnancy risk was related to the cycle day of intercourse. Women with BMI >25 kg/m^2 should be offered a copper IUD as first-line care or UPA if immediate copper IUD insertion is unavailable or declined by the patient.

Side Effects

In a recent study of 1,104 women with an average age of 24.5 years, old, adverse effects were reported in 54% of participants.[30] Most of side effects (94%) were rated as mild or moderate and were mostly headaches, dysmenorrhea, nausea, fatigue, dizziness, abdominal pain, and back pain (in order of frequency). Only one severe adverse event was associated with the use of EC in that study: a case of dizziness that resolved after 24 hours. Onset of next menses after EC occurred a mean 2.1 days (SD 8.2) *later* than expected in the UPA group, but duration of bleeding was not affected by UPA use. In women with available data on cycle length, menses occurred within 7 days of expected time in 769 (76%) of 1,013 women in the UPA group. The most frequently reported side effects for the Yuzpe method, nausea and vomiting, occur in 13% to 29% of women treated with LNG and UPA for EC compared to 50% having nausea and 20% having vomiting when COCs were used for EC.[24] Routine use of the antinausea medication, meclizine, 1 hour before the first ECP dose was studied and decreased nausea and vomiting associated with the Yuzpe method[41]; antinausea medication is generally considered unnecessary when using LNG or UPA for EC.[24]

⬤ LEVONORGESTREL PILLS FOR EC

Types
NextChoice

Manufactured by Watson Pharmaceuticals, Inc., this product is currently available in pharmacies and health centers and contains one tablet with 1.5 mg of LNG. This generic EC is currently priced around 10% to 20% lower than Plan B OneStep ($35 to $60).

LNG Tablets

Manufactured by Perrigo Pharmaceuticals, Inc., it is currently available in Rite Aid Pharmacies and other locations nationwide. Two tablets each, 0.75 mg LNG, this generic EC is currently priced around 10% to 20% lower than Plan B OneStep ($35 to $60).

Plan B OneStep

Manufactured by Teva Pharmaceuticals and currently available in pharmacies and health centers. The single-tablet dose contains 1.5 mg LNG. It is available OTC, and no prescription or ID is needed to purchase it regardless of age. Cost is about $35 to $60. One tablet is taken orally as soon as possible within 72 hours after unprotected intercourse.

Both NextChoice and LNG tablets are "dual labeled" for both prescription and OTC usage with the following restrictions: prescription for those 16 years and younger, OTC for those aged 17 years and older. In pharmacy access states, a pharmacist can write the prescription. "Pharmacy access" means specially trained pharmacists can decide if EC is medically appropriate for the adolescent requesting it and can prescribe or dispense ECPs under a collaborative agreement protocol. The States that currently have pharmacy access in place include Alaska, California, Hawaii, Maine, Massachusetts, New Hampshire, New Mexico, Vermont, and Washington State.[39]

Both NextChoice and Levonorgestrel tablets contain 2 tablets, each of 0.75 mg LNG. The first tablet should be taken orally as soon as possible within 72 hours after unprotected intercourse, and the second tablet should be taken 12 hours after the first dose. A recent meta-analysis from Cochrane reviewed data from three different trials showed that the efficacies of LNG 1.5-mg single-dose and 0.75-mg two-dose regimens 12 hours apart were similar.[29] Another double-blind randomized multicenter trial conducted in China[42] compared two regimens of LNG split-dose administrated at 24 hours or 12 hours apart showed that the two regimens had similar overall effectiveness (RR 0.98; 95% CI 0.53 to 1.82). Although not statistically significant, the 24-hour single-dose regimen appeared more effective than the 12-hour split-dose regimen among high-risk women. This is of particular importance for adolescents, among whom adherence may be more difficult.

Specific Advantages

OTC availability of LNG EC pills has dramatically increased women's access. Pharmacy access reduces barriers in many ways: not requiring appointments; being open evening, weekends, and holidays; offering OTC EC to men; prescribing EC to undocumented women immigrants and women Medicaid clients who otherwise cannot afford OTC ECPs, and women needing a prescription for their private insurance to cover the cost of ECPs.

Mechanism of Action

LNG EC delays ovulation and fertilization and may inhibit implantation, but it is not effective once implantation has begun. James Trusell and collaborators in their review in 2014 noted that literature shows so far that "early treatment with ECPs containing only LNG has been shown to impair the ovulatory process and luteal function.[26] The literature reviewed by Trusell and collaborators describes no effect on the endometrium was found in earlier studies, but in another study LNG taken before the LH surge altered the luteal phase secretory pattern of glycodelin in serum and the endometrium. However, this finding was not confirmed in two later studies explicitly designed to assess endometrial glycodelin expression. The second of these studies also found no effect on other endometrial receptivity biomarkers or PRs. In another study, LNG taken before the LH surge increased prematurely serum and intrauterine concentrations of glycodelin at the time of ovulation; since glycodelin inhibits fertilization, this result may indicate an additional mechanism of action when ovulation is not inhibited.

Side Effects

Studies have shown similar side effects for LNG and for UPA when used for EC. Reported complaints include fatigue, breast tenderness, headache, lower abdominal pain, dizziness, and diarrhea. As mentioned, LNG and UPA cause nausea and emesis in less users than the Yuzpe method.[20] In the study conducted by Glasier in 2010, the onset of next menses after EC occurred a mean 1.2 days (7.9), earlier than expected in the LNG group, but duration of bleeding was not affected by EC. In women with available data on cycle length, menses occurred within 7 days of expected time in 731 (71%) of 1,031 women in the LNG group compared to 769 (76%) of 1,013 women in the UPA group.[30] In 69 women with a reported stable menstrual cycle length of 24 to 34 days, bleeding patterns following EC administration in the follicular ($n = 26$), periovulatory ($n = 14$), and luteal ($n = 29$) phase were studied. Data obtained in this limited number of women indicated that EC administered before the onset of the LH surge inhibits ovulation and hastens the end of the current menstrual cycle. Thereafter, the menstrual cyclicity is "reset" and proceeds normally in the subsequent cycle. In contrast, EC administered after the onset of the LH peak has no effect on ovulation and consequently on cycle characteristics.

Repeated Use

Pregnancy risk increases with repeated acts of unprotected intercourse, especially after EC use. When women have multiple episodes of unprotected sexual intercourse, EC effectiveness decreases even when EC is used after every incident of unprotected intercourse. A copper IUD provides women with the best protection because all future episodes of intercourse will be protected. Some clinicians have worried that because UPA delays, rather than inhibits ovulation, that women might be at greater risk of pregnancy if they have subsequent unprotected intercourse after taking UPA compared to women who take LNG. However, the evidence does not support this.

REFERENCES

1. Curtin SC, Abma JC, Ventura SJ. *Pregnancy rates for U.S. women continue to drop*, NCHS Data Brief No. 136. December 2013. Available at http://www.cdc.gov/nchs/data/databriefs/db136.pdf.
2. United Nations. *Demographic yearbook 2012*. New York, NY: United Nations, 2010. Available at http://unstats.un.org/unsd/demographic/products/dyb/dyb2.htm. Accessed June 12, 2014.
3. Martinez G, Copen CE, Abma JC. Teenagers in the United States: sexual activity, contraceptive use, and childbearing, 2006–2010 National Survey of Family Growth. *Vital Health Stat* 2011;23:1–35.
4. Finer LB, Zolna MR, Shifts in intended and unintended pregnancies in the United States, 2001–2008. *Am J Public Health* 2014;104 (Suppl 1):S43–S48.
5. O'Neil-Callahan M, Peipert JF, Zhao Q, et al. Twenty-four-month continuation of reversible contraception. *Obstet Gynecol* 2013;122(5):1083–1091.
6. Kost K, Singh S, Vaughan B, et al. Estimates of contraceptive failure from the 2002 National Survey of Family Growth. *Contraception* 2008;77(1):10–21.
7. Centers for Disease Control and Prevention. *United States, selected practices recommendations for contraceptive use*. Atlanta, GA: Centers for Disease Control and Prevention, 2013. Available at www.cdc.gov/reproductivehealth/Unintended Pregnancy/USSPR.htm. Accessed June 2014.
8. Centers for Disease Control and Prevention. *United States Medical Eligibility Criteria (US MEC) for contraceptive use*. Atlanta, GA: Centers for Disease Control and Prevention, 2010. Available at http://www.cdc.gov/reproductivehealth/Unintended Pregnancy/USMEC.htm.
9. The American College of Obstetricians and Gynecologists, Women's Health Care Physicians. *Committee on Adolescent Health Care LARC Working Group*, Committee Opinion Number 539. October 2012.
10. McNicholas C, Peipert JF. Long-acting reversible contraception for adolescents. *Curr Opin Obstet Gynecol* 2012;24(5):293–298.
11. AAP Policy. Contraception for adolescents. *Pediatrics* 2014;134:e1244–e1256.
12. Finer LB, Jerman J, Kavanaugh ML. Changes in use of long-acting contraceptive methods in the United States, 2007–2009. *Fertil Steril* 2012;98:893–897.
13. United Nations, Department of Economic and Social Information and Policy Analysis, Population Division. *World contraceptive use*. 2011. Available at http://www.un.org/esa/population/publications/contraceptive2011/wallchart_front.pdf. Accessed May 8, 2014.
14. Russo JA, Miller E, Gold MA. Myths and misconceptions about long-acting reversible contraception (LARC). *J Adolesc Health* 2013;52(4, Suppl):S14–S21.
15. Daniels K, Mosher WD, Jones J. *Contraceptive methods women have ever used: United States, 1982–2010*, National Health Statistics Report No. 62. Hyattsville, MD: National Center for Health Statistics, February 14, 2013.
16. Funk S, Miller MM, Mishell Jr DR, et al. Safety and efficacy of Implanon, a single-rod implantable contraceptive containing etonogestrel. *Contraception*. 2005;71(5):319–26.
17. Guazzelli CA, de Queiroz FT, Barbieri M, et al. Etonogestrel implant in postpartum adolescents: bleeding pattern, efficacy and discontinuation rate. *Contraception* 2010;82(3):256–259.
18. Jones J, Mosher W, Daniels K. Current contraceptive use in the United States, 2006–2010, and changes in patterns of use since 1995. *Natl Health Stat Report* 2012;(60):1–25.
19. Brownell EA, Fernandez ID, Fisher SG, et al. The effect of immediate postpartum depot medroxyprogesterone on early breastfeeding cessation. *Contraception* 2013;87(6):836–843.
20. Singhal S, Sarda N, Gupta S, et al. Impact of injectable progestogen contraception in early puerperium on lactation and infant health. *J Clin Diagn Res* 2014;8:69–72.
21. ManchikantiA, Grimes DA, Lopez LM, et al. Steroid hormones for contraception in women with sickle cell disease. *Cochrane Database Syst Rev* 2007;(2):CD006261.
22. Mattson RH, Cramer JA, Darney PD, et al. Use of oral contraceptives by women with epilepsy. *JAMA* 1986;256:238–240.
23. Speroff L, Fritz MA. *Clinical gynecologic endocrinology and infertility*. Philadelphia, PA: Lippincott Williams & Wilkins, 2011.
24. Hatcher RA, Trussell J, Nelson AL, et al. *Contraceptive technology*. 20th revised ed. New York, NY: Contraceptive Technology Communications, 2011.
25. Department of Reproductive Health, World Health Organization. *Medical eligibility criteria for contraceptive use*. 4th ed. Geneva: WHO Press, 2009.
26. Trussell J, Raymond EG. Emergency contraception: a last chance to prevent unintended pregnancy. 2014. Available at ec.princeton.edu/questions/ec-review.pdf. Accessed June 2014.
27. Meyer JL, Gold MA, Haggerty CL. Advance provision of emergency contraception among adolescent and young adult women: a systematic review of literature. *J Pediatr Adolesc Gynecol* 2011;24:2–9.
28. Committee On Adolescence. Emergency contraception. *Pediatrics* 2012;130(6):1174–1182.
29. Cheng L, Che Y, Gülmezoglu AM. Interventions for emergency contraception. *Cochrane Database Syst Rev*. 2012;(8):CD001324.
30. Glasier AF, Cameron ST, Fine PM, et al. Ulipristal acetate versus levonorgestrel for emergency contraception: a randomised non-inferiority trial and meta-analysis. *Lancet* 2010;375(9714):555–562.
31. Cleland K, Zhu H, Goldstuck N, et al. The efficacy of intrauterine devices for emergency contraception: a systematic review of 35 years of experience. *Hum Reprod* 2012;27:1994–2000.
32. Richardson AR, Maltz FN. Ulipristal acetate: review of the efficacy and safety of a newly approved agent for emergency contraception. *Clin Ther* 2012;34:24–36.
33. Creinin MD, Schlaff W, Archer DF, et al. Progesterone receptor modulator for emergency contraception: a randomized controlled trial. *Obstet Gynecol* 2006;108(5):1089–1097.
34. American College of Obstetricians and Gynecologists. ACOG Practice Bulletin No. 112: emergency contraception. *Obstet Gynecol* 2010;115:1100–1109.
35. Trussell J, Schwarz EB. Emergency contraception. In: Hatcher RA, Trussell J, Nelson AL, et al., eds. Contraceptive technology. 20th revised ed. New York, NY: Ardent Media, 2011:113–145.
36. Lowe RF, Prata N. Hemoglobin and serum ferritin levels in women using copper-releasing or levonorgestrel-releasing intrauterine devices: a systematic review. *Contraception* 2013;87:486–496.
37. Veldhuis HM, Vos AG, Lagro-Janssen AL. Complications of the intrauterine device in nulliparous and parous women. *Eur J Gen Pract* 2004;10:82–87.
38. Harper CC, Speidel JJ, Drey EA, et al. Copper intrauterine device for emergency contraception: clinical practice among contraceptive providers. *Obstet Gynecol* 2012;119:220-226. doi: 10.1097/AOG.0b013e3182429e0d.
39. Office of Population Research & Association of Reproductive Health Professionals. 2014. http://ec.princeton.edu/questions/state-pharmacy-access-list.html. Accessed March 16, 2014.
40. Glasier A, Cameron ST, Blithe D, et al. Can we identify women at risk of pregnancy despite using emergency contraception? Data from randomized trials of ulipristal acetate and levonorgestrel. *Contraception* 2011;84:363–367.
41. Raymond EG, Creinin MD, Barnhart KT, et al. Meclizine for prevention of nausea associated with use of emergency contraceptive pills: a randomized trial. *Obstet Gynecol*. 2000;95(2):271-277.
42. Ngai SW, Fan S, Li S, et al. A randomized trial to compare 24 h versus 12 h double dose regimen of levonorgestrel for emergency contraception. *Hum Reprod* 2005;20:307–311.

📶 **ADDITIONAL RESOURCES AND WEBSITES ONLINE**

42

Barrier Contraceptives and Spermicides

Michelle Forcier

Barrier methods of contraception include male condom, female condom (FC), cervical cap, cervical shield, sponge, and diaphragm. The addition of vaginal spermicides in the forms of gel, cream, foam, suppository, and film may offer some additional contraceptive benefits for these barrier methods. Both barrier methods and spermicides have fewer systemic side effects than hormonal contraceptive methods, but are significantly less efficacious, and are rarely recommended as the sole method of contraception for patients who wish to avoid an unwanted pregnancy. Barrier methods of contraception are most efficacious when used in addition to significantly more effective long-acting reversible contraceptive (LARC) implants or hormonal methods. Dual methods, that include either male or FCs, also provide superior protection against sexually transmitted infections (STIs) for adolescents and young adults (AYAs) who elect to be sexually active. Barrier methods may both prevent physical contact and retain seminal fluids, thus effective for prevention of STIs, and block sperm from ascending into the uterus and upper tract. Barriers and spermicides are nonprescription and sometimes easier for AYAs to access over the counter. When patients elect to use barrier methods as their sole contraceptive, providers should offer detailed counseling and prescriptions for emergency contraception to improve potential contraceptive efficacy.

MALE CONDOMS

Condoms, the oldest and most common method of barrier contraception, still serve as a major form of birth control in the US, despite consistently higher failure rates than most other current contraceptive methods. Condoms are commonly used by AYAs, with data from 2006 to 2010 indicating that 96% of females use condoms followed by 57% withdrawal and 56% combined contraceptive pill.[1] Self-reports of frequent use of condoms are encouraging, from the perspective of STI prevention and public health campaign efforts to reduce human immunodeficiency virus (HIV). However, the validity of self-reported condom use is suspect as studies demonstrate significant discordance between self-reports of 100% condom use and indicators of sperm presence in the vaginal tract.[2]

Data from the 2011 National Survey of Family Growth (NSFG) survey suggest that condoms are used at sexual debut in 68% of female teens, with younger teens (<14 years) less likely to use condoms (53% of females, 71% males) than older teens (17 to 18 years), including 80% and 86% of females and males, respectively. There appear to be no differences in condom use at first sexual encounter by race and ethnicity. Condoms are reported as a dual method in 15% of teens, with non-Hispanic White female teenagers having the highest rates of dual method use.[1] Dual method rates may also be associated with nulliparity, insured status, and later sexual debut (>16 years).[3]

According to the 2014 NSFG report, 47.4% of women aged 15 through 24 use some form of contraception. Similar percentages of women aged 15 to 24 (10.1%) and 25 to 34 (11.5%) were using condoms. Rates of condom use for contraception are similar among Hispanic, Black and White youth aged 15 through 24 at 9%.[4] In the high school sample from the 2013 Youth Risk Behavior Survey, a median of 53% females and 64% males used condoms at last intercourse.[5] Among college students, the recent National College Health Assessment (NCHA) data suggest that similar use of condoms exists among young adults. Sixty-eight percent of college males and 61.6% of college females reported using condoms during last intercourse.[6]

Condoms for STI Prevention

Condom use has risen since the 1980s, related to public health campaigns to promote HIV prevention. Condoms are most protective for STIs transmitted in genital fluids that can be exchanged during penile intercourse. Condoms may also offer protection from bacterial exposure during oral and anal receptive sex as well as skin-to-skin viral transmission of disease. Latex and polyurethane condoms are impermeable to *Chlamydia trachomatis*, *Neisseria gonorrhoeae*, trichomoniasis, syphilis, hepatitis B and C, and HIV. Consistent use of condoms in heterosexual couples reduced transmission of HIV seroconversion by 80% or incidence 1.14/100 person-years "always" users versus 5.75/100 person-years for "never" users.[7] Condoms also provide some measure of skin-to-skin barrier protection against viruses such as herpes simplex virus (HSV) and human papillomavirus (HPV). Consistent and correct condom use demonstrated a 70% reduction in HPV transmission, improved clearance of HPV infection, decreased risk of genital warts and cervical cancer, and regression of cervical intraepithelial neoplasia.[8]

An updated 2013 American Academy of Pediatrics policy statement on condom use for AYAs readdresses these issues, recommending that pediatric providers:

- Encourage communication between parents and adolescents about sexual activity and sex education with guidance from the American Academy of Pediatrics Bright Futures
- Provide parent educational programs to create skills and incentives to talk to adolescent children about condom use

- Improve condom availability in their medical home and in the community[9]

Uses of Male Condoms
Contraceptive Use

1. As a primary method of birth control, alone or in conjunction with a spermicide, a female barrier, hormonal method, or intrauterine contraception
2. As a backup method of contraception after a late start with a hormonal method, or whenever two or more combined oral contraceptive pills or one progestin-only pill have been missed
3. As a barrier contraceptive, used as part of the fertility awareness method (FAM) of contraception during vulnerable days of the woman's cycle

Noncontraceptive Uses

1. To reduce transmission of STIs
2. To blunt sensation, to treat premature ejaculation
3. To reduce cervical antisperm antibody titers in women with associated infertility
4. To reduce allergic reaction in women with sensitivity to sperm

Types of Male Condoms

Latex condoms are most commonly used in the US. These are marketed in a variety of shapes and sizes, but typically measure 170 mm long and 50 mm wide, and 0.03 to 0.10 mm thick. Additional features such as ribbing, lubricants (spermicides, silicone, water-based gels), colors, scents, and tastes are marketing strategies, but are not linked to efficacy. In the past, sex educators promoted a "one-size-fits-all" concept to discourage some males from refusing to wear condoms because of self-reports of large penis size. More recent data suggest that size matters, and improved fit may improve condom use. In a sample of almost a thousand heterosexual men and women, 38.3% reported condom fit or feel problems that included decreased sensation, lack of naturalness, condom size complaints, decreased pleasure, and pain and discomfort.[10] Condoms that fit poorly are more than two times more likely to break, slip, or interfere with erection, orgasm, and sexual pleasure. Additionally, males with poorly fitting condoms are twice as likely to remove a condom during intercourse than males with well-fitting condoms.[11] Polyurethane condoms are made with nonbiodegradable materials that are stronger and less likely to be damaged by handling, petroleum lubricants, or shelf life. However, polyurethane condoms continue to be less popular than their latex counterparts as they are more expensive, less elastic and form fitting, and 2 to 5 times more likely to break or slip.[12]

Natural or skin (lamb cecum) condoms are as effective as latex or polyurethane condoms for pregnancy prevention, but not recommended for STI protection. Skin condoms have larger pores (up to 1,500 nm in diameter) that may allow HIV and hepatitis B virus transmission across these membranes. Skin or natural

---

The male condom is a sheath of plastic or rubber that fits snugly over the erect penis. It blocks the man's sperm from entering the woman's body. It also covers the penis to help protect the man and the woman from getting sexually transmitted infections from each other. The male condom can be used with other contraceptives. It can be used with other birth control methods such as birth control pills, shots, implants, spermicide, and diaphragms. It should not be used with the female condom. On average, if 100 couples use condoms for a year, 12 will become pregnant. Correct and more consistent use can reduce the risk of pregnancy even more.

- Use a condom every time you have sex. Keep a few handy.
- Put the condom on before there is any genital contact.
- Open the package carefully.
- Unroll the condom all the way to the base of the penis.
- Squeeze the air out of the top of the condom to make room for the ejaculate.
- Make sure your partner is well lubricated. Use spermicide or water-based or silicon-based lubricants. Do **not** use petroleum-based lubricants with latex condoms.
- If the condom tears or starts to slip off during sex, grasp the rim of the condom against the penis and withdraw the penis. The man should wash his hands and his penis. The woman should wash her hands and her labia (do **not** douche). If spermicide is available, the woman should insert spermicide into her vagina according to product directions. She should also use emergency contraception as soon as possible. If the couple wants to have sex again, use a new condom.
- Right after ejaculation, while the penis is still firm, the rim of the condom could be gently pressed against the penis as it is removed from the vagina.
- Check the used condom for any breaks or tears. If breaks or tears are noticed follow instructions above regarding spermicide and emergency contraception. Tie up the end and throw it away.

DOs and DON'Ts:

Do use a new condom each time you have sex	Don't reuse a condom
Do use a condom made of latex or polyurethane	Don't use lambskin or fake plastic condoms
Do change your condom if you have oral or anal sex before you have intercourse	Don't use the same condom for different sex practices or different sex partners
Do check the expiration date of the condom	Don't use a condom after the expiration date
Do place the condom before the penis touches her genitals	Don't let the penis touch her genitals before the condom goes on
Do use water-based lubricants if needed, such as spermicide, K-Y jelly	Don't use the petroleum-based products, such as Vaseline, oils, vaginal creams for infection treatment
Do hold the condom rim against the penis and pull them out together before the penis starts to soften or after ejaculation	Don't let the penis become soft inside her vagina—the condom can fall off
Do check the condom for tears, then tie it off and throw it away	Don't ever wash the condom and recycle it
Do keep emergency contraception and spermicide ready in case something happens and the condom does not work well	Don't wait until you need it, because emergency contraception works better the sooner you use it

FIGURE 42.1 The male condom—patient information sheet.

condoms may not prevent STIs and are therefore not recommended for teens and young adults at high risk for STIs.[13] Despite demonstrated drawbacks, nonlatex condoms remain an important barrier method for persons with sensitivities or allergies to latex.

Mechanism of Action

Condoms are sheaths that by covering the penis block transmission of semen, as well as other skin-to-skin infections. Condoms are regulated medical devices subject to testing by the US Food and Drug Administration (FDA). Latex condoms manufactured in the US are tested electronically for holes before packaging. Consumer Reports regularly tests the US manufactured condom models for strength, reliability, and perforation. All models passed minimum standards for reliability, holes, and packaging with additional features not affecting failure or score. Consumer Reports did not find a single perforation in their "smart picks" selection of condoms even though industry standards do permit a limited number of defects per batch.[12]

Effectiveness

Condoms are currently the most efficacious way to prevent STIs in sexually active AYAs, but are inferior with respect to birth control in comparison to newer and LARC methods. The US Selected Practice Recommendations for Contraceptive Use, 2013, does not reference a content section for condoms as a sole method of contraception, reflecting a shift highlighting condom use as a superior method for STI prevention, but inferior method for pregnancy prevention.[14,15]

Contraception counseling for all sexually active couples optimally focuses on dual methods such as hormonal or implant contraceptives for maximal pregnancy prevention supported by concurrent use of condoms to provide STI protection. The combination optimizes reproductive health outcomes in all sexually active AYAs. Estimates of dual method prevalence vary widely, with US rates consistently lower than Western Europe. Dual method research has focused on adolescent populations with associations including sociodemographics (age, race/ethnicity, education), risk perception, types of relationships, number of partners, relationship length, partner support of condoms, and exposure to HIV counseling and prevention.[16] A 2013 study of 15- to 24-year-olds attending US family planning clinics demonstrated that one-third of AYAs reported condom use, with 5% dual method users. Women who used condoms before hormonal contraception and believed that their partner supported condom use were more likely to use dual methods over time.[17]

Perfect use is estimated with two condoms breaking per 100 condoms used. However, real life condom efficacy requires proper technique and application with each and every coitus. Condom failure rates are estimated between 15% and 21%, with only half of users continuing the method at 1 year.[15,18] Condom failure typically results from lack of correct and consistent use as opposed to device failure in most instances.[19]

Improving Condom Success

Correct and consistent condom use over time is the key to efficacy. High rates of STIs in young women of color have led to a number of condom studies in this population. In one study of high risk African American women, aged 15 to 21, nearly 75% used condoms inconsistently.[20] In another study of 824 sexually active students at historically Black colleges (51.8% female, 90.6% heterosexuals), 526 (63.8%) reported condom use at last coitus.[21]

Factors associated with decreased condom use include spontaneous intercourse with more casual sexual partners, not feeling at risk for HIV, lack of family connectedness, experience of interpersonal violence, and use of alcohol or other substances.[22–27] Factors that have been linked to improved condom use include peer influence, knowledge about condom use and STI prevention, easy access to condoms (including carrying condoms on their person), and more open communication both with family and partners.[23,26]

Behavioral interventions that have been tailored to address cultural characteristics of individual populations have been effective in promoting condom use, but are not effective in promoting abstinence.[28,29]

A 2013 Cochrane review demonstrated that multiple sessions of social cognitive and health belief models over time were more likely to prevent second pregnancies and improve consistent condom use and use during last sex.[29]

Multiple studies have demonstrated condom availability programs effectiveness in the US including improved condom use and condom acquisition/condom carrying, delayed sexual initiation among youth, and reduced incident STIs.[30–33] Comprehensive sex education programs increase condom and contraceptive use. Two-thirds of 48 comprehensive sex education programs demonstrated significant effects improving condom use.[27] Behavioral interventions that have been tailored to address cultural characteristics of individual populations have been effective in promoting condom use, but are not effective in promoting abstinence.[28] A 2013 Cochrane review demonstrated that multiple sessions of social cognitive and health belief models over time were more likely to prevent second pregnancies and improve consistent condom use and use during last sex.[29]

Improving consistent and correct use of condoms is essential to their ultimate effectiveness. Studies indicate that condom errors vary across time and populations assessed.[19] Common errors that impair effectiveness include using condom during only part of penetrative activities; using incorrect placement techniques, including not squeezing air from the tip or leaving room at the tip; putting a condom on upside down; using lubricants that decrease condom integrity; and not removing the condom correctly. Studies demonstrate common issues with uncomfortable feel or fit, erectile dysfunction, slipping, leaking, or breaking are common and deterrents to regular use.

The following are some recommended tips for discussing *correct and consistent condom use*: (Fig. 42.1)

- Ensure safe storage conditions (heat, expiration dates) along with privacy and easy access.
- Plan how to integrate condom use during intercourse.
- Follow techniques for opening and removing the condom from its package, as many as half of condom breaks occur before penetration.
- Correct direction for unrolling condom, pinching tip to allow slack or remove air from reservoir, and pulling condom down over entire length of penis.
- Continue to check placement of condom during the whole period of intercourse to assess slippage and integrity of device.
- Use new condom for each orifice (oral, vaginal, anal).
- Use only water-based or silicone lubricants applied to external surface of the condom, vulva or vagina (petroleum-based lubricants or medications can destroy condom integrity in less than a minute allowing viral or sperm transmission).
- Correct condom removal includes grasping the rim of the condom at the base of the penis and carefully pulling off the condom while the penis is still partially erect or firm.
- Inspect for signs of breakage or spillage. If concerned, consider emergency contraception or spermicide.

Advantages

- Readily available without prescription and in many school, pharmacy, or retail settings
- Relatively inexpensive costing between $0.50 and $1.50 each
- Portable and easily carried by men and women for easy access in many settings
- Male partner is included in contraception and family planning participation
- Visible proof of protection during each act of coitus
- Most importantly, our currently most effect method of STI prevention[7,8,12]

Disadvantages

- One of the least effective methods of contraception
- Requires availability and application with each coitus
- May be perceived as invasive, interruptive, and unnatural
- Requires cooperation of male partner
- May diminish sensation and pleasure

Side Effects of Male Condoms

While condoms may be less effective than other hormonal or inserted forms of birth control, there are no restrictions on the use of latex condoms with any medical condition except true latex allergy.[15] Although many women report irritation and discomfort with condom use, this is more likely due to lack of lubrication or irritation from spermicide rather than a true latex allergic reaction. True latex allergies are estimated in less than 5% of the general population, but may be higher in health care providers and youth with spina bifida. Nonlatex polyurethane condoms are recommended for those with true latex allergy.

Future Developments

Condom development, or building a better condom, has been of international interest for both effective STI prevention and easy access, inexpensive contraception. The Bill and Melinda Gates Foundation in 2008 made a Grand Challenges Exploration call for a Next Generation of Condom, which has subsequently led to a second round call to innovation in September of 2013.[34] The Gates Foundation is sponsoring a variety of innovations that may create a condom device that men and women would actually prefer to use over unprotected sex. Multipurpose Prevention Technologies (MPTs) are also in the pipeline as combination products that potentially offer both contraception and STI prevention, but are likely years away from FDA approval and availability. The University of Washington is developing condoms made of electrospinning, using nanosized medication polymers to create a tightly woven barrier fabric that additionally delivers medication to kill sperm and sources of both viral and bacterial infection. The Origami Male Condom (OMC) is the first nonrolled pre-engineered silicone condom, which creates reciprocating motion for the penis inside the internally lubricated condom. The prefabricated design avoids the rolling process and can be placed over the penis in a single movement. This condom will be reviewed by the FDA, the World Health Organization (WHO), and the European Union C-Mark to gain approval and meet regulatory safety standards. This device is undergoing clinical trials in collaboration with the Department of Research at the California Family Health Council and expected to reach the market in 2015. Of note, Origami makes an Anal Condom (OAC) for both males and females who engage in receptive anal intercourse and provides a receptive partner control to use a condom without partner negotiations. This condom will likewise go through similar regulatory reviews and is in clinical trials in Boston in collaboration with the research department at The Fenway Institute. The Origami brand's innovation has been recognized in 2013 by the Bill & Melinda Gates Foundation as innovative example for reinventing the condom.

FEMALE CONDOMS

The FC came into use in the 1980s, but still only accounts for less than 1% of all condom use worldwide. Very few adolescents elect to use the FC, with 1.5% reporting ever using. As with male condoms, use is inconsistent and often incorrect, decreasing its potential usefulness.[1] The FC1 female condom was first made from polyurethane (before 2009), but has evolved into the FC2 nitrile sheath, which is less expensive, as well as less noisy than its earlier counterpart. This 17-cm sheath, 7.8-cm width device is inserted into the vagina with a ring and closed end deep toward the cervix. The open end has a flexible ring that remains outside the entrance to the vagina. FCs are not sensitive

to petroleum-based products, and the sheath contains a silicone lubricant on the inside. The FC can be used with additional lubricants, but should not be used with the latex male condom, because each device can compromise the integrity of the other. A version of a natural latex FC is available in other countries, but is not FDA approved.[34]

Data on the attitudes and use of the FC in AYAs in the US are limited. Much of the work has focused on sex workers in underdeveloped countries so that women can self-administer barrier STI and pregnancy prevention. One study using focus groups of New York City urban youth aged 15 to 20 years suggested that young women identified correctly that the FC is woman controlled, while young males often focused on sexual feeling and pleasure. The authors recommended that focusing on contraceptive effectiveness, lack of side effects, and availability may be important when discussing the FC.[34] The majority of current studies looking at contraceptive behaviors in US AYAs do not include data about FC use. Older studies report very low ever use and likely even lower consistent use, with most young couples preferring to use male condoms.

Efficacy

Typical first-year failure rates of 21% are considerably higher than the 5% perfect-use failure; this is due to users' ability to use consistently and correctly each and every time over time.[18] The FC offers protection against STIs similar to its male counterpart and has been of research interest for HIV prevention in underdeveloped countries, sex workers, and women at high risk for HIV exposure.

Advantages

- Like the male condom, there are usually no contraindications or medically complex conditions that would contraindicate FC use.
- The polyurethane is not sensitive to petroleum-based products. Additional lubrication applied within the condom helps reduce breakage related to friction and allows for less device-related noise.
- For woman whose partner refuses to wear condoms, the FC offers another option, though again may be perceived as diminishing sensation and pleasure for both parties.

Disadvantages

- Coitus dependent
- Technically difficult to insert
- More expensive than male condoms.

All factors contribute to its infrequent use in AYAs. In addition to being more technically complicated for correct vaginal insertion, couples should check placement throughout the entirety of coitus. Excessive friction can break the condom or invert the condom on withdrawal. Additional lubrication applied within the FC can help reduce this risk and also reduces the noise the device may make during intercourse. For AYAs, efficacy related to correct and consistent use depends on extensive education, hands-on practice, and significant motivation. As with male condoms, providers should offer EC in advance to all FC users.

Instructions for insertion and use are shown (Fig. 42.2).While a wearer may insert the FC up to 8 hours before intercourse, both the woman and her partner need to maintain its correct position during sex to prevent it from getting pushed off or into the vagina.

Future Developments

Relatively new models of the FC appear to be noninferior to the FDA-approved FC2 model. Newer models with variations in design were developed to provide women with greater and individual choices. FCs made of latex and nitrile are less expensive and noisy options to polyurethane FC. Models available in other countries include Reddy and VA w.o.w Condom, which are latex and use a soft, polyurethane

The Female Condom

What is the female condom?

The female condom is a thin, soft, loose-fitting pouch with two flexible rings at either end. One ring helps hold the device in place inside the woman's vagina over the end of the womb (cervix), while the other ring rests outside the vagina.

Outer ring lies against the labia (lips of the vulva)

Inner ring is used for insertion; helps hold female condom in place

How does it work?

The female condom is made of polyurethane, a type of plastic. The plastic condom covers the inside of the vagina, cervix, and area around the opening to the vagina. The device acts as a barrier to help prevent pregnancy and the transmission of germs that can cause sexually transmitted diseases (STDs), including human immunodeficiency virus (HIV) and acquired immunodeficiency syndrome (AIDS). The device can be inserted by the woman up to 8 hours before sex.

How to insert the female condom

1. Find a comfortable position. You may want to stand up with one foot on a chair, squat with knees apart, or lie down with legs bent and knees apart.
2. Hold the female condom with the open end hanging down. Squeeze the inner ring with your thumb and middle finger.
3. Holding the inner ring squeezed together, insert the ring into the vagina and push the inner ring and pouch into the vagina past the pubic bone.
4. When properly inserted, the outer ring will hang down slightly outside the vagina. During intercourse, when the penis enters the vagina, the slack will lessen.

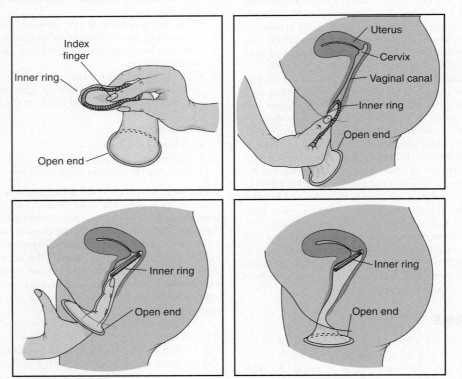

FIGURE 42.2 The female condom.

Remember:

The female condom may be hard to hold or slippery at first. Before you use one for the first time during sex, practice inserting one to get used to it. Take your time. Be sure to insert the condom straight into the vagina without twisting the pouch.

During Sex

1. It's helpful to use your hand to guide the penis into the vagina inside the female condom.
2. The ring may move from side to side or up and down during intercourse. This is OK.
3. If the female condom seems to be sticking to and moving with the penis rather than resting in the vagina, stop and add more lubricant to the inside of the device (near the outer ring) or to the penis.

How to remove the female condom after intercourse

1. Squeeze and twist the outer ring to close it.
2. Pull the female condom out gently.
3. Throw the condom away in the garbage. Do not flush down the toilet.
4. Do not wash out and use again.

Special Reminders

- Use a new female condom with every act of intercourse.
- Use it every time you have intercourse.
- Read and follow the directions carefully.
- Do not use a male and female condom at the same time.
- Be careful not to tear the condom with fingernails or sharp objects.
- Use enough lubricant.

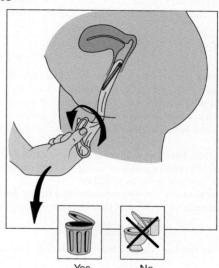

Yes   No

Latex condoms for men are highly effective at preventing STDs, including HIV infection (AIDS), if used properly. If your partner refuses to use a male latex condom, use a female condom to help protect yourself and your partner.

FIGURE 42.2 *(Continued).* The female condom.

sponge to hold it in place inside the vagina and the oil-based lubricants should not be used with latex-based FC as they can damage latex. The VA received the CE mark for distribution in the European Union and is being reviewed by the WHO. PATH's Woman's Condom makes insertion easier using a rounded cap, which dissolves once it is put in place. The US studies are in effect at present. The Cupid FC condom is WHO approved and available in South Africa, Mozambique, Indonesia, India, and other countries, and is cheaper than the FC2. FC choices are expanding—new models have low failure rates and are acceptable to users. The Natural Sensation Panty Condom is worn like underwear, with the condom built into the panty design. FC choices are expanding with newer models having low failure rates and acceptable to users. MFTs continue to create dual use devices and are exploring electrospinning technologies that use fibers from liquid spermicides and viro-bactericides to create FC. The Origami Female Condom (OFC) is a prefabricated mold allowing rapid insertion and sensation both inside and outside the condom.

CONTRACEPTIVE SPONGE

The contraceptive sponge was approved in 1983, removed from the US market in 1994, and then returned in 2005. This device is available over the counter, is relatively easy to insert, and can be inserted long before coitus. The sponge is donut-shaped, one-size-fits-all,

soft polyurethane foam device inserted over the cervix and acts as a physical barrier to sperm penetrating the upper tract. The device is moistened with water and then slid back into the posterior vagina where a small concavity fits against the cervix to provide immediate effective contraception. It contains a slow release of 125 to 150 mg of nonoxynol-9 so that no additional spermicides are needed over the 24-hour time frame and may provide protection for multiple acts of coitus. The sponge should stay in place for 6 hours after coitus and then can be removed at anytime thereafter. When the woman wishes to remove the sponge, she gently grasps a small polyester loop and pulls it out. Women are warned against leaving the sponge in for great than 24 hours because of risk of toxic shock syndrome.

Mechanism of Action

The primary contraceptive action of the sponge is provided by the spermicidal activity of nonoxynol-9, which is impregnated in the polyurethane foam. The sponge releases 125 to 150 mg of nonoxynol-9 slowly over a 24-hour period. The sponge also traps and absorbs semen and acts as a physical barrier between sperm and the cervical os.

Efficacy

As with any other coitus method, the sponge has higher typical-use failure rates than many other methods. Failure rates of 16% in

IX

nulliparous women compared to 32% in parous women are associated with the fit and barrier effect with a more patulous gravid cervix.[18] Nulliparous and parous perfect-use rates are higher at 9% and 20%, respectively.

As with other barrier devices, the sponge is available without a prescription, controlled by the female, and may be inserted before and used for multiple acts of sex. Young women electing to use the sponge must intentionally place it before intercourse and be comfortable touching their vagina and inserting and removing the device. Its local action eliminates any concerns regarding systemic hormonal side effects. There are few contraindications to use of the sponge, and these may include allergy to sponge components (polyurethane, metabisulfite, and nonoxynol-9), prior toxic shock syndrome, and current menstruation. Up to 4% of users experience odor, itching, burning, redness, or a rash with its use. Local irritation is most likely due to sensitivity to detergent effects of the spermicide.

Patient Education

Insertion

- Remove the sponge from its package and hold it with the "dimple" side facing up and the loop hanging down.
- Moisten with approximately two tablespoons of water and squeeze the sponge a few times until it becomes sudsy.
- Fold the sides of the sponge upward with a finger on each side to support it.
- While in a standing, lying, or squatting position gently introduce the sponge into the vagina and using one or two fingers push the sponge upward as far as it will go.
- Check the position of the sponge by running a finger around the edge of the sponge to make sure that the cervix is covered.

Removal

- Wait 6 hours after the last act of intercourse before removing the sponge.
- Insert one finger into the vagina until the loop is felt.
- If the loop cannot be felt, bear down, lie on your back on the bed with your knees up against your chest, squat down in a low position, or sit on the toilet and tilt your pelvis forward (so that the small of your back is rounded) to bring the sponge closer to the vaginal opening.
- Hook one finger into the loop then gently and slowly pull the sponge out.
- Check to make sure the sponge is intact; if it is torn, remove all pieces from the vagina.
- Discard sponge.

Contraindications

- History of toxic shock syndrome
- Allergy or sensitivity to polyurethane foam, nonoxynol-9, or metabisulfite, or allergy to sulfa
- During menstruation

Advantages

- Lack of hormonal side effects or medical contraindications
- Allows for spontaneity after insertion; can be used over repeated acts of intercourse
- Available without a prescription or fitting by health care personnel; one size fits all
- Female-controlled method; does not require partner participation
- May be more comfortable to wear than other barrier methods such as the diaphragm
- Easy to use and not "messy"

Disadvantages

- Relatively high failure rate

- AYAs must be comfortable touching genitals in order to insert device
- Spermicide may cause vaginal, vulvar, or penile irritation. As many as 4% of users will experience a sensitivity reaction to the sponge that can lead to itching, burning, redness, or a rash. Although this may be due to nonoxynol-9, other components of the sponge such as the preservative may be the source of the sensitivity reaction.
- Sponge can become discolored or malodorous in the presence of vaginitis.
- Can be difficult to remove
- Not recommended for use during menses

Future Developments

Three brands of contraceptives sponges are currently marketed: Today (US), Pharmatex (France, Quebec), and Protectaid (Canada, Europe). Pharmatex and Protectaid may eventually be FDA approved. Protectaid contains active ingredients 6.25 mg of nonoxynol-9, 6.25 mg of benzalkonium chloride, and 25 mg of sodium cholate; Pharmatex contains 60 mg of benzalkonium chloride. MPTs using sponge-like devices are also in the pipeline as combination products that potentially offer both contraception and STI prevention, but are likely years away from FDA approval and availability.

⬤ CERVICAL SHIELD

The cervical shield (Lea's Shield) (Fig. 42.3) was approved in 2002 and is available by prescription. This cervical shield is a one-size-fits-all device to block sperm from entering the cervix and upper tract. The device is oval with a small concave cup that fits over the cervix, with the remainder of the device filling the proximal vagina. A small one-way valve allows both air and menses to be released from behind the device. This device provides barrier protection by covering the cervix in its entirety, and is even more effective with the additional application of spermicide. The shield differs from its barrier prescription counterparts (cap and diaphragm) in two important ways. First, the shield is held in place by its physical volume and the muscles of the vaginal wall compared to the cap, which is held in place by the cervix, the diaphragm, and the pubic bone. Second, the cervical shield is independent of cervical or vaginal size, and therefore it does not require fitting by a provider. Because of the one-way valve design, this method can be used as contraception during menses, although some resources

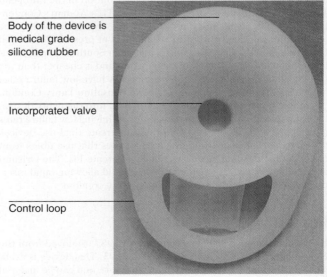

Body of the device is medical grade silicone rubber

Incorporated valve

Control loop

FIGURE 42.3 The Lea's Shield.

advise against this practice. Composed of silicone rubber, it is non-allergenic, washable, and reusable for multiple acts of intercourse over a period of 48 hours. It can be worn hours before intercourse and should remain in place for at least 8 hours post-coitus, but correct positioning should be reconfirmed before sex.

Efficacy

Like other barrier methods, efficacy is dependent on correct and consistent use. Reported failure rates range from 4% to 15% per year. Efficacy is also improved by the addition of spermicide with each coitus. Like the sponge, the shield is more effective in nulliparous women, but differs from the diaphragm and cap in that it seems to provide more protection than these methods in multiparous women. Although the shield is not included in the Center for Disease Control Medical Eligibility Contraceptive Guidelines (CDC MEC) comparative list for efficacy and continuation, other studies estimate up to an 11% failure rate per year.[35]

Insertion of Lea's Shield

Like other barrier methods, women must be comfortable manually inserting and removing the device from the vagina. Prior to intercourse, the cup is filled with spermicide and then the device is pushed into the proximal vagina.

- Apply a small amount of spermicide in the bowl of the device.
- Gently squeeze the shield and insert into the vaginal bowl first as high as it will go.
- Check to make sure that the entire cervix is covered by the bowl.

Removal of Lea's Shield

- Insert a finger into the vagina, grasp and twist the control loop to break the suction, and gently remove.
- The shield should be washed thoroughly with mild liquid soap for approximately 2 minutes, dried, and then stored.

Advantages

- There are few contraindications to using this device and no systemic effects.
- Effective for up to 48 hours; additional doses of spermicide are not required for multiple acts of intercourse.
- May be placed early and is usually not detected by the partner
- May offer some reduction of STI risk, especially for cervical and upper genital tract infections

Disadvantages

- Requires a clinician visit to obtain a prescription
- Requires training in placement, removal, cleaning, and storage and may be difficult or uncomfortable insert and remove
- Replacement every 1 to 3 years

CERVICAL CAP AND DIAPHRAGM

The cervical cap and diaphragm are prescription-only devices that require fitting by a medical provider. Like other barrier methods, they block the cervix and prevent sperm from ascending to the upper tract. These methods are rarely used by AYAs, but are of interest to reproductive health scientists because they have the potential to protect against STIs and HIV when used in combination with antimicrobial spermicides.

The cap (FemCap) (Fig. 42.4) is smaller than the diaphragm and made of nonallergenic silicone. It comes in three sizes (22 mm, 26 mm, and 30 mm) that are fit based on obstetrical history, and not by physical examination. The small 22-mm rim is recommended for nulliparous women, the medium for women with prior pregnancy, but no vaginal delivery, and the 30-mm rim for users whose cervix has experienced vaginal delivery. The cap is filled with spermicide, most of it on the side of the cap facing away from

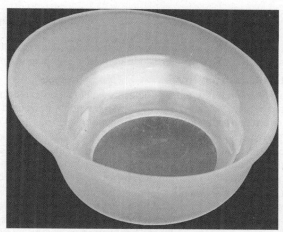

FIGURE 42.4 The FemCap. (Courtesy of FemCap, Inc., and Alfred Shihata, MD.)

the cervix and into the vagina, which may reduce cervical irritation. The device may be used for multiple acts of coitus for up to 48 hours, with checking required to ensure proper placement with each act.

The diaphragm is a latex or silicone cup, which is fit with a spring mechanism rim that secures the device and covers the cervix. It has a semiflexible ring that helps hold the device, anchoring it with the pubic bone. Spermicide is placed within the cup on the side that comes in contact with the cervix. There are four styles of diaphragms available in a range of sizes (50 to 105 mm). Sizing is determined by rim size and increases by 5 mm until a full seal is obtained. An *arcing spring* diaphragm is the easiest to insert, folding for insertion, and then springing open to secure itself with the pubic bone (Fig. 42.5). This design has the strongest rim and is useful for women with all levels of vaginal muscle tone, including those with weak muscle tone. It can be used in women with a retroverted uterus, cystocele, or rectocele. Two devices, coil and flat spring, can be inserted using an introducer. Coil spring is useful for women with firm to average vaginal tone, while the flat spring is thinner and more comfortable in women with firm vaginal tone. A wide seal rim is the fourth type and has limited availability.

Effectiveness

Effectiveness of the cervical cap is not included in the CDC MEC, but appears to be less effective than its counterpart, the diaphragm, with a failure rate estimated at 23%.[35]

Diaphragm typical-use failure rate is 16%, with perfect use estimated at 6%.[16] A diaphragm is more likely to dislodge in women who have extreme uterine ante- or retroversion, as well as in women who prefer to be on top during sex. Diaphragm effectiveness requires additional vaginal spermicide with each act of coitus after that 6-hour window, with the diaphragm left in place for a full 6 hours after last coitus. Emergency contraception should be considered if a diaphragm is removed or dislodged prior to these 6 hours post-coitus.

AYAs can use caps and diaphragms, but are often unable to anticipate intercourse and are more uncomfortable touching the vulva and vagina for correct insertion, making these unusual methods of choice for teens. These devices require additional care and maintenance, with soap and water washes, followed by a soak in an alcohol solution, and cornstarch coating prior to storage in a cool and dry environment.

Contraindications to Use

- History of toxic shock syndrome
- Allergy to latex or spermicidal agents

Diaphragm Patient Information and Instructions

The diaphragm is a shallow, dome-shaped cup made of soft rubber. It is inserted into the vagina and placed securely over the cervix. It must be used with spermicidal cream or jelly. The diaphragm prevents pregnancy by providing a barrier between the sperm and uterus.

Instructions to patients
Check diaphragm for tears or holes by holding it up to a bright light and stretching the rubber slightly. Always use with contraceptive cream or jelly. Hold the diaphragm with the dome down and squeeze a tablespoon of cream or jelly into the dome and spread it around the dome and onto the rim with your finger.

To insert your diaphragm, stand with one foot propped up (i.e., on the toilet seat), squat, or lie on your back. Press the edges of the diaphragm together with one hand. With your other hand, spread the lips of your vagina and insert the diaphragm into your vagina. Push the diaphragm downward and back along the back wall of your vagina as far as it will go. Then tuck the front rim of the diaphragm up along the roof of your vagina behind the pubic bone.

Check the placement of your diaphragm by sweeping your index finger across the diaphragm to make sure the cervix is completely covered by the soft rubber dome and that the front rim of the diaphragm is snugly in place behind your pubic bone. (The cervix will feel like the tip of your nose.) When properly placed, the diaphragm will neither cause discomfort nor interfere with sex. The diaphragm and contraceptive cream or jelly can be inserted up to 6 hours before intercourse. If 6 hours have passed since insertion and the time intercourse occurs, put another applicator full of jelly or cream into your vagina without removing the diaphragm.

A new application of spermicidal cream or jelly is necessary with each additional act of intercourse. Do not remove the diaphragm. Use the plastic applicator to insert the jelly or cream in front of the diaphragm.

The diaphragm must be left in place for 6 to 8 hours after the last time you have intercourse, but never leave the diaphragm in place for more than 24 hours. Do not douche.

To remove the diaphragm
To remove the diaphragm, place your index finger behind the front rim of the diaphragm and pull down and out. Sometimes squatting and pushing with your abdominal muscles (i.e., bearing down as though you were having a bowel movement) helps to hook your finger behind the diaphragm. After use, the diaphragm should be washed with soap and water, rinsed thoroughly, and dried with a towel. Store it in its plastic container. You may dust it with cornstarch. Do not use talcum, perfumed powder, Vaseline, baby oil, or contraceptive foam, as they may damage the diaphragm. Inspect the diaphragm (especially around the rim) for holes or defects.

Side effects
Occasionally, the spermicidal cream or jelly has been found to be irritating. Changing to another brand should resolve the problem. Some patients have reported bladder symptoms or urinary tract infections with use of the diaphragm. Rare cases of toxic shock syndrome have been reported in users of the diaphragm. Contact your physician if you have:

- Fever above 38.3° C (101 °F)
- Diarrhea
- Vomiting
- Muscle aches
- Rash (sunburnlike)

FIGURE 42.5 Sample instruction sheet for diaphragms. (Courtesy of Teenage Health Center, Children's Hospital of Los Angeles, Los Angeles, California.)

- Recent pregnancy, before renormalization of anatomy
- Inability of patient to correctly insert and remove diaphragm

Tips to Improve Success of Method
- Correct fitting of device (see later discussion)
- Detailed, hands-on instruction for patient education (see later discussion)
- Careful monitoring of diaphragm between uses to identify any defects (see later discussion)
- Careful selection of patient
  - Offer only to motivated woman willing to touch her genitals and to use the device with *every* act of intercourse
  - Avoid offering to a woman with a markedly anteverted or retroverted uterus (diaphragm tends to dislodge)
  - Discourage coital positions that compromise stability of diaphragm, particularly the female superior position

Correct Fitting of Diaphragm
Diaphragms are rarely used today, even in specialized family planning centers. A diaphragm must be fit properly to be effective. The diagonal length of the vaginal canal from the posterior aspect of the symphysis pubis to the posterior vaginal fornix is measured during the bimanual examination and measured against a diaphragm rim. A diaphragm is inserted and checked using the correct size (one size smaller than the first diaphragm felt or perceived by the patient). The diaphragm should touch the lateral vaginal walls, cover the cervix, and fit snugly between the posterior vaginal fornix and behind the symphysis pubis. A diaphragm that is too large may buckle and permit sperm to bypass the diaphragm. A diaphragm that is too small may slip out of place. The health care provider should appreciate that the adolescent may be tense during initial fitting, causing the fitting of a smaller diaphragm than would be required if the adolescent were relaxed.

Patient Education
Insertion of the FemCap
- Apply approximately $\frac{1}{4}$ teaspoon of spermicide in the bowl, spread a thin layer over the outer brim, and insert $\frac{1}{2}$ teaspoon between the brim and the dome.
- Gently squeeze the cup and insert it into the vagina with the bowl facing upward and the longer brim entering first.
- Push the cap down toward the rectum and back as far as it can go.
- Check to make sure that the cap completely covers the cervix.

Removal of the FemCap
- To remove the cap, squat and bear down.
- Push the tip of a finger against the dome cap to break the suction.
- Grasp the removal strap with the tip of your finger and gently remove the device.
- Wash the cap thoroughly with a mild soap then rinse it with tap water. Allow the cap to air dry or gently pat it dry with a clean, soft towel and store.

Insertion and Removal of Diaphragm
Patient education programs should include the following.
- Demonstration of insertion and removal techniques: After being shown how to place the diaphragm, the teen should insert and remove it at least once in the office and have the placement checked by the provider.
- Detailed guidance about use of spermicide
  - Coat the inner surface of the diaphragm with spermicidal gel. One application is effective for up to 6 hours.
  - Add additional spermicide with the applicator if intercourse is delayed beyond 6 hours or if additional acts of coitus are anticipated. Additional doses must be placed into the vagina; the diaphragm should not be removed to add spermicide.
  - Apply an extra dose immediately if the diaphragm is dislodged during intercourse, and consider using emergency contraception.
- Removal instructions
  - Wait at least 6 hours after the last episode of coitus to remove the device.
  - Remove before 24 hours of use to reduce the risk of toxic shock syndrome.
- Concrete instructions about cleaning and storage of device: Recommend washing device in soap and water, then soaking it in an alcohol solution (70% isopropanol or 80% ethanol) for at least 20 minutes after each application. Coat the device with cornstarch or another agent to prevent contamination or cracking, and store it in a dry container.
- Return for refitting of the diaphragm every 1 to 2 years, after every pregnancy, and after any 10% to 20% change in body weight.

Advantages
- Reduced risks of STIs, including HIV
- May be placed in anticipation of coitus

Disadvantages
- Requires professional sizing and is available only by prescription
- Requires motivation and extensive education for proper use
- Requires preparation and access to supplies; therefore, it may limit spontaneity and may not meet the impulsive needs of the adolescent
- May be considered messy, especially for multiple acts of intercourse
- Not an acceptable method if either partner is allergic to spermicide or latex
- There is a small risk of toxic shock syndrome associated with poorly timed or prolonged use.
- The diaphragm increases the risk of cystitis by increasing the count of enteric organisms within the vagina.

Future Developments
The SILCS intravaginal barrier is a one-size-fits-all diaphragm made of silicone, designed to be easier to use, and intended for sale over the counter. The BufferGel Duet is a disposable, one-size-fits-all polyurethane diaphragm prefilled with a microbicide and contraceptive.

VAGINAL SPERMICIDES
The common active ingredient of spermicides is nonoxynol-9, a surfactant and organic compound used in various cosmetic and cleaning products. Benzalkonium chloride and sodium choate are spermicidal agents active in some contraceptive sponges. The inert base blocks or absorbs sperm, and the chemically active ingredient breaks down sperm cell membranes. Lemon juice, lactic acid, and neem plant oils are anecdotally spermicidal, but there are no data supporting the effectiveness of these methods.

Types of Spermicides
Spermicides come in a variety of forms (gels, films, foams, and suppositories) (Table 42.1). Spermicides vary in application, onset, and duration of use. Most spermicides are active for 1 hour unless used with additional barrier methods. Foam is one of the most commonly used spermicides with the benefit of being instantly efficacious. Gels, films, and suppositories need approximately 15 minutes to coat the cervix and become effective.

HIV researchers have long been interested in exploring the in vitro virucidal and bactericidal activity of vaginal spermicides. At present, clinical data do not support its use in this way. A number of studies have consistently demonstrated that nonoxynol-9 does not reduce risk of HIV and other STI transmission. The detergent effects of nonoxynol-9 seem to cause local epithelial irritation and sloughing exposing the submucosal and creating a portal of entry for HIV and other STIs. A case-control study of sex workers in Africa has demonstrated that multiple daily use (>3.5 times/day) increases the risk of HIV.[36] Benzalkonium can likewise work as an irritant in the vagina and negatively impact normal lactobacillus flora.

Efficacy
Typical-use failure rates are estimated at 29%. Less than half of women continue to use this method a year out. Correct and consistent use of spermicides has a slightly lower perfect-use failure rate of 18%.[18] Use with adjunct barrier methods improves effectiveness. Spermicides have low efficacy compared to most other methods. As a nonprescription method, with few systemic side effects and additional local lubricant effect, spermicides may offer some benefits to AYAs. Messiness, need to apply in advance of each coitus, and changes in odor and taste may be unpleasant for some AYAs. Along with lack of efficacy, the risk for STI transmission risk should make spermicides a less desirable option in this age-group. The CDC does not recommend the use of spermicide alone or as a lubricant for condoms. Condoms lubricated with spermicides are no more effective than other lubricated condoms in protecting against the transmission of HIV and other STIs.[8] Use of nonoxynol-9 is associated with breakdown of the protective genital epithelium, which has been associated with increased risk for transmission of HIV infection.

Condoms lubricated with nonoxynol-9 are not recommended for STI and HIV prevention. Spermicide-coated condoms cost more, have a shorter shelf life than other lubricated condoms, and have been associated with urinary tract infection in young women.

TABLE 42.1
Examples of Various US Brand Spermicides

Manufacturer	Brand Name of Nonoxynol-9	Delivery System	Dose
Ortho	Conceptrol	Gel	4% 100 mg/applicator
NcNeil	Delfen II	Jelly	2% 0.1 gm
Blairex Lab.	Encare	Suppository	100 mg
J and J Products	Gyncol II	Jelly	150 mg
Apothecus Pharm.	VCF	Film Foam	28% 12.5%

The CDC does recommend condom use, even with spermicide, if there is no other option available. Petroleum- or oil-based products (mineral oil, baby oil, vegetable oil, Vaseline, cold creams, hand moisturizers) degrade and weaken latex after as little as a minute of contact. Water- or silicone-based lubricants do not react with latex and can decrease friction, irritation, and breakage, thus making them a relatively more useful adjunct to condoms than spermicides

Mechanism of Action

The components of spermicidal agents include an inert base (foam, cream, or jelly), which holds the spermicidal agent and blocks sperm from entering the cervical os. Spermicides destroy sperm by breaking down the outer cell membrane.

Contraindications

- Allergy or sensitivity to spermicidal agents or to the ingredients in the base
- Inability to use due to vaginal abnormalities or inability to master the insertion technique

Advantages

- No proven systemic side effects
- Readily available without prescription
- Overall, convenient, easy-to-learn method for teenagers
- May be used by women with or without involvement of partner
- May provide lubrication
- May be useful as a backup method for other contraceptives

Disadvantages

- Relatively high failure rate
- Considered messy by some teenagers (some forms)
- Must be used only a short time before intercourse is started
- Requires 10 to 15 minutes for activation (some formulations)
- Requires that woman be comfortable with touching her genitals
- Unpleasant taste if oral-genital sex is involved
- May cause a local allergic reaction

Future Developments

The need for vaginal agents that are contraceptive and protective against HIV and other STIs is increasingly compelling. Much of current research and development activity is centered on developing an agent with these properties.

⬤ CONCLUSION

Barrier methods may offer some measure of contraception for AYAs, but are neither less efficacious nor easier to use than many other forms of birth control such as continuous hormonal or injectable contraceptives. The most important function of barrier methods for many AYAs may be the protection they offer against STI, including HIV. When offering sexual health counseling, it may be more beneficial to separate out superior family planning and contraceptive options from barrier methods, which offer most benefit for STI prevention. Dual method use, along with patient readiness and careful partner selection, offers a four-fold approach to more responsible sexual decision making.

REFERENCES

5. Martinez G, Copen CE, Abma JC. Teenagers in the United States: sexual activity, contraceptive use, and childbearing, National Survey of Family Growth 2006–2010. *Vital Health Stat* 2011;23(31). Available at http://www.cdc.gov/nchs/data/series/sr_23/sr23_031.pdf. Accessed October 15, 2013.
6. Rose E, Diclemente RJ, Wingood GM, et al. The validity of teens' and young adults' self-reported condom use. *Arch Pediatr Adolesc Med* 2009;163:61–64.
7. Tyler CP, Whiteman MK, Kraft JM, et al. Dual use of condoms with other contraceptive methods among adolescents and young women in the United States. *J Adolesc Health* 2013;54(2):169–175.
8. Daniels K, Daugherty J, Jones J. *Current contraceptive status among women aged 15–44: United States, 2011–2013*, NCHS Data Brief No. 173. Hyattsville, MD: National Center for Health Statistics, 2014.
9. Kann L, Kincher S, Shanklin SL, et al. Youth risk behavior surveillance—United States, 2013. *MMWR Surveill Summ* 2014;63 (Suppl 4):1–168.

10. American College Health Association. *National College Health Assessment II: undergraduate students reference group executive summary Spring 2014*. Hanover, MD: American College Health Association, 2014.
11. Weller S, Davis K. Condom effectiveness in reducing heterosexual HIV transmission. *Cochrane Database Syst Rev* 2002;(1):CD003255. doi:10.1002/14651858. CD003255.
12. www.cdc.gov/condomeffectiveness/latex.html. Accessed October 25, 2013.
13. American Academy of Pediatrics (AAP). Committee on Adolescence. Policy statement: condom use by adolescents. *Pediatrics* 2013;132:973–981.
14. Crosby RA, Milhausen RR, Mark KP, et al. Understanding problems with condom fit and feel: an important opportunity for improving clinic-based safer sex programs. *J Prim Prev* 2013;34:109–115.
15. Crosby RA, Yarber WL, Graham CA, et al. Does it fit okay? Problems with condom use as a function of self-reported poor fit. *Sex Trans Infect* 2010;86:36–38.
16. http://www.consumerreports.org/cro/shopping/december-2009/sex-and-the-super-market/overview/index.htm. Accessed October 25, 2013.
17. Steiner MJ, Warner L, Stone KM, et al. Condoms and other barrier methods for prevention of STI/HIV infection, and pregnancy. In: Holmes KK, Sparling PF, Stamm WE, eds. *Sexually transmitted diseases*. 4th ed. New York, NY: MacGraw-Hill, 2008.
18. Division of Reproductive Health, National Center for Chronic Disease Prevention and Health Promotion, Centers for Disease Control and Prevention. U.S. selected practice recommendations for contraceptive use, 2013: adapted from the World Health Organization selected practice recommendations for contraceptive use, 2nd edition. *MMWR Recomm Rep* 2013;62 (RR-05):1–60.
19. Centers for Disease Control and Prevention. U.S. medical eligibility criteria for contraceptive use, 2010. *MMWR Recomm Rep* 2010;59 (RR-4):1–86.
20. Higgins JA, Cooper AD. Dual use of condoms and contraceptives in the USA. *Sex Health* 2012;9:73–80.
21. Goldstein RL, Upadhyay UD, Raine TR. With pills, patches, rings, and shots: who still uses condoms? A longitudinal cohort study. *J Adolesc Health.* 2013;52:77–82.
22. Trussell J. Contraceptive efficacy. In: Hatcher RA, Trussell J, Nelson AL, et al., eds. *Contraceptive technology*. 19th ed. New York, NY: Ardent Media, 2007.
23. Sanders SA, Yarber WL, Kaufman EL, et al. Condom use errors and problems: a global view. *Sex Health* 2012;9:81–95.
24. Voisin DR, Hotton A, Tan K, et al. A longitudinal examination of risk and protective factors associated with drug use and unsafe sex among young African American females. *Child Youth Serv Rev* 2013;35:1440–1446.
25. El Bcheraoui C, Sutton MY, Hardnett FP, et al. Patterns of condom use among students at historically Black colleges and universities: implications for HIV prevention efforts among college-age young adults. *AIDS Care* 2013;25:186–193.
26. Secor-Turner M, McMorris B, Sieving R, et al. Life experiences of instability and sexual risk behaviors among high-risk adolescent females. *Perspect Sex Reprod Health* 2013;45:101–107.
27. Staras SA, Livingston MD, Maldonado-Molina MM, et al. The influence of sexual partner on condom use among urban adolescents. *J Adolesc Health* 2013;53:742–748.
28. Manlove J, Ikramullah E, Terry-Humen E. Condom use and consistency among male adolescents in the United States. *J Adolesc Health* 2008;43:325–333.
29. Tschann JM, Flores E, de Groat CL, et al. Condom negotiation strategies and actual condom use among Latino youth. *J Adolesc Health* 2010;47:254–262.
30. Rice E. The positive role of social networks and social networking technology in the condom-using behaviors of homeless young people. *Public Health Rep* 2010;125:588–595.
31. Kirby DB, Laris BA, Rolleri LA. Sex and HIV education programs: their impact on sexual behaviors of young people throughout the world. *J Adolesc Health* 2007;40:206–217.
32. von Sadovszky V, Draudt B, Boch S. A systematic review of reviews of behavioral interventions to promote condom use. *Worldviews Evid Based Nurs* 2014;11(2):107–117. doi:10.1111/wvn.12017.
33. Lopez LM, Tolley EE, Grimes DA, et al. Theory-based interventions for contraception. *Cochrane Database Syst Rev* 2013;(8):CD007249.
34. Charania MR, Crepaz N, Guenther-Gray C, et al. Efficacy of structural-level condom distribution interventions: a meta-analysis of U.S. and international studies, 1998–2007. *AIDS Behav* 2011;15:1283–1297.
35. Wretzel SR, Visintainer PF, Pinkston Koenigs LM. Condom availability program in an inner city public school: effect on the rates of gonorrhea and chlamydia infection. *J Adolesc Health.* 2011;49:324–326.
36. Condom Distribution Programs, Diffusion of Effective Behavioral Interventions project (DEBI). Available at http://www.effectiveinterventions.org/en/HighImpact Prevention/StructuralInterventions/CondomDistribution/HealthDepartment Programs.aspx. Accessed January 31, 2014.
37. De Rosa CJ, Jeffries RA, Afifi AA. Improving the implementation of a condom availability program in urban high schools. *J Adolesc Heatlh.* 2012;51:572–579.
38. Beksinska M, Smit J, Joanis C, et al. Female condom technology: new products and regulatory issues. *Contraception* 2011;83:316–321.
39. McNaught J, Jamieson MA. Barrier and spermicidal contraceptives in adolescence. *Adolesc Med Clin* 2005;16:495–515.
40. World Health Organization. WHO/CONRAD technical consultation on nonoxynol-9, World Health Organization, Geneva, 9–10 October 2001: summary report. *Reprod Health Matters* 2002;10:175–181.
41. Develop the Next Generation of Condom. Available at http://www.grandchallenges.org/Explorations/Topics/Pages/NextGenerationCondomRound12.aspx. Accessed January 31, 2014.
42. Latka MH, Kapadia F, Fortin P. The female condom: effectiveness and convenience, not "female control," valued by U.S. urban adolescents. *AIDS Educ Prev* 2008;20:160–170.

🛜 **ADDITIONAL RESOURCES AND WEBSITES ONLINE**

43

Contraceptive Pills, Patches, Rings, and Injections

Anita L. Nelson

KEY WORDS

- Contraceptive patches
- Contraceptive vaginal rings
- Depot medroxyprogesterone acetate (DMPA)
- Injectable contraceptives
- Oral contraceptives

Despite the availability of top-tier contraceptive options (such as intrauterine devices [IUDs] and implants) and the professional endorsement of their use as first-line contraceptive choices for adolescent and young adult (AYA) women, combined oral contraceptives (COCs) remain the most frequently used reversible method in the US, especially among women under 26 years of age. Newer delivery systems of estrogen-containing hormonal contraception (transdermal patches and vaginal rings) have also enjoyed great popularity among young women. Injectable contraception was extremely important in reducing adolescent pregnancy rates in the 1990s, but subsequently, lost favor as a result of the unfortunate black box warning about bone loss. Progestin-only pills are underutilized in all age groups.

This chapter will address practical issues about the selection, initiation, and continuation of each of these methods and will provide suggestions to help AYAs using these methods become more successful contraceptors. Much of the content will be based on two evidence-based guidelines from the US Centers for Disease Control and Prevention (CDC), which have significantly streamlined access to birth control, standardized contraceptive practices, and simplified identification of candidates for each method.[1,2] These documents have freed practitioners from the theoretical concerns and the restrictions imposed by product labels and have provided current recommendations that enable at-risk women of all ages to choose from a more complete array of contraceptive methods. It should be noted that in these documents younger age does not enter into any consideration for use of these methods. The only age group that presents any medical concern for any method is women over 35. Therefore, recommendations made for women in this chapter apply to both adolescent women and young adult women unless otherwise specified. In the past, adolescent women had the highest rates of unintended pregnancy. Today, it is women in their early 20s who have the highest rates, so combining these two groups is logical not only from a clinical perspective but also from a public health standpoint.

The first of these publications was the US Medical Eligibility Criteria (see Figure 41.1), which rated the safety of each method for women with a wide variety of medical problems.[1] Many sexually active AYAs today have serious medical problems (e.g., obesity, tobacco addiction, migraine headaches) that need to be considered when offering contraception. The effectiveness of each method must also be factored into the calculation of safety, particularly because women in this age group are more fertile and, therefore, are more apt to become pregnant and to suffer significant pregnancy complications. When grouped by first-year failure rates in typical use, the methods discussed in this chapter fall into what is considered to be second-tier contraceptive methods, that is those that fall between the top-tier long-acting reversible contraceptive methods and all the other methods in the third tier (barrier and behavioral methods).

The second document that forms the foundation for this chapter's recommendations is the CDC's Selected Practice Recommendations for Contraception, 2013.[2] This publication removed many of the traditional, unnecessary practices that had previously created barriers to women's contraceptive success.

There are over 90 contraceptive pills on the US market, as well as the transdermal patch, vaginal ring, and two injectables. Rather than list each product with its ingredients, this chapter will provide a brief discussion of the characteristics of each group of hormones, followed by generalizations designed to help clinicians find their ways through this cornucopia of choices.

CONTRACEPTIVE FORMULATIONS BY HORMONE

Estrogens

There are only three forms of estrogen currently found in COCs. The transdermal and vaginal delivery systems use only one estrogen.

Mestranol is the oldest estrogen and is used only in older oral contraceptives. It is a prodrug (a compound that, on administration, undergoes chemical conversion to an active pharmacological agent) that requires hepatic conversion to create its active form ethinyl estradiol (EE). In general, ingestion of 50 µg mestranol will yield 35 to 40 µg EE. Monophasic pills with 50 µg mestranol are still marketed. There is no advantage to using formulations with this estrogen; the less predictable estrogen dose may be a disadvantage.

EE is found in virtually all US combined hormonal contraceptives (CHCs). EE is fairly resistant to hepatic metabolism and, therefore, maintains therapeutic systemic levels throughout the day to provide adequate endometrial support. Because it is so potent and long acting, EE profoundly impacts hepatic production of a wide array of carrier proteins, increasing binding globulins (e.g., sex hormone–binding globulin (SHBG), corticosteroid-binding globulin, thyroid-binding globulin), lipid components (increasing high-density lipoprotein-cholesterol and triglycerides), and coagulation factors (increasing factors in the extrinsic cascade and deceasing antifibrinolytic molecules). Together, these can impact the risks, particularly of thrombosis, with some minor impacts on metabolic profiles.

Estradiol valerate is found in one US birth control pill. The valerate ester is cleaved during intestinal absorption; the resulting estradiol is rapidly converted along familiar pathways to weaker estrogens, such as estrone (E1). In Europe, there is a monophasic formulation containing estradiol. These estrogens have considerably less hepatic impact than EE, but surrogate measures, such as antithrombin-III levels, are not reliable predictors of important clinical outcomes, such as thrombosis. Thus, longer-term studies are needed to determine the clinical significance of the differences between EE and estradiol.

Progestins

The progestin component of combined hormonal birth control methods provides most of the contraceptive effects. There are some distinctions among these groups of progestins, but they all provide solid pregnancy protection. Their differences are manifested more in potential side effect profiles.[3]

Norethindrone, norethindrone acetate, and ethynodiol diacetate are the progestins that have been used in oral contraceptives since the 1960s; they have a long record of safety and efficacy. In a survey of pill users from 2006 to 2010, 20% said they used pill brands with these progestins.[4] Although derived from a C-19 scaffolding (19-nortestosterone), pills with these progestins rarely cause noticeable androgenic side effects. The progestin-only pill in the US has low doses of norethindrone (0.35 mg). The only clinical issue with this progestin is its relatively short half-life (8 hours), which can translate clinically into higher rates of unscheduled bleeding and spotting, especially in low-dose combined formulations with traditional 21 active pills per packet.

Norgestrel and levonorgestrel are much more potent and longer-lasting progestins introduced to provide better cycle control, particularly when combined with lower doses of estrogens. Levonorgestrel is used in pills taken by 19% of women, in the progestin-releasing IUDs and in some contraceptive implants offered overseas.[4] The issue with these progestins is that they are more strongly androgenic; in preclinical studies, these progestins induce greater growth in ventral rat prostate. Clinically, this may be reflected in women by acne, oily skin, and facial hair growth. While these cosmetic impacts may not be well tolerated by a minority of users of this class of progestin, stronger androgenicity may cancel some of the estrogen-induced hepatic impacts. Studies, especially in populations with relatively high prevalence of Factor V Leiden mutations, have suggested that combined pills with these progestins may be associated with lower risk of thrombosis.[5]

Norgestimate and desogestrel were introduced in the US in an attempt to decrease androgenicity of the progestin while maintaining long half-life. In Europe, *gestodene* is also available. The first pill with a US Food and Drug Administration (FDA)-approved noncontraceptive benefit (i.e., treatment of mild-to-moderate cystic acne) contained norgestimate. The progestin in the patch (norelgestromin) is a primary metabolite of norgestimate. In the 2006 to 2010 survey, over 30% of pill users took pills containing norgestimate and another 8% used desogestrel-containing pills.[4] The main metabolite of desogestrel (etonogestrel) is the progestin used in both the vaginal contraceptive ring and in the contraceptive implant. While these progestins themselves are not prothrombotic, it has been suggested that in CHC products, they may be associated with slightly increased risk of thrombosis because they do not mute the impact of EE on hepatic production of coagulation factors.[6]

Drospirenone (DRSP) differs from other synthetic progestins in that its pharmacological profile is closer to natural progesterone. DRSP is an analog of the potassium-sparing diuretic, spironolactone. At the 3 mg doses found in oral contraceptives, it exhibits both anti-androgenic and anti-mineralocorticoid impacts equivalent to 25 mg spirolactone. Its anti-mineralocorticoid properties counteract the estrogen-stimulated renin–angiotensin–aldosterone system, which helps explain its benefits in reducing the physical and emotional symptoms of premenstrual dysphoric disorder

(PMDD). This effect is also why it should not be coadministered with drugs that increase serum potassium levels. As a mild anti-androgenic compound, DRSP enables the fullest expression of the estrogen component of the pill and, therefore, is particularly useful on-label for treatment of acne and off-label for treatment of hirsutism. However, DRSP may also permit an increase in the risk of thrombosis. Although studies have produced widely divergent results, the FDA amended the labeling of pills with DRSP to say "Based on presently available information, DRSP-containing COCs may be associated with a higher risk of venous thromboembolism (VTE) than COCs containing the progestin levonorgestrel or some other progestins."[7] In recent years, use of DRSP-containing pills has diminished, but in the 2006 to 2010 survey, 17% of pill users reported taking pills with this progestin.[4]

Newer progestins, such as the currently available *dienogest*, and possible future candidates such as *nomegestrol acetate* so significantly suppress the endometrium that they can provide good cycle control when coupled with estradiol in lieu of EE. The multiphasic formulation containing dienogest is the only oral contraceptive that is FDA-approved for the treatment of heavy menstrual bleeding.

Medroxyprogesterone acetate is a derivative of progesterone, not testosterone, and has two different formulations as microcrystals suspended in an aqueous solution for contraception as intramuscular or subcutaneous injections.

Progestin-only pills—There is only one such product available in the US at this time, although many generic versions are sold. Each pill contains 0.35 mg norethindrone. The pack contains 28 active pills and no placebo pills. These pills are the safest of all available oral contraceptives; they have few contraindications and are as effective as combination pills in typical use.

Special Features and Additives of Oral Contraceptives

- Some formulations add iron supplements to the placebo pills.
- Two formulations include levomefolate calcium in each pill to raise serum folate levels to a therapeutic range in an attempt to reduce risk of neural tube defects should pregnancy occur while a woman is taking pills or shortly after she stops taking them.
- One formulation is chewable.

Formulations/Delivery Systems for CHCs
Combined Oral Contraceptives
COC options include:

a. Dosing patterns in single-pill packets vary in the following patterns:
   Monophasic formulations—each active pill has the same doses of hormones as all the other active pills. Monophasic formulations may simplify missed pill instructions.
   Multiphasic formulations—the dose of estrogen and/or progestin in different active pills varies. Multiphasic formulations reduce the total hormonal exposure over a cycle and may be useful in controlling unscheduled bleeding seen with some monophasic formulations.
b. Number of active pills and placebo pills in traditional 28-pill packs varies:
   21/7: classic pattern of 21 active pills and 7 placebo pills
   21/2/5: 21 active pills, 2 placebo pills, and 5 tablets with 10 µg EE
   24/4: 24 active pills, 4 placebo pills
   24/2/2: 24 active pills, 2 placebos, 2 low-dose estrogen-only pills
c. Extended-cycle formulations
   84/7: 84 active pills followed by 7 placebo pills or
   84/7: 84 active pills followed by 7 tablets each with 10 µg EE

Vaginal Contraceptive Ring

Labeled for use as a 21-day device that is then removed for 7 days to recreate the 21/7 pattern of traditional COC, the ring actually contains sufficient hormonal reserve for 6 weeks for both

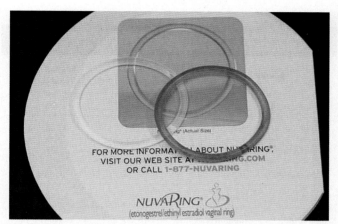

FIGURE 43.1 Examples of vaginal contraceptive rings highlight their small size and flexible shape.

normal-weight and obese women (Fig. 43.1).[8] Therefore, it can also be prescribed as an extended-cycle (continuous) once-a-month method. Over a 24-hour period, the amount of progestin released from the ring (area under the curve) is equivalent to that absorbed from oral contraceptives, but area under the curve for EE is half of that seen with oral contraceptives. Thus, the amount of estrogen absorbed via the ring is substantially less. Despite the lower levels of estrogen, cycle control with the ring was found to be superior to that of COCs.[9] The most recent FDA review of this issue concluded that the risk of VTE with the ring was equivalent to COCs.

Instructions for ring use are quite straightforward; use requires that the consumer feel comfortable touching herself. Tampon users are often the most willing to try this method. For women who have any difficulty placing the ring, a smooth-ridge tampon insertion tube can be used (after removal of the tampon) to place the ring flat against the vaginal walls anywhere in the upper vagina. In that position, only 30% of partners report they can detect the ring's presence during coitus and only a fraction of those women need to remove the ring for partner comfort. Women need to remember that in order to maintain efficacy, the ring may be removed for no more than 3 hours in any 24-hour period. The pouch that the ring comes in serves as a temporary storage area and also should be used to dispose of the ring at the end of its useful life. The ring increases vaginal secretions, which can be helpful to provide lubrication during intercourse and it increases lactobacillus numbers, which reduces recurrences of bacterial vaginosis.[10]

Transdermal Contraceptive Patch

To date, the contraceptive patch is a unique product with EE and norelgestromin (metabolite of norgestimate). The user applies one patch per week at different sites on her abdomen, back, chest (not breasts) or on her upper arm for three consecutive weeks followed by one patch-free week. Occasionally, extending the use of consecutive active patches for a few weeks for specific indications is reasonable, but ongoing extended-cycle use is not recommended. Only one study has investigated the safety and efficacy of 12 weeks of uninterrupted use; it found that serum levels of EE increased with time. In the clinical trials, greater numbers of women of all ages reported correct use with the patch than with the pill, but the greatest improvement was found in women aged 18 to 19. With initial use, breast tenderness was noted in 20% of women, but in subsequent cycles, patch users reported this no more frequently than COC users.

The patch has been associated with a higher risk of VTE, which was plausible because 24-hour area-under-the-curve levels of EE with the patch are about 60% higher than those found with use of 35 μg oral contraceptives. Although epidemiological studies have not consistently reported higher rates of VTE, the product

label suggests that patch users might face greater VTE risks than by lower-dose pill users, but those VTE risks are lower than those faced by women in pregnancy.

Depot Medroxyprogesterone Acetate

There are two branded formulations of depot medroxyprogesterone acetate (DMPA) in the US—one administered intramuscularly (IM) (DMPA 150 mg IM) and one that is given subcutaneously (Sub-Q) (DMPA 104 mg/0.6 cc Sub-Q). These products differ not only in amount of DMPA and the intended site of injection, but also in the buffers used in the injection fluid. As a result, the two formulations are not interchangeable with each other, nor are they interchangeable with the 425 mg/mL DMPA product used in chemotherapy. Generic products exist for the IM version. Efficacy for either DMPA is not affected by body mass index (BMI). Reinjections are scheduled every 11 to 13 weeks for the DMPA-IM and every 12 to 14 weeks for the DMPA Sub-Q. Serum levels of medroxyprogesterone acetate remain detectable in some users as late as 7 to 9 months after injection. There is slow absorption (not steady state) of DMPA from the injection site; some metabolites are biologically active and are stored within the adipose tissue. Return to fertility averages 7 to 9 months after injection; it is independent of the number of injections the woman has had, but is generally slower in women with more adiposity.

Efficacy

There are two important measures of contraceptive efficacy:

"Perfect Use" Failure Rate

Estimates of the potential pregnancy protection afforded with correct and consistent use of a method during the first year of use ("perfect use" failure rate). This statistic is derived from data from clinical trials after adjustments have been made for inconsistent use. For DMPA, the Pearl index (failure rate) with correct and consistent use is 0.2%, while all the other second-tier methods have failure rates with correct and consistent use of 0.3%.

Typical Use Failure Rate

The first-year failure rates with typical use are obtained from the National Survey of Family Growth—a detailed survey conducted every 5 years. First-year typical use failure rates for each of these second-tier methods are much higher than those seen in clinical trials. For the injection DMPA, the first-year typical use failure rate is 6%, while the typical use failure rates of all the other hormonal methods in this category are 9%. It is important to note that, contrary to common belief, the failure rates in typical use for the progestin-only pills are no higher than those found with the estrogen-containing pills. On the other hand, it might be expected that with the convenience of non-daily dosing, the patch and ring would have lower failure rates than the daily pills, but data have not yet substantiated that hypothesis. The gap between the pregnancy protection that is possible with each of these methods and what is actually achieved demonstrates the impact of inconsistent use (Table 43.1).

Other Considerations

Impact of Formulation on Effectiveness: Recent work suggests that some formulations of COCs may be more effective in typical use than others; extended-cycle formulations have lower failure rates than 24/4 formulations and the 24/4 formulations have lower failure rates than traditional 21/7 formulations.[11]

Impact of BMI on Effectiveness: The potential efficacy of pills and vaginal rings is not reduced in women with higher BMI,[12,13] even though absorption of progestin has been shown to be slower in obese women compared to normal-weight women.[14] The explanation for the fact that some studies showed higher failure rates among obese

TABLE 43.1

Real-Life Utilization of Second-Tier Methods[38,39]

- 57% of established pill users miss at least three pills per pack
- Women typically use pills only 8 cycles out of 10
- Only a quarter of new start pill, patch, or ring users obtains "timely refills" during the first 12 mo of use
- One in 5 new start DMPA users returns "on time" for reinjection for 12 mo (3 reinjections)
- Methods for which the patient perceives a noncontraceptive benefit are used more consistently

TABLE 43.2

Impact of Enzyme-Inducing Anticonvulsants on Systemic Levels of Sex Steroids[40]

Drug	Brand Name	EE Reduction (%)	Progestin Reduction (%)
Carbamazepine	Tegretol	42	58
Felbamate	Felbatol	13	42
Oxcarbazine	Trileptal	48	32
Phenobarbital	Generic	64–72	None
Phenytoin	Dilantin	49	42
Topiramate	Topamax	15–33	None

women may rest in the observation that obese women were significantly more likely not to take their pills than were lighter women. When the study findings were adjusted for pill use, obese women had no higher rates of ovulation than the normal-weight women.[15] The efficacy of the patch may be significantly diminished in women weighing more than 198 pounds.

Mechanisms of Action

What These Methods to Not Do

- None of these methods is an abortifacient.
- None disrupts an established pregnancy.
- There is also no convincing evidence that any of these methods interferes with implantation of a fertilized egg, although these methods all induce changes in the endometrium that affect bleeding patterns.

What These Methods Do to Prevent Pregnancy

Overall, progestins provide contraception by several different mechanisms, depending on the dose, potency of the progestins, and the delivery system used.

- Every progestin consistently thickens cervical mucus, which blocks sperm penetration into the upper genital tract.
- Progestins also alter tubal transport time, which slows transit of both the ovum and sperm.
- Ovulation inhibition varies with each method:
  - Progestin-only pills available in the US prevent ovulation in 40% to 60% of cycles.
  - Mid-dose birth control pills/patches/rings suppress ovulation in >90% of cycles.
  - DMPA provides almost complete ovulation suppression.
- Estrogen, which is generally added for cycle control, may also blunt follicular stimulating hormone release.

Drug–Drug Interactions

Drugs that induce hepatic enzymes can alter the serum concentration of estrogen and/or progestin of these contraceptives, which may increase failure rates or result in excessive circulating hormone levels. It should be noted that the only drug known to affect DMPA efficacy is aminoglutethimide. There is also the possibility that sex steroids could influence the metabolism of other drugs and alter their efficacy. Other potential mechanisms for drug–drug interactions, such as enterohepatic recirculation or induction of binding globulins, have either no or insignificant clinical impacts compared to the background interindividual variability observed in the absorption and metabolism of these compounds.

Anticonvulsants

This is the most common class of drugs known to have reciprocal impacts on progestin and estrogen. Many of these drugs are used for other indications, such as treatment of bipolar disease, neuropathic pain, migraines, and posttraumatic stress syndrome. Barbiturates (phenobarbital and primidone), phenytoin, carbamazepine, felbamate, and topiramate all decrease circulating levels of both estrogen and progestin in oral contraceptives,

pills, and patches (**Table 43.2**). If a COC is selected for women using enzyme-inducing anticonvulsants, formulations with at least 35 µg EE and shortened or no pill-free intervals should be used. DMPA concentrations are not significantly affected by any of these drugs and may be a better contraceptive option. Many of the newer anticonvulsant drugs do not induce hepatic enzyme activity (**Table 43.3**) and, therefore, do not affect estrogen or progestin levels. Lamotrigine presents unique challenges. While lamotrigine does not affect the levels of contraceptive hormones, lamotrigine's own metabolic clearance is significantly increased by estrogens and circulating levels of lamotrigine are reduced to 41% to 64% of those seen without estrogen-containing contraceptives. This means that the dose of lamotrigine, when used as monotherapy, must be significantly increased (i.e., doubled) while the woman is taking active pills, to avoid breakthrough seizures. The doses need to be decreased significantly when she stops pill use, to avoid overdosing. For this reason, the number of pill-free days needs to be minimized between cycles. Individual monitoring is needed to calculate the doses of lamotrigine each woman will need when on CHC. Other methods, such as DMPA, appear safer to use. Of note, therapies that combine a non–enzyme-inducing anticonvulsant, such as valproic acid, with lamotrigine do not require any dosing modifications for lamotrigine when the woman uses estrogen-containing contraceptives.

Anti-tuberculosis Drugs

Rifampin alone or in combination with other anti-tuberculosis agents is a very potent inducer of CYP450, which increases hepatic clearance of both estrogen and progestin. It also increases SHBG to reduce circulating levels of biologically active contraceptive hormones. Ovulation rates in COC users taking rifampin have

TABLE 43.3

Non-Enzyme-Inducing Anticonvulsants

Drug	Brand Name
Ethosuximide	Zarontin
Levetiracetam	Keppra
Tiagabine	Gabitril
Valproic acid	Depakene, Depakote
Clonazepam	Klonopin
Galanin, Pregabalin	Lyrica

been noted to be as high as 50%. Other options, such as DMPA or IUDs, are more appropriate. Rifampin is used in some settings to treat methicillin-resistant *Staphylococcus aureus*. At a minimum, backup contraception should be used during rifampin therapy and for at least one month following completion of that therapy.

Antiretroviral Agents

The various classes of drugs in this category have different impacts of hepatic enzyme activity. As a general rule, the US Medical Eligibility Criteria for Contraceptive Use (see Figure 41.1) rate the nucleoside reverse transcription inhibitors as Category 1 (no restriction) for all hormonal methods, but the non-nucleoside reverse transcriptase inhibitors (NNRTIs) as Category 2 (advantages of using the method generally outweigh the risks) for all tier 2 hormonal methods except DMPA (Category 1). The possible exception is the NNRTI Efavirenz; it may require higher doses of contraceptives. Ritonavir-boosted protease inhibitors are Category 3 (risks usually outweigh the advantages of using method) for all tier 2 methods except DMPA, which remains at Category 1.

Herbal Medicines

The most significant agent to consider in this group is St. John's Wort (Hypericum perforation), which is a strong inducer of CYP3A4 and of the transmembrane transporter P-glycoprotein. Even after only a brief exposure, St. John's Wort significantly increases both unscheduled bleeding and pregnancy. DMPA is the only tier 2 method that is unaffected by this botanical agent.[16]

Other Important Interactions

Other potentially important drug interactions deserve mention. Women using high doses of vitamin C or acetaminophen may have higher circulating levels of EE. On the other hand, griseofulvin and modafinil may reduce CHC efficacy. In women using a CHC method, clearance of the following drugs may be reduced, so *higher* systemic levels may result: warfarin, chlordiazepoxide, alprazolam, diazepam, nitrazepam, theophylline, prednisone, caffeine, cyclosporine, and tacrolimus. On the other hand, clearance of the following drugs may be increased in the face of CHC use resulting in *lower* systemic levels: temazepam, salicylic acid, paracetamol, morphine, and clofibric acid. Other issues that need to be considered are secondary impacts. For example, since fractures occur in 30% to 50% of chronic glucocorticoid steroid users, should there be concerns about DMPA use in these women?[17] Immunosuppressive agents can cause hypertension. Can women on these agents with well-controlled hypertension use a CHC?[18] Progestins contribute to insulin resistance; DMPA has the highest levels of circulating progestin so can women with additional risk factors for diabetes or for developing diabetic complications use DMPA? The answer to each of these questions is generally yes, but it is prudent to evaluate the woman's other contraceptive options before recommending these agents.

Drospirenone

A special mention must be made that DRSP-containing contraceptives should be used with caution in women who have medical conditions that predispose them to hyperkalemia. In general, these conditions themselves contraindicate use of any estrogen-containing products. Women who, on a daily basis, use long-term medications that place them at risk for hyperkalemia (e.g., nonsteroidal anti-inflammatory drugs) should have their serum potassium levels tested once for reassurance about two weeks after initiating DRSP-containing contraceptives. If that potassium level is normal, no further testing is needed.

Safety

Progestin-only products (progestin-only pills and DMPA injections) are safe for virtually all women. This can be seen in the fact that there are few Category 4 (condition that represents an unacceptable health risk if the contraceptive method is used) medical

conditions that prohibit their use (see Figure 41.1). The only absolute contraindication to progestin-only pills or injections is current or recent (<5 years) breast cancer. Category 3 conditions are also limited to severe manifestations of diseases, such as diabetes, hypertension, cardiovascular disease, hepatocellular carcinoma, stroke, or systemic lupus erythematosus. However, often progestin-only methods are the only viable options left to women with these problems who do not want to use copper IUD.

Combination Pills

The addition of estrogen to progestin markedly increases the numbers of potential types of serious adverse events, although their absolute incidence is low. The most significant of these serious events relates to arterial and VTE—myocardial infarction, pulmonary embolism, and stroke. Estimates are that the risk of death from myocardial infarction in a healthy young nonsmoking pill user is about 1 in a million,[19] which is roughly the risk of being hit by lightning. Other studies of COC users have found that the risk of thrombotic stroke and myocardial infarction increased by a factor of 0.9 to 1.7 with 20 mcg EE contraceptives and by 1.3 to 2.3 with higher doses of EE, with relatively small differences in risk according to progestin type.[20]

VTE risk in adolescents is even lower than the general population, but 5% to 10% of total contraceptive-related VTE events occur among teens because of the high frequency of CHC use in this group.[21] As the FDA points out, the absolute VTE risks are increased for users of an estrogen-containing CHC compared to nonusers, but the rates during pregnancy are even greater, especially during the postpartum period. For new users, the FDA-commissioned study found that pills with DRSP may be associated with high risk for VTE and arterial thromboembolism (ATE) compared to other CHCs, but the patch and ring did not.[22] A large prospective Phase IV study of 33,295 new users of oral contraceptives or the contraceptive ring followed for two to four years found that the adjusted hazard ratio for ring users compared to pill users to be 0.8 (95% confidence interval (CI): 0.5 to 1.5) for VTE and 0.7 (95% CI: 0.2 to 7.3) for ATE.[23]

The FDA also noted that the risk of VTE with COC use is greatest with initiation of a COC or restarting the same or a different COC (following a four-week or greater pill-free interval). This has significant implications for counseling women about ways to reduce their risks with use of estrogen-containing methods—messages that seem counterintuitive. Unless a woman plans to entirely discontinue her use of the method, it is actually safer for her to continue to use it rather than to interrupt its use (skip a month or two of pills). The increase in risk of thromboembolism due to use of estrogen-containing contraceptives is not permanent; it gradually disappears after the method has been discontinued.

Many young women have risk factors, such as hypertension, obesity, dyslipidemia, tobacco addiction, type 2 diabetes, and migraine headaches with aura, which tend to increase their baseline risks for thromboembolic and other adverse events. These factors must be considered when selecting a method with the AYAs and should always be put into the context of the effectiveness of her other available options (her risk of pregnancy with other method use).

There are other serious health risks that have been associated with use of COC. Estimates of their relative and absolute risks (**Table 43.4**) are derived only for populations of all users (not only younger women) and, in many cases, they also reflect the impact of older, higher-dose formulations. Even though these risk estimates may seem inflated, they prove the point that these methods are safer than pregnancy. This is in stark contrast to patients' perceptions. In a recent survey, 76% of women rated oral contraceptives as more hazardous to a woman's health than pregnancy.[24]

Long-term safety of pill use has been well established. In the final Oxford Family Planning Report, ever-oral contraceptive use was not associated with any increase in breast cancer or

TABLE 43.4

Serious Adverse Effects Associated with Oral Contraceptive Use for Women of Reproductive Age

Adverse Effects	Relative Risk	Absolute Risk
Cholelithiasis	2×	1:1,250
Thrombophlebitis	3×	1:10,000
Stroke	4×	1:30,000
Hepatic adenoma	500×	1:30,000
Mild hypertension	2–3×	<1:20

Courtesy of Paul Brenner, M.D., University of Southern California.

TABLE 43.5

Hormones Implicated with Specific Side Effects

Estrogen-Related	Progestin-Related	
Estrogenic	Progestogenic	Androgenic
Nausea and vomiting	Fatigue	Noncyclic weight gain
Edema, leg cramps	Depression	Oily skin
Bloating	Bloating	Hirsutism
Cervical ectropion	Mastalgia	Acne
Visual changes or vascular headaches	Increased breast size	Decreased breast size
Telangiectasia, melisma	Venous dilation, pelvic congestion	Decrease in libido
		Increased appetite

nonreproductive system cancer, but past COC use significantly reduced the risk of ovarian and endometrial cancer. Perhaps because of selection bias, cervical cancer risk is increased, but was on par with the risk associated with high parity.[25] In the long-term follow-up of the cohort studied for decades in the Royal College General Practitioners' Oral Contraceptive Study, it was shown that ever OC users had a decreased risk in all-cause mortality as well as decrease in cardiovascular diseases.[26] Many of these women had used high-dose pills—much higher than modern formulations. Although selection bias may color these results, at least these studies show no increased risks in any long-term health outcome for pill users.

Side Effects

Attributable Side Effects

Bleeding pattern changes are clearly altered by hormonal contraceptives. CHCs are unquestionably responsible for increased unscheduled bleeding, especially with inconsistent use and with early use. DMPA initially causes considerable unscheduled bleeding and spotting, but many women achieve amenorrhea between the third and fourth injection. Facial melasma and darkening of skin pigment elsewhere are also direct effects of estrogen stimulation. Eversion of the cervical ectropion is also to be expected with pharmacologic dose of estrogens. Dry eye symptoms are mentioned more often by women who wear contact lens and use oral contraceptives. Menstrual migraine symptoms may be exacerbated by monthly withdrawal from the pharmacologic levels of EE associated with CHC use. Progestins relax vascular tension, so more venous varicosities may be attributable to exposure to those compounds.

Nocebo Effects

This new term, nocebo effects, has been applied to a group of side effects that have been inappropriately assigned to CHC use. Product labeling and over 50 years of clinical practice claim that other adverse events such as nausea, vomiting, headache, weight changes, mood changes, and persistent mastalgia are due to hormonal contraceptive use. However, placebo-controlled studies (done for non-contraceptive indications) clearly demonstrate that at a population level, these side effects occur at no higher rates and no greater intensity in CHC users than in placebo users.[27] Furthermore, since counseling women about the risks of developing such side effects with oral contraceptives undoubtedly increases the likelihood that the women will experience those problems, it has been concluded that counseling women about those risks is unwarranted and is probably unethical.[27] While this may be a controversial (although evidence-based) conclusion, it is clear that none of these side effects will occur with hormonal contraception with the frequency or intensity that is seen in pregnancy.

It may be difficult in this day and age to dissuade women from anticipating side effects they "know" happen with the pill.

Additionally, at the individual level, some women may be more sensitive to exogenous hormones than others, so it would be helpful to suggest pill formulations that might reduce her symptoms. **Table 43.5** lists the hormones (estrogen, progestin, or androgen) and the associated complaints in an effort to help guide the clinician in pill selection.

DMPA and Side Effects

Weight gain with DMPA may fall into a different category. The original data linking weight gain to DMPA use did not adjust for the background increase in expected weight gain in the study population. This is particularly true of weight gain seen in adolescents. In the only prospective, double-blind, placebo-controlled study of DMPA and weight changes, DMPA users showed no weight gain, no change in appetite, and no change in resting metabolic rate. However, excessive weight gain has been variably seen in retrospective studies. One important observation is that younger women, who experience at least 5% weight gain with initial DMPA use, are apt to continue gaining weight with continued DMPA use and need at least targeted counseling.[28]

The *bone density loss* that prompted the FDA black box warning limiting DMPA use to 2 years has been now found to be reversible and generally not clinically significant for healthy women of any age.[29]

HIV Infection: A potential association seen in some South African studies between DMPA use and increased transmission of HIV infection has not been supported by all similar studies, but underscores the need to encourage dual method use for at-risk DMPA users.

Noncontraceptive Benefits

Young women are often acutely troubled by irregular menses, androgen excess challenges, and dysmenorrhea, and they wish to preserve their fertility and reduce their risk for serious health problems (cancer) in the future. Hormonal contraception can contribute to each of these objectives.[30]

Menstrually Related Symptoms Reduced

Cyclic use of COC, patches, and vaginal rings makes scheduled bleeding more predictable, decreases blood loss, and reduces dysmenorrhea.[31] Mittelschmerz is eliminated in most women because ovulation is inhibited in virtually all cycles. The multiphasic pill with dienogest and estradiol valerate is FDA-approved for the treatment of idiopathic heavy menstrual bleeding. These benefits are particularly important to women with bleeding disorders, endometriosis, and primary dysmenorrhea. Painful menses is the most common reason why women younger than 25 years of age miss days of school and work.[32] Premenstrual tension symptoms are generally reduced by any of these agents, but only the low-dose DRSP COC is FDA-approved for the treatment of PMDD.

DMPA and extended-cycle use of COCs or vaginal rings are most effective in controlling menstrual symptoms. The Sub-Q DMPA formulation is an FDA-approved treatment for the symptoms of endometriosis. DMPA and extended-cycle use of CHCs also are helpful in treating medical problems, which tend to exacerbate with menses—such as menstrual migraines, catamenial seizures, asthma attacks, and catamenial porphyria.

Improvement in Acne, Hirsutism, and Other Androgen Excess Problems

The FDA has approved three brands of CHC for the treatment of mild-to-moderate cystic acne. Other estrogen-containing formulations reduce ovarian production of androgens and increase SHBG to decrease circulating unbound testosterone levels. Hirsutism scores drop slowly with CHC use, so maximum effect may not be seen for up to 2 years. Estrogen-containing contraceptives may also help women with hidradenitis suppurativa reduce their numbers of outbreaks.

Reduction in the Risk of Endometrial and Ovarian Cancers

Endometrial cancer is the most common reproductive system malignancy. Precursor lesions can develop in young women with anovulatory cycles (infrequent menses), especially if they are obese. Provision of progestin significantly reduces these risks. Even a few years of COC use can reduce incidence of endometrial carcinoma by 40%, and longer-duration use provides greater protection. This protection lasts for 20 years beyond the time of last hormone use.

CHC is the only medical intervention with strong evidence that appears to reduce the risk of ovarian carcinoma. Women with BRCA-1 mutations benefit greatly from its use. This protection is increased with longer duration of use and endures for at least 15 years.[33]

Other Health Benefits

Anemia is reduced because menstrual blood loss is diminished. Women with sickle cell anemia experience significant reduction in the number of acute sickle crises with DMPA (70% reduction) and with COCs (50% reduction) and their remaining crises tend to be less severe. Long-term COC use has been associated with decrease in benign breast disorders of all types except atypical hyperplasia.

Method Initiation

Required Pretesting

Patient counseling is the most critical element in helping the adolescent or young adult woman achieve contraceptive success and a high rate of method continuation. More time must be dedicated to education during patient visits. The Selected Practice Recommendation for Contraception, 2013 separates routine well-women care from examinations and tests that may be needed before initiation of a contraceptive method.[2] This approach is intended to reduce barriers to birth control and may be particularly important to AYAs who may delay seeking contraception because they are apprehensive about having a pelvic examination. Key to the success of this approach, however, is a complete medical history to identify women who might need additional testing before starting a given hormonal method. According to these new guidelines for healthy women, no examinations or testing is needed prior to initiation of DMPA injections or progestin-only pills and only blood pressure measurements are recommended before prescribing estrogen-containing methods to women whose medical histories do not reveal health problems. It may be prudent to measure the woman's weight and to calculate her BMI in order to monitor changes she may attribute to her method in the future.

All methods in this group can be initiated anytime in a woman's cycle when it is reasonably certain she is not pregnant. Backup methods are needed for 7 days if a method is started more than five days after the first day of the woman's last menstrual period. Emergency contraception (EC) may be added, if needed. If ulipristal acetate is used for EC, provide 14 days of backup. Also consider delaying CHC initiation until the woman's next menses. Following first- or second-trimester pregnancy loss/termination, any of these methods may be started promptly within seven days without need for backup method. Following term delivery, progestin-only methods may be started prior to discharge home, even in breast-feeding women.[34] Timing of initiation of estrogen-containing methods in both breast-feeding and non–breast-feeding women is determined by their risk factors. Healthy women can start those methods at 21 days postpartum, even if they are breast-feeding.[35] However, women who are obese, immobile, delivered by C-section, as well as those who experienced hemorrhage or preeclampsia, required transfusion, or are tobacco smokers should wait until 42 days postpartum to start using estrogen-containing methods.[1] Progestin-only pills can provide an excellent bridge until combined hormonal methods can be started.

Practice Recommendations for Each of the Second-Tier Methods

Practice recommendations to enhance young women's success with contraceptive pills, patches, and vaginal rings are summarized in **Table 43.6**. Corresponding recommendations for DMPA users are outlined in **Table 43.7**. It should be expected that some adolescents or young adult women will forget pills or delay patch or ring placement and removal; recommendations for management of missed doses of CHCs are highlighted on **Table 43.8**. For those using progestin-only pills, the rules are easier to remember: If the woman is more than 3 hours late in taking a progestin-only pill, she needs to take her pill at once and use a backup method for at least 2 days after she restarts her pills. EC may be needed if she has had unprotected intercourse in the last 5 days.

Young women are particularly at risk for acquiring sexually transmitted infections (STIs), both because of their increased biological susceptibility and their behaviors. Always remind women who choose to use these second-tier methods that condom use for STI risk reduction is very important. It is estimated that only 5% of women aged 15 to 24 years use dual methods. Counseling can have a temporary impact, but that will wane if not sustained at each visit by clinician reinforcement.[36]

TABLE 43.6

Practice Recommendations: Pills, Patches, Rings[41,42]

- All second-tier method tips
  - Quick start/same day start for each method
  - Order adequate supplies to last 12 months and provide at once
    - For more than four vaginal rings, advise refrigeration
  - No routine follow-up visit needed for low-risk patients
    - Patient may return for problems or change in medication
    - Adolescents and women with medical conditions may be seen more frequently
  - Help woman plan ahead
    - Where to store supplies (privacy, access)
    - How to remember to use (computer apps helpful)
  - Provide EC for contraceptive "insurance" routinely
  - Encourage use of male condoms for STI risk reduction

Additional contraceptives
- Ring tips: Place with emptied tampon introducer
  - Avoid applicators with sharp edges
  - Okay to use rings with tampons or menstrual cups
- Patch tip:
  - Use baby oil or vegetable oil to remove adherent material at old patch site

TABLE 43.7
DMPA Clinical Pearls[43-45]

- Use Quick Start/Same Day injection protocol to initiate or reinject
  - Grace period for reinjection is 4 wk beyond label-recommended date
  - Administer any day in the cycle when patient not pregnant
    - Combine with EC, backup method for 7 d and repeat pregnancy test in 2–3 wk if recent coitus. If Ulipristal acetate used for EC, use 14 d of backup method
- Routine pregnancy testing is unwarranted if asymptomatic patient returns on time for reinjection
- Inject IM DMPA with Z pattern. Do not massage injection site
  - Inject in deltoid or gluteus muscles
    - If obese, use spinal needle if gluteal site is used
- Inject SQ DMPA in abdomen or thigh. Consider teaching self-injection
  - Warn about possible skin puckering with Sub-Q formulations
- Ignore black box warning
  - Provide DMPA to identified candidate (USMEC) of any age, for any duration until menopause
- Related issues
  - Provide LNG-EC by advance prescription; many women return for reinjection late
  - Encourage condoms for STI protection

TABLE 43.8
Recommendations for Late or Missed Dose(s) of CHCs

	How Long Late/Missed Dose?		
# COCs to take now	<24 Hours **1**	24–48 Hours **2[a]**	>48 Hours **2[a]**
Patch instruction	Reattach current patch or replace with new patch	New patch	New patch
Ring instruction	Replace current ring	Replace current ring	Replace current ring
Next dose COC	Usual time	Usual time	Usual time
Patch change	Usual day	Usual day	Usual day
Ring change	Usual date	Usual date	Usual date
Backup needed	No	7 d	7 d of uninterrupted active method use
EC needed if coitus in last 5 days	No	Yes, if missed method earlier in cycle too	Yes, especially if in first week of use

Vomiting or diarrhea with pill <48 hours requires no changes. If gastrointestinal problem persists >48 hours, follow instructions for >48 missed doses and use backup for 7 days of consecutive method use after symptoms resolve
[a]May take two pills at once

With any hormonal method, unscheduled bleeding or spotting can be a bothersome side effect. Menstrual calendars with pad counts can be helpful to monitor patterns. Obtaining accurate bleeding information has become so much easier with specific apps to help women record that data. **Table 43.9** outlines management suggestions for helping women who are experiencing this problem; this can be used in conjunction with appropriate counseling. Of course, other causes of bleeding must be considered. In

TABLE 43.9
Unscheduled Bleeding or Spotting Management Suggestions[46-49]

- **DMPA**
  - Recommend: Ibuprofen 800 mg orally every 8 h for 5 d if bleeding not tolerated
  - Shorten interval for reinjection (10 wk) if bleeding occurs late in injection cycle
  - Consider low-dose CHC for 1–2 cycles if NSAIDs not helpful (especially vaginal ring)

- **Extended-cycle pills or vaginal rings**
  - Prophylactically give doxycycline SR 40 mg once daily to shorten time to amenorrhea
  - Allow 2–4 d of pill interruption (after 3 wk consistent CHC use) if bleeding not acceptable. Restart pills again once flow started in that 2–4-d window
  - Alternatively, double up on pills for 1–2 d if not good time to bleed
  - Consider ibuprofen 800 mg orally every 8 h for 5 d if bleeding not tolerated

- **Cyclic pills**
  - Check for inconsistent pill use or tobacco use
  - For bleeding that occurs late in pill pack: provide formulation with higher doses of progestin in last pills
  - For bleeding that occurs early in pill pack: provide formulation with higher doses of estrogen or lower doses of progestin in first pills in pack
  - For midcycle bleeding: shorten pill-free interval or provide triphasic pills with midcycle hormone dose increases

this population, pregnancy, cervical infections, and inconsistent method use are all frequent causes of abnormal bleeding that need specific attention. Smokers have high rates of unscheduled bleeding with estrogen-containing methods and may benefit even more from using patches or rings in lieu of daily dosing methods.

Amenorrhea typically does not reflect an underlying health problem in healthy adolescents and young women who are users of an extended-cycle pill, vaginal ring, or DMPA. In many instances it can be healthier than her natural cycling or even than scheduled bleeding episodes with conventional pill use. However, many young women feel uncomfortable with it and worry that it indicates that they are infertile or that they will bleed heavily when they do menstruate. Counseling about the benefits of amenorrhea can be most effective when we know what most concerns the young woman about absence of bleeding.

New Developments

There may be some new options in this class of methods. For example, stronger progestin-only pills; monophasic-containing nomegestrol acetate, also known as NOMAC-containing combination pills; once-a-week contraceptive patch with levonorgestrel and lower doses of EE; combination once-a-month injections; a single vaginal ring able to provide one year's supply of contraception; and a progestin-only vaginal ring; are all in various stages of development and testing. The American College of Obstetrics and Gynecology has recommended that all oral contraceptives be made available over the counter.[37] An important and less controversial step would be to make progestin-only pills available without prescription since they are safe and easier to use.

REFERENCES

1. *US medical eligibility criteria updated 2013.* Available at http://www.cdc.gov/reproductivehealth/UnintendedPregnancy/USSPR.htm. Accessed February 25, 2014.
2. *US selected practice recommendations for contraception, 2013.* Available at http://www.cdc.gov/mmwr/preview/mmwrhtml/rr6205a1.htm. Accessed March 4, 2014.
3. Lawrie TA, Helmerhorst FM, Maitra NK, et al. Types of progestogens in combined oral contraception: effectiveness and side-effects. *Cochrane Database Syst Rev* 2011;(5):CD004861.
4. Hall KS, Trussell J. Types of combined oral contraceptives used by US women. *Contraception* 2012;86(6):659–665.

5. Lidegaard Ø, Milsom I, Geirsson RT, et al. Hormonal contraception and venous thromboembolism. *Acta Obstet Gynecol Scand* 2012;91(7):769–778.

6. Martínez F, Avecilla A. Combined hormonal contraception and venous thromboembolism. *Eur J Contracept Reprod Health Care* 2007;12(2):97–106.

7. *US Food and Drug Administration—Yasmin labeling.* Available at http://www.fda.gov/Safety/MedWatch/SafetyInformation/ucm211766.htm. Accessed February 25, 2014.

8. Dragoman M, Petrie K, Torgal A, et al. Contraceptive vaginal ring effectiveness is maintained during 6 weeks of use: a prospective study of normal BMI and obese women. *Contraception* 2013;87(4):432–436.

9. Dieben TO, Roumen FJ, Apter D. Efficacy, cycle control, and user acceptability of a novel combined contraceptive vaginal ring. *Obstet Gynecol* 2002;100(3):585–593.

10. De Seta F, Restaino S, De Santo D, et al. Effects of hormonal contraception on vaginal flora. *Contraception* 2012;86(5):526–529.

11. Howard B, Trussell J, Grubb E, et al. Comparison of pregnancy rates in users of extended and cyclic combined oral contraceptive (COC) regimens in the United States: a brief report. *Contraception* 2014;89(1):25–27.

12. McNicholas C, Zhao Q, Secura G, et al. Contraceptive failures in overweight and obese combined hormonal contraceptive users. *Obstet Gynecol* 2013;121(3):585–592.

13. Dinger JC, Cronin M, Möhner S, et al. Oral contraceptive effectiveness according to body mass index, weight, age, and other factors. *Am J Obstet Gynecol* 2009;201(3):263.e1–e9.

14. Edelman AB, Carlson NE, Cherala G, et al. Impact of obesity on oral contraceptive pharmacokinetics and hypothalamic-pituitary-ovarian activity. *Contraception* 2009;80(2):119–127.

15. Westhoff CL, Torgal AT, Mayeda ER, et al. Predictors of noncompliance in an oral contraceptive clinical trial. *Contraception* 2012;85(5):465–469.

16. Borrelli F, Izzo AA. Herb-drug interactions with St John's wort (*Hypericum perforatum*): an update on clinical observations. *AAPS J.* 2009;11(4):710–727.

17. Paulen ME, Folger SG, Curtis KM, et al. Contraceptive use among solid organ transplant patients: a systematic review. *Contraception* 2010;82(1):102–112.

18. Pietrzak B, Bobrowska K, Jabiry-Zieniewicz Z, et al. Oral and transdermal hormonal contraception in women after kidney transplantation. *Transplant Proc* 2007;39(9):2759–2762.

19. Schwingl PJ, Ory HW, Visness CM. Estimates of the risk of cardiovascular death attributable to low-dose oral contraceptives in the United States. *Am J Obstet Gynecol* 1999;180(1, Pt 1):241–249.

20. Lidegaard Ø, Løkkegaard E, Jensen A, et al. Thrombotic stroke and myocardial infarction with hormonal contraception. *N Engl J Med* 2012;366(24):2257–2266.

21. O'Brien SH. Contraception-related venous thromboembolism in adolescents. *Semin Thromb Hemost* 2014;40(1):66–71.

22. Sidney S, Cheetham TC, Connell FA, et al. Recent combined hormonal contraceptives (CHCs) and the risk of thromboembolism and other cardiovascular events in new users. *Contraception* 2013;87(1):93–100.

23. Dinger J, Möhner S, Heinemann K. Cardiovascular risk associated with the use of an etonogestrel-containing vaginal ring. *Obstet Gynecol* 2013;122(4):800–808.

24. Nelson AL, Rezvan A. A pilot study of women's knowledge of pregnancy health risks: implications for contraception. *Contraception* 2012;85(1):78–82.

25. Vessey M, Yeates D. Oral contraceptive use and cancer: final report from the Oxford-Family Planning Association contraceptive study. *Contraception* 2013;88(6):678–683.

26. Hannaford PC, Iversen L, Macfarlane TV, et al. Mortality among contraceptive pill users: cohort evidence from Royal College of General Practitioners' Oral Contraception Study. *BMJ* 2010;340:c927.

27. Grimes DA, Schulz KF. Nonspecific side effects of oral contraceptives: nocebo or noise? *Contraception* 2011;83(1):5–9.

28. Bonny AE, Secic M, Cromer B. Early weight gain related to later weight gain in adolescents on depot medroxyprogesterone acetate. *Obstet Gynecol* 2011; 117(4):793–797.

29. Harel Z, Johnson CC, Gold MA, et al. Recovery of bone mineral density in adolescents following the use of depot medroxyprogesterone acetate contraceptive injections. *Contraception* 2010;81(4):281–291.

30. Maguire K, Westhoff C. The state of hormonal contraception today: established and emerging noncontraceptive health benefits. *Am J Obstet Gynecol* 2011;205 (4, suppl):S4–S8.

31. Davis AR, Westhoff C, O'Connell K, et al. Oral contraceptives for dysmenorrhea in adolescent girls: a randomized trial. *Obstet Gynecol* 2005;106(1):97–104.

32. Davis AR, Westhoff CL. Primary dysmenorrhea in adolescent girls and treatment with oral contraceptives. *J Pediatr Adolesc Gynecol* 2001;14(1):3–8.

33. Havrilesky LJ, Moorman PG, Lowery WJ, et al. Oral contraceptive pills as primary prevention for ovarian cancer: a systematic review and meta-analysis. *Obstet Gynecol* 2013;122(1):139–147.

34. Brownell EA, Fernandez ID, Fisher SG, et al. The effect of immediate postpartum depot medroxyprogesterone on early breastfeeding cessation. *Contraception* 2013; 87(6):836–843.

35. Espey E, Ogburn T, Leeman L, et al. Effect of progestin compared with combined oral contraceptive pills on lactation: a randomized controlled trial. *Obstet Gynecol* 2012;119(1):5–13.

36. Goldstein RL, Upadhyay UD, Raine TR. With pills, patches, rings, and shots: who still uses condoms? A longitudinal cohort study. *J Adolesc Health* 2013; 52(1):77–82.

37. ACOG Committee Opinion No. 544: Over-the-counter access to oral contraceptives. *Obstet Gynecol* 2012;120(6):1527–1531.

38. Potter L, Oakley D, de Leon-Wong E. Measuring compliance among oral contraceptive users. *Fam Plann Perspect* 1996;28(4):154–158.

39. Nelson AL, Westhoff C, Schnare SM. Real-world patterns of prescription refills for branded hormonal contraceptives: a reflection of contraceptive discontinuation. *Obstet Gynecol* 2008;112(4):782–787.

40. Thorneycroft I, Klein P, Simon J. The impact of antiepileptic drug therapy on steroidal contraceptive efficacy. *Epilepsy Behav* 2006;9(1):31–39.

41. Lopez LM, Newmann SJ, Grimes DA. Immediate start of hormonal contraceptives for contraception. *Cochrane Database Syst Rev* 2012;12:CD0062.

42. Castaño PM, Bynum JY, Andrés R, et al. Effect of daily text messages on oral contraceptive continuation: a randomized controlled trial. *Obstet Gynecol* 2012;119(1):14–20.

43. Steiner MJ, Kwok C, Stanback J. Injectable contraception: what should the longest interval be for reinjection? *Contraception* 2008;77(6):410–414.

44. Williams RL, Hensel DJ, Fortenberry JD. Self-administration of subcutaneous depot medroxyprogesterone acetate by adolescent women. *Contraception* 2013;88(3):401–407.

45. Kaunitz AM, Grimes DA. Removing the black box warning for depot medroxyprogesterone acetate. *Contraception* 2011;84(3):212–213.

46. Abdel-Aleem H, d'Arcangues C, Vogelsong KM, et al. Treatment of vaginal bleeding irregularities induced by progestin only contraceptives. *Cochrane Database Syst Rev* 2007;(4):CD003449.

47. Dempsey A, Roca C, Westhoff C. Vaginal estrogen supplementation during Depo-Provera initiation: a randomized controlled trial. *Contraception* 2010;82(3):250–255.

48. Kaneshiro B, Edelman A, Carlson NE, et al. A randomized controlled trial of sub-antimicrobial-dose doxycycline to prevent unscheduled bleeding with continuous oral contraceptive pill use. *Contraception* 2012;85(4):351–358.

49. Sulak PJ, Smith V, Coffee A, et al. Frequency and management of breakthrough bleeding with continuous use of the transvaginal contraceptive ring: a randomized controlled trial. *Obstet Gynecol* 2008;112(3):563–571.

🛜 **ADDITIONAL RESOURCES AND WEBSITES ONLINE**

IX

44 Intrauterine Devices and Long-acting Reversible Contraception

Michelle Forcier

KEY WORDS

- Contraception
- Hormonal implant
- Intrauterine device (IUD)
- Intrauterine system
- Long-acting reversible contraception (LARC)

Long-acting reversible contraceptive (LARC) is an umbrella term for provider-inserted methods, which once placed provide superior protection against unintended pregnancy. LARCs, such as intra-uterine devices (IUDs) and progestin contraceptive implants, have a major advantage over other birth control methods as they minimize problems with adherence and maximize continuation rates. Family planning experts have recommended LARCs as a first-line contraceptive for women of all ages, including adolescents and nulliparous young women, since 2007. However, LARCs continue to be an underutilized method of contraception despite a long history of efficacy, safety, and ease of use for women of all ages. Fewer than 1 in 10 young women less than 25 years of age take advantage of these easy-to-use, extremely effective methods. Providers, and patients, who wish to avoid early or unintended pregnancy, can benefit from improved counseling on the option of these LARC devices.

TYPES

Long-acting reversible contraception includes a variety of "set and forget" methods of contraception. These forgettable contraceptives are typically provider-inserted devices that last over many years, but, once removed, are quickly and completely reversible, offering women a flexible and responsive means of family planning. LARCs offer adolescents and younger women a means of contraception that is as effective as more permanent sterilization procedures, but keeps a young woman's future reproductive options fully intact without sparing efficacy. Adolescent and young adult (AYA) women are at high risk for early and unintended pregnancy. Therefore, LARCs have been recommended as a top-tier method for teens since 2007.[1]

Because LARCs are functionally user independent, typical and perfect use failure rates are essentially the same, eliminating problems with adherence and misuse (Fig. 44.1). Additionally, LARC users demonstrate consistently higher continuation rates than short-acting methods across all ages. At present, there are four Food and Drug Administration (FDA)-approved devices in the US, with many more options available internationally. Two FDA-approved IUDs include levonorgestrel (LNG) intrauterine system (LNG-IUD, Mirena, Bayer Healthcare Pharmaceuticals, 2000) and CuT380A IUD (CU-IUD, Paragard, Duramed Pharmaceuticals,

1984). Both have been in use and well studied for over 20 years. In 2013, the FDA approved an additional LNG device, Skylar (Bayer Healthcare Pharmaceuticals) onto the US market. The etonorg-estrel (ENG) progesterone-only implant (formerly Implanon, now Nexplanon, Merck Pharmaceuticals) was FDA-approved in 2006, and is another inserted device that is placed in the subdermal tissues of the nondominant upper arm. All four methods can be safely used in teens and nulliparous young adults, and should be considered first-line options for young women wanting to avoid unintended pregnancy. While use of LARCs is increasing in the US, and in particular among younger women, providers miss opportunities for educating, counseling, and recommending these options as the most effective methods of contraception for AYA women.[2]

MECHANISM

The ENG is a single 4 cm by 2 mm flexible ethylene vinyl acetate copolymer rod that is inserted subdermally (Fig. 44.2). The newer ENG device, Nexplanon, has an improved inserter that limits the placement depth, and prevents deep or intramuscular insertions. Nexplanon contains 15 mg barium sulfate, making it radiopaque and easier to detect with x-ray, especially important for verifying location during the removal procedure. ENG's active ingredient is 68 mg ENG, which is slowly released over 3 years. Peak serum ENG concentrations reach 800 pg/mL, with a gradual decrease to less than 200 pg/mL by year 3. As with other progesterone contraceptive methods, ENG inhibits ovulation, thickens cervical mucous, and thins the endometrial lining. Its overall pearl index is estimated at 0.38%, indicating a less than 1% failure rate.[3] While FDA approved its use for 3 years, there are indications that the ENG has demonstrated effectiveness (0 pregnancies) for up to 4 years.[4] LN-IUDs are approved for 3 (Skylar) to 5 years (Mirena) of use (Fig. 44.3). As with the ENG device, Mirena seems to have excellent efficacy for up to year seven. Similarly, the CU-IUD (Paragard) is approved for 10 years, but additional efficacy has been demonstrated up to 12 years or longer.[5]

IUDs are not abortifacients and do not interrupt an implanted pregnancy. IUDs do not work by suppressing endogenous estrogen and progesterone hormone production; thus, ovulation may continue. In general, IUDs are toxic to sperm and oocytes; gametes are rendered inactive or ineffective, and do not fertilize or form viable embryos.[6] CU-IUDS create an intrauterine sterile foreign body reaction with cytotoxic inflammatory mediators destroying sperm and ova, inhibiting motility, disconnecting head–tail, inhibiting acrosomal enzyme and capacitation, impairing penetration of the zona pellucida, and with increased local prostaglandin levels,

Effectiveness of Family Planning Methods

Most Effective	Reversible		Permanent		How to make your method most effective
	Implant	**Intrauterine Device (IUD)**	**Male Sterilization** (Vasectomy)	**Female Sterilization** (Abdominal, Laparoscopic, Hysteroscopic)	After procedure, little or nothing to do or remember.
Less than 1 pregnancy per 100 women in a year	0.05 %*	LNG - 0.2 % Copper T - 0.8 %	0.15 %	0.5 %	**Vasectomy and hysteroscopic sterilization:** Use another method for first 3 months.
	Injectable	**Pill**	**Patch**	**Ring**	**Diaphragm**	**Injectable:** Get repeat injections on time.
6-12 pregnancies per 100 women in a year	6 %	9 %	9 %	9 %	12 %	**Pills:** Take a pill each day. **Patch, Ring:** Keep in place, change on time. **Diaphragm:** Use correctly every time you have sex.

Male Condom 18 % **Female Condom** 21 % **Withdrawal** 22 % **Sponge** 24 % parous women 12 % nulliparous women

Fertility-Awareness Based Methods

JANUARY

24 %

Spermicide 28 %

18 or more pregnancies per 100 women in a year

Least Effective

Condoms, sponge, withdrawal, spermicides: Use correctly every time you have sex.

Fertility awareness-based methods: Abstain or use condoms on fertile days. Newest methods (Standard Days Method and TwoDay Method) may be the easiest to use and consequently more effective.

* The percentages indicate the number out of every 100 women who experienced an unintended pregnancy within the first year of typical use of each contraceptive method.

CS 242797

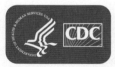

U.S. Department of Health and Human Services Centers for Disease Control and Prevention

CONDOMS SHOULD ALWAYS BE USED TO REDUCE THE RISK OF SEXUALLY TRANSMITTED INFECTIONS.

Other Methods of Contraception

Lactational Amenorrhea Method: LAM is a highly effective, temporary method of contraception.

Emergency Contraception: Emergency contraceptive pills or a copper IUD after unprotected intercourse substantially reduces risk of pregnancy.

Adapted from World Health Organization (WHO) Department of Reproductive Health and Research, Johns Hopkins Bloomberg School of Public Health/Center for Communication Programs (CCP). Knowledge for health project. Family planning: a global handbook for providers (2011 update). Baltimore, MD; Geneva, Switzerland: CCP and WHO; 2011; and Trussell J. Contraceptive failure in the United States. Contraception 2011;83:397–404.

FIGURE 44.1 Contraceptive efficacy, Centers for Disease Control and Prevention Medical Eligibility Criteria. Summary table of contraceptive efficacy. Percentage of women experiencing an unintended pregnancy during the first year of typical use and the first year of perfect use of contraception and the percentage continuing use at the end of the first year. United States. (From Trussell J. Contraceptive efficacy. In Hatcher RA, Trussell J, Nelson AL, et al., eds. *Contraceptive technology.* 20th ed. New York, NY: Ardent Media, 2011.)

additionally impairing ova fertilizability. The LNG-IUD creates thick impenetrable mucous, a thin atrophic lining, inflammatory effects, and impaired tubal motility. The CU-IUD T-shaped polyethylene frame is wrapped in copper wire and contains barium sulfate in the stem to render it radiopaque. Copper ions act as a functional spermicide, which both renders gametes inactive and creates an environment unsuitable for fertilization. With a pearl index of 0.8 and estimated 100% efficacy as an emergency contraception (EC) method, CU-IUD is an extremely effective FDA-approved method of contraception for all ages.[6]

LNG, like its copper counterpart, is a nonsystemic hormonal method, creating a local intrauterine environment hostile to gametes and fertilization. The larger (32 mm × 32 mm) T-shaped polyethylene Mirena contains 52 mg LNG, which is slow released at a rate of 20 mg per day over 5 years, with an overall pearl index of 0.7%. By year 5, the daily progestin dose decreases by 50%, but the device has demonstrated effectiveness up to 7 years.[7] LNG is released directly into the uterine body for largely paracrine rather than systemic effects. Serum progestin levels are about half that of

ENG implant users and one-tenth of oral LNG users.[8] The smaller (28 mm × 30 mm) Skylar IUD contains 13.5 mg LNG with a release rate of 14 µg/day and decline to 5 µg/day after 3 years. Ovulation may be suppressed in some women, but is not the main mechanism of action, with between 45% and 75% of women ovulating on the 52 mg device, and almost all women ovulating on the lower-dose LNG-IUD. Ovulation on the lower-dose LNG-IUD may result in less amenorrhea and more regular menses, which can be a desired effect for some women.[8]

These "set it and forget it," long-acting, completely and immediately reversible forms of birth control offer patients improved adherence and greater likelihood of continuation over time, making LARC an ideal form of contraception for AYAs, and all-age women wishing to delay or prevent unwanted pregnancy and parenthood. The less than 1% failure rate for LARCs remains the same across both younger and older age groups, while women younger than age 21 years have twice the risk of contraceptive failure, as they use more short-acting methods compared to their older peers.[9] As the inherent characteristics of inserted methods

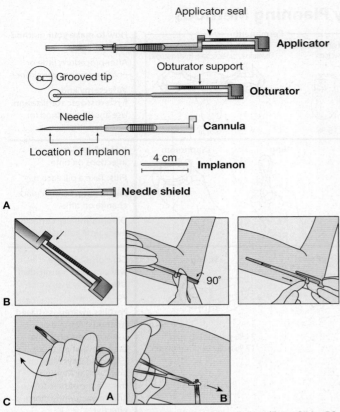

FIGURE 44.2 Insertion of Implanon contraceptive device. (From Gibbs RS, Karlan BY, Haney AF, et al. *Danforth's obstetrics and gynecology.* 10th ed. Philadelphia, PA: Lippincott Williams & Wilkins, 2008.)

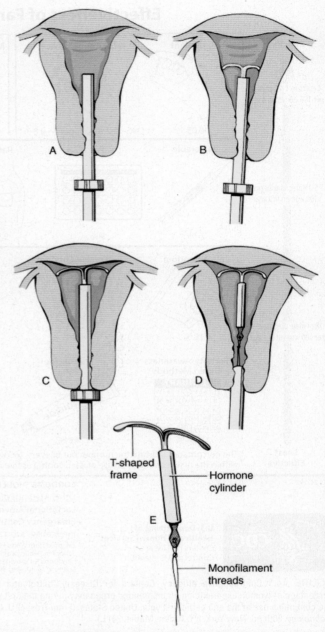

FIGURE 44.3 Image of a Mirena IUD. (Adapted from Gibbs RS, Karlan BY, Haney AF, et al. *Danforth's obstetrics and gynecology.* 9th ed. Philadelphia, PA: Lippincott Williams & Wilkins, 2003; In: Curtis M, Linares ST, Antoniewicz L, eds. *Glass' office gynecology.* 7th ed. Philadelphia, PA: Wolters Kluwer Health, 2014.)

eliminate problems with misuse and adherence, method initiation and continuation become the critical elements in promoting their usefulness for pregnancy prevention in younger populations.

Despite many years of accrued safety and efficacy data, LARC initiation rates continue to be remarkably low in the relatively resource-rich setting as the US. Data published in 2010, and again in 2012 indicate that less than 1 in 10 women will have ever used a LARC method.[2,10] Despite low overall uptake, LARC use is trending upward in all US women, increasing from 2.4% in 2002 to 8.5% in 2009.[2] Older teens, aged 15 to 19, are less likely to use LARC (4.5%) than young adults, aged 20 to 24 (8.3%). Of LARC use in young women, IUDs predominate with the ENG implant comprising only 0.5% use in the adolescent age group.[11] Users of all ages report the confidence in efficacy and no interruption during the act of sex as important reasons for choosing LARCs, with high levels of user satisfaction reported across studies.[12]

Issues Affecting Efficacy—Initiation

Despite proven safety, efficacy, ease of use, and improved adherence, low rates of initiation limit LARC usefulness in US AYA sexually active populations.[2,9,13] Young women are more likely to ever use LARC with the following associated characteristics:

- Earlier age of sexual debut
- Increasing age and parity, cohabitation or marriage
- High IUD knowledge

Women less likely to use LARCs (and IUDs) include those with:

- lower education;
- external locus of control;
- foreign language; and
- sex outside of marriage (≥4 sexual partners, widowed, divorced, or separated).

Socioeconomic status as a predictive factor for LARC use varies across studies. A history of an adolescent pregnancy was associated with ever use of injected depot medroxyprogesterone (DMPA), but not IUD.[10]

As in cases of other health-related decisions, provider recommendation and confidence is among the reasons women select IUDs and ENG. Family planning experts have promoted LARCs as a first-line method of contraception for women of all ages for many years.[1] Despite excellent efficacy and safety profiles, many providers still do not recommend LARC use in AYAs. A 2012 study of pediatricians, nurse practitioners, social workers, and health educators in

New York City school-based health centers showed that only 55% of respondents were likely to recommend an IUD.[14] Only 77% believed that IUDs were safe for adolescents, with decreasing rates of provider confidence and recommendation associated with recent sexually transmitted infections (STIs), remote pelvic inflammatory disease (PID), nonmonogamous relationship, or nulliparity, all representing patient characteristics that are no longer contraindications to IUD insertion. In this study, over half of the professionals were also biased in believing that time required for counseling about LARC would be more excessive than for short-acting methods.

In addition to improving provider knowledge, confidence, and recommendations, another barrier to effective youth contraception is point of access at the facility level. Youth-oriented contraceptive programs may improve LARC uptake by offering improved inserter competence and accessibility, flexible hours, and open appointments, with additional social networking and education outreach in the community.[9] Youth-friendly programs have included facilities such as Planned Parenthood and Title X, and other specialty reproductive health–focused programs demonstrated increased rates of LARC use in younger women. Facility obstacles for LARC use in younger patients include device and insertion cost, inconvenience of clinic appointment and hours, provider misconceptions and lack of recommendation, and limited support and training for time of visit and in-clinic LARC insertion.

Both health systems and providers have ample room to improve access and offer evidence-based, patient-centered counseling, eliminating outdated and inaccurate information, in order to improve LARC initiation and continuation (Table 44.1). Medical costs associated with LARC contraceptive use are far superior to other forms of shorter-acting hormonal contraception.[15]

Insert methods are safe, relatively painless, and simple procedures that are well tolerated in outpatient settings. Side effects are limited, with satisfaction levels consistently higher in LARC than short-acting method users. While LARCs clearly offer superior first-line contraception, providers must balance evidence and enthusiasm with patient autonomy and patient-centered care. Determining each young woman's family planning needs and goals requires a contraceptive plan responsive to lifestyle, avoiding undesired side effects. To counsel adequately, providers must keep an open mind, as well as actively listen and engage adolescents to form and assume ownership of their own contraceptive planning and outcomes.

Initiation—Balancing Risk of Pregnancy with Quick Start

Initiation of LARC contraceptives need not be hindered or delayed depending on patient history and attitudes about pregnancy.[16-18] FDA Pharmaceutical Inspectorate indicates that LARC methods

TABLE 44.1

Pros and Cons of LARC Contraception: Provider Highlights for Patient-Centered Counseling

	ENG	LNG-IUD	CU-IUD
Upfront cost[a]	$400–$800 includes exam, implant, and insertion	$500–1,000 includes IUD, medical exam, the insertion of the IUD	
	Office visit (CPT 99213) $73.33 implant insertion (CPT 11981), $150.91 implant removal (CPT 11982), $181.28 Protection lasts 3–4 y	Office visit (CPT 99213), $73.33 IUD insertion (CPT 58300), $126.62 IUD removal (CPT 58301), $143.07 Protection lasts 5–7 y	
Cost over time[a]	LARCs' higher initial acquisition costs offset within 1 y by lower contraceptive failure rates and consequent pregnancy costs, making them the least expensive reversible (hormonal) contraceptives		
Covered by Medicaid	Yes	Yes	Yes
Programs for financial assistance	No	Yes	No
Insertion	Upper arm, does not involve pelvic exam Simple procedure, few additional materials needed	Requires bimanual and speculum pelvic exam Requires additional clinic materials (tenaculum, sponge forceps, sound, dilators)	
Removal	Slightly more difficult than insertion Requires curved scalpel and curved forceps Less bleeding with lidocaine + epinephrine	Decrease complication risks with experience, uterine position, and number of insertions/year Decrease perforation risks with ultrasound guidance during insertion, location, and assist with removals	
Menstrual effects	Irregular menses	90% reduction in menstrual blood loss 50% amenorrhea, 1 y 80% amenorrhea, 2 y	Regular menses Heavier more painful menses
Pain	Local pain at insertion site, with some possible bruising	Immediate post-insertion cramping, bleeding Partner may complain of penile discomfort with string if cut too short	
	No vaginal changes	Some increased risk vaginitis	
Expulsion risks	No difference in expulsion by age Patients can play with and break device	Slightly increased risk of expulsion in younger nulliparous patients Partners may sabotage birth control and pull device out	

[a]Medical costs associated with contraceptive use were based on the Current Procedural Terminology (CPT) codes and prices based on an analysis of the Thomson Reuters MarketScan Commercial Claims and Encounters Database 2011.
Crespi S, Kerrigan M, Sood V. Budget impact analysis of 8 hormonal contraceptive options. *Am J Manag Care* 2013:19(7):e249–e255.

should only be inserted within 5 days of last menstrual period (LMP), with a negative pregnancy test, and reasonable certainty that the patient is not pregnant. Family planning experts offer more flexible guidelines for starting LARCs as long as there is a reasonable certainty that the AYA is not pregnant. Determining potential for very early pregnancy that may not be detectable by urine human choriogonadotropic hormone testing includes inquiring about date or time of last unprotected sex (i.e., sex without birth control or a condom). If coitus occurred within 5 days, EC may be offered (see Chapter 41). If unprotected sex occurred more than 14 days prior, and the pregnancy test is negative, providers may confidently insert both ENG and IUDs. Patients who are starting LARC after the 5-day window of the LMP should be strongly encouraged to use backup protection or abstain from intercourse for 7 days while the method takes effect.

If there is some possibility of fertilization and/or early implantation, some family planning experts have three options:

- recommend abstinence for 2 to 4 weeks and reschedule for LARC insertion
- start another short-acting contraceptive and reschedule LARC insertion, or
- provide LARC insertion at time of visit with plan for continued family planning follow-up.

If there are questions about pregnancy status, it can be easier to manage subdermal ENG, which still may be inserted, with a follow-up pregnancy test in 3 weeks. If the patient is pregnant, there are no demonstrated teratogenic effects of progesterone on fetal development. The patient may elect to continue the pregnancy with removal of the ENG or terminate the pregnancy while maintaining her ENG implant.

It is less desirable to insert an IUD if a patient may have a very early pregnancy given some increased risks of spontaneous abortion and other poor pregnancy outcomes. However, if a young woman desires urgent IUD placement, an IUD may be inserted with the understanding and consent that the IUD could affect ongoing pregnancy and increase the risk of miscarriage. For patients who are clear that they would elect pregnancy termination, an IUD may be placed with careful follow-up, with subsequent pregnancy testing in 3 to 4 weeks. Abortion suction procedure would remove both the pregnancy and the IUD at the same time. Patients could elect to replace their IUD at the time of abortion if they choose.

Providers may recommend LARC insertion immediately after abortion or postpartum unless there are concerns about endometrial infection or puerperal sepsis. There are no longer restrictions about timing of insertion or post-cesarean section. Women >21 days postpartum or 7 days post-abortion require additional backup methods again for 7 days following insertion. Counseling young women about these options before or with their pregnancy management may increase initiation and prevent another unintended pregnancy.

Issues Affecting Efficacy—Continuation

Continuation rates are an additional factor in LARC methods potential to decrease unintended pregnancy rates in all ages, including high-risk populations such as teens. Adolescents are more likely to stop *all* contraceptive methods compared to their older adult counterparts, contributing to overall higher contraceptive failure rates in young women.[19] Continuation rates at 1 year out for short-acting methods have been as low as 11% patch, 16% DMPA, and 30% vaginal ring and pills.[20] In contrast, LARC continuation rates were found to be as high as 72% to 86%, significantly greater than continuation rates of short-acting methods over multiple studies.[21,22] Another report found a 22-fold method failure (unintended pregnancy rates) with short-acting contraceptives than with LARC. Younger women (<21 years) were at two times the risk of unintended pregnancy using short-acting contraceptives, but had equivalent risk with LARC as in older populations.[23]

Providing additional perspective about initiation and continuation, the large prospective cohort CHOICE Project (Saint Louis, Missouri) evaluated contraceptive use patterns in women of all ages when misinformation and financial inequities were eliminated. Sixty-four percent of the initial 658 adolescents in this study chose a LARC method at baseline, with 63% of teens electing to start ENG.[24] Rates of continuation for adolescents and young women (85% LNG-IUS; 80% for ENG) were similar to adult counterparts at one year. Adolescent continuation rates for CU-IUD were lower (72%), but still much higher than short-acting methods.

ADVANTAGES

The most time-intensive aspect of LARCs, as with most other aspects of AYA care including family planning, includes detailed counseling about what to expect and how best to manage post-insertion side effects. Focusing on advantages of LARC, with careful preparation for side effects, may improve patient acceptance, satisfaction, and continuation (Table 44.1). Patient counseling on benefits of LARC should focus on:

- Efficacy—<1% failure rate, which is far superior to all other forms of contraception
- Safety—Has been recommended as safe first-line contraceptive for adolescents, nulliparous young adults, and any woman desiring safe, effective contraception
  - No associations with changes in future fertility—For teens and young adults concerned about future fertility, focus should be shifted to healthy lifestyles, weight and nutrition, substance use, and prevention of STIs. Neither IUD nor ENG has been linked to any problems with future fertility.[25]
- Ease of use—Once inserted, patients do not need to "do" anything to assure contraceptive effectiveness.
- Immediate reversibility—Once removed, these methods are quickly and completely reversible. Return to ovulation and fertility can occur as early as 7 to 14 days after removal.

Additional medical indications, patient factors, and device features may improve recommendation, initiation, and continuation of LARCs. Noncontraceptive benefits may help determine method selection for young teens anticipating future sexual activity and looking to initiate contraception before first intercourse.

CU-IUD Especially Indicated for

- FDA indicated for EC and represents the most effective EC method available (see Chapter 41). There are essentially no failures if initiated within the indicated 5-day time frame. Patient weight and time out from exposure do not decrease this method's EC efficacy.
  - Some women elect to continue and keep a CU-IUD in place for long-term contraception.
  - Many younger women continue to decline CU-IUD for EC. Possible reasons may be unstated ambivalence regarding pregnancy, as well as undesirable future menstrual effects.
- Concerns about pregnancy with amenorrhea—allows women who have strong preferences regarding ongoing monthly menses
- Concerns and desire to avoid use of medications or hormones
- Long-acting, long-term contraception—lasting 10 years or more.

LNG-IUD 52 mg (Mirena) Can Be Recommended for

- Menorrhagia—There is FDA approval for treatment of menometrorrhagia in all ages and may be especially useful in women with menorrhagia related to bleeding diatheses (see Chapter 48).
- Endometriosis, hyperandrogenism, and endometrial hyperplasia—relative to local uterine progestin effects

may offer additional benefit for women with: endometriosis, hyperandrogenism, and endometrial hyperplasia[26,27]

- Dysmenorrhea—May be less effective for premenstrual systemic symptoms as it does not suppress endogenous progesterone and estrogen secretion[27]
- HIV infection—Safety and efficacy of IUDs generally outweigh risks for women with and do not increase risk of viral shedding, overall complications, infection rates, or morbidity.[16,17]
- Both Cu and LNG IUDs, unlike oral contraceptive pills, have fewer medication interactions—no restrictions with antimicrobials and anticonvulsants, including lamotrigine; no known interactions between antiretrovirals (ARVs) and IUDs.[16]

ENG with Additional Benefits

- Ease of insertion—does not require a vaginal and uterine exam, and speculum insertion for placement
- Dysmenorrhea—Off-label management for heavy prolonged menses
- Obese women—ENG does not appear to affect appetite in the same way that DMPA does in young overweight women. As weight gain is a concern for many young women starting contraception, lack of impact on appetite and weight gain makes ENG an attractive option for many AYAs.
- Medical conditions such as
  - Hyperlipidemia—Earlier studies have long demonstrated that ENG has little effect on metabolic and coagulation parameters.
  - Bleeding diatheses (thrombophilias or hemorrhagic disorders)—Earlier studies show no impact on coagulation parameters.
  - Osteopenia or future high risk of osteoporosis—Unlike DMPA, current research indicates that ENG does not appear to diminish bone mineral density, making it a safe and effective option for women at risk for future osteoporosis.
  - Other medications—No interactions or impact when used with anticonvulsants (phenytoin, carbamazepine, oxcarbapezine, primidine, topiramate, and barbiturates), and ARVs such as ritonavir-boosted protease inhibitors, nonrifampicin, and rifabutin.[16,17]

DISADVANTAGES

Contraindications

There are few absolute contraindications for use of LARCs in all women, including adolescents and young nulliparous adults. The Centers for Disease Control and Prevention (CDC) (see Figure 41.1) and the World. Health Organization offer regularly updated Medical Eligibility Criteria for Contraceptive Use for reference when assessing comorbid conditions that may preclude safe use of LARCs (see Figure 41.1).[1,16] Absolute contraindications include the following:

- Active PID—For women with PID, recommendations are to leave the IUD in place and treat around it.[16,28]
- Ongoing, desired pregnancy—If an IUD user is determined to be pregnant, she must be evaluated for possible ectopic pregnancy. IUDs decrease risk of ectopic pregnancy (0 to 0.5 per 1,000 women years) compared to women not using birth control (3.25 to 5.25 per 1,000 women years); however, if a woman with an IUD becomes pregnant, it is more likely to be ectopic.
- Women with intrauterine pregnancy are at risk for spontaneous abortion, septic abortion, preterm delivery, and

chorioamnionitis if the IUD is left in place.[16,17,28,29] IUD removal decreases these risks somewhat, especially if the IUD strings are visible and the device is removed as soon as possible.[18]

- Allergic reactions to device components
- Wilson's disease (Cu-IUD)
- Uterine cavity size (<6 cm or >10 cm) or significant structural abnormalities—IUDs are not typically recommended in women with extremely small or large uteri (<6 cm >10 cm) or with anatomic uterine abnormalities, as there is a greater risk of expulsion.

The FDA Patient Information warns against using IUDs with these conditions, but recommendations may be tailored according to the individual and the evidence supporting the Centers for Disease Control Medical Eligibility Contraceptive Guidelines (see Figure 41.1). Most adolescents and young women are unlikely to have contraindications or medical conditions that preclude LARC use so that for almost all women, the advantages of using LARCs outweigh any risks, with the exception of placing a new IUD into an actively infected or pregnant uterus.

Adverse Events and Side Effects

- **Pain**—LARC insertion is no more painful or difficult in young women than in older counterparts. LARC insertion is generally well tolerated in the outpatient clinic setting.[30]
  - Decreasing anxiety is another means of improving pain management in the younger patient and can be accomplished with small in-clinic doses of an oral anxiolytic or other behavioral interventions.
  - Careful preprocedure preparation, such as setting up the instruments and keeping instruments out of the patient's field of vision, may also minimize anxiety.
  - A calm, compassionate bedside assistant can provide verbal distraction, guide relaxation breathing, offering safe and comfortable setting.
- **IUD**—Reassuring women that the majority of young women with IUDs report minimal to moderate pain with insertion is important
  - Adequate pain management can be individualized.[31] There is no strong evidence that pre-insertion administration of nonsteroidal anti-inflammatory drugs (NSAIDs) such as ibuprofen or naproxen, paracervical or intracervical lidocaine blocks, or other interventions help decrease pain with cervical dilation and fundal placement of device.
    - For younger adolescents and nulliparous women, the internal os may be tighter than in parous women, requiring cervical dilation prior to insertion. For these patients, careful and painless local injection of lidocaine in the cervix may minimize pain associated with dilating the internal cervical os and gain patient confidence that the procedure will be tolerable.
  - There is no use for misoprostol in softening or decreasing insertion pain. Misoprostol does have significant undesirable gastrointestinal side effects.
- **Psychogenic Pain, Anxiety Associated with Pelvic— Bimanual and Speculum Exam**—Some young, immature, or developmentally delayed sexually active teens cannot tolerate the bimanual exam or placement of the speculum necessary before IUD insertion. To promote positive regard and improve acceptance and continuation of the device, conscious sedation can offer optimal pain and anxiolytic control for certain teens who may not tolerate the exam and speculum. Conscious sedation for IUD placement may also be helpful for younger teens who are not yet sexually active, but who strongly desire initiating intrauterine contraception prior to sexual debut or for LARC noncontraceptive benefits.

TABLE 44.2

ENG Insertion Tips

The ENG is preloaded in a sterile and disposable inserter device. The package insert and ENG provider training materials can provide detailed instructions for insertion technique.
1. The nondominant upper arm is the preferred site for insertion
2. Insertion site is measured and marked at 6–10 cm from the medial epicondyle in the sulcus between the biceps and triceps. Measure and mark with the patient in both the upright and supine position to assure placement. Marking the lidocaine injection site 1 cm proximal to the actual device insertion, and marking the expected 4 cm length of the device, assure painless and correct placement
3. The skin is cleaned with antiseptic and sterilely draped
4. Providers then inject 3–5 cc 1% lidocaine proximal to the insertion point and along the insertion tract. Allow the lidocaine to take effect and test for sensation prior to device insertion
5. The ENG obturator is introduced at a 30-degree angle and then advanced in subdermal tissue until the obturator needle is completely within the subdermal tissue. Introduction of the obturator requires firm but gentle forward pressure and tenting to assure correct placement
6. The ENG obturator is pulled back, releasing the implant, with a simple sliding motion of the release tab
7. The device is palpated to ensure correct placement
8. The insertion area and local antiseptic are cleaned with sterile saline, dried, and the insertion site is secured with Steri-Strips that remain in place until they fall off with normal use. Providers may apply a pressure dressing. Patients are advised to leave the pressure dressing in place for 24 h according to FDA training protocols

- **ENG**—Many younger or not yet sexually active patients opt for ENG as the insertion procedure does not require a pelvic and speculum exam.
  - Patients may be reassured that ENG insertion is preceded by a generous local lidocaine block that will be painful for about 10 seconds, but will afterward ensure excellent pain control thereafter.
  - The actual insertion time from skin entry to removal of insertion device takes 5 to 10 seconds (Fig. 44.2, **Table 44.2**).
  - Implant removals may be more complicated and take more time, depending on the depth of placement, encapsulation around the rod, and provider experience. Lidocaine, with a small amount of epinephrine, may help decrease bleeding with removal.
- Insertion Complications
  - **IUD**—Providers can minimize insertion errors and complications by being well prepared for most contingencies before and during the insertion. Having the range of potential surgical adjuncts bedside during the procedure allows controlled responses to situational factors.
    - Flexible plastic endometrial biopsy catheters, which have been to be safer than their larger metal counterparts, are used to sound and assess uterine size prior to insertion.
    - Silver nitrate or monsels solution can help stop bleeding from puncture wounds at tenaculum sites.
    - Cervical dilators, such as Pratt dilators 13 to 21, can be helpful in gently enlarging a tight internal os before device placement.
  - A thorough understanding of pelvic anatomy and confidence with assessing the position of the uterus is essential to avoid perforation and assure correct IUD placement.
  - Ultrasound can guide cervical dilation, assure correct fundal placement, and assist IUD removal when the strings are no longer visible on speculum exam.
  - Ultrasound guidance is not necessary for insertion, but is very useful in training settings as direct visualization can decrease perforation and complications. IUD insertion complications are most commonly related to provider experience with fewer complications occurring when providers perform more than 75 uterine procedures on an annual basis.
  - Expulsion
    - ENG is rarely expulsed, but there are reports of device breakage. Younger users of the ENG implant should be counseled against "playing" with their insert as regular flexing and bending of the implant is associated with

breakage. Continued efficacy may be an issue if the integrity of the device is impaired.
  - Expulsion rates of IUDs are estimated at 5% and are slightly higher in adolescent populations, but should not be considered a barrier in offering adolescents IUDs.[32,33]
  - Greater risk of IUD expulsion is associated with younger age, nulliparity, and previous IUD expulsion.
- **ENG**—There are very few insertional complications or adverse events associated with the new ENG inserter device. The newer device helps limit depth of insertion, avoiding placement deep into the muscle.

Misinformation with STIs and LARCs
Despite many years of reliable evidence, many providers still refuse to offer LARCs, and especially IUDs, to young women because of concerns regarding increasing PID and infertility risks.

- Risk of developing PID with an IUD is the same as the risk without an IUD.[25]
- There is a slightly increased risk of PID during the first 20 days of IUD use, most likely related to preexisting *Chlamydia trachomotis* or *Neisseria gonorrhoeae* infection at time of insertion.[34] PID rates are 9.7 per 1,000 women years, 1 to 20 days after insertion (see Chapter 58). Rates return to baseline in the general population (1.4 per 1,000 women years) on day 21 onward.[34]
- There are no recommendations for prophylactic antibiotic treatment in the general population.[35]
- However, in populations at risk for STIs, which includes AYA women 25 years of age or younger, providers may screen for STIs or treat empirically according to clinical indicators. Unknown STI status in asymptomatic women should not preclude same-day insertion. Providers may offer prophylactic antibiotic treatment for *Chlamydia trachomotis* or testing for cervicitis during insertion. Prophylactic treatment of *Chlamydia trachomotis* reduces PID rates and return visits in populations at high risk for disease.[35]
- Providers can be reassured that *Chlamydia trachomotis*-positive patients are unlikely to develop PID after insertion if treated in a timely manner.
- Providers can leave an IUD in place with the diagnosis of cervicitis or PID *after* insertion, provided there is clinical improvement with treatment in 48 hours.[35]
- Again, pre- and postoperative counseling should focus on dual method, condom use, partner negotiation, and other behavioral means of preventing STIs.

Common and Expected Side Effects
Irregular Uterine Bleeding

Pre-insertion counseling on post-insertion changes in menstrual bleeding is likely the most important aspect in preparing young women for continuation of LARC. Women should be counseled that many women experience a change in periods and irregular menstrual bleeding the first 3 months post-insertion.

- CU-IUD—Young women using the CU-IUD can expect regular, but heavier menses. For a minority of youth, avoiding amenorrhea and having a regular period make this their method of choice, but more often, the predicted CU-IUD effect on menstrual periods makes this a less desirable choice for young women.
- LNG-IUD 52 mg (Mirena) tends to lesson menses with a 90% reduction in all menstrual bleeding, with 50% of patients experiencing amenorrhea at one year post-insertion.
- LNG-IUD 14.5 mg smaller (Skylar) will experience bleeding patterns similar to Mirena but with more break through bleeding as well as increased likelihood of ongoing lighter periods.[36]
- ENG—The following changes in menstrual bleeding are observed: infrequent bleeding (33%), amenorrhea (21%), intermittent prolonged bleeding (17%), and frequent bleeding (6%), with the menstrual bleeding pattern in the first 3 months predicting future patterns.[37]
- While irregular bleeding may be a normal and expected immediate side effect, supporting young women and helping them tolerate this effect is important for continuation rates.

Treating Expected Abnormal Uterine Bleeding

Historically, NSAIDs, estrogen/progestin pills, and doxycycline have been used to manage problematic irregular bleeding although this practice is not evidence based. Limited clinical trial data suggest that, compared with placebo, mefenamic acid, mifepristone in combination with ethinyl estradiol or doxycycline, and doxycycline alone decrease the length of bleeding episodes in implant users.[38] A Cochrane review of 15 trials showed that NSAIDS (naproxen, suprofen, mefenamic acid, ibuprofen, indomethacin, flufenamic acid, alclofenac, and diclofenac) were effective in reducing menstrual blood loss and pain associated with IUD use.[39]

GUIDELINES FOR PATIENTS

Counseling and Consent

As with all medications, open discussion that puts benefits and risks in perspective is essential for effective contraception counseling. LARC insertion is a relatively simple outpatient surgical procedure. Pre-insertion consent reviews the insertion procedure, and more importantly, counsels on expected benefits and side effects of these long-acting devices. Key elements in counseling and consent include a discussion of:

1. Selection of a method that most meets their needs and goals, while avoiding least desirable side effects;
2. Insertion technique, with specific surgical risks of pain, bleeding, expulsion, perforation, and infection, along with ways providers can help avoid or manage these issues;
3. Immediate aftercare, including expected early side effects, ways to manage side effects, and adverse events that would require a follow-up; and
4. Long-term follow-up for continued contraception care and additional anticipatory guidance for safe, healthy sexual and reproductive health.

ENG Insertion

- Patient-centered counseling and preparation
  - Serious adverse events reported in 5% with none judged as drug related[3]
- Common complaints are bleeding and pain at insertion site immediately after insertion, which are usually managed with pressure, re-dressing, and oral medication.
- Clinicians must be trained for insertion competency according to FDA guidelines.
  - Time for insertion from the skin entry to complete insertion was 1 minute or less. It should be noted that this does not include the time for preparation or anesthetic injection and onset of action. Practical insertion time is from 5 to 10 minutes depending on the situational variables (inserter experience, patient need for reassurance, and clinic infrastructure for preparation).
- The ENG implant comes packaged in a preloaded, sterile, disposable inserter.
- To prevent any risk for unintended pregnancy, the ENG implant is FDA recommended to be inserted during the first 5 days of a woman's menstrual cycle, immediately post-abortion, or postpartum.
- The device is placed 6 to 8 cm above the medial epicondyle along the medial aspect of the nondominant upper arm, in the sulcus between the biceps and the triceps.
- The skin is cleansed with an antiseptic and 1 to 5 cc of 1% lidocaine is placed at the trochar insertion point and can be places along the planned insertion track of the device.
- The trochar, with implant loaded, is introduced directly under the skin and subdermal layer, tenting the skin until the needle hub is at the level of the skin. Stabilizing the base, the needle is smoothly retracted, leaving the implant behind.
- The implant remains invisible for most women, but it is easy to palpate. It is important to palpate the area immediately after the removal of the insertion needle to confirm implant placement.
- Pressure is applied to the skin incision site for hemostasis.
- A Steri-Strip is placed to close the incision along with a pressure dressing.
- Routine precautions should be provided for post-insertion care for bruising, minor bleeding, and pain after insertion.

ENG Removal

- Removal rates were higher for amenorrhea, occasional spotting or bleeding, and regular menses than for prolonged or continuous bleeding.
- In clinical trials, ENG showed high contraceptive efficacy, palpability before removal, short removal times, and few removal complications.
- Age, race, BMI, parity, prior contraception method, and postpartum and breast-feeding status did not predict bleeding or removal for bleeding risk.
- The implant was visible on x-ray and palpable before removal with a mean removal time of 2 to 4 minutes, using "pop-out" method or grasping the implant with a small hemostat and removing it through a small incision. Fibrosis around the implant is the most common removal complication.
- Removal of ENG implants is distinctly more straightforward than the removal of the LNG capsules (Norplant) for several reasons: single implant, stiffer rod, less fibrous capsule formation.
  - The digital extrusion or "pop-out" technique is encouraged for removal. In the "pop-out" technique, the rod is first palpated, marked, and removal site cleansed.
  - A small amount of local anesthetic is infused beneath the distal tip of the rod. A 2-mm incision parallel to the rod is made parallel at the distal tip of the implant.
  - Then pressure is applied at the proximal end, pushing the rod toward the incision until it pops out, at which time it can be grasped with fingers or forceps.
  - Instrument removal with noncrushing clamps also may be utilized.

IUD Insertion

IUD insertion requires a pelvic bimanual and speculum exam. Patients may benefit from pre-insertion NSAIDs (800 mg ibuprofen or 500 mg naproxen). Patients benefit from verbal distraction techniques to decrease anxiety and improve procedure tolerance as with other pelvic exam procedures.

- The bimanual exam assesses for uterine size, placement (anteverted, midline, retroverted), and location of cervix. It will also inform the examiner about cervical motion tenderness or other palpable pelvic abnormalities.
- The speculum exam allows for visualization of the external cervical os, paracervical block, and tenaculum grasp for maintaining traction with insertion.
- Insertion requires measuring or sounding the uterus to determine adequate uterine size (6 to 10 cm) and direction of placement.
- Both IUDs have slightly **different** intrauterine insertion techniques but both aim for fundal placement for maximal efficacy.
- IUD removal is generally a 5- to 10-second procedure by which the strings are grasped with locking forceps and the IUD is gently pulled out from the cervical os.

Patient Preparation and Education before IUD Insertion

1. What is IUD?—IUD is a small plastic device that is placed in the uterus (womb).
2. How is IUD placed?—IUD is inserted in the doctor's office. It does not require surgery but sometimes a local anesthetic is used to numb the cervix (the opening to the uterus) and make inserting IUD more comfortable.
3. How does IUD work?—IUD appears to work primarily by preventing fertilization of an egg by sperm. The copper in the ParaGard IUD probably has an antisperm effect, and the progestin hormones in the medicated IUD blocks sperm from entering the womb.
4. Are there different types of IUD?—In the US, currently, there are two types of IUD available. One contains copper, and the other contains the hormone LNG. Both are shaped like the letter T and are approximately 11/4 in tall. Each has a thread or "tail" on the end, which allows the woman to check that the device is in place and also makes removal easier. The copper IUD is effective for up to 12 years. The LNG-IUS can be used for up to 5 years.
5. How effective is IUD?—IUD is one of the most effective forms of reversible birth control. Both the copper T380-A IUD and the LNG-IUS are more than 99% effective at preventing pregnancy in the first year of use.
6. Are there side effects?—With the copper T-380A IUD, the most common side effects are increased menstrual flow and cramps, which may be reduced by use of an over-the-counter pain medication such as ibuprofen. These side effects lessen after the first few months. With the LNG-IUD, irregular spotting and bleeding are common in the first 3 to 6 months, but after that a woman's periods decrease dramatically and may stop altogether. Absence of a period is not dangerous and does not mean that the blood is "building up inside." Rather, the lining of the uterus is so thin that there is very little or no tissue to be shed each month.
7. Is IUD safe?—IUD is safe and has been recommended for young women, never-been-pregnant women, and all women desiring effective birth control for many years now.
8. What are the benefits of IUD?—IUD is a safe, effective, easy-to-use, and cost-effective form of contraception. There is no need to remember to use the method every day or with every act of sex.

Remember

1. IUD does not protect against STIs. If you may be at risk for STIs and have IUD, use a latex or polyurethane condom to help protect yourself against infection.
2. If you ever have fever, pelvic pain, severe cramping, heavy vaginal bleeding, or a foul-smelling vaginal discharge, contact your clinician immediately. These may be signs of a serious infection or pregnancy or a warning that your IUD may be coming out.
3. If you have any symptoms of pregnancy, contact your provider immediately.
4. Do not remove IUD yourself or tug on the strings.
5. If you have any problems or questions, call your provider.

FUTURE DEVELOPMENTS

There continues to be excitement about the role LARC can play in improving contraceptive efficacy for women of all ages. Recent data strongly support the first-line role LARCs may have for AYA women for whom adherence and continuation are problematic. The family planning community has made continued progress in contraceptive research and development addressing both efficacy and side effects to improve uptake and user satisfaction. Concerns over the adverse effects of hormonal contraceptives have led to research and development of new combinations with improved metabolic profile. Recent developments include use of smaller devices, changes in hormonal content (newer progestins, estradiol), and progesterone antagonists and receptor modulators to block ovulation and prevent follicular rupture. Multipurpose prevention technologies are investigating combination products that potentially offer both contraception and STI prevention, but are not likely to be on the market for many years.[40]

CONCLUSION

LARCs represent a state-of-the-art, first-line contraceptive option for adolescents and women of all ages. Health care providers for AYA women should be confident and encouraging of their use given their safety, efficacy, and ease of use. Promoting improved patient knowledge, access, and support for long-term use of these contraceptives may improve initiation and continuation rates in youth, which may directly impact unintended early pregnancy. Providers may offer these safe, most effective methods as the first line of contraception for all sexually active youth and young women at risk for unintended pregnancy.

REFERENCES

1. ACOG Committee Opinion, Committee on Adolescent Health Care: Long Acting Reversible Contraception Work Group. Adolescents and long-acting reversible contraceptives: implants and intrauterine devices. *Obstet Gynecol* 2012;120: 983–988.
2. Finer LB, Jerman J, Kavanaugh ML. Changes in use of long acting contraceptive methods in the United States, 2007–2009. *Fertil Steril* 2012;98: 893–897.
3. Mommers E, Blum GF, Gent TG, et al. Nexplanon, a radiopaque etonogestrel implant in combination with a next-generation applicator: 3-year results of a noncomparative multicenter trial. *Am J Obstet Gynecol* 2012;207:388.e1–e6.
4. Affandi B, Korver T, Geurts TB, et al. A pilot efficacy study with a single-rod contraceptive implant (Implanon) in 200 Indonesian women treated for greater than or equal to 4 years. *Contraception* 1999;59:167–174.
5. Sivin I. Utility and drawbacks of continuous use of a copper T IUD for 20 years. *Contraception* 2007;75 (6, suppl):S70–S75.
6. Trussell J. Contraceptive efficacy. In Hatcher RA, Trussell J, Nelson AL, et al., eds. *Contraceptive technology.* 20th ed. New York, NY: Ardent Media, 2011.
7. Sivin I, Stern J, Coutinho E, et al. Prolonged intrauterine contraception: a seven-year randomized study of the levonorgestrel 20 mcg/day (LNg 20) and the Copper T380 Ag IUDS. *Contraception* 1991;44:473–480.
8. Dean G, Schwarz EB. Intrauterine contraceptives (IUCs). In: Hatcher RA, Trussell J, Nelson AL, et al., eds. *Contraceptive technology.* 20th ed. New York, NY: Ardent Media, 2011:147–191.
9. Xu X, Macaluso M, Frost J, et al. Characteristics of users of intrauterine devices and other reversible contraceptive methods in the United States. *Fertil Steril* 2011;96:1138–1144.

10. Whitaker AK, Dude AM, Neustadt A, et al. Correlates of use of long-acting reversible methods of contraception among adolescent and young adult women. *Contraception* 2010;81:299–303.

11. Mosher WD, Jones J. Use of contraception in the United States: 1982–2008. *Vital Health Stat 23* 2010;29:1–44.

12. Kavanaugh ML, Jerman J, Ethier K, et al. Meeting the contraceptive needs of teens and young adults: youth-friendly and long-acting reversible contraceptive services in U.S. family planning facilities. *J Adolesc Health* 2013;52:284–292.

13. Dempsey AR, Billingsley CC, Savage AH, et al. Predictors of long-acting reversible contraception use among unmarried young adults. *Am J Obstet Gynecol* 2012;2006:526.e1–e5.

14. Kohn JE, Hacker JG, Rousselle MA, et al. Knowledge and likelihood to recommend intrauterine devices for adolescents among school-based health center providers. *J Adolesc Health* 2012;51:319–324.

15. Crespi S, Kerrigan M, Sood V. Budget impact analysis of 8 hormonal contraceptive options. *Am J Manag Care* 2013;19:e249–e255.

16. Center for Disease Control and Prevention. U.S. Medical eligibility criteria for contraceptive use. *MMWR* 2010;59 (RR04):1–6.

17. Center for Disease Control and Prevention. U.S. selected practice recommendations for contraceptive use, 2013. *MMWR* 2013;62:10–60.

18. American College of Obstetricians and Gynecologists. ACOG Practice Bulletin No. 121: Long-acting reversible contraception: Implants and intrauterine devices. *Obstet Gynecol* 2011;118:184–196.

19. Blanc AK, Tsui AO, Croft TN, et al. Patterns and trends in adolescents' contraceptive use and discontinuation in developing countries and comparisons with adult women. *Int Perspect Sex Reprod Health* 2009;35:63–71.

20. Raine TR, Foster-Rosales A, Upadhyay UD, et al. One-year contraceptive continuation and pregnancy in adolescent girls and women initiating hormonal contraceptives. *Obstet Gynecol* 2011;117:363–371.

21. Rosenstock JR, Peipert JF, Madden T, et al. Continuation of reversible contraception in teenagers and young women. *Obstet Gynecol* 2012;120:1298–1305.

22. O'Neil-Callahan M, Peipert JF, Zhao Q, et al. Twenty-four-month continuation of reversible contraception. *Obstet Gynecol* 2013;122:1083–1091.

23. Winner B, Peipert JF, Zhao Q, et al. Effectiveness of long-acting reversible contraception. *N Engl J Med* 2012;366:1998–2007.

24. Mestad R, Secura G, Allsworth JE, et al. Acceptance of long-acting reversible contraceptive methods by adolescent participants in the Contraceptive CHOICE Project. *Contraception* 2011;84:493–498.

25. Hov GG, Skjeldestad FE, Hilstad T. Use of IUD and subsequent fertility—follow-up after participation in a randomized clinical trial. *Contraception* 2007;75:88–92.

26. Bednarek PH, Jensen JT. Safety, efficacy and patient acceptability of the contraceptive and non-contraceptive uses of the LNG-IUS. *Int J Womens Health* 2010;9:45–58.

27. American College of Obstetricians and Gynecologists. ACOG Practice Bulletin No. 110. Noncontraceptive uses of hormonal contraceptives. *Obstet Gynecol* 2010;115:206–218.

28. Centers for Disease Control and Prevention. Sexually transmitted treatment guidelines. *MMWR* 2010;59 (RR-12).

29. Brahmi D, Steenland MW, Renner RM, et al. Pregnancy outcomes with an IUD in situ: a systematic review. *Contraception* 2012;85:131–139.

30. Meirik O, Brache V, Orawan K, et al. WHO Study Group on contraceptive implants for women. A multicenter randomized clinical trial of one-rod etonogestrel and two-rod levonorgestrel contraceptive implants with nonrandomized copper-IUD controls: methodology and insertion. *Contraception* 2013;87:113–120.

31. Allen RH, Bartz D, Grimes DA, et al. Interventions for pain with intrauterine device insertion. *Cochrane Database Syst Rev* 2009;(3):CD007373. doi: 10.1002/14651858.CD007373.

32. Deans EI, Grimes DA. Intrauterine devices for adolescents: a systematic review. *Contraception* 2009;79:418–423.

33. Board of the Society of Family Planning. Use of the Mirena LNG-IUS and Paragard CuT380A intrauterine devices in nulliparous women. *Contraception* 2010;81:367–371.

34. Mohllajee AP, Curtis KM, Peterson HB. Does insertion and use of an intrauterine device increase the risk of pelvic inflammatory disease among women with sexually transmitted infection? A systematic review. *Contraception* 2006;73:145–153.

35. Grimes DA, Lopez LM, Schulz KF. Antibiotic prophylaxis for intrauterine contraceptive device insertion [Original publication 1999]. *Cochrane Database Syst Rev* 1999;(3):CD001327. doi:10.1002/14651858.CD001327.

36. Gemzell-Danielsson K, Schellschmidt I, Apter D. A randomized, phase II study describing the efficacy, bleeding profile, and safety of two low-dose levonorgestrel-releasing intrauterine contraceptive systems and Mirena. *Fertil Steril* 2012;97:616–622.e1–e3.

37. Darney P, Patel A, Rosen K, et al. Safety and efficacy of a single-rod etonogestrel implant (Implanon): results from 11 international clinical trials. *Fertil Steril* 2009;91:1646–1653.

38. Weisberg E, Hickey M, Palmer D, et al. A randomized controlled trial of treatment options for troublesome uterine bleeding in Implanon users. *Hum Reprod* 2009;24:1852–1861.

39. Grimes DA, Hubacher D, Lopez LM, et al. Non-steroidal anti-inflammatory drugs for heavy bleeding or pain associated with intrauterine-device use [Review]. *Cochrane Database Syst Rev* 2006;(4):CD006034. doi:10.1002/14651858.CD006034.pub2.

40. Sitruk-Ware R, Nath A. Contraception technology: past, present and future. *Contraception* 2013;87:319–330.

ADDITIONAL RESOURCES AND WEBSITES ONLINE

IX

PART XII

Other Reproductive System and Breast Disorders

CHAPTER 45

Gynecologic Examination of the Adolescent and Young Adult Female

Sarah Pitts
Merill Weitzel

KEY WORDS

- Gynecologic examination
- Pap test

THE GYNECOLOGIC EXAMINATION

A gynecological examination is an essential component of the health care of female patients from birth onward. Reassuring and educating girls about their normal external anatomy is as important as addressing the concerns and needs of an adolescent or young adult woman in advance of her first internal examination.

INDICATIONS FOR GYNECOLOGIC EXAMINATIONS

Indications

The indications for a complete or modified gynecologic examination vary with the patient's complaint. A 13-year-old girl presenting for a physical examination can be reassured that external structures appear healthy and normal. A virginal 15-year-old girl with complaint of white vaginal discharge may be evaluated by obtaining a sample to differentiate physiologic discharge from a *Candidal* vaginitis. In contrast, a sexually active 20-year-old woman with lower abdominal pain and vaginal discharge deserves a complete pelvic examination (Table 45.1).

Providers should separate the provision of contraceptive services from gynecologic examinations. Such an examination should not be a barrier to the provision of hormonal contraceptives unless a patient is requesting an intrauterine device (IUD). It cannot be emphasized enough that physical examination of the

TABLE 45.1

Indication for Modified or Complete Pelvic Examination

Female over 21 y of age
Symptoms of vaginal or uterine infection
Menstrual disorders including amenorrhea, dysfunctional uterine bleeding, severe dysmenorrhea, or mild to moderate dysmenorrhea unresponsive to therapy
Undiagnosed lower abdominal pain
Sexual assault (modified to collect the appropriate information and samples)
Suspected pelvic mass
Request by the adolescent or young adult

external genitals should be a routine part of preventive care for girls and women alike, but not if the patient is resistant or uncomfortable, or if such an examination is in conflict with their cultural or religious beliefs. Patients and parents should also be informed that a bynecologic examination and Papanicolaou test (Pap test) are not the same. While external genital examination is routine from birth onward, there are several indications for a modified or complete internal pelvic examination in addition to cervical cancer screening. These include symptoms of a vaginal or uterine infection, menstrual disorders, pelvic pain, sexual assault, suspected pelvic mass, or request by the patient.

Cervical Cancer Screening

Cervical cancer screening[1,2] or a Pap test should be initiated at 21 years of age in most cases. Exceptions to this rule include sexually active adolescents with acquired HIV who should be screened twice in the year following diagnosis and annually thereafter as recommended by the US Centers for Disease Control and Prevention (CDC). There are no studies to support similar recommendations in women immunosuppressed from other causes (e.g., transplant recipients), and the American College of Obstetricians and Gynecologists (ACOG) recommends screening at 21 years of age in such populations. Screening assesses cellular changes of the cervix that may put a woman at risk for cancer associated with prior genital exposure to the human papillomavirus (HPV). ACOG recommends Pap tests every 3 years without co-testing for HPV strains in women younger than 30 years. Should abnormal cytologic changes be noted, reflex HPV testing and/or colposcopy is warranted. Chapter 50 provides a detailed review of Pap tests and management.

Sexually Transmitted Infection Screening

Screening for sexually transmitted infections (STIs)[3] should be conducted once a female patient has had a sexual experience, including genital to genital, or mouth to genital contact, penetrative vaginal contact (digital, penile, or foreign body), or penetrative anal contact. While urine-based screening tests for *Chlamydia trachomatis* and/or *Neisseria gonorrhoeae* exist, nucleic acid amplification testing (NAAT) of the vagina or cervix may be more sensitive. Without a genital complaint, asymptomatic sexually active adolescent and young adult (AYA) women under the age of 21 years do not require an internal gynecologic examination, but a thorough external examination is highly recommended. Screening urine or a vaginal swab for *C. trachomatis*, and also for *N. gonorrhoeae* depending on the local prevalence, is recommended annually in asymptomatic sexually active patients.

OBTAINING THE HISTORY

Building rapport and developing a trusting relationship with the adolescent or young adult prior to examining her is important. In order to reduce patient anxiety, it is essential that the office setting be comfortable and friendly. Creating an environment in which private and confidential matters can be discussed without judgment and with reassurance is of the upmost importance. This may require a special waiting area for AYA, evening clinic hours, and age-appropriate reading materials. Front desk staff, clinical assistants, nurses, and providers should be trained to address confidentiality and the unique psychosocial needs of AYAs. While parents are welcome and often essential in providing key pieces of history or support during gynecologic examinations, a separate time and space to interview the patient privately and to answer her questions is essential. Confidentiality and its limits must be addressed early in all clinical encounters with patients and parents (see Chapter 4).[4,5] Doing so will encourage more open discussions and better care.

The history should include a gynecologic assessment, general health history, review of systems, and information on risk behaviors. The HEEADSSS psychosocial screening framework as outlined in Chapter 4 can be used. Answers to these questions must be obtained confidentially. Some adolescents, and even some young adults, may feel more comfortable if most of the history is obtained with a parent in the room. A few moments of privacy are all that is needed to obtain pertinent negatives about risk behaviors, safety, and sexual activity. It is not uncommon for AYAs to feel uncomfortable discussing such topics. Acknowledging this and normalizing questions or concerns about sexual health can put a young person at ease and facilitate the discussion.

It is essential to know what the patient's reason for the visit is and whether there is any expectation for a gynecologic examination. If possible, doing this early on in the history can help allay fears and put the patient at ease. It is also important to gauge a patient's understanding of menstrual periods, sexuality, and genital hygiene. Providing proper education during the interview and normalizing the patient's questions and concerns help build rapport. Establishing a trusting relationship makes the gynecologic examination more comfortable.

It is not uncommon for a patient presenting with one apparent goal of care to report a gynecologic concern later in the encounter or to be in denial of an important gynecologic need. Therefore, the sexual history should be part of structured questioning preceded by the statement, "I routinely ask all my patients these screening questions." Complete gynecologic histories should include the following:

1. Menstrual history—age at menarche and date of last menstrual period; duration of menses and interval between periods or intermenstrual staining, number of pads or tampons changed in a day to assess amount of flow; dysmenorrhea—severity on 10-point scale and extent of missed school, work, or activities; premenstrual symptoms;
2. History of vaginal discharge—characteristics and associated symptom;
3. Sexual history—type of sexual contact, consensual versus coerced, number of partners, sex of partners, age at first sexual intercourse; contraceptive methods used, preferences and fertility goals; prior STIs; prior pregnancies;
4. Prior Pap test screening—any difficulties with the examination or abnormalities found through testing?
5. Family history—any history of uterine abnormalities or gynecologic cancers?

GYNECOLOGIC EXAMINATION

An external genital examination should be part of an annual examination for all female patients. The patient should give her consent and be made to feel that she is in control and can stop the examination at any point to ask questions or, if need be, to stop the examination entirely. A handheld mirror to permit viewing of the genitalia can be helpful and educational for some patients. For a first internal gynecologic examination, the clinician should acknowledge that some patients may feel nervous. Explain that it takes only two or three minutes to perform. Patients should be given the choice of whether to have a support person in the room during the examination. Generally, male providers have a female chaperone present for pelvic examinations. Female providers may or may not have a chaperone depending on the setting and patient preference.

Having the appropriate gynecologic equipment readily accessible is essential (Table 45.2). Before the patient changes into a gown, indicate the reasons why the gynecologic examination is important for evaluating her chief complaint. It is also good to talk about ways in which the patient might relax and feel in control. The use of imagery, deep breathing, and other relaxation techniques may be helpful in the anxious patient. Patients should also be reassured that adequate drapes will be used to maintain privacy during the examination. Before the examination begins, it is helpful to review the main steps in the examination. Each step will then be explained again as the actual examination is performed. The steps are as follows for the gynecologic examination:

1. Make sure that the patient has emptied her bladder before the examination.
2. Ask the patient to undress from the waist down and to cover herself with a sheet. If additional examinations are to be performed at the same time, such as a breast examination, then the patient would need to undress completely and wear a gown.
3. Cover the patient to the waist with the sheet. Have her lie supine on the examination table, feet resting on the ankle supports. Instruct the patient to bend her knees and slide her buttocks to the end of the table toward her feet. Elevating the head of the table 30 degrees is optional; it can provide the adolescent with an increased sense of control as it allows improved eye contact with the clinician.
4. Ask the patient to relax her knees to your hands which are held out at either side. Do not pry her legs apart.

TABLE 45.2
Gynecologic Examination Equipment

Examination table with ankle supports
Gowns, sheets
Light source (speculum light or lamp)
Specula: Metal—Pederson or Huffman or plastic (medium and small)
Chlamydia and *N. gonorrhoeae* screening tests (e.g., NAATS for urine, vagina, or cervix)
Cotton swabs
Tubes or slides for wet mounts
10% KOH and saline for wet mounts
pH paper
Spatula and cytobrush (or cytobroom) for Pap test
Pap kits for ThinPrep or other Pap systems
Water-soluble lubricating jelly
Warm water source
Nonsterile gloves
Handheld mirror (use is optional and up to the patient)
Tissues
Tampons and sanitary napkins
Rapid pregnancy test kits
Microscope or access to a laboratory for specimen review

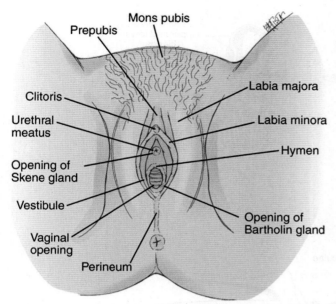

Mons pubis
Prepubis
Clitoris
Urethral meatus
Opening of Skene gland
Vestibule
Vaginal opening
Perineum
Labia majora
Labia minora
Hymen
Opening of Bartholin gland

FIGURE 45.1 External genitalia of the pubertal female. (From Weber JR. *Nurse's handbook of health assessment.* 8th ed. Philadelphia, PA: Lippincott Williams & Wilkins, 2013.)

5. The sheet should be adjusted so that eye contact is maintained with the patient, the patient's legs are still covered, and the perineum is adequately visualized.

6. Inspect the external genitalia (Fig. 45.1).
   a. Note pubic hair distribution and sexual maturity rating.
   b. Inform the patient before touching her thighs, and then again before grasping each labia lightly between forefinger and thumb and retracting gently in a downward angle, separating the labia to examine the external structures.
   c. Assess for signs of erythema, inflammation, nevi, warts, or other lesions over the perineum, thighs, mons, labia, and perianal region. Check the size of the clitoris, which is typically 2 to 4 mm wide. The Skene glands are two small glands located just inside the urethra and are usually not visible. Bartholin glands are the two small mucus-secreting glands located just outside the hymeneal ring at the 5 and 7 o'clock positions and should not be enlarged, red, or tender.
   d. The hymen should be carefully inspected for estrogen effect (light pink, thickened), for congenital anomalies (septate, imperforate, microperforate), and for transections that might result from consensual or nonconsensual sexual intercourse. With gentle retraction, the anterior vagina may be visible and again the estrogen effect can be observed—pink mucosa, white vaginal secretions.
   e. Obtaining samples: For patients who have never been sexually active but who need wet mounts to evaluate vaginal discharge, saline-moistened or dry cotton-tipped applicators can be inserted intravaginally to obtain samples without the use of a speculum. Routine NAAT testing in an asymptomatic patient using a vaginal swab can be obtained similarly.

7. Speculum examination: The correct size of speculum should be selected, and metal speculum should be warmed, if possible, before insertion. Depending on the Pap test system used, it may or may not be fine to use a lubricant on the speculum, but warm water is always safe to use. If the hymenal opening is small, a Huffman (Huffman-Graves) speculum ($\frac{1}{2} \times 4\frac{1}{2}$ in.) is used to visualize the cervix. For the sexually active patient, a Pederson speculum ($\frac{7}{8} \times 4\frac{1}{2}$ in.) or occasionally a Graves speculum ($\frac{3}{8} \times 3\frac{3}{4}$ in.) is appropriate (Fig. 45.2). A small or medium plastic speculum with an attached light source is also useful for facilitating the examination. For a given patient, the provider must decide if it would be beneficial and educational to show the patient the speculum prior to use or if it would induce unnecessary fear. A one-finger, gloved (water-moistened) examination performed first may make subsequent speculum insertion and finding of the cervix easier. To avoid surprising the patient during the speculum examination, touch the speculum to the thigh first and tell the patient that you are going to place the speculum into the vagina. The speculum should be inserted posteriorly in a downward direction to avoid the urethra (Fig. 45.3).
   a. Observe the vaginal walls for signs of estrogenization, inflammation, adherent discharge or lesions.
   b. Inspect the cervix. The stratified squamous epithelium of the external os is usually a dull pink color. There is often a more erythematous area of columnar epithelium surrounding the cervical os, called a *cervical ectropion*. The junction between the two types of mucosa is called the *squamocolumnar junction*, and it is particularly important that this area be sampled during the Pap test screening. This ectropion may persist throughout the adolescent years, especially in hormonal contraceptive users. Mucopurulent discharge from the cervix characterizes cervicitis, typical of infections with *N. gonorrhoeae, C. trachomatis,* and herpes virus. Small, pinpoint hemorrhagic spots on the cervix, so-called "strawberry" cervix, can occur rarely with *Trichomonas* infections. The cervix should be examined for any lesions or polyps. Any abnormal growth on the cervix should be referred for further evaluation and colposcopy.
   c. To assess signs and symptoms of vaginitis, swabs for wet mounts and pH can be obtained from the vagina and then rolled in one or two drops of saline on one slide (for *Trichomonas,* white cells, or "clue cells") and in one drop of 10% potassium hydroxide (KOH) (for pseudohyphae) on another slide. A swab should also be applied to pH paper.
   d. If indicated, obtain a Pap test of the cervix. This should include at least a 360-degree rotation of the spatula in contact with the cervix, with care taken to sample the "transition zone" or squamocolumnar junction. Nylon cytobrushes are also commonly used in addition to the spatula, thereby ensuring the collection of cells from the endocervical canal.
   e. Tests for STIs: Tests for *N. gonorrhoeae* and/or *C. trachomatis* include NAATs, DNA probes, immunoassays, and cultures. Vaginal and endocervical *Chlamydia* NAAT screening have slightly higher sensitivity than urine screening.[6]
   f. Remove the speculum being careful not to pinch the vaginal side walls.

8. Bimanual examination (Fig. 45.4): The bimanual vaginal-abdominal examination involves the insertion of one or two gloved, lubricated fingers into the vagina while the other hand is placed on the abdomen. If this is her first bimanual examination, it is worthwhile having the patient practice relaxing her abdominal muscles first. Remind the patient that you will be examining her uterus and ovaries and ask her to communicate any feelings of discomfort she may be experiencing during the examination.
   a. Palpation of the vagina and cervix: Check for masses along the side walls and posterior cul-de-sac, and on the cervix and any tenderness with cervical motion.
   b. Palpation of the uterus: Assess the size, the position of the uterus, and any masses or tenderness. Pushing backward on the cervix causes the uterus to move anteriorly, allowing for its palpation with the abdominal hand.
   c. Gently explore the posterior fornix and the rectouterine pouch (pouch of Douglas) for masses, fullness, and tenderness.

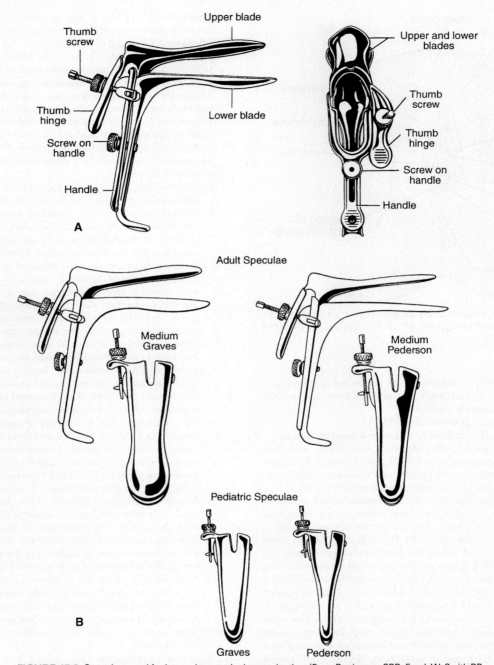

FIGURE 45.2 Speculum used for internal gynecologic examination. (From Beckmann CRB, Frank W, Swith RP, et al. *Obstetrics and gynecology.* 5th ed. Philadelphia, PA: Lippincott Williams & Wilkins, 2006.)

   d. Palpation of the adnexa: Assess for any masses, tenderness, or abnormalities of the ovaries or the adnexal area. To palpate these structures, insert the examining fingers into each lateral fornix, positioning them slightly posteriorly and high. Sweep the abdominal examining hand downward over the internal fingers. Normal ovaries are usually <3 cm long and are rubbery.

   e. If there is a history of significant pelvic pain or an adnexal mass is felt, a rectovaginal–abdominal examination can help complete the evaluation of the adnexa or uterus and the rectum, anus, and posterior cul-de-sac. A rectovaginal–abdominal examination is performed with the index finger in the vagina, the middle finger in the rectum, and the other hand on the abdomen. The examination permits evaluation of the uterosacral ligaments and cul-de-sac as well as the mobility of the uterus. It is important to inform the patient that she may experience an urge to defecate, but she will not. The rectovaginal septum should be thin and pliable, and the pelvic floor should be free of masses and tenderness. On indication, stool retrieved can be tested for occult blood.

9. At the completion of the examination, offer the patient a box of tissues to be used to remove the lubrication from her perineum after you leave the room. Some patients may require assistance in sliding up the table before taking their feet out of the ankle supports. Instruct the patient to dress fully and

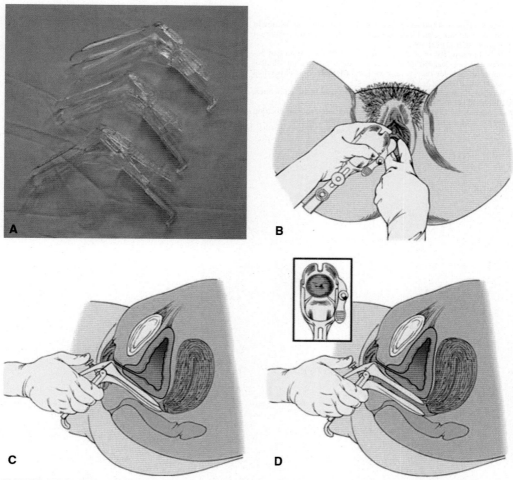

FIGURE 45.3 Insertion of speculum. (From Weber JR. *Nurse's handbook of health assessment.* 8th ed. Philadelphia, PA: Lippincott Williams & Wilkins, 2013.)

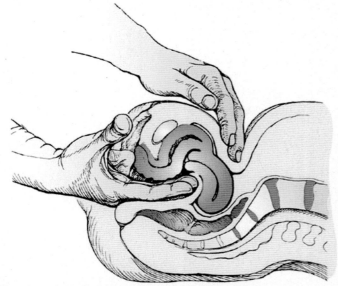

FIGURE 45.4 Bimanual examination. (From Gibbs RS, Karlan BY, Haney AF, et al. *Danforth's obstetrics and gynecology.* 10th ed. Philadelphia, PA: Lippincott Williams & Wilkins, 2008.)

return to the office for a discussion of your findings and plan. Before the practitioner leaves the room, the patient should be in a sitting position and draped.

During the post-examination discussion, the patient should be congratulated for her cooperation, and the importance of the findings of the examination (positive or negative) should be discussed in relation to her chief complaint. All questions should be answered, and any therapies or further tests required should be outlined. This is an important time for discussion of the patient's concerns about normal anatomy and physiology, contraception (including emergency contraception), and sexuality. During this discussion, it is important for the examiner to listen carefully, remembering that patients may not communicate all their concerns initially. At the conclusion of the discussion, the parent or partner can be invited to join the health care provider and the patient. With the patient's consent, the parent can be informed of the results of the examination and the treatment plan. Maintaining confidentiality is essential to preserving the provider–patient relationship. Parents should be encouraged to ask questions and to voice concerns.

Helping AYAs through their gynecologic visit sets the stage for reproductive health care throughout life. The gynecologic visit is an ideal opportunity to provide education, listen to concerns, assess medical and psychosocial complaints, and promote a healthy future. The examination also allows the clinician an opportunity to impart a positive attitude about the female body and to stress the importance of health maintenance.

REFERENCES

1. American College of Obstetricians and Gynecologists. Cervical cancer screening in adolescents: screening, evaluation, and management. ACOG Committee Opinion No.463. *Obstet Gynecol* 2010;116(2):469.
2. Saslow D, Solomon D, Lawson HW, et al. American Cancer Society, American Society for Colposcopy and Cervical Pathology, and American Society for Clinical Pathology screening guidelines for the prevention and early detection of cervical cancer . *CA Cancer J Clin* 2012;62(3):147.
3. Workowski KA, Berman S. Sexually transmitted diseases treatment guidelines, 2010. *MMWR* 2010;59(RR-12):1–116.
4. Ford C, English A, Sigman G. Confidential health care for adolescents: position paper of the society for adolescent medicine. *J Adol Health* 2004;35:160.
5. Thrall JS, McCloskey L, Ettner SL, et al. Confidentiality and adolescents' use of providers for health information and for pelvic examinations. *Arch Pediatr Adolesc Med* 2000;154:885.
6. Papp JR, Schachter J, Gaydos CA, et al. Recommendations for the laboratory-based detection of *Chlamydia trachomatis* and *Neisseria gonorrhoeae*—2014. *MMWR* 2014;63(2):1–24.

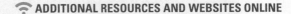 **ADDITIONAL RESOURCES AND WEBSITES ONLINE**

CHAPTER 46

Normal Menstrual Physiology

Sari L. Kives
Nicole Hubner

This chapter reviews normal menstrual physiology, and the next several chapters discuss common menstrual abnormalities in adolescents and young adults (AYAs).

The development of the menstrual cycle depends on the maturation of the hypothalamic–pituitary–ovarian (HPO) axis that occurs during puberty. A coordinated sequence of events is required for cyclic menses to occur, beginning with the hypothalamic secretion of gonadotropin-releasing hormone (GnRH). In response to GnRH, the pituitary secretes follicle-stimulating hormone (FSH) and luteinizing hormone (LH), and the ovaries secrete estrogen, progesterone, activin, and inhibins.[1] The endometrium of the uterus responds to estrogen and progesterone with endometrial growth and differentiation. In the absence of fertilization, this process culminates in menses.[2]

Growth acceleration can be the first sign of puberty, followed by thelarche (breast budding), then pubarche (presence of pubic hair), and finally menarche (the onset of menses).[3] Menarche occurs on average 2.6 years after the onset of puberty and after the peak of growth has passed.[3] In the US, the median age of menarche is 12.34 years, and in approximately two-thirds of girls, it occurs at a sexual maturity rating (SMR) of 4. The timing of menarche occurs approximately 2.3 years after thelarche. In the first 2 years after menarche, 55% to 82% of cycles are anovulatory.[4] Menarche is followed by approximately 5 to 7 years of increasing regularity as the cycles shorten to reach the usual reproductive pattern.[3]

The exact trigger of menarche is unknown. We know that both inhibitory and excitatory neurotransmitters, as well as peptides, modulate the activity of the HPO axis. The axis is inactive from late infancy continuing through childhood secondary to central inhibitory mechanisms suppressing GnRH secretion, and to a lesser extent the high sensitivity to low levels of gonadal steroid feedback. At gonadarche, the HPO axis is reactivated in response to metabolic signals from the periphery. FSH and LH levels rise followed by a gradual increase in estradiol concentrations, which stimulates breast development. The increase in pulsatile LH secretion occurs first at night, during sleep, but gradually extends throughout the day. At midpuberty, estrogen production increases sufficiently to stimulate endometrial proliferation, ultimately resulting in menarche.[3] Evidence suggests that menarche may be associated with achieving a critical body weight of 46 to 47 kg and a minimum fatness level of 17%, although this point has generated controversy.

The maintenance or restoration of menstruation is thought to require a minimum of 22% body fat.[5]

DEFINITION OF MENSTRUAL CYCLE

The duration of a menstrual cycle is from the first day of one menstrual period to the first day of the next period. A typical menstrual cycle has fluctuating levels of pituitary hormones (FSH and LH), stimulating ovarian follicular, ovulatory, and luteal phases, with concurrent growth and differentiation of the endometrium (proliferative and secretory phases) (Fig. 46.1).[6]

GnRH is secreted in a pulsatile fashion by a specialized network of hypothalamic neurons termed "the GnRH pulse generator." GnRH stimulates both LH and FSH synthesis and pulsatile secretion by pituitary gonadotropes.[7] At the beginning of the menstrual cycle, low levels of estradiol initiate positive feedback on hypothalamic GnRH to stimulate pituitary secretion of FSH and LH. At higher levels, estradiol and progesterone provide negative feedback and suppress FSH and LH, thereby preventing further follicular recruitment. Neurotransmitters (e.g., dopamine, norepinephrine) and endorphins (opioids) also play a role in modulating GnRH secretion.[2] Menstrual irregularities that occur with weight loss, stress, exercise, and drugs may be secondary to the effect of these entities on the hypothalamus.[8]

The menstrual cycle is best understood by reviewing these three descriptive phases—the follicular phase, the ovulatory phase, and the luteal phase.

Follicular Phase
The duration of the follicular phase is the major determinant of cycle length, usually lasting 14 days (range 7 to 22 days). This phase begins with the onset of menses and ends with ovulation.

1. The corpus luteum from the previous cycle involutes, resulting in decreasing levels of estradiol and progesterone. The low levels stimulate the hypothalamic release of GnRH, which increases the pituitary release of FSH and LH.
2. FSH stimulates the recruitment of ovarian follicles.
3. LH stimulates ovarian theca cells to produce androgens, which are then converted to estrogens in the ovarian granulosa cells under the influence of FSH. Estradiol increases FSH binding to granulosa cell receptors, leading to amplification of the FSH effect, allowing one follicle to predominate. Although the gonadotropins act synergistically, FSH primarily affects follicular growth and LH mainly stimulates ovarian steroid biosynthesis.
4. Estrogen drives the proliferative phase of the endometrium. Estradiol increases the production of growth factors that stimulate proliferation within the glandular and stromal

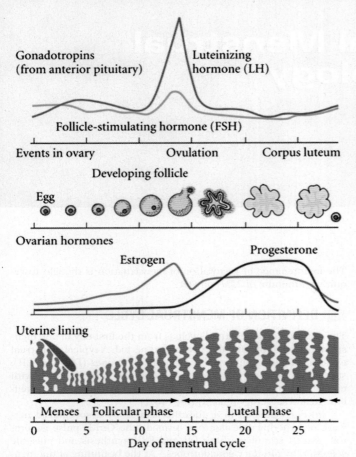

FIGURE 46.1 Normal menstrual cycle. (From Gilbert SF. *Developmental biology*. 10th ed. Sunderland: Sinauer, 2013, with permission)

compartments of the endometrium. The height of the endometrium increases from approximately 1 mm at menstruation to 5 mm at ovulation. Estrogen upregulates the number of estrogen and progesterone receptors in endometrial cells.

5. In response to rising estradiol levels in the middle and late follicular phase, FSH release begins to fall.[2]

Ovulatory Phase

1. An estradiol surge triggers the midcycle LH surge, which induces ovulation approximately 10 to 16 hours later. An estradiol level ≥200 pg/mL for at least 2 days is needed to induce ovulation.[2] A small preovulatory rise in progesterone is required to induce the FSH surge.
2. A mature follicle releases an oocyte and becomes a functioning corpus luteum.

Luteal Phase

The luteal phase begins with ovulation and ends with the menstrual flow. This phase is more constant, lasting approximately 14 ± 2 days, reflecting the life of the corpus luteum.

🛜 **ADDITIONAL RESOURCES AND WEBSITES ONLINE**

1. The corpus luteum produces large amounts of progesterone, as well as increased levels of estrogen. Granulosa cells utilize low-density lipoprotein (LDL) cholesterol as a substrate for progesterone synthesis. A serum progesterone level >3 ng/mL is presumptive evidence of ovulation. Rising levels of estrogen and progesterone lead to falling levels of FSH and LH.
2. Progesterone antagonizes the action of estrogen by reducing estrogen receptor sites and increasing conversion of estradiol to estrone, a less potent estrogen. Progesterone halts the growth of the endometrium and stimulates differentiation into a secretory endometrium preparing for implantation. Increased tortuosity of the glands and spiraling of the blood vessels histologically characterize the secretory endometrium.
3. Local progesterone suppresses follicular development in the ipsilateral ovary so that ovulation in the following month may occur in the contralateral ovary.
4. The cervical mucus becomes thick during the luteal phase, owing to the influence of progesterone.
5. Unless there is fertilization with subsequent production of human chorionic gonadotropin, the corpus luteum involutes after approximately 10 to 12 days. Sloughing of the endometrium occurs secondary to the loss of estrogen and progesterone. Local prostaglandins cause vasoconstriction and uterine contractions.[2]
6. The decreased levels of estrogen and progesterone lead to increased levels of FSH and LH, providing the positive feedback loop required to initiate another menstrual cycle.

● CONCLUSION

Menarche is the onset of menses and commencement of orderly cyclic hormonal changes. Normal menstrual cycles require an orchestrated sequence of events to occur between the hypothalamus, pituitary, ovaries, and the endometrium. Abnormal menstrual cycles are not uncommon and require appropriate clinical assessment and evaluation to determine etiology.

● ACKNOWLEDGMENTS

This chapter is based on Normal Menstrual Physiology from the 5th Edition authored by Sari L. Kives and Judith A. Lacy.

REFERENCES

1. Silberstein SD, Merriam GR. Physiology of the menstrual cycle. *Cephalalgia* 2000;20:148–154.
2. Neinstein LS. Menstrual problems in adolescents. *Med Clin North Am* 1990;74:1181–1203.
3. Fritz MA, Speroff L, eds. *Clinical gynecologic endocrinology and infertility*, 8th ed. Philadelphia, PA: Wolters Kluwer Health/Lippincott Williams & Wilkins, 2011.
4. Emans SJH, Laufer MR, eds. *Emans, Laufer, Goldstein's pediatric & adolescent gynecology*, 6th ed. Philadelphia, PA: Lippincott Williams & Wilkins, 2012.
5. Frisch RE, McArthur JW. Menstrual cycles: fatness as a determinant of minimum weight for height necessary for their maintenance or onset. *Science* 1974;185:949–951.
6. Gilbert SF. *Developmental biology*, 10th ed. Sunderland: Sinauer, 2013.
7. McCartney CR, Gingrich MB, Hu Y, et al. Hypothalamic regulation of cyclic ovulation: evidence that the increase in gonadotropin-releasing hormone pulse frequency during the follicular phase reflects the gradual loss of the restraining effects of progesterone. *J Clin Endocrinol Metab* 2002;87:2194–2200.
8. Gordon CM. Functional hypothalamic amenorrhea. *N Engl J Med* 2010;363:365–371.

CHAPTER 47

Dysmenorrhea and Premenstrual Disorders

Paula K. Braverman

KEY WORDS

- Drospirenone
- Dysmenorrhea
- Endometriosis
- Leukotriene
- Nonsteroidal anti-inflammatory drug (NSAID)
- Premenstrual dysphoric disorder (PMDD)
- Premenstrual syndrome (PMS)
- Prostaglandin

Female adolescents and young adults (AYAs) commonly experience menstrual dysfunction. Both dysmenorrhea and premenstrual disorders (PMDs) (premenstrual syndrome [PMS] and premenstrual dysphoric disorder [PMDD]) affect women to some extent during their lifetime. Research into the etiology of these menstrual disorders has led to improved therapies. Experts have also been moving toward consensus opinion for the diagnosis of PMDs in order to facilitate clinical diagnosis and research into therapeutic options. This chapter reviews the epidemiology, etiology, clinical presentation, diagnosis, and treatment options currently available for these menstrual disorders.

DYSMENORRHEA

The term "primary dysmenorrhea" refers to pain associated with the menstrual flow, with no evidence of organic pelvic disease. "Secondary dysmenorrhea" refers to pain associated with menses secondary to organic disease such as endometriosis or outflow tract obstruction.[1]

Etiology

Prostaglandins

Prostaglandins are formed in the secretory endometrium. Phospholipids from cell membranes are converted into arachidonic acid, the fatty acid precursor for prostaglandin synthesis. Prostaglandin E_2 (PGE_2) and $PGF_2\alpha$, which are formed through the cyclooxygenase pathway, are the key prostaglandins involved in dysmenorrhea, although $PGF_2\alpha$ is considered the most important. $PGF_2\alpha$ induces myometrial contractions, vasoconstriction, and ischemia and mediates pain sensation, whereas PGE_2 causes vasodilation and platelet disaggregation. There are two enzymes in the cyclooxygenase system. The COX-1 enzyme has homeostatic functions, including gastrointestinal mucosal integrity, renal and platelet function, and vascular hemostasis. COX-2 is induced by inflammation.[1,2] It has been noted that:

1. Locally, prostaglandins cause uterine contractions, but they enter the systemic circulation and cause associated symptoms such as headache, nausea, vomiting, backache, diarrhea, dizziness, and fatigue.

2. Exogenous administration of PGE_2 and $PGF_2\alpha$ produce myometrial contractions and pain similar to dysmenorrhea.
3. Anovulatory cycles are associated with lower prostaglandin levels in the menstrual fluid and usually no dysmenorrhea. Because many cycles in the first 2 years after menarche are anovulatory, many adolescents do not experience dysmenorrhea from the outset. Rather, it occurs more frequently 1 to 3 years after menarche.
4. Patients with dysmenorrhea have higher levels of prostaglandins in the endometrium.
5. Most of the prostaglandins are released in the first 48 hours of menstruation, correlating with the most severe symptoms.
6. Prostaglandin inhibitors decrease dysmenorrhea.

This evidence supports the hypothesis that primary dysmenorrhea is related to prostaglandins released during menses, which seem to be increased during ovulatory cycles. It is postulated that women with dysmenorrhea may be more sensitive to prostaglandins. The upregulation of COX-2 expression and subsequent production of prostaglandin levels have also been shown to be present in secondary dysmenorrhea caused by endometriosis.[1,2]

Leukotrienes

Leukotrienes (LT) which mediate the inflammatory response are produced from arachidonic acid through the lipoxygenase pathway. LT receptors are present in uterine tissue, and a correlation has been found between LT C_4 and D_4 (two types of LT) levels and the severity of symptoms in primary dysmenorrhea.[2,3]

Other Factors

A meta-analysis showed that age (<30 years), low body mass index, smoking, earlier menarche (<12 years), longer cycles, heavy menstrual flow, nulliparity, and psychological symptoms were associated with dysmenorrhea.[4]

Epidemiology

Dysmenorrhea is a significant cause of lost work and school hours in adolescent girls and young adult women. Various studies worldwide have shown the following[3,5]:

1. About 48% to 93% of all postpubescent females have some degree of dysmenorrhea; between 5% and 42% of these females describe the pain as severe; and 14% miss two or more days of school per month.
2. Reports of school absence increase with more severe symptoms; dysmenorrhea also affects other activities, including sports, socialization, and sleep.
3. Approximately 10% to 50% of women lose work days due to dysmenorrhea, which has socioeconomic impact.

Many AYA women do not report dysmenorrhea symptoms to a clinician.

1. A survey of 12- to 21-year-olds in an urban adolescent clinic found that only 2% reported receiving information about menstruation from a health care provider.[6]
2. Many adolescents use nonpharmacologic self-treatment (rest, heat, exercise, massage, special food or drink, attempts at distraction) and insufficient doses of over-the-counter medications.[5,7,8]

Clinical Manifestations

Primary dysmenorrhea usually begins within 1 to 3 years of menarche and is associated with the establishment of ovulatory cycles. Although the pain usually begins within a few hours of starting menses, it may also start several days before the onset of menses. Local symptoms include pain that is spasmodic in nature and is strongest in the lower abdomen, with radiation to the back and anterior aspects of the thighs. In most cases, the pain resolves within 24 to 48 hours, but sometimes the symptoms may persist further into the menstrual cycle. Associated systemic symptoms can include nausea or vomiting, fatigue, mood change, dizziness, diarrhea, backache, and headache.[1]

Differential Diagnosis

Gynecologic Causes

These include endometriosis, pelvic inflammatory disease, benign uterine tumors (fibroids), intrauterine devices, anatomic abnormalities (congenital obstructive mullerian malformations, outflow obstruction), pelvic adhesions, ovarian cysts, masses or torsion, and pregnancy complications (miscarriage, ectopic pregnancy).

1. **Endometriosis** (Fig. 47.1) is characterized by the presence of endometrial glands and stroma outside of the uterus. These implants are commonly located in various locations throughout the pelvis. This condition is not as rare in adolescents as previously thought. In addition to being the most common pathologic condition in adolescents with chronic pelvic pain, it is considered a progressive disease that increases in prevalence and severity with age. Endometriosis has been diagnosed by laparoscopy in 19% to 73% of adolescents being evaluated for chronic pelvic pain and in 50% to 70% of adolescents not

responsive to oral contraceptive pills (OCPs) and nonsteroidal anti-inflammatory drugs (NSAIDs).[1,9]

The symptoms of endometriosis in adolescents include chronic pelvic pain, which may be cyclic or acyclic. Cyclic pain alone is found in only 9.4% of adolescents.[9] This is in contrast to adults who are more likely to have cyclic pain. Other associated symptoms can include dyspareunia; irregular menses; bowel symptoms such as rectal pain, nausea, constipation, diarrhea, and pain on defecation; and urinary symptoms such as dysuria, urgency, and frequency.

On examination, a tender or nodular cul-de-sac or tender uterosacral ligaments may be found. However, adolescents may not have the classic thickened nodular sacrouterine ligaments. Endometriosis should be considered in patients with dysmenorrhea who do not respond to a combination of OCP and NSAID, as well as those with associated bowel or urinary function symptoms. This diagnosis is also more common when there is a positive family history for endometriosis, and there is a high rate of concordance in monozygotic twins. The inheritance is believed to be polygenic and multifactorial.[1,2]

2. **Anatomical abnormalities** include congenital obstructive müllerian malformations, outflow obstruction. Obstructive müllerian abnormalities predispose the patient to endometriosis.

Nongynecologic Causes

These include gastrointestinal disorders (inflammatory bowel disease, irritable bowel syndrome, constipation, lactose intolerance), musculoskeletal pain, genitourinary abnormalities (cystitis, ureteral obstruction, calculi), and psychogenic disorders (history of abuse, trauma, psychogenic complaints).

Diagnosis

History

1. **Menstrual history:** Primary dysmenorrhea usually starts 1 to 3 years after menarche, most commonly begins between the ages of 14 and 15 years. Secondary dysmenorrhea should be considered if the pain starts with the onset of menarche or after the age of 20 years. AYAs should be asked about the degree of pain and the amount of impairment in school, work, and

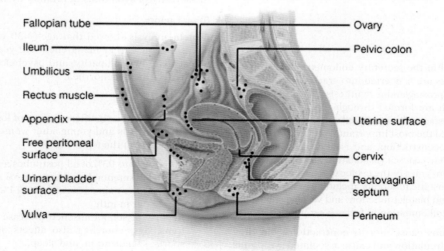

Common sites of endometriosis

Fallopian tube — Ileum — Umbilicus — Rectus muscle — Appendix — Free peritoneal surface — Urinary bladder surface — Vulva — Ovary — Pelvic colon — Uterine surface — Cervix — Rectovaginal septum — Perineum

FIGURE 47.1 Endometriosis. (From Endometriosis. In *Lippincott's Nursing Advisor 2012.* Philadelphia, PA: Lippincott Williams & Wilkins, 2012.)

other activities. Any previous use of therapeutic modalities and their effectiveness should be ascertained.

2. **Other history:** Additional questions should include prior sexually transmitted infections (STIs) and sexual activity; a review of systems related to the gastrointestinal, genitourinary, and musculoskeletal systems; and a psychosocial history to assess stress, substance abuse, and sexual abuse.

Physical Examination

Examine the pelvis for evidence of endometriosis, endometritis, fibroids, uterine or cervical abnormalities, or adnexal masses and tenderness. However, if the teen or young adult is not sexually active and the history is typical for dysmenorrhea, a pelvic examination is indicated only if the symptoms do not respond to standard medical therapy. Examination limited to a cotton swab inserted into the vagina can help rule out a hymenal abnormality or vaginal septum without performing a speculum examination. The musculoskeletal examination should focus on range of motion of the hips and spine to assess for tenderness and limitation in motion.

Laboratory Tests

A complete blood count and a determination of the erythrocyte sedimentation rate should be done if pelvic inflammatory disease or inflammatory bowel disease is suspected. Sexually active AYAs should be tested for STIs and pregnancy. A urinalysis and urine culture will help diagnose urinary tract problems. If a müllerian abnormality is suspected, ultrasonography or magnetic resonance imaging (MRI) will define the anatomy. If evaluation of the genitourinary, gastrointestinal, and musculoskeletal systems fails to reveal a cause of the pain, and if the pain is severe and intractable despite treatment with antiprostaglandins and oral contraceptives, laparoscopy should be considered.

Therapy

The two most effective treatments for primary dysmenorrhea are NSAIDs and hormonal contraceptives.

Education

The patient should be educated and reassured that the problem is physiological and can be helped. The importance of education has been demonstrated repeatedly in studies demonstrating that adolescents have a knowledge deficit about available treatment modalities and how to use them most effectively.[5,7]

Nonsteroidal Anti-inflammatory Drugs

NSAIDs are the primary modality of therapy; 80% of dysmenorrhea can be relieved with these medications. Because much of primary dysmenorrhea is secondary to prostaglandin-mediated uterine hyperactivity, prostaglandin inhibitors can alleviate menstrual cramps and associated systemic symptoms. Many NSAIDs have been found effective in alleviating menstrual cramps.[1,2] Some of these drugs and their typical doses are found in **Table 47.1**.

Over-the-counter ibuprofen and naproxen are available, but because these over-the-counter medications come in lower doses than the prescription formulations, a larger number of tablets may be needed for effectiveness. The medications should be started either as soon as possible when the symptoms of dysmenorrhea occur or to coincide with the first sign of menstruation. It is not necessary to start before the onset of menses, but if there is early vomiting with severe pain, starting a few days prior to menses may be helpful.[1] Usually, these medications are needed only for 1 to 3 days. After one of the NSAIDs is started, it should be tried for two or three menstrual cycles before being judged ineffective. At that time, a trial of a different prostaglandin inhibitor should be tried.

With the outlined doses of NSAIDs used for short periods, side effects are usually minimal. The NSAIDs in **Table 47.1** inhibit both the COX-1 and COX-2 enzymes. However, selective COX-2

TABLE 47.1

Common Medications Used to Treat Dysmenorrhea

Drug (Trade Name)	Initial Dose (mg)	Following Dose (mg)
Propionic acids		
Ibuprofen (Motrin)	400	400 q4–6h
Naproxen (Naprosyn)	500	250 q6–8h
Naproxen sodium (Anaprox)	550	275 q6–8h
Fenamates		
Mefenamic acid (Ponstel)	500	250 q6h

inhibitors will have less gastrointestinal side effects and may also be preferred in patients with coagulation disorders related to platelet function. Because of drug recalls, the only COX-2 inhibitor available at the time of this printing is celecoxib. The dosing is 400 mg as a loading dose, followed by 200 mg every 12 hours.[2] These medications are more expensive, potentially more toxic, and not necessarily superior in efficacy to less expensive, nonselective NSAIDs.

Hormonal Therapies

If the patient wishes contraception or the pain is severe and not responsive to NSAIDs, oral contraceptives can be tried. The maximal effect may not become apparent for several months.

1. Combined oral contraceptives (COCs) inhibit ovulation and lead to an atrophic decidualized endometrium, resulting in decreased menstrual flow and prostaglandin and leukotriene release.
2. OCPs are also useful to treat endometriosis because they decrease endometrial proliferation and thereby decrease total local prostaglandin and leukotriene production. A 2009 Cochrane review of randomized clinical trials concluded that OCPs provide pain relief compared to placebo for primary dysmenorrhea, with low dose pills (35 μg or less) being most effective.[10] No significant differences were found between different pill formulations with respect to progestin content, but the studies were limited. When assessing other combined hormonal contraceptive methods, the vaginal ring appears to be better than the transdermal patch for dysmenorrhea.[2,5] If cyclic hormonal contraception is ineffective, continuous combination hormonal therapy can be tried.[1,5,9] Extended cycling may be particularly helpful. Several extended cycling OCP formulations are commercially available, and continuous therapy with the vaginal ring appears to be more effective than the transdermal patch.[5]
3. Long-acting reversible contraception (LARC) methods have also been effective for both primary and secondary dysmenorrhea. Injectable depot medroxyprogesterone acetate (Depo-Provera), the levonorgestrel intrauterine system (LNG IUS), and the subdermal progestin rod have all been shown to improve symptoms of dysmenorrhea, while Depo-Provera and the LNG IUS have been shown to be effective for endometriosis.[5,8]

Other Hormonal Modalities

1. Gonadotropin-releasing hormone (GnRH) agonists with utilization of add-back therapy to prevent side effects related to hypoestrogenic state (including bone loss) have been tried in severe cases of endometriosis unresponsive to other modalities. Caution should be used in patients younger than 16 years because of concerns about compromised bone density accrual.[9]

Other Nonhormonal Modalities

Nonhormonal modalities with possible benefit include vitamin B_1 and magnesium supplements.[11] Other dietary regimens or supplements could not be recommended based on the 2009 Cochrane review. Transcutaneous nerve stimulation[12] and acupuncture[13] require further study.

PREMENSTRUAL DISORDERS

The term "premenstrual disorders" is used to describe an array of predictable physical, cognitive, affective, and behavioral symptoms that occur cyclically during the luteal phase of the menstrual cycle and resolve with menstruation followed by a symptom-free interval until the next time of ovulation.[14] Evidence has accumulated that PMD is not a single condition, but a set of interrelated symptom complexes and pathophysiologic events that begin with ovulation.[15] Universal classification of PMD has been lacking, and terminology in the literature includes *PMS* and *PMDD*.[14] Symptoms of PMS and PMDD overlap, although PMDD focuses more on problems with mood and symptoms that are more severe.[16] Some published opinions[15] have suggested that there is a broad spectrum of impairment and that rather than differentiating PMS from PMDD, the latter should be categorized as severe PMS. Most recently, a consensus group of international experts was established (the International Society for Premenstrual Disorders [ISPMDs])[14] and published criteria defining *Core PMD* which encompasses both PMS and PMDD. Although there is a growing literature on PMD in adolescents, most of the research has focused on adult women (with women in their 20s commonly included in discussions of women in older age-groups). Reference is made in the text when specific information is being discussed about the adolescent or young adult age-group.

Epidemiology

The perceived impact of premenstrual symptoms on activities of daily living (ADL) does not vary significantly across countries or cultures, and the mental and physical symptoms have equal impact.[17] The exact prevalence of PMD is unknown, in part because of differences in definitions and classification, but estimates among AYAs and adult women are similar.[18,19] The age range for peak intensity of PMD symptoms is the 20s to 30s.[17,19] While mild premenstrual symptoms are common among AYAs and adult women, severe symptoms affecting ADL occur less frequently.

1. About 80% to 95% of menstruating AYAs and adult women have some degree of symptoms before menses, which in many cases are mild physiologic symptoms not significantly affecting ADL.[14,17,19]
2. About 20% to 40% have moderate to severe symptoms affecting ADL, which meet criteria for PMS[14,18]
3. About 3% to 8% are most severely affected and meet criteria for PMDD.[14,18]

Risk Factors

Risk factors for PMD include genetic factors.[20,21] There are no significant differences in personality profile or level of stress in women with PMS compared with asymptomatic women. However, women with PMS may not handle stress as well or have an impaired stress response.[20,21] Studies have also shown an association with traumatic events such as a physical and emotional trauma, and abuse.[18,20,21] Comorbidities are found with psychiatric disorders, including depression, anxiety, and seasonal affective disorders.[19–21]

Pathophysiology

The exact mechanism of PMD is unknown. Current hypotheses revolve around gonadal sex steroids and central neurotransmitters, as well as brain function.[18,20–23]

1. Alterations in neurotransmitters: γ-aminobutyric acid (GABA) and serotonin have been implicated
   a. GABA is the key inhibitory neurotransmitter regulating anxiety and stress. Metabolites of progesterone (e.g.,

allopregnanolone) positively modulate GABA. Studies show women with PMD have reduced GABA functional receptor sensitivity and, in some studies, lower concentrations of allopregnanolone during the luteal phase.
   b. Symptoms of reduced serotonin transmission and PMD overlap. Serotonergic function is altered in the luteal phase of women with PMD. Ovarian sex steroids impact serotonergic activity, with progesterone decreasing serotonin availability.
2. Brain function: Neuroimaging studies with positronic emission tomography and functional MRI have demonstrated differences in brain activity and neurotransmitter concentration in women with PMD as compared to controls.
3. Hormonal factors: Women with PMD are felt to be more sensitive to normal cyclical hormonal fluctuations. There are no differences from controls in the absolute levels of estrogen, progesterone, testosterone, and adrenal, pituitary, and thyroid hormones; however, the timing of hormone secretion may be abnormal.

Clinical Manifestations

More than 150 symptoms have been described in literature, ranging from mild symptoms to those severe enough to interfere with normal activities. Data analysis from community-based studies of women from 14 countries found that physical symptoms are most commonly reported. Various emotional and physical symptoms include the following[17]:

a. Emotional symptoms: depressed mood, anger, irritability, mood swings, restlessness, tension, confusion, social withdrawal, sleep disturbances, poor concentration, lack of energy
b. Physical symptoms: lack of energy, breast tenderness, abdominal bloating, swelling of extremities, weight gain, changes in appetite/food cravings, headaches, joint-muscle-back pain, cramps, and abdominal pain

Diagnosis

The diagnosis relies on the history of cyclic symptoms. No specific physical findings or laboratory tests have proved useful. Although universally accepted, specific diagnostic criteria have not been historically established among the various sources defining PMD, including the World Health Organization's International Classification of Diseases, American College of Obstetricians and Gynecologists, the National Institute of Mental Health, and the *Diagnostic and Statistical Manual of Mental Disorders*, 5th edition, (DSM-5). Three important findings are usually needed to make a diagnosis of PMD:

1. Symptoms must occur in the luteal phase and resolve within a few days of onset of menstruation. Symptoms should not be present in the follicular phase.
2. The symptoms must be prospectively documented over several menstrual cycles and not caused by other physical or psychological problems.
3. Symptoms must be recurrent and severe enough to disrupt normal activities.

The ISPMD criteria published in 2011 divided PMD into *Core PMD* and *Variant PMD*. *Core PMD* fulfills the three findings outlined above.[14] Symptoms must be prospectively found in at least two menstrual cycles and cause significant distress or impairment in daily functioning such as work, school, and interpersonal relationships. Unlike the DSM (which requires five of eleven specific somatic or affective symptoms with a minimum of one affective symptom) or American College of Obstetricians and Gynecologists criteria (which requires one of ten specific somatic or affective symptoms), there is no delineation of specific symptoms (somatic or psychological) or criteria for the number of symptoms needed to make the diagnosis. *Variant PMD* includes (1) premenstrual exacerbation of underlying psychological or somatic disorders; (2) symptoms occurring with nonovlutaory ovarian activity; (3) progesterone-induced symptoms (use of exogenous progestogens); and (4) PMDs without menstruation (hysterectomy with preservation of ovaries).

While various validated assessment tools have been developed, the prospectively administered Daily Record of Severity of Problems is among the most commonly used. In general, retrospective assessments are not considered diagnostic, but the Premenstrual Symptoms Screening Tool (PSST) has been shown to be useful for initial screening during clinical consultation. This self-rated retrospective questionnaire has been revised for use in adolescents.[24] If a validated tool is not used, a calendar can be helpful in the diagnosis and in monitoring AYAs after the start of any therapy. Prospective recording should be done for at least 2 to 3 months to document that symptoms are occurring cyclically in the luteal phase. One author recommends daily rating of the five worst symptoms on a four point scale from 0 (none) to 3 (severe) along with menstrual bleeding.[19]

The *DSM-5*[16] lists specific criteria for PMDD as a new diagnostic category rather than in the appendix. It is important to remember that the symptoms cannot represent exacerbation of an existing medical condition or psychiatric disorder although those disorders may co-occur with PMDD. Symptoms of certain medical disorders (e.g., seizures, migraine headaches, irritable bowel syndrome, asthma, allergies) may also exacerbate during menstruation.

Therapy

No single treatment is universally accepted as effective. Studies have yielded conflicting results with many therapies, and most trials have not been well controlled. Treatments have included the following: lifestyle changes, education, stress management, aerobic exercise, vitamin and mineral supplementation, herbal preparations, dietary manipulation, suppression of ovulation, selective serotonin reuptake inhibitors (SSRIs), and medications to suppress physical and psychological symptoms.[18,19,22,23,25,26]

Nonpharmacologic Treatment

To date, the strongest evidence for nonpharmacologic treatment of PMD exists for calcium, chasteberry, and cognitive-behavioral therapy (CBT).

1. Calcium (1,200 mg/day in divided doses) has been reported to reduce physical and emotional symptoms of PMS. Calcium homeostasis fluctuates during the menstrual cycle, and hypocalcemia has been associated with affective changes.[18] High intake of calcium and vitamin D has been associated with a reduced risk of developing PMS.[19,22,23]
2. *Vitex agnus-castus* (chasteberry) has been found to be superior to placebo in reducing somatic and psychological PMD symptoms with few side effects.[18,19,22,25,26]
3. CBT works by improving coping strategies and modifying maladaptive thinking. Utilizing CBT appears to result in longer long-term efficacy for PMD symptoms than fluoxetine alone.[19,22]

Other Nonpharmacologic Therapies

1. Lifestyle changes: Although lifestyle changes have not been definitively proven in controlled studies, exercise and stress management practices can improve overall feelings of well-being and aerobic exercise may reduce mood symptoms and bloating.[19,22] Education regarding menstrual physiology and the relationship of changing hormones to symptoms can help with understanding of symptoms and may improve self-management.[19]
2. Vitamin and mineral supplementation, herbal preparations, and dietary manipulation: There have been some positive outcomes for complementary and alternative therapies. However, although some show promise, more research needs to be carried out to recommend definitively any of these therapies.

   a. *Ginkgo biloba* (ginkgo leaf extract) and *Crocus sativus* (saffron) were cited as deserving additional evaluation by the ISPMD.[22]
   b. Mood and carbohydrate food craving improved in randomized trials evaluating the intake of simple and complex carbohydrates. Carbohydrates may increase tryptophan, which is a precursor to serotonin.[18,22]
   c. Vitamin E, magnesium, and vitamin B_6 have mixed or equivocal results.[18,22,26]
   d. Other dietary recommendations: Recommendations have been made based on observations that included eliminating high-sodium foods and caffeine, as well as eliminating refined and processed carbohydrates. However, these have not been adequately studied to date to assess efficacy for PMS.[22]
   e. Other complementary therapies including acupuncture, Qi therapy, reflexology, massage, krill oil, lavender oil, Chinese herbs, transmagnetic stimulation, sleep deprivation, and light therapy need more investigation.[18,22]
   f. Evening primrose oil and St. John's wort are not more effective than placebo.[25]

Suppression of Ovulation

Because PMD appears to be a cyclic disorder of menses occurring in the luteal phase, suppression of ovulation has been used as a therapy.

1. COCs: Although combined OCP prevents ovulation, data on their effectiveness are mixed and they primarily impact somatic symptoms. Mood symptoms in some individuals with PMD may actually worsen with use of OCP.[22,23] One pill with a new progestogen (drospirenone) is approved by the US Food and Drug Administration (FDA) for the severe symptoms of PMDD. Drospirenone has spironolactone antimineralocorticoid and antiandrogenic properties. The 24/4 formulation OCP containing drospirenone and 20 µg of ethinyl estradiol demonstrated improvement in both mood and physical symptom scores in subjects with PMDD. Possible reasons for efficacy of this new formulation include the lower estrogen dose, as well as improved follicular suppression. The maintenance of a more stable hormonal environment due to the longer number of days on hormone may also be helpful (e.g., 24 rather than 21 days).[27] A Cochrane review of five trials concluded that although this OCP formulation may be helpful for severe symptoms of PMDD, more studies are needed to see whether it is effective for longer than three cycles, in women with less severe symptoms, and whether it is superior to other OCPs.[28]
2. Continuous hormonal therapy with COC can also be considered to suppress cyclic changes and endogenous sex hormone variability; however, some studies have shown mixed results.[29]
3. High-dose estrogen patch: Suppression of ovulation with high-dose estrogens (patch) is effective, but must be accompanied by administration of progesterone to prevent endometrial hyperplasia. Since adding progesterone may make PMD symptoms worse, some clinicians have used the levonorgestrel-releasing IUS to deliver progesterone to the endometrium and minimize systemic absorption. Use of this IUS has not been specifically studied for this purpose.[18,22,23]
4. GnRH: Most studies have shown benefit from the use of GnRH, but the hypoestrogenic effects with loss of bone density are concerning, especially for adolescents, and therefore limit its use. GnRH with add-back therapy with estrogen and progesterone can be considered when other modalities have failed. However, add-back regimens may cause a recurrence in PMD symptoms, and there are no long-term studies in adolescents.[19,23]
5. Danazol: An androgen analog and gonadotropin inhibitor can reduce premenstrual symptoms, but is rarely used because of masculinization and other side effects.[18,22]

6. Bilateral salpingo-oophorectomy would not be considered in adolescents. If done for severe and debilitating symptoms in an adult woman, estrogen replacement would be needed until natural menopause would have occurred.[22,23]

Medications to Suppress Symptoms

1. *Prostaglandin inhibitors:* NSAIDs have been used to treat PMS, particularly for the physical symptoms. They can be started during the luteal phase after ovulation.[1]
2. *Spironolactone*, an aldosterone receptor agonist, may be helpful in patients with breast tenderness and bloating. Doses of 100 mg/day on day 12 of the menstrual cycle until the onset of menses have been used.[19,22]

Psychotropic Medications (SSRIs)

SSRIs are the drugs of choice and first-line therapy for severe PMS/PMDD in adult women, including young adult women. Efficacy of SSRIs has been shown in randomized placebo-controlled trials and affirmed in a Cochrane review.[30] Fluoxetine, sertraline, and paroxetine are FDA approved for PMDD, and also escitalopram and the serotonin-norepinephrine reuptake inhibitor venlafaxine have also been shown to be effective.[18] Placebo-controlled studies in adult women have shown that they are effective for 50% to 90% of patients and can improve both physical symptoms and mood.[18,22] Unlike in adults, fluoxetine is not considered first-line therapy for adolescents with PMDD, and there is a paucity of studies in this age-group.[19]

1. SSRIs used intermittently only during the luteal phase (i.e., 14 days before onset of menses) rather than continuously are equally effective for symptom reduction.[18,30] Some more recent studies have also have demonstrated some success with symptom-onset dosing by taking the SSRI a few days before or with the onset of symptoms and stopping with the onset or a few days after menses start.[18]
2. Unlike treatment for depression, symptoms improve within 24 to 48 hours of initiating therapy, and there are no reports of discontinuation symptoms when SSRIs are used intermittently for PMDD.
3. Low doses are usually effective (**Table 47.2**), although higher doses may be more effective with intermittent dosing.[18]
4. The most common adverse effects include insomnia, gastrointestinal disturbances, and fatigue. Other side effects include dizziness, sweating, and sexual function disturbances, but these medications are usually well tolerated.

Anxiolytics and Other Antidepressants

These medications are second-line therapies that may be useful if there is anxiety and irritability as primary PMD symptoms. Suggested therapies have included benzodiazepines (especially alprazolam), clomipramine, and buspirone. In general, other antidepressants are less effective than SSRIs. These medications can be given in the luteal phase rather than continuously.[22]

TABLE 47.2
Doses of FDA Approved SSRIs for Premenstrual Dysphoric Disorder

Name of Drug	Dose	Schedule
Fluoxetine	10–20 mg/d	Intermittent
Sertraline	50–150 mg/d	Intermittent
Paroxetine	10–30 mg/d	Intermittent

Adapted from Rapkin AJ, Lewis EI. Treatment of premenstrual dysphoric disorder. *Women's Health* 2013;9:537–556.

1. Buspirone is a partial serotonin receptor agonist.
2. Clomipramine, a tricyclic antidepressant, is a nonselective inhibitor of serotonin reuptake.
3. Alprazolam affects the GABA receptor complex.

None of these medications would be recommended for routine use in adolescents, but only for use in selected adolescents with severe symptoms unresponsive to other treatment modalities.

⬤ SUMMARY

Choice of treatment modalities may vary by the age of the patient and severity of symptoms. The ISPMD consensus statement does not propose a specific treatment algorithm, but suggests that the treatment modality be based on the patient's choice. Rapkin proposes the following when considering treatment for PMD in AYAs[18,19]:

1. If there are mild/moderate symptoms, supportive therapy with good nutrition, complex carbohydrates, aerobic exercise, calcium supplements, and possibly chasteberry fruit may be helpful.
2. If physical symptoms predominate, a drospirenone containing OCP could be considered first line for hormonal suppression, while high-dose transdermal estrogen along with a progestin can be considered as a first- or second-line choice.
3. When mood symptoms predominate, SSRI therapy is first line in young adult women. An anxiolytic can be used for specific symptoms not relieved by the SSRI medication. In adolescents although not necessarily first choice, SSRIs can be used with careful monitoring.
4. GnRH agonists are considered third-line therapy after other steps have failed.
5. Hysterectomy and bilateral oophorectomy would be a choice of last resort and not considered in adolescents.

REFERENCES

1. Emans SJ, Laufer MR. *Pediatric & adolescent gynecology.* 6th ed. Philadelphia, PA: Wolters Kluwer/ Lippincott Williams & Wilkins, 2012.
2. Harel Z. Dysmenorrhea in adolescents and young adults: from pathophysiology to pharmacological treatments and management strategies. *Expert Opin Pharmacother* 2008;9:2661–2672.
3. Zahradnik H-P, Hanjalic-Beck A, Groth K. Nonsteroidal anti-inflammatory drugs and hormonal contraceptives for pain relief from dysmenorrhea: a review. *Contraception* 2010;81:185–196.
4. Latthe P, Mignini L, Grav R, et al. Factors predisposing women to chronic pelvic pain: systematic review. *BMJ* 2006;332(7544):749. doi:10.1136/bmj.38748.697465.55.
5. Allen LM, Lam AC. Premenstrual syndrome and dysmenorrhea in adolescents. *Adol Med State of the Art Rev* 2013;23:139–163.
6. Houston AM, Abraham A, Huang Z, et al. Knowledge, attitudes, and consequences of menstrual health in urban adolescent females. *J Pediatr Adolesc Gynecol* 2006;19:271–275.
7. O'Connell K, Davis AR, Westhoff C. Self treatment among adolescent girls with dysmenorrhea. *J Pediatr Adolesc Gynecol* 2006;19:285–289.
8. Sanfilippo J, Erb T. Evaluation and management of dysmenorrhea in adolescents. *Clin Obstet Gynecol* 2008;51:257–267.
9. American College of Obstetrics and Gynecology. ACOG Committee on adolescent health care. Committee opinion No 310. Endometriosis in adolescents. *Obstet Gynecol* 2005;105:921.
10. Wong CL, Farquhar C, Roberts H, et al. Oral contraceptive pill for primary dysmenorrhoea. *Cochrane Database Syst Rev* 2009;(4):CD002120. doi:10.1002/14651858.CD002120.pub3.
11. Proctor M, Murphy PA. Herbal and dietary therapies for primary and secondary dysmenorrhoea. *Cochrane Database Syst Rev* 2001;(2):CD002124. doi:10.1002/14651858.CD002124. (republished with same conclusion 2009)
12. Proctor M, Farquhar C, Stones W, et al. Transcutaneous electrical nerve stimulation for primary dysmenorrhoea. *Cochrane Database Syst Rev* 2002;(1):CD002123. doi:10.1002/14651858.CD002123. (republished with same conclusions 2010)
13. Smith CA, Zhu X, He L, et al. Acupuncture for dysmenorrhoea. *Cochrane Database Syst Rev* 2011;(1):CD007854. doi:10.1002/14651858.CD007854.pub2. (republished with same conclusion 2012)
14. O'Brien PMS, Backstrom T, Brown C, et al. Towards a consensus on diagnostic criteria, measurement and trial design of the premenstrual disorders; the ISPMD Montreal consensus. *Arch Womens Ment Health* 2011;14:13–21.
15. Johnson SR. Premenstrual syndrome, premenstrual dysphoric disorder, and beyond: a clinical primer for practitioners. *Obstet Gynecol* 2004;104:845.
16. American Psychiatric Association. *Diagnostic and Statistical Manual of mental disorders, DSM-5.* 5th ed. Washington, DC: American Psychiatric Publishing, 2013.
17. Dennerstein L, Lehert P, Heinemann K. Epidemiology of premenstrual symptoms and disorders. *Menopause Int* 2012;18:48–51.
18. Rapkin AJ, Lewis EI. Treatment of premenstrual dysphoric disorder. *Women's Health* 2013;9:537–556.

19. Rapkin AJ, Mikacich JA. Premenstrual dysphoric disorder and severe premenstrual syndrome in adolescents. *Pediatr Drugs* 2013;15:191–202.
20. Cunningham J, Yonkers KA, O'Brien S, et al. Update on research and treatment of premenstrual dysphoric disorder. *Har Rev Psychiatry* 2009;17: 120–137.
21. Epperson CN, Steiner M, Harlage SA, et al. Premenstrual dysphoric disorder: evidence for a new category for DSM-5. *Am J Psychiatry* 2012:169:465–475.
22. Nevatte T, O'Brien PMS, Backstrom T, et al. ISPMD consensus on the management of premenstrual disorders. *Arch Womens Ment Health* 2013;16: 279–291.
23. Rapkin AJ, Akopians AL. Pathophysiology of premenstrual syndrome and premenstrual dysphoric disorder. *Menopause Int* 2012;18:52–59.
24. Steiner M, Peer M, Palova E, et al. The premenstrual symptoms screening tool revised for adolescents (PSST-A): prevalence of severe PMS and premenstrual dysphoric disorder in adolescents. *Arch Womens Ment Health* 2011;14:77–81.
25. Dante G, Facchinetti F. Herbal treatments for alleviating premenstrual symptoms: a systematic review. *J Psychosomatic Obstet Gynecol* 2011;32: 42–51.
26. Whelan AM, Jurgens TM, Naylor H. Herbs, vitamins and minerals in the treatment of premenstrual syndrome: a systematic review. *Can J Clin Pharmaol* 2009;16: e407–e429.
27. Yonkers KA, Brown C, Pearlstein TB, et al. Efficacy of a new low-dose oral contraceptive with drospirenone in premenstrual dysphoric disorder. *Obstet Gynecol* 2005;106:492.
28. Lopez LM, Kaptein AA, Helmerhorst FM. Oral contraceptives containing drospirenone for premenstrual syndromes. *Cochrane Database Syst Rev* 2012;(2):CD006586. doi:10.1002/14651858.CD006586.pub4.
29. Freeman EW, Halbreich U, Grubb GS, et al. An overview of four studies of a continuous oral contraceptive (levonorgestrel 90 mcg/ ethinyl estradiol 20 mcg) on premenstrual dysphoric disorder and premenstrual syndrome. *Contraception* 2012;85:437–445.
30. Marijoribanks J, Brown J, O'Brien PMS, et al. Selective serotonin reuptake inhibitors for premenstrual syndrome. *Cochrane Database Syst Rev* 2013;(6):CD001396. doi: 10.1002/14651858.CD001396.pub3.

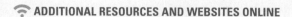 **ADDITIONAL RESOURCES AND WEBSITES ONLINE**

XII

48

Abnormal Uterine Bleeding

Laurie A.P. Mitan
Beth I. Schwartz

Abnormal uterine bleeding (AUB) is a common menstrual problem during adolescence. When severe, it can result in life-threatening anemia. Even when mild, it is usually both a concern and a nuisance for the adolescent or young adult. In 2011, the International Federation of Gynecology and Obstetrics recommended discontinuation of the popular term dysfunctional uterine bleeding and the use of a new classification system for causes of AUB in nonpregnant women known by the acronym PALM-COEIN (polyp, adenomyosis, leiomyoma, malignancy and hyperplasia, coagulopathy, ovulatory dysfunction, endometrial, iatrogenic, and not yet classified)[1,2] (**Table 48.1**). The etiology of AUB is quite different in the adolescent and young adult (AYA) compared to that of the older adult. Uterine fibroids and malignancy are the leading diagnoses in the older adult, but are rare in women under age 39. This chapter will focus mainly on AUB that falls into the COEIN subtypes, with ovulatory dysfunction being the leading cause in AYAs.

DEFINITIONS

1. Normal menstrual cycles occur every 21 to 40 days, with 2 to 8 days of bleeding and 20 to 80 mL of blood loss per cycle.

TABLE 48.1

AUB Classification System for Nonpregnant Women of Reproductive Age, Known by the Acronym PALM-COEIN

PALM: Structural Etiologies	COEIN: Nonstructural Etiologies
Polyp (AUB-**P**)	Coagulopathy (AUB-**C**)
Adenomyosis (AUB-**A**)	Ovulatory (AUB-**O**)
Leiomyoma (AUB-**L**)	Endometrial (AUB-**E**)
Malignancy and hyperplasia (AUB-**M**)	Iatrogenic (AUB-**I**)
	Not yet classified (AUB-**N**)

Modified from Munro MG, Critchley HOD, Broder MS, et al. FIGO classification system (PALM-COEIN) for causes of abnormal uterine bleeding in nongravid women of reproductive age. *Int J Gynecol Obstet* 2011;113:3–13.

2. Up to 80% of menstrual cycles are anovulatory in the first year after menarche. Cycles become ovulatory on average by 20 months after menarche.
3. Menorrhagia, prolonged or heavy uterine bleeding that occurs at regular intervals, is now known as AUB/heavy menstrual bleeding.[1]
4. Metrorrhagia, uterine bleeding that occurs at irregular intervals, is now referred to as AUB/intermenstrual bleeding.[1]
5. Oligomenorrhea is uterine bleeding that occurs at prolonged intervals of 41 days to 3 months, but is of normal flow, duration, and quantity, and is discussed in Chapter 49.

EVALUATION

The evaluation of any patient with bleeding begins with an assessment of hemodynamic stability. The next objective is to determine the site of bleeding (e.g., gastrointestinal, urinary, vaginal, cervical, or uterine). Once the site of bleeding is found to be uterine, the evaluation focuses on determination of its cause.

History

The history should be obtained from the adolescent or young adult and, if possible, the parent or guardian. The sexual history should be obtained from the patient alone.

1. Menstrual history: Age at menarche, cycle regularity, cycle duration, flow by number of pads or tampons over a 24-hour period, need to double up products or change products overnight, "gushing" or "flooding" sensation, frequency of bleeding through products, interference with daily activities including absences from school or work, dysmenorrhea, symptoms of anemia.[3]
2. Sexual history: Age at coitarche, use of condoms, contraception, pregnancies, deliveries, miscarriages, abortions, past sexually transmitted infections (STIs)/pelvic inflammatory disease, number of partners, new partner, vaginal discharge, known exposure to an STI. A history of sexual abuse, genital trauma, or foreign body is also essential to ascertain.
3. History of systemic illness, anemia, iron deficiency, frequent nose bleeds, easy bleeding or bruising, excessive bleeding after surgery or dental procedures, history of blood transfusions, recent changes in weight, eating, exercise, stress, or medications
4. Endocrine history: Symptoms suggestive of hypothyroidism (e.g., fatigue, weight gain), hyperthyroidism (e.g., palpitations, weight loss), or hyperandrogenism (e.g., hirsutism, severe acne), and exogenous hormone use
5. Family history: AUB, bleeding diathesis, infertility, diabetes mellitus
6. Medications: Recent use of hormone contraception, antipsychotics, or anticonvulsants

Physical Examination

Vital signs should include date of last menstrual period, height, weight, body mass index, and blood pressure and heart rate in supine, sitting, and standing positions to detect orthostatic changes. Thorough physical exam should note sexual maturity rating of breasts and pubic hair, as well as presence or absence of galactorrhea. Pelvic examination should be considered in sexually active patients to screen for STIs. However, it is unnecessary in virginal teens whose clinical presentation is otherwise consistent with anovulatory bleeding.

Laboratory Tests

Laboratory testing may not be necessary in the adolescent with mild anovulatory bleeding associated with physiological immaturity. Depending on the history and physical examination, other patients may require some of the following laboratory evaluation[1]:

1. Pregnancy test: A urine pregnancy test should be done in all patients if there is any question of sexual activity. If the urine test result is positive, a quantitative serum pregnancy test should be performed. In cases of possible ectopic pregnancy (see Chapter 53), gynecology referral is recommended.
2. Complete blood cell count and ferritin to assess for anemia, thrombocytopenia, and iron deficiency if there is a history of heavy or frequent bleeding.[4]
3. STI screening: Screening for gonorrhea, chlamydia, and trichomonas infections is indicated for all AYAs who have ever been sexually active (see Chapters 56 and 57).
4. Thyroid function tests for all patients with moderate to severe menorrhagia
5. For those who screen positive for a possible bleeding disorder by history, a coagulation screen, including prothrombin time, partial thromboplastin time, and a von Willebrand (vW) profile (vW factor antigen, vW factor/ristocetin cofactor activity, factor VIII activity), should be conducted.[5] There is no evidence for obtaining a PFA-100.[6] Hematology consultation is recommended for any abnormal laboratory results.
6. Follicle-stimulating hormone, luteinizing hormone, testosterone (total and free), dehydroepiandrosterone-sulfate, and 17-hydroxyprogesterone if there are clinical signs of hyperandrogenism (see Chapter 49).
7. Pelvic ultrasonography may be helpful in situations in which structural pathology is suspected or to measure endometrial stripe thickness to help guide therapy.
8. Endometrial biopsy is not indicated in adolescents. It may be considered in adults aged 19 to 39 who fail medical management, especially in patients with conditions that cause endometrial hyperplasia, such as polycystic ovary syndrome (PCOS) (see Chapter 49).[1]

THERAPY

The severity and cause of the bleeding will guide the management. Severe bleeding with hemodynamic instability, regardless of cause, requires immediate intervention with intravenous fluids and/or blood transfusion. AYAs without underlying cardiovascular disease usually respond quickly to intravenous fluids and supplemental iron therapy, without the need for transfusion. Severe anemia that developed over months of abnormal bleeding is better tolerated than the same level of anemia that developed over hours or days of acute bleeding. Bleeding secondary to pregnancy or infection requires prompt treatment of the underlying condition. Bleeding secondary to a systemic problem, such as a clotting abnormality or thyroid dysfunction, may require short-term hormonal therapy identical to that for anovulatory bleeding until the systemic problem is brought under control.

Ovulatory Dysfunction (AUB-O)

Immaturity of the hypothalamic–pituitary–ovarian (HPO) axis is the leading cause of AUB during adolescence. After menarche, anovulation is associated with 50% to 80% of bleeding episodes during the first 2 years, with decreasing rates over time.[7] Excess estrogen can stimulate the endometrium to proliferate in an undifferentiated manner and to shed at irregular intervals in the absence of adequate progesterone to provide endometrial stabilization. However, despite these high rates of anovulation with HPO axis immaturity, the negative feedback of estrogen on the HPO axis protects most adolescents from AUB. Even when ovulation does not occur, estrogen production usually declines before the endometrium becomes excessively thickened, and withdrawal bleeding occurs. Most anovulatory cycles, therefore, tend to be fairly regular, and the bleeding limited in duration and quantity. Frequently PCOS (see Chapter 49), and less commonly late-onset congenital adrenal hyperplasia (see Chapter 49), also present in this age-group with AUB.

The treatment approach to anovulatory menstrual bleeding depends on the hemoglobin value, hemodynamic stability, the patient's emotional tolerance, and potential need for contraception if the teen or young adult is sexually active. Studies comparing progestin regimens, with or without estrogen for bleeding control, have failed to produce clear evidence for one specific regimen. Decades of clinical experience suggest the following:

1. Light to moderate flow, hemoglobin level of at least 12 g/dL: Reassurance, multivitamin with iron, menstrual calendar, reevaluation within 3 months
2. Ongoing moderate flow, hemoglobin level of 10 to 12 g/dL: Begin a 35-µg combined oral contraceptive pill to be taken every 6 to 12 hours for 24 to 48 hours until the bleeding stops, along with an antiemetic if necessary for nausea. Oral iron therapy should be initiated as early as possible but may not be tolerated during the first 2 days of high-dose hormonal therapy. Nonsteroidal anti-inflammatory drugs (NSAIDs) can be used as adjunctive therapy, along with the oral contraceptive to decrease both bleeding and, when present, dysmenorrhea. Taper the oral contraceptive to one pill daily by day 5. Begin a new 28-day pill packet and inform the patient that a withdrawal bleed is likely during the week of placebo pills. Continue the combined oral contraceptive for 3 to 6 months. This regimen should not be used in patients with an absolute contraindication to estrogen therapy.[8] Alternatively, progestin-only oral medications have been used with success to manage active bleeding: norethindrone acetate 5 mg, once to three times daily or medroxyprogesterone 10 mg, once to three times daily for several weeks or months.[9]
3. Heavy flow, hemoglobin level <10 g/dL: If the patient is hemodynamically stable, reliable, and able to tolerate an oral contraceptive, management is as stated earlier. Otherwise, hospitalization is indicated until the bleeding stops. A 50-µg combined oral contraceptive every 6 hours may be necessary to control the bleeding in some patients. If the bleeding does not slow within two doses of the 50-µg pill, add conjugated estrogen intravenously (25 mg every 6 hours for a maximum of six doses). Then taper the oral contraceptive to one pill daily by day 7. High-dose progestins or tranexamic acid are alternative therapies.[9–12] The levonorgestrel intrauterine device is also effective. Endometrial curettage is rarely necessary.[2]

Abnormal Uterine Bleeding Secondary to Hormonal Contraception (AUB-I)

Exogenous estrogen and/or progestins, whether intended for contraception or replacement therapy, may cause anovulation and irregular bleeding. If a uterus is present, unopposed estrogen is associated with an increased risk for endometrial carcinoma. In most postpubertal patients, the regimen therefore should include both estrogen and a progestin administered cyclically or in a fixed daily dose. Among patients using hormonal contraception, irregular bleeding is more common with progestin-only than combined estrogen–progestin methods due to increased endometrial atrophy.

1. Persistent bleeding on a 20-μg combined oral contraceptive pill may stop when a higher-dose estrogen (e.g., 30 to 35 μg) pill is prescribed.
2. Persistent bleeding on a 30- to 35-μg pill may require a full withdrawal bleed and change to a different progestin. A 50-μg pill is rarely needed.
3. Persistent bleeding on progestin-only contraceptives can be managed with short-term addition of conjugated estrogen (1.25 to 2.50 mg daily for 5 to 7 days), if not contraindicated, and/or NSAIDs. Although this will stop the bleeding acutely, the likelihood of subsequent spotting is increased because of estrogen-induced endometrial proliferation.
4. Persistent breakthrough bleeding on a long-acting contraceptive method (e.g., hormonal implanted rod or intrauterine device) may be due to irregular endometrial proliferation. Although much of this bleeding is expected to improve over time, patients may benefit from a short course of a high-dose progestin (i.e., norethindrone acetate 5 mg for 30 days) to induce accelerated endometrial thinning.

Bleeding Diatheses (AUB-C)

Evaluation for common bleeding diatheses, such as von Willebrand disease and idiopathic thrombocytopenia, should be considered as above. AUB is also common in patients receiving chemotherapy or other interventions that alter bone marrow production, platelet function, or clotting factor synthesis. The management of bleeding in these patients attempts to decrease menstrual frequency or induce endometrial atrophy. Options are[5]:

1. Combined oral contraceptive pills, used in cyclic or extended-cycle fashion. This option should be used with caution in patients undergoing chemotherapy due to the theoretical increased risk of venous thromboembolic events due to malignancy in conjunction with estrogen use.
2. Progestin-only pills, either in typical contraceptive doses (i.e., norethindrone 35 μg daily) or in higher doses (i.e., norethindrone acetate 5 mg or medroxyprogesterone 10 mg), to achieve amenorrhea
3. Depot medroxyprogesterone 150 mg intramuscularly every 11 to 12 weeks can be used to achieve amenorrhea in many adolescents and young women. Due to its high frequency of irregular bleeding initially, this may not be the best option for those who need more acute or reliable menstrual regulation or suppression.
4. The levonorgestrel intrauterine device can be used to achieve decreased overall bleeding with improved amenorrhea rates over time.[13] Although it has not been FDA approved for use in women under age 18 years, it has been successfully used off-label in this population. In patients who are not sexually active, placement in the operating room may be required.
5. Gonadotropin-releasing hormone agonists (e.g., leuprolide acetate) can be used to achieve longer-term amenorrhea in selected patients. Owing to its hypoestrogenemic side effects, including association with a low bone mineral density, this option should be used for more than 6 months only in certain patient populations, such as those undergoing chemotherapy.[14] Add-back therapy is usually indicated for use over 6 months.[15]

REFERENCES

1. The American College of Obstetricians and Gynecologists; Committee on Practice Bulletins—Gynecology. Practice bulletin no. 128: diagnosis of abnormal uterine bleeding in reproductive-aged women. *Obstet Gynecol* 2012;120(1):197–206.
2. The American College of Obstetricians and Gynecologists; Committee on Practice Bulletins—Gynecology. Practice bulletin no. 136: management of abnormal uterine bleeding associated with ovulatory dysfunction. *Obstet Gynecol* 2013;122(1):176–185.
3. Philipp CS, Faiz A, Dowling NF, et al. Development of a screening tool for identifying women with menorrhagia for hemostatic evaluation. *Am J Obstet Gynecol* 2008;198:163.e1–e8.
4. Hurskainen R, Grenman S, Komi I, et al. Diagnosis and treatment of menorrhagia. *Acta Obstet Gynecol Scand* 2007;86(6):749–757.
5. American College of Obstetricians and Gynecologists Committee on Adolescent Health Care; American College of Obstetricians and Gynecologists Committee Gynecologic Practice. ACOG. Committee Opinion No. 451: Von Willebrand disease in women. *Obstet Gynecol* 2009;114(6):1439–1443.
6. Naik S, Teruya J, Dietrich JE, et al. Utility of platelet function analyzer as a screening tool for the diagnosis of von Willebrand disease in adolescents with menorrhagia. *Pediatr Blood Cancer* 2013;60(7):1184–1187.
7. ACOG Committee on Adolescent Health Care. Menstruation in girls and adolescents: using the menstrual cycle as a vital sign. Committee Opinion number 349. *Obstet Gynecol* 2006;108(5):1323–1328.
8. Centers for Disease Control and Prevention. U.S. Medical eligibility criteria for contraceptive use, 2010: adapted from World Health Organization Medical eligibility criteria for contraceptive use, 4th edition. *MMWR* 2010;59 (RR-4).
9. American College of Obstetricians and Gynecologists. Management of acute abnormal uterine bleeding in nonpregnant reproductive-aged women. *Obstet Gynecol* 2013;121(4):891–896.
10. Dhananjay BS, Nanda SK. The role of sevista in the management of dysfunctional uterine bleeding. *J Clin Diagn Res* 2013;7:132–134.
11. Lukes AS, Moore KA, Muse KN, et al. Tranexamic acid treatment for heavy menstrual bleeding. A randomized controlled trial. *Obstet Gynecol* 2010;116(4):865–875.
12. Gray SH, Emans SJ. Abnormal vaginal bleeding. In: Emans SJ, Laufer MR, eds. *Emans, Laufer, Goldstein's pediatric & adolescent gynecology.* 6th ed. Philadelphia, PA: Wolters Kluwer Health/Lippincott Williams & Wilkins, 2012:159–167.
13. Lethaby AE, Cooke I, Rees M. Progesterone or progestogen-releasing intrauterine systems for heavy menstrual bleeding. *Cochrane Database Syst Rev* 2005;(4):CD002126.
14. Quaas AM, Ginsburg ES. Prevention and treatment of uterine bleeding in hematologic malignancy. *Eur J Obstet Gynecol Reprod Biol* 2007;134:3–8.
15. Chwalisz K, Surrey E, Stanczyk FZ. The Hormonal profile of norethindrone acetate: rationale for add-back therapy with gonadotropin-releasing hormone agonists in women with endometriosis. *Reprod Sci* 2012;19(6):563–571.

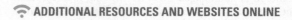 **ADDITIONAL RESOURCES AND WEBSITES ONLINE**

Amenorrhea, the Polycystic Ovary Syndrome, and Hirsutism

Amy Fleischman
Catherine M. Gordon

INTRODUCTION

Primary amenorrhea is defined by a lack of menses by 14 years without secondary sexual characteristics or lack of menses by 16 years. Secondary amenorrhea is the lack of menses for 6 months, or the duration of three prior cycles. The causes of primary and secondary amenorrhea include specific genetic abnormalities, enzymatic defects, and structural abnormalities. The hypothalamus, pituitary and/or gonads may be affected. Decreased energy availability due to reduced intake or increased exercise is a common cause of hypothalamic amenorrhea. Polycystic ovary syndrome (PCOS) is another common cause of irregular menses. This syndrome consists of clinical and laboratory hyperandrogenism and dysregulated menses, and may include typical ovarian structural changes. Metabolic abnormalities are commonly associated with this syndrome. Hirsutism, increased body hair in females, is a common manifestation of PCOS, but may also be seen in other conditions causing hyperandrogenism. This chapter will review the causes, evaluation, and treatment of amenorrhea, PCOS, and hirsutism.

AMENORRHEA

Definition

Normal Menstrual Timing

- The average age of menarche for the American adolescent remains at 12.7 years, with a 2 standard deviation range of 11 to 15 months. Although a large cohort study demonstrated earlier thelarche in some ethnic groups compared to prior studies, and an average range of thelarche of 8.8 to 9.7 years (8.8 years in Black; 9.3 years in Hispanics; 9.7 years in Whites and Asian girls), there have been no definitive trials demonstrating earlier menarche.[1]
- Ninety-five to ninety-seven percent of females reach menarche by age 16 years and 98% by 18 years.
- There is an average of 2 years between the start of thelarche, the first sign of puberty, and the onset of menarche.
- The onset of menarche is fairly constant in adolescent development, with approximately two-thirds of females reaching

menarche at a sexual maturity rating (SMR) of 4. Menarche occurs at SMR 2 in 5% of girls, SMR 3 in 25%, and not until SMR 5 in 10%.

- Ninety-five percent of teens have attained menarche 1 year after attaining SMR 5.
- Although anovulatory cycles are common in the first few years after menarche, thereafter, menstrual cycles are typically less than 45 days in healthy adolescent girls.[2]

Amenorrhea

Primary Amenorrhea

1. No episodes of spontaneous uterine bleeding by the age of 14 years with secondary sexual characteristics absent
2. No episodes of spontaneous uterine bleeding by age 16 years regardless of normal secondary sexual characteristics (chronological criteria)
3. No episodes of spontaneous uterine bleeding, despite having attained SMR 5 for at least 1 year or despite the onset of breast development 4 years previously (developmental criteria).
4. No episodes of spontaneous uterine bleeding by age 14 years in any individual with clinical stigmata of or genotype consistent with Turner syndrome

Secondary Amenorrhea

After previous uterine bleeding, no subsequent menses for 6 months or a length of time equal to three previous cycles.

Etiology

Primary Amenorrhea without Secondary Sexual Characteristics (Absent Breast Development), but with Normal Genitalia (Uterus and Vagina)

1. Genetic or enzymatic defects causing gonadal (ovarian) failure (hypergonadotropic hypogonadism): A growing number of primary amenorrhea cases are attributable to a genetic cause.
   - *Turner syndrome, Turner mosaicism, or related genotypes* (45, X; 45, XX/X; 45, XY/X, or structurally abnormal X chromosome): most common genetic causes of hypogonadism. Stigmata are variable in mosaicism, but classically include short stature (height usually <60 in); streaked gonads; hypogonadism; and somatic anomalies (webbed neck, short fourth metacarpal, cubitus valgus, coarctation of the aorta) (see Fig. 49.1).
   - *Premature ovarian insufficiency:* Etiologies can include autoimmunity and enzymatic or genetic abnormalities. The etiology may be important in directing further evaluation and in counseling families. For example, a carrier of a premutation in the FMR1 gene (fragile X gene) in a female can manifest as ovarian insufficiency while future generations would be at risk for severe mental retardation among males.

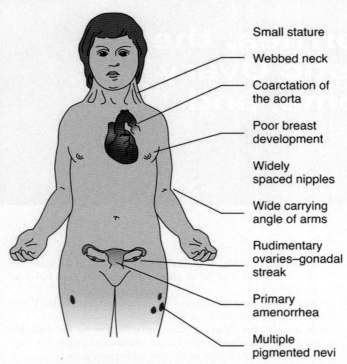

Small stature

Webbed neck

Coarctation of the aorta

Poor breast development

Widely spaced nipples

Wide carrying angle of arms

Rudimentary ovaries–gonadal streak

Primary amenorrhea

Multiple pigmented nevi

FIGURE 49.1 Clinical features of Turner syndrome. (From Rubin R, Strayer DS, Rubin E. *Rubin's pathology.* 6th ed. Philadelphia, PA: Lippincott Williams & Wilkins, 2011.)

Evidence of autoimmunity, such as ovarian and/or adrenal antibodies, suggests the need to evaluate adrenal status and consider clinical evidence of other autoimmune diseases such as hypothyroidism, hypoparathyroidism, or type 1 diabetes mellitus. Rarer mutations have been identified that manifest as premature ovarian insufficiency and thus may play a role in amenorrhea such as EIF4ENIF1.[3]

• *17α-hydroxylase deficiency with 46, XX karyotype*: These individuals have normal stature, lack of secondary sexual characteristics, hypertension, and hypokalemia. Laboratory test results show an elevated progesterone, low 17-hydroxyprogesterone (17-OHP), and elevated serum deoxycorticosterone level. Mild cases may present without electrolyte abnormalities.

2. Pituitary/hypothalamic gonadotropin insufficiency (hypogonadotropic hypogonadism): With the discovery of multiple factors contributing to GnRH activation, idiopathic hypogonadotropic hypogonadism (IHH) (Kallmann, normosmic IHH) has been shown to have multiple genetic contributors. Mutations in KAL1, FGFR1, FGF8, PROK2, PROKR2, and Kisspeptin1, in addition to GnRH1, GnRH receptor, TAC3, TAC3R, and CHD7, among others, have been linked to hypogonadism. This active field continues to evolve, and novel factors and genetic mutations continue to be reported.

Primary Amenorrhea with Normal Breast Development, but Absent Uterus

1. *Complete androgen insensitivity*: In these XY-karyotype individuals, the Wolffian ducts fail to develop and external female genitalia are present. The underlying defect is a mutation in the androgen receptor, rendering it insensitive to testosterone's actions. Because müllerian inhibitory factor (MIF) continues to be secreted by the Sertoli cells of male gonads, the müllerian ducts regress, and there is lack of formation of internal female genitalia. Internally, there may be normal male gonads and fibrous müllerian remnants. At puberty, if the gonads remain

present, the low levels of endogenous gonadal and adrenal estrogens, unopposed by androgens, may result in breast development. Because of the end-organ insensitivity to androgens, the teen develops sparse or absent pubic and axillary hair despite marked elevations in serum testosterone concentrations.

2. *Congenital absence of uterus/agenesis* is often associated with agenesis of the vaginal canal, or Mayer–Rokitansky–Küster–Hauser syndrome. These young women have a 46 XX karyotype and ovaries. They may experience cyclic breast and mood changes. They present with secondary sexual characteristics and normal female testosterone concentrations. They may also have associated renal, skeletal, or other congenital anomalies.

Primary Amenorrhea with No Breast Development and No Uterus

This condition is extremely rare. The individual usually has a 46, XY karyotype, elevated gonadotropin levels, and low-normal female testosterone levels. These individuals produce enough MIF to inhibit development of female internal genital structures, but not enough testosterone to develop male internal and external genitalia. The causes include the following:

1. 17,20-Lyase deficiency
2. Agonadism, including no internal sex organs
3. 17α-Hydroxylase deficiency with 46, XY karyotype: may present with hypertension.

Primary and Secondary Amenorrhea with Normal Secondary Sexual Characteristics (Breast Development) and Normal Genitalia (Uterus and Vagina)

1. Hypothalamic causes
   • *Idiopathic hypogonadotropic hypogonadism,* as outlined above, mild cases can cause primary and secondary amenorrhea with normal secondary sexual characteristics
   • *Medications and drugs:* Particularly phenothiazines; oral, injectable, or transdermal contraceptives; glucocorticoids; and heroin.
   • *Other endocrinopathies:* Hyperthyroidism or hypothyroidism, prolactinoma, and cortisol excess
   • *Stress:* Common in adolescents and young adults (AYAs) and may relate to family, school, or peer problems
   • *Exercise:* Athletes, particularly runners, gymnasts, competitive divers, figure skaters, and ballet dancers, have higher rates of amenorrhea and higher rates of low energy availability, sometimes associated with disordered eating. Sports that may place athletes at higher risk for this condition include those that emphasize leanness, such as dance or gymnastics, or those that use weight classification, such as martial arts. The "female athlete triad," a term coined in 1992, has been more recently redefined by the American College of Sports Medicine[4] to include a spectrum of energy availability, menstrual irregularity, and bone health. This spectrum notes that young women can have low energy availability due to under-eating, over-exercise, or both.[2]

   The prevalence of secondary amenorrhea in adult athletes ranges broadly depending on the sport studied. As many as 18% of female recreational runners, 50% of competitive runners training 80 miles/week, and 47% to 79% of ballet dancers may be amenorrheic.[5,6] The prevalence of secondary amenorrhea in the teen athlete also varies based on the sport studied. A study of 170 girls participating in 8 sports from 6 high schools in California demonstrated that 23.5% had menstrual irregularities (17.1% had oligomennorhea, 5.3% secondary amenorrhea, and 1.2% primary amenorrhea).[7]

   The pulsatile nature of luteinizing hormone (LH), and normal menstrual function, appears to be dependent on energy availability (caloric intake minus energy expenditure). Low energy availability may result in a hypometabolic state that can include the metabolic alterations, hypoglycemia, hypoinsulinemia, euthyroid sick syndrome, hypercortisolemia, and suppression of the total secretion and amplitude of the diurnal rhythm of leptin.[2] Leptin, a hormone secreted by fat tissue, has been shown to be a permissive factor in menstruation, likely due to its correlation with adequate fat mass.[8] Although both amenorrheic athletes and regularly menstruating athletes have reduced LH pulsatile secretions and 24-hour mean leptin levels, amenorrheic runners have more extreme suppression and disorganization of LH pulsatility. The level of energy availability needed to maintain normal reproductive function is not known for a given individual. However, recent studies have used 30 kcal/kg of lean body mass, as there are demonstrable metabolic and bone effects that occur below this amount.[9]

Low levels of estradiol (E_2) may be present, which have been implicated as the cause of bone loss, placing these young women at increased risk of stress fractures. The condition may be reversible with weight gain or with lessening of the intensity of exercise. However, there is also evidence that this loss of bone density may be partially irreversible despite resumption of menses, estrogen replacement, or calcium supplementation. There remain many unanswered questions about exercise-induced amenorrhea, especially related to whether hormonal therapy or vitamin/mineral supplementation is beneficial in minimizing skeletal loss in this population. This is an active area of research, with preliminary data suggesting that transdermal estrogen[10] and combined therapy with dehydroepiandrosterone and estrogen/progestin may be beneficial.[11]

- *Weight loss:* This group includes AYAs with simple weight loss and those with anorexia nervosa. In both patients with anorexia nervosa and patients with simple weight loss, the mechanism of amenorrhea appears to be hypothalamic derangement. This alteration appears to be more severe in AYAs with anorexia nervosa. The E_2 levels in patients with weight loss and anorexia nervosa can vary from low to normal. Consequently, such individuals may or may not respond to progesterone withdrawal with uterine bleeding. The AYAs with amenorrhea and severe weight loss are also at risk for decreased bone density, and treatment of this metabolic consequence in anorexia nervosa is also an active area of research.
- *Chronic illnesses:* Certain chronic illnesses can affect the hypothalamic–pituitary axis. Examples include cystic fibrosis and chronic renal disease.
- *Hypothalamic failure:*
  - Idiopathic
  - Lesions: include craniopharyngioma, tuberculous granuloma, and other tumors and infectious etiologies.
2. Pituitary causes
  - *Non-neoplastic lesions resulting in hypopituitarism:* Sheehan syndrome (pregnancy related), Simmonds disease (non-pregnancy-related), aneurysm, or empty sella syndrome
  - *Tumors:* Adenoma or carcinoma
  - *Idiopathic*
  - *Infiltrative:* Hemochromatosis
3. Ovarian causes
  Premature ovarian insufficiency: Menopause occurring at younger than 35 years. This can be a genetically determined process (see above section: Amenorrhea), or associated with autoantibodies directed against ovarian tissue, sometimes in association with thyroid and adrenal autoantibodies. This can also be iatrogenic, such as in individuals who received chemotherapy and/or radiation therapy for cancer as children or adolescents.
4. Hyperandrogenism: PCOS, congenital adrenal hyperplasia (CAH), or androgen-producing tumor. These etiologies are discussed in detail below.
5. Uterine causes: Uterine synechiae (Asherman syndrome)
6. Pregnancy

Diagnosis

The evaluation of amenorrhea can be pursued with a thorough history, physical examination, and performance of several laboratory tests in a logical sequence. Too often, AYAs are subjected to an expensive "shotgun" approach to evaluation. It is essential to rule out the diagnosis of pregnancy before conducting an extensive evaluation. Figures 49.2 and 49.3 review the evaluation of primary and secondary amenorrhea.

History

History should include the following:

1. Systemic diseases: Diseases associated with secondary amenorrhea include, but are not limited to, anorexia nervosa, systemic illness such as inflammatory bowel disease and diabetes mellitus, as well as central processes such as pituitary adenoma. A history of thyroid dysfunction is particularly important, because even mild thyroid dysfunction can lead to menstrual abnormalities.
2. Family history, including ages of parental growth and development, mother's and sisters' ages at menarche, as well as a family history of thyroid disease, diabetes mellitus, eating disorders, or menstrual problems
3. Past medical history including any significant childhood illnesses
4. Pubertal growth and development, including breast and pubic hair development, and the presence of a growth spurt
5. Menstrual history
6. History of androgen excess such as significant acne or hair growth, suggesting PCOS, or other ovarian or adrenal abnormality
7. Emotional status
8. Medications: Including illicit drugs (heroin and methadone, for example, can cause menstrual dysfunction)
9. Nutritional status and recent weight changes
10. Exercise history, particularly for sports that might predispose to amenorrhea
11. Sexual history, contraception, and symptoms of pregnancy

Physical Examination

The physical examination should include the following:

1. Check for signs of systemic disease or malnutrition.
2. Evaluate for SMR: This is important for evaluating progress in secondary sexual characteristics, because most adolescents are not menarcheal until SMR 4, and 95% are menarcheal by 1 year after SMR 5.
3. Check height and weight.
4. Check for signs of androgen excess such as acne or hirsutism.
5. Check for signs of thyroid dysfunction, including examination of thyroid gland, skin, and hair.
6. Check for signs of insulin resistance such as acanthosis nigricans (hyperpigmented velvety skin changes on neck, axillae, or other intertriginous areas) (Fig. 49.4).
7. Check for phenotype consistent with Turner syndrome: Webbed neck, low-set ears, broad shield-like chest, short fourth metacarpal, and increased carrying angle of the arms (Fig. 49.1).
8. Test for anosmia in females with primary or secondary amenorrhea when considering anosmic hypogonadotropic hypogonadism (Kallmann syndrome).
9. Breast examination: Check for estrogenized texture and for galactorrhea.
10. Pelvic examination: Search for a stenotic cervix, vaginal agenesis, imperforate hymen, transverse vaginal septum, absent uterus, or enlarged uterus suggesting pregnancy. An external genital examination is a critical component of the workup. A full pelvic examination may not be necessary if the teen is not sexually active, and the history or physical examination may reveal the cause of amenorrhea.

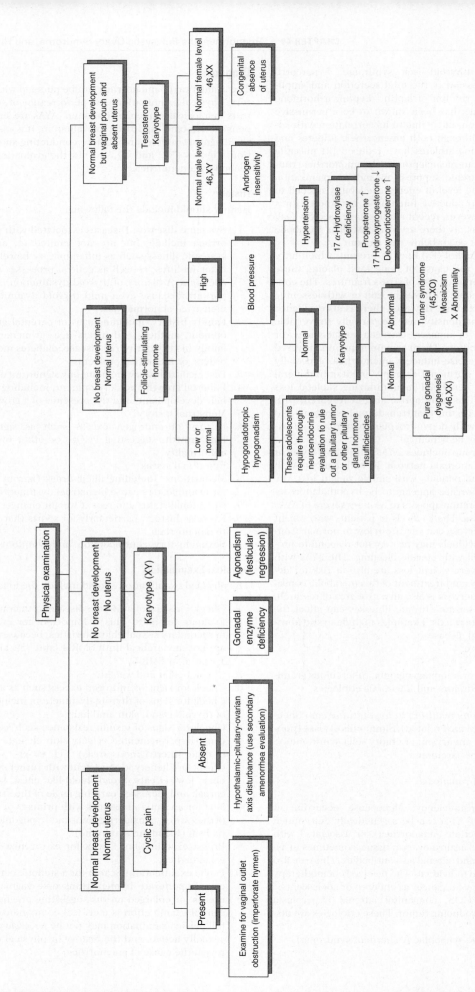

FIGURE 49.2 The evaluation of primary amenorrhea.

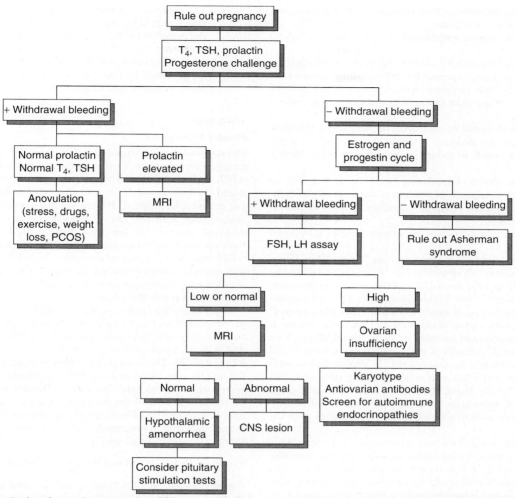

FIGURE 49.3 The evaluation of secondary amenorrhea. TSH, thyroid-stimulating hormone; PCOS, polycystic ovary syndrome; MRI, magnetic resonance imaging; FSH, follicle-stimulating hormone; LH, luteinizing hormone; CNS, central nervous system.

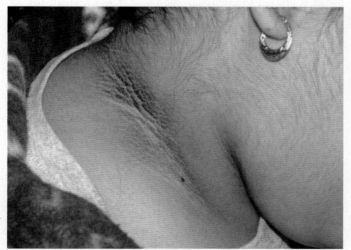

FIGURE 49.4 Acanthosis nigricans. Linear, alternating dark and light pigmentation becomes more apparent when the skin is stretched. (From Goodheart HP. *Goodheart's photoguide of common skin disorders.* 2nd ed. Philadelphia, PA: Lippincott Williams & Wilkins, 2003.)

Laboratory Evaluation

The laboratory evaluation for AYAs can begin with evaluation of LH, follicle-stimulating hormone (FSH), and estradiol to establish whether primary hypogonadism or hypogonadotropic hypogonadism is the cause.

1. Evaluation for primary and secondary amenorrhea with normal secondary sexual characteristics:
   a. If evidence of galactorrhea is present, the adolescent should be evaluated, as described in Chapter 55. If clinical hyperandrogenism is present, see discussion below on PCOS.
   b. Pregnancy should always be considered and ruled out.
   c. Diabetes mellitus and hypothyroidism should be considered, and if clinically indicated should be ruled out with measurements of blood glucose and/or thyroid function studies.
   d. Uterine synechiae, or Asherman syndrome, should be considered if there is a history of dilation and curettage, or endometritis. This condition may cause partial or total obliteration of the uterine cavity. If this problem is suggested by the history, a gynecological referral for evaluation by hysteroscopy or hysterosalpingography is indicated.

If the results of the aforementioned evaluation are negative, the workup should proceed as follows:

Administer progesterone withdrawal test or "challenge" (5-10 day course)

- A *positive response to progesterone* correlates with circulating E_2 levels adequate to prime the endometrium, as seen with either hypothalamic–pituitary dysfunction or PCOS. A positive response ranges from minimal brown staining to normal menstrual flow.
  - Prolactin level should be measured, because this is the most sensitive test for pituitary microadenomas. Rarely, a patient who responds to progesterone withdrawal can have a microadenoma.
  - In addition, thyroid-stimulating hormone and a free or total T_4 with a measure of binding protein should be measured to rule out the possibility of either primary or central hypothyroidism.
  - The laboratory evaluation of hyperandrogenism is outlined below.
- If there is *no response to progesterone*, then either hypothalamic–pituitary dysfunction or ovarian insufficiency is likely. A high FSH level indicates ovarian insufficiency, whereas a normal or low FSH level suggests a hypothalamic–pituitary disturbance. If ovarian insufficiency is suspected, a karyotype, antiovarian antibodies, and screening for autoimmune endocrinopathies may be done. In addition, more rare causes, such as fragile X premutation carrier status and galactosemia, should be considered. If hypothalamic–pituitary failure is suspected, magnetic resonance imaging (MRI) scans of the brain, visual fields, and a pituitary hormonal evaluation are warranted. An MRI should always be considered in a female patient with a history of headaches or visual changes.
- Individuals with weight loss, anorexia nervosa, heavy substance abuse, or excessive exercise may or may not respond to progesterone withdrawal. If they do not experience bleeding within 10 to 14 days of discontinuing the progesterone, it is indicative of low E_2 levels and further evaluation may be warranted.
2. Evaluation for primary amenorrhea with either absent uterus or absent secondary sexual characteristics:
   a. A physical examination and potentially radiographic studies will divide the teens into three groups:
      - Absent uterus, normal breasts
      - Absent breasts, normal uterus
      - Absent breasts, absent uterus

      In general, breast development should be at least at stage SMR 4 to be considered indicative of full gonadal function. A breast stage of SMR 2 or SMR 3 may indicate adrenal function alone without gonadal function.
   b. If the examination reveals normal breast development, but an absent uterus and blind vaginal pouch, a karyotype and a test for serum testosterone concentrations are indicated.
      - XX karyotype plus female testosterone concentration: Congenital absence of uterus
      - XY karyotype plus male testosterone concentration: Androgen insensitivity
   c. If the examination reveals absent secondary sexual characteristics, but a normal uterus:
      - A low or normal FSH level suggests a hypothalamic or pituitary abnormality, and a full pituitary evaluation is indicated.
      - A high FSH level and a blood pressure within the reference range suggest a genetic disorder or gonadal dysgenesis. A karyotype should be ordered.
      - A high FSH level and hypertension suggest 17α-hydroxylase deficiency. This is confirmed by an elevated progesterone level, low 17α-hydroxyprogesterone level, and an elevated serum deoxycorticosterone level.
   d. The absence of both breast development and uterus or vagina is very rare. These findings suggest gonadal failure and the presence of MIF secretion from a testis. This could arise from anorchia occurring after MIF activity was present or an enzyme block, such as a 17,20-lyase defect. The evaluation should include LH, FSH, progesterone, and 17-OHP measurements, and a karyotype.

Treatment
Primary Amenorrhea

Hypogonadotropic Hypogonadism: Therapy should begin with estrogen replacement. A transdermal patch can be used starting at 0.025 mg/day of estradiol, or cut to initiate lower doses, and used nightly and advanced slowly over time. Half of the 0.3 mg Premarin pill can also be utilized. Recent studies support improved safety and efficacy with the use of transdermal estrogen preparations, avoiding effects of the first pass through the liver.[12] Patients who have already reached an acceptable adult height can receive up to 0.625 mg/day of conjugated estrogens (Premarin) or 0.05 to 0.1 mg of estradiol via transdermal patch. High doses of estrogen should be avoided early to prevent premature epiphyseal closure in girls who have not yet reached final adult height.

A typical maintenance schedule would be 0.625 to 1.25 mg/day of conjugated estrogens on days 1 through 25 of each month or twice-weekly estrogen patch application of 0.05 to 0.1 mg of estradiol, with 10 mg of medroxyprogesterone acetate (Provera) on days 12 through 25. The progestin is added to induce withdrawal bleeding and thereby avoid endometrial hyperplasia. This schedule can be repeated each month. The dose of estrogen may vary depending on the individual and the estrogen response, but usually does not exceed 1.25 mg/day of conjugated estrogens or 0.1 mg/day of transdermal estrogen. If pregnancy is desired, pulsatile GnRH via pump therapy is a therapeutic option.

Pituitary Defect: Hormonal therapy, as outlined above.

Genetic Abnormalities Leading to Gonadal Defects: Hormonal therapy, as outlined above. If a Y chromosome is present, gonadal removal is usually necessary because of the risk of gonadoblastoma development. If a 46, XX karyotype is present, then the gonadal tissue should be visualized to assess whether more than a streaked gonad is present to evaluate if the tissue is at increased risk for tumor progression. With complete gonadal dysgenesis, these individuals are universally sterile. However, with an intact uterus, the individual may be able to bear children after donor oocyte implantation and hormonal support.

Enzymatic Defects

17α-hydroxylase Deficiency: Both glucocorticoid and estrogen–progesterone replacement are needed.

17,20-lyase Deficiency: Estrogen–progesterone replacement is needed.

Androgen Insensitivity: All intra-abdominal gonads associated with a Y chromosome have a relatively high potential for malignancy and should be removed. The appropriate timing for removal should be individualized for each patient. After the gonads are removed, maintenance estrogen therapy is needed. The adolescent should be informed that she may require vaginoplasty to have normal sexual function. The discussion about infertility and the abnormal sex chromosome should be done with additional counseling support as needed.

Congenital Absence of the Uterus: Because these adolescents have normal-functioning ovaries, they do not require hormonal replacement therapy. They may require a vaginoplasty for normal sexual function and an MRI or intravenous pyelogram to rule out renal anomalies. These adolescents must be informed that they cannot carry a pregnancy, but may be able to have genetic offspring with the assistance of a surrogate. Therefore, they may require additional support and counseling.

Primary and Secondary Amenorrhea with Normal Secondary Sexual Characteristics

1. PCOS (see detailed discussion below)
2. Hypothalamic–pituitary dysfunction
   a. Alleviate the precipitating cause, if known.
   b. Hormonal therapy with progestins to induce uterine bleeding every 1 to 2 months and/or estrogen and progestin therapy is recommended.
3. Hypothalamic–pituitary failure
   a. The cause must be evaluated and corrected if possible.
   b. Replacement therapy with cyclic conjugated estrogens and progestins, as outlined above, is recommended.
4. Ovarian insufficiency
   These AYAs also require cyclic estrogen and progestin therapy.
5. Uterine synechiae: This problem requires referral to a gynecologist for possible transhysteroscopic lysis of the adhesions.

Amenorrhea Associated with Weight Loss

In young women with amenorrhea associated with weight loss, bone mineral density (BMD) loss can occur soon after amenorrhea develops. The efficacy of estrogen replacement therapy, with provision of oral versus transdermal preparations, in this setting is an area of continued debate. Estrogen likely has beneficial effects on bone and other tissues, but other supplemental therapies appear to be needed, in addition to the estrogen replacement. Experimental therapies, such as low-dose androgen supplementation (dehydroepiandrosterone [DHEA] or testosterone), insulin-like growth factor I (IGF-I), or growth hormone, and bisphosphonates, are gaining further support in the literature.[11,13–15] Many adolescents who recover from anorexia nervosa at a young age (younger than 15 years) have regional (lumbar spine and femoral neck) bone deficits. The longer the duration of anorexia nervosa and/or weight loss, the less likely the BMD will return to a normal range.

The Female Athlete Triad

Female AYAs who participate regularly in athletics may develop the female athlete triad, which includes low energy availability due to a high level of physical activity, which is sometimes accompanied by disordered eating, menstrual dysfunction (typically oligomenorrhea), and decreased BMD as discussed above.

Treatment considerations for athletes with amenorrhea include the following:

a. Most bone mineralization in female adolescents occurs by the middle of the second decade of life.
b. Premature bone demineralization occurs in young women with hypothalamic dysfunction that manifests as either amenorrhea or oligomenorrhea in the setting of participation in athletics or dance, and eating disorders.
c. Regular menses and fertility should return with a decrease in the intensity of activity. An AYA with significant menstrual dysfunction attributed to exercise should be encouraged to increase her caloric intake and modify excessive exercise activity.
d. Calcium intake should be increased to 1,500 mg/day in these young women with efforts made to optimize dietary calcium intake.
e. Vitamin D deficiency should be avoided, and supplemental vitamin D of 600 to 1,000 IU provided daily.
f. Hormonal therapy remains an area of active study. Studies have suggested that transdermal estrogen may be more beneficial to bone health in this population[10] compared to oral estrogen therapy. In addition, combined therapy with DHEA and low-dose combined oral contraceptive pills has demonstrated a positive effect on BMD.[11] Androgens, estrogens, growth hormone, IGF-1, and bisphosphonates are being

tested in clinical trials, with some demonstrating improvements in bone health.
g. The practitioner should evaluate these individuals, as outlined previously, to eliminate the possibility of pregnancy, thyroid dysfunction, prolactinoma, or a disorder of androgen excess. It should not be assumed that amenorrhea is simply secondary to exercise.

🔵 THE PCOS AND HIRSUTISM

Definition

PCOS is a disorder of the hypothalamic–pituitary–ovarian system, giving rise to temporary or persistent anovulation and androgen excess. The syndrome was originally described in 1935 by Stein and Leventhal as amenorrhea, hirsutism, and obesity associated with enlarged cystic ovaries. For many years, there was an emphasis on the morphological changes in the ovary. However, enlarged polycystic ovaries may occur in healthy women and up to 30% of healthy adolescent girls, and in females with other conditions such as Cushing syndrome and CAH. In addition, women with other classic features of PCOS may have ovaries of normal size. A 1990 US NIH consensus conference identified key features for the diagnosis of PCOS—hyperandrogenism, menstrual dysfunction, clinical evidence of hyperandrogenism, and the exclusion of CAH. Probable criteria for PCOS included insulin resistance and perimenarchal onset.

The 2003 Rotterdam consensus workshop defined PCOS more broadly, recognizing ovarian dysfunction as the primary component, without mandatory anovulation. The revised definition included two of the three following criteria with the exclusion of other etiologies of hyperandrogenism:

- Oligo- and/or anovulation
- Clinical and/or biochemical signs of hyperandrogenism
- Polycystic ovaries by ultrasonography.

The Androgen Excess and PCOS Society in 2008 broadened the definition to include clinical and/or biochemical hyperandrogenism (most reliably hirsutism and an elevated free testosterone) and ovarian dysfunction. Evaluation of ovarian morphology was suggested and other causes of hyperandrogenism were to be ruled out. The consensus definitions are broad, allowing for a clinical and biochemical diagnosis of a wide spectrum of phenotypes. More recent research criteria have included abnormal response to GnRH stimulation, dexamethasone suppression testing, and adrenocorticotropic hormone (ACTH) stimulation testing.[16] Reaching an accurate diagnosis is particularly important because PCOS increases metabolic and cardiovascular risks, which are linked to insulin resistance and compounded by obesity. Androgen excess can result in laboratory changes including decreased high-density lipoprotein cholesterol (HDL-C) level. Insulin resistance and its associated risks are also present in nonobese women with PCOS.

PCOS is one of the most common endocrine disorders, affecting approximately 5% to 10% of premenopausal women, and is the most common cause of hyperandrogenism in women and adolescents. True prevalence rates are difficult to study due to referral biases and variable phenotypes. The use of a large health plan database in California allowed for the review of records of almost 150,000 adolescent girls and found a prevalence of 1.14%, ranging from 0.9% in White girls to 1.3% in Black and Hispanic White girls.[17]

Etiology

Endocrine Findings

PCOS is characterized by menstrual irregularities ranging from amenorrhea or oligomenorrhea, to abnormal uterine bleeding. An androgen-excess state is present, leading to hirsutism and acne with rare mild virilization.

Hyperandrogenism:
- Androstenedione and dehydroepiandrosterone sulfate (DHEAS): Elevated serum levels
- Testosterone: Often minimally elevated serum levels are seen, with elevated free (unbound) testosterone.

Source of excess androgens: The source may be secretion from the ovaries, the adrenal gland, or both, in women with a primary diagnosis of PCOS. Two other sources contribute to androgen excess:

a. Androstenedione is converted peripherally in adipose tissue to testosterone.
b. There is a decrease in binding of testosterone to sex hormone–binding globulin (SHBG). Healthy females have approximately 96% of their testosterone bound to SHBG, where it is inactive, whereas patients with PCOS have only 92% of their testosterone bound; therefore, there is a larger percentage of free and active testosterone in patients with PCOS.

Pathophysiology

The exact initiating cause of PCOS is not known, but may be related to the following:

1. Abnormal hypothalamic–pituitary function
2. Abnormal ovarian function
3. Abnormal adrenal androgen metabolism
4. Insulin resistance: Insulin resistance may exist in both obese and lean women with PCOS, and the hyperinsulinism that ensues may promote the hyperandrogenic state.

Factors leading to the development of PCOS include the following:

1. Insulin resistance at the time of puberty contributing to a relative hyperinsulinemic state. The rates of insulin resistance and glucose intolerance found in adolescent girls with PCOS are similar to the rates in adult women, of up to 30%.[18]
2. Insulin and IGF-1 have mitogenic effects on the ovaries, causing theca cell hyperplasia, which leads to excessive androgen production. Hyperinsulinemia has been directly correlated with a decrease in hepatic production of insulin-like growth factor–binding protein 1 (IGFBP1). The decrease in bound IGF-1 results in an increase in free IGF-1. The increase in IGF-1 and the decrease in IGFBP1 have both been found to correlate with increases in adrenal and ovarian androgens, resulting in the clinical presentation of premature adrenarche and PCOS.[19] Therefore, both high IGF-1 levels and low IGFBP1 levels may correlate with early insulin resistance and be pathophysiologically and clinically linked to the progression to PCOS and insulin resistance.
3. The increased ovarian androgen levels cause follicular atresia, impairing E2 production.
4. The combination of theca cell hyperplasia and arrested follicular maturation constitutes the typical histological features of PCOS.
5. Because not all adolescents ultimately develop PCOS, it is thought that there is a genetic factor involved. Genetic studies of family clusters have shown a high incidence of affected relatives, with high inheritance rates.[20] However, chromosomal studies of patients with PCOS have suffered from lack of consensus in diagnosis, overlap with obesity, and inconsistent findings. Some recent studies have supported the association with certain gene polymorphisms, but a specific genetic profile has yet to be validated.
6. Valproate can also induce menstrual disturbances, polycystic ovaries, and hyperandrogenism.[21] In a study of 238 women with epilepsy, 43% of the women using valproate had polycystic ovaries. In those women using valproate before reaching age 20 years, 80% had polycystic ovaries or hyperandrogenism.

Clinical Consequences

PCOS can present with many symptoms:

1. *Anovulation:* Anovulation is a key feature. Usually, the anovulation in PCOS is chronic and presents as either oligomenorrhea or amenorrhea of perimenarcheal onset. Some women who report normal menses may be anovulatory. Few women with PCOS have normal ovulatory function.
2. *Polycystic ovaries:* The ovaries in patients with PCOS are usually enlarged, pearly white, sclerotic with multiple (20 to 100) cystic follicles. Normally, follicles develop to approximately 19 to 20 mm and then ovulation occurs. In AYAs with PCOS, multiple follicles develop, but only to approximately 9 to 10 mm in size. Histologically, the ovaries have the same number of primordial follicles, but the number of atretic follicles is doubled. Also, there is an absence of corpora lutea. The polycystic ovary is a sign, not a disease entity on its own. The typical histological changes of the polycystic ovary can be seen in ovaries of any size. A sonographic spectrum exists within patients with PCOS, and polycystic ovaries on ultrasound are not by themselves sufficient for diagnosis of PCOS.
3. *Hyperandrogenism/hirsutism:* Hyperandrogenism is a key feature of PCOS. Hyperandrogenism in PCOS is primarily ovarian in origin, although adrenal androgens may contribute. Hirsutism is defined as increased growth of terminal (long, coarse, and pigmented) hair in a young woman, more than is cosmetically acceptable in a certain culture. The condition commonly refers to an increase in length and coarseness of the hair, in a male pattern, including predominantly midline hair of the upper lip, chin, cheeks, inner thighs, lower back, and periareolar, sternal, abdominal, and intergluteal regions. The effects of sex hormones and other factors on hair development and distribution can be more easily understood by considering the pilosebaceous unit (Fig. 49.5). The clinical manifestations of androgen excess vary depending on end-organ sensitivity to androgens. Hirsutism can result either from overproduction or increased sensitivity of hair follicles to androgens. Terminal hair growth is stimulated by the increased conversion of testosterone to dihydrotestosterone (DHT) from excess 5α-reductase within this unit or the presence of more numerous hair follicles. Androgens are synthesized from the ovary or adrenals from steroidogenic pathways within each gland (Fig. 49.6). Clinical hirsutism may not occur in all women with PCOS, but women with PCOS have elevated blood androgen levels.
4. *Obesity:* Originally, obesity was regarded as a classic feature, but its presence is extremely variable and not mandatory for diagnosis. Approximately 40% to 50% of women and adolescents with PCOS are obese. Obesity in women with PCOS is usually of the android type, with increased waist–hip ratios. The obesity with PCOS also worsens insulin resistance and increases cardiovascular risk. In obese women, weight loss may improve and/or cure the signs and symptoms of PCOS.
5. *Infertility:* Although infertility is usually not of concern to the adolescent patient, the risk is significantly elevated due to anovulation.
6. *Cancer risk:* There is an increased risk for cancer of the endometrium due to prolonged unopposed estrogen stimulation of the endometrial lining from chronic anovulation. There may also be an increased risk of breast cancer associated with chronic anovulation during the reproductive years.
7. *Elevated lipoprotein profile:* The abnormalities in women with PCOS include elevated levels of cholesterol, triglycerides, and low-density lipoprotein cholesterol (LDL-C) and lower levels of HDL-C and apolipoprotein A-1. Although hyperandrogenism plays some role in these changes, hyperinsulinemia (insulin resistance) and increased inflammatory cytokines probably have a larger effect.
8. *Insulin resistance and hyperinsulinemia:* Both are well-recognized features of PCOS and associated with many of the late complications of PCOS. Approximately 50% of women with PCOS are insulin resistant. Although insulin resistance is

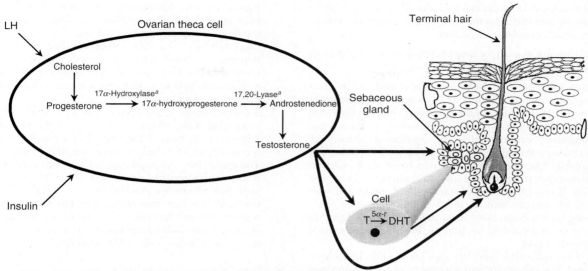

FIGURE 49.5 Effect of ovarian androgens on the pilosebaceous unit. Within the ovarian theca cell, insulin and LH may stimulate cytochrome P-450c17α activity, resulting in increased 17α-hydroxylase and 17,20-lyase activity, as denoted by *asterisks* above. These two enzymes comprise the P-450c17α complex. Ovarian testosterone, along with DHT from 5α-reductase within the pilosebaceous unit, stimulates the androgen receptors at the hair follicle and sebaceous glands. Hirsutism and acne can result. (From Gordon CM. Menstrual disorders in adolescents: excess androgens and the polycystic ovary syndrome. *Pediatr Clin North Am* 1999;46:519–543, with permission.)

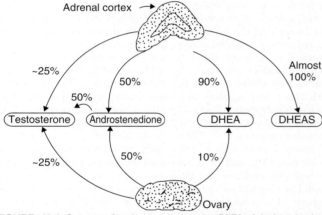

FIGURE 49.6 Sources of androgens in women. DHEA, dehydroepiandrosterone; DHEAS, dehydroepiandrosterone sulfate. (From Emans SJ. Androgen abnormalities in the adolescent girl. In: *Pediatric and adolescent gynecology*. 5th ed. Philadelphia, PA: Lippincott Williams & Wilkins, 2005:301, with permission.)

associated with obesity, it can also be found in normal-weight women with PCOS.

9. *Impaired glucose tolerance and diabetes*: Women and adolescents with PCOS are at increased risk for impaired glucose tolerance and overt type 2 diabetes mellitus because of the insulin resistance.

10. *Cardiovascular disease*: Because of the prevalence of the risk factors listed previously, women with PCOS may be at long-term risk for increased cardiovascular disease. Adult women with PCOS have an estimated sevenfold risk of myocardial infarction.[22] In addition, these young women can also have increased levels of plasminogen-activator inhibitor 1, which inhibits fibrinolysis and is a risk factor for myocardial infarction.[23]

Differential Diagnosis

1. Familial hirsutism and/or increased sensitivity to normal androgen levels
2. Androgen-producing ovarian and adrenal tumors
3. Cushing syndrome: Cushing syndrome is usually excluded by history and physical examination, and if needed, a 24-hour

urine collection for free cortisol, midnight salivary cortisol, or an overnight dexamethasone suppression test can be done.

4. CAH: A late-onset 21-hydroxylase deficiency can mimic PCOS. The diagnosis of CAH is based on elevated morning serum 17-OHP level, or stimulated level after ACTH infusion.

Diagnosis

Criteria for the diagnosis of PCOS include the following (**Table 49.1**):

1. *Irregular menses:* Chronic anovulation with a perimenarcheal onset of menstrual irregularities is classic and can present as oligomenorrhea, primary or secondary amenorrhea.
2. *Hyperandrogenism with or without skin manifestations:* Biochemical or clinical evidence of androgen excess. Serum-free

TABLE 49.1

Prevalence of Major Clinical Features of Polycystic Ovary Syndrome

	Goldzieher and Axelrod (1963)[a]	Balen et al. (1995)[b]	Carmina and Lobo (1996)[c]
No. of patients	1,079	1,741	240
Amenorrhea	51%	19.2%	16%
Oligomenorrhea	NR	47%	64%
Polymenorrhea	NR	2.7%	4%
Normal menses	12%	29.7%	15%
Hirsutism	69%	66.2%	70%
Acne	NR	34.7%	11.2%
Obesity	41%	38.4%	43.7%
Acanthosis nigricans	—	2.5%	2.1%

[a]Compilation of data from 187 published studies. Polycystic ovary syndrome (PCOS) was diagnosed on the basis of clinical data and the laparoscopic diagnosis of polycystic ovaries.
[b]Patients were diagnosed on the basis of ultrasonographic findings alone.
[c]PCOS was diagnosed on the basis of hyperandrogenic chronic anovulation (unpublished data).
From Lobo RA. Polycystic ovary syndrome. In: Lobo RA, Mishell DR, Shoupe D, et al., eds. *Infertility, contraception and reproductive endocrinology*. Malden, MA: Blackwell Science, 1997, with permission.

testosterone level is the best marker for ovarian causes of hyperandrogenism and DHEAS is the best marker of adrenal sources.

3. *Absence of other androgen disorders*

The following are not needed for diagnosis, but are supportive evidence of the diagnosis:

1. *Polycystic ovaries*: The Androgen Excess and PCOS Society updated recommendations in 2013 regarding ultrasound evaluation.[24] The meta-analysis and expert opinion concluded that follicle number per ovary in adult women (≥25) was the best diagnostic criteria using high-resolution ultrasound. Ovarian volume should be used if high-resolution studies are not available. The use of anti-Mullerian hormone concentrations to assess ovarian function instead of ultrasound has been proposed. However, the lack of standardized assays and variability in adolescents limit the utility at this time.

2. *Increased body weight*: Body mass index (BMI) >30 kg/m² in adults or >85th percentile in children, based on standardized CDC growth curves

3. *Elevated LH and FSH levels*: Although LH and FSH levels have been used, the sensitivity and specificity of these hormones are low.

4. Prolactin: Most individuals with PCOS have reference-range levels of prolactin, although 20% have mildly elevated levels.[23] Prolactin may augment adrenal androgen secretion in this subset of patients.

Therapy

1. Medroxyprogesterone acetate (10 mg) can be given for 10 days every 1 to 3 months to induce withdrawal bleeding, or estrogen and progestins can be given as oral contraceptive pills or estradiol patch with progesterone administered orally. The addition of spironolactone can be considered for significant clinical hyperandrogenism unresponsive to estrogen/progestin therapy.

2. Insulin-sensitizing agents, specifically metformin, should be considered as first-line therapy, particularly in adolescent girls with clinical (acanthosis nigricans, Fig. 49.4) or biochemical evidence of hyperinsulinism.

3. Weight loss in obese girls with PCOS reduces insulin resistance and insulin levels, thereby reducing testosterone secretion and PCOS symptoms. Lifestyle modification with dietary and activity interventions should be the initial intervention in obese women with PCOS. However, weight loss is difficult to achieve. Older AYAs with morbid obesity (BMI >40 kg/m²) or BMI >35 kg/m² and secondary complications, such as hypertension, sleep apnea, cardiovascular disease, and PCOS, may be candidates for medication use and/or surgical therapy.

4. Infertility is usually not a concern in the adolescent patient. However, when fertility is desired, clomiphene citrate and/or metformin therapy may be used to stimulate ovulation. Exogenous gonadotropins are also used in research and clinical practice.

Therapy for Hirsutism

Therapies outlined above including estrogen and progestin, weight loss, and metformin may improve hirsutism. Other therapies include:

1. *Cosmetic approaches*: Camouflaging with heavy makeup, bleaching, and removal with physical methods such as shaving, plucking, or waxing. Chemical depilatories are designed to use on specific body locations. Electrolysis or thermodestruction of the hair follicle retards regrowth for days to weeks and can permanently remove hair. Photothermodestruction with a laser is expensive but can offer long periods between regrowth and can lead to permanent hair loss. All of these methods can cause skin irritation, folliculitis, and pigment abnormalities.

2. *Topical therapy*: Eflornithine hydrochloride 13.9% cream has been approved by the US Food and Drug Administration for the treatment of unwanted facial hair. The agent is an irreversible inhibitor of L-ornithine decarboxylase, an enzyme that is important in controlling hair growth and proliferation. The agent slows and miniaturizes hairs that are present. Side effects can include rash and stinging, and occurred in <10% of patients in early trials.

3. *Anti-androgenic agents:* Spironolactone works primarily by competing at the androgen receptor peripherally, and also inhibits 5α-reductase. The starting dose is usually 50 mg/day and is typically effective between approximately 75 and 200 mg/day. The medication can be increased by 25 mg every 1 to 2 weeks. However, the maximal response is not seen for 6 months to 1 year. Side effects are minimal but can include dry mouth, diuresis, fatigue, menstrual spotting, and hyperkalemia on laboratory evaluation. The drug is contraindicated during pregnancy, because it can lead to feminization of the male fetus. Therefore, an oral contraceptive should be prescribed simultaneously.

Screening and Therapy for Metabolic Abnormalities

Because of the potential for abnormal glucose tolerance (insulin resistance) and hyperlipidemia, it is important to evaluate these factors in adolescents with PCOS and to consider therapeutic interventions. Many clinicians and scientists favor the treatment of insulin resistance in women with PCOS with insulin-sensitizing medications because the reduction of hyperandrogenism by hormonal therapy does not correct the underlying hyperinsulinism. The use of insulin-sensitizing agents such as metformin may reduce the risk of hyperinsulinism, type 2 diabetes, and the metabolic syndrome.[25] In addition, the reduction in hyperinsulinism has been shown to induce ovulation and regulation of menstrual cycling.[26] Studies have shown that the use of metformin in young adolescents with PCOS may regulate menstrual cycling and reduce the clinical hyperandrogenic effects. In addition, metformin may be able to prevent the development of the PCOS phenotype in young girls with premature adrenarche.[27] These remain areas of active research.

Young women with PCOS should have their cholesterol, triglycerides, LDL, and HDL measured, according to the guidelines for high-risk children and adolescents. In addition, these women should be checked and followed for impaired glucose tolerance and diabetes. The screening evaluation for abnormal glucose metabolism is an area of continued debate. The current American Diabetes Association recommendations[28] for pediatric diabetes screening include the evaluation of a fasting blood sugar every 2 years, beginning at age 10 years or puberty, in all children who are overweight, as defined by a BMI of greater than the 85th percentile for age and sex, weight for height >85th percentile, or weight >120% of ideal for height plus any two of the designated risk factors:

• Family history of type 2 diabetes mellitus in a first- or second-degree relative
• High-risk race/ethnicity (native American, African American, Hispanic, Asian/Pacific Islander)
• Signs of insulin resistance or conditions associated with insulin resistance (acanthosis nigricans, hypertension, dyslipidemia, PCOS).

PCOS is listed as a condition associated with insulin resistance, and therefore, the diagnosis of PCOS in an adolescent who is obese and has a family history of diabetes or a high-risk ethnicity meets the criteria for a fasting blood glucose screening. However, there is growing evidence that lean adolescents with PCOS may also be at risk for insulin resistance and that both lean and obese girls with PCOS may benefit from oral glucose tolerance testing (oral glucose challenge of 1.75 g/kg up to a maximum of 75 g). The use of HgbA1C (≥6.5%), as a screening tool for diabetes, was agreed upon by an International Expert Committee in 2009. However, the use of HgbA1C remains controversial in this population. The absence of obesity and acanthosis nigricans does not rule out insulin resistance in the presence of clinical hyperandrogenism. Diagnosis and continued monitoring of these individuals may reduce the risk of metabolic and cardiovascular disease. Reduction in insulin resistance is important, and diet and exercise are critical first-line steps. Insulin-sensitizing medications may prove beneficial, but a consensus regarding guidelines for their usage has not been reached to date for adolescents with PCOS. Patients with PCOS should be treated medically for diabetes mellitus and hyperlipidemia as standard for adolescent patients.

HIRSUTISM

Differential Diagnosis

The differential diagnosis for hirsutism is presented in **Table 49.2**, with data obtained from an original sample of more than 1,000 women.[29] Note that PCOS is the most common cause of androgen excess and one of the most common endocrine abnormalities in female adolescents and young women. Other causes may include:

1. Idiopathic hirsutism
2. Ovarian causes
   a. Tumor: Sertoli–Leydig cell tumor, lipoid cell tumor, hilar cell tumor
   b. Pregnancy: Luteoma
3. Adrenal causes
   a. CAH: 21-hydroxylase or 11-hydroxylase deficiency, classic or nonclassic, late onset
   b. Tumors: Adenomas and carcinomas
   c. Cushing syndrome

4. Nonandrogenic causes of hirsutism
   a. Genetic: Racial, familial
   b. Physiological: Pregnancy, puberty, postmenopausal
   c. Endocrine: Hypothyroidism, acromegaly
   d. Porphyria
   e. Hamartomas
   f. Drug-induced: Drugs that cause hirsutism by increasing androgenic activity include testosterone, DHEAS, danazol, corticotropin, high-dose corticosteroids, metyrapone, phenothiazine derivatives, anabolic steroids, androgenic progestin, and acetazolamide. Nonandrogenic drugs that can cause hirsutism include cyclosporine, phenytoin, diazoxide, triamterene-hydrochlorothiazide, minoxidil, hexachlorobenzene, penicillamine and psoralens, and minoxidil. Valproate is also associated with menstrual disturbances and hyperandrogenism.
   g. Syndromes: Hurler syndrome, de Lange syndrome

Indications for Further Evaluation

1. Rapid onset of signs and symptoms
2. Virilization
3. Symptoms suggesting Cushing syndrome (e.g., weight gain, slow linear growth, weakness, or hypertension)

Evaluation
Physical Examination

1. Extent of hirsutism: Grading systems are available that enable a clinician to quantitate the degree of hirsutism in a patient. The Ferriman–Gallwey hirsutism scoring system (**Fig. 49.7**)[30] enables clinicians to quantify the extent of hirsutism

TABLE 49.2

Differential Diagnosis of Clinically Apparent Androgen Excess

Diagnosis	Sample (%)	Key History/Examination Findings	Additional Testing
Polycystic ovary syndrome (PCOS)	82.0	±Irregular menses, slow-onset hirsutism, obesity, infertility, diabetes, hypertension, family history of PCOS, diabetes	Fasting glucose, insulin and lipid profile, blood pressure (BP), ultrasonography positive for multiple ovarian cysts
Hyperandrogenism with hirsutism, normal ovulation	6.8	Regular menses, acne, hirsutism without detectable endocrine cause	Elevated androgen levels and normal serum progesterone in luteal phase
Idiopathic hirsutism	4.7	Regular menses, hirsutism, possible overactive 5 α-reductase activity in skin and hair follicle	Normal androgen levels, normal serum progesterone in luteal phase
Hyperandrogenic insulin-resistant acanthosis nigricans (HAIR-AN)	3.1	Brown velvety patches of skin (acanthosis nigricans), obesity, hypertension, hyperlipidemia, strong family history of diabetes	Fasting glucose and lipid profile, BP, fasting insulin level >80 µIU/mL or insulin level >300 on 3-h glucose tolerance test
21-Hydroxylase nonclassic adrenal hyperplasia (late-onset CAH)	1.6	Severe hirsutism or virilization, strong family history of CAH, short stature, signs of virilization, more common in Ashkenazi Jews of Eastern European descent	17-OHP level before and after ACTH stimulation test elevated, CYP21 genotyping
Hypothyroidism	0.7	Fatigue, weight gain, history of thyroid ablation and untreated hypothyroidism, amenorrhea	TSH elevated
Hyperprolactinemia	0.3	Amenorrhea, galactorrhea, infertility	Prolactin elevated
Androgenic secreting neoplasm	0.2	Pelvic masses, rapid-onset hirsutism or virilization	Pelvic ultrasonography or abdomen/pelvic CT scan
Cushing syndrome	0	Hypertension, buffalo hump, purple striae, truncal obesity	Elevated BP, positive urinary 24-hour free cortisol, salivary cortisol, and/or dexamethasone suppression test

ACTH, adrenocorticotpic hormone; TSH, thyroid-stimulating hormone; CT, computed tomography; 17-OHP, 17-hydroxyprogesterone.

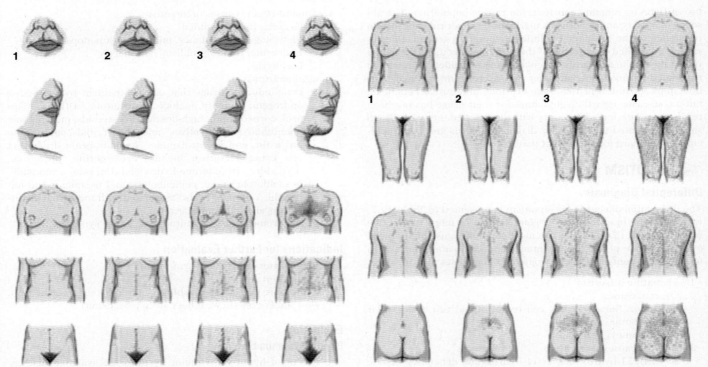

FIGURE 49.7 Ferriman–Gallwey hirsutism scoring system. Each of the nine body areas most sensitive to androgen is assigned a score from 0 (no hair) to 4 (frankly virile), and these separate scores are summed to provide a hormonal hirsutism score. (Reproduced from Hatch R, Rosefield RL, Kim MH, et al. Hirsutism: implications, etiology, and management. *Am J Obstet Gynecol* 1981;140:815–830, ©Elsevier)

by circling an individual's appearance on a flow sheet and recording the total score on the patient's chart. These scores can be helpful for making comparative assessments between visits and for appraising the efficacy of a particular therapy. Some terminal hair on the lower abdomen, face, and around the areola is normal, but hair on the upper back, shoulders, sternum, and upper abdomen suggests more marked androgen activity.

2. Stigmata of Cushing syndrome (e.g., truncal obesity, striae, posterior fat pad)
3. Signs of virilization: Check clitoral diameter or index. A clitoral diameter >5 mm is abnormal. The clitoral index is the product of the vertical and horizontal dimensions of the glans. The normal range is 9 to 35 mm^2; a clitoral index >100 mm^2 suggests virilization.

Laboratory Evaluation

The goals of the laboratory evaluation include demonstrating androgen excess and locating the source of the excess.

1. Measuring androgen excess
   a. Plasma testosterone (free and total)
   b. DHEAS: Levels >700 µg/dL suggest significant adrenal androgen production. An adrenal tumor must be ruled out. Rarely, PCOS, CAH, or an ovarian tumor will result in levels this high.
   c. 17-OHP: This hormone should only be measured in the morning (ideally between 7 and 9 a.m.). This is characteristically elevated in patients with CAH due to 21-hydroxylase deficiency. One can also measure 11-deoxycortisol in the morning to rule out 11-hydroxylase deficiency if suspected clinically.
2. Locating the source of androgen excess
   a. If male levels of testosterone or very elevated DHEAS levels are obtained, or a mass is felt on examination, perform an ultrasonography or MRI scan of adrenal glands and ovaries.

b. If elevated androgen levels and signs suggest hypercortisolism, perform a screening for Cushings: 24-hour urine for free cortisol or midnight salivary cortisol. This can be followed by a dexamethasone suppression test.
   • An ovarian source is suggested by cortisol suppression, but a lack of androgen suppression. An ultrasonography of the ovaries is helpful in this instance.
   • Cushing syndrome or an adrenal tumor is suggested by lack of cortisol suppression.
c. If 17-OHP level is elevated, perform an ACTH stimulation test. This is helpful in differentiating normal and idiopathic hirsute females from those with late-onset CAH due to incomplete 21-hydroxylase deficiency.

To perform the test measure a baseline 17-OHP and repeat a serum level 60 minutes after 0.25 mg of ACTH is administered intravenously. This test can also be used to rule out less common forms of late-onset CAH due to 11-hydroxylase or 3β-hydroxysteroid dehydrogenase deficiency by measuring the appropriate adrenal hormone values pre- and poststimulation.

Therapeutic considerations for hirsutism are discussed above under PCOS therapy.

REFERENCES

1. Biro FM, Greenspan LC, Galvez MP, et al. Onset of breast development in a longitudinal cohort. *Pediatrics* 2013;132(6):1019–1027.
2. Gordon CM. Clinical practice. Functional hypothalamic amenorrhea. *N Engl J Med* 2010;363(4):365–371.
3. Kasippillai T, MacArthur DG, Kirby A, et al. Mutations in eIF4ENIF1 are associated with primary ovarian insufficiency. *J Clin Endocrinol Metab* 2013;98(9): E1534–E1539.
4. Nattiv A, Loucks AB, Manore MM, et al. American College of Sports Medicine position stand. The female athlete triad. *Med Sci Sports Exerc* 2007;39(10): 867–1882.
5. American Academy of Pediatrics. Committee on Sports Medicine and Fitness. Medical concerns in the female athlete. *Pediatrics* 2000;106(3):610–613.
6. Goodman LR, Warren MP. The female athlete and menstrual function. *Curr Opin Obstet Gynecol* 2005;17(5):466–470.

7. Nichols JF, Rauh MJ, Lawson MJ, et al. Prevalence of the female athlete triad syndrome among high school athletes. *Arch Pediatr Adolesc Med* 2006;160(2):137–142.
8. Welt CK, Chan JL, Bullen J, et al. Recombinant human leptin in women with hypothalamic amenorrhea. *N Engl J Med* 2004;351(10):987–997.
9. Reed JL, De Souza MJ, Williams NI. Changes in energy availability across the season in Division I female soccer players. *J Sports Sci* 2013;31(3):314–324.
10. Misra M, Katzman D, Miller KK, et al. Physiologic estrogen replacement increases bone density in adolescent girls with anorexia nervosa. *J Bone Miner Res* 2011;26(10):2430–2438.
11. DiVasta AD, Feldman HA, Giancaterino C, et al. The effect of gonadal and adrenal steroid therapy on skeletal health in adolescents and young women with anorexia nervosa. *Metabolism* 2012;61(7):1010–1020.
12. Kenigsberg L, Balachandar S, Prasad K, et al. Exogenous pubertal induction by oral versus transdermal estrogen therapy. *J Pediatr Adolesc Gynecol* 2013;26(2):71–79.
13. Gordon CM, Grace E, Emans SJ, et al. Effects of oral dehydroepiandrosterone on bone density in young women with anorexia nervosa: a randomized trial. *J Clin Endocrinol Metab* 2002;87(11):4935–4941.
14. Grinspoon S, Thomas L, Miller K, et al. Effects of recombinant human IGF-I and oral contraceptive administration on bone density in anorexia nervosa. *J Clin Endocrinol Metab* 2002;87(6):2883–2891.
15. Miller KK, Grieco KA, Klibanski A. Testosterone administration in women with anorexia nervosa. *J Clin Endocrinol Metab* 2005;90(3):1428–1433.
16. Rosenfield RL, Mortensen M, Wroblewski K, et al. Determination of the source of androgen excess in functionally atypical polycystic ovary syndrome by a short dexamethasone androgen-suppression test and a low-dose ACTH test. *Hum Reprod* 2011;26(11):3138–3146.
17. Christensen SB, Black MH, Smith N, et al. Prevalence of polycystic ovary syndrome in adolescents. *Fertil Steril* 2013;100(2):470–477.
18. Palmert MR, Gordon CM, Kartashov AI, et al. Screening for abnormal glucose tolerance in adolescents with polycystic ovary syndrome. *J Clin Endocrinol Metab* 2002;87(3):1017–1023.
19. Ibanez L, Dimartino-Nardi J, Potau N, et al. Premature adrenarche—normal variant or forerunner of adult disease? *Endocr Rev* 2000;21(6):671–696.
20. Legro RS. The genetics of polycystic ovary syndrome. *Am J Med* 1995;98(1A):9S–16S.
21. Isojarvi JI, Laatikainen TJ, Pakarinen AJ, et al. Polycystic ovaries and hyperandrogenism in women taking valproate for epilepsy. *N Engl J Med* 1993;329(19):1383–1388.
22. Lobo RA, Carmina E. The importance of diagnosing the polycystic ovary syndrome. *Ann Intern Med* 2000;132(12):989–993.
23. Luciano AA, Chapler FK, Sherman BM. Hyperprolactinemia in polycystic ovary syndrome. *Fertil Steril* 1984;41(5):719–725.
24. Dewailly D, Lujan ME, Carmina E, et al. Definition and significance of polycystic ovarian morphology: a task force report from the Androgen Excess and Polycystic Ovary Syndrome Society. *Hum Reprod Update* 2014;20(3):334–352.
25. Knowler WC, Barrett-Connor E, Fowler SE, et al.; Diabetes Prevention Program Research Group. Reduction in the incidence of type 2 diabetes with lifestyle intervention or metformin. *N Engl J Med* 2002;346(6):393–403.
26. Baillargeon JP, Iuorno MJ, Nestler JE. Insulin sensitizers for polycystic ovary syndrome. *Clin Obstet Gynecol* 2003;46(2):325–340.
27. Ibanez L, Valls C, Marcos MV, et al. Insulin sensitization for girls with precocious pubarche and with risk for polycystic ovary syndrome: effects of prepubertal initiation and postpubertal discontinuation of metformin treatment. *J Clin Endocrinol Metab* 2004;89(9):4331–4337.
28. American Diabetes Association. Type 2 diabetes in children and adolescents. *Pediatrics* 2000;105(3, Pt 1):671–680.
29. Azziz R, Sanchez LA, Knochenhauer ES, et al. Androgen excess in women: experience with over 1000 consecutive patients. *J Clin Endocrinol Metabol* 2004;89(2):453–462.
30. Ferriman D, Gallwey JD. Clinical assessment of body hair growth in women. *J Clin Endocrinol Metab* 1961;21:1440–1447.

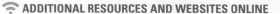 **ADDITIONAL RESOURCES AND WEBSITES ONLINE**

50 Pap Smears and Abnormal Cervical Cytology

Anna-Barbara Moscicki

PREVALENCE OF ABNORMAL CYTOLOGY

The prevalence of abnormal cytology peaks in adolescent and young adult (AYA) women in the US, with rates ranging from 3% to 14%.[1] This is not surprising since this parallels the peak prevalence of human papillomavirus (HPV) of around 25% to 41% in the US and European women under 25 years of age.[2,3] The high rates of HPV and abnormal cytology underscore the vulnerability of young women to HPV. It is estimated that over 60% of young sexually active women will acquire HPV at least once within 3 to 5 years after the onset of sexual intercourse.[4] Repeated infections are also common in young women, with 70% to 80% acquiring second and third infections within 3 years of the initial infection.[5] Infection with multiple HPV types is also common. Fortunately, most of these infections and their corresponding abnormal cytologies spontaneously regress.[1]

The majority of the abnormal cytology is low-grade squamous intraepithelial lesions (LSILs), which are considered benign changes due to HPV infection. These lesions are found to be associated with both low (nononcogenic) and high (oncogenic) risk HPV types.[6] High-grade squamous intraepithelial lesions (HSILs) are considered true precancer lesions. Although the rates of these are substantially lower than those of LSILs in adolescents and young women, the prevalence of both of these lesions peaks in young adult women less than 30 years of age.[1] The prevalence of cytologic LSIL and HSIL among 21- to 24-year-olds is 6.5% and 0.7%, respectively, and among 25- to 29-year-olds is 3.8% and 0.4%.[7] Because of the insensitive nature of cytology, the actual rates of histologic HSIL[8] are higher. Studies that incorporate colposcopy and biopsy show that the rate of histologic HSIL is higher than cytology. In one large study, the prevalence of histologic HSIL was 1.3% and 2.1% in 21 to 24 and 25- to 29-year-olds, respectively.[7] The natural history of HSIL is also influenced by age. HSIL in young women is much more likely to regress spontaneously than in older women. One study of AYA women aged 13 to 24 years of age showed that 70% of biopsy-proven HSIL regressed over 3 years.[9] Of those HPV 16/18 associated, 50% regressed. Several other studies of young women showed similar results.[10] Although the reasons for this are not completely clear, it is likely that HSIL develops relatively quickly after infection in cells vulnerable to dysplasia. Consequently, HSIL in a young woman likely represents a relatively recent abnormality when the chances of clearance are the greatest. HSIL detected in an older woman is far more likely due to a long-term persistent infection of which the immune system fails to clear.[11]

VULNERABILITY OF THE CERVIX TO HPV

The importance of the cervical transformation zone (TZ) in cancer development has long been recognized. It is useful to review the formation of this zone and the natural history of HPV in understanding abnormal cervical changes.[12]

In Utero and Prepuberty

During embryological development, the müllerian ducts give rise to the fallopian tubes, uterus, and vagina. These structures in the fetus are lined by immature cuboidal epithelium (which becomes columnar epithelium) from the uterus to the hymenal ring. The urogenital sinus epithelium grows up the vaginal vault and replaces the native epithelium up to the ectocervix with squamous epithelium. This replacement is usually incomplete, creating an abrupt squamocolumnar junction (SCJ) on the ectocervix. Squamous metaplasia is a process during which undifferentiated columnar cells transform themselves into squamous epithelium. However, the process is relatively quiescent until puberty, resulting in little changes to the SCJ during childhood. The area of columnar epithelium seen on the ectocervix is referred to as *ectopy*.

Pubertal Metaplastic Changes

With puberty, the pH level of the vagina drops and this is thought to be secondary to rising levels of estrogen, which enhances glycogen production of the squamous cells, which in turn provides a source of energy for the vaginal flora, specifically lactobacilli. Lactobacilli convert glycogen to lactic acids, resulting in a lowered pH level. This new acidic environment most likely contributes to the augmentation of the squamous metaplastic process, resulting in relatively rapid replacement of columnar epithelium by squamous epithelium, hence referred to as the TZ (Fig. 50.1).

The TZ is a relatively fluid area of definition, because it represents the area between the original SCJ and the current SCJ. By the early 30s, most women have had substantial replacement of their columnar epithelium, resulting in little to no visible ectopy. Although squamous metaplasia continues, it is now found well inside the endocervical canal.

Squamous epithelium is generally 60 to 80 cell layers thick and appears smooth and pink covering the vagina and a portion of the ectocervix. *Columnar epithelium* is a single-layer, mucus-producing, tall epithelium extending between the endometrium and the squamous epithelium. This thin layer results in a red

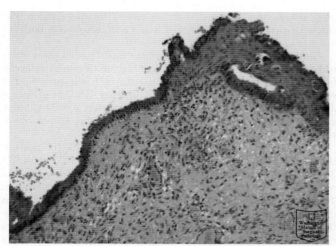

FIGURE 50.1 Replacement of cervical columnar epithelium by squamous epithelium (the transformation zone). From Humphrey PA, Dehner LP, Pfeifer JD. Washington Manual of Surgical Pathology. Philadelphia: Lippincott Williams & Wilkins, 2008.

appearance due to its increased vascularity and has an irregular surface with long papillae and deep clefts. During puberty, the TZ is a combination of squamous and columnar epithelium as well as metaplastic tissue. Hallmarks of metaplasia seen on magnification include fusion of the villi causing a loss of translucency to the columnar epithelium. Eventually the papillary structures are lost, and the new surface takes on a less translucent appearance more similar to squamous epithelium. As this process is somewhat piecemeal, the examiner can often see reminants of columnar epithelium in small pockets. When these openings become completely closed by squamous epithelium, the mucus-secreting epithelium may continue to produce mucus. If that mucus becomes inspissated, the gland dilates and a *nabothian cyst* results. Nabothian cysts eventually self-destruct from the pressure of the inspissated mucus.

Metaplasia and HPV Infections

The vulnerability of the cervix to HPV infections is most likely related to the process of squamous metaplasia.[13] This association reflects the natural life cycle of HPV and its dependence on host cell proliferation and differentiation, both characteristics of squamous metaplasia. Initial HPV infections are thought to occur by invasion of cells of the basal epithelium. Disruption of the epithelium by inflammation or trauma may cause an increased risk for infection with HPV. Differentiation of these basal cells to well-differentiated squamous epithelial cells supports HPV replication by allowing expression of certain viral proteins at different layers of differentiation. The expression of the oncogenic proteins E_6 and E_7 in turn causes histological changes, which include abnormal cell proliferation, and the appearance of abnormal mitotic figures, both features of SIL. Features that are mild in nature and restricted to the basal and parabasal areas are referred to as LSIL. When these features become more extensive and extend into the upper half of the epithelium, the changes are referred to as HSIL. These changes coincide with increased expression of the oncogenes E_6 and E_7. Consequently, both LSIL and HSIL are pathological changes due to HPV infection.

⬤ CERVICAL DYSPLASIA

Impact of Cofactors

HPV infection is clearly the causative factor for cervical SIL and cancer, and sexual behavior is the strongest risk for HPV infections specifically reporting new sexual partner or having a

nonmonogamous relationship.[5,14] Acquiring other sexually transmitted infections (STIs) also increases the risk, which may represent a break in the cervical barrier due to inflammation caused by the STI or reflects the "at risk" partner. Condom use also shows some protection against HPV acquisition underscoring important counseling messages to young women.

Causes of cervical cancer are more complex. Because the rates of HPV are 100 to 700 times more common than invasive cancers, it is assumed that HPV is necessary but not sufficient for the development of cancer. Most HPV infections are quickly eliminated by the host's innate and adaptive immune responses.[15,16] Innate responses are likely responsible for rapid clearance, whereas cell-mediated immune responses are important in clearing established infections as well as offering protection from re-exposure. This immune response is likely responsible for the observation that with age the prevalence of HPV declines. In comparison, lack of an adequate immune response results in persistence of HPV infection, and in turn, HPV persistence is a strong risk for the development of HSIL and cervical cancer.[11] In a study of young women, HPV 16 persistence at 2 years was associated with a 50% risk of CIN 3 within 12 years.[11] HPV persistence is a common problem among persons with immunodeficiencies including human immunodeficiency virus (HIV) infection.[17]

Another factor associated with cancer development is tobacco exposure. Even when adjusted for numbers of sex partners, women who smoke have a higher risk of developing cervical SIL and invasive cancers than nonsmokers.[18] Other risk factors implicated include *Chlamydia trachomatis* infections, multiparity, and history of prolonged oral contraceptive use.[1,19–21] Final molecular events leading to cancer have not been defined, but include viral integration into the host chromosome and activation of telomerase to lengthen chromosomes and avoid physiologic cell senescence.[22]

Cervical Screening Tests

Because HPV infections are common in young women and rarely ever become cancerous during this period, screening for cervical cancer in this age-group is not cost effective and leads to inappropriate treatment and potential harm.[23] The most recent guidelines for the initiation and frequency of cervical cancer screening recommend using either the Pap smear or liquid-based cytology (Table 50.1) and to start screening at age 21 years with screening at 3-year intervals.[24,25] For HIV-infected women, screening should begin once sexually active. At 30 years of age, screening can also include co-testing with HPV DNA. The power of HPV testing in older women is the negative predictive value—that is if HPV is not present, then there is no cancer. HPV testing is not recommended in younger women since the high rates of infection and low cancer risk result in a test with an extremely low positive predictive value. With these less frequent screening recommendations, it is important to continue annual STI screening.

Recently, the FDA approved a commercial HPV DNA test for primary cervical cancer screening for women ages 25 and older.[26] If a woman is HPV 16/18 positive, referral to colposcopy is recommended. If the woman is positive for non-16/18 high-risk (HR) HPV, then triage to cytology is recommended with referral to colposcopy if cytology is found to have atypical squamous cells of undetermined significance (ASC-US) or worse. If cytology is normal, then the HPV test is repeated in one year. If the HPV test is negative, then routine screening in 3 years is recommended. The recommendations to start this screening at 25 years of age are controversial.

The follow-up evaluation required for benign Pap smear findings not associated with neoplastic changes is shown in Table 50.2. Current triage practices for abnormal cytology changes in young adult women are outlined in the following sections.[27]

Recommendations for Young Adult Women (21 to 24 Years)

HPV Testing: General Considerations

HR HPV testing is not recommended in young women under the age of 25 years including triage for ASC-US or in follow-up of abnormal

TABLE 50.1

Guidelines for Initiation and Frequency of Cervical Cancer Screening: Select US Organizations

Criteria	American Cancer Society (2012)	US Preventative Services Task Force (2012)
Begin screening	21 y	21 y
Screening interval		
Cytology (conventional or liquid-based)	Every 3 y	Every 3 y
Women aged ≥30 y		
HPV and cytology co-testing	Every 5 y[a] (preferred)	Every 5 y[a] (acceptable)
Cytology alone	Every 3 y (acceptable)	Every 3 y (acceptable)

[a]If HPV DNA negative and normal cytology.

TABLE 50.2

Follow-Up Evaluation Recommendations for Abnormal Pap Smear Findings

Pap Smear Finding	Recommendation
Insufficient quantity	Repeat Pap smears in 2–3 mo
Poor specimen	Repeat Pap smears in 2–3 mo
Air-drying artifact	Repeat Pap smears in 2–3 mo
No endocervical cells	No need to repeat Pap smear if patient has had normal test results previously and is compliant with therapy; if not, repeat in 2–3 mo
Endometrial cells	Normal if near menses or while using oral contraceptives or intrauterine devices; otherwise, recall and evaluate for endometritis
Trichomoniasis	Recall patient, perform sexually transmitted infection evaluation, and treat patient and partner
Yeast	Review chart; if no symptoms, no need to follow up
Inflammation	Consider recent coitus, infection
Reactive, reparative changes	Identify irritant, if possible; essentially normal

cytology. The one exception to this rule was in follow-up of young women for CIN 2, 3 (see below).

ASC-US and LSIL on Cytology

A recent publication highlighted data from a large database of over 1 million women, which found that among 21- to 24-year-old women, the 5-year cumulative risk of CIN 3+ after LSIL or ASC-US/HPV positive was lower among the 21- to 24-year-olds than women aged 25 to 29 or 30 to 64 years (3% to 4.4% versus 5% to 7% versus 5.2% to 6.8%, respectively) leading to different strategies by age-group.[28] ASC-US/HPV negative had extremely low risk of CIN 3+ in all age-groups. In addition, the risk of CIN 3+ among women with ASC-US not taking HPV status into account was only slightly lower than ASC-US/HPV positive in the young women. The rate of invasive cancer during this period was 0.03% among the 21- to

24-year-olds, underscoring the rare risk of missing cancer. The similar natural histories for ASC-US and LSIL resulted in both being managed similarly.

Guidelines recommended that women aged 21 to 24 years of age with ASC-US or LSIL have repeat cytology at 12-month intervals for 2 years. HPV testing or immediate referral to colposcopy is not recommended. If at any of the follow-up visits, HSIL or greater is diagnosed, referral to colposcopy is recommended. If at 24 months, a diagnosis of ASC-US or higher is made, referral to colposcopy is recommended.

Since the risk of CIN 3+ is higher among ASC-US/HPV positive than HPV negative, HPV testing is acceptable. Since the risk of CIN 3+ is extremely low, similar observation as discussed above is recommended if the HPV test is positive—that is, repeat cytology at 12-month intervals for 2 years. Immediate referral to colposcopy is not recommended. If the two consecutive cytology visits are negative, the woman can be returned to routine screening. If the reflex HPV testing is performed and is negative, it is recommended that the woman return to routine screening every 3 years.

It is recommended that adult women (25 years+) with ASC-US/HPV positive or LSIL are referred to colposcopy. If ASC-US is not triaged with HPV testing, then a repeat cytology is recommended in 12 months. If persistent ASC-US or greater, referral to colposcopy is recommended; http://www.asccp.org/Guidelines-2/Management-Guidelines-2.

ASC-H and HSIL

Women with ASC suggestive of HSIL (ASC-H) and HSIL cytology reports are managed similar to adults by immediate referral to colposcopy. This is because women aged 21 to 24 have similar CIN 3+ risks as older women with these cytologic diagnosis. Management of young women with ASC-H and HSIL differs from older women in that immediate loop electrocautery excision procedure (LEEP) without histologic confirmation of CIN 3 is not acceptable. This is because many young women are likely to have regression of HSIL. When no lesion is seen, random biopsy and ECC are recommended.

When CIN 2+ is not identified by histology in young women with ASC-H and HSIL, observation is recommended by colposcopy and cytology at 6-month intervals up to 24 months, provided the examination is adequate and endocervical assessment is negative or CIN 1. If at any follow-up visit CIN 2, 3 is identified, the woman should be managed per CIN 2, 3 guidelines (see below), which can also be an observation. If during follow-up high-grade lesions are seen on colposcopy or HSIL persists at 1 year, re-biopsy is recommended. If HSIL persists at the 24-month follow-up by cytology, histology, or colposcopy, a diagnostic excisional procedure is recommended (i.e., LEEP/loop excision of the TZ). A diagnostic excisional procedure is also recommended for this age-group if the colposcopy is unsatisfactory (i.e., assessment of the TZ is unsatisfactory) or ungraded CIN or CIN 2+ is identified on endocervical sampling. Women can return to routine screening after two consecutive visits with negative cytology and no evidence of high-grade colposcopy lesions. http://www.asccp.org/Guidelines-2/Management-Guidelines-2.

Management of Histologic LSIL (CIN 1)

Because over 90% of CIN 1 will regress spontaneously in young and adult women, treatment of CIN 1 is not recommended at any age. Follow-up of histologically diagnosed CIN 1 depends on the referral cytology. If CIN 1 is diagnosed after ASC-US/LSIL cytology, follow-up is similar to those recommended for ASC-US/LSIL cytology with cytology at 12-month intervals. ASC-H or HSIL at any visit warrants referral back to colposcopy. ASC-US or LSIL can be followed unless persistent at 24 months where referral to back to colposcopy is recommended. After two consecutive negative tests, routine screening is recommended. If CIN 1 is diagnosed after ASC-H or HSIL referral and there is adequate colposcopy, observation with colposcopy and cytology is recommended as above as for ASC-H and HSIL cytology. If inadequate colposcopy or ungraded CIN or CIN 2+ is seen on endocervical sampling, a diagnostic excisional procedure is recommended; http://www.ascep.org/Guidelines-2/Management-Guidelines-2.

Management of Histologic HSIL (CIN 2, 3)

Since a significant proportion of young women will show regression of CIN 2, 3 lesions,[9] it is recommended that if the colposcopic assessment is adequate, observation is preferred and treatment is optional. Of note, the new histologic terminology uses the similar terms as cytology: LSIL for CIN 1 and HSIL for CIN 2 or 3.[8,29] When HSIL/CIN 2 is specified, observation is preferred, and when HSIL/CIN 3 is specified or colposcopy is inadequate, treatment is recommended. Observation is similar as described for HSIL cytology with colposcopy and cytology performed at 6-month intervals for 12 months. If the lesion progresses to CIN 3 or greater by colposcopy or HSIL is persistent at 1 year, repeat biopsy is recommended. If CIN 2, 3 persists at 24 months, treatment is recommended. After two consecutive negative cytology results, an additional co-test (HPV and cytology) is recommended. This is the one exception where HPV testing is recommended in young women. This is because the sensitivity of HPV is greater than cytology alone in detecting CIN 3+ lesions. Women with CIN 2, 3 have the highest risk of CIN 3+, regardless of age. If co-testing is negative, then repeat co-testing is recommended in 3 years. Colposcopy referral is recommended if either of the co-tests are abnormal.

Cervical cancer screening for women aged 30 and older can be found at www.ascep.org. These guidelines do not include HIV-infected adolescents because progression to HSIL is common.[30]

Therapy for Cervical Dysplasia

The principle in developing a treatment plan is that cervical dysplasia, specifically HSIL, is treated to prevent progression to cancer. If the lesions are confined to the ectocervix, a wide range of treatment options is available (**Table 50.3**).

1. Avoid both diagnostic and treatment steps at same procedure: One practice to be avoided, particularly in young women, is to combine the diagnostic and treatment steps by performing colposcopic examination to rule out invasion and excising the T-zone by a LEEP without biopsy confirmation. This practice is inappropriate. Approximately 90% of such referred adolescents have no HSIL found on the specimen on undergoing a LEEP, and the cost exceeds the benefit for patients without dysplasia with regard to side effects.[31] As can be seen in **Table 50.3**, each of the major treatment modalities has minimal adverse impacts when used once. However, because recurrent lesions may develop and require further treatment, the cumulative effects of multiple treatments (particularly LEEP) must be considered. A recent meta-analysis showed that excisional therapy has a higher rate of premature labor and low birth weight.[32] Ablative treatment for small lesions (less than 2 quadrants) may be preferable in young women with adequate colposcopy. Ablative therapy has less risk on future fertility than excisional procedures. Excisional therapy can also be targeted to the lesion itself, thus avoiding large excisions.

2. Screen for STIs: In general, screening for STIs before cryotherapy or LEEP is recommended to avoid the complications of PID. Because of the benign nature of histological CIN 1 in all ages, it is recommended that CIN 1 be observed and not treated. Observation of CIN 2 in compliant adolescents is also allowed (www.ascep.org and American College of Obstetricians-Gynecologists ACOG Committee Opinion, 2006).[33]

3. Smoking cessation advice: All women with dysplasia who smoke should be encouraged to stop smoking. Advise them that continued tobacco use increases susceptibility to cancer.

4. Condom Use: Condom use has been shown to decrease acquisition and enhance LSIL regression, so condom use should be encouraged.[34]

There is no recommendation to stop hormonal contraception during treatment. It is also not recommended to screen male partners of women with abnormal Pap smears for HPV infections because few studies have demonstrated HPV disease in this group.

Recommendations for treatment of cervical lesions change over time and differ based on the patient's age and other risk factors. Clinicians involved in the treatment of cervical lesions should refer to the American Society for Colposcopy and Cervical Pathology Web site where consensus recommendations are updated as they become available: http://www.ascep.org/consensus.html.

1. Prevention with HPV vaccines: HPV vaccines have been shown to have high efficacy in preventing HPV infection and its associated SIL, specifically if given before the onset of sexual activity. However, good efficacy was shown up to the age of 26 years in women and men.

TABLE 50.3		
Cervical Dysplasia Treatment Regimen Response Rates		
	Cryotherapy	**LEEP**
Response rate		
Single (%)	80	95
Repeated (%)	95	95
Advantages	Simple office-based procedure	SCJ on ectocervix
	Inexpensive	Can tailor to lesion
	Only mildly painful	Provides specimen for pathology
Disadvantages	Watery vaginal discharge for 4–6 wk	Expensive, more painful
	May not be as effective for large lesions or those that extend well onto the ectocervix	Bleeding complications Premature rupture of membrane in future
	New SCJ on endocervix	
	No specimen for pathology	
	Stenosis	

LEEP, loop electrocautery excision procedure; SCJ, squamocolumnar junction.

REFERENCES

1. Moscicki AB, Schiffman M, Burchell A, et al. Updating the natural history of human papillomavirus and anogenital cancers. *Vaccine* 2012;30 (suppl 5): F24–F33.
2. Forman D, de Martel C, Lacey CJ, et al. Global burden of human papillomavirus and related diseases. *Vaccine* 2012;30 (suppl 5):F12–F23.
3. Kjaer SK, Munk C, Junge J, et al. Carcinogenic HPV prevalence and age-specific type distribution in 40,382 women with normal cervical cytology, ASCUS/LSIL, HSIL, or cervical cancer: what is the potential for prevention? *Cancer Causes Control* 2014;25(2):179–189.
4. Winer RL, Feng Q, Hughes JP, et al. Risk of female human papillomavirus acquisition associated with first male sex partner. *J Infect Dis* 2008;197(2): 279–282.
5. Moscicki AB, Ma Y, Jonte J, et al. The role of sexual behavior and human papillomavirus persistence in predicting repeated infections with new human papillomavirus types. *Cancer Epidemiol Biomarkers Prev* 2010;19(8):2055–2065.
6. Guan P, Howell-Jones R, Li N, et al. Human papillomavirus types in 115,789 HPV-positive women: a meta-analysis from cervical infection to cancer. *Int J Cancer* 2012;131(10):2349–2359.
7. Wright TC Jr, Stoler MH, Behrens CM, et al. The ATHENA human papillomavirus study: design, methods, and baseline results. *Am J Obstet Gynecol* 2012;206(1):46 e1–e11.
8. Darragh TM, Colgan TJ, Cox JT, et al. The Lower Anogenital Squamous Terminology Standardization Project for HPV-associated lesions: background and consensus recommendations from the College of American Pathologists and the American Society for Colposcopy and Cervical Pathology. *J Low Genit Tract Dis* 2012;16(3):205–242.

9. Moscicki AB, Ma Y, Wibbelsman C, et al. Rate of and risks for regression of cervical intraepithelial neoplasia 2 in adolescents and young women. *Obstet Gynecol* 2010;116(6):1373–1380.

10. Monteiro DL, Trajano AJ, Russomano FB, et al. Prognosis of intraepithelial cervical lesion during adolescence in up to two years of follow-up. *J Pediatr Adolesc Gynecol* 2010;23(4):230–236.

11. Kjaer SK, Frederiksen K, Munk C, et al. Long-term absolute risk of cervical intraepithelial neoplasia grade 3 or worse following human papillomavirus infection: role of persistence. *J Natl Cancer Instit* 2010;102(19):1478–1488.

12. Moscicki AB, Singer A. The cervical epithelium during puberty and adolescence. In: Jordan JA, Singer A, eds. *The cervix.* 2nd ed. Malden: Blackwell, 2006:81–101.

13. Hwang LY, Ma Y, Shiboski SC, et al. Active squamous metaplasia of the cervical epithelium is associated with subsequent acquisition of human papillomavirus 16 infection among healthy young women. *J Infect Dis* 2012;206(4):504–511.

14. Moscicki AB, Ma Y, Farhat S, et al. Redetection of cervical human papillomavirus type 16 (HPV16) in women with a history of HPV16. *J Infect Dis* 2013;208(3):403–412.

15. Daud II, Scott ME, Ma Y, et al. Association between toll-like receptors expression and human papillomavirus type 16 persistence. *Int J Cancer* 2011;128(4):879–886.

16. Farhat S, Nakagawa M, Moscicki AB. Cell-mediated immune responses to human papillomavirus 16 E6 and E7 antigens as measured by interferon gamma enzyme-linked immunospot in women with cleared or persistent human papillomavirus infection. *Int J Gynecol Cancer* 2009;19(4):508–512.

17. Moscicki AB, Ellenberg JH, Fahrat S, et al. HPV persistence in HIV infected and uninfected adolescent girls: risk factors and differences by phylogenetic types. *J Infect Dis* 2004;190(1):37–45.

18. Roura E, Castellsague X, Pawlita M, et al. Smoking as a major risk factor for cervical cancer and pre-cancer: results from the EPIC cohort. *Int J Cancer* 2014;135(2):453–466.

19. Smith JS, Bosetti C, Munoz N, et al. Chlamydia trachomatis and invasive cervical cancer: a pooled analysis of the IARC multicentric case-control study. *Int J Cancer* 2004;111(3):431–439.

20. Smith JS, Green J, Berrington de Gonzalez A, et al. Cervical cancer and use of hormonal contraceptives: a systematic review. *Lancet* 2003;361(9364):1159–1167.

21. Arnheim Dahlstrom L, Andersson K, Luostarinen T, et al. Prospective seroepidemiologic study of human papillomavirus and other risk factors in cervical cancer. *Cancer Epidemiol Biomarkers Prev* 2011;20(12):2541–2450.

22. Galloway DA, Gewin LC, Myers H, et al. Regulation of telomerase by human papillomaviruses. *Cold Spring Harb Symp Quant Biol* 2005;70:209–215.

23. Sasieni P, Castanon A, Parkin DM. How many cervical cancers are prevented by treatment of screen-detected disease in young women? *Int J Cancer* 2009;124(2):461–464.

24. Moyer VA. Screening for cervical cancer: U.S. Preventive Services Task Force recommendation statement. *Ann Intern Med* 2012;156(12):880–891, W312.

25. Saslow D, Solomon D, Lawson HW, et al. American Cancer Society, American Society for Colposcopy and Cervical Pathology, and American Society for Clinical Pathology screening guidelines for the prevention and early detection of cervical cancer. *Am J Clin Pathol* 2012;137(4):516–542.

26. Huh WK, Ault KA, Chelmow D, et al. Use of primary high-risk human papillomavirus testing for cervical cancer screening: interim clinical guidance. *Gynecol Oncol* 2015;136(2):178–182.

27. Massad LS, Einstein MH, Huh WK, et al. 2012 updated consensus guidelines for the management of abnormal cervical cancer screening tests and cancer precursors. *Obstet Gynecolo* 2013;121(4):829–846.

28. Katki HA, Schiffman M, Castle PE, et al. Five-year risk of CIN 3+ to guide the management of women aged 21 to 24 years. *J Low Genit Tract Dis* 2013; 17 (5, suppl 1):S64–S68.

29. Waxman AG, Chelmow D, Darragh TM, et al. Revised terminology for cervical histopathology and its implications for management of high-grade squamous intraepithelial lesions of the cervix. *Obstet Gynecol* 2012;120(6):1465–1471.

30. Moscicki AB, Ellenberg JH, Crowley-Nowick P, et al. Risk of high grade squamous intra-epithelial lesions in HIV infected adolescents. *J Infect Dis* 2004;190(8):1413–1421.

31. Sadler L, Saftlas A, Wang W, et al. Treatment for cervical intraepithelial neoplasia and risk of preterm delivery. *JAMA* 2004;291:2100–2106.

32. Kyrgiou M, Koliopoulos G, Martin-Hirsch P, et al. Obstetric outcomes after conservative treatment for intraepithelial or early invasive cervical lesions: systematic review and meta-analysis. *Lancet* 2006;367(9509):489–498.

33. ACOG Committee Opinion. Evaluation and management of abnormal cervical cytology and histology in the adolescent. Number 330. *Obstet Gynecol* 2006;107(4):963–968.

34. Hogewoning CJ, Bleeker MC, van den Brule AJ, et al. Condom use promotes regression of cervical intraepithelial neoplasia and clearance of human papillomavirus: a randomized clinical trial. *Int J Cancer* 2003;107(5):811–816.

🛜 **ADDITIONAL RESOURCES AND WEBSITES ONLINE**

Vaginitis and Vaginosis

Sherine Patterson-Rose
Paula K. Braverman

- Bacterial vaginosis
- Trichomonas vaginalis
- Vaginitis
- Vulvovaginal candidiasis

VAGINA: NORMAL STATE

Vaginal Flora

Before the onset of puberty, the vagina is colonized with various bacterial species ranging from fecal flora to skin flora, resulting in a vaginal pH of >4.7. After puberty, the estrogen-stimulated epithelial cells produce more glycogen, and lactobacilli become predominant, comprising >95% of the normal flora. Metabolism of glycogen to lactic acid by the lactobacilli contributes to the lowering of the vaginal pH to <4.5 and helps to maintain a vaginal environment that appears to protect the individual from colonization by more pathogenic organisms. Some lactobacilli also produce hydrogen peroxide, a potential microbicide.[1]

Vaginal Secretions

Physiologic discharge may begin 6 to 12 months before menarche; these secretions may be copious but are not associated with odor or pruritus. During the menstrual cycle, changes can be noted in vaginal secretions, including little to no secretions to sticky white or clear profuse secretions. These secretions are a normal result of the changing hormonal milieu of the menstrual cycle.[1]

VULVOVAGINITIS IN PREPUBERTAL FEMALES

Most vulvovaginitis in prepubertal females is related to poor hygiene, tight clothing, or nonabsorbent underpants. Patients should be counseled regarding hygienic measures, and antibiotics should be prescribed only if a predominant organism is identified by culture. Usually, the organisms involved are either normal flora (i.e., lactobacilli, diphtheroids, streptococci, and *Staphylococcus epidermidis*) or gram-negative enteric organisms (i.e., *Escherichia coli*). Any sexually transmitted infection (STI) should prompt an investigation for sexual abuse.[1]

VULVOVAGINITIS AND VAGINOSIS IN PUBERTAL FEMALES: GENERAL APPROACH

Etiology

The three most common types of vaginitis are bacterial vaginosis (BV), vulvovaginal candidiasis (VVC), and *Trichomonas vaginalis* (TV). Other causes of discharge include hormonal contraceptives (estrogen effect), chemical irritants, foreign bodies (i.e., tampons), trauma, allergies, and poor hygiene. From the patient's perspective, vaginal discharge secondary to cervicitis from *Neisseria*

gonorrhoeae or *Chlamydia trachomatis* can be indistinguishable from discharge secondary to vaginitis.

Evaluation

1. *History:* It should include type, duration, and extent of symptoms (i.e., discharge, pruritus, odor, dyspareunia, dysuria, rash, pain); relation of symptoms to menses; frequency and type of sexual activity, and number of sexual partners; previous STIs; contraceptive history; medications, especially antibiotics and steroids; use of deodorants, soaps, lubricants, or douches; and history of immunosuppression.
2. *Examination:* It should include inspection of color, texture, origin (vaginal or cervical), adherence, and odor of the vaginal discharge; inspection of the perineum, vulva, vagina, and cervix for erythema, swelling, lesions, atrophy, trauma, and foreign bodies; and palpation of the introitus, uterus, and adnexa for tenderness or masses (Fig. 51.1).
3. *Laboratory:*
   a. The pH value of vaginal secretions is sampled from the anterior vaginal fornix or lateral vaginal wall. Cervical mucosa should not be sampled due to its higher pH of approximately 7.0.
   b. A saline wet mount should be examined under dry high power. Normal findings include <5 to 10 WBCs per high-power field or ≤1 WBC per epithelial cell, as well as lactobacilli. Abnormal findings include presence of "clue cells" (Fig. 51.2), defined as epithelial cells covered with bacteria and demonstrating indistinct borders and intracellular debris, as well as trichomonads. Motility of trichomonads decreases with time; thus, immediate inspection of wet mount is advised.
   c. A potassium hydroxide (KOH) slide should be prepared, and an immediate fishy, amine odor is called a positive "whiff test" and is suggestive of BV. Under dry high power, abnormal findings are yeast buds and pseudohyphae.
   d. Rapid or point-of-care tests (POCTs) for TV, VVC, and BV should be considered particularly when microscopy is not available in the office setting.
   e. In women with discharge, testing for *C. trachomatis* and *N. gonorrhoeae* is advised.

Table 51.1 outlines the causes of vaginitis in adolescents and young adults (AYAs).

BACTERIAL VAGINOSIS

BV is the most frequent cause of abnormal vaginal discharge and odor in postpubertal females. It is not a true vaginitis as it is not characterized by a marked inflammatory response of the vaginal mucosa, thus the term "vaginosis."

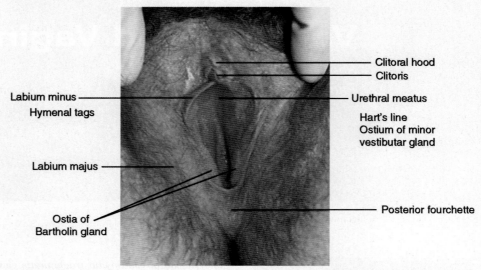

FIGURE 51.1 Normal vulva. (From Edwards L, Lynch PJ. *Genital dermatology atlas*. 2nd ed. Philadelphia, PA: Lippincott Williams & Wilkins, 2010.)

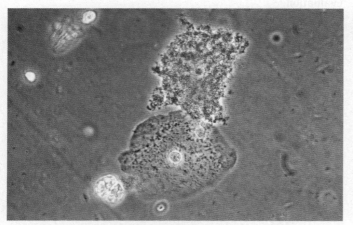

FIGURE 51.2 Clue cell. This photomicrograph of a vaginal smear specimen depicts two epithelial cells, a normal cell, and an epithelial cell with its exterior covered by bacteria, giving the cell a roughened, stippled appearance known as a "clue cell." Clue cells are a sign of bacterial vaginosis. (Image couresty of M. Rein and the Centers for Disease Control and Prevention Public Health Image Library ID 14574. Available at http://phil.cdc.gov/phil.)

Etiology

The BV syndrome consists of the replacement of normal lactobacilli in the vagina with *Gardnerella vaginalis*, anaerobic bacteria (i.e., *Bacteroides* sp, *Mobiluncus* sp), and *Mycoplasma hominis*. Lactobacilli help maintain an acid pH level that prevents the growth of *G. vaginalis* and anaerobic bacteria. In BV, there is loss of lactobacilli, leading to an elevated pH level, and high concentrations of *G. vaginalis*, anaerobes such as *Bacteroides* and *Mobiluncus* sp, and genital mycoplasmas.[2]

Epidemiology

1. Prevalence: Data show an overall prevalence of the disease of 29%; among those 14 to 19 years old the prevalence is 23%, and among those 20 to 29 years old the prevalence increases to 31%.[3]
2. Transmission: There continues to be controversy about the possibility of BV being transmitted sexually. Although BV has a higher prevalence among sexually active AYAs, it can also be found in females who are not sexually active. In addition, while the use of condoms seems to be a protective factor, treatment of partners does not prevent reoccurrence of the disease process.[2]

TABLE 51.1

Vaginal Discharge in the AYAs

Condition	Signs and Symptoms	Diagnosis in the Office Setting
Physiologic discharge	Clear gray discharge, no offensive odor, no burning or itching	Wet prep: Epithelial cells with no or few polymorphonuclear cells; no pathogens
Vulvovaginal candidiasis (VVC)	Curd-like discharge, intense burning, pruritus, usually no odor, often associated vulvitis	KOH/wet prep: budding yeast and pseudohyphae
Trichomoniasis	Pruritus; malodorous, frothy, yellow-green discharge; dysuria; rarely, abdominal pain	Wet prep: pear-shaped organism with motile flagella, point-of-care test
Bacterial Vaginosis (BV)	Homogenous, malodorous, gray-white discharge; usually mild or no pruritus or burning	Wet prep: epithelial cells covered with gram-negative rods, few polymorphonuclear leukocytes, pH >4.5
Retained tampon	Malodorous discharge, local discomfort	History and physical examination, history of exposure to deodorant spray or scented tampons
Irritant vaginitis	Vaginal discharge, erythema	History and physical examination

3. Predisposing factors: BV is associated with Black race/ethnicity, increased frequency of douching, cigarette smoking, and increased number of lifetime sex partners.[3]

Clinical Manifestations

1. Presentation: Up to 50% of cases are asymptomatic. Symptoms include vaginal pruritus and discharge, more noticeable after intercourse or after menses. The discharge is classically homogeneous, thin, and grayish-white, with a "fishy" odor.[2]
2. Examination may reveal the typical discharge adhering to the vaginal walls and odor.

3. Complications: BV is linked to serious sequelae including pelvic inflammatory disease (PID), increased human immunodeficiency virus (HIV) acquisition and transmission, infertility, and postsurgical/postabortal infection. Obstetric complications include chorioamnionitis, premature rupture of membranes, preterm labor, postpartum endometritis, and postabortal infection.[2]

Diagnosis

1. The Amsel criteria are used for clinical diagnosis. *Three* of the four clinical symptoms and signs are required: (1) homogeneous, grayish-white discharge; (2) vaginal pH level >4.5; (3) positive whiff test; and (4) wet prep showing "clue cells," that comprise at least 20% of the epithelial cells.[2]
2. Commercial tests are available including Affirm VP III, an automated DNA probe assay for detecting *G. vaginalis*;[4] OSOM BVBlue (Sekisui Diagnostics), a 10-minute Clinical Laboratory Improvement Amendments (CLIA)-waived chromogenic diagnostic test based on the presence of elevated sialidase enzyme activity, which is produced by bacterial pathogens including Gardnerella;[5] and Pip Activity TestCard (Quidel Corporation), a proline-aminopeptidase that detects proline iminopeptidase (PIP) activity found with *G. vaginalis* and *Mobiluncus* spp.[6] Sensitivities and specificities for these test are 95% / 100%, 90.3% / 96.6%, and 91.6% / 97.67%, respectively, compared to Gram stain and/or the Amsel criteria.[4–6]

Therapy

1. For nonpregnant patients, recommended regimens are metronidazole 500-mg oral tablet twice daily for 7 days, metronidazole 0.75% gel 5 g intravaginally once daily for 5 days, or clindamycin 2% cream 5 g intravaginally daily for 7 days. Cure rates for all these regimens are 75% to 85%. Alternative treatments include tinidazole and oral clindamycin regimens. Please see the Centers for Disease Control and Prevention [CDC][7] guidelines for the most updated information (www.cdc.gov). Patients should be warned to avoid ingestion of alcohol within 3 days of taking oral metronidazole because of the possibility of disulfiram-like reaction with nausea, vomiting, and flushing. In addition, clindamycin cream is oil based and might weaken latex condoms and diaphragms for 5 days after use.
2. Recurrent BV occurs in 20% to 30% of cases within 3 months. The treatment recommended by the CDC[7] is an initial 7-day course of oral or intravaginal metronidazole or clindamycin. For reoccurrence, re-treatment with the same regimen and use of a different treatment regimen are both acceptable. Suppression therapy then follows with a 4- to 6-month course of metronidazole gel twice a week.[7]
3. Symptomatic pregnant women in any trimester should be treated with either metronidazole 500-mg oral tablet twice a day for 7 days; metronidazole 250 mg orally three times daily for 7 days; or clindamycin 300 mg orally twice a day for 7 days.[7] It is not recommended to screen asymptomatic women at low risk for premature delivery. Evidence is insufficient in comparing the risk and benefits of screening asymptomatic women at high risk for premature delivery.[7,8]
4. HIV-infected women may receive the same regimens as non-HIV-infected women.
5. Treatment of asymptomatic women with BV before hysterectomy is recommended by American Congress of Obstetrics and Gynecology.[9]
6. *Counseling:* Patients should be advised to avoid douching and reduce the number of sex partners. Treatment of male partners is not helpful, but female sex partners should be evaluated for BV. Follow-up is not necessary unless symptoms persist.

⬤ VULVOVAGINAL CANDIDIASIS

VVC is the second most common form of vaginitis after BV. A major issue in diagnosis is distinguishing true infection from nonpathogenic colonization.

Etiology

VVC is usually caused by *Candida albicans* (85% to 95% of clinical cases) and occasionally by other *Candida* sp, *Torulopsis* sp, or other yeasts.[10]

Epidemiology

1. Prevalence: The overall prevalence of VVC is unknown; however, an estimated 75% of women experience at least one episode of VVC during their lifetime; 40% to 45% will have a recurrence, and approximately 5% will have recurrent vulvovaginitis candidiasis, defined as ≥4 episodes in a 12-month period.[10]
2. Transmission: Although VVC is usually not sexually acquired or transmitted, evidence exists that sexual contact plays a role in transmission in some patients.[10] Approximately 20% of male partners have asymptomatic penile colonization. Symptomatic male partners might present with balanitis.[7]
3. Predisposing factors: Immunosuppressive states (uncontrolled diabetes mellitus, HIV infection, or therapy with steroids or immunosuppressive agents), pregnancy, and use of antibiotics in women colonized with *Candida*;[11] behavioral factors (orogenital sex, douching);[10] innate host factors, including genetic predispositions and decreased local vaginal immune responses (such as those seen with nonsecretors of Lewis antigens or impaired *Candida* antigen-specific immunity).[7,11,12] There are conflicting studies regarding the possible increased risk of infection with contraceptives, including estrogen containing oral contraceptives, condoms, and the contraceptive sponge. Studies have also shown increased *Candida* carriage in users of the intrauterine device (IUD).[11]

Clinical Manifestations

1. Presentation: Patients may experience nonspecific symptoms of intense burning, vulvar pruritus, erythema, external dysuria, dyspareunia, and discharge. The discharge may worsen before menses and classically appears white, odorless, and "cottage cheese–like."[10]
2. Examination may reveal the classic discharge and erythematous vulva with fissures, excoriations, edema, and satellite lesions.[10]

Diagnosis

1. Diagnosis is supported by wet prep or KOH findings of yeast buds and pseudohyphae (Fig. 51.3) (sensitivity 65% to 85%) and a normal pH of <4.5.[10]
2. Cultures may be useful in cases of recurrent VVC, but are not used for routine diagnosis because asymptomatic colonization is common.[10]
3. A rapid test for *Candida* antigens in vaginal discharge is commercially available. The Affirm VP III is a DNA probe that can provide results for detecting *Candida* in less than 1 hour. Sensitivity and specificity are 81%/98.2%.[4]
4. VVC is classified as "uncomplicated" when there are infrequent episodes with mild-to-moderate symptoms due to *C. albicans* in nonimmunocompromised women; VCC is classified as "complicated" when there is recurrent VVC consisting of four or more episodes in 12 months, or severe symptoms, or due to nonalbicans species, or in immunocompromised pregnant women.[7]

Therapy

1. Uncomplicated cases in nonpregnant patients can be treated by:
   a. Topical, intravaginal agents: Short-course topical formulations (i.e., single dose and regimens of 1 to 3 days) effectively treat uncomplicated VVC. Topical azoles such as clotrimazole, miconazole, and terconazole are more effective than nystatin. Please see the CDC treatment guidelines for a more comprehensive list of topical treatment options (www.cdc.gov).[7]
   b. Oral agent: Fluconazole 150-mg oral tablet, one tablet in a single dose. Patients often prefer single-dose oral therapy over intravaginal therapy because of convenience and ease of use.[7]

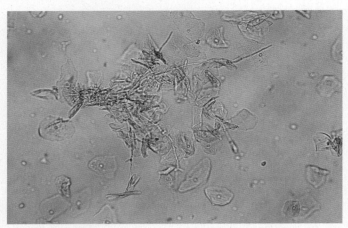

FIGURE 51.3 Vaginal candidiasis. This photomicrograph of a wet-mounted vaginal smear specimen reveals the presence of *C. albicans* in a patient with vaginal candidiasis. (Image courtesy of Dr. Stuart Brown and the Centers for Disease Control and Prevention Public Health Image Library ID 15675. Available at http://phil.cdc.gov/phil.)

2. Pregnancy: Seven-day therapy with topical azole medications can be used during pregnancy. Oral agents should be avoided.[7]

3. Severe VVC or immunocompromised host: Cases with severe symptoms and signs have lower clinical cure rates with short-course medications. Treating with either 7 to 14 days of topical azoles or oral fluconazole 150 mg once and then repeating the same dose in 3 days is advised.[7]

4. HIV infection: Same as non-HIV-infected women. However, cases of clinically severe VVC may be treated as discussed in the section on severe VVC.[7] Prompt treatment of VVC in HIV-infected patients is especially advised because of potential for increased transmission of HIV to their sexual partners. Since recurrence is not uncommon in immunocompetent individuals, HIV testing should only be considered in women with recurrent VVC who have risk factors for HIV infection.[10]

5. Recurrent VVC: Predisposing factors for infection should be reduced and vaginal cultures obtained to guide therapy. For recurrent *C. albicans* VVC, prescribe the routine short courses for uncomplicated infection or 7 to 14 days of topical treatment or oral therapy every 3 days for three total doses. Maintenance therapy consists of weekly oral medications for 6 months (see CDC guidelines for more details). About 30% to 50% of women will have recurrent disease after maintenance therapy is discontinued.[7]

6. Nonalbicans *Candida* species: Optimal treatment is unknown; however, consider 7 to 14 days of a nonfluconazole azole drug (oral or topical) as first-line therapy. For recurrence, CDC recommends 600 mg of boric acid in a gelatin capsule intravaginally daily for 2 weeks. If symptoms recur, consider referral to a specialist.[7]

7. Counseling: Partners are not routinely treated unless the male partner has symptoms and signs of balanitis. Follow-up is not necessary for individuals who become asymptomatic after treatment.[7]

TRICHOMONIASIS

Etiology
TV infection of the vaginal epithelium is caused by protozoa with four anterior flagella and one posterior flagellum.

Epidemiology
1. Prevalence: The overall prevalence of the disease among reproductive age women 14 to 49 is estimated at 3.1%. The prevalence among female AYAs varies with studies ranging from

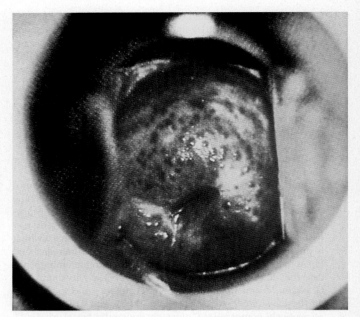

FIGURE 51.4 Strawberry cervix due to a TV infection. With TV, the cervical mucosa may reveal punctuate hemorrhages with accompanying vesicles or papules, also known as strawberry cervix. (Image courtesy of Centers for Disease Control and Prevention Public Health Image Library ID 5240. Available at http://phil.cdc.gov/phil.)

2.3% to 25% among 20 to 29 years old and from 2.1% to 22.8% among those less than 20 years. Difference in prevalence varies with the study population examined.[13–17]

2. Transmission: The organism is almost always sexually transmitted. Although rare, transmission can occur via nonsexual contaminated formites, mutual masturbation, and perinatal transmission.[18] Trichomonads can infect sites in addition to the vagina, for example, the urethra, Bartholin gland, Skene glands, and the endocervix.[18]

3. Predisposing factors: Risk factors similar to that of other STIs including high-risk sexual behaviors.

Clinical Manifestations
1. Presentation: Up to 25% to 50% of females are asymptomatic. Nonspecific symptoms include pruritus, dysuria, dyspareunia, lower abdominal pain, and postcoital bleeding. Discharge is seen in 50% of cases, and is classically diffuse, frothy, yellow or green, and occasionally (10%) malodorous.[18]

2. Examination may reveal edema and excoriation of the external genitalia; frothy, foul-smelling vaginal discharge; erythematous, edematous, and granular vaginal walls; bartholinitis; and, rarely, PID. Cervicitis ("strawberry cervix") (Fig. 51.4) consists of erosions or petechiae of the cervix and is seen in only 2% of cases.[18]

3. Complications: According to a review article by Meites,[19] evidence links *Trichomonas* infection to an increased rate of HIV acquisition and transmission, an increased rate of PID in HIV-infected women, and an increase in perinatal morbidity.

Diagnosis
1. Wet prep is commonly used when a microscope is available in the office setting, but sensitivity is 50% to 70% at best. Trichomonads appear as flagellated pear-shaped motile organisms similar in size to polymorphonuclear leukocytes (Fig. 51.5). The whiff test is often positive on KOH prep, and vaginal pH is >4.5.[18]

2. Cultures: Culture of *Trichomonas* via Diamonds' medium or with the use of the InPouch culture system was previously considered gold standard for diagnosis because of high sensitivity

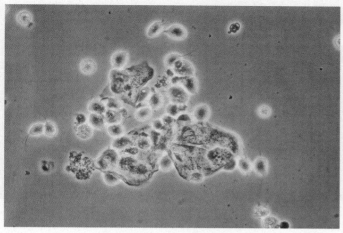

FIGURE 51.5 TV protozoan parasites. This photomicrograph of a wet-mounted vaginal discharge specimen reveals numbers of TV protozoan parasites. (Image courtesy of Joe Miller and the Centers for Disease Control and Prevention Public Health Image Library ID 14500. Available at http://phil.cdc.gov/phil.)

and specificity.[18] However, due to the technical challenges of culture and length of time to diagnosis, nucleic acid–based techniques are more commonly used.

3. Nucleic Acid Amplification Test (NAAT): APTIMA (GenProbe, San Diego, CA) is a transcription-mediated amplification assay that can detect *Trichomonas* from clinician-collected vaginal and endocervical swabs, liquid endocervical cytology media, and urine specimens. Sensitivity ranges from 95.3% to 100% and specificity between 98.9% and 99.6% compared to wet mount and culture, respectively.[20]

4. Rapid/POCTs: There are two US Food and Drug Administration-approved methods for rapid testing of vaginal samples. The OSOM *Trichomonas* POCT Rapid Test yields results in 10 minutes,[21] and the Affirm VP III yields results in 60 minutes. Sensitivity is >83% and specificity is >99%, for both tests compared to culture.[4]

5. Liquid-based cytology versus conventional pap: Due to their poor sensitivity, neither conventional pap (50%) nor liquid-based cervical cytology (61%) is ideal for the diagnosis of *Trichomonas*. However, since the specificity of liquid-based cytology reaches 99%, positive results should be treated.[19]

Therapy

1. Nonpregnant patients should receive metronidazole 2 g orally in a single dose or tinidazole 2 g orally in a single dose. The alternative regimen is metronidazole 500-mg tablet twice a day for 7 days. Patients allergic to nitroimidazoles should receive desensitization, since no other medication classes are effective.[7] Patients should be warned to avoid ingestion of alcohol within 3 days of taking these medications because of the possibility of disulfiram-like reaction with nausea, vomiting, and flushing.

2. Treatment failure: If failure occurs with either regimen, the adolescent or young adult should be retreated with metronidazole 500 mg twice daily for 7 days. If failure occurs again, the patient can be treated with tinidazole or metronidazole 2 g PO daily for 5 days. Some TV strains demonstrate decreased susceptibility to medications, but high-level resistance is rare. Any suspicion of resistance to metronidazole should be reported to the CDC for discussion of further susceptibility, testing, and recommendations.[7]

3. Pregnancy: *Trichomonas* treatment in pregnancy has not been shown to reduce perinatal morbidity but may increase the possibility of prematurity or low both weight. In asymptomatic females, consider delaying treatment until >37 weeks; in symptomatic patients, treatment should be considered. Recommended treatment includes 2 g of metronidazole in one oral dose. Data have shown no association between teratogenicity and metronidazole use during pregnancy.[7]

4. HIV infection: As a single 2 g dose of metronidazole is not as effective; women should be treated with 500 mg orally twice a day for 7 days.[7]

5. Counseling: Routine treatment of partners is recommended. Patients should also avoid sexual contact until the patient and all partners have completed medications and are asymptomatic. Follow-up is not necessary for individuals who become asymptomatic after treatment. Due to high rates of reinfection, consider rescreening 3 months after initial treatment.[7]

OTHER CAUSES OF VAGINAL DISCHARGE

1. *Physiologic discharge:* normal overall increase in vaginal secretions 6 to 12 months before menarche and just before each menses[1]

2. *Extravaginal lesions:* may cause staining of the underwear and perception of a discharge[1]

3. *Irritant vaginitis:* related to tampons, pads, douches, deodorants, powders, scented toilet paper, bubble baths, laundry detergents, fabric softeners, swimming pools, spermicides, and others[1]

4. *Foreign bodies:* forgotten tampons and others[1]

ACKNOWLEDGMENTS

This chapter is based on Chapter 55 from the 5th edition, authored by Loris Y. Hwang and Mary-Ann B. Shafer.

REFERENCES

1. Braverman PK. Urethritis, vulvovaginitis, and cervicitis. In: Long SS, Pickering LK, Prober CG, eds. *Principles and practice of peadiatric infectious diseases.* 4th ed. New York, NY: Elsevier Saunders, 2012: 353–363.
2. Hillier SL, Marrazzo JM, Holmes KK. Bacterial vaginosis. In: Holmes K, Sparling PF, Stamm W, et al. eds. *Sexually transmitted diseases.* 4th ed. New York, NY: The McGraw-Hill Companies, Inc., 2008:737–768.
3. Koumans EH, Sternberg M, Bruce C, et al. The prevalence of bacterial vaginosis in the United States, 2001–2004; associations with symptoms, sexual behaviors, and reproductive health. *Sex Transm Dis* 2007;34(11):864–869.
4. Becton, Dickinson. *Affirm VPIII microbial identification test.* Package Insert. Available at http://www.bd.com/ds/technicalCenter/inserts/670160JAA(201008).pdf.
5. Sekisui Diagnostics. *OSOM BVBlue test.* Product Insert.
6. Quidel Corporation. *QuickVue advance G. vaginalis test.* Product Insert.
7. Workowski KA, Berman S. Sexually transmitted diseases treatment guidelines, 2010. *MMWR Recomm Rep* 2010;59(RR-12):1–110.
8. U.S. Preventive Services Task Force. *USPSTF A-Z topic guide.* Available at http://www.uspreventiveservicestaskforce.org/uspstf/uspstopics.htm.
9. ACOG Committee on Practice Bulletins—Gynecology. ACOG practice bulletin No. 104: antibiotic prophylaxis for gynecologic procedures. *Obstet Gynecol* 2009;113(5):1180–1189.
10. Sobel JD. Vulvovaginal candidiasis. In: Holmes K, Sparling PF, Stamm W, et al. eds. *Sexually transmitted diseases.* 4th ed. New York, NY: The McGraw-Hill Companies, 2008:823–838.
11. Sobel JD. Vulvovaginal candidosis. *Lancet* 2007;369(9577):1961–1971.
12. Jaeger M, Plantinga TS, Joosten LA, et al. Genetic basis for recurrent vulvo-vaginal candidiasis. *Curr Infect Dis Rep* 2013;15(2):136–142.
13. Sutton M, Sternberg M, Koumans EH, et al. The prevalence of *Trichomonas vaginalis* infection among reproductive-age women in the United States, 2001–2004. *Clin Infect Dis* 2007;45(10):1319–1326.
14. Satterwhite CL, Torrone E, Meites E, et al. Sexually transmitted infections among US women and men: prevalence and incidence estimates, 2008. *Sex Transm Dis* 2013;40(3):187–193.
15. Miller WC, Swygard H, Hobbs MM, et al. The prevalence of trichomoniasis in young adults in the United States. *Sex Transm Dis* 2005;32(10):593–598.
16. Ginocchio CC, Chapin K, Smith JS, et al. Prevalence of *Trichomonas vaginalis* and coinfection with *Chlamydia trachomatis* and *Neisseria gonorrhoeae* in the United States as determined by the Aptima *Trichomonas vaginalis* nucleic acid amplification assay. *J Clin Microbiol* 2012;50(8):2601–2608.
17. Meites E, Llata E, Braxton J, et al. *Trichomonas vaginalis* in selected U.S. sexually transmitted disease clinics: testing, screening, and prevalence. *Sex Transm Dis* 2013;40(11):865–869.
18. Hobbs MM, Sena AC, Swygard H, et al. *Trichomonas vaginalis* and Trichomoniasis. In: Holmes K, Sparling PF, Stamm W, et al. eds. *Sexually transmitted diseases.* 4th ed. New York, NY: The McGraw-Hill Companies, 2008:771–794.
19. Meites, E. Trichomoniasis—the "neglected" sexually transmitted disease. *Infect Dis Clin North Am* 2013;27(4):755–764.
20. Gen Probe. *APTIMA Trichomonas vaginalis assay.* Package insert. Available at http://www.gen-probe.com/pdfs/pi/503684-EN-RevA.pdf.
21. Sekisui Diagnostics. *OSOM Trichomonas rapid test.* Product Insert. Available at http://www.sekisuidiagnostics.com/pdf/OSOM_Trich_181_PI.pdf.

XII

 ADDITIONAL RESOURCES AND WEBSITES ONLINE

Pelvic Masses

Paula J. Adams Hillard

A pelvic mass may be identified during a routine screening examination, or it can be discovered during an evaluation for abdominopelvic pain or abnormal bleeding. It may also be an incidental finding at the time of imaging for an unrelated medical concern. The list of likely diagnoses of a pelvic mass for prepubertal, adolescent and young adult (AYA) females is different than that for older women, although there may be some overlap.[1] Table 52.1 lists a number of conditions that may be diagnosed as a pelvic mass in women of reproductive age.

 CONGENITAL ANOMALIES

Uterine Defects: Incomplete Fusion

Anatomical genital anomalies, which typically present as a pelvic mass during adolescence, are rare, but they can have profound

TABLE 52.1

Conditions Diagnosed as a Pelvic Mass in Women of Reproductive Age

Full urinary bladder
Urachal cyst
Sharply anteflexed or retroflexed uterus
Pregnancy—intrauterine, tubal, abdominal
Ovarian or adnexal masses
    Functional cysts
    Paratubal cyst
    Tuboovarian abscess/complex
    Neoplastic tumors
        Benign
        Malignant
Appendiceal abscess
Uncommon and rare conditions in AYAs
    Pelvic kidney
    Diverticular abscess
    Carcinoma of the colon, rectum, appendix
    Carcinoma of the fallopian tube
    Retroperitoneal tumors (anterior sacral meningocele)
    Uterine sarcoma or other malignant tumors
    Metastatic tumors (lymphoma or leukemia)

implications for future reproductive capability.[2] It is uncommon, but not unheard of for nonobstructing anomalies to present in young adulthood. Embryologically, the uterus is formed by fusion of paramesonephric ducts in the midline (Fig. 52.1). If lateral fusion is incomplete, then a uterine didelphys may form with two separate uterine halves (each with its own cervix, corpus, attached fallopian tube and ovary, and possibly vaginal canal) (Fig. 52.2). On examination, one of the two uteri may be mistaken for an adnexal mass. If uterine fusion is partial, there may be a bicornuate uterus or blind uterine horn. There may be a unilateral obstructed horn, and if functional endometrium is present within this obstructed horn, severe cyclic pain can occur. The diagnosis can be suggested on the basis of a screening pelvic ultrasound examination. If a developmental anomaly is suspected on ultrasound examination, magnetic resonance imaging (MRI) is the best technique for clarifying genital anomalies.[3] Renal and skeletal anomalies are common in conjunction with uterine lateral fusion defects.[4]

The vagina also forms in two parts, and defects typically occur as a result of failure of longitudinal fusion or canalization. If the upper and lower vaginal portions do not fuse, then a transverse vaginal septum forms. Similarly, if the solid core of tissue at the junction of the vaginal plate and the urogenital sinus not canalize completely, the woman can have an imperforate hymen or vaginal agenesis. If a uterus with functional endometrium is present along with a transverse vaginal septum or imperforate hymen, menstrual fluid accumulates within the patent portion of the vagina (hematocolpos) and within the uterus (hematometra), which then presents as a "pelvic mass" (Fig. 52.3). Imperforate hymen is the most frequent obstructive anomaly of the female genital tract, but estimates of its frequency vary from 1 case per 1,000 population to 1 case per 10,000 population.[5]

Uterovaginal Agenesis

Women with uterovaginal agenesis—Mayer–Rokitansky–Küster–Hauser syndrome—may have uterine remnants that may or may not contain functioning endometrium, which can cause pain, and a mass that is diagnosed with ultrasonography or MRI.

Müllerian Duct Remnants

Another class of anatomical congenital anomalies that can create pelvic masses arises from remnants of the mesonephric/müllerian duct system or mesovarium that should have degenerated in utero in the presence of antimüllerian hormone. At least 25% of adult women have small remnants of these systems. These remnants can be present in the lateral adnexa as paraovarian cysts or paratubal cysts (Fig. 52.4). They are often multiple and can vary in size from <1 cm to 20 cm. Along the lateral wall of the vagina or uterus, these remnants present as Gartner duct cysts. These müllerian

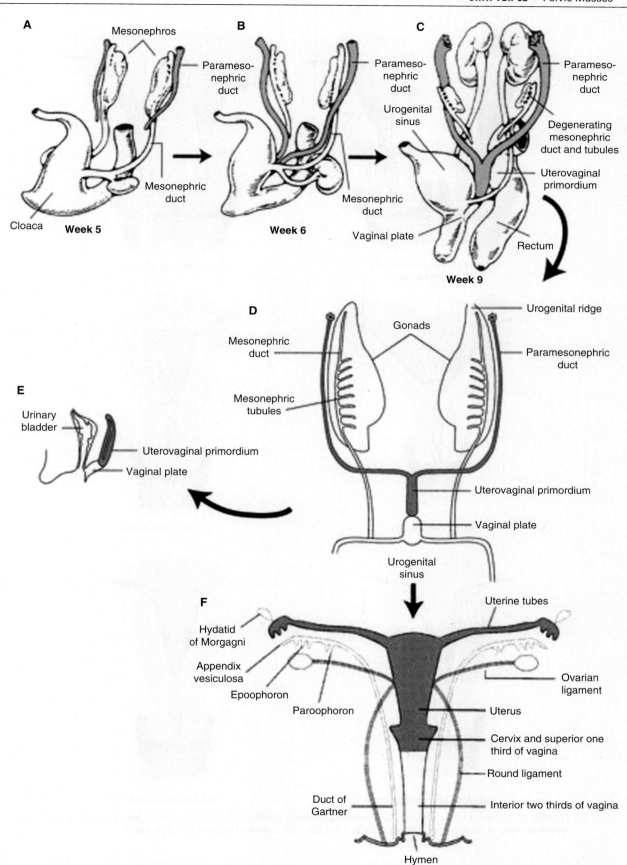

FIGURE 52.1 Development of uterus from paired paramesonephric ducts. (From Dudek RW. *BRS embryology*. 5th ed. Philadelphia, PA: Lippincott Williams & Wilkins, 2010.)

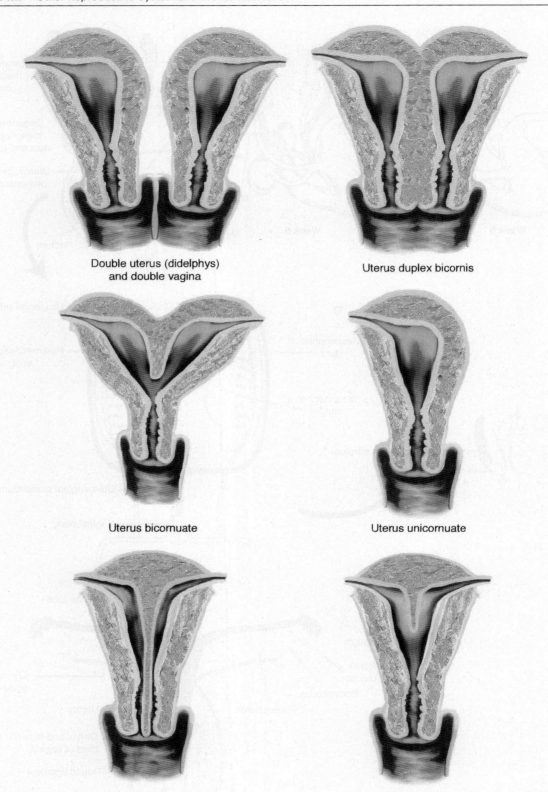

FIGURE 52.2 Uterine fusion abnormalities. (From Baggish MS, Valle RF, Guedj H. *Hysteroscopy: visual perspectives of uterine anatomy, physiology and pathology.* 3rd ed. Philadelphia, PA: Lippincott Williams & Wilkins, 2007.)

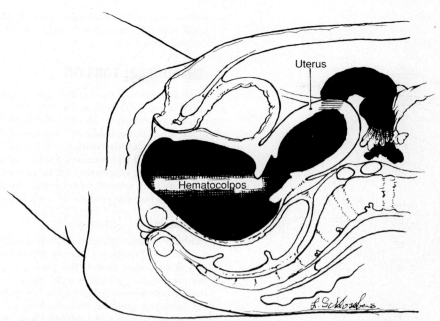

FIGURE 52.3 Hematocolpos, hematometra, hematosalpinx due to imperforate hymen. (From Rock JA, Jones HW. *Te Linde's operative gynecology.* 10th ed. Philadelphia, PA: Lippincott Williams & Wilkins, 2008.)

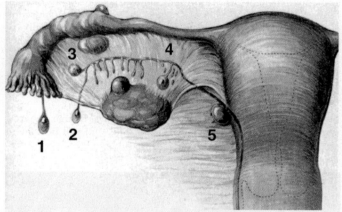

FIGURE 52.4 Paratubal cysts from embryologic remnants. (From Dudek RW. *BRS embryology.* 5th ed. Philadelphia, PA: Lippincott Williams & Wilkins, 2010.)

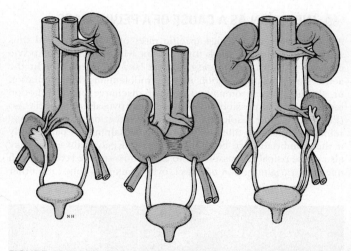

FIGURE 52.5 Pelvic kidney, horseshoe kidney, and supernumerary kidney. (Courtesy of Neil O. Hardy, Westpoint, CT.)

remnants are rarely symptomatic; however, torsion of an adnexal mass can occur, and persistent larger masses may be confused with an ovarian neoplasm.

Urachal Cysts and Pelvic Kidneys

Urachal cysts, although rare, can be found along the midline above the bladder and can be confused with other pelvic masses. A pelvic kidney must also be included in the differential diagnosis (Fig. 52.5). Any other structure in the pelvis, such as a full bladder or hard stool in the bowel, can be confused with a pelvic mass.

PREGNANCY PRESENTING AS PELVIC MASS

The possibility of an intrauterine pregnancy enlarging the uterus or an ectopic pregnancy (see Chapter 53) causing an abdominal or adnexal mass must be considered in the differential diagnosis of every young woman with secondary sexual characteristics (Fig. 52.6). A sensitive urine pregnancy test can reliably rule out a clinically

significant pregnancy. However, in many instances, the test is not ordered because the provider does not consider it likely that the adolescent or young adult has been sexually active. Adolescents may be unwilling or unable to disclose their history of sexual activity for a variety of reasons—they may fear disappointing their parents or the clinician; they may have insufficient knowledge or awareness of pregnancy-related symptoms; they may deny the possibility of pregnancy; the clinician may not have established or discussed provisions of confidentiality; or the question may not have been asked in a sensitive manner in a private setting. Both sexual abuse and early consensual sexual activity may occur, resulting in pregnancy. If pregnancy testing is a routine order, then its use in any individual case does not require justification. The consequences of missing a pregnancy-related cause of pain, bleeding, or asymptomatic pelvic mass justify routine pregnancy testing in all young women presenting with pain, amenorrhea, abnormal bleeding, or a pelvic mass.[6]

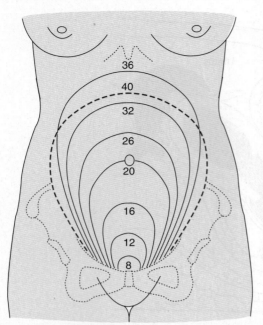

FIGURE 52.6 Pregnancy with fundal height corresponding to gestational age. (From Beckmann CRB, Ling FW, Smith RP et al. *Obstetrics and gynecology.* 5th ed. Philadelphia, PA: Lippincott Williams & Wilkins, 2006.)

INFECTION AS A CAUSE OF A PELVIC MASS

AYAs have the highest age-specific rates of chlamydia, and thus are at risk for upper track involvement with salpingitis or pelvic abscess (tuboovarian abscess [TOA]) (see Chapter 58)[7]. In the acute stage, pelvic infection may be indolent in its presentation or, alternatively, accompanied by fever, discharge, cervical motion tenderness, and possibly adnexal masses (pyosalpinges or TOAs) (Fig. 52.7). After resolution of the acute infection, the tubes may remain dilated and filled with fluid (hydrosalpinges), particularly if their fimbriae have been sealed. Treated pelvic abscesses may also cause palpable masses due to adhesions—pelvic scarring with matting or agglutination of bowel, ovary, fallopian tube, and other

structures. Other infectious causes of pelvic masses include an appendiceal abscess or (rarely in young girls) diverticulitis or Meckel diverticulum.

ADNEXAL TORSION

Adnexal torsion involves the acute rotation of adnexal structures, and is a cause of acute pelvic pain, which may be accompanied by nausea and vomiting. The diagnosis may be missed if the possibility of torsion is not considered.[8] Torsion of the normal adnexa can occur; however, torsion is more likely to occur when an adnexal mass rotates around its vascular pedicle. Once rotated, the venous flow to the mass is obstructed while arterial flow continues, inflating the mass until arterial flow is compressed (Fig. 52.8). The adnexal structures become edematous and ultimately gangrenous.

Diagnosis

Findings on examination include peritoneal signs with rebound tenderness. Typical findings on ultrasound examination with Doppler flow studies include the presence of a mass, edema, adnexal asymmetry, and absent venous and/or arterial flow; unfortunately, these findings are neither perfectly sensitive nor specific, and clinical judgment must be used, including a high index of suspicion.[8] Consultation with a gynecologist is essential, as adnexal torsion is a surgical emergency.

Treatment

Treatment consists of untwisting the adnexa, even if hemorrhage and apparent necrosis are present, as ovarian preservation is almost always possible. This can usually be performed laparoscopically. Excision of the cyst can be performed laparoscopically, or may be delayed and performed as an interval procedure once edema has resolved. Every attempt should be made to preserve the involved ovary.

UTERINE NEOPLASMS

In AYA women, uterine neoplasms are quite rare. Benign leiomyomas (fibroids) may cause abnormal bleeding, and will be evident on pelvic imaging.

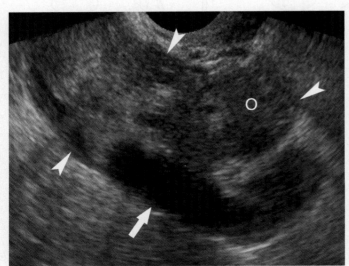

FIGURE 52.7 Tuboovarian abscess. Ultrasound of the pelvis shows complex mass (*arrowheads*) around the ovary (*O*) and dilated tube (*arrow*). (From Brant WE; Helms CA. *Brant and Helms solution.* Philadelphia, PA: Lippincott Williams & Wilkins, 2006.)

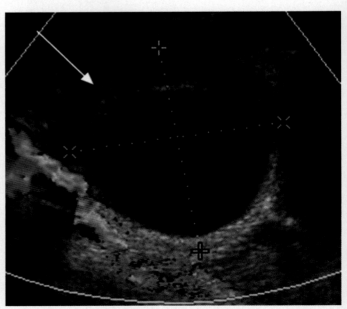

FIGURE 52.8 Ovarian torsion. Ultrasound with ovarian cyst with no Doppler flow. (From Shirkhoda A. *Variants and pitfalls in body imaging.* 2nd ed. Philadelphia, PA: Lippincott Williams & Wilkins, 2010.)

BENIGN OVARIAN MASSES

Benign ovarian masses include *functional ovarian cysts, endometriomas, and benign ovarian neoplasms.* Whenever an ovarian mass is diagnosed in an adolescent female or prepubertal child, every effort must be made to preserve the reproductive function, whether the mass is physiologic or neoplastic, benign, or malignant.[9] **Table 52.2** lists benign ovarian tumors. **Figure 52.9** provides a plan for management of pelvic masses in premenarchal and adolescent girls.

Physiologic (Functional) Ovarian Cysts

Functional ovarian cysts include *follicular cysts, corpus luteum (CL) cysts, and theca lutein cysts.* All are benign and usually do not cause symptoms or require surgical management. Functional cysts result from expansion of the cavity of a preovulatory follicle (follicular cyst) or CL, and are associated with the disordered function of the pituitary–ovarian axis. The incidence of functional ovarian cysts in adolescents or young adults is not well established, but most follicular cysts are asymptomatic, and they are frequently an incidental finding on pelvic imaging (**Fig. 52.10AB**). CL cysts can be painful. Theca lutein cysts—the least common type of functional cyst—result from human chorionic gonadotropin (hCG) stimulation, producing bilateral follicular cystic ovarian enlargement. They occur in patients with gestational trophoblastic disease (molar pregnancies and choriocarcinoma) and multiple pregnancies and regress with the removal of the pregnancy-associated hCG production.

1. **Follicular cysts**: The most common type of functional ovarian cyst is a follicular cyst. Follicular cysts are unilocular and simple without internal structure and range in size from 3 to 15 cm in diameter, but rarely exceed 8 cm (**Fig. 52.11**). Follicular cysts can be seen in prepubertal girls, and they

TABLE 52.2
Benign Ovarian Tumors

Functional
    Follicular
    Corpus luteal
    Theca lutein

Neoplastic
    Germ cell
        Benign cystic teratoma (dermoid)
    Epithelial
        Serous cystadenoma
        Mucinous cystadenoma
    Sex cord–stromal tumor
        Fibroma
        Adenofibroma
        Brenner tumor

Other
    Endometrioma

typically resolve over time. Management depends on symptoms, patient age, menarchal status, cyst size and character, as well as associated medical conditions. Torsion or rupture may occur, causing pain, and misdiagnosis is common.[10] In AYAs, follicular cysts usually resolve spontaneously in 4 to 8 weeks unless the patient is taking progestins (e.g., levonorgestrel intrauterine system or depot medroxyprogesterone acetate [DMPA]), which can slow follicular atresia and require a longer time for resolution. In general, conservative management of cysts smaller than 8 cm in a premenopausal woman is recommended. Persistent ovarian masses are more likely to be neoplastic and should prompt consideration of surgical

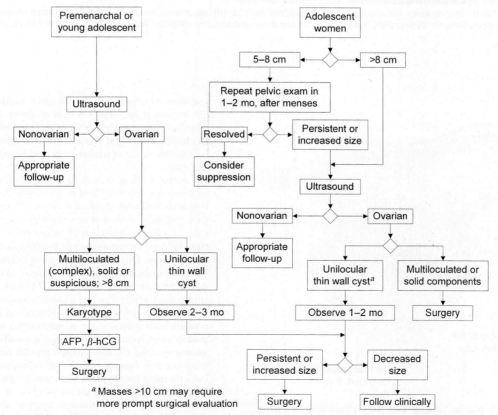

FIGURE 52.9 Management of pelvic masses in prepubertal, adolescent, and young adult women. AFP, α-fetoprotein; hCG, human chorionic gonadotropin.

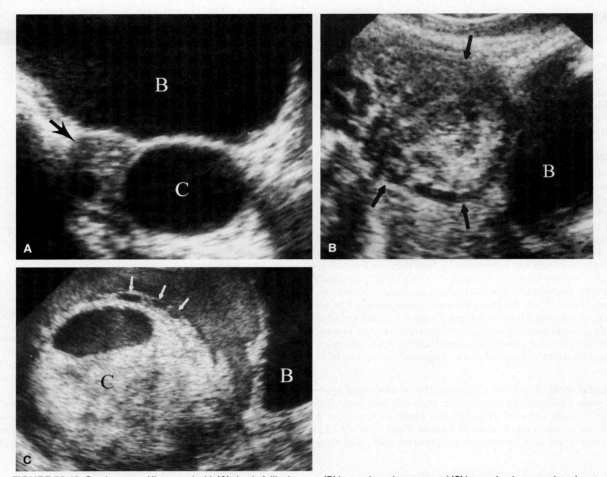

FIGURE 52.10 Ovarian cysts. Ultrasound with **(A)** simple follicular cyst, **(B)** hemorrhage into cyst, and **(C)** hemorrhagic corpus luteal cyst in patient on warfarin. (From Brant WE, Helms CA. *Brant and Helms solution*. Philadelphia, PA: Lippincott Williams & Wilkins, 2006.)

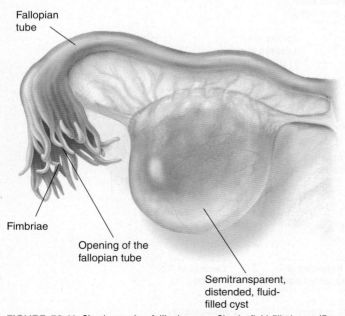

Fallopian tube

Fimbriae

Opening of the fallopian tube

Semitransparent, distended, fluid-filled cyst

FIGURE 52.11 Simple ovarian follicular cyst. Simple fluid-filled cyst (From Lippincott. *Pathophysiology made incredibly visual!* 2nd ed. Philadelphia, PA: Lippincott Williams & Wilkins 2011.)

excision. Decisions about whether surgical excision of ovarian masses is required are best made by gynecologic surgeons who have experience with adolescent and pediatric patients.[11] Decisions about the type of surgical intervention are guided by the suspicion of malignancy and imaging characteristics of the mass.

2. **CL cysts**: A CL cyst is defined as a "cyst" if it exceeds 3 cm in diameter, but they can reach larger dimensions. They may be associated with delayed menses. CL cysts are less common than follicular cysts but are clinically more significant because they can be associated with acute pain (due to bleeding into the enclosed cystic space) or rupture, leading to acute hemoperitoneum. This can be a surgical emergency, particularly if the patient is anticoagulated. A cyst may rupture during intercourse late in the cycle (days 21 to 26); although rare, rupture can also follow pelvic examination, strenuous exercise, or trauma. Pain can occur in the absence of trauma. Patients presenting with pain and an adnexal mass on ultrasound examination may require gynecologic consultation to differentiate an unruptured CL cyst, which should be managed medically, from torsion, hemoperitoneum, or appendicitis—acute surgical emergencies. Typical ultrasonographic findings include a mixed echogenic adnexal mass (Fig. 52.10C). Doppler flow ultrasonographic studies can suggest the possibility of torsion with decreased venous and/or arterial flow. Because oral contraceptives suppress follicular development and ovulation,

they reduce the risk of functional cysts in a dose-dependent manner. Administration of oral contraceptives to induce cyst regression is no more effective than an observation period with no hormonal therapy, although it will suppress the development of subsequent functional cysts.[12]

Endometriomas and Endometriosis

Endometriosis is a condition in which ectopic endometrium is present outside of the uterus. The presence of ovarian endometriosis can result in the formation of an ovarian endometrioma. There is a broad range of ultrasound appearances of endometriomas—diffuse, low-level internal echoes occur in most endometriomas, and hyperechoic wall foci and multilocularity also suggest the diagnosis of an endometrioma (Fig. 52.12).

Endometriosis has historically been considered to be a condition affecting adult women; however, it is receiving increasing recognition as a cause of pelvic pain in adolescents.[13] Although the prevalence of endometriosis in adolescents is not well established, there is a familial incidence, and endometriosis can be demonstrated in up to 40% to 50% of adolescents undergoing laparoscopy because of chronic pelvic pain unresponsive to the use of hormonal manipulation, such as oral contraceptives and nonsteroidal anti-inflammatory drugs (NSAIDs). Endometriomas are also rare in adolescents, who typically have early stage or mild disease.

Clinical manifestations include worsening dysmenorrhea, premenstrual or acyclic pelvic pain, and deep dyspareunia. On pelvic examination, findings of diffuse or localized tenderness, particularly in the cul-de-sac posterior to the uterus, diminished uterine motility (a result of adhesion formation particularly between the uterus and the sigmoid), cervical motion tenderness (from adhesions), and possibly an ovarian mass (endometrioma) are suggestive of endometriosis.

Adolescents rarely have the "classic" finding of uterosacral nodularity. Because laparoscopy provides a definitive diagnosis of suspected endometriosis, AYAs with pelvic pain or dysmenorrhea that is unresponsive to NSAIDs and oral contraceptives should be referred to a gynecologist for consideration of surgical confirmation.[14]

Benign Ovarian Neoplasms

Benign ovarian neoplasms typically are unilocular and cystic, without solid components, papillations, vascular septae, or ascites.[15] AYAs with persistent cystic ovarian masses on ultrasonography

following 6 to 8 weeks of observation may have an ovarian neoplasm and should be referred to a gynecologist for surgical management. Benign cystic teratomas (dermoid cysts) are the most common ovarian neoplasm in adolescents. Any woman with a plain film x-ray or an ultrasonogram showing characteristics suspicious of this tumor (bone, teeth, or fat components) should also be referred for gynecologic surgical evaluation (Fig. 52.13). Solid masses of any size are suspicious for a malignant tumor, and should lead to prompt referral.

Benign Germ Cell Tumors

Benign cystic teratomas (dermoid cysts) are the most common benign ovarian neoplasm of adolescent and reproductive years.[11] Dermoid cysts include all three germ cell layers. They are generally thick-walled cysts and may be filled with sebaceous material and hair; they may also contain cartilage, teeth, or other tissues such as thyroid (Fig. 52.14). These embryologic elements produce characteristic findings on ultrasonography that can suggest the likelihood of a benign cystic teratoma. Malignant transformation occurs in

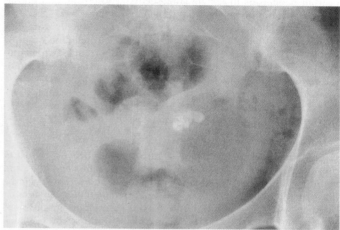

FIGURE 52.13 AP x-ray of pelvis with teeth and radiolucent fat in a benign cystic ovarian teratoma (dermoid cyst). (Courtesy of Hal Grass, DC, Denver, CO.)

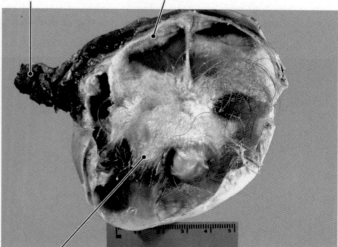

Fimbriated end of fallopian tube

Wall of cyst lined by skin

Mass of hair and sebaceous material

FIGURE 52.14 Benign ovarian cystic teratoma (dermoid cyst). (From McConnell TH. *Nature of Disease*. 2nd Ed. Philadelphia, PA: Lippincott Williams & Wilkins, 2013.)

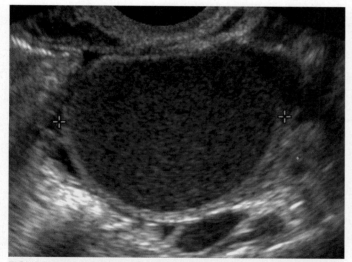

FIGURE 52.12 Endometrioma. Transvaginal sonogram shows adnexal cyst with homogeneous internal echoes. Appearance is similar to a hemorrhagic cyst, but an endometrioma will not resolve over approximately 2 cycles. (From Brant WE, Helms CA. *Brant and Helms solution*. Philadelphia, PA: Lippincott Williams & Wilkins, 2006.)

less than 2% of dermoid cysts in women of all ages and is rare in adolescents. Dermoid cysts vary in size from millimeters to quite large, but the vast majority of dermoids are smaller than 10 cm. On examination, they are unilateral (approximately 10% are bilateral), very mobile, anteriorly positioned, and nontender adnexal masses. Benign cystic teratomas are usually asymptomatic. The risk of torsion with dermoid cysts is approximately 15%, and it occurs more frequently than in other ovarian tumors in general, perhaps because of the high fat content of most dermoid cysts, allowing them to float within the abdominal and pelvic cavity. An ovarian cystectomy is almost always possible rather than an oophorectomy, even if it appears that only a small amount of ovarian tissue remains. Preserving a small amount of ovarian cortex in a young patient with a benign lesion is preferable to the loss of the entire ovary. AYAs with ultrasonography suggesting a dermoid should be referred to a gynecologic surgeon who appreciates the importance of ovarian conservation.

Benign Epithelial Neoplasia

Serous or mucinous cystadenomas account for 10% to 20% of benign ovarian neoplasms in female adolescents. These tumors are typically uni- or multiloculated, fluid-filled cystic masses (Fig. 52.15). Serous cystadenomas may not be recognized as a neoplasm; cyst aspiration without removal of the entire cyst (including multiple loculated areas and cyst wall) may result in recurrence. Benign mucinous cystadenomas have smooth, lobulated surfaces with multiloculations filled with viscous mucoid material (Fig. 52.16); these masses can reach very large dimensions (Fig. 52.17). Surgical removal of these adenomas is necessary for tissue diagnosis and to prevent symptoms from an enlarging mass or torsion.

Sex Cord–Stromal Tumors

Overall, these tumors are relatively rare, but they occur with higher prevalence in premenarchal girls than in adolescents or adults, and comprise 10% to 20% of childhood ovarian tumors. They may be hormonally active. Granulosa cell tumors and theca cell tumors produce estrogen, whereas Sertoli–Leydig cell tumors produce androgens with or without estrogen. As a result of this sex steroid production, sex cord–stromal tumors can cause precocious puberty, menstrual abnormalities, endometrial hyperplasia or carcinoma, or hirsutism, acne, and virilization. These signs should prompt pelvic imaging for diagnosis which typically reveals a solid or mixed solid and cystic mass (Fig. 52.18). Pure granulosa cell tumors are highly malignant, whereas mixed tumors behave less aggressively. Prognosis is excellent with unilateral salpingo-oophorectomy and appropriate surgical staging for the 95% of tumors that are unilateral.

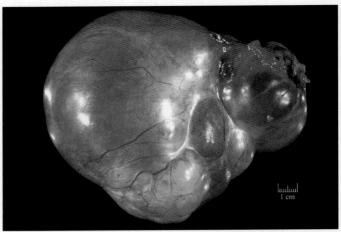
FIGURE 52.16 Mucinous cystadenoma with multiple loculations. (From Reichert RA. *Diagnostic gynecologic and obstetric pathology*. Philadelphia, PA: Lippincott Williams & Wilkins, 2011.)

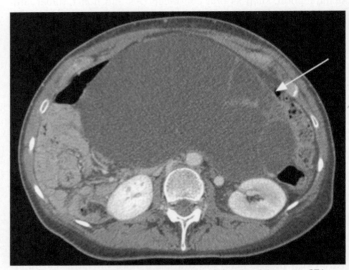
FIGURE 52.17 Large mucinous cystadenoma filling the abdomen on CT imaging. (From Shirkhoda A. *Variants and pitfalls in body imaging*. 2nd ed. Philadelphia, PA: Lippincott Williams & Wilkins, 2010.)

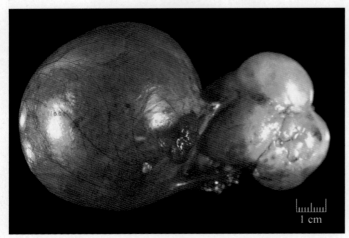
FIGURE 52.15 Intact serous cystadenoma as thin-walled cyst. (From Reichert RA. *Diagnostic gynecologic and obstetric pathology*. Philadelphia, PA: Lippincott Williams & Wilkins, 2011.)

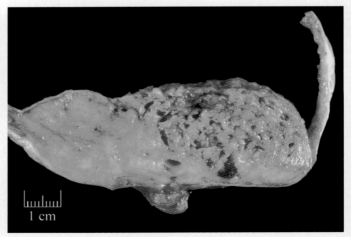
FIGURE 52.18 Granulosa cell tumor with section through solid and spongy portion of cystic and solid ovarian mass. (From Reichert RA. *Diagnostic gynecologic and obstetric pathology*. Philadelphia, PA: Lippincott Williams & Wilkins, 2011.)

MALIGNANT OVARIAN MASSES

Ovarian cancer is rare in adolescents, younger girls, and young adults. Only slightly more than 1% of all ovarian cancers occur in women younger than 20.[16] Ovarian cancers are more common in White women at all ages than in Black women.[17] With increasing age from childhood through young adulthood, there is a progression from germ cell to epithelial call malignancies.[17] Ultrasound features of an ovarian mass that are a cause of concern for malignancy include solid consistency, large size, complex appearance (not entirely cystic), internal loculations, internal or external excrescences, and ascites.[18] Efforts to preserve fertility are important considerations in the management of ovarian malignancies in adolescents.

Malignant Germ Cell Tumors

In women younger than 20 years, one-half to two-thirds of all ovarian tumors are of germ cell origin and one-third of those tumors are malignant. Germ cell tumors of all types, including dermoids, are seen with slightly greater frequency in the third decade of life compared to during adolescence, but secondary malignant change in teratomas remains uncommon in women under 30.[19] Malignant germ cell tumors include dysgerminoma, mixed germ cell tumor, endodermal sinus tumor, immature teratoma, embryonal tumor, choriocarcinoma, and polyembryoma. Because some ovarian neoplasms secrete protein tumor markers, including α-fetoprotein (AFP), hCG, carcinoembryonic antigen (CEA), lactate dehydrogenase (LDH), and others, measurement of these substances can be considered in making a diagnosis of an ovarian tumor and in following up malignant tumors for recurrence and clinical response.[20] CA-125 is a tumor marker for epithelial ovarian cancer, and while useful in evaluating adnexal masses in postmenopausal women it is not very specific, and in adolescents and premenopausal women it may be elevated with many other benign gynecologic conditions.

Dysgerminomas comprise 50% of all ovarian germ cell malignancies (Fig. 52.19). About 5% to 10% of these tumors occur in phenotypically female patients with disorders of sex differentiation (DSD). The presence of a Y chromosome is associated with a risk of malignancy, although the degree of risks is related to the type of DSD; bilateral gonadectomy is recommended if the risk is high.[21]

Malignant Epithelial Tumors

Although these tumor types are the most common type of ovarian malignancy in adult women, they are rare in adolescents.[22] Less than 5% of ovarian epithelial tumors in adolescents are invasive malignancies. In these patients, appropriate surgical staging, cytoreductive surgery, and chemotherapy are required, as in adults; conservative management in early stage disease may allow the preservation of fertility.[23] These patients require ongoing management by a gynecologic oncologist. Included in this group of neoplasias are serous cystadenocarcinoma, mucinous cystadenocarcinoma, and endometrial cystadenocarcinoma. In adolescents, approximately 7% of epithelial tumors will be borderline malignancies, which can be managed in conjunction with a gynecologic oncologist, with conservative surgery (unilateral salpingo-oophorectomy), careful assessment of the contralateral ovary, and appropriate staging procedures.[24] Epithelial borderline tumors become more common in the third decade of life, compared to during adolescence.[19]

Genetic Risk of Epithelial Ovarian Cancers

Approximately 15% of ovarian cancer is associated with the genetic mutations in the breast cancer gene 1 (*BRCA-1*), although other cancer susceptibility genes are now being identified.[25] Families with multiple family members with breast and/or ovarian cancer should be offered referral to specific familial cancer centers for genetic counseling and potential testing. Although the optimal age at which genetic testing should be performed has not been well established, professional guidelines recommend against testing minors, and many clinicians recommend offering counseling and testing in young adulthood.[26,27] Some reports of interviews with mutation carriers and their adult offspring indicate that improved health behaviors during adolescence and young adulthood may result from disclosure of hereditary risks for adult cancers.[27,28]

Other Carcinomas

In young women, the more common metastatic lesions of the ovary include lymphomas and leukemias.

Minimizing the Risks of Ovarian Masses and Malignancies

Hormonal contraception minimizes the risks of functional ovarian masses in a dose-dependent manner[12] AYAs who have had an oophorectomy, an ovarian cystectomy, or an ovarian neoplasm may benefit from the use of oral contraceptive pills to minimize the risks of developing a subsequent functional cyst. Oral contraceptives minimize the risks that a sole-remaining ovary will develop a functional ovarian cyst and be vulnerable to surgical extirpation. In adolescents with a previous malignancy who are being monitored for recurrence, the development of a functional cyst will almost invariably lead to patient and parental anxiety, additional diagnostic testing, and even potential surgical exploration. Therefore, suppression of ovarian functional cysts can be particularly beneficial.

Combination oral contraceptives are associated with a 30% to 60% reduction in the risk of epithelial ovarian malignancies.[29] Preventing ovarian cancer is seldom a motivating factor for adolescents; however, when combined with the contraceptive and other noncontraceptive benefits of oral contraceptives, such as decreased acne, dysmenorrhea, menorrhagia, and ovarian cysts, this benefit may provide additional motivation for ongoing oral contraceptive use to teens and their families.

REFERENCES

1. Hillard PJA. Benign diseases of the female reproductive tract. In: Berek JS, ed. *Berek & Novak's gynecology*. Philadelphia, PA: Wolters Kluwer Health/Lippincott Williams & Wilkins, 2012.
2. Spence J, Gervaize P, Jain S. Uterovaginal anomalies: diagnosis and current management in teens. *Curr Womens Health Rep* 2003;3(6):445–450.
3. Church DG, Vancil JM, Vasanawala SS. Magnetic resonance imaging for uterine and vaginal anomalies. *Curr Opin Obstet Gynecol* 2009;21(5):379–389.
4. Hall-Craggs MA, Kirkham A, Creighton SM. Renal and urological abnormalities occurring with Mullerian anomalies. *J Pediatr Urol* 2013;9(1):27–32.
5. Hillard PA. Imperforate Hymen. eMedicine. 2013.
6. Hillard APJ, Deitch HR. Menstrual disorders in the college age female. *Pediatr Clin North Am* 2005;52(1):179–197, ix–x.
7. Workowski KA, Berman S. Sexually transmitted diseases treatment guidelines, 2010. *MMWR Recomm Rep* 2010;59(12):1–110.
8. Breech LL, Hillard PJ. Adnexal torsion in pediatric and adolescent girls. *Curr Opin Obstet Gynecol* 2005;17(5):483–489.
9. Kirkham YA, Kives S. Ovarian cysts in adolescents: medical and surgical management. *Adolesc Med* 2012;23(1):178–191, xii.

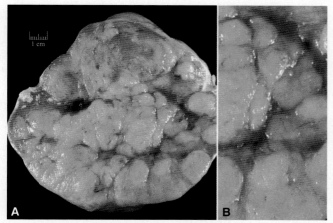

FIGURE 52.19 Dysgerminoma with solid lobulated appearance. (From Reichert RA. *Diagnostic gynecologic and obstetric pathology*. Philadelphia, PA: Lippincott Williams & Wilkins, 2011.)

10. Pomeranz AJ, Sabnis S. Misdiagnoses of ovarian masses in children and adolescents. *Pediatr Emerg Care* 2004;20(3):172–174.
11. Hernon M, McKenna J, Busby G, et al. The histology and management of ovarian cysts found in children and adolescents presenting to a children's hospital from 1991 to 2007: a call for more paediatric gynaecologists. *BJOG* 2010;117(2):181–184.
12. Grimes DA, Jones LB, Lopez LM, et al. Oral contraceptives for functional ovarian cysts. *Cochrane Database Syst Rev* 2011;9:CD006134.
13. Steenberg CK, Tanbo TG, Qvigstad E. Endometriosis in adolescence: predictive markers and management. *Acta Obstet Gynecol Scand* 2013;92(5):491–495.
14. Laufer MR, Sanfilippo J, Rose G. Adolescent endometriosis: diagnosis and treatment approaches. *J Pediatr Adolesc Gynecol* 2003;16(3, suppl):S3–S11.
15. Barroilhet L, Vitonis A, Shipp T, et al. Sonographic predictors of ovarian malignancy. *J Clin Ultrasound* 2013;41(5):269–274.
16. Young JL Jr, Cheng Wu X, Roffers SD, et al. Ovarian cancer in children and young adults in the United States, 1992–1997. *Cancer* 2003;97(10, suppl):2694–2700.
17. Wu X, Groves FD, McLaughlin CC, et al. Cancer incidence patterns among adolescents and young adults in the United States. *Cancer Causes Control* 2005;16(3):309–320.
18. Stepanian M, Cohn DE. Gynecologic malignancies in adolescents. *Adolesc Med Clin* 2004;15(3):549–568.
19. Young RH. Ovarian tumors and tumor-like lesions in the first three decades. *Semin Diagn Pathol* 2014;31(5):382–426.
20. Deligeoroglou E, Eleftheriades M, Shiadoes V, et al. Ovarian masses during adolescence: clinical, ultrasonographic and pathologic findings, serum tumor markers and endocrinological profile. *Gynecol Endocrinol* 2004;19(1):1–8.
21. Looijenga LH, Hersmus R, de Leeuw BH, et al. Gonadal tumours and DSD. *Best Pract Res Clin Endocrinol Metab* 2010;24(2):291–310.
22. Hazard FK, Longacre TA. Ovarian surface epithelial neoplasms in the pediatric population: incidence, histologic subtype, and natural history. *Am J Surg Pathol* 2013;37(4):548–553.
23. Kajiyama H, Shibata K, Suzuki S, et al. Fertility-sparing surgery in young women with invasive epithelial ovarian cancer. *Eur J Surg Oncol* 2010;36(4):404–408.
24. du Bois A, Ewald-Riegler N, de Gregorio N, et al. Borderline tumours of the ovary: a cohort study of the Arbeitsgmeinschaft Gynakologische Onkologie (AGO) Study Group. *Eur J Cancer* 2013;49(8):1905–1914.
25. Pennington KP, Swisher EM. Hereditary ovarian cancer: beyond the usual suspects. *Gynecol Oncol* 2012;124(2):347–353.
26. Laufer MR, Goldstein DP. *Benign and malignant ovarian masses. Pediatric and adoelscent gynecology.* 5th ed. Philadelphia, PA: Lippincott Williams & Wilkins; 2005:685-728.
27. Bradbury AR, Patrick-Miller L, Pawlowski K, et al. Should genetic testing for BRCA1/2 be permitted for minors? Opinions of BRCA mutation carriers and their adult offspring. *Am J Med Genet C Semin Med Genet* 2008;148c(1):70–77.
28. Bradbury AR, Patrick-Miller L, Pawlowski K, et al. Learning of your parent's BRCA mutation during adolescence or early adulthood: a study of offspring experiences. *Psychooncology* 2009;18(2):200–208.
29. Grimbizis GF, Tarlatzis BC. The use of hormonal contraception and its protective role against endometrial and ovarian cancer. *Best Pract Res Clin Obstet Gynaecol* 2010;24(1):29–38.

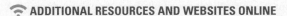

ADDITIONAL RESOURCES AND WEBSITES ONLINE

53

Ectopic Pregnancy

Melissa Mirosh
Mary Anne Jamieson

KEY WORDS

- Ectopic pregnancy
- Methotrexate
- Quantitative β-hCG
- Salpingectomy
- Salpingostomy
- Transvaginal ultrasound

ECTOPIC PREGNANCY

Ectopic pregnancy in the adolescent population is fortunately uncommon. Teens usually have not had enough exposures to infection or other intra-abdominal pathologies to acquire tubal damage and then conceive with resultant ectopic pregnancy. However, patients in their 20s are more likely to have encountered these risk factors. Ectopic pregnancy should be a consideration when any reproductive age female presents with new onset of abnormal uterine vaginal bleeding or abdominal/pelvic pain and a positive pregnancy test.

Incidence and Prevalence

1. *Rate and anatomic location*: The overall risk of ectopic pregnancy is 2%. This rate has been stable for many years, but is elevated from previous decades.[1] This is only an approximation because there are many miscarriages, abortions, and medically treated ectopic pregnancies that are not reported. Ectopic pregnancies occur almost exclusively in the oviduct (95.5%), while 1.3% are abdominal and approximately 3% are cervical or ovarian. Within the tube itself, 70% of ectopic pregnancies are located in the ampullary region, 12% are isthmic, 11% are fimbrial, and 2.4% are interstitial.[2]
2. *Trends*: Although the rate of ectopic pregnancy has remained unchanged, the chance of dying from one has decreased, most likely due to increased detection of early pregnancy. From 1980–1984 to 2003–2007, the ectopic pregnancy mortality rate declined from 1.15 to 0.50 deaths per 100,000 live births (a drop of 56.6%) in the US.[3] The risk of death from ectopic pregnancy in the United Kingdom also fell between 1999–2002 and 2006–2008.[4]
3. *Age:* Ectopic pregnancy occurs throughout the reproductive age spectrum. A review from California found a low rate of 12.5 per 1,000 reported pregnancies in women aged 15 to 19 compared to a higher rate of 42.5 per 1,000 pregnancies in women aged 40 to 49.[5]
4. *Race:* Ectopic pregnancies are more frequently seen in Black women (8%) compared to White women (4%). This demographic trend is also seen with respect to overall maternal

mortality. This discrepancy is unexplained at present, although it is consistent with the higher sexually transmitted infection (STI) rate and lower socioeconomic status seen in the Black population in the US.[3,6]

Etiology and Risk Factors

There are many factors associated with an increased risk of developing an ectopic pregnancy. Fallopian tube pathology is the leading cause and includes untreated or recurrent STIs or pelvic inflammatory disease (PID), previous ectopic pregnancy, tubal surgery, or intra-abdominal pathology or infection (ruptured appendix, inflammatory bowel disease, etc.)[7] Although the absolute risk of ectopic pregnancy is lower with the use of an intrauterine device (IUD) (explained by low rate of contraceptive failure), the risk of ectopic pregnancy is elevated should a pregnancy occur with an IUD in situ.[8] Other associated risks include infertility and fertility therapy,[9] smoking, increasing age, tubal ligation failure, and diethylstilbestrol exposure.

Differential Diagnosis

In addition to ectopic pregnancy, the differential diagnosis for a teen or young adult presenting with acute abdominal or pelvic pain is best divided into obstetric, gynecologic, and nongynecologic categories.

1. Obstetric
   a. Normal intrauterine pregnancy
   b. Hemorrhagic corpus luteum
   c. Spontaneous or threatened abortion
2. Gynecologic
   a. Adnexal torsion
   b. Hemorrhagic ovarian cyst
   c. Symptomatic or ruptured ovarian cyst
   d. PID
3. Nongynecologic
   a. Appendicitis
   b. Renal colic
   c. Inflammatory bowel disease
   d. Gastroenteritis
   e. Severe constipation
   f. Musculoskeletal pain

Clinical Presentation

Symptoms can range from mild cramping and vaginal spotting to frank hemorrhagic shock. However, the classic triad of vaginal bleeding, delayed menses, and severe lower abdominal pain associated with tubal rupture is now a fairly infrequent presentation, because early diagnosis is more typical.

Acute Presentation: Classic, Ruptured Ectopic Pregnancy

1. The patient who presents with an acutely ruptured ectopic pregnancy would typically exhibit symptoms of pain and hemodynamic instability. Pelvic pain may be extreme, sharp, or stabbing in nature, and shoulder tip pain can be associated with hemoperitoneum. Dizziness, lightheadedness, and loss of consciousness may occur from hypotension. Some women may present with symptoms related to gastrointestinal distress (e.g., nausea, vomiting, and diarrhea), and these should not be discounted as a possible ectopic pregnancy. Menses may be abnormal or absent, and this may not seem unusual as teens often have irregular bleeding patterns.

2. Classic signs of a ruptured ectopic pregnancy:
   a. Vital signs: The patient may be in shock with rapid thready pulse, hypotension, and change in mental status.
   b. Abdomen will be tender to palpation, possibly even rigid, with marked rebound tenderness.
   c. Bimanual examination: Cervical motion tenderness is apparent with a slightly enlarged and globular uterus. Often, a pelvic mass is not palpable, due to limitations of the examination or because the rupture has eliminated the bulging mass in the fallopian tube.

3. Laboratory tests: Laboratory testing requirements are minimal and are necessary only to confirm pregnancy, prepare for surgery, and rule out other pathologies.
   a. Pregnancy testing: Sensitive qualitative urine pregnancy test results should be positive. A baseline quantitative serum β-human chorionic gonadotropin (β-hCG) will allow monitoring of pregnancy resolution.
   b. The "three Cs of hemorrhage":
      • Complete blood cell (CBC) count—including hemoglobin and hematocrit
      • Crossmatch—blood group and screen to prepare for possible transfusion, as well as Rh typing to determine the need for Rh immunoglobulin
      • Coagulation factors—if blood loss has been significant, patients may have evidence of disseminated intravascular coagulation and consideration should be given to appropriate laboratory testing.
   c. Ultrasonography: If the patient is hemodynamically unstable, an ultrasound is not indicated and should not delay a patient's surgery. If ultrasonography is performed, however, the most remarkable finding will be free fluid and clots in the pelvis; blood may fill the entire abdominal cavity. If there is a positive pregnancy test, a corpus luteum ovarian cyst may be seen and the endometrium thickened with decidual material. In fact, a hemorrhagic corpus luteum cyst is the other main consideration in the differential diagnosis, particularly if the pregnancy is too early to be identified visually. The presence of an intrauterine pregnancy essentially rules out ectopic pregnancy in an adolescent or young adult because heterotopic pregnancy is extremely rare without assisted reproductive technologies. It is not necessary to visualize the pregnancy in the tube, and the absence of a uterine pregnancy on ultrasonography is not necessarily diagnostic of an ectopic pregnancy. In the context of an acute and unstable presentation, the final diagnosis will usually be confirmed at the time of surgery.

4. Therapy: Fluid resuscitation should be started immediately and performed aggressively. Blood transfusion can also be initiated if appropriate. The primary method of management is surgery, both for diagnostic and therapeutic purposes. If the patient is Rh negative, she requires Rh immunoglobulin perioperatively. In the operating room (OR), effort should be made in an adolescent or young adult to preserve the fallopian tube, if possible. If a hemorrhagic corpus luteum is the cause of the bleeding, then if at all possible the ovary should be preserved.

If an oophorectomy is required, progesterone supplementation should be instituted until 10 to 12 weeks gestation if the patient wishes to continue the intrauterine pregnancy.

Subacute Presentations

An adolescent or young adult with a positive pregnancy test result who presents with cramping, abnormal vaginal spotting or bleeding, and lower abdominal/adnexal pain should be suspected of having an ectopic pregnancy, particularly if the diagnosis is supported by physical findings of cervical motion tenderness, a closed cervix, adnexal tenderness, and (possibly) an adnexal mass. The workup and treatment depend on the adolescent's or young woman's risk factors and her pregnancy intentions.

The initial diagnosis of a clinically suspected ectopic pregnancy in the hemodynamically stable patient begins with a complete history and physical examination, lab work, and transvaginal ultrasound imaging. The timing of her last normal menstrual period, positive pregnancy test, or previous ultrasound imaging is potentially helpful; however, the definitive management will be based on current transvaginal ultrasound and serial quantitative β-hCG levels. The lab work should include CBC count (for white blood cell [WBC], hemoglobin [Hgb], and hematocrit), blood typing and screening to determine Rh status, and a serum quantitative β-hCG. The adolescent patient may need an explanation for the role of transvaginal ultrasonography as she may be hesitant to have a probe inserted vaginally.

Laboratory and Imaging Evaluation

The properties and limitations of each diagnostic test should be recognized to appropriately use each of them in the workup.

1. β-hCG: Typically, β-hCG levels will double every 2 days in a normal first-trimester intrauterine gestation. Only 15% of normal pregnancies will fail to have this appropriate increase in β-hCG levels. The smallest increase over 48 hours that can still be associated with a continuing intrauterine pregnancy is 53%.[10] If β-hCG measurements are unchanged or increasing abnormally, the pregnancy is nonviable, regardless of location. Pregnancies that have inappropriately low β-hCG levels are more likely to be ectopic. Serial β-hCG measurements can be extremely helpful in determining the fate of these pregnancies.

2. Ultrasonography: Ultrasound studies at appropriate β-hCG levels are usually diagnostic, and often the definitive method of pregnancy dating and localization. Transvaginal ultrasound is highly accurate at identifying ectopic pregnancy, with sensitivities and specificities ranging from 87% to 99%.[11] This may require more than one assessment depending on the clinical picture. There is still debate over what β-hCG cutoff should be used as the discriminatory level (the lowest concentration of β-hCG that is associated with a visible normal intrauterine gestation), but this level is generally considered to be above 1,500 to 2,000 IU/L when using a transvaginal ultrasound probe. Above this level of serum β-hCG, a normal intrauterine gestational sac should be seen.[12] Although an intrauterine pregnancy may be detected at lower levels, the possibility that the pregnancy in question is intrauterine cannot be excluded until the β-hCG levels reach the discriminatory range. If no intrauterine gestation is seen, then an ectopic pregnancy should be strongly suspected. If transabdominal scanning is the only method available, the β-hCG cutoff should be 6,500 IU/L.[13]

Outpatient Follow-Up—Using Serial β-hCG Levels

1. Declining β-hCG levels: If the β-hCG levels are declining by 50% to 66% every 3 days, it is likely that the patient has experienced a complete resolution of the pregnancy. The β-hCG levels must be followed up until they are undetectable (based on local laboratory values).

2. Increasing β-hCG levels: If the β-hCG levels are increasing by at least 66% every 2 to 3 days, they should be followed up in a mildly symptomatic patient until they reach the discriminatory zone and the diagnosis can be made ultrasonographically. If the patient becomes increasingly symptomatic before reaching the discriminatory zone, laparoscopic investigation may be considered. It is useful to discuss with the patient whether the pregnancy is wanted. A dilation and curettage (D&C) can be performed at the time of laparoscopy if the pregnancy is discovered to be intrauterine. If the pregnancy is wanted, consider delaying insertion of the uterine manipulator until an ectopic gestation is confirmed.

3. Abnormally changing β-hCG levels: If the β-hCG levels are declining or rising at an inappropriate rate, the pregnancy (either intrauterine or ectopic) is likely nonviable. However, this does not differentiate between a miscarriage and an ectopic pregnancy.

   a. If her β-hCG levels are above the discriminatory level, an ultrasound should be obtained to localize the pregnancy. If it is not within the endometrial cavity, the pregnancy is likely ectopic.

   b. If her β-hCG levels are less than the discriminatory range, it is important to assess the patient's desire for pregnancy. If she does not wish to continue with the pregnancy, medical termination can be offered without definitively locating the pregnancy. This commonly involves methotrexate followed by misoprostol to evacuate the uterus. Some advocate for the use of a D&C to provide a tissue diagnosis of an abnormal intrauterine pregnancy. The presence of trophoblastic villi and a rapid drop in β-hCG levels rule out an ectopic pregnancy.[14]

Other Diagnostic Modalities

1. Serum progesterone levels: The 1998 meta-analysis of Mol et al.[15] examined the use of a single serum progesterone level for diagnosing ectopic pregnancy. It was not helpful in determining either the potential for viability or the location of the pregnancy.

2. Culdocentesis to determine if there is blood in the cul-de-sac is rarely used today. It has been replaced by ultrasonic imaging.

Management

Issues Unique to Adolescents

1. Access to care and follow-up: There are several factors in the evaluation and treatment of ectopic pregnancy that are unique to, or should be emphasized in, adolescents and young adult women. These patients may present later in gestation because of denial of pregnancy or fear of consequences. They may have trouble accessing the medical system or are unable to seek help due to lack of transportation or money. Once in your office, establishing an accurate history is often difficult as menstrual cycles can be irregular and these patients may be poor historians.

2. Confidentiality and consent for treatment: One must be aware of the local legislation with respect to informed consent for minors. In many regions, health care providers can provide medical care to an adolescent who understands the nature of the diagnosis and/or treatment, without necessarily involving a parent or guardian. Teens may have a particular need for confidentiality which must be respected. On the other hand, health care providers should make every effort to negotiate with the teen to involve a parent or a guardian in such an important issue as the diagnosis and treatment of an ectopic pregnancy. Young adults may be able to provide consent, but confidentiality could be an issue particularly with respect to insurance coverage.

Approaches to Management

In the adolescent or young adult with an ectopic pregnancy, treatment should generally be fertility sparing and take into account the challenges that some adolescents may have with follow-up recommendations.

1. *Surgical approach*: Most young women diagnosed with an ectopic pregnancy will be treated surgically through laparoscopy or laparotomy. The majority of these cases can be done laparoscopically, even with significant hemorrhage.[16] Although a recent Cochrane review concluded that the laparoscopic route was less successful than laparotomy for complete resolution of trophoblastic tissue, laparoscopy remains the cornerstone of treatment, owing to its decreased operative time, hospital stay, and recovery times.[17]

   Conservative or radical treatment? The most common surgical procedures are salpingostomy and salpingectomy. In theory, the benefit of removing the affected tube is an almost guaranteed resolution of the ectopic pregnancy, while treating conservatively preserves the potential for fertility with that tube (which is crucial in younger patients, including the adolescent or young adult). Salpingostomy has a higher risk of persistent trophoblastic tissue, but this can be improved by adding a single dose of methotrexate postoperatively.[18]

   There are some patients in whom salpingectomy is the preferred method of treatment. These would include cases of intractable hemorrhage, recurrent ectopic pregnancy in the same tube, or in women who have completed childbearing. The latter two scenarios seldom occur in the adolescent or young woman. One aspect to consider before removing the affected tube is the state of the contralateral tube. If the patient wishes to conserve her chances for spontaneous conception, the unaffected tube must appear normal. If it is abnormal or damaged, salpingostomy for the ectopic pregnancy would be recommended.

2. *Medical therapy*: Early diagnosis of ectopic pregnancy using laboratory tests and sensitive imaging techniques has significantly reduced the mortality and morbidity of this condition. It has also enabled the use of outpatient medical therapy in lieu of surgical intervention, which in time has reduced hospitalization costs and surgical complications. Methotrexate has become the established medical method of treatment for patients diagnosed with an unruptured ectopic pregnancy. It is a folic acid antagonist and, therefore, exerts its effect on rapidly dividing cells.

   Single-dose and multidose protocols are available for methotrexate use. A large meta-analysis found that although a multidose regimen is more successful (92.7% versus 88.1%), the overall success of medically treating an ectopic pregnancy with any method of methotrexate is 89%.[19] One study reviewed a group of 55 adolescents who had successfully used the single-dose method and were able to follow the strict follow-up protocols. In this group of teens, the success rate of methotrexate for ectopic pregnancy resolution was 85%.[20]

   Methotrexate therapy is more likely to be successful if the initial β-hCG level is <4,000 IU/L and fetal cardiac activity is not seen. Indicators predictive of failure included visible extrauterine yolk sac on ultrasonography and previous ectopic pregnancy.[21] Patients must be counseled about the possibility of treatment failure (and possible tubal rupture) and the signs and symptoms that may indicate complications and necessitate return to hospital. Because it is common for abdominal pain to occur as the ectopic pregnancy resolves 24 to 48 hours after administration of methotrexate, the differentiation of "normal" from "abnormal" pain can be challenging and may result in additional emergency room visits for reassessment and reassurance.

   The dose used for treating ectopic pregnancy, usually 50 mg/m², is much lower than that used for cancer chemotherapy. Many different regimens of methotrexate delivery have been employed for treatment of ectopic pregnancy, including oral, intramuscular, and local injection (under laparoscopic or ultrasound guidance). **Tables 53.1** and **53.2** list exclusion criteria and a logarithm for methotrexate use.

TABLE 53.1
Methotrexate Therapy for Ectopic Pregnancy—Exclusion Criteria

Patient characteristics:
  Hemodynamically unstable
  Unable to comply with follow-up visit schedule or to return if complications develop
  Immunocompromised (WBC count <3,000)
  Anemia (hemoglobin <8 g/dL)
  Active pulmonary disease
  Renal compromise (creatinine clearance >1.3 mg/dL)
  Hepatic compromise (elevated liver function test results; aspartate aminotransferase >50 IU/L)
  Hematological dysfunction
  Thrombocytopenia

β-hCG characteristics:
  Most institutions exclude levels >10,000 mIU/ng

Ultrasonography findings:
  Gestational sac (maximum density of entire mass) >3.5–4.0 cm[a]
  Fetal cardiac motion[a]
  Excessive fluid in cul-de-sac consistent with hemorrhage

[a]Relative contraindication.

TABLE 53.2
Systemic Methotrexate Treatment Algorithm

Treatment Day	Investigation/Management
1	Patient eligible for methotrexate therapy
	Labs: Quantitative β-hCG, renal function tests, liver function tests, CBC count, blood type and screen
	Methotrexate administered in 50 mg/m² dose intramuscularly
	Patient care instructions, including anticipated symptoms and analgesia
4	Labs: Quantitative β-hCG
7	Labs: Quantitative β-hCG, renal and liver function tests, CBC count
	Compare β-hCG levels from day 4 and 7: If the decline in value is ≥15%, continue to monitor β-hCG until they resolve. If the decline is <15%, a second methotrexate dose is needed.
	Consider surgical treatment if the patient becomes hemodynamically unstable, has increasing pain and/or falling hematocrit, or if there is an ineffective response to methotrexate.

hCG, human chorionic gonadotropin; CBC, complete blood cell.

Because the doses are so much lower than that used for chemotherapy, the common side effects of methotrexate observed at higher dosages (e.g., nausea, vomiting, stomatitis, and diarrhea) are rarely seen with doses used to treat ectopic pregnancies. Rarely, reversible leukopenia or transient hair loss may be seen.

3. *Other medical modalities*: Other medical interventions have included injecting the embryo with methotrexate, hypertonic saline, or prostaglandins. Although successful, these methods are more cumbersome and invasive compared to oral or intramuscular methotrexate, and therefore, are much less frequently used.[17,22]

4. *Treatment of unusual ectopic pregnancy sites*: As mentioned previously, ectopic pregnancies are rarely located outside the fallopian tubes. There are a number of individual case reports documenting surgical and medical management of pregnancies located on ovaries, surgical scars, omentum, and the cervix. The method of treatment for pregnancies in these sites is usually systemic or local methotrexate under ultrasound guidance,[23] as surgical treatment would be technically difficult or dangerous due to uncontrollable bleeding or poor surgical access.

5. *Expectant management*: Expectant management is reasonable for a certain subset of young women presenting with ectopic pregnancy. These patients are usually asymptomatic and generally have a β-hCG level below 1,500 IU/L, which is falling spontaneously. They also need to be reliable, as losing a patient to follow-up could be disastrous. Under these circumstances, approximately 70% of patients will have successful resolution of their ectopic pregnancy without intervention.[24] Those who have spontaneous resolution of their ectopic pregnancies also tend to have a good chance of return to normal fertility. A review by Buster et al. found similar reproductive outcomes after surgical, medical, or expectant management.[25] Unfortunately, the need to assess carefully these patients over the course of several weeks, especially if they develop pain, may result in the need for repeated clinical visits. Adolescents should be considered on an individual basis as candidates for conservative management because for many teens the follow-up and surveillance requirements will be too compliance demanding.

Follow-up

Women treated with methotrexate or expectant management will require weekly (or more frequent) quantitative β-hCG determinations until the levels become undetectable. Table 53.3 outlines specific guidelines for following up a patient treated with methotrexate. For patients undergoing surgical management, the typical protocol is to check the quantitative β-hCG level on the first postoperative day, followed by weekly tests until the β-hCG level is undetectable. With tube-sparing surgery, approximately 8% of women will have persistent trophoblastic tissue; so it is prudent to ensure that the β-hCG levels return to normal, and another pregnancy should be prevented until that time.[26]

Persistent Disease

If persistent disease is diagnosed, further treatment is necessary. If surgical treatment was used initially, methotrexate should probably be used as second line as long as the patient is not continuing to bleed from the ectopic pregnancy. If methotrexate was used initially, options include surgical treatment or repeat methotrexate. Rarely, expectant management can be considered, but would again require a well-informed, compliant patient.

Contraception

It is important to provide effective contraception during the recovery period, not only to prevent a second pregnancy from complicating the β-hCG results, but also to allow the tubal tissue time to heal, thereby presumably reducing the risk of a second ectopic pregnancy in rapid succession. Waiting until the β-hCG levels "zero out" before starting contraception puts a woman in jeopardy for pregnancy because ovulation often precedes complete β-hCG clearance. Assuming the adolescent or young adult is not seeking to conceive, every effort should be made to offer and provide reliable and acceptable contraception after a failed pregnancy (intrauterine or ectopic) or any pregnancy for that matter.

TABLE 53.3
Systemic Methotrexate Follow-Up Instructions

To patients:

Avoid sexual intercourse (may rupture ectopic pregnancy)

Avoid sun exposure (photosensitivity reaction possible)

Avoid consuming gas-producing foods—leeks, beans, corn, cabbage (abdominal bloating may worsen)

No alcohol

No ibuprofen, naproxen, aspirin, or other nonsteroidal anti-inflammatory agents

No penicillin

No prenatal vitamins or folate supplements

Return to clinic in 4 d for repeat tests of the pregnancy hormone β-human chorionic gonadotropin

Be aware that in the next few days, you may experience sharp abdominal pain and some cramping. This discomfort should be self-limited, but if you feel dizzy or weak, or if the pain does not resolve, have someone take you to the emergency room immediately. There is a small chance that the pregnancy could rupture through the tube and you would need immediate surgery.

Your next period may be particularly heavy.

To providers:

No need for vaginal examination

Rh Considerations

Unsensitized Rh-negative women should be given an appropriate dose of Rh immunoglobulin (50 to 120 µg if gestational age <12 weeks; 300 µg if >12 weeks) promptly.[27,28] Although very occasionally the blood type of the "father" is used to determine whether an Rh-negative woman receives immunoglobulin, it is always prudent to treat the Rh-negative adolescent anyway, because of the uncertainty that may exist with respect to paternity.

FERTILITY AFTER TREATMENT OF ECTOPIC PREGNANCY

One randomized controlled trial has been published comparing fertility outcomes after medical, conservative (salpingostomy), and radical (salpingectomy) treatment for ectopic pregnancy. No significant difference was found between each method of treatment and the rate of intrauterine pregnancy 2 years after treatment ranged from 64% to 71%.[29] One study comparing medical and surgical treatment of younger women aged 18 to 28 had an intrauterine pregnancy rate of 60% to 69% at 2 years ($p = 0.942$).[30]

On average, ectopic pregnancies recur in 10% of patients.[2,29] Some studies suggest a higher recurrence rate for patients treated with salpingostomy,[31] while others show no difference.[29] Given this relatively high rate of recurrence, an early ultrasound is recommended for any subsequent pregnancies to confirm the location of the pregnancy.

Regardless of the method of treatment, adolescent or young adult patients patients who have had only one ectopic pregnancy can be reassured that their chances of having an intrauterine pregnancy in the future are excellent. The method of treatment can therefore be tailored to the needs of the individual patient.

REFERENCES

1. Chang J, Elam-Evans LD, Berg CJ, et al. Pregnancy related mortally surveillance—United States, 1991–1999. *MMWR Surveill Summ* 2003;52:1–9.
2. Bouyer J, Coste J, Fernandez H, et al. Sites of ectopic pregnancy: a 10 year population-based study of 1800 cases. *Hum Reprod* 2002;17:3224.
3. Creanga AA, Shapiro-Mendoza CK, Bish CL, et al. Trends in ectopic pregnancy mortality in the United States: 1980–2007. *Obstet Gynecol* 2011;117(4):837–843.
4. Centre for Maternal and Child Enquiries (CMACE). Saving mothers' lives: reviewing maternal deaths to make motherhood safer: 2006–08. The eighth report on confidential enquiries into maternal deaths in the United Kingdom. *Br J Obstet Gynaecol* 2011;118 (suppl 1):1–203.
5. Van Den Eeden SK, Shan J, Bruce C, et al. Ectopic pregnancy rate and treatment utilization in a large managed care organization. *Obstet Gynecol* 2005;105:1052.
6. Centers for Disease Control and Prevention; Workowski KA, Berman SM. Sexually transmitted diseases treatment guidelines, 2006. *MMWR Recomm Rep* 2006;4;55(RR-11):1.
7. Barnhart KT. Clinical practice. Ectopic pregnancy. *N Engl J Med* 2009;361:379–87.
8. Weir E. Preventing pregnancy: a fresh look at the IUD. *Can Med Assoc J* 2003;169:585.
9. Clayton HB, Schieve LA, Peterson HB, et al. Ectopic pregnancy risk with assisted reproductive technology procedures. *Obstet Gynecol* 2006;107:595–604.
10. Barnhart K, Sammel MD, Chung K, et al. Decline of serum human chorionic gonadotropin and spontaneous complete abortion: defining the normal curve. *Obstet Gynecol* 2004;104:975.
11. Kirk E, Bottomley C, Bourne T. Diagnosing ectopic pregnancy and current concepts in the management of pregnancy of unknown location. *Hum Reprod Update* 2014;20(2):250–261.
12. Condous G, Okaro E, Khalid A, et al. The accuracy of transvaginal ultrasonography for the diagnosis of ectopic pregnancy prior to surgery. *Hum Reprod* 2005;20:1404.
13. Kadar N, Bohrer M, Kemmann E, et al. The discriminatory human chorionic gonadotropin zone for endovaginal sonography: a prospective, randomized study. *Fertil Steril* 1994;61:1016.
14. Seeber BE, Barnhart KT. Suspected ectopic pregnancy. *Obstet Gynecol* 2006;107(2, Pt 1):399.
15. Mol BW, Lijmer JG, Ankum WM, et al. The accuracy of single serum progesterone measurement in the diagnosis of ectopic pregnancy: a meta-analysis. *Hum Reprod* 1998;13:3220.
16. Takeda A, Manabe S, Mitsui T, et al. Management of patients with ectopic pregnancy with massive hemoperitoneum by laparoscopic surgery with intraoperative autologous blood transfusion. *J Minim Invasive Gynecol* 2006;13(1):43–48.
17. Hajenius PJ, Mol F, Mol BW, et al. Interventions for tubal ectopic pregnancy [Review]. *Cochrane Database Syst Rev* 2007;24;(1):CD000324.
18. Mol F, Mol BW, Ankum WM, et al. Current evidence on surgery, systemic methotrexate and expectant management in the treatment of tubal ectopic pregnancy: a systematic review and meta-analysis. *Hum Reprod Update* 2008;14(4): 309–319.
19. Barnhart KT, Gosman G, Ashby R, et al. The medical management of ectopic pregnancy: a meta-analysis comparing "single dose" and "multidose" regimens. *Obstet Gynecol* 2003;101:778.
20. McCord ML, Muram D, Lipscomb GH, et al. Methotrexate therapy for ectopic pregnancy in adolescents. *J Pediatr Adolesc Gynecol* 1996;9:71.
21. Lipscomb GH, Givens VA, Meyer NL, et al. Previous ectopic pregnancy as a predictor of failure of systemic methotrexate therapy. *Fertil Steril* 2004;81:1221.
22. Yao M, Tulandi T, Falcone T. Treatment of ectopic pregnancy by systemic methotrexate, transvaginal methotrexate, and operative laparoscopy. *Int J Fertil Menopausal Stud* 1996;41(5):470.
23. Doubilet PM, Benson CB, Frates MC, et al. Sonographically guided minimally invasive treatment of unusual ectopic pregnancies. *J Ultrasound Med* 2004;23:359.
24. Craig LB, Khan S. Expectant management of ectopic pregnancy. *Clin Obstet Gynecol* 2012;55(2):461–470.
25. Buster JE, Krotz S. Reproductive performance after ectopic pregnancy. *Semin Reprod Med* 2007;25(2):131–133.
26. Bangsgaard N, Lund CO, Ottesen B, et al. Improved fertility following conservative surgical treatment of ectopic pregnancy. *Br J Obstet Gynaecol* 2003;110(8): 765.
27. American College of Obstetrics and Gynecology. ACOG Practice Bulletin. Prevention of Rh D alloimmunization. Clinical management guidelines for obstetrician-gynecologists. *Int J Gynaecol Obstet* 1999;66:63.
28. Fung Kee Fung K, Eason E, Crane J, et al. Prevention of Rh alloimmunization. *J Obstet Gynaecol Can* 2003;25:765.
29. Fernandez H, Capmas P, Lucot JP, et al; GROG. Fertility after ectopic pregnancy: the DEMETER randomized trial. *Hum Reprod* 2013;28(5):1247–1253.
30. Turan V. Fertility outcomes subsequent to treatment of tubal ectopic pregnancy in younger Turkish women. *J Pediatr Adolesc Gynecol* 2011;24(5):251–255.
31. Yao M, Tulandi T. Current status of surgical and nonsurgical management of ectopic pregnancy. *Fertil Steril* 1997;67(3):421–433.

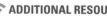 ADDITIONAL RESOURCES AND WEBSITES ONLINE

XII

Men's Health

William P. Adelman

- Epididymitis
- Hydrocele
- Male genital examination
- Men's health
- Scrotal masses
- Scrotal swelling
- Spermatocele
- Testicular self-examination
- Testicular torsion
- Varicocele

MALE GENITAL EXAMINATION

Examination of the male genitalia is a crucial part of the examination of the teenager and young adult. It is necessary to assess growth and development, to identify common variants and abnormalities, and is recommended by national organizations as part of adolescent and young adult (AYA) primary care.[1–4] It is a relatively easy examination to learn because the male genitalia are readily accessible for palpation and the anatomy is straightforward (Fig. 54.1). Once the anatomy is understood, a history and physical examination are often all that are required to make an accurate diagnosis. If the anatomy of the presenting condition is unclear, due to inability to perform a complete examination or loss of usual landmarks, ultrasonography is a simple, noninvasive method to clarify

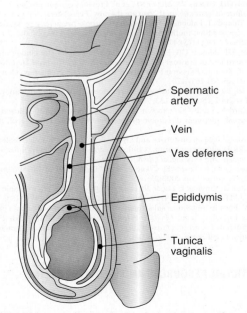

FIGURE 54.1 Male genitalia showing inguinal area, spermatic cord, epididymis, and testis.

Spermatic artery

Vein

Vas deferens

Epididymis

Tunica vaginalis

anatomy. Before beginning the examination, the examiner should make sure that his or her gloved hands are warm.[5,6]

Inspection

Inspect the pubic hair area and underlying skin noting sexual maturity rating (SMR).[5,7] Next, inspect the groin and inner aspect of thighs, followed by the penile meatus, prepuce, glans, corona, and shaft (Fig. 54.2). It is best to have the uncircumcised patient retract his own foreskin. Uncircumcised males have higher prevalence rates of pearly penile papules as well as ulcerative sexually transmitted infections (STIs). Pink, pearly penile papules are benign, uniform-sized papules that arise most commonly along the corona, during SMR 2 or 3, in as many as 15% of teenagers (Fig. 54.3). Inspect the scrotum and recognize that contraction of the dartos muscle of the scrotal wall produces folds or rugae, most prominent in the younger adolescent. An underdeveloped scrotum may indicate an ipsilateral undescended testicle. With a retractile testicle, the scrotum is normally developed. Finally, inspect the testes—the left testis is usually lower than the right. Check for enlargement (tumor, infection, hydrocele, or hernia) or asymmetry, suggesting atrophy or cryptorchidism on one side or unilateral enlargement as seen in tumor. Check for a "transverse lie" or "horizontal lie" of the testis, suggesting a "bell clapper deformity" (Fig. 54.4) and increased risk for torsion.

Palpation

Palpate the inguinal area, spermatic cord, epididymis, testes, and external inguinal ring. Check for lymphadenopathy or hernia in the inguinal area. In order to palpate the spermatic cord, apply gentle traction on the testis with one hand and palpate the structures of the cord with the index or middle finger and thumb of the opposite hand. The vas deferens feels like a smooth, rubbery tube and is the most posterior structure in the spermatic cord. Thickening and irregularity of the vas deferens may be caused by infection. Check for a varicocele (dilated pampiniform plexus of veins) within the spermatic cord. The epididymis lies along the posterolateral wall of the testis. The head of the epididymis attaches at the superior pole of the testis. The epididymis becomes the vas deferens and leaves the testis as part of the spermatic cord. The easiest way to find the epididymis is to follow the vas deferens toward its junction with the tail of the epididymis. Tenderness, induration, and swelling in this area usually indicate epididymitis. A well-localized, nontender, spherical enlargement of the epididymal head is a spermatocele. Palpate the testes to check size, shape, and presence of tenderness or masses. The adult testes are approximately 4 to 5 cm long and 3 cm wide but vary from one person to another. Stabilize the testis with one hand and use the other hand's thumb and first two fingers to palpate the entire surface. The testes should be roughly the same

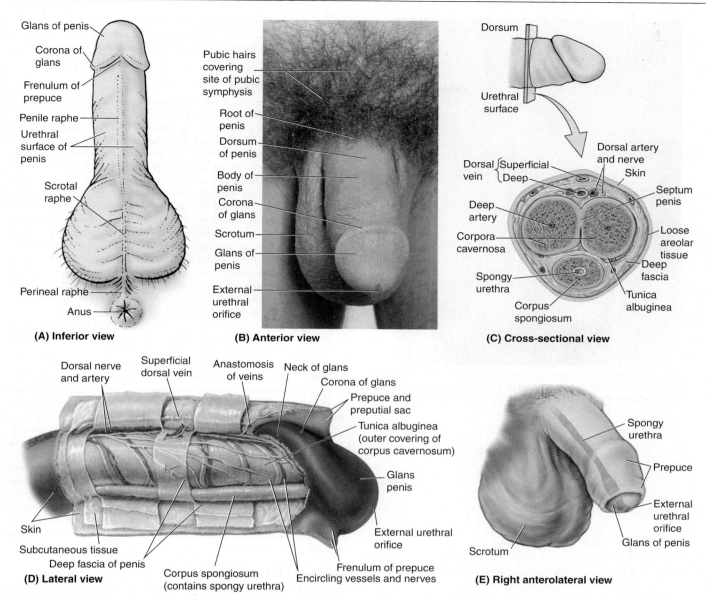

FIGURE 54.2 Penis and scrotum. **A:** The urethral surface of the circumcised penis is shown. **B:** The dorsum of the circumcised penis and the anterior surface of the scrotum are shown. The penis comprises a root, body, and glans. **C:** The penis contains three erectile masses: two corpora cavernosa and a corpus spongiosum (containing the spongy urethra). **D:** The skin of the penis extends distally as the prepuce, overlapping the neck and corona of the glans. **E:** An uncircumcised penis. (From Moore KL, Dalley AF, Agur AM. *Clinically Oriented Anatomy.* 6th ed. Baltimore: Wolters Kluwer Health, 2010.)

size (within 2 mL in volume), and volumes vary according to pubertal stage. Testicular volume could be quantified with the use of an orchidometer or by ultrasound. *Any induration within the testis is suspicious of testicular cancer until proved otherwise.* The appendix testis, present in 90% of males, can sometimes be palpated at the superior pole of the testis. Palpate the external inguinal ring by sliding your index finger along the spermatic cord above the inguinal ligament while having the patient cough or strain to check for a hernia.

CRYPTORCHIDISM

Cryptorchidism refers to an undescended testis that cannot be drawn into the scrotum.[8]

Epidemiology

Cryptorchidism is the most common genitourinary disorder of childhood, with a prevalence of 0.7% after 9 months of age.

Diagnosis

When a testis is not palpable in the scrotum, gentle massage should be performed along the line of descent from the anterosuperior spine, medially, and downward to the pubic tubercle. If the testis is not truly undescended, it should become palpable in the scrotum. If cryptorchidism is present, the teen should be examined for stigmata of associated disorders (i.e., Noonan, Klinefelter, or Kallmann syndrome or trisomy 13, 18, or 21).[1,5]

Complications

Infertility

Sperm production in the cryptorchid testis may be significantly impaired compared with normal testicular function, regardless of patient age at the time of discovery.

Malignancy

About 5% to 12% of all malignant testicular tumors occur in males with a history of an undescended testis. The relative risk of tumors

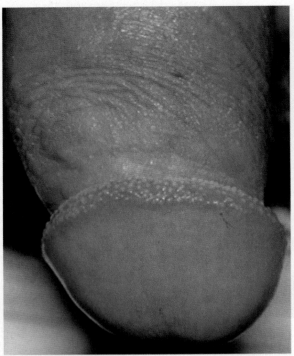

FIGURE 54.3 Pearly penile papules. (Reproduced with permission from Goodheart HG. *Photoguide to common skin disorders: diagnosis and management.* 3rd ed. Philadelphia, PA: Lippincott Williams & Wilkins, 2009.)

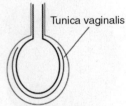

FIGURE 54.4 Bell clapper deformity. (From Shah SS, Frank G, Diallo A. Inpatient pediatrics work-up. Philadelphia, PA: Lippincott Williams & Wilkins, 2009.)

in such individuals is increased approximately 10 to 40 times that of a male without cryptorchidism. Moreover, the risk is increased even if the testis is brought down into the scrotum.

Therapy

Therapy for cryptorchidism in teenagers should be corrective surgery. These teens should be aware of the increased risk of testicular cancer and may be taught testicular self-examination.

 SCROTAL SWELLING AND MASSES

Evaluation

The general approach to the adolescent or young adult with a scrotal mass or a painful scrotum (Fig. 54.5) includes a directed history, physical examination, and laboratory testing.[5,9]

History

The adolescent or young adult should be questioned regarding the presence and prior history of genitourinary anomalies, pain, trauma, change in testicular or scrotal size, and sexual activity. Abrupt onset of pain is suggestive of torsion; gradual onset suggests epididymitis or orchitis; lack of pain suggests a tumor or cystic mass. Torsion is often preceded by episodes of mild pain. Reactive

hydroceles are common secondary to trauma, orchitis, testicular cancer, and epididymitis, and are noted as changes in the scrotum. Epididymitis in adolescence and young adulthood is usually sexually transmitted.

Physical Examination

Inspection of the testes can differentiate torsion from infection. In torsion, the affected testis is often higher than on the contralateral side. With infections, the affected testis is often lower. In torsion, the affected testis and often the contralateral testis lie horizontally instead of in the usual vertical position, secondary to the congenital defect involved, and the epididymis is usually displaced anteriorly, as the testis twists on its vascular pedicle. Careful palpation of the testicular surfaces, the epididymis and cord (posterior structures), and the head of the epididymis (superior structure) can further identify the cause of the painful mass. Isolated swelling and tenderness of the epididymis suggest epididymitis. A tender, pea-sized swelling at the upper pole of the testis suggests torsion of the appendix testis. Generalized swelling and tenderness of both the testis and the epididymis can be found in either testicular torsion or epididymitis with orchitis. Presence of a cremasteric reflex makes torsion unlikely. However, it is often present in torsion of the appendix testis. Prehn's sign, the relief of pain with elevation of the testis, suggests epididymitis. Lack of pain relief with elevation of the testis is not a reliable test for torsion. Nausea or vomiting with testicular pain is usually caused by torsion.

If a painless mass is present (Fig. 54.5), palpate to assess its location and then transilluminate the mass. Important findings on physical examination include the following: a mass within the testis is a tumor until proved otherwise; a mass palpable separate from the testis is unlikely to be a tumor; a "bag of worms" or "squishy tube" along the left spermatic cord is a varicocele; a mass located near the head of the epididymis, above and behind the testis is probably a spermatocele; a mass anterior to or surrounding the testis is probably a hydrocele; or a mass that is separate from the testis/epididymis, enlarges with straining (Valsalva), and is reducible is probably a hernia. Transilluminate the mass with a light source. Clear transillumination suggests a hydrocele or a typical spermatocele, whereas absence of transillumination suggests a testicular tumor or, if the mass is separate from the testis/epididymis, a hernia or a large spermatocele.

Laboratory Evaluation

A painful scrotum, or dysuria, a urine dipstick test that is positive for leukocyte esterase, or the presence of leukocytes on microscopy (especially if there are >20 white blood cells/high-power field) is suggestive of epididymitis rather than torsion. If a reasonable suspicion of torsion exists, emergent urology consultation is warranted. One should not delay this referral by ordering diagnostic tests, as the primary therapy should be surgical exploration.

Differential Diagnosis

When confronted with a painless scrotal mass or swelling (Fig. 54.5), important conditions to consider include hydrocele, spermatocele, varicocele, hernia, testicular tumor, and idiopathic scrotal edema. When addressing a painful scrotal mass or swelling, the differential diagnosis should include torsion of spermatic cord, torsion of appendix testis, epididymitis, orchitis, trauma with hematoma, incarcerated hernia, Henoch–Schonlein syndrome, cellulitis or infected piercing, hymenoptera sting or insect bite, and testicular torsion with bleeding or infarction.

TORSION

Etiology

Testicular torsion is a twisting of the testis and spermatic cord, which results in venous obstruction, progressive edema, arterial

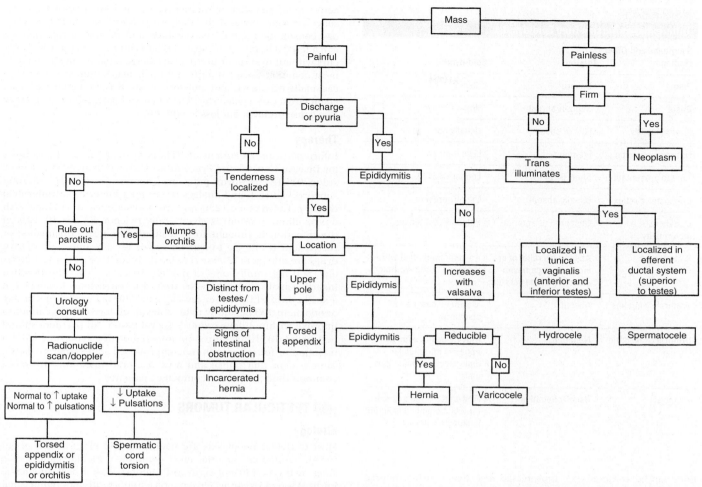

FIGURE 54.5 Diagnostic approach to scrotal masses. (Adapted from Schlossberger N. Male reproductive health: I. Painful scrotal masses. *Adolesc Health Update* 1992, 4:1; Klein BL, Ochsenschlager DW. Scrotal masses in children and adolescents: a review for the emergency physician. *Pediatr Emerg Care* 1993;9:351.)

compromise, and, eventually, testicular infarction. Normally, the testes are covered anteriorly with a mesothelial structure, the tunica vaginalis. In some males, the tunica vaginalis is abnormally enlarged and engulfs the testes. This causes the testis to lie like a "bell clapper" in the scrotal cavity (Fig. 54.4). With this deformity, a testis can twist on the spermatic cord, compromising circulation. Aside from torsion at the spermatic cord, appendages of the testes or of the epididymis can occasionally undergo torsion (Fig. 54.6A).

Epidemiology

Two-thirds of cases occur between 12 and 18 years, with incidence peaking at 15 to 16 years. The risk of developing torsion by age 25 is estimated to be approximately 1 in 160.

Clinical Manifestations

The onset of testicular torsion is usually abrupt, and 50% of teenagers have had brief prior episodes of scrotal pain. Pain may be isolated to the scrotum or may radiate to the abdomen, and nausea or vomiting may occur. Physical examination shows a tender and swollen testis, where the affected side is higher than the contralateral side because of the elevation from the twisted spermatic cord. In contrast, in inflammatory conditions, the affected side is often lower.

The epididymis, if palpable, is often out of the usual posterolateral location. The affected testis and often the contralateral testis lie in a horizontal plane rather than in the normal vertical plane. The cremasteric reflex, fever, and scrotal redness are usually absent.

Diagnosis

Testicular torsion is a surgical emergency. The diagnosis of torsion should be suspected in any adolescent or young adult with a painful swelling of the scrotum. If the history (acute onset of pain, nausea or vomiting, prior episodes of pain, lack of fever, lack of dysuria, or urethral discharge) and physical examination (patient in distress, high-riding testis, horizontal position of testis, generalized swelling of the testis) are consistent with torsion, a urology consultation should be obtained immediately and decisions made for further testing or direct surgical exploration (Fig. 54.5).

Therapy

Therapy involves immediate surgery. Saving testicular function depends on early surgical intervention. If surgery is performed within 6 hours of symptom onset, recovery is the rule; if surgery is performed between 6 and 12 hours, 62% of patients have recovery of testicular function. After 12 hours, the success rate falls to 20% to 38% and after 24 hours, only up to 11% of testes survive.

⬤ EPIDIDYMITIS

Etiology

Epididymitis is an inflammation of the epididymis caused by infection or trauma. In sexually active men younger than 35 years, it is most frequently caused by *Chlamydia trachomatis* or *Neisseria gonorrhoeae*. Epididymitis due to *Escherichia coli* or other bowel

TABLE 54.1

Differentiating Torsion from Epididymitis

Symptoms and Other Findings	Torsion	Epididymitis
Pain	Severe	Severe
Onset	Sudden/abrupt	Hours to days
Prior episodes	50% of cases	Usually not
Nausea or vomiting	Frequent	Less frequent
Time to presentation	Short (<24 h)	Longer (>24 h)
Cremasteric reflex	Usually absent	Usually present
Epididymal abnormality	Obscured or anterior	Palpable and tender
Prehn's sign	Absent: No relief of or increase in pain with elevation of the scrotum	Present: Pain relief with elevation of the scrotum
Urethral symptoms	Absent	May have dysuria, discharge
Urethral Gram stain	Negative	May be positive for gram-negative intracellular diplococci or white blood cells
Urinalysis	Usually negative	First-catch urine positive for white blood cells and/or leukocyte esterase

flora can be secondary to unprotected insertive anal intercourse. Sexually transmitted epididymitis usually is accompanied by urethritis, which often is asymptomatic.[10] Non–sexually transmitted epididymitis may be caused by instrumentation, surgery, catheterization, or anatomical abnormalities. Epididymitis can be difficult to differentiate from torsion (**Table 54.1**).

Epidemiology

Epididymitis is uncommon in prepubertal males and in non–sexually active males without a history of genitourinary tract abnormalities.

Diagnosis

The diagnosis is suggested when a sexually active adolescent or young adult presents with subacute onset of pain in the hemiscrotum, inguinal area, or abdomen, with epididymal swelling and tenderness, a reactive hydrocele, urethral discharge, dysuria, possibly fever, and pyuria (**Fig. 54.6B**). Approximately two-thirds of individuals see a physician after 24 hours of pain—later than those who have testicular torsion. Swelling of the epididymis alone is more common with epididymitis than with torsion of the testes (59% versus 15%). The laboratory evaluation should include a nucleic acid amplification test on a urine sample or an intraurethral swab for *N. gonorrhoeae* and *C. trachomatis* or a culture of intraurethral exudate. Examination of a first-void urine for leukocytes and syphilis serology, and human immunodeficiency virus (HIV) testing are appropriate.

Absence of urethral discharge, leukocytes on a Gram-stained endourethral swab specimen, or pyuria (including a negative urine dip for leukocyte esterase) would necessitate an urgent urology consultation, as the likelihood of torsion increases. If one of the preceding tests is abnormal but the teen or young adult has any risk factors suggesting torsion (i.e., prepubertal or non–sexually

active teen, elevated or rotated testes, history of prior pain episodes, or acute onset with rapid progression), an immediate urology consultation should be obtained and further testing may be considered. Orchitis can cause similar symptoms, but it usually occurs without dysuria or urethral discharge. Mumps infection is the most common cause. Mumps orchitis is usually unilateral and occasionally occurs without a history of parotitis. Other viruses (e.g., adenovirus, Coxsackie virus, ECHO virus, Epstein–Barr virus) may also cause orchitis, but less commonly.

Therapy

Information on treatment of STIs is available from the Centers for Disease Control and Prevention (CDC) at http://www.cdc.gov/std/tg2015/tg-2015-print.pdf (see Chapters 56 to 62).[10] Scrotal support, bed rest, and analgesics are an adjunct to antimicrobial therapy. Ceftriaxone (250 mg) intramuscularly once along with doxycycline (100 mg) is given orally twice a day for 10 days. If the infection is thought to be caused by enteric organisms, or the patient is allergic to ceftriaxone or tetracyclines, alternative drugs are ofloxacin (300 mg) twice daily for 10 days, or levofloxacin (500 mg) orally once a day for 10 days. Men who practice insertive anal sex should be treated with ceftriaxone 250 mg IM in a single dose PLUS either levofloxacin 500 mg orally once a day or ofloxacin 300 mg orally twice a day, both for 10 days. Failure to improve within 3 days requires reevaluation. All partners should be treated. In HIV/acquired immunodeficiency syndrome (AIDS) infection or for other immunocompromised states, therapy is the same except that fungal and mycobacterial infections are more common than in immunocompetent patients.

⬤ TESTICULAR TUMORS

Etiology

Most testicular neoplasias are malignant and of germ cell origin (95%). Seminomas are the most common testicular cancer of a single cell type (40% of germ cell tumors), with a peak incidence in the 25- to 45-year age-group; nonseminoma tumors (embryonal cell, choriocarcinoma, teratoma, yolk sac, and mixed forms) peak in the 15- to 30-year age-group (**Fig. 54.6C**).[11]

Epidemiology

Testicular tumors are the most common solid tumor in males aged 15 to 35 years, with an incidence of 1.4 to 12 per 100,000 males. Testicular cancer is 4.5 times more common among White men compared to African American men, and more than twice that of Asian American men. The risk for Hispanics is between that of Asians and non-Hispanic Whites. The risk of a testicular tumor is increased 10 to 40 times in a teenager with a history of cryptorchidism.

Diagnosis

The diagnosis of tumor should be suspected in any male with a firm, circumscribed, painless area of induration within the testis that does not transilluminate. Swelling is noted in up to 73% of cases at presentation, but is usually considered asymptomatic by the patient. Testicular pain is the presenting symptom in 18% to 46% of patients who have germ cell tumors.

Therapy

Therapy involves a direct biopsy for confirmative diagnosis and cell type. Definitive therapy involves a coordinated effort among the urologist, the primary care specialist, and the oncologist.

⬤ HYDROCELE

Etiology

This mass is actually a collection of fluid between the parietal and visceral layers of the tunica vaginalis, which lies along the anterior

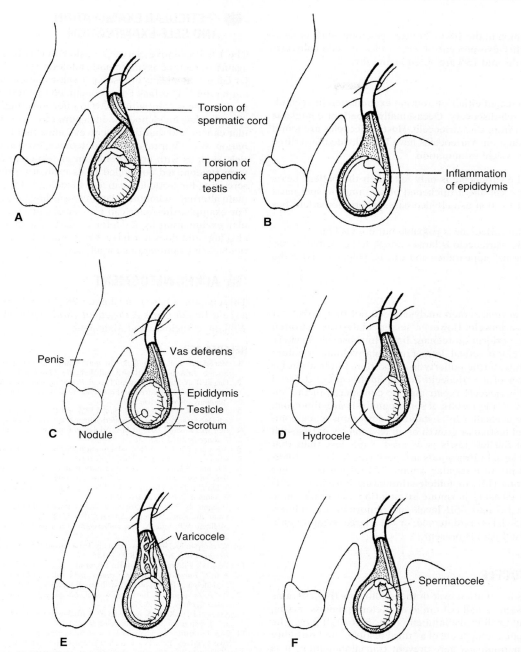

FIGURE 54.6: A: Torsion. **B:** Epididymitis. **C:** Testis tumor. **D:** Hydrocele. **E:** Varicocele. **F:** Spermatocele. (From Kapphahn C, Schlossberger N. Male reproductive health: I. Painful scrotal masses. *Adolesc Health Update* 1992;4:1.)

surface of the testicle and is a remnant of the processus vaginalis—the embryonic sleeve through which the testes descend. If the processus vaginalis remains fully open, an inguinal hernia will result. If a small opening remains, a hydrocele will form in the scrotum (Fig. 54.6D). If an opening remains proximally but is closed distally before the scrotum, a hydrocele of the spermatic cord will form.

Diagnosis

A hydrocele is usually a soft, painless, fluctuant, scrotal mass that is anterior to the testis, transilluminates, and appears cystic on ultrasonography. Hydroceles often decrease in size by morning and increase in size by evening. Long-standing hydroceles are usually benign. The presence of a new hydrocele should alert the examiner to check for a possible underlying cause such as a hernia, testicular tumor, trauma, or infection.

Therapy

No therapy is required for an asymptomatic long-standing hydrocele. Indications for surgical treatment include a painful or tense hydrocele that might reduce circulation to the testis, a bulky mass that is uncomfortable, an embarrassment for the adolescent or young adult, or a hydrocele associated with a hernia (a communicating hydrocele).

VARICOCELE

Etiology

A varicocele, or dilated scrotal veins, results from increased pressure and incompetent venous valves in the internal spermatic veins (Fig. 54.6E), and is most often noted on the left side.

Epidemiology

Varicocele is common in the 10- to 20-year age-group, with a prevalence of 15%. Eighty-five percent of varicoceles are clinically evident on the left side, and 15% are noted bilaterally.

Diagnosis

Varicoceles are detected either on routine examination or secondary to a patient's self-discovery. Occasionally, a patient complains of an ache or pain from the varicocele. Most varicoceles are found on physical examination. Varicoceles have been divided into three grades based on physical examination:

- Grade 1—The varicocele is only felt when the patient bears down. It may feel like a thickened or asymmetric spermatic cord. The distension usually decreases when the patient lies down.
- Grade 2—The varicocele is palpable but not visible.
- Grade 3—The varicocele is large enough to be visible. It has a "bag of worms" appearance and can be palpated above the testes.

Therapy

A patient with a normal semen analysis need not be referred for treatment of his varicocele. However, semen analysis is not often a practical test to perform on teenage boys. In those cases where semen analysis is not practical, loss of testicular volume or failure of the testis to grow during puberty is a traditional indication for surgical correction of a varicocele during adolescence. Referral to a urologist for varicocele repair may be considered in the following instances[12,13]: (1) results of semen analysis are abnormal; (2) testicular size is smaller by 2 standard deviations when compared with normal testicular growth or an asymmetry exists such as the volume of the left testis is at least 3 mL less than that of the right, or if serial ultrasounds are performed, then a difference exists of >2 mL in testicular volume; (3) response of either luteinizing hormone (LH) or follicle-stimulating hormone (FSH) to gonadotropin-releasing hormone stimulation is supranormal, or nonstimulated LH and FSH levels are abnormal; (4) bilaterally palpable varicoceles are detected; or (5) a large, symptomatic varicocele or scrotal pain is present.

SPERMATOCELE

A spermatocele is a retention cyst of the epididymis that contains spermatozoa. Most are small (<1 cm in diameter), painless, cystic, freely movable, and will transilluminate (Fig. 54.6F). If large, the patient may present complaining of a "third testicle," and turbidity from increased spermatozoa may prevent transillumination. It is usually felt as a smooth, cystic sac located above and posterior to the testis, at the head of the epididymis. No therapy is indicated, unless it is large enough to annoy the patient, in which case a urologist may excise it.

ADDITIONAL RESOURCES AND WEBSITES ONLINE

TESTICULAR EXAMINATION AND SELF-EXAMINATION

The US Preventive Services Task Force (USPSTF) recommends against screening asymptomatic adolescents and adults for testicular cancer by means of testicular self-examination or clinician examination.[14] The Task Force concluded that testicular examination as a cancer screen is unlikely to offer meaningful health benefits given the low incidence and high cure rate of even advanced testicular cancer and that there is no evidence that teaching self-examination would improve health outcomes, even among those at high risk, such as with cryptorchidism or testicular atrophy. Evidence from randomized controlled trials evaluating the effectiveness of screening for testicular cancer is lacking.[15] Despite this, there remain alternate recommendations regarding testicular examination. For example, the American Cancer Society recommends a testicular examination by a doctor as part of a routine cancer-related checkup and does not have a recommendation about regular testicular self-examinations for all men.[16]

ACKNOWLEDGMENT

This chapter is based on Chapter 28 "Scrotal Disorders" from *Adolescent Health Care. A Practical Guide*, fifth edition, authored by William P. Adelman and Alain Joffe.

REFERENCES

1. Marcell AV, Bell DL, Joffe A. The male genital examination: a position paper of the Society for Adolescent Health and Medicine. *J Adolesc Health* 2012;50(4):424–425.
2. Hagan JF Jr, Shaw JS, Duncan P, et al. *Bright futures: guidelines for health supervision of infants, children and adolescents*. 3rd ed. Elk Grove Village, IL: American Academy of Pediatrics, 2008.
3. Marcell AV, Wibbelsman C, Seigel WM and the Committee on Adolescence. Male adolescent sexual and reproductive health care. *Pediatrics* 2011;128:e1658–e1676.
4. Bell DL, Breland DJ, Ott MA. Adolescent and young adult male health: a review. *Pediatrics* 2013;132:535.
5. Adelman WP, Joffe A. The adolescent male genital examination: what's normal and what's not. *Contemp Pediatr* 1999;16:76.
6. Adelman WP, Joffe A. Genitourinary issues in the male college student: a case-based approach. *Pediatr Clin North Am* 2005;52:199.
7. Teichman JMH, Thompson IM, Elston DM. Noninfectious Penile Lesions. *Am Fam Physician* 2010;81(2):167–174.
8. Docimo SG, Silver RI, Cromie W. The undescended testicle: diagnosis and management. *Am Fam Physician* 2000;62(9):2037–2044.
9. Adelman WP, Joffe A. The adolescent with a painful scrotum. *Contemp Pediatr* 2000;17:111.
10. Workowski KA, Bolan GA. Sexually Transmitted Diseases Guidelines, 2015. *MMWR Recomm Rep* 2015;64(RR-3):1–135.
11. Bosl GJ, Feldman DR, Bajorin DF, et al. Cancer of the testis. In: DeVita VT, Hellman S, Rosenberg SA, eds. *Cancer: principles and practice of oncology*. 9th ed. Philadelphia, PA: Lippincott Williams & Wilkins, 2011:1280–1301.
12. Gat Y, Zukerman Z, Bachar GN, et al. Adolescent varicocele: is it a unilateral disease? *Urology* 2003;62:742.
13. Evers JLH, Collins JA. Assessment of efficacy of varicocele repair for male subfertility: a systematic review. *Lancet* 2003;361:1849.
14. U.S. Preventive Services Task Force. Screening for testicular cancer: U.S. Preventive Services Task Force reaffirmation recommendation statement. *Ann Intern Med* 2011;154:483–486. Available at http://www.uspreventiveservicestaskforce.org/uspstf/uspstest.htm Accessed February 7, 2014.
15. Ilic D, Misso ML. Screening for testicular cancer. *Cochrane Database Syst Rev* 2011;16:CD007853.
16. American Cancer Society. *Testicular cancer*. Available at http://www.cancer.org/acs/groups/cid/documents/webcontent/003142-pdf.pdf. Accessed February 23, 2014.

CHAPTER 55

Breast Disorders and Gynecomastia

Holly C. Gooding
Amy D. DiVasta

KEY WORDS

- Breast cyst
- Breast development
- Breast imaging
- Fibroadenoma
- Galactorrhea
- Gynecomastia
- Macromastia
- Mastalgia
- Mastitis
- Prolactinoma

While serious breast disorders are rare during adolescence and young adulthood, breast complaints and anxieties regarding normal development are common (Table 55.1).[1] Health care providers must understand normal breast development and its variations, common breast complaints including breast masses, galactorrhea, and gynecomastia, and warning signs of serious disease. When evaluating breast complaints, key historical features assist the clinician (Table 55.2).

NORMAL DEVELOPMENT

Breast tissue begins as ectoderm-derived mammary bands apparent in embryos 4 mm in length. By the time of birth, breast glands in newborns are still rudimentary. Until puberty, male and female breast development is equivalent. During puberty, the breast goes through several developmental stages in response to an increase in sex hormones as outlined in Chapter 2.

The milk-producing alveolus, or terminal duct, is the primary unit of the breast. Ten to 100 alveoli make up a lobule, which drains into lactiferous ducts that merge to form a sinus beneath the nipple. The fibrous tissue stroma surrounds and supports the lobules and ducts. Other structures in the breast include lymphatics, fat tissue, and nerves.[2]

Women of reproductive age tend to have breasts with a nodular texture representing the glandular units/lobules of the breast. During each menstrual cycle, these units undergo proliferative changes under hormonal stimulation. This nodularity can increase, particularly with lobular enlargement and edema that may occur toward the end of

menstrual cycles. This process may vary from a feeling of breast fullness to distinct masses, the latter suggestive of a pathological process.

CONGENITAL ANOMALIES

Aberrant Breast Tissue

Failure of the primordial milk crest to regress leads to the persistence of breast tissue along the milk line in 2% to 6% of women.

1. *Polythelia*: accessory nipple; the most common congenital breast anomaly in males and females. Not associated with other congenital anomalies
2. *Polymastia*: presence of accessory breast tissue along the milk line
3. *Supernumerary breast*: presence of a nipple and underlying breast tissue. May be associated with renal anomalies

If the diagnosis is uncertain from clinical exam, ultrasonography or biopsy can be done. No excision is needed unless the mass increases in size or the patient has cosmetic concerns.

TABLE 55.1
Common Breast Complaints in Female Adolescents

Congenital Anomalies	Disorders of Development	Benign Breast Disease
Polythelia	Asymmetry	Mastalgia
Polymastia	Macromastia	Nipple discharge
Supernumerary breast	Hypoplasia	Mastitis
Amastia	Tuberous breast	Abscess
Inverted nipple	deformity	Mass
	Gynecomastia	

TABLE 55.2
Historical Features Key to Evaluate Breast Complaints in Adolescent/Young Adult Females

1. History of symptoms: Duration, timing, relationship of symptoms with menses. If pain is present, what are the exacerbating and alleviating factors? Has there been any breast discharge, skin change, trauma, or change in breast size?
2. Change in size of mass: Masses that change in size with menstrual cycles may be cysts; those that do not are more likely solid masses. Sudden increase in growth is a concerning sign
3. Medication history: Recent initiation of certain medications could explain mastodynia (estrogen/progesterone oral contraceptivel) or nipple discharge
4. History of trauma to the breast
5. Past medical history: Certain factors increase the risk of malignancy. Chest wall radiation increases the risk of subsequent breast cancer. A history of malignancy that can metastasize to the breast (lymphoma, rhabdomyosarcoma) should raise concern. Any patient with a history of cancer must be followed up carefully for evidence of recurrence, including breast cancer recurrence
6. Family history: First-degree family members affected by cancer increase a patient's risk; the age of these family members should be carefully documented. Screening for breast disease should begin 10 years before the age at which the youngest close relative was diagnosed. Patients with strong family histories of breast cancer, especially if bilateral disease or in conjunction with ovarian or endometrial cancer, should be referred for genetic counseling

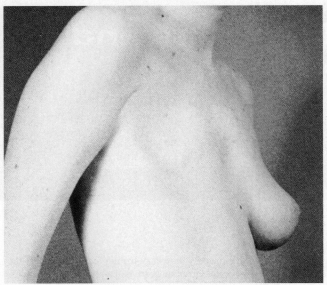

FIGURE 55.1 A 14-year-old girl with Poland syndrome. Note the right-sided amastia. (From Shamberger RC. Chest wall deformities. In: Shields TW, ed. *General thoracic surgery*. 4th ed. Baltimore: Williams & Wilkins, 1994:529–557.)

Absence of Breast Tissue (Amastia and Athelia)

1. Amastia, absence of breast tissue, results from complete involution of the mammary ridge. Amastia is a rare, usually unilateral abnormality. Iatrogenic amastia can occur if the developing breast undergoes surgical procedures such as biopsy. *Poland syndrome* presents with amastia, ipsilateral rib anomalies, webbed fingers, and radial nerve palsies. Amastia can be extremely disturbing to adolescents and young adults (AYAs), but can be surgically corrected (Fig. 55.1).[3] Athelia is the absence of the nipple on one or both sides, and can be corrected surgically.[3]

⬤ DISORDERS OF BREAST DEVELOPMENT

Breast Asymmetry

Some degree of breast asymmetry and differential rates of breast growth are normal. Breast asymmetry may also be caused by a large mass that distorts the normal breast tissue, such as a giant fibroadenoma; these masses are typically evident during a routine breast examination. Pseudoasymmetry is also a possibility, resulting from deformities of the rib cage such as a pectus excavatum. If the physical examination is normal other than the asymmetry, the appropriate treatment is reassurance. Most asymmetry seen during early puberty will resolve completely by adulthood. After sexual maturity rating (SMR) 4, however, significant asymmetry is unlikely to resolve on its own. Plastic surgical correction can be offered to those with marked asymmetry or significant distress.[4] In the discussion with the patient and her family, the health care provider must be sensitive to the adolescent's desire to be "normal" and not appear different than her peers. What may seem like a trivial issue to an adult may provoke shame and embarrassment in an adolescent.

Macromastia

Macromastia, or breast overgrowth, can be associated with many physical and psychological symptoms. Macromastia is more than a cosmetic concern; its potential negative impact should not be underestimated.[5] The cause of macromastia is not well understood, but may represent an abnormal response of the breast to normal hormonal stimulation, especially by estrogen. Obesity and macromastia are closely related, but the relationship is complex.

1. Clinical manifestations: Physical complaints include back and shoulder pain, postural changes, breast discomfort, mood disturbances, intertrigo, and limited ability to participate in physical activity. Adolescents are also concerned about self-image, difficulty finding clothing that fits, and unwanted social attention.
2. Diagnosis: Evaluation should include a thorough examination and ultrasound if needed to rule out any underlying mass.
3. Management: Patients should be fit for a supportive, comfortable bra. Weight loss may help to improve symptoms for obese patients. For persistent symptoms, reduction mammoplasty is performed in adolescents who have completed breast growth to prevent the need for a second procedure. Adolescents report a high rate of both satisfaction and symptom relief following surgery.[6] Patients should be referred to a plastic surgeon with experience in treating teens, and who are sensitive to the teens' particular body image concerns.

Breast Hypoplasia

Breast hypoplasia, or undergrowth of breast tissue, may also be present in adolescence. Underlying causes include iatrogenic injury, trauma, malnutrition, aggressive athletic activity, or an idiopathic condition. Other disorders in the differential diagnosis include premature ovarian failure, androgen excess (from tumor or exogenous anabolic steroid use), and chronic diseases (diabetes mellitus, inflammatory bowel disease) that lead to weight loss. Workup consists of a careful physical examination, as well as search for underlying causes. Treatment is targeted at the underlying primary disorder. Idiopathic breast hypoplasia can be addressed by a plastic surgeon.

Tuberous Breast Deformity

Tuberous breast deformity (Fig. 55.2) is a rare disorder of breast development. Patients present with long, narrow, ptotic breasts that appear to be the result of an overdevelopment of the nipple-areolar complex with an underdevelopment of the breast mound. Treatment of choice is plastic surgery; reassurance is also an option for milder cases.

⬤ BENIGN BREAST DISEASE

Mastalgia

Breast pain can be a distressing problem and affects up to 50% of reproductive-age young women.[2] *Mastalgia* can be cyclic pain

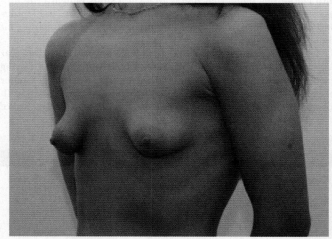

FIGURE 55.2 Tuberous breast deformity. Note the overdevelopment of the superior aspect and nipple-areolar complex on the right. (Courtesy of David A. Horvath, MD.)

(worse immediately before menses) or noncyclic pain (*masto-dynia*). Common causes include premenstrual fibrocystic changes, exercise, infection, early pregnancy, or medications such as oral contraceptives. The evaluation should include a breast assessment and a pregnancy test. Once the diagnosis of mastalgia or masto-dynia has been made, treatment includes analgesics (nonsteroidal anti-inflammatory drugs), good bra support (both night and day if needed), and reassurance. Most breast pain resolves spontaneously within 3 to 6 months. Oral contraceptives may improve or worsen breast pain, possibly in a dose-related manner. Evening primrose oil and vitamin E have shown some efficacy in small trials.

Breast Infection

Mastitis or breast abscesses present with an acute history of a red inflamed breast. Predisposing conditions include pregnancy, lactation, recent cessation of breast-feeding, preexisting cyst/ductal ectasia (see below), and breast trauma.

1. Clinical manifestations: Constitutional symptoms (malaise, fever) may occur. Physical examination reveals an edematous erythematous breast, possibly with purulent discharge (Fig. 55.3). A discrete abscess may be palpated as an area of fluctuance.
2. Diagnosis: Any purulent breast drainage or nipple discharge should be sent for culture. Abscess can be confirmed with ultrasound if necessary.
3. Management: For simple mastitis, treat with antibiotics for 7 to 10 days and warm compresses. Antibiotic therapy should be targeted at the most likely pathogens (*Staphylococcus aureus*, streptococci, enterococcus). Dicloxacillin or amoxicillin-clavulanic acid provides adequate coverage of skin pathogens. For penicillin-allergic patients, clindamycin is a good choice. If patients are breast-feeding, expression of milk from the affected side should continue to prevent milk stasis. Infants can continue breast-feeding from the affected side.
4. Abscess: Patients should be reexamined within several days to confirm response to therapy. Persistent infection despite antibiotic therapy should be evaluated with re-examination of the breast and ultrasonography for an underlying abscess. Abscess drainage can be attempted in the office with a large-bore needle. If needle aspiration is unsuccessful or if the abscess re-accumulates, the patient should be referred for incision and drainage. Incisions should be as small as possible to limit resulting distortion. Material obtained at aspiration or incision and drainage should be cultured. Infections that fail to respond to adequate antibiotic therapy should also be referred for surgical management. These patients should be screened

for underlying immunosuppressive disease that may interfere with their ability to clear the infection, like diabetes mellitus or human immunodeficiency virus infection.

Nipple Discharge

Nipple discharge can be caused by endocrine disorders, as well as breast pathology. The first step in the evaluation is to distinguish the discharge itself. Milky discharge suggests galactorrhea (see further details below). Non-milky discharge (watery, serous, purulent, serosanguinous, bloody) usually indicates an underlying breast or nipple problem, with the following etiologies most common in AYAs[7]:

1. Contact dermatitis: Local contact dermatitis of the nipple can give rise to serous, purulent, or bloody discharge. Culprits include soap, clothes, clothing detergent, or lotion used by the patient. Treatment is identification and discontinuation of the offending agent, with topical steroid cream for symptom relief.
2. Infection: Purulent discharge indicates infection. Culture the discharge, and treat with appropriate antibiotics and warm compresses. If the infection fails to respond to antibiotic therapy, incision and drainage may be indicated.
3. Montgomery tubercles: The periareolar glands of Montgomery will occasionally drain fluid through ectopic openings on the areola. Discharge is usually serous or serosanguinous. Ultrasound can confirm the clinical suspicion through visualization of the retroareolar cyst. Discharge will resolve spontaneously.
4. Mammary duct ectasia: Ductal ectasia refers to dilation of the mammary ducts as well as periductal inflammation. No clear etiology is known. Discharge is usually serous or serosanguinous. Ultrasound can confirm the diagnosis. Treatment includes reassurance and supportive care; mastitis risk may be slightly increased.[8]
5. Intraductal papilloma: These rare, benign, proliferative tumors often present with bloody discharge from a single duct. They represent a focal hyperplasia of the ductal epithelium invaginating into the duct on a vascular stalk. Disruption of this stalk leads to the bloody discharge. If the proliferation of duct epithelium grows large enough, it creates a palpable mass. Although an infrequent finding in AYAs, a palpable mass associated with a bloody nipple discharge has a 95% probability of being an intraductal papilloma, even in teens. Ultrasound and potentially ductogram should be performed. Any abnormality found should be excised. Bloody discharge is usually not related to underlying carcinoma in the AYA age-group.

⬤ GALACTORRHEA

Galactorrhea is the secretion of milk or a milk-like fluid from the breast in the absence of parturition or beyond 6 months postpartum in a non-breast-feeding woman or man. It is usually bilateral, may occur intermittently or persistently, and may be spontaneous or expressed. Other types of discharge do not suggest galactorrhea (see other causes of nipple discharge above).

Prolactin secretion from lactotrophs of the anterior pituitary gland (Fig. 55.4) is necessary for normal lactation. Dopamine binds to lactotrophs, and inhibits prolactin secretion. Transection or compression of the pituitary stalk increases prolactin secretion by interfering with dopaminergic pathways. Prolactin secretion is also increased by stress, suckling, sleep, and intercourse.

Etiology

In women, most galactorrhea is caused by hyperprolactinemia from prolactinomas (benign anterior pituitary neoplasms that secrete prolactin through lactotroph hyperplasia) or secondary to medications (Table 55.3). Less common causes of hyperprolactinemia include:[9]

1. Hypothalamic and infundibular lesions, including cranio-pharyngiomas, infiltrative disorders, and damage to the

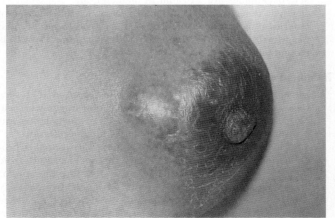

FIGURE 55.3 Mastitis. (From Sweet RL, Gibbs RS. *Atlas of infectious diseases of the female genital tract.* Philadelphia, PA: Lippincott Williams & Wilkins, 2005.)

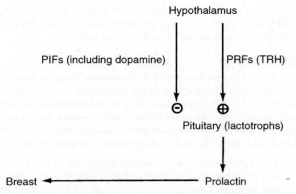

FIGURE 55.4 Schema of prolactin control. PIF, prolactin-inhibiting factors; PRF, prolactin-releasing factors; TRH, thyrotropin-releasing hormone.

TABLE 55.4	
Interpretation of Serum Prolactin Concentrations	
Prolactin Concentration (ng/mL)	**Suggested Diagnosis**
<25	Normal
25–150	Non–prolactin-secreting tumor Dysfunction of dopaminergic pathway
150–250	Microprolactinoma
>500	Macroprolactinoma

TABLE 55.3	
Medications Causing Hyperprolactinemia	
Antipsychotics	***Antihypertensive agents***
Risperidone	Verapamil
Olanzapine	α-Methyldopa
Butyrophenones (haloperidol)	Reserpine
Phenothiazines	
	Gastrointestinal medications
Antidepressants	Metoclopramide
Tricyclic antidepressants	Domperidone
Monoamine oxidase inhibitors	
Selective serotonin reuptake	***Other medications***
inhibitors	Opiates and opiate antagonists
	Estrogens
	Anesthetics
	Anticonvulsants
	Antihistamines (H2)
	Dopamine-receptor blockers

infundibulum from surgery or head trauma (inhibition of counterregulatory dopamine release)
2. Primary hypothyroidism (increased thyrotropin-releasing hormone stimulates lactotrophs)
3. Acromegaly or Cushing disease
4. Renal failure (decreased prolactin clearance) or liver failure (decreased dopamine synthesis)

Infrequently, galactorrhea can occur with normal prolactin concentrations in women with unexplained hypersensitivity to prolactin, or those who engage in frequent breast stimulation.

Diagnosis

Evaluation should start with a carefully drawn serum prolactin level. Prolactin secretion is pulsatile, and is augmented by stress, eating, and breast stimulation. Levels should be drawn in the morning in a fasting, nonexercised state without prior breast manipulation (no tight-fitting clothes or breast examination). If results are abnormal, the test should be repeated (Table 55.4).

Additional evaluation includes a pregnancy test, thyroid-stimulating hormone (TSH), blood urea nitrogen, and creatinine.[10] Persistent hyperprolactinemia with no known underlying etiology or prolactin >200 ng/mL requires a pituitary brain magnetic resonance imaging (MRI) with contrast to evaluate for an intracranial lesion. Patients with incidentally discovered elevated prolactin levels in the absence of symptoms should be assessed for

macroprolactinemia, a large-molecule circulating prolactin that is less bioactive, and often does not require further diagnostic testing or treatment. If a discrepancy exists between a large pituitary tumor and mildly elevated prolactin levels, blood samples should undergo serial dilution to eliminate a laboratory artifact that can occur with certain assays that leads to falsely low prolactin levels (the "hook effect").

Medication-Induced Hyperprolactinemia

A full medication list should be queried to identify any potential pharmacological causes (Table 55.3). If possible, the offending drug should be changed or discontinued. If prolactin levels fail to decrease within 2 weeks after discontinuation, an intracranial mass should be considered. Alternative medications with lower potential to elevate prolactin levels should be considered. In patients with antipsychotic-induced hyperprolactinemia, dopamine agonist therapy is not recommended.[11] Prolactin levels are less likely to normalize in this setting, and the underlying psychosis may be exacerbated. Patients with hypogonadism or low bone mass related to medication-induced hyperprolactinemia should be treated with estrogen or testosterone if the causative medication cannot be stopped.

Classification of Prolactinomas

1. Microadenomas are <10 mm in diameter, and do not cause any local symptoms. They rarely grow (<10% chance of increasing in size). Treatment is not needed if estradiol levels are within the reference range, menses are normal, and galactorrhea is absent/tolerable unless the young woman wants to conceive. Restoration of gonadal function and prevention of decreased bone mineral density (BMD) can be accomplished with a dopamine agonist to lower prolactin levels or estrogen replacement therapy.
2. Macroadenomas are >10 mm in diameter, and can cause visual field defects, headaches, neurological deficits, and loss of anterior pituitary function. They have a significant potential for growth, and initial treatment with dopamine agonists is recommended.

Treatment of Prolactinomas

1. Dopamine agonists decrease prolactin secretion and synthesis. Therapeutic goals include resolution of galactorrhea, correction of visual field defects, reversal of amenorrhea, improvement of sexual function, and resolution of infertility.[12]
   a. Cabergoline is the most effective therapy to normalize prolactin levels and shrink pituitary tumors. The Endocrine Society recommends cabergoline as first-line therapy for prolactinomas.[12] Initial doses of 0.25 mg PO twice weekly should be prescribed, increasing to 0.5 to 1 mg twice weekly as needed. Only 3% of patients are unable to tolerate the drug because of side effects, which include headache, dizziness, and nausea. High doses of cabergoline (≥3

mg daily) have been associated with an increased risk of cardiac valve regurgitation, but standard doses of cabergoline for hyperprolactinemia do not appear to cause clinically significant valvular disease.[13] Although there are no known detrimental fetal effects, current recommendations are to discontinue the drug 1 month before attempting conception.

   b. Bromocriptine is also effective in lowering prolactin levels and reducing tumor size, although less so than cabergoline.[14] Initial dosing is 1.25 mg PO at bedtime, increased to 2.5 to 5 mg twice a day as needed. Side effects include nausea, vomiting, and dizziness in 12% of patients. When bromocriptine is used to restore fertility, and stopped when pregnancy is confirmed, there is no increased risk of spontaneous abortions, ectopic pregnancies, or congenital malformations.

   c. Pergolide is a dopamine agonist approved in the US for the treatment of Parkinson disease. It is used outside the US for treatment of hyperprolactinemia.

2. Combined estrogen/progestin oral contraceptives (COCs): Women with a microadenoma who are amenorrheic may be treated with COCs in lieu of dopamine agonist therapy. COC therapy restores menses and prevents hypogonadal effects. Patients treated with COCs for two years have not shown an increase in tumor size.

3. Transphenoidal surgery is rarely required and reserved for AYAs who are resistant to or intolerant of dopamine-receptor agonists, or have invasive macroprolactinomas with compromised vision.[10] Prolactin levels normalize in approximately 70% of all patients who have been operated on for microprolactinomas, and in 30% with macroprolactinomas. However, the recurrence risk is 20% to 50%.

4. Radiation has been used rarely in patients with aggressive tumors that do not respond to dopamine agonists or surgery.

Monitoring of Prolactinomas

1. Estrogen status should be closely monitored because of the known risk of low BMD associated with hypoestrogenic amenorrhea. BMD may improve with therapy, but does not return to normal. Fracture risk may be increased in adult patients even before a diagnosis of a prolactinoma is confirmed. Baseline BMD measurement by dual-energy x-ray absorptiometry should be considered in patients with hyperprolactinemia and amenorrhea.

2. Periodic prolactin measurement should begin 1 month after therapy initiation to guide dosing, and repeated 1 to 3 months after each change in dosage. Once normal prolactin levels are achieved, prolactin should be measured every 6 to 12 months[12].

3. A dedicated pituitary MRI should be done 1 year after diagnosis for microadenomas, or 3 months after diagnosis for macroadenomas. Repeat MRI with any increase in symptoms or serum prolactin level.

4. Visual field examinations should be performed for all patients with a macroadenoma potentially impinging on the optic chiasm.

5. If a patient wishes to conceive, bromocriptine should be the initial treatment to induce ovulation. Barrier contraceptives should be used until two normal menstrual cycles have occurred. Bromocriptine should be discontinued after the first missed menstrual cycle/confirmation of pregnancy. Microadenomas rarely grow during pregnancy; macroadenomas that do not undergo surgery or irradiation prior to pregnancy enlarge in 31% of cases. The Endocrine Society does not recommend performing serum prolactin measurements during gestation, given the expected changes in prolactin during pregnancy. Similarly, routine pituitary MRI is not recommended during pregnancy unless new symptoms (headache, visual change)

develop. If symptomatic growth of prolactinomas occurs during pregnancy, bromocriptine therapy is recommended.

6. Once patients achieve 2 years of normal prolactin levels and no visible tumor remains on MRI, dopamine agonist withdrawal may be attempted. The risk of recurrence after withdrawal is 26% to 69%, and correlates with the degree of prolactin elevation at diagnosis as well as tumor size. Recurrence is most likely in the first year after therapy is stopped. Serum prolactin should be measured every 3 months for the first year, and annually thereafter or if symptoms recur. Pituitary MRI should be repeated if the prolactin increases.

BREAST MASSES IN FEMALES

While the presence of a breast mass typically causes concern during adolescence and young adulthood, breast masses are overwhelmingly benign (**Table 55.5**). Malignancies comprise less than 1% of excisional biopsies performed. In addition to appropriately establishing the cause of a mass, practitioners must reassure AYAs and their parents that malignant disease is highly unlikely.

Evaluation of a Breast Mass

Evaluation should include a detailed history outlining the location, duration, growth pattern, and characteristics of the mass (**Table 55.2**). Family history should determine if there is a predisposition to breast problems. Physical examination should characterize the mass: size, shape, firmness, location, and associated findings. Ultrasound is indicated for lesions that are irregular, firm, immobile, difficult to assess, or associated with overlying skin changes.[15] Mammography is not helpful in AYA women as the breast density of these patients obscures pathological findings. Current strategies seek to establish a diagnosis without surgical excision, saving patients with benign lesions from an unnecessary surgery.

Fibroadenomas

1. Fibroadenomas are the most common benign surgical breast mass in AYAs, comprising 60% to 90% of benign breast lesions. These well-circumscribed fibroepithelial lesions are uniformly smooth and sharply demarcated from surrounding tissue. Fibroadenomas are most common in 15- and 16-year-olds, and twice as common in African Americans.[16]

2. Clinical manifestations: Round or oval firm mass distinct from the rest of the breast that can be multiple and/or bilateral. Giant fibroadenomas (fibroadenomas >5 to 10 cm) occur more frequently in teens and in African Americans.

3. Diagnosis can be made clinically. Ultrasound can be used to confirm a fibroadenoma, which appears as a hypoechoic lesion with smooth round distinct borders, wider than tall.

4. Management: Since most fibroadenomas spontaneously regress, surveillance is a reasonable therapeutic option. Expectant management includes serial examination and perhaps ultrasonography every 6 months. Patients should be advised that the fibroadenoma will likely regress, but may grow,

TABLE 55.5		
Breast Masses in Adolescence		
Benign Breast Masses—Common	**Benign Breast Masses—Rare**	**Malignant Breast Masses—Extremely Rare**
Fibroadenoma	Intraductal papilloma	Adenocarcinoma
Cyst	Juvenile papillomatosis	Cystosarcoma
Abscess	Tubular/lactational adenoma	Rhabdomyosarcoma
	Cystosarcoma phyllodes (benign)	Angiosarcoma
		Lymphoma
		Cystosarcoma phyllodes (malignant)
		Adenocarcinoma

XII

especially with subsequent pregnancy. If the lesion is large or the patient/family is anxious, fibroadenomas can be removed via excision or cryoablation. *Giant fibroadenomas* may distort the affected breast and should the patient desire removal, simple surgical excision should be performed, sparing as much normal compressed breast tissue as possible. Plastic surgical assistance should be considered to correct the resulting deformity.

Cysts

1. Breast cysts can present as multiple breast masses, or increasing size or tenderness of a mass associated with menses.
2. Clinical manifestations: A firm, well-circumscribed mass distinct from the surrounding breast is found.
3. Diagnosis: Ultrasonography reveals a round, well-demarcated hypoechoic structure with fluid content.
4. Management: Cysts will usually resolve spontaneously over weeks to months. If a breast cyst persists and is symptomatic, it can be treated with fine-needle aspiration (FNA) of fluid and resolution of the mass. Simple cysts can recur and can easily be reaspirated. Symptomatic cysts that recur after multiple aspirations should be referred for simple excision.

Fibrocystic Breast Changes

Fibrocystic changes occur in approximately 50% of all women clinically, and 90% histologically, and can lead to complaints of multiple masses or nodularity, with cyclic pain increasing with menses. The mean age at diagnosis is 15 to 17 years. The pathophysiology is unknown, but may be related to an imbalance of estrogen/progesterone. Risk factors include consumption of animal fats and alcohol and higher body weight.[17]

1. Clinical manifestations: Nodularity is apparent on exam, most commonly in the upper outer quadrant of the breasts. A diffuse cord-like thickening and lumpiness is present; the exam will change over time. Tenderness and swelling are more common a week before menstruation, and are often relieved by menstruation.
2. Diagnosis is primarily by clinical exam. Ultrasonography fails to reveal a single underlying mass; it may show areas of increased fibrous tissue or microcysts.
3. Management: Mild analgesics, supportive bras, and a trial of COCs have been effective for symptoms. While oral danazol or tamoxifen have been utilized in adults with severe symptoms, these medications have not been studied in teens.

Juvenile Papillomatosis

1. Juvenile papillomatosis is a rare, benign proliferative tumor that presents as a firm, well-circumscribed mass with multiple cysts separated by fibrous septa, usually affecting patients <30 years of age.[18]
2. Clinical manifestations: Patients present with a unilateral, solitary, painless breast mass clinically consistent with a fibroadenoma.
3. Management: The clinical significance of juvenile papillomatosis involves controversy over whether it is associated with concurrent or subsequent carcinoma. The patients at highest risk are those who (1) have a family history of breast cancer; (2) have atypical proliferative lesions; (3) have bilateral or multifocal lesions; or (4) have a recurrence of juvenile papillomatosis. For these reasons, treatment is wide surgical excision and close clinical follow-up.

Phyllodes Tumors

1. Phyllodes tumors (also called cystosarcoma phyllodes) are benign or malignant tumors comprising only 1% of breast neoplasms in AYAs, but are the most common malignant lesion in this age-group.

2. Clinical manifestations: A painless, rapidly growing mass that is large upon presentation. Skin changes overlying the mass are common.
3. Management: Wide local resection with achievement of negative margins is the surgical goal. These tumors do not metastasize to axillary lymph nodes but can metastasize to lung and bone.

BREAST MALIGNANCY

Primary breast cancer is extremely rare in AYAs. Data from the Surveillance Epidemiology and End Results program of the National Cancer Institute from 1972 to 2008 suggest a rate of 0.08 new breast cancers per 100,000 girls younger than age 20 years in the US. Other population studies have found an annual age-adjusted incidence of breast cancer of 3.2 per million in patients under age 25 (with all documented cases occurring in those ages 20 to 24 years).[19] The more common malignant tumors found in AYAs are secondary or metastatic, including rhabdomyosarcoma, cystosarcoma phyllodes, or lymphoma. Tumors that metastasize to the breast include rhabdomyosarcoma, lymphoma, and neuroblastoma. Patients with a breast biopsy showing rhabdomyosarcoma should be screened for occult primary disease outside the breast, as metastatic disease is more common than primary breast rhabdomyosarcoma.

Probably the most important genes that lead to striking family clusters of breast cancer are mutations of BRCA1 and BRCA2, which account for almost 80% of hereditary breast cancer and approximately 5% to 6% of all breast cancers. Although these mutations are rare in the general population (5 to 50 per 100,000), they may occur in approximately 1% of all Jewish women of Ashkenazi descent. For individuals whose personal or family history suggests a hereditary predisposition to breast cancer, genetic screening should be considered. Decisions around genetic screening are difficult, and should be carried out with the help of a qualified genetic counselor.[20] Screening for mutations should not occur until a time the information would be helpful. While an 18-year-old can legally pursue genetic testing, neither screening nor follow-up recommendations will change regardless of the results, as cancer risk associated with BRCA1/2 rarely manifests before the late 20s. At age 25 years, things change. At 25 years, annual mammography, breast MRI, and clinical breast exams are recommended for surveillance. Thus, the optimal time to pursue genetic testing time is at this age.

Patients with a history of radiation therapy to the chest are at increased risk of developing a second primary cancer of the breast at a young age, and require careful monitoring. Estrogen-containing contraceptives should be avoided when possible in these patients with a history of chest radiation.[21] In contrast, no recent data support an association between increased risk of breast cancer when comparing users with controls in healthy patients or patients with nongenetic family history of breast cancer. Studies of breast cancer risk with COC in carriers of the BRCA 1 and 2 mutations are mixed.[22]

PHYSICAL EXAMINATION OF THE BREAST

A thorough and careful breast examination is essential to the evaluation of any breast complaint. Clinicians must be sensitive to the patient's potential feelings of embarrassment or modesty. The patient should be informed of the parts of the exam, and given the opportunity to be accompanied by a parent or friend. If she declines, a female chaperone should be offered by the examiner, especially if he is male. Optimal examination occurs within a week of completion of menses, when the breast is least tender. If an examination is indeterminate, repeating it at a different point in her menstrual cycle may be informative.

Inspection should be performed with the adolescent or young adult in an upright position to assess for asymmetry, breast distortion, or skin conditions. Palpation should occur in a systematic manner to cover the entire breast in an orderly fashion. Regional lymph nodes should also be assessed. The areola should be compressed to elicit nipple discharge; if found, note the color, and from where it appeared (nipple, periphery of areola). Masses should be measured, and their consistency and mobility evaluated. The analogy of a clock face can be used to describe the offending area of breast abnormality.

Breast Self-Examination

The American Cancer Society states that "breast self-examination (BSE) is an option for women starting in their 20s." Clinical breast exam by a trained professional is recommended at least every 3 years starting at age 20. BSE has not been shown to improve survival in breast cancer and may increase anxiety and depression in all patients who believe they find an abnormality.[23] However, we believe BSE is beneficial for establishing a life-long habit of patients investing in their own breast health. BSE should begin earlier in those with history of previous radiation to the chest, a history of malignancy that may metastasize to the breast, or a family history of BRCA1/2 mutations.

BREAST IMAGING AND BIOPSY

Breast Imaging

Ultrasonography is superior in characterizing masses in AYAs, and can distinguish a cystic mass from a solid one.[24] It cannot distinguish a benign solid mass from a malignant one. MRI may offer additional characterization of breast masses above that of ultrasound, but indications are still being determined. Mammography is of limited utility in the AYA breast. The dense fibroglandular tissue leads to poor-quality images and poor sensitivity. Mammography should not be used in patients <age 30 years unless specifically recommended for follow-up of other imaging by a radiologist skilled in evaluating ultrasound and MRI images obtained from AYAs.

Breast Biopsy

AYAs rarely need breast biopsies given the benign nature of the vast majority of masses found in this age-group. However, FNA and core-needle biopsy may be considered in rare circumstances, such as young adults with a history of prior chest radiation or malignancy, hard masses with irregular borders, axillary lymphadenopathy, or a persistent solid mass with concerning features on ultrasound or MRI.[25] FNA is also used to manage breast cysts. If an aspiration obtains nonbloody cyst fluid, the lesion is a benign cyst and no further treatment is needed. Cytology on the cyst fluid is not indicated unless it is bloody. If FNA reveals a solid mass, a core biopsy can be obtained to characterize the mass. Given the rarity of the need for these procedures even in young adults, patients should be referred to a breast center with experience treating AYAs.[26]

Once cytological or core biopsy results have been obtained, all three pieces of the diagnostic triad must be reviewed—physical examination, imaging, and biopsy. If all three concur the mass is benign, the patient may safely decline further intervention. She should be followed up with serial examinations and ultrasonograms, every 6 months to a year, to establish stability of the lesion.[27] Any sudden growth should raise suspicion of malignant transformation. If any one piece of the diagnostic triad is not in concordance, the lesion must be excised.

GYNECOMASTIA

Gynecomastia refers to an increase in the glandular and stromal tissue of the male breast. When identified during puberty, it is usually benign and transient. Gynecomastia can also be due to a serious underlying disorder or can persist long enough that the adolescent seeks treatment.[28]

Epidemiology

Transient gynecomastia affects 40% to 60% of adolescent males.[29] It usually occurs 1.2 years after a boy reaches SMR 2 genital development, and peaks in prevalence at age 14. Approximately 4% of males will have severe gynecomastia (breast tissue >4.0 cm in diameter or the size of an average mid-pubertal female breast) that persists into adulthood.

Etiology

The exact etiology of gynecomastia remains unknown. Male breast tissue reacts to the balance between estrogens (which stimulate breast tissue development) and androgens (which antagonize breast development), and increase in estrogen relative to testosterone can lead to gynecomastia. In cases where serum hormones are within the reference range, heightened sensitivity of the breast tissue to hormones may be responsible for the breast enlargement. Mechanisms to account for an increase in estrogen or a decrease in androgen activity include[30]:

1. Increase in serum estrogen concentrations
   a. Increased estradiol secretion from testes (e.g., Leydig cell tumors) or from adrenal tumors
   b. Excessive extraglandular conversion of androgens to estrogens by aromatase (overproduction of adrenal precursors that are converted into estrone, overproduction of testicular precursors that are converted to estradiol, or enhancement of extraglandular aromatase activity due to hyperthyroidism, liver disease, increased body fat, medication or drug use, or persistence of the fetal form of aromatase)
   c. Increased bioavailability of estrogen due to a decrease in the amount of estrogen bound to sex hormone–binding globulin (SHBG)
   d. Exogenous intake of estrogens (oral intake or use of topical estrogens)
2. Decrease in serum androgen concentrations
   a. Impairment of testicular production in Leydig cells: primary hypogonadism (anorchia, Klinefelter syndrome), secondary hypogonadism (disordered hypothalamus or pituitary), congenital enzyme defects, drug-induced inhibition of enzymes needed in testosterone synthesis, or chronic stimulation of Leydig cells by high levels of human chorionic gonadotropin (hCG)
   b. Hyperestrogenic states suppressing luteinizing hormone (LH) and testosterone secretion
   c. Increased hepatic clearance of androgens
   d. Decrease in bioavailability of testosterone due to increases in SHBG with liver disease or hyperestrogenic states
3. Alterations of estrogen and androgen receptors
   a. Androgen-receptor deficiency states (androgen insensitivity syndromes)
   b. Drug interference with androgen receptors (spironolactone, flutamide, or cimetidine)
   c. Drugs that mimic estrogens and stimulate estrogen-receptor sites (digoxin and phytoestrogens in some marijuana preparations)

Clinical Manifestations

Most cases of gynecomastia are bilateral. Classification includes the following:

1. Type I—one or more subareolar nodules, freely movable
2. Type II—breast nodules beneath areola but also extending beyond the areolar perimeter
3. Type III—resembles breast development of SMR 3 in girls

Types I and II are associated with a firm, rubbery consistency of the breasts whereas type III has a consistency similar to that of the female breast. Types I and II gynecomastia are usually associated with tenderness on palpation or when clothing touches the breast.

True gynecomastia should be distinguished from pseudogynecomastia caused by adipose tissue over the pectoral muscles in some obese males or prominent musculature in some physically fit adolescent boys, and from breast masses due to cancer, dermoid cysts, lipomas, hematomas, or neurofibromas.[31]

Physical Examination

Examine the patient in the supine position, with his hands behind his head; the examiner then places the thumb and forefinger at opposing margins of the breast. In gynecomastia, as the fingers are brought together, rubbery or firm breast tissue can be felt as a freely movable, and occasionally tender, disk of tissue concentric to the areola. In pseudogynecomastia, no discrete mass is felt. In other conditions such as a lipoma or dermoid cyst, the mass is usually eccentric to the areola. Physical examination should also be performed to exclude other causes of gynecomastia including hypogonadism, thyroid dysfunction, testicular mass or atrophy, and liver disease.

Diagnosis

Pubertal gynecomastia can be presumed as the etiology of the breast enlargement in adolescents who (a) present with a unilateral or bilateral, subareolar, rubbery or firm mass; (b) are not using any medications or drugs possibly associated with gynecomastia (**Table 55.6**); (c) have a normal testicular examination; and (d) lack any evidence of renal, hepatic, thyroid, or other endocrine disease. No further tests are necessary but the patient should be reevaluated in 6 months. If medication or drug use is suspected, it should be discontinued and the adolescent reexamined in 1 month. At that time, breast tenderness, if present, should decrease and breast size may decrease.

If an endocrine disorder is suspected, the practitioner should order measurements of serum hCG, LH, testosterone, and estradiol with further workup of abnormal results as follows[30]:

1. Elevated hCG concentration: Perform testicular ultrasonography. The presence of a mass suggests a testicular germ cell tumor. A normal sonogram suggests an extragonadal germ cell tumor or hCG-secreting neoplasm; a chest film and abdominal computed tomography (CT) are indicated.
2. Decreased testosterone and elevated LH concentrations suggest primary hypogonadism, including Klinefelter syndrome or testicular atrophy caused by mumps orchitis.
3. Decreased testosterone and normal/low LH concentrations suggest secondary hypogonadism. Prolactin should be measured and a pituitary MRI obtained if prolactin is elevated.
4. Elevated testosterone and LH concentrations suggest androgen resistance, although TSH should also be measured as hyperthyroidism can increase LH concentrations.
5. Elevated estradiol with low/normal LH concentrations: Perform testicular ultrasonography. A testicular mass indicates a likely Leydig or Sertoli cell tumor. The absence of a mass should prompt an adrenal CT or MRI to assess for adrenal neoplasm. If none are found, an increase in extraglandular aromatase activity is likely.
6. Normal concentrations of hCG, LH, testosterone, and estradiol indicate idiopathic gynecomastia.

Management

Underlying causes of gynecomastia should be treated as appropriate, including discontinuation of causative medications. In most individuals with mild to moderate pubertal gynecomastia, only reassurance is needed. Most cases will improve or resolve within 12 to 18 months. A small percentage of cases (<10%) may persist into adulthood. There has been no proven relationship between gynecomastia and the development of breast cancer in males.

Medical therapy should be reserved for those individuals who have more than mild to moderate gynecomastia and who are

TABLE 55.6

Medications Causing Gynecomastia

Hormones	***Cardiovascular drugs***
Estrogens	Verapamil, nifedipine
Testosterone	α-Methyldopa
Anabolic steroids	Digoxin
Chorionic gonadotropin	Captopril, enalapril
	Minoxidil
Antiandrogens	
Spironolactone	***Antibiotics***
Flutamide	Ketoconazole
Cyproterone	Metronidazole
Psychoactive agents	***Gastrointestinal agents***
Phenothiazines	Cimetidine
Atypical antipsychotic agents	Ranitidine
Tricyclic antidepressants	Omeprazole
Diazepam	Metoclopramide
Haloperidol	
	Others
Drugs of Abuse	Antiretroviral drugs
Marijuana	Cancer chemotherapeutics
Alcohol	Phenytoin
Amphetamines	Penicillamine

significantly concerned about the condition. Several drugs have been tried to reduce gynecomastia, including androgens (testosterone, dihydrotestosterone, and danazol), antiestrogens (clomiphene, tamoxifen, and raloxifene), and aromatase inhibitors (testolactone, anastrozole, letrozole, and formestane). No drug is approved by the US Food and Drug Administration for the treatment of adolescent gynecomastia, and studies using these medications in adolescents are limited. Lawrence et al. (2004) reviewed their experience in managing 38 patients with persistent pubertal gynecomastia using either tamoxifen (10 to 20 mg twice daily) or raloxifene (60 mg daily) for 3 to 9 months.[32] Mean reduction in breast diameter was 2.1 cm with tamoxifen versus 2.5 cm with raloxifene. Overall improvement was comparable (tamoxifen, 86%; raloxifene, 91%) but more raloxifene-treated patients (86%) than tamoxifen-treated patients (41%) had at least a 50% reduction in breast size. However, the study was neither randomized nor blinded and there was no true control group. In older adolescents with moderate to severe gynecomastia associated with psychological sequelae, or in patients with persistent gynecomastia >1 year in whom spontaneous resolution is unlikely, surgical treatment is preferable. Recent surgical advances include the use of ultrasonic liposuction.

● SUMMARY

Breast complaints in AYAs commonly include discomfort (mastalgia), developmental variations (asymmetry), developmental anomalies (hypo- or hyperplasia), nipple discharge, and gynecomastia. Medications are common causes of both galactorrhea and gynecomastia. Health care providers should reassure AYAs and their families regarding the spectrum of normal development, and appropriately intervene when anomalies occur. Clinicians should not hesitate to involve mental health experts and plastic surgeons when appropriate. Masses in this age-group are uncommon; malignant masses are rare. Persistent masses require evaluation. Physical examination, fine-needle biopsy, and ultrasound imaging provide diagnostic information in a minimally invasive manner.

REFERENCES

1. ACOG Committee on Adolescent Health Care. ACOG Committee Opinion No. 350, November 2006: Breast concerns in the adolescent. *Obstet Gynecol* 2006;108(5):1329–1336.
2. Santen RJ, Mansel R. Benign breast disorders. *N Engl J Med* 2005;353(3):275–285.
3. Sadove AM, van Aalst JA. Congenital and acquired pediatric breast anomalies: a review of 20 years' experience. *Plast Reconstr Surg* 2005;115(4):1039–1050.

4. Eidlitz-Markus T, Mukamel M, Haimi-Cohen Y, et al. Breast asymmetry during adolescence: physiologic and non-physiologic causes. *Isr Med Assoc J* 2010;12(4): 203–206.

5. Cerrato F, Webb ML, Rosen H, et al. The impact of macromastia on adolescents: a cross-sectional study. *Pediatrics* 2012;130(2):e339–e346. doi:10.1542/peds. 2011-3869.

6. Singh KA, Losken A. Additional benefits of reduction mammaplasty: a systematic review of the literature. *Plast Reconstr Surg* 2012;129(3):562–570.

7. Morrogh M, Park A, Elkin EB, et al. Lessons learned from 416 cases of nipple discharge of the breast. *Am J Surg* 2010;200(1):73–80.

8. McHoney M, Munro F, Mackinlay G. Mammary duct ectasia in children: report of a short series and review of the literature. *Early Hum Dev* 2011;87(8):527–530.

9. Huang W, Molitch ME. Evaluation and management of galactorrhea. *Am Fam Physician* 2012;85(11):1073–1080.

10. Catli G, Abaci A, Bober E, et al. Clinical and diagnostic characteristics of hyperprolactinemia in childhood and adolescence. *J Pediatr Endocrinol Metab* 2013;26(1/2):1–11.

11. Holt RIG, Peveler RC. Antipsychotics and hyperprolactinaemia: mechanisms, consequences and management. *Clin Endocrinol (Oxf)* 2011;74(2):141–147.

12. Melmed S, Casanueva FF, Hoffman AR, et al. Diagnosis and treatment of hyperprolactinemia: an Endocrine Society clinical practice guideline. *J Clin Endocrinol Metab* 2011;96(2):273–288.

13. Auriemma RS, Pivonello R, Perone Y, et al. Safety of long-term treatment with cabergoline on cardiac valve disease in patients with prolactinomas. *Eur J Endocrinol* 2013;169(3):359–366.

14. Dos Santos Nunes V, El Dib R, Boguszewski CL, et al. Cabergoline versus bromocriptine in the treatment of hyperprolactinemia: a systematic review of randomized controlled trials and meta-analysis. *Pituitary* 2011;14(3):259–265.

15. Salzman B, Fleegle S, Tully AS. Common breast problems. *Am Fam Physician* 2012;86(4):343–349.

16. Jayasinghe Y, Simmons PS. Fibroadenomas in adolescence. *Curr Opin Obstet Gynecol* 2009;21(5):402–406.

17. Frazier AL, Rosenberg SM. Preadolescent and adolescent risk factors for benign breast disease. *J Adolesc Health* 2013;52(5, suppl):S36–S40.

18. Patterson SK, Jorns JM. A case of juvenile papillomatosis, aka "Swiss cheese disease." *Breast J* 2013;19(4):440–441.

19. Simmons PS, Jayasinghe YL, Wold LE, et al. Breast carcinoma in young women. *Obstet Gynecol* 2011;118(3):529–536.

20. Werner-Lin A, Hoskins LM, Doyle MH, et al. Cancer doesn't have an age: genetic testing and cancer risk management in BRCA1/2 mutation-positive women aged 18–24. *Health (London)* 2012;16(6):636–654.

21. Patel A, Schwarz EB. Cancer and contraception. Release date May 2012. SFP Guideline #20121. *Contraception* 2012;86(3):191–198.

22. Moorman PG, Havrilesky LJ, Gierisch JM, et al. Oral contraceptives and risk of ovarian cancer and breast cancer among high-risk women: a systematic review and meta-analysis. *J Clin Oncol* 2013;31(33):4188–4198.

23. Gaskie S, Nashelsky J. Clinical inquiries. Are breast self-exams or clinical exams effective for screening breast cancer? *J Fam Pract* 2005;54(9):803–804.

24. Bock K, Duda VF, Hadji P, et al. Pathologic breast conditions in childhood and adolescence: evaluation by sonographic diagnosis. *J Ultrasound Med* 2005;24(10): 1347–1354; quiz 1356–1357.

25. Ezer SS, Oguzkurt P, Ince E, et al. Surgical treatment of the solid breast masses in female adolescents. *J Pediatr Adolesc Gynecol* 2013;26(1):31–35.

26. Vargas HI, Vargas MP, Eldrageely K, et al. Outcomes of surgical and sonographic assessment of breast masses in women younger than 30. *Am Surg* 2005;71(9): 716–719.

27. Harvey JA, Nicholson BT, Lorusso AP, et al. Short-term follow-up of palpable breast lesions with benign imaging features: evaluation of 375 lesions in 320 women. *Am. J. Roentgenol* 2009;193(6):1723–1730.

28. Nuzzi LC, Cerrato FE, Erickson CR, et al. Psychosocial impact of adolescent gynecomastia: a prospective case-control study. *Plast Reconstr Surg* 2013;131(4): 890–896.

29. Johnson RE, Murad MH. Gynecomastia: pathophysiology, evaluation, and management. *Mayo Clin Proc* 2009;84(11):1010–1015.

30. Braunstein GD. Clinical practice. Gynecomastia. *N Engl J Med* 2007;357(12): 1229–1237.

31. Rosen H, Webb ML, DiVasta AD, et al. Adolescent gynecomastia: not only an obesity issue. *Ann Plast Surg* 2010;64(5):688–690.

32. Lawrence SE, Faught KA, Vethamuthu J, et al. Beneficial effects of raloxifene and tamoxifen in the treatment of pubertal gynecomastia. *J Pediatr* 2004;145(1): 1–76.

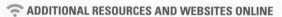 **ADDITIONAL RESOURCES AND WEBSITES ONLINE**

PART XIII

Sexually Transmitted Infections

CHAPTER 56

Overview of Sexually Transmitted Infections

J. Dennis Fortenberry

GENERAL OVERVIEW

From a clinical and public health perspective, sexually transmitted infections (STIs) are visible tracks marking the developmental trails of sexuality through adolescence into young adulthood. Sexuality itself occupies an uncomfortable, ambiguous position among the health challenges of adolescence and young adulthood—the appropriate experiential elements of healthy sexual learning balanced against the threats posed by STIs that may reverberate through the lifespan.

The key clinical considerations of adolescent and young adult (AYA) sexual health include issues of sexuality, discussions during clinical visits that identify knowledge, attitudes, and behaviors that increase or reduce risk of acquiring an STI, immunization, screening by physical examination and laboratory testing, treatment of identified infections, and counseling for partner treatment and prevention of new infections. Annual attention to these issues is recommended and some experts suggest even more frequent risk-reduction counseling and screening, particularly in AYAs with prior infections or in those involved in higher STI risk sexual behaviors.[1] STI screening provides an opportunity to discuss human immunodeficiency virus (HIV) testing and prevention.

STIs are associated with significant disease burden among AYAs.[2] Rates of both gonorrhea and chlamydia genital infections in the US are highest among 20- to 24-year-olds, closely followed by 15- to 19-year-olds. Chlamydia rates are about 3% among 15- to 25-year-old women, but may be 6% or more among non-Hispanic Black women. Chlamydia prevalence decreases when aggressive community-wide screening and treatment policies are implemented. *Trichomonas vaginalis* rates are up to 14% in young women and 3% to 5% in asymptomatic young men. Serological studies show positivity rates for herpes simplex virus type 2 (HSV-2) of up to 40% for some groups of AYAs; most do not have symptomatic infection. HSV type 1 is now a common cause of genital herpes among AYAs. Evidence for human papillomavirus (HPV) infection may be seen in up to one-third of some clinical samples. Three vaccines for some HPV types are commercially available. Clinician recommendation is an important element for acceptance of HPV vaccination by parents, adolescents, and by young adults.[3] These HPV vaccines—along with hepatitis B vaccines—are associated with significant decreases in infections, transmissions to others, and adverse outcomes caused by sexually transmitted viruses.

The elevated risk for some STIs in AYAs is almost certainly multifactorial in origin, and may change as adolescents transition into young adulthood.[4] Developmental susceptibility of the reproductive tract of young women, the substantial rates of sex partner infections, and inconsistent or incorrect condom use are potential contributors. Socioenvironmental risks such as high endemic STI rates, sexual and physical abuse, social chaos, poverty, drug trafficking and use, and inadequate health care access also contribute and may be more powerful explanations of STI risk than developmental or individual behaviors.

Diagnostic tests for many STIs, particularly gonorrhea and chlamydia, have been revolutionized by nucleic acid amplification test (NAAT) and hybrid capture (HC) techniques. NAAT and HC techniques have replaced culture diagnosis in many areas, and have the advantage of automated, high throughput systems that maintain relatively low testing costs. NAAT and HC have the added advantage of use of urine or vaginal samples, as well as traditional cervical, urethral, and anal samples.

APPROACHES TO STI DIAGNOSIS, TREATMENT, AND PREVENTION

STIs constitute a diverse set of etiologic agents most often transmitted through one or more of the between-person interactions called "sex." Behaviors identified as "sex" are quite diverse, however, and it is important to remember that no single behavior—including penile-vaginal intercourse—is universally endorsed as "sex."[5] It is likely that some patients do not accurately answer clinicians' questions about sexual activity. It is also likely, however, that many clinicians simply fail to ask at all, fail to ask the right question, or do not allow sufficient time for a response. A recent study showed that 36 seconds was the average time spent by physicians in discussing sexual issues in health maintenance visits.[6]

The various etiologic agents of STIs vary in terms of specific types of sexual contact associated with transmission, the tissue or organ typically infected, ease of diagnosis, and outcomes of treatment. The diversity of organisms and their diagnostic approaches and treatments appropriately require focused attention in the organism- or condition-specific chapters that follow. However, the relative specificity of organisms for some tissues create symptoms and signs that allow a narrower differential diagnosis and more focused diagnostic testing (**Table 56.1**). Several additional issues for STI diagnosis, treatment, and prevention are summarized below.

TABLE 56.1

STIs by Presenting Symptom

1. Urethral discharge/dysuria
   a. *Neisseria gonorrhoeae*
   b. *Chlamydia trachomatis*
   c. *Ureaplasma urealyticum*
   d. Herpes genitalis
   e. *Trichomonas vaginalis*
   f. *Mycoplasma genitalium*
   g. Epstein–Barr viruses
   h. Adenoviruses

2. Vaginal discharge
   Vaginal site of infection:
   a. *Candida* species
   b. *T. vaginalis*
   c. Bacterial vaginosis
   Cervical site of infection:
   a. *N. gonorrhoeae*
   b. *C. trachomatis*
   c. Herpes genitalis
   d. *M. genitalium*

3. Genital ulcer/lymphadenopathy
   a. Herpes genitalis
   b. *Treponema pallidum*
   c. *Haemophilus ducreyi*
   d. *C. trachomatis* (LGV types)
   e. *Calymmatobacterium granulomatis*

4. Genital growths
   a. Human papillomavirus (genital warts)
   b. Molluscum contagiosum
   c. Condyloma latum (secondary syphilis)

5. Abdominal/pelvic pain
   a. PID

6. Anorectal pain/discharge/bleeding
   a. *N. gonorrhoeae*
   b. *C. trachomatis*
   c. *Shigella* species
   d. *Campylobacter* species
   e. *Entamoeba histolytica*
   f. *Giardia lamblia*

7. Scrotal pain
   a. *N. gonorrhoeae*
   b. *C. trachomatis*
   c. Coliform/enteric bacteria

8. Throat pain/Pharyngitis
   a. *N. gonorrhoeae*
   b. *C. trachomatis*

9. Hepatitis
   a. Hepatitis A and B virus
   b. Cytomegalovirus
   c. *T. pallidum*

10. Arthralgia/arthritis
    a. *N. gonorrhoeae*
    b. Hepatitis B virus

11. Pruritus
    a. *Pthirus pubis*
    b. *Sarcoptes scabiei*
    c. *T. pallidum*

12. Flu-like or mononucleosis syndrome
    a. Cytomegalovirus
    b. Herpes genitalis
    c. Hepatitis A and B virus
    d. Human immunodeficiency virus (HIV)

Self-sampling/Self-testing

Vaginal samples are preferable to urine for diagnosis of common STIs such as chlamydia and gonorrhea. However, urine samples are often easier to obtain and are more acceptable than clinician-obtained vaginal or anal samples. Self-obtained vaginal or anal samples are a useful alternative, typically performing as well as clinician-obtained samples, and may be especially useful for screening. Many young women find self-obtained vaginal samples to be preferable to clinical-obtained ones, although pictorial guides and staff support may be necessary.[7] Meatal swab samples in young men have excellent diagnostic performance characteristics in some studies but this sample type has not yet been widely evaluated or recommended.

Commercially obtained self-testing kits for HIV are now available. In 2012, US Food and Drug Administration approved the retail sale of an over-the-counter, self-administered "at-home" HIV test kit (OraQuick; OraSure Inc.). This test uses a saliva collection technique and allows users to complete testing, interpret results, and use consumer support materials for counseling, confirmatory testing, and linkage to care. Although beyond the out-of-pocket affordability for many young people, these tests provide private and less stigmatized alternatives to HIV testing in clinics or other venues.[8]

A variety of mobile phone applications have been developed to provide direct information for youth about STIs and to provide links to local youth-friendly services. Uptake of these applications has been limited, and evaluations have not shown substantial impact on testing and treatment rates. Barriers include lack of availability across platforms, limited appeal to specific user groups, and lack of locally relevant information.[9]

Screening

Clinical identification of STIs among AYAs is complicated by the lack of urogenital symptoms or clinical signs to guide STI testing. Routine screening of persons meeting age, gender, or behavior characteristics allows testing of persons with appreciable risk of infection while limiting the testing of lower-risk persons.

Chlamydia Screening

The Centers for Disease Control & Prevention (CDC) recommends annual chlamydia screening for sexually active women aged 15 to 25 years. Chlamydia screening of young men is not recommended in the absence of risk indicators such as sexual contact with an infected partner, or incarceration in a detention facility.

Gonorrhea Screening

Routine testing for asymptomatic gonorrhea is recommended only for AYAs with risk indicators although these tests are often paired with chlamydia NAAT. HIV screening is recommended for all AYAs at least once.

Syphilis Screening

Syphilis screening is often paired with HIV screening and is recommended for AYAs diagnosed with other STIs, or risk indicators such as commercial sex work or injection drug use.

Point-of-Care STI Tests

Rapid STI tests that are relatively simple to perform are now available for relatively common STIs such as trichomonas. However, point-of-care diagnostic tests for chlamydia or gonorrhea have poor performance characteristics at this time. Point-of-care tests have the obvious advantage of allowing treatment at the time of testing, reducing the need for subsequent contact to deliver results and arrange treatment.[10]

Extragenital Infections

Changes in the prevalence of noncoital sexual behaviors, whether with different-sex or same-sex partners, as well as improved diagnostic tests have expanded our understanding of the frequency and clinical significance of oropharyngeal and anorectal STIs.

Oropharynx

The oropharynx is a site of both infection and transmission of common STIs, including *Chlamydia trachomatis*, *Neisseria gonorrhoeae*, *Treponema pallidum*, HSV-1, HPV, and HIV. Patterns of orogenital sex in populations likely determine prevalence.[11] Most oropharyngeal STIs are asymptomatic although *T. pallidum* and HSV-1 are particularly likely to cause symptomatic and observable lesions. Selective rather than routine screening for oropharyngeal *C. trachomatis* or *N. gonorrhoeae* is recommended.

Anus and Rectum

Anal and rectal infections may accompany genital STIs, represent an isolated infection site, or represent an initial entry site for infection. Some anal infections likely represent spread from contiguous genital sites, so that history of receptive anal intercourse is often not elicited. *C. trachomatis*, *N. gonorrhoeae*, *T. pallidum*, HSV-1 and 2, and HPV cause localized infections, and HIV may initially infect rectal mucosa before leading to systemic infection. NAAT screening of genital sites will not identify anal and rectal infections so that sexual history or symptoms should guide clinical decisions about anal and rectal testing. Youth may not understand that genital STI screening does not detect anal infections.

HPV is a common anal STI that is now almost 100% preventable. HPV vaccination clearly reduces anal HPV infection in AYA women and men, significantly reduces the incidence of perianal warts and, over time, the incidence of anal cancers. Anal cellular dysplasia may be seen in a small proportion of young men and women with history of receptive anal intercourse: screening with high-resolution anoscopy and anal cytology is increasingly used for high-risk men and women, but routine screening of AYAs is currently not recommended.[12]

Emerging Issue—*Mycoplasma genitalium*

Mycoplasma genitalium was identified in the early 1980s and has been associated as both a sole pathogen or as a coinfection organism.[13]

Males

M. genitalium is a recognized cause of male urethritis (about 15% to 20% of nongonococcal urethritis and about 30% of persistent or recurrent urethritis). The prevalence is likely higher than gonorrhea and lower than chlamydia.

Women

It is less definitively studied to have a pathogenic role in women but the organism can be found in the vagina, cervix, and endometrium. While *M. genitalium* is usually asymptomatic, it has been found in 10% to 30% of individuals with clinical cervicitis and it is found in the cervix or endometrium of 2% to 22% of those women with pelvic inflammatory disease (PID). There is suggestive evidence that this organism can cause PID.

Clinical

- There is lack of a characteristic clinical syndrome.
- Clinicians should suspect *M. genitalium* in individuals with persistent or recurrent urethritis and also consider it in those with persistent or recurrent cervicitis/PID.

Diagnosis

- Organism is slow growing and culture can take up to six months.
- NAAT testing is the preferred method of diagnoses, but at the moment some labs do not have a commercially available FDA-approved diagnostic test.

Treatment

- Doxycycline 100 mg b.i.d. × 7 days ineffective (31% cure rate)
- Azithromycin 1 g single dose is preferred over doxycycline but resistance is rapidly increasing (85% cure rate). Alternative dosing is azithromycin 500 mg once and then 250 mg every day for four days.
- Moxifloxacin (400 mg daily × 7, 10 or 14 days) has been successful (approximately 100%) in small clinical trials.
- In PID cases that fail to respond to recommended PID treatment regimens, one might consider *M. genitalium* and thus potentially treat with moxifloxacin 400 mg/day × 14 days.

STI TREATMENT

We recommend that all STI treatments follow the *Sexually Transmitted Diseases Treatment Guidelines* revised every four years by the CDC (http://www.cdc.gov/std/treatment/). These treatment guidelines are evidence-based and also address issues of specific relevance to adolescents. Full guidelines can be downloaded as well as printable treatment summaries and an application for smartphones (see references and additional readings for links). New information in the updated guidelines include (1) alternative treatment regimens for *N. gonorrhoeae*; (2) use of NAAT for the diagnosis of trichomoniasis; (3) alternative treatment options for genital warts; (4) the role of *M. genitalium* in urethritis/cervicitis and treatment-related implications; (5) updated HPV counseling messages; (6) new section on the management of transgender individuals; (7) annual testing for hepatitis C in persons with HIV infection; (8) updated recommendations for diagnostic evaluation of urethritis; and (9) retesting to detect repeat infection.[13] Readers seeking treatment advice are referred directly to these resources, as well as the individual chapters that follow.

Partner Notification

Untreated partners represent a major source of reinfection for successfully treated adolescents: up to 30% of young women with treated chlamydia infections may have a second infection within three months. Infections such as chlamydia and gonorrhea are reportable to local health departments in almost all jurisdictions. However, partner-tracing services for these infections are often reserved only for specific types of patients. Simply advising patients of the need for partner treatment is effective in only a minority of cases. Provision of more detailed printed partner information is more effective than simple verbal advice, especially for youth who prefer to notify partners themselves. Exploration of the possibility of partner violence in response to notification should be explored at this time.

Patient-delivered partner treatment (sometimes called expedited partner services) is the practice of provision of medications or prescriptions for patient delivery to partners. This approach has been shown to reduce rates of chlamydia and gonorrhea reinfection among AYA women, but may be ineffective for prevention of trichomonas reinfections.[14] Provision of partner treatment is supported by a position paper of the Society for Adolescent Health and Medicine, but legal endorsement of the practice varies by state. Updated state-by-state information is available at http://www.cdc.gov/std/ept/legal/default.htm. Emergence of appreciable rates of gonococcal resistance to orally administered antibiotics has limited application of patient-delivered medication for partners of patients with gonorrhea. Patient-delivered treatment is not recommended for men with same-sex partners.

REFERENCES

1. Walker J, Tabrizi SN, Fairley CK, et al. *Chlamydia trachomatis* incidence and re-infection among young women--behavioural and microbiological characteristics. *PLoS One* [Electronic Resource]. 2012;7(5):e37778.
2. Satterwhite CL, Torrone E, Meites E, et al. Sexually transmitted infections among US women and men: prevalence and incidence estimates, 2008. *Sex Transm Dis* 2013;40(3):187–193.
3. Holman DM, Benard V, Roland KB, et al. Barriers to human papillomavirus vaccination among us adolescents: a systematic review of the literature. *JAMA Pediatr* 2014;168(1):76–82.
4. Torrone E, Papp J, Weinstock H; Centers for Disease Control and Prevention. Prevalence of *Chlamydia trachomatis* genital infection among persons aged 14–39 years—United States, 2007–2012. *MMWR* 2014;63(38):834–838.
5. Byers ES, Henderson J, Hobson KM. University students' definitions of sexual abstinence and having sex. *Arch Sex Behav* 2009;38(5):665–674.
6. Alexander SC, Fortenberry JD, Pollak KI, et al. Sexuality talk during adolescent health maintenance visits. *JAMA Pediatr* 2014;168(2):163–169.
7. Fielder RL, Carey KB, Carey MP. Acceptability of sexually transmitted infection testing using self-collected vaginal swabs among college women. *J Am Coll Health* 2013;61(1):46–53.
8. Bilardi JE, Walker S, Read T, et al. Gay and bisexual men's views on rapid self-testing for HIV. *AIDS Behav* 2013;17(6):2093–2099.
9. Muessig KE, Pike EC, Legrand S, et al. Mobile phone applications for the care and prevention of HIV and other sexually transmitted diseases: a review. *J Med Internet Res* 2013;15(1):e1.
10. Tucker JD, Bien CH, Peeling RW. Point-of-care testing for sexually transmitted infections: recent advances and implications for disease control. *Curr Opin Infect Dis* 2013;26(1):73–79.
11. Karlsson A, Osterlund A, Forssen A. Pharyngeal *Chlamydia trachomatis* is not uncommon any more. *Scand J Infect Dis* 2011;43(5):344–348.
12. Smyczek P, Singh AE, Romanowski B. Anal intraepithelial neoplasia: review and recommendations for screening and management. *Int J STD AIDS* 2013;24(11):843–851.
13. Workowski KA, Bolan GA. Sexually Transmitted Diseases Treatment Guidelines, 2015. *MMWR Recomm Rep* 2015;64(RR-3):1–135.
14. Hogben M, Kidd S, Burstein GR. Expedited partner therapy for sexually transmitted infections. *Curr Opin Obstet Gynecol* 2012;24(5):299–304.

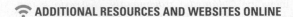 **ADDITIONAL RESOURCES AND WEBSITES ONLINE**

Gonorrhea and Chlamydia

Margaret J. Blythe

Gonococal and chlamydial genital infections are sexually transmitted infections (STIs) frequently diagnosed in adolescents and young adults (AYAs) having the potential for serious complications.

ETIOLOGY

Gonorrhea is an STI caused by *Neisseria gonorrhoeae,* which has the following characteristics:

1. Small, intracellular gram-negative cocci, arranged in pairs (diplococci) typically located within or associated with polymorphonuclear (PMN) leukocytes
2. Physical contact required for transmission, specifically contact of mucosal surfaces; no evidence that infection can be transmitted by inantimate objects or outside of host
3. Differentiated from other strains, such as *N. meningitidis* and *N. lactamica,* through use of laboratory techniques as growing on chemically defined media (auxotyping), serotyping (monoclonal antibodies specific for various epitopes on outer membrane protein), antimicrobial susceptibilities, and genotyping
4. Possesses a number of structures on the outer membrane contributing to pathogenesis, such as reduction modifiable protein (prevents bactericidal activity), porin B protein (insertion into host cell membrane), lipooligosaccharide (tissue toxin), Opa protein (adherence), and pili (adherence to host tissue)
5. Evades host defenses by antigenic variation of many of the structures on the outer membrane.[1]

Chlamydia is an STI caused by *Chlamydia trachomatis,* which has the following characteristics:

1. Serovars B, D, E, F, G, H, I, J, K found in genital infections such as urethritis, cervicitis, salpingitis, proctitis, and newborn/adolescent conjunctivitis and serovars L1, L2, L3 in lymphogranuloma venereum
2. Unique developmental cycle lasting between 48 and 72 hours: initial attachment and ingestion of the infectious particle (the elementary body) into the host cell, reorganization into a *reticulate body,* replication, transformation to new infectious elementary bodies, and release, most often resulting in the destruction of the host cell
3. Pathogenesis of non-LGV serovars related to being obligate intracellular parasites limited to infection within the squamocolumnar–columnar epithelial cells with resulting cellular death, an inflammatory response and tissue damage; pathogenesis of LGV serovars related to systemic effects such as lymphoproliferative disease with associated capability to replicate within macrophages
4. Immune response induces both a neutralizing antibody and a T cell–mediated immune response, which neutralizes chlamydial infectivity. *C. trachomatis* has a heat shock protein (cHSP60) 50% homologous to human HSP60. Scarring of the fallopian tubes in pelvic inflammatory disease (PID) is thought to be a result of repeated infections and the hypersensitivity reactions specifically related to these shared proteins[2]

EPIDEMIOLOGY

Gonorrhea

Incidence

Gonorrhea is the second most frequently reported disease in the US after *C. trachomatis* infections. Approximately 333,004 cases were reported in 2013 or 106.1/100,000, slightly down from 2012 (106.7) (**Table 57.1**).

TABLE 57.1

Cases and Incidence of Gonorrhea in the US, 1977 to 2013

	1977	1997	2000	2002	2006	2009	2012	2013
Cases	1,002,219	327,665	363,136	351,852	358,366	301,174	334,826	333,304
Incidence per 100,000	456.0	120.2	128.7	122.0	119.7	98.1	106.7	106.1

Adapted from Centers for Disease Control and Prevention. *Sexually transmitted disease surveillance 2013.* Atlanta: US Department of Health and Human Services; 2014. Available at http://www.cdc.gov/std/stats13/tables/1.htm

Trends

National rates decreased by 74% from 1977 to 1997 (122.4/100,000). The rate recorded in 2009 (98.1/100,000) was the lowest rate ever reported by the Centers for Disease Control and Prevention (CDC). Since 2009, the gonorrhea rate has increased slightly each year, with a slight decrease in 2013 representing a 9.6% increase overall into 2012.[3]

Risk Groups

a. *Age/Gender:* Highest rates in 2013 were in women 20 to 24 (541.6/100,000) and 15 to 19 years old (459.2). Young men 20 to 24 years old had the highest rate (459.4) while among young men 15 to 19 years old, the rate was 220.9. From 2012 to 2013 gonorrhea rates for 15- to 19-year-olds decreased by 13% for females and 8.9% for males, while decreasing by 4.7% for 20- to 24-year-old females and increasing 1.3% for 20- to 24-year-old males.[4]

b. *Ethnicity/Gender:* Rates vary dramatically among AYAs of different racial/ethnic backgrounds and in various practice settings. Incidence in Blacks, Hispanics, and Native Americans is disproportionately high compared with Whites and Asians. Historically, rates for Blacks have been the highest for both males and females in the 15- to 24-year-old age-groups. For these two age-groups in 2013, the lowest rate recorded for males was for 15- to 19-year-old Asians (21.7/100,000) while the highest rate was among 20- to 24-year-old Black males (1,734.5/100,000). The lowest rate recorded for females was for 15- to 19-year-old Asian females (40.2/100,000) while the highest rate was among 20- to 24-year-old Black females (1949.1/100,000).[5]

Geography

The decision by providers to "routinely screen" for gonorrhea in teens and young adults may be made on the prevalence of disease in the area of country in which the teen resides. Wide variation occurs based on region of country, state, and even city. Outside of the South and Southeast, the highest reported rates of gonorrhea are reported in the District of Columbia (DC) (391.1) and Alaska (154.3). Examples of states in the south include Louisiana (188.4), Alabama (173.7), and Mississippi (170.7). These rates compare to the lowest rates in Western states such as Wyoming (11.5), Idaho (13.2), and Montana (22.3) and in the Northeast (New Hampshire [9.2] and Vermont [15.5]).[6]

Chlamydia Trachomatis
Incidence

Chlamydia is the most frequently reported disease in the US with 1,401,906 infections reported to the CDC in 2013, yielding a rate of 446.6/100,000. This represents a slight decrease of 1.5% from 2012 (453.3). However, the trend since 1990 (160.2/100,000) has been a steady increase (**Table 57.2**).

Trends

National rates have increased steadily since 1984, when reporting for chlamydia began; more widespread testing with more sensitive techniques has resulted in population rates increasing from 1984 to 2013 (from 6.5/100,000 to 446.6 in 2013).[7]

Risk Groups

a. *Age/Gender:* Highest rates in 2013 were in women 20 to 24 years (3621.1/100,000) and 15 to 19 years (3043.3); although substantially lower for young men, the highest rates are also in the 20- to 24-year-old age-group (1325.6) while for young men 15 to 19 years, the rate is 715.2/100,000. From 2012 to 2013, the chlamydia rates for young adult 20- to 24-year-old men remained about the same in 2013 compared to 2012 (1322.8) and decreased by about 9% for adolescent males. At the same time, the rates for 15- to 19-year-old women in 2013 decreased by 8.7% compared to 2012 and remained the same for 20- to 24-year-old women.[8]

b. *Ethnicity/Gender:* Rates vary dramatically among AYAs from different racial/ethnic backgrounds and practice settings. Incidence in Blacks, Hispanics, and Native Americans is disproportionately high compared with Whites and Asians. Different from gonorrhea, rates among females are 2 to 6 times higher than among males of similar age-group and racial/ethnic backgrounds. Similar to gonorrhea, for these two age-groups in 2013, the lowest rate recorded for males was for 15- to19-year-old Asians (71.5/100,000) while the highest rate was among 20- to 24-year-old Black males (3282.5/100,000). The lowest rate recorded for females was among 15- to 19-year-old Asian females (503.2/100,000) while the highest rate was among 20- to 24-year-old Black females (7342.7/100,000).[9]

Geography

Regardless of place of residence, "routine" annual screening of sexually active 15- to 24-year-old females for chlamydia is recommended, with inconsistent recommendations for screening sexually active 15- to 24-year-old males. The CDC recommends routine screening of "high-risk" males such as those attending adolescent clinics, school-based clinics, correctional systems, Job Corps, and the military.[10,11] Variation in reported rates of chlamydia occurs as a function of the likelihood of testing, reporting, and in what part of the country residence occurs.[12]

Prevalence of Gonorrhea and Chlamydia

1. Reported prevalence rates will vary depending on the population and anatomical sites screened for gonorrhea and chlamydia (**Table 57.3**).
    a. *Opportunities for screening:* At a STI clinic, routine testing of men who have sex with men (MSM) and high-risk females occurred at oropharyngeal, anorectal, and urogenital sites. Results indicated that 6.3% (154/2436) of men were positive for gonorrhea and 10.4% (254/2436) were positive for chlamydia at one or more of the sites; 76% (117/154) of positive samples for gonorrhea were at the anorectal/oropharyngeal sites while 68.5% (174/254) for chlamydia. For women, 3.1% (41/1321) were positive for gonorrhea with 58.5% (24/41) of positive samples anorectal/oropharyngeal; for chlamydia, 7% (92/1321) were positive with 22.8% (21/92) anorectal/oropharyngeal.[13]

TABLE 57.2

Cases and Incidence of Chlamydia in the US, 1984 to 2013

	1984	1997	2000	2002	2004	2006	2009	2012	2013
Cases	7594	537,904	709,452	834,555	929,462	1,030,911	1,244,180	1,422,976	1,401,906
Incidence per 100,000	6.5	205.5	251.4	289.4	316.5	344.3	405.3	456.7	446.6

Adapted from Centers for Disease Control and Prevention. *Sexually transmitted disease surveillance 2013.* Atlanta: US Department of Health and Human Services; 2014. Available at http://www.cdc.gov/std/stats13/tables/1.htm

TABLE 57.3

Reported Prevalence Rates for Gonorrhea and Chlamydia by Population and Anatomical Site Screened

Population	GC (%)	CT (%)	No.	Author
Males *MSM*				
STI Clinics				
Urethral	1.5	3.3	2436	Van Liere
Anogenital	3.7	7.9		et al., 2013
Pharyngeal	3.4	1.1		
Pharyngeal	7.0	2.3	3949	Park et al., 2012
Community Clinics				
Urethral	0.4	2.3	3398	Marcus
Anogenital	3.6	7.8	7061	et al., 2011
Pharyngeal	5.0	1.9		
Pharyngeal	4.0–5.5	1.4		Park et al., 2012
Heterosexual/ Bisexual/Gay				
Job Corps	0.9 (0.0–2.6)	8.0 (2.7–13.0)		CDC, 2011
Detention Clinics	0.7 (0.0–6.0)	6.3 (0.4–19.1)		
Internet	1	13	501	Chai et al., 2010
STI Clinics	14.5 (2.8–21.0)	11.3 (6.5–23.1)		CDC, 2011
Females				
STI clinics				
Genital	1.3	5.4	1321	Van Liere
Anogenital	0.9	4.8		et al., 2013
Pharyngeal	2.3	1.4		
Family-planning Clinics	0.7 (0.0–3.5)	8.4 (3.8–14.3)		CDC, 2011
Job Corps	1.0 (0.0–4.9)	10.3 (4.1–18.7)		CDC, 2011
Detention Clinics	3.4 (0.0–9.6)	13.5 (3.7–27.7)		CDC, 2011
Emergency Dept.	3.5	19.7	236	Goyal et al., 2012
Internet		9.1	1203	Gaydos et al., 2009
NHANES	2.5	7.1	404	Forhan, 2009

One study suggests that fellatio performed by women resulted in a urethral infection rate of 3.5% for chlamydia and 3.1% for gonorrhea, when no other type of sexual contact was acknowledged.[14]

b. **National studies:** Chlamydia prevalence among sexually active females aged 14 to 24 years is nearly three times the prevalence among those aged 25 to 39 years (NHANES 1999–2008, unpublished data, 2011). Prevalence among non-Hispanic Blacks is approximately five times the prevalence among non-Hispanic Whites.[15] Among sexually active females aged 14 to 19 years, chlamydia prevalence is 7.1%

overall, and for gonorrhea 2.5%.[16] Estimated prevalence of gonorrhea in NHANES from 1999 to 2008 among 14- to 25-year-old females and males (0.40%; 95% confidence interval [CI], 0.20% to 0.72%) is similar to estimated 0.43% (95% CI, 0.29% to 0.63%) prevalence among 18- to 26-year-olds in the National Longitudinal Study of Adolescent Health in 2001 to 2002.[17,18]

c. **MSM:** Among asymptomatic MSM, 83.8% of gonorrhea and chlamydia infections would be missed if only urethral screening occurred. The fewest infections would be missed by screening the rectum and pharynx, thus helping reduce the risk of human immunodeficiency virus (HIV) acquisition and transmission.[19] In one analysis, 62.7% of pharyngeal gonorrhea and 57.8% of pharyngeal chlamydia infections were in MSM who did not have a concurrent urogenital or rectal gonorrhea or chlamydia infection.[20] One study reported results from screening for gonorrhea and chlamydia in 5539 MSM attending STI clinics and 895 men attending gay men's health center; routine screening of urethral, anogenital, and pharyngeal sites found that 64% of gonococcal infections (574) were non-urethral sites as were 53% of chlamydia infections (452). Overall, of the three sites and the two infections, the highest rates and sites of infection were gonorrheal pharyngeal (9.4%) and chlamydial anogenital (8.8%). Highest rates of any infections were found in the ≤24-year-old age-group for gonorrhea (17.3%) and chlamydia (15.4%).[21] An editorial addressing screening for chlamydia and gonorrhea in MSM indicated that 47% to 84% of chlamydial infections and 38% to 65% of gonorrhea infections would be missed if only urethral specimens were obtained.[22]

d. **STI clinics:** Across the participating STI sites, the median site-specific gonorrhea prevalence was 14.5% (range by site: 2.8% to 21.0%) while the median site-specific chlamydia prevalence was 11.3% (range by site: 6.5% to 23.1%).[23]

STD Surveillance Network examines the number of cases of gonorrhea and characteristics of the population to better develop strategies for control. Across all sites in 2011, 21.6% of gonorrhea cases were estimated to be among MSM, 31.0% among men having sex with women (MSW), and 47.4% among women.

STI clinics remain the most common reporting source of gonorrhea for men but for women, private physicians or health maintenance organizations were the most common. Among women, 7.7% of chlamydia cases reported were from STI clinics, while 23.6% of cases reported from men were from an STI clinic.[24]

e. **Family-planning clinics** in the US serving 15- to 24-year-old females: In 2011, median state-specific rate for chlamydia was 8.4% (range Vermont 3.8% to Mississippi 14.3%). In 2011, the median state-specific gonorrhea test positivity among women aged 15 to 24 years screened in selected family-planning clinics was 0.7% (range: 0.0% to 3.5%).[25]

f. **National Job Corps:** Among women in 2011 entering the program in 46 states, the DC, and Puerto Rico, the median state-specific chlamydia prevalence was 10.3% (range: 4.1% to 18.7%), while for men, median state-specific chlamydia prevalence was 8.0% (range: 2.7% to 13.0%). Among women entering the program, the median state-specific gonorrhea prevalence in 2011 was 1.0% (range: 0.0% to 4.9%), while for men, the median state-specific gonorrhea prevalence was 0.9% (range: 0.0% to 2.6%).[26]

g. **Juvenile detention facilities:** In 2011, of the 49 clinics reporting that serve teens in detention centers, the median facility-specific chlamydia positivity for females was 13.5% (range: 3.7% to 27.7%) while the median gonorrhea positivity was 3.4% (range: 0.0% to 9.6%). For males, the median facility-specific chlamydia positivity was 6.3%

(range: 0.4 to 19.1%); the median gonorrhea positivity was 0.7% (range: 0.0% to 6.0%).[26]

h. *Emergency departments:* Of the 236 symptomatic (e.g., vaginal discharge) 14- to 19-year-old female patients tested, 19.7% were positive for chlamydia, 9.9% trichomononas, and 3.5% gonorrhea.[27]

i. *Nonclinical outreach testing:* Specific program in the US demonstrated high prevalence rate of chlamydia: 9.1% overall, with 15.3% of females 15 to 19 and 11.1% of 20- to 24-year-olds infected.[28] Rates of infection were higher than those in family-planning clinics. Similar program for males indicated that 1% had tested positive for gonorrhea and 13% for chlamydia.[29] A review was published of 25 programs predominantly in Australia and US targeting 15- to 29-year-olds, MSM, and sex workers. Median testing rate was 79.6% with median gonorrhea rate 2.6% and chlamydia 7.7%. Participation rate was highest among those gathering in community service centers (e.g., homeless shelters) and social venues (e.g., bars, clubs). Lowest participation rates were in street/public sites.[30]

Systematic review and meta-analysis of studies suggest that home-based testing enhances uptake of STI screening when compared to clinic testing for gonorrhea and chlamydia for 14- to 50-year-old females.[31]

j. *The Health Care Effectiveness Data and Information Set:* Among sexually active women aged 16 to 24 years in commercial plans, chlamydia screening increased from 23.1% in 2001 to 45.1% in 2012; the screening rate among sexually active women aged 16 to 24 years covered by Medicaid increased from 40.4% to 57.1%.[32]

Host

Humans are the only natural host for *N. gonorrhoeae* and *C. trachomatis.*

Transmission

Transmission is virtually exclusively through oral, vaginal, or anal sexual contact except for occasional conjunctival mucosal infection from cross contamination with infected secretions.

Clinical Manifestations

Clinical manifestations of *N. gonorrhoeae* are similar to those caused by *C. trachomatis,* and both *C. trachomatis* and *N. gonorrhoeae* can occur together in the same individual. Susceptible sites are usually mucosal columnar epithelial areas or surfaces. The spectrum of infections includes the following:

1. *Asymptomatic gonorrheal and chlamydial infections* in males and females:
   a. Majority of male urethral infections are asymptomatic in the general population and may persist for months if untreated; if symptoms occur, chlamydial infections are more likely milder than gonorrhea.
   b. Most endocervical infections for females in general population are asymptomatic, but may have symptoms that are relatively short term and/or may be mistaken for symptoms of another infectious process, such as urinary tract infections and/or other causes of vaginal discharge.
   c. Asymptomatic rectal and pharyngeal infections are a major reservoir of infections, particularly for MSM. Infection with non-LGV immune types of chlamydia as well as gonorrhea may result in asymptomatic proctitis.
   d. Estimates are that over 90% of pharyngeal gonorrhea infections are asymptomatic.
   e. Asymptomatic infections can involve the following for males and females:
      • Urethra
      • Endocervix (females only)
      • Rectum
      • Pharynx

2. *Symptomatic* uncomplicated infections may result in the following:
   a. Urethritis
   b. Cervicitis
   c. Proctitis
   d. Pharyngitis
   e. Bartholinitis
   f. Conjunctivitis

3. *Local complications* include the following:
   a. PID
   b. Epididymitis
   c. Bartholin gland abscess
   d. Infection of male accessory sex glands presenting as periurethritis: seminal vesicles, bulbourethral glands (Cowper glands), and/or prostate gland
   e. Perihepatitis: Complication of salpingitis (Fitz–Hugh–Curtis syndrome)

4. *Systemic complications* for gonorrhea and chlamydia might include the following:
   a. Disseminated gonococcal infection (DGI)
   b. Arthritis–dermatitis syndromes
   c. Gonococcal meningitis
   d. Gonococcal endocarditis

Genitourinary Infections

The most common clinical manifestation of gonorrhea and chlamydia is a genitourinary infection.

Males

1. Urethritis
   a. Gonococcal
      • Incubation period: Ranges from 1 to 14 days with most men symptomatic 2 to 5 days after exposure
      • Symptoms: Urethral discharge, dysuria, meatal pruritus
      • Clinical findings: Profuse purulent urethral discharge (25% scanty, minimally purulent discharge), urethral edema, and erythema
      • Spontaneous resolution over several weeks without treatment
   b. Chlamydial
      • Incubation period: 7 to 21 days
      • Symptoms: Dysuria, mild to moderate discharge
      • Clinical findings: Minimal urethral discharge or no findings

2. Both infections can spread and cause *epididymitis*
   a. More than two-thirds of AYAs with epididymitis have gonorrhea and/or chlamydia.
   b. Urethral symptoms may or may not be present.
   c. Scrotal pain and tenderness, usually unilateral with swelling and erythema
   d. Pain in the inguinal area and flank pain in severe cases
   e. Pain, tenderness, or swelling of the lower pole of the epididymis, which can spread to the head of the epididymis

3. A limited number of studies have examined transmissibility of either or both infections but suggest that the majority of males exposed to an infected female partner will be infected.[33,34]

Females

Signs and symptoms are less specific in females than in males for both gonorrhea and chlamydial infections. If symptomatic, the female may complain of vaginal discharge, dysuria, or frequency. Common local problems include the following:

1. *Endocervicitis:*
   a. Most often asymptomatic for both infections
   b. May present with increased vaginal discharge, irregular bleeding, and dysuria

c. Findings on exam may include mucopurulent endocervical discharge, endocervical friability with bleeding, and erythema and edema of an area of ectopy.

d. May persist for weeks or months without symptoms or spontaneously resolve

2. *Urethritis*:
    a. Most often asymptomatic for both infections
    b. Urinary symptoms as dysuria, urinary frequency
    c. Infrequently exudate from urethra, urethral redness, or swelling
    d. Lack of suprapubic pain

3. *Bartholinitis/Bartholin gland abscess*: Purulent exudate from Bartholin gland may be either or both infections; abscess presents as labial pain and swelling. With gonorrhea infections, occasionally purulent exudate may be expressed also from the urethral or periurethral glands.[34]

4. Spread of infection can extend into the following areas:
    a. *Endometritis*: Endometrial biopsy findings of polymorphonuclear leukocytes, plasma cells, and lymphocytes migrating among epithelial cells, stroma, and glands.[35]
    b. *Fallopian tubes*: PID or salpingitis (Chapter 58) refers to infections including endometritis, tuboovarian abscess, pelvic peritonitis. Estimates are that in about 10% to 20% of untreated females with acute urogenital gonorrhea and 10% of those with chlamydial cervicitis, organisms will ascend to cause PID. Patients with gonococcal-associated PID compared to chlamydial-associated PID or nongonococcal, nonchlamydial–associated PID may be more ill and febrile at clinical presentation with shorter period of abdominal pain.[35]
    c. *Perihepatitis* (Fitz–Hugh–Curtis syndrome): Presents as right-upper-quadrant pain, fever, nausea, and vomiting; majority of cases associated with chlamydial infection rather than gonorrheal infections.
    d. *Ovary*: Tuboovarian abscess

Extragenital Sites

1. Pharyngitis
    a. Pharyngeal involvement is usually asymptomatic in >90% of infected individuals.
    b. Gonorrhea pharyngitis may be manifested by a sore throat 3 to 7 days after exposure and occasionally with fever and cervical adenopathy; chlamydial pharyngitis has not been well studied.
    c. Fellatio is a more effective mode of transmission than cunnilingus. Pharyngeal infection may be a significant cause of urethral gonorrhea in MSM.
    d. Spontaneous elimination of the organism can occur in 12 weeks.
    e. Infected individuals may be at risk for dissemination of gonorrhea.[34]

2. Proctitis
    a. Most anorectal infections in males and females are asymptomatic.
    b. Rectal gonorrhea can produce the following symptoms:
        • Minimal anal pruritus with mucous
        • Mucopurulent anal discharge
        • Rectal bleeding
        • Anorectal pain
        • Tenesmus
        • Constipation
    c. Proctoscopic examination may show a normal appearance with some mucous when either infection present or a range of findings including painless mucopurulent discharge with patchy, generalized erythema of rectal mucosa **or** purulent exudate, erythema, edema, friability, or other inflammatory changes of the rectal mucosa.
    d. The differential diagnosis for infections involving the first 5 to 10 cm of the rectum (proctitis) includes gonorrhea,

chlamydia (non-LGV), herpes, and syphilis. Inflammation extending more than 15 cm (proctocolitis) is usually caused by *Shigella, Campylobacter, Entamoeba histolytica, Chlamydia* (LGV serotypes), or *Salmonella*. Non-LGV serotypes of chlamydia appear to act as parasites infecting only the squamocolumnar epithelial cells, while LGV types act as a systemic infection, specifically of the lymphoid tissue, capable of infecting and replicating even within macrophages.[33]

3. *Conjunctivitis*: Gonococcal ophthalmia usually occurs in newborns 2 to 5 days after birth with no prophylaxis; conjunctivitis has been reported in physicians, laboratory technicians, and the general adult population, presumably when direct contact of the organism or infected secretions with the eye occurs. Chlamydial inclusion conjunctivitis can be a result of contact with infected genital secretions in the general population or by neonates at birth. Serovars B, Ba, D→K cause STIs while serovars A→C are the etiologic agents of trachoma.[36]

Arthritis–Dermatitis Syndrome
Disseminated Gonococcal Infection

Less than 1% of individuals with gonorrhea develop disseminated disease (DGI), characterized by fever, dermatitis, acute arthritis, tenosynovitis, or a combination of findings. Joint pain and skin lesions are the most common presenting symptoms. Certain strains of *N. gonorrhoeae* are more likely to disseminate. These strains tend to cause asymptomatic urogenital or pharyngeal infection and are more resistant to complement-mediated bactericidal activity in serum. DGI is more common in females, with a 4:1 ratio of female:male. In about half the women, symptoms occur within 7 days of the last menstrual period. Inherited complement deficiency may be a risk factor as are other diseases that lower complement levels, such as lupus erythematosus.[34]

1. Purulent arthritis: Purulent arthritis is the most common systemic complication of *N. gonorrhoeae* and usually occurs within 1 month of exposure. Approximately 25% to 50% of patients complain of pain in a single joint. The knee is the most common site of purulent gonococcal arthritis but may involve the wrist, metacarpophalangeal joints, and ankle. Monoarticular septic arthritis may present without preceding dermatitis or tenosynovitis.

2. Migratory polyarthralgias/arthritis: Others have migratory polyarthralgia or asymmetrical polyarticular arthritis involving the knees, wrists, small joints of hands, ankles, and elbows with not enough fluid to aspirate. Knees are the most frequently involved joints, but all joints, including the hip and shoulder, have been affected. Sacroiliac, temporomandibular, and sternoclavicular joints are rarely involved. Estimates are that 30% to 40% of patients with DGI will develop overt arthritis.

3. Tenosynovitis: Tenosynovitis, involving the extensor and flexor tendons and sheaths, may affect the hands and fingers and less likely the lower extremities.

4. Fever, chills, and leukocytosis are common but 40% are afebrile.

5. Approximately 90% will have a skin rash:
    a. Variable presentations:
        • *Hemorrhagic lesions* presenting as purpura and necrotic centers
        • *Vesiculopapular lesions* on an erythematous base
    b. All lesions begin as *erythematous papules* with hemorrhagic lesions located most often on palms and soles, while others progress from papules to vesicles to pustules.
    c. Frequently painful, asymmetrical lesions over extremities near the joints, palms, soles of feet, and occasionally on trunk and rarely on face.

d. Lesions more likely on distal extremities and less than 30 in number.
6. Diagnosis:
   a. Positive blood cultures in 20% to 30% of patients, but cultures should be done in the first few days of the illness.
   b. Joint cultures are rarely positive with polyarticular presentation. For monoarticular presentation, the affected joint's synovial fluid may appear turbid, with predominance of PMN cells and low glucose. Positive cultures from skin, blood, and/or joints occur in less than 50% of cases. PCR has been used on joint fluid to make the diagnosis.
   c. Gram stain results and cultures are usually negative from skin.
   d. Elevated peripheral white counts occur in the majority and elevation of sedimentation rate in most.
   e. In more than 80% of DGI patients, gonococci have been identified from a primary infected anogenital or pharyngeal mucosal surface of the patient or patient's partner(s) despite negative blood, skin, and joint fluid cultures.
7. Differential diagnosis of gonococcal arthritis
   a. Infections: Meningococcemia, bacteremias, endocarditis, infectious arthritis, and infectious tenosynovitis.
   b. Seronegative arthritides: Reiter syndrome, ankylosing spondylitis, psoriatic arthritis, rheumatoid arthritis, rheumatic fever, Lyme disease, bacterial endocarditis
   c. Lupus erythematosus
   d. Allergic reaction to drugs[34]

Sexually Acquired Reactive Arthritis (Reiter Syndrome)

This refers to a syndrome of urethritis, conjunctivitis, and seronegative spondyloarthritis:

1. Triggered by a reaction associated with urogenital infection (most often chlamydia infection) or enteric infections (*Shigella, Yersinia, Campylobacter,* and *Salmonella*).
2. Estimates are that 1% to 3% of men will develop reactive arthritis following genital infection with *C. trachomatis.*
3. Seventy-five percent to ninety percent of men with Reiter syndrome are positive for HLA B27 and antibody studies in men with Reiter syndrome suggest that 80% have had chlamydia.
4. Systemic manifestations of the disease occur about 1 month after infection; conjunctivitis occurs within a few weeks of arthritis and urethritis.
5. Primary lesion of keratoderma blennorrhagicum begins as a dull red papule that rapidly forms a hyperkeratotic yellow surface. Lesions coalesce into plaques and may have a circinate collarette of scale with some pustular lesions. Lesions are most often on the soles of the feet, legs, hands, fingers, nails, and scalp.
6. If lesions appear on penis, they are moist, red erosions that merge to form circinate balanitis in uncircumcised males and hard crusts and plaques in circumcised males. Mucocutaneous lesions of keratoderma blennorrhagicum and circinate balanitis develop in 15% and 36% of patients, respectively.
7. Ocular manifestations are mainly mild, bilateral mucopurulent conjunctivitis that resolves spontaneously within 10 days. Approximately one-third may develop unilateral uveitis along with the conjunctivitis, which presents acutely with diffuse redness around the border of the cornea and sclera accompanied by pain and photophobia. Inflammation may diminish over three months but reoccurrence is not uncommon.

Differences and similarities between DGI and sexually acquired reactive arthritis are summarized in **Table 57.4.**[33,36]

Other Sites of Dissemination

1. Mild hepatitis: Found in up to 50% of patients, but not usually clinically suspected and usually follows bacteremia of DGI

TABLE 57.4

Comparison of Acute Gonococcal Arthritis and Acute Reiter Syndrome

Characteristic	Acute Gonococcal Arthritis (%)	Acute Reiter Syndrome (%)
Back pain	0	20
Urethritis	28	76
Migratory arthralgias	83	10
Chills	33	0
Temperature >39.4°C	27	39
Skin lesions	Isolated papules and pustules on extremities and trunk	Circinate balanitis; keratoderma of shaft of penis. Asymptomatic oral macular lesions on palate, buccal mucosa
Sacroiliac involvement	3	30
Wrist involvement	67	30
Heel involvement	7	67
Antigen HLA-B27	Usually negative	>90 positive

2. Gonococcal meningitis: Rare complication that can be clinically indistinguishable from other meningococcal infections
3. Rare cardiac manifestations: Myopericarditis, heart block, endocarditis
4. Other: Osteomyelitis, pneumonia

Screening Options for the Detection of Gonorrhea and Chlamydia

A careful sexual history dictates anatomic sites where screening should occur, including potentially pharyngeal, rectal, urethral for males and pharyngeal, rectal, vaginal for females.

Gonococcal and Chlamydial Urethritis: Males

1. Gram-negative intracellular diplococci on smear of urethral exudates:
   a. If positive, sufficient for diagnosis of gonorrhea
   b. Sensitivity and specificity of Gram stains for infected male urethra is 90% to 95% and 95% to 100%, respectively if symptomatic and 50% to 70% and 95% to 100% if asymptomatic.
2. If *Gram stain* result is negative or not done or urethral exudate not present, and *culture* is the only test available, obtain a specimen from anterior urethra:
   For gonorrhea and chlamydia:
   a. Gonorrhea: Use a sterile calcium alginate urethral swab inoculating a modified Thayer–Martin medium culture plate (chocolate [blood] agar), which has antibiotics added to suppress other organisms that "normally" colonize the sites. Chlamydia: use a Dacron swab to obtain samples and place in sucrose buffered media for transport.
   b. Cultures (for gonorrhea) obtained from other sites normally colonized by other organisms (i.e., rectum, pharynx, or endocervix) should be cultured on selective medium (Thayer–Martin) and/or for chlamydia-buffered transport media as well.
   c. Cultures obtained from sterile areas (i.e., blood, spinal fluid, or synovial fluid) can be plated onto nonselective, chocolate agar (gonorrhea).

d. For gonorrhea, organisms have to be inoculated directly on medium, transported in warm 36°C to 37°C environment with 5% to 10% carbon dioxide, while for chlamydia, the vial of transport media needs to be placed on ice for transportation.

e. Growth of oxidase-positive, gram-negative diplococci on selective media is sufficient evidence for a diagnosis of gonorrhea; samples of transport media need to be placed on tissue culture for growth, isolation, and identification of chlamydia.

f. Carbohydrate tests to discriminate types of Neisseria show that *N. gonorrhoeae* metabolizes only glucose; other Neisseria species metabolize other sugars (such as lactose, maltose, sucrose, and/or fructose). Culture sensitivity is 92.7% in symptomatic and 46.2% in asymptomatic men but 100% specific.[37] Using tissue culture to identify patients infected with chlamydia, especially with LGV, has a low rate of yield.

3. *Nucleic acid amplification tests (NAATs) available* for gonorrhea and chlamydia: *Abbott* real-time CT/NG; *Becton Dickinson* BD ProbeTec ET CT/GC (SDA); *Becton Dickinson* BD ProbeTecTM CT/GC QX amplified DNA assays; *Cepheid* CT/NG Xpert Rapid PCR Test; *Gen Probe* APTIMA COMBO 2 Assay (AC2); *Roche* COBAS CT/NG Test (PCR).[38]

a. Urine is the preferred sample type for testing or screening men using NAATs, especially if asymptomatic.

b. First-catch urine is recommended sample type and is equivalent to urethral swab.

c. Urethral swab specimens in some studies are less sensitive than urine, especially in asymptomatic populations; urethral swab specimens and male urine were equivalent in specificity.[39]

d. Point-of-care testing on urine samples for chlamydia and gonorrhea for males now allows results in <2 hours. When compared to two currently approved NAATs, point-of-care testing for chlamydia on male urine resulted in sensitivity of 97.5% and specificity ≥99.4% and for gonorrhea, sensitivity on male urine was 98.0% with specificity ≥99.4%.[40]

Gonococcal and Chlamydial Endocervicitis: Females

1. If *cultures* are the only tests available, they should be obtained from the endocervical canal and inoculated on Thayer–Martin medium to diagnose gonorrhea, and specific transport media for chlamydia:

a. Do not use a lubricant during the pelvic examination, as this may be toxic to the organisms.

b. Place a swab in the cervical os for 20 to 30 seconds and rotate. A single culture is 80% to 95% sensitive in detecting gonorrhea.

c. If anorectal sex has occurred, a separate swab can be used in the anal canal. Approximately 5% of females have positive culture from this site only. The swab can be inserted approximately 2 cm, avoiding fecal mass, and moved side to side for 20 to 30 seconds.

d. Gram stain smears from the endocervix for gonorrhea are not recommended. Such smears are only 50% to 70% sensitive in uncomplicated endocervical infection.

2. NAATs

a. Patient- or provider-collected vaginal swabs are equal or superior to endocervical swabs or urine when processed with NAATs for the detection of *C. trachomatis* and *N. gonorrhoeae* in women.

b. Vaginal swab specimens are as sensitive as cervical swab specimens and there is no difference in specificity. Cervical samples are acceptable when pelvic examinations are done, but vaginal swab specimens are preferred.[41,42]

c. Cervical sample specimens are acceptable for NAAT when combined with Pap in the same sample, such as liquid cytology. Some liquid cytology samples are more likely to result in inhibition of amplification or even contamination. One study of samples from 1838 subjects found the sensitivity and specificity of a Pap test method of screening for CT to be 94.1% and 99.8%, respectively, and for GC to be 95.3% and 99.95%, respectively, when compared to one of the NAATs, with similar results reported in both high- and low-risk populations.[43]

d. First-catch female urine, while acceptable, may have reduced performance and detect 10% fewer infections when compared to genital swab samples.[39]

e. Point-of-care testing on endocervical/vaginal/urine samples of women for gonorrhea and chlamydia allows results in <2 hours. When compared to two currently approved NAAT tests, sensitivities of 97.4% for endocervical, 98.7% for vaginal, and 97.6% for urine of women for chlamydia were obtained with specificity of ≥99.4%. For gonorrhea for women, the sensitivities for endocervical and vaginal samples were 100.00% and for urine 95.6%. Specificity for gonorrhea on all samples was ≥99.4%.[40]

Anorectal Gonorrhea and Chlamydia: Males and Females

1. *Culture*: Follow directions above if rectal cultures for gonorrhea are to be obtained.

2. NAATs: NAATs have superior performance to culture for the detection of rectal infections caused by *C. trachomatis* and *N. gonorrhoeae*. Due to "target selection" of the available assays, the sensitivity and specificity vary among NAATs when testing rectal and pharyngeal specimens for *C. trachomatis* and *N. gonorrhoeae*.

a. US Food and Drug Administration has not cleared NAATs for use for anorectal samples but laboratories can establish performance specifications to satisfy regulations for Clinical Laboratory Improvement Amendment (CLIA) compliance before reporting results for patient management. Currently, NAATs cannot differentiate non-LGV from LGV chlamydia.

b. *Studies*: In one study of 377 patients, test sensitivities for detection of gonorrhea ranged from 66.7% to 71.9% for culture to 100% for TMA (Transcription Mediated Amplification). Specificities were 99.7% to 100% for culture and greater than 95.5% for all three NAATs. Test sensitivities for chlamydia ranged from 36.1% to 45.7% for culture and among NAATs from 91.4% to 95.8% for PCR and 100% for TMA. Specificities of the NAATs ranged from 95.6% to 98.5% (two of three tests negative) and 88.8% to 91.8% (three of three tests were negative). In another study of 1,110 MSM, sensitivity of culture for rectal samples for gonorrhea was 43%, 78% for SDA (Strand Displacement Amplification), and 93% for AC2 (Aptima Combo2); performance for detecting rectal chlamydia included sensitivity of 27% for culture, 63% for SDA, and 93% for AC2. Specificities of SDA and AC2 were 99.4% for both organisms.[44–46]

In one study using 409 anorectal samples, the performance of the rapid test for chlamydia and gonorrhea was compared to another NAAT for test performance; sensitivity for chlamydia was 86% and specificity 99%, while for gonorrhea, 91.1% and 100%, respectively.[52]

Evaluations of self-obtained rectal swabs compared to provider obtained are comparable in sensitivity and specificity when using NAATs. NAATs are superior to culture for detection of chlamydia and gonorrhea in rectum.[46]

c. NAATS are more sensitive than culture for the detection of gonococal and chlamydial anorectal infections and are the recommended tests.[47]

3. *Gram stains*: Cultures may still be used for both gonorrhea and chlamydia but Gram stains for gonorrhea are not suitable as anal swabs are only 40% to 60% sensitive and 95% to 100% specific.

4. Recommendations: Anorectal gonorrhea and chlamydia infections are frequently asymptomatic and can be often present in

the absence of urethral gonorrhea or chlamydia, reinforcing the need to screen at the exposed anatomic sites. CDC recommends at least yearly screening for rectal gonorrhea and chlamydia for MSM who have had receptive anal intercourse during the preceding year.[48,49]

Gonococcal Pharyngitis: Males and Females

NAATs have superior performance to culture for the detection of pharyngeal infections caused by *C. trachomatis* and *N. gonorrhoeae*, but the sensitivity and specificity vary among NAATs when testing pharyngeal specimens. Pharyngeal specimens being assessed for *N. gonorrhoeae* should be tested using a NAAT that has been shown to be minimally affected by commensal *Neisseria* spp.[47]

1. CDC recommends at least yearly screening for pharyngeal gonorrhea for MSM who have participated in receptive oral intercourse during the preceding year.
2. CDC recommends screening at 3- to 6-month intervals for MSM who have multiple or anonymous partners, have sex in conjunction with illicit drug use, or have sex partners who participate in those activities.
3. Currently, CDC does not recommend routine screening for pharyngeal chlamydia, but two studies indicate that NAAT outperforms culture.[50]
4. As with anal infection, NAAT detection techniques may be used if a lab has a CLIA waiver; cultures may be used but Gram stains to diagnose pharyngeal gonorrhea are not appropriate.[45]
5. In one study of 1,110 MSM, sensitivity of culture for oropharyngeal GC was 41%, 72% for SDA, and 84% for AC2. PCR had poor specificity and thus was not included.[48–51]

Systemic Infection with Gonorrhea

1. Screen samples from the urethra, endocervix, pharynx, rectum, and/or conjunctiva.
2. Screen using cultures from skin lesions, synovial fluid, or blood.

◖ THERAPY

Recommendations for treatment of gonorrhea and chlamydia reflect that strains of *N. gonorrhoeae* resistant to traditional treatment are rising, that these two infections often coexist, and that serious complications can arise from both infections.

Resistance

Neisseria gonorrhoeae

In 1986, the Gonococcal Isolate Surveillance Project (GISP) was established to monitor trends in antimicrobial susceptibilities of strains of *N. gonorrhoeae* in the US. From 2006 to 2011 the percentage of isolates of *N. gonorrhoeae* with increasing minimal inhibitory concentration (MIC) ≥0.25 µg/mL to cefixime went from 0.1% to 1.5%.[53] The percentage with elevated ceftriaxone MICs (≥0.125 µg/mL) increased from 0.1% in 2006 to 0.3% to 0.4% in 2009 and remained stable through early 2012.[53]

From 1992 until early 2009, only 0.04% of samples had MICs ≥8 µg/mL for azithromycin, indicating reduced susceptibility. In later 2009, 5 of 55 (9.1%) *N. gonorrhoeae* isolates obtained from men with symptomatic urethritis tested in a West coast STI clinic had high azithromycin MICs: three with 8 µg/mL and two with 16 µg/mL.[54]

The prevalence of resistance remained high for penicillin (11.2% to 13.2%), tetracycline (16.7% to 22.8%), and ciprofloxacin (9.6% to 14.8%).[53] Certain epidemiologic characteristics (e.g., being an MSM or an intravenous drug user) are associated with increased risk for infection with relatively resistant *N. gonorrhoeae*, as these characteristics result in shared transmission within a limited population.[55]

These patterns in increasing resistance led to changes in recommendations to treatment for gonorrhea in 2012.[56]

Chlamydia trachomatis

Questions regarding azithromycin treatment failures with currently recommended regimens continue to be debated in the literature and surveillance for new variants of chlamydia discussed.[57,58]

Coinfection

1. Nationally representative sample of 18- to 26-year-olds: 0.3% of the population had both gonorrhea and chlamydia. For those with gonorrhea, 70% had chlamydia. For those with chlamydia, 7.9% had gonorrhea.[22]
2. In an STI clinic population, the prevalence of chlamydia in those with diagnosed or contact of gonorrhea was 20% for men and 42% for women. Among patients with gonorrhea, the chlamydia prevalence was higher among men younger than 25 years than older (27% versus 13%) and also among women younger than 25 years than older (54% versus 20%).[59]
3. Of youth in juvenile detention facilities with gonorrhea, 54% of females and 51% of males were coinfected with chlamydia.[60]
4. Another study of family-planning attendees indicated that approximately 40% of those with gonorrhea were also infected with chlamydia.[61]

Treatment Recommendations for *Neisseria gonorrhoeae* and *Chlamydia trachomatis*

1. Uncomplicated gonococcal infections of the cervix, urethra, and rectum
   a. Recommended regimen
      • **Ceftriaxone** 250 mg in a single intramuscular dose
      PLUS
      • **Azithromycin** 1 g orally in a single dose or **doxycycline** 100 mg orally twice daily for 7 days*
   b. Alternative regimens
      If ceftriaxone is not available:
      • **Cefixime** 400 mg in a single oral dose
      PLUS
      • **Azithromycin** 1 g orally in a single dose or **doxycycline** 100 mg orally twice daily for 7 days*
      PLUS
   c. Test-of-cure in 1 week
      If the patient has severe cephalosporin allergy:
      • **Azithromycin** 2 g in a single oral dose
      PLUS
   d. Test-of-cure in 1 week
      • Uncomplicated gonococcal infections of the pharynx
   e. Recommended regimen
      • **Ceftriaxone** 250 mg in a single intramuscular dose
      PLUS
      • **Azithromycin** 1 g orally in a single dose or **doxycycline** 100 mg orally twice daily for 7 days*

   *Because of the high prevalence of tetracycline resistance among GISP isolates, particularly those with elevated minimum inhibitory concentrations to cefixime, the use of azithromycin as the second antimicrobial is preferred.

2. Uncomplicated chlamydial infections of the cervix, urethra, and rectum
   a. Recommended regimen
      • **Azithromycin** 1 g orally in a single dose or
      • **Doxycycline** 100 mg orally twice a day for 7 days
   b. Alternative Regimens
      • **Erythromycin** base 500 mg orally four times a day for 7 days

- **Erythromycin ethylsuccinate** 800 mg orally four times a day for 7 days
- **Levofloxacin** 500 mg orally once daily for 7 days
- **Ofloxacin** 300 mg orally twice a day for 7 days[62]

3. Treatment and education of patient and of sex partners
   a. All AYAs exposed to gonorrhea and chlamydia should be examined, screened for infection, and treated presumptively, as should sex partner(s) of patients diagnosed with these infections.
   b. Treatment should be given for both chlamydia and gonorrhea if the diagnosis was gonorrhea and/or if chlamydia status unknown; if chlamydia was diagnosed, then treatment for that infection should occur.
   c. Teens and young adults should be instructed to avoid sexual intercourse until they and their partners are cured.
   d. No sexual intercourse for 7 days after one-dose treatment and no longer having symptoms

   OR

   e. No sexual intercourse until 7 days of therapy completed and no longer having symptoms.[62]
   f. Partner treatment, including expedited partner treatment (EPT)

      Sex partners of patients with *N. gonorrhoeae* and/or *C. trachomatis* infection whose last sexual contact with the patient was within 60 days before onset of symptoms or diagnosis of infection in the patient should be evaluated and treated for *N. gonorrhoeae* and *C. trachomatis* infections. If a patient's last sexual intercourse was >60 days before onset of symptoms or diagnosis, the patient's most recent sex partner should be treated. Patients should be instructed to abstain from sexual intercourse until therapy is completed and until they and their sex partners no longer have symptoms.

      For heterosexual patients with gonorrhea whose partners' treatment cannot be ensured or is unlikely, delivery of antibiotic therapy for gonorrhea and/or chlamydia by the patients to their partners can be considered. Use of this approach should always be accompanied by efforts to educate partners about symptoms and to encourage partners to seek clinical evaluation. For male patients informing female partners, educational materials should include information about the importance of seeking medical evaluation for PID (especially if symptomatic). Possible undertreatment of PID in female partners and possible missed opportunities to diagnose other STIs are of concern and have not been evaluated in comparison with patient-delivered therapy and partner referral. *This approach should not be considered a routine partner management strategy in MSM because of the high risk for coexisting undiagnosed STIs or HIV infection.*
      - EPT is permissible in 34 states.
      - EPT is potentially allowable in 10 other states, Puerto Rico, and DC.
      - EPT is prohibited in six states including Florida, Kentucky, Michigan, Ohio, Oklahoma, and West Virginia.
      - EPT is not routinely recommended for MSM as high risk for coexisting infections including HIV infection in partners.[63]

4. Follow-up: Routine follow-up cultures are not needed for persons treated for *uncomplicated* gonorrhea or chlamydia. Patients should be told to return for an examination if symptoms or signs persist after therapy. Clinicians should advise patients with gonorrhea and/or chlamydia to be retested 3 months after treatment. If patients do not seek medical care for retesting in 3 months, providers are encouraged to test these patients whenever they next seek medical care within the following 12 months, regardless of whether the patients believe that their sex partners were treated. Most treatment failures are due to reinfection either by untreated partner or exposure to new partner(s). Retesting is distinct from test-of-cure to detect therapeutic failure, which is not recommended.[62]

5. Pharyngeal gonococcal infection: Gonococcal infection of the pharynx may be more difficult to eradicate than urogenital and anorectal sites. Few regimens have consistent cure rates >90%.
   a. Recommended regimen
      - **Ceftriaxone** 250 mg IM in a single dose

      PLUS

      - **Azithromycin** 1 g PO in a single dose or **Doxycycline** 100 mg PO b.i.d. for 7 days
      - Cefixime or any other oral cephalosporin is not considered effective for pharyngeal infection.

   *Currently, there is no specific recommendation for treatment of chlamydial pharyngitis.

6. Treatment of uncomplicated gonorrhea and/or chlamydia in pregnant patients: Pregnant patients should be screened for gonorrhea, chlamydia, and syphilis at the first prenatal care visit, with tests repeated in the third trimester. Tetracyclines (i.e., doxycycline) and quinolones for chlamydia should be avoided during pregnancy. *N. gonorrhoeae* infection should be treated with the recommended cephalosporin ceftriaxone 250 mg IM and coverage for chlamydia with one of the regimens listed below. Treatment for chlamydia should include only one of the following regimens.
   a. Recommendations for chlamydial infections
      - Azithromycin 1 g orally, single dose or
      - Amoxicillin 500 mg orally three times daily for 7 days
   b. Alternative regimens for chlamydial infections
      - Erythromycin base 500 mg orally four times a day for 7 days or
      - Erythromycin base 250 mg orally four times a day for 14 days or
      - Erythromycin ethylsuccinate 800 mg orally four times a day for 7 days or
      - Erythromycin ethylsuccinate 400 mg orally four times a day for 14 days

Note: Erythromycin estolate is contraindicated during pregnancy because of drug-related hepatotoxicity.

7. Allergy, intolerance, and adverse reactions: Reactions to first-generation cephalosporins occur in approximately 5% to 10% of persons with a history of penicillin allergy and occur less frequently with third-generation cephalosporins. *In those persons with a history of penicillin allergy, the use of cephalosporins is contraindicated only in those with a history of a severe reaction to penicillin (e.g., anaphylaxis, Stevens–Johnson syndrome, and toxic epidermal necrolysis).*

   Because data are limited regarding alternative regimens for treating gonorrhea among persons who have severe cephalosporin allergy, providers treating such patients should consult infectious disease specialists. **Azithromycin 2 g** orally is effective against uncomplicated gonococcal infection.[62]

8. HIV infection: Teens and young adults infected with HIV and *N. gonorrhoeae* and/or *C. trachomatis* should receive the same treatment as those not infected with HIV.

9. Acute salpingitis: See Chapter 58 for discussion and treatment of PID.

10. Acute epididymitis (for either or if both infections suspected; see Chapter 54 for a more detailed discussion)
    a. Ceftriaxone 250 mg IM once

XIII

PLUS

b. Doxycycline 100 mg b.i.d. for 10 days

11. DGI: Hospitalization for intravenous treatment is recommended for initial therapy.

a. Recommended regimen
- Ceftriaxone 1 g IM or IV every 24 hours

b. Alternative regimens
- Cefotaxime 1 g IV every 8 hours or
- Ceftizoxime 1 g IV every 8 hours

*All of the preceding regimens should be continued for 24 to 48 hours after improvement begins, at which time therapy may be switched to the following oral regimens to complete at least 1 week of antimicrobial therapy.

- Cefixime 400 mg orally twice daily OR
- Cefixime suspension 500 mg twice daily orally (25 cc twice daily) OR
- Cefpodoxime 400 mg orally twice daily

**Persons treated for DGI should be treated presumptively for concurrent *C. trachomatis* infection.

***Patients should be instructed to refer their sex partners for evaluation and treatment.

12. Gonococcal meningitis and endocarditis: These serious complications require high-dose intravenous therapy with an antibiotic effective against the causative strain. The recommended initial regimen is 1 to 2 g of ceftriaxone IV every 12 hours. Although optimal duration is not known, most authorities treat gonococcal meningitis for 10 to 14 days and endocarditis for at least 4 weeks.

*Patients should be instructed to refer their sex partners for evaluation and treatment.

13. Gonococcal/Chlamydial conjunctivitis: For adolescents and children weighing >20 kg, the treatment includes ceftriaxone (1 g IM once), and eye irrigation with buffered ophthalmic solution should be performed once to help clear the discharge followed by careful eye examination, including slit-lamp examination. Simultaneous infection with *C. trachomatis* should be considered possible and simultaneous treatment for this infection should include:

a. Azithromycin (20 mg/kg once [maximum 1 g]) or
b. Erythromycin base (50 mg/kg/day [maximum 1,000 mg daily]) or ethylsuccinate (50 mg /kg/day [maximum 1,600 mg daily]), divided into 4 doses for 14 days

14. Dosing in adolescence: Adolescents who weigh <45 kg should be treated as follows:

a. For uncomplicated gonococcal and/or chlamydial vulvovaginitis, cervicitis, urethritis, pharyngitis, and proctitis
- Ceftriaxone 125 mg IM once

PLUS

- Azithromycin (20 mg/kg once [maximum 1 g]) *or*
- Erythromycin base (50 mg/kg per day [maximum 1,000 mg daily]) or ethylsuccinate (50 mg /kg per day [maximum 1,600 mg daily]), divided into 4 doses for 14 days

b. For bacteremia or arthritis secondary to gonorrhea
- Ceftriaxone (50 mg/kg as a single dose [maximum 1 g] IV/IM for 7 days)

c. For gonococcal meningitis
- Ceftriaxone (50 mg/kg as a single daily dose [maximum 2 g] IV/IM for 10 to 14 days)

* Adolescents weighing >45 kg should be treated with the adult doses, as already outlined.

**Adolescents with documented gonorrhea and/or chlamydia but "no history" of sexual activity should be carefully evaluated for sexual abuse.[62]

Prevention

Male Latex Condoms

Trends in condom use at last sex using most recent national data suggest a statistically nonsignificant increase at 20.8%.[64] Male latex condoms are effective in preventing the sexual transmission of HIV infection and can reduce the risk for other STIs (i.e., gonorrhea, chlamydia, and trichomonas). Studies that evaluate behaviors associated with condom use to protect from STIs must include *both reported consistent and correct use*.[65–67] For MSW, errors for condom use included not using one, not using a new one, contact with sharp objects, condoms drying and not staying on, and breakage and slippage during and after sex.[66,68] Breakage or slippage, nonuse, and partial use (delayed use or late application) were often described by HIV-negative MSM reporting anal sex within partnerships.[69]

Public Health Issues

1. High prevalence rates of gonorrhea and chlamydia in AYAs, particularly among minority youth, as compared with other age-groups
2. Large number of asymptomatic gonococcal and chlamydial infections in both AYA males and females
3. Large reservoirs of gonorrheal and chlamydial rectal and pharyngeal infections in MSM currently not being identified and appropriately treated, increasing risk of HIV transmission
4. Rapid emergence of antibiotic-resistant strains of gonorrhea and perhaps chlamydia
5. Lack of effective prevention strategies to control these infections.

REFERENCES

1. Sparling PF. Biology of *Neisseria gonorrhoeae*. In: Holmes K, Sparling P, Stamm W, et al., eds. *Sexually transmitted diseases*. 4th ed. New York, NY: The McGraw-Hill Co. 2008: 607–626.
2. Schachter J, Stephens RS. Biology of *Chlamydia trachomatis*. In: Holmes K, Sparling P, Stamm W, et al., eds. *Sexually transmitted diseases*. 4th ed. New York, NY: The McGraw-Hill Co. 2008: 555–574.
3. Centers for Disease Control and Prevention. *STD surveillance 2013*. Available at http://www.cdc.gov/std/stats13/default.htm. Accessed January 15, 2015.
4. Centers for Disease Control and Prevention. *STD surveillance 2013*. Available at http://www.cdc.gov/std/stats13/surv2013-print.pdf. Accessed January 18, 2015.
5. Centers for Disease Control and Prevention. *STD surveillance 2013*. Available at http://www.cdc.gov/std/stats13/surv2013-print.pdf. Accessed February 04, 2015.
6. Centers for disease Control and Prevention. *STD surveillance 2013*. Available at http://www.cdc.gov/std/stats13/tables/13.htm. Accessed February 04, 2015.
7. Centers for disease Control and Prevention. *STD Surveillance 2013*. Available at http://www.cdc.gov/std/stats13/tables/1.htm. Accessed February 04, 2015.
8. Centers for Disease Control and Prevention. *STD Surveillance 2013*. Available at http://www.cdc.gov/std/stats13/chlamydia.htm. Accessed February 04, 2015.
9. Centers for Disease Control and Prevention. *STD surveillance 2013*. Available at http://www.cdc.gov/std/stats13/tables/11b.htm. Accessed February 04, 2015.
10. United States Preventive Tasks Force. *Screening for chlamydial infection*. June 2013. Available at http://www.uspreventiveservicestaskforce.org/uspstf/uspschlm.htm#update. Accessed January 13, 2014.
11. Centers for Disease Control and Prevention. Division of STD Prevention. *Male Chlamydia screening consultation*. Atlanta, Georgia. March 28–29, 2006. Meeting Report 2007. Available at http://www.cdc.gov/std/chlamydia/chlamydiascreening-males.pdf. Accessed January 13, 2014.
12. Centers for Disease Control and Prevention. *STD Surveillance 2013*. Available at http://www.cdc.gov/std/stats12/tables/2.htm; http://www.cdc.gov/std/stats12/tables/6.htm. Accessed February 17, 2014.
13. Van Liere G, Hoeve CJPA, Dukers-Muijrers NHTM. Evaluation of the anatomical site distribution of *Chlamydia* and *Gonorrhoea* in men who have sex with men and in high risk women by routine testing: cross-sectional study revealing missed opportunities for treatment strategies. *Sex Transm Infect* 2014;90(1):58–60. doi: 10.1136/sextrans-2013-051248.
14. Marcus JL, Kohn RP, Barry PM, et al. *Chlamydia trachomatis* and *Neisseria gonorrhoeae* transmission from the female oropharynx to the male urethra. *Sex Transm Dis* 2011;38:372–373.
15. Centers for Disease Prevention. *Grand Rounds*. Available at http://www.cdc.gov/mmwr/preview/mmwrhtml/mm6012a2.htm#fig1. Accessed February 17, 2014.
16. Forhan SE. Prevalence of sexually transmitted infections among female adolescents aged 14 to 19 in the United States. *Pediatrics* 2009;124:1505–1512.
17. Torrone EA. Prevalence of *Neisseria gonorrhoeae* among persons 14–39 years of age, United States, 1999–2008. *Sex Transm Dis* 2013;40:202–205.
18. Miller WC, Ford CA, Morris M, et al. Prevalence of chlamydial and gonococcal infections among young adults in the united states. *JAMA* 2004;291:2229–2236.
19. Marcus JL, Bernstein KT, Kohn RP, et al. Infections missed by urethral only screening for *Chlamydia* or *Gonorrhea* detection among men who have sex with men. *Sex Transm Dis* 2011;38:922–924.

20. Park J, Marcus JL, Pandori M, et al. Sentinel surveillance for pharyngeal *Chlamydia* and *Gonorrhea* among men who have sex with men—San Francisco 2010. *Sex Transm Dis* 2012;39:482–484.
21. Kent CK, Chaw JK, Wong W, et al. Prevalence of rectal, urethral, and pharyngeal *Chlamydia* and *Gonorrhea* detected in 2 clinical settings among men who have sex with men: San Francisco, California, 2003. *Clin Infect Dis* 2005;41:67–74.
22. Schachter J, Philip SS. Testing men who have sex with men for urethral infection with *Chlamydia trachomatis* and *Neisseria gonorrhoeae* is only half the job, and we need the right tools. *Sex Transm Dis* 2011;38:925–927.
23. Centers for Disease Control and Prevention. *STD surveillance 2011*. Available at http://www.cdc.gov/STD/stats11/Surv2011.pdf. Accessed January 13, 2014.
24. Centers for Disease Control and Prevention. *STD surveillance 2011*. Available at http://www.cdc.gov/std/stats11/gonorrhea.htm; http://www.cdc.gov/STD/stats11/Surv2011.pdf. Accessed January 13, 2014.
25. Centers for Disease Control and Prevention. *STD Surveillance 2011*. Available at http://www.cdc.gov/std/chlamydia2011/national-figB.htm; http://www.cdc.gov/std/chlamydia2011/statesB.htm; http://www.cdc.gov/std/stats11/gonorrhea.htm. Accessed January 14, 2014.
26. Centers for Disease Control and Prevention. *STD Surveillance 2011*. Available at http://www.cdc.gov/std/stats11/adol.htm. Accessed January 14, 2014.
27. Goyal M, Hayes K, Mollern C. Sexually transmitted infection prevalence in symptomatic adolescent emergency department patients. *Pediatr Emerg Care* 2012;28:1277–1280.
28. Gaydos CA, Barnes M, Aumakhan B, et al. Can E-techonology through the internet be used as a new tool to address the *Chlamydia trachomatis* epidemic by home sampling and vaginal swabs? *Sex Transm Dis* 2009;36;577–580.
29. Chai SJ, Aumakhan B, Barnes M, et al. Internet-based screening for sexually transmitted infections to reach nonclinic populations in the community: risk factors for infection in men. *Sex Transm Dis* 2010;37:756–763.
30. Hengel B, Jamil MS, Mein JK, et al. Outreach for *Chlamydia* and *Gonorrhea* screening: a systematic review of strategies and outcomes. *BMC Public Health* 2013;13:1040.
31. Odesanmi TY, Wasti SP, Odesanmi OS, et al. Comparative effectiveness and acceptability of home-based and clinic-based sampling methods for sexually transmissible infections screening in females aged 14–50 years: a systematic review and meta-analysis. *Sex Health* 2013;10:559–569.
32. National Committee on Quality Assurance. Available at http://www.ncqa.org/tabid/136/default.aspx. Accessed January 13, 2014.
33. Stamm W. *Chlamydia trachomatis* infections of the adult. In: Holmes K, Sparling P, Stamm W, et al., eds. *Sexually transmitted diseases*. 4th ed. NewYork, NY: The McGraw-Hill Co, 2008:575–593.
34. Hook E, Handsfield HH. Gonococcocal infections in the adult. In: Holmes K, Sparling P, Stamm W, et al., eds. *Sexually transmitted diseases*. 4th ed. NewYork, NY The McGraw-Hill Co, 2008:627–645.
35. Paavonen J, Westrom L, Eschenback D. Pelvic inflammatory disease. In: Holmes K, Sparling P, Stamm W, et al., eds. *Sexually transmitted diseases*. 4th ed. NewYork, NY The McGraw-Hill Co, 2008:1017–1050.
36. Lynn W, Lightman S. Ocular infections associated with sexually transmitted diseases and HIV/AIDS. In: Holmes K, Sparling P, Stamm W, et al., eds. *Sexually transmitted diseases*. 4th ed. NewYork, NY: The McGraw-Hill Co, 2008:1227–1244.
37. Martin DH, Cammarata C, Van Der Pol B, et al. Multicenter evaluation of Amplicor and automated Cobas Amplicor CT/NG tests for *Neisseria gonorrhoeae*. *J Clin Microbiol* 2000;38:3544–3549.
38. Centers for Disease Control and Prevention. *Recommendations for the laboratory-based detection of Chlamydia trachomatis and Neisseria gonorrhoeae—2014*. Available at http://www.cdc.gov/mmwr/preview/mmwrhtml/rr6302a1.htm. Accessed April 28, 2014.
39. Centers for Disease Control and Prevention. *Expert Consultation Meeting, 2009. Recommendations for the laboratory-based detection of Chlamydia trachomatis and Neisseria gonorrhoeae-2014*. Available at http://www.cdc.gov/mmwr/preview/mmwrhtml/rr6302a1.htm. Accessed April 28, 2014.
40. Gaydos CA, Van Der Pol B, Jett-Goheen M, et al; Hook EW III; CT/NG Study Group. Performance of the Cepheid CT/NG Xpert Rapid PCR test for detection of *Chlamydia trachomatis* and *Neisseria gonorrhoeae*. *J Clin Microbiol* 2013;51:1666–1672.
41. Schachter J, McCormack WM, Chernesky MA, et al. Vaginal swabs are appropriate specimens for diagnosis of genital tract infection with *Chlamydia trachomatis*. *J Clin Microbiol* 2003;41:3784–3789.
42. Cosentino LA, Landers DV, Hillier SL. Detection of *Chlamydia trachomatis* and *Neisseria gonorrhoeae* by strand displacement amplification and relevance of the amplification control for use with vaginal swab specimens. *J Clin Microbiol* 2003;41:3592–3596.
43. Martens MG, Fine P, Fuller D, et al. Clinical evaluation of a new pap test-based method for screening of *Chlamydia trachomatis* and *Neisseria gonorrhoeae* using liquid based cytology media. *Southern Med J* 2013;106:506–512.
44. Bachmann LH, Johnson Re, Cheng H, et al. Nucleic acid amplification tests for diagnosis of *Chlamydia trachomatis* and *Chlamydia trachomatis* rectal infections. *J Clin Microbiol* 2010;48:1827–1832.
45. Association of Public Health Laboratories. *Expert consultation meeting summary report: laboratory diagnositc testing for Chlamydia trachomatis and Neisseria gonorrhoeae* [APHL web site]. Atlanta, GA: APHL, 2009. Available at http://www.aphl.org/aphlprograms/infectious/std/Documents/ID_2009Jan_CTGCLab-Guidelines Meeting-Report.pdf.
46. Moncada J, Schachter J, Liska S, et al. Evaluation of self-collected glans and rectal swabs from men who have sex with men for detection of *Chlamydia trachomatis* and *Neisseria gonorrhoeae* by use of nucleic acid amplification test. *J Clin Microbiol* 2009;47:1657–1662.
47. Centers for Disease Control and Prevention. *Recommendations for the laboratory-based detection of Chlamydia trachomatis and Neisseria gonorrhoeae—2014*. Available at http://www.cdc.gov/mmwr/preview/mmwrhtml/rr6302a1.htm. Accessed April 28, 2014.
48. Centers for Disease Control and Prevention. 2009. Available at http://www.cdc.gov/mmwr/preview/mmwrhtml/mm5826a2.htm.
49. Centers for Disease Control and Prevention. 2006. Available at http://www.cdc.gov/mmwr/preview/mmwrhtml/rr5511a1.htm. Accessed April 28, 2014.
50. Schachter J, Moncada J, Liska S, et al. Nucleic acid amplification tests in the diagnosis of chlamydia and gonococcal infections of the oropharynx and rectum in men who have sex with men. *Sex Transm Dis* 2008;35:637–642.
51. Bachmann LH, Johnson Re, Cheng H, et al. Nucleic acid amplification tests for diagnosis of *Neisseria gonorrhoeae* and *Chlamydia trachomatis* pharyngeal infections. *J Clin Microbiol* 2009;47:902–907.
52. Goldenberg SD, Finn J, Seduzi E, et al. Performance of the GeneXpert CT/NG assay compared to that of the Aptima AC2 assay for detection of *Chlamydia trachomatis* and *Neisseria gonorrhoeae* by use of residual Aptima samples. *J Clin Microbiol* 2012;50:3867–3869.
53. Centers for Disease Control and Prevention. *Neisseria gonorrhoeae* with reduced susceptibility to Azithromycin—San Diego County, California, 2009. *MMWR* 2011;60(18):579–581. Available at http://www.cdc.gov/mmwr/preview/mmwrhtml/mm6018a2.htm?s_cid=mm6018a2_w. Accessed January 13, 2014.
54. Kirkcaldy RD, Kidd S, Weinstock HS, et al. Trends in antimicrobial resistance in *Neisseria gonorrhoeae* in the USA: the gonococcal isolate surveillance project (GISP), January 2006–June 2012. *Sex Transm Infect* 2013;89:iv5–iv10.
55. Hook E, Van der Pol B. Evolving gonococal antimicrobial resistance: research priorities and implications for management. *Sex Transm Infect* 2013;89:iv60–iv62.
56. Centers for Disease Control and Prevention. Update to CDC's *sexually transmitted diseases treatment guidelines, 2010*: oral cephalosporins no longer a recommended treatment for gonococcal infections. *MMWR* 2012;61(31):590–594. Available at http://www.cdc.gov/mmwr/preview/mmwrhtml/mm6131a3.htm?s_cid=mm6131a3_w#tab. Accessed January 13, 2014.
57. Horner H, Ramachandran P, Steece R, et al. Is there evidence of the new variant *Chlamydia trachomatis* in the United States? *Sex Transm Dis* 2013;40:352–353.
58. Won H, Ramachandran P, Steece R, et al. Is there evidence of the new variant *Chlamydia trachomatis* in the United States? *Sex Transm Dis* 2013;40:352–353.
59. Lyss SB, Kamb ML, Peterman TA, et al. *Chlamydia trachomatis* among patients infected with and treated for *Neisseria gonorrhoeae* in sexually transmitted disease clinics in the United States. *Ann Intern Med* 2003;139:178–185.
60. Kahn RH, Mosure DJ, Blank S, et al. Jail STD prevalence monitoring project. *Chlamydia trachomatis* and *Neisseria gonorrhoeae* prevalence and coinfection in adolescents entering selected US juvenile detention centers, 1997–2002. *Sex Transm Dis* 2005;32:255–259.
61. Einwalter LA, Ritchie JM, Ault KA, et al. *Gonorrhea* and *Chlamydia* infection among women visiting family planning clinics: racial variation in prevalence and predictors. *Perspect Sex Reprod Health* 2005;37:135–140.
62. Workowski KA, Bolan GA. Sexually transmitted diseases treatment guidelines, 2015. *MMWR Recomm Rep* 2015;64(RR-3):1–113. Available at http://www.cdc.gov/std/tg2015/default.htm. Accessed July 25, 2015.
63. Centers for Disease Control and Prevention. *Expedited partner treatment. 2013.* Available at http://www.cdc.gov/std/ept/default.htm. Accessed January 13, 2014.
64. Anderson JE, Warner L, Maurizio M. Condom use among adults at last sexual intercourse, 1996–2008: an update from national survey data. *Sex Transm Dis* 2011;38:919–921.
65. Holmes KK, Levine R, Weaver M. Effectiveness of condoms in preventing sexually transmitted infections. *Bull World Health Organ* 2004;82:454–461.
66. Crosby R, Shrier LA, Charnigao RJ, et al. A prospective event-level analysis of condom use experiences following STI testing among patients in three US cities. *Sex Transm Dis* 2012;39:756–760.
67. Crosby R, Charnigao RJ, Weathers C, et al. Condom effectiveness against non-viral sexually transmitted infections: a prospective study using electronic diaries. *Sex Transm Infect* 2012;88:484–489.
68. D'Anna LH, Korosteleva L, Warner L, et al. The Respect Group. Factors associated with codom use problems during vaginal sex with main and nonmanin partners. *Sex Transm Dis* 2012;39:687–693.
69. D'Anna LH, Margolis AD, Warner L, et al. Condom use problems during anal sex among men who have sex with men (msm): findings from the Safe in the City study. *AIDS Care* 2012;24:1028–1038.

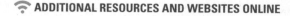 **ADDITIONAL RESOURCES AND WEBSITES ONLINE**

58

Pelvic Inflammatory Disease

Lydia A. Shrier

DEFINITION

Pelvic inflammatory disease (PID) is an ascending polymicrobial infection of the female upper genital tract and includes endometritis, parametritis, salpingitis, oophoritis, tuboovarian abscess (TOA), peritonitis, and perihepatitis.

ETIOLOGY

Risk Factors

1. Age: Adolescent and young adult (AYA) women account for up to one-third of cases of PID; the peak incidence is among 20- to 24-year-olds.[1]
   a. Cervical ectropion: The erythematous ring around the cervical os, commonly seen in adolescents, is the transitional zone between the columnar and squamous epithelium and is highly susceptible to sexually transmitted infections (STIs).
   b. Cervicitis with *Neisseria gonorrhoeae* or *Chlamydia trachomatis*: Among women with gonococcal or chlamydial cervicitis, approximately 10% to 20% develop PID, with higher rates being reported among high-risk adolescents.[2]
   c. Sexual and other health-risk behaviors: AYAs who frequently engage frequently engage in behaviors associated with increased rates of STIs and PID, including unprotected and/or frequent intercourse, multiple sex partners, intercourse during menses, smoking, alcohol, and other drug use.[3]
   d. Age at first intercourse: Risk for PID is more common among women who had coitarche before the age of 15 or 16 years.[3]
2. Previous PID: A history of previous PID increases the risk of subsequent PID.[3,4]
3. Race: Black AYAs have an increased risk of PID compared to non-Black AYAs.[3,5]
4. Contraceptive methods
   a. Condoms: Inconsistent use is associated with two to three times the risk of PID.[6]
   b. Oral contraceptives: Associated with increased risk of infection with chlamydia, and possibly gonorrhea,[7] but not with risk of PID.[6]
   c. Medroxyprogesterone acetate: May reduce the risk of PID,[3] although the association has not been consistently observed.[6]
   d. Intrauterine device (IUD): The risk of PID following insertion of the current generation of IUDs is low, even in the presence of cervicitis,[8] and generally restricted to the first 3 weeks after insertion.
5. Bacterial vaginosis (BV): May facilitate ascension of organisms pathogenic for PID to the upper genital tract. Anaerobic bacteria associated with BV have been found in the upper genital tract of women with acute PID,[9] but longitudinal studies have not consistently supported an association between BV and subsequent PID.[10,11]
6. Menses: May be associated with increased risk of ascending infection because of cervical mucus plug loss, endometrial shedding, menstrual blood (a good culture medium), and/or myometrial contractions, resulting in reflux of blood into the fallopian tubes.

Microbiology

PID is a polymicrobial infection. *N. gonorrhoeae* and *C. trachomatis* have been identified in the lower or upper genital tract in up to two-thirds of PID cases[12]; adolescents with PID are more likely than adults to be infected with these organisms.[13] PID also involves genital mycoplasmas, and aerobic and anaerobic bacteria comprising endogenous vaginal flora.

1. *N. gonorrhoeae:* Found in the upper and/or lower genital tract of 11% to 33% of women with PID[9,14–16] and associated with a dramatic presentation.[17]
2. *C. trachomatis:* Recovered from the upper and/or lower genital tract in up to 44% of women with PID.[9,14–16] Chlamydial PID presents more subtly than gonococcal PID, which may delay care, contributing to worse reproductive health outcomes.[18]
3. Genital mycoplasmas (*Mycoplasma genitalium, Mycoplasma hominis, Ureaplasma urealyticum*): M. genitalium has been found in the upper and/or lower genital tract of 7% to 14% of women with nongonococcal, nonchlamydial PID[14,19] and may be more common among women <25 years of age.[20]
4. *Bacteroides* species and other anaerobes: More than 60% of women with PID have evidence of upper tract infection with anaerobic organisms.[21]
5. Other endogenous vaginal flora (*Escherichia coli, Haemophilus influenzae, Streptococcus* species, and other facultative bacteria).

Pathogenesis

1. Following lower tract infection, commonly with *N. gonorrhoeae* or *C. trachomatis,* anaerobes, facultative bacteria, and genital mycoplasmas supplant vaginal lactobacilli.
2. Inflammatory disruption of the cervical barrier facilitates ascension of the inciting pathogens and other microorganisms from the vagina into the normally sterile uterus.
3. Decreased tubal motility secondary to inflammation results in collection of fluid (hydrosalpinx) or pus (pyosalpinx) within the tube.
4. Spillage of infected contents from the tubes into the peritoneal cavity may result in the following:
   a. Peritonitis
   b. Perihepatitis (Fitz-Hugh–Curtis syndrome): Infected material tracks along the paracolic gutter. Inflammation of the hepatic capsule and diaphragm causes right upper quadrant pain and referred right subscapular pain. Perihepatitis is relatively uncommon in adolescents with PID (4%[22] to 7%[16]).
   c. TOA: Develops if resolution of upper tract infection is delayed or if previous tubal scarring occludes the tube. The abscess can form in the tube or between the tube and ovary. TOA may be found in 26% of hospitalized adolescents,[23] but rates may be much lower among adolescents treated as outpatients.[24] Incidence of TOA in young adult women with PID has not been reported separately from that in older women.
   d. Adhesions: Scar tissue in the tube, between the tube and ovary, or in the peritoneal cavity leads to infertility, ectopic pregnancy, and chronic abdominal or pelvic pain.

⬤ PRESENTING SIGNS AND SYMPTOMS

The classic presentation—lower abdominal or pelvic pain, abnormal vaginal and/or cervical discharge, fever and chills, leukocytosis, and increased erythrocyte sedimentation rate (ESR)—is seen in only approximately one in five laparoscopically verified cases of PID. Subclinical infection likely accounts for most cases.

1. Pelvic or abdominal pain: Constant, cramping, exacerbated by walking and intercourse.
2. Abnormal vaginal bleeding: Approximately one-third to one-half of AYAs with PID report painful irregular, prolonged, and/or heavy vaginal bleeding.[17]
3. Abnormal vaginal discharge: Reported by more than 50% of AYAs with PID.[17,24]
4. Gastrointestinal symptoms: An ileus may result in anorexia, nausea, or vomiting.

Other history, signs, and symptoms consistent with PID include dysuria or urinary frequency, symptom onset within 1 week of menses, and a sexual partner with recent urethritis.

Findings on Physical Examination

1. Vital signs: Only 1 in 6 to 1 in 7 women with PID present with fever,[12] likely due to the increasing proportion infected with *C. trachomatis* and *M. genitalium*, particularly young women.[16,17] Tachycardia secondary to pain and fever is common.
2. Abdomen: Lower abdominal tenderness, with or without rebound and guarding
3. Pelvic examination
   a. Abnormal vaginal or cervical discharge
   b. Friable, inflamed cervix
   c. Cervical motion tenderness (present in >80% of patients with PID)
   d. Adnexal tenderness (unilateral or bilateral)
   e. Palpation of an adnexal mass (5% to 60%), may be unilateral or bilateral
   f. Uterine tenderness (common)

Laboratory and Radiologic Evaluation

No single test is diagnostic of PID. The following tests should be considered in the evaluation:

1. White blood cell (WBC) count: Elevated in 30% to 67% of patients with PID, but may be normal in mild to moderate PID.[17] WBC count is generally elevated with perihepatitis,[22] but is often normal with a TOA.
2. ESR and/or C-reactive protein (CRP): Elevated ESR and CRP levels are common in women with PID and predict the presence of TOA,[25] but they may be normal in mild to moderate disease. Elevated CRP correlates with disease severity.[26]
3. Saline wet mount of vaginal secretions: Leukocytes in vaginal secretions may support the diagnosis. BV is present in most women with PID,[12,17] and its diagnosis warrants the inclusion of anaerobic coverage in the treatment. It is also important to evaluate for concurrent vaginitis (e.g., from *Trichomonas vaginalis*).
4. Microbiologic tests: Presumptive diagnosis and treatment of PID should not await microbiologic test results. Positive results support but do not confirm, and negative results do not eliminate the diagnosis of PID.
   a. Specimens should be collected before initiating antibiotic therapy.
   b. Endocervical specimens should be evaluated using nucleic acid amplification tests (NAATs) for *N. gonorrhoeae* and *C. trachomatis,* but not for organisms that normally colonize the vagina.
5. Urinalysis and urine culture: For possible urinary tract infection/pyelonephritis.
6. Urine pregnancy test: If positive, an ectopic pregnancy must be considered, but a positive pregnancy test does not exclude the diagnosis of PID.
7. HIV testing
8. Syphilis testing: In women with signs or symptoms of syphilis or particularly high risk.
9. Pelvic ultrasonography: Used if the clinician cannot adequately assess the adnexa, palpates an adnexal mass, or questions the presence of an ectopic pregnancy or TOA.
10. Laparoscopy: Indicated diagnostically in the patient who does not respond to antibiotic therapy and therapeutically in the patient with a persistent TOA.

⬤ DIAGNOSIS

Timely and accurate diagnosis of PID is essential to preventing sequelae. The positive predictive value of a clinical diagnosis of PID, using laparoscopic diagnosis as the gold standard, ranges from 65% to 90%. Because missing the diagnosis of PID exposes the patient to risk of complications and sequelae, the minimum criteria required to make the diagnosis of PID are by intent sensitive, but not specific. Thus, it is important to consider the entire clinical picture, evaluate alternative diagnoses carefully, and examine additional criteria to avoid the consequences of misdiagnosing PID, including delay of appropriate treatment, unnecessary antibiotics, psychological stigma, clinician bias toward making future diagnoses of PID, and financial burden. The differential diagnosis is broad (Table 58.1).

Empirical treatment should be initiated in sexually active young women with pelvic or lower abdominal pain if any of the minimum criteria is present and no other cause(s) for the illness can be identified (Table 58.2). Additional criteria enhance diagnostic specificity, but are not required to make the diagnosis. The clinician must have a high index of suspicion for PID in young women.

⬤ THERAPY

PID requires treatment with broad-spectrum antibiotics. At a minimum, treatment regimens should include coverage for

---

TABLE 58.1

Differential Diagnosis of PID

Gastrointestinal	Gynecological
Appendicitis	Corpus luteum cyst
Cholecystitis	Dysmenorrhea
Cholelithiasis	Ectopic pregnancy
Constipation	Endometriosis
Diverticulitis	Mittelschmerz
Gastroenteritis	Ovarian
Hernia	Cyst
Inflammatory bowel disease	Torsion
Irritable bowel syndrome	Tumor
Urological	Pregnancy
Cystitis	Ectopic
Nephrolithiasis	Spontaneous, septic, *or*
Pyelonephritis	threatened abortion
Urethritis	Postabortion endometritis
Musculoskeletal	Rheumatologic/autoimmune
	Psychiatric

TABLE 58.2

CDC Diagnostic Criteria for PID

Minimum criteria (initiate treatment in sexually active women under the age of 26 complaining of lower abdominal or pelvic pain when one or more clinical signs are present and no other diagnosis is apparent)
    Cervical motion tenderness, *or*
    Uterine tenderness, *or*
    Adnexal tenderness

Additional criteria (support a diagnosis of PID)
    Oral temperature >101°F (>38.3°C)
    Abnormal cervical or vaginal mucopurulent discharge
    Presence of abundant numbers of WBCs on saline microscopy of vaginal secretions
    Elevated ESR
    Elevated CRP level
    Laboratory documentation of cervical infection with *N. gonorrhoeae* or *C. trachomatis*

Definitive criteria (warranted in selected cases)
    Endometrial biopsy with histopathologic evidence of endometritis
    Transvaginal sonography or magnetic resonance imaging techniques showing thickened, fluid-filled tubes with or without free pelvic fluid or tuboovarian complex, or Doppler studies suggesting pelvic infection (e.g., tubal hyperemia)
    Laparoscopic abnormalities consistent with PID

TABLE 58.3

CDC-Recommended Parenteral Antibiotic Regimens for PID

Cefotetan 2 g IV every 12 h *or* cefoxitin 2 g IV every 6 h
plus doxycycline 100 mg PO or IV every 12 h *or*
Clindamycin 900 mg IV every 8 h
plus gentamicin loading dose IV or IM (2 mg/kg of body weight), followed by a maintenance dose (1.5 mg/kg) every 8 h (single daily dosing 3–5 mg/kg may be substituted)
Alternative: Ampicillin/sulbactam 3 g IV every 6 h *plus* doxycycline 100 mg PO *or* IV every 12 h
Parenteral therapy can be discontinued 24 h after clinical improvement. Therapy should be continued with doxycycline 100 mg PO twice a day *or* clindamycin 450 mg PO four times a day to complete a total of 14 d of therapy.

TABLE 58.4

CDC-Recommended Intramuscular/Oral Regimens

Ceftriaxone 250 mg IM in a single dose or cefoxitin 2 g IM and probenecid 1 g PO concurrently in a single dose *or* another parenteral third-generation cephalosporin
plus doxycycline 100 mg PO twice a day for 14 d
with or without metronidazole 500 mg PO twice a day for 14 d

---

infection with *N. gonorrhoeae* and *C. trachomatis*, regardless of the test results. Many experts also recommend coverage of anaerobes (**Tables 58.3** and **58.4**).[21]

Centers for Disease Control and Prevention (CDC) criteria for hospitalization of women with suspected PID are as follows[27]:

1. Surgical emergencies such as appendicitis cannot be excluded.
2. Pregnancy
3. Poor response to oral antimicrobial therapy
4. Inability to follow or tolerate an outpatient oral regimen
5. Severe illness, nausea and vomiting, or high fever
6. TOA

Other reasons to consider hospitalization in AYAs with suspected PID include age <15 years, abortion/other gynecologic surgery within previous 14 days, a previous PID episode, immunodeficiency, and extenuating medical or social circumstances that may preclude appropriate outpatient treatment. Among both younger and older women with mild to moderate PID, reproductive outcomes do not differ between inpatient and outpatient treatment.[12,13]

Regardless of treatment setting, the following recommendations should be considered:

1. Patients should be educated about the importance of completing a full 14-day course of antibiotics. The duration of treatment does not depend on the result of any laboratory test.
2. All sex partners within the preceding 60 days require treatment for *C. trachomatis* and *N. gonorrhoeae* infections, regardless of patient or partner microbiologic test results.
3. Nonsteroidal anti-inflammatory drugs are recommended for abdominal pain or cramping.
4. Single-dose azithromycin (used for chlamydial cervicitis or urethritis) has not been effective for PID treatment. There has been promising research on multidose regimens, but at present evidence is insufficient to routinely recommend azithromycin for PID.
5. IUDs do not need to be removed in women with acute PID.[27]
6. Patients and their partners should be advised to abstain from sexual intercourse until they have completed treatment and their symptoms have resolved.

Patients who do not improve within 72 hours require further evaluation, parenteral antibiotic therapy, and/or surgical intervention.[27] If a parenteral regimen is used:

1. Intravenous doxycycline should be avoided because of pain and venous sclerosis.
2. Cephalosporins other than cefotetan or cefoxitin are less active against anaerobes and are not recommended.[27]
3. Parenteral therapy may be discontinued 24 hours after clinical improvement. Therapy should continue with doxycycline orally to complete 14 days of therapy. When treating severe PID, including TOA, adding clindamycin or metronidazole to continued therapy with doxycycline is recommended to optimize anaerobic coverage.[21,27]

If the baseline *C. trachomatis* and/or *N. gonorrhoeae* tests are positive, repeated screening for reinfection is recommended 3 to 6 months after the completion of therapy.[27]

SEQUELAE

Adolescent and adult women do not differ in risk for adverse outcomes following PID.[13] However, adolescents treated for PID are more likely to have subsequent STIs and shorter time to recurrent PID and pregnancy,[13] and warrant particularly close follow-up.

1. Recurrence: Reported rates vary widely, but at least one in five women with PID will experience another episode.[4] Risk is inversely correlated with treatment of contacts.
2. Infertility: PID is the most common cause of tubal factor infertility. Risk of infertility following one episode is as high as 18% among women with mild to moderate PID.[12] Risk of infertility is higher with severe PID[28] and with recurrence (risk almost doubles with each successive episode).[4] While it is important to counsel an adolescent about the risk of infertility from PID, if the risk of possible infertility is overemphasized, the adolescent may assume that she is unable to conceive and not use effective contraception.
3. Ectopic pregnancy: One episode of PID may increase risk of ectopic pregnancy 6- to 10-fold,[28] although there may not be increased risk with mild to moderate disease.[12]
4. Chronic pelvic pain: More than 40% of women with mild to moderate PID experience subsequent chronic pelvic pain.[13] Women with recurrent PID have more than four times the risk of chronic pelvic pain, compared to women with a single episode.[4]

PREVENTION

1. Primary prevention involves education about STI prevention and annual screening for *C. trachomatis* and *N. gonorrhoeae* in all sexually active women under the age of 25.[27]
2. Secondary prevention focuses on preventing or ameliorating complications and sequelae among AYAs who have been diagnosed with PID, and should include partner counseling and treatment.
3. Tertiary prevention helps to decrease the risk of morbidity following an episode of PID.
   a. Consistent condom use reduces the risk of recurrent PID and infertility by 50% and 60%, respectively.[29]
   b. Optimizing screening for subsequent STIs is important in preventing PID sequelae, especially chronic pelvic pain.[4,13]

REFERENCES

1. Grodstein F, Rothman KJ. Epidemiology of pelvic inflammatory disease. *Epidemiology* 1994;5:234–242.
2. Risser WL, Risser JM, Benjamins LJ. Pelvic inflammatory disease in adolescents between the time of testing and treatment and after treatment for gonorrheal and chlamydial infection. *Int J STD AIDS* 2012;23:457–458.
3. Ness RB, Smith KJ, Chang C-CH, et al. Prediction of pelvic inflammatory disease among young, single, sexually active women. *Sex Transm Dis* 2006;33:137–142.
4. Trent M, Bass D, Ness RB, et al. Recurrent PID, subsequent STI, and reproductive health outcomes: findings from the PID evaluation and clinical health (PEACH) study. *Sex Transm Dis* 2011;38:879–881.
5. Goyal M, Hersh A, Luan X, et al. National trends in pelvic inflammatory disease among adolescents in the emergency department. *J Adolesc Health* 2013;53:249–252.
6. Ness RB, Soper DE, Holley RL, et al. Hormonal and barrier contraception and risk of upper genital tract disease in the PID Evaluation and Clinical Health (PEACH) study. *Am J Obstet Gynecol* 2001;185:121–127.
7. Morrison CS, Turner AN, Jones LB. Highly effective contraception and acquisition of HIV and other sexually transmitted infections. *Best Pract Res Clin Obstet Gynaecol* 2009;23:263–284.
8. Mohllajee AP, Curtis KM, Peterson HB. Does insertion and use of an intrauterine device increase the risk of pelvic inflammatory disease among women with sexually transmitted infection? A systematic review. *Contraception* 2006;73:145–153.
9. Haggerty CL, Hillier SL, Bass DC, et al. Bacterial vaginosis and anaerobic bacteria are associated with endometritis. *Clin Infect Dis* 2004;39:990–995.
10. Ness RB, Hillier SL, Kip KE, et al. Bacterial vaginosis and risk of pelvic inflammatory disease. *Obstet Gynecol* 2004;104:761–769.
11. Ness RB, Kip KE, Hillier SL, et al. A cluster analysis of bacterial vaginosis-associated microflora and pelvic inflammatory disease. *Am J Epidemiol* 2005;162:585–590.
12. Ness RB, Soper DE, Holley RL, et al. Effectiveness of inpatient and outpatient treatment strategies for women with pelvic inflammatory disease: results from the Pelvic Inflammatory Disease Evaluation and Clinical Health (PEACH) Randomized Trial. *Am J Obstet Gynecol* 2002;186:929–937.
13. Trent M, Haggerty CL, Jennings JM, et al. Adverse adolescent reproductive health outcomes after pelvic inflammatory disease. *Arch Pediatr Adolesc Med* 2011;165:49–54.
14. Cohen CR, Mugo NR, Astete SG, et al. Detection of *Mycoplasma genitalium* in women with laparoscopically diagnosed acute salpingitis. *Sex Transm Infect* 2005;81:463–466.
15. Trent M, Ellen JM, Walker A. Pelvic inflammatory disease in adolescents: care delivery in pediatric ambulatory settings. *Pediatr Emerg Care* 2005;21:431–436.
16. Shrier LA, Moszczenski SA, Emans SJ, et al. Three years of a clinical practice guideline for uncomplicated pelvic inflammatory disease in adolescents. *J Adolesc Health* 2000;27:57–62.
17. Short VL, Totten PA, Ness RB, et al. Clinical presentation of *Mycoplasma genitalium* infection versus *Neisseria gonorrhoeae* infection among women with pelvic inflammatory disease. *Clin Infect Dis* 2009;48:41–47.
18. Ness RB, Soper DE, Richter HE, et al. Chlamydia antibodies, chlamydia heat shock protein, and adverse sequelae after pelvic inflammatory disease: the PID Evaluation and Clinical Health (PEACH) Study. *Sex Transm Dis* 2008;35:129–35.
19. Haggerty CL, Totten PA, Astete SG, et al. *Mycoplasma genitalium* among women with nongonococcal, nonchlamydial pelvic inflammatory disease. *Infect Dis Obstet Gynecol* 2006;2006:30184.
20. Short VL, Totten PA, Ness RB, et al. The demographic, sexual health and behavioural correlates of *Mycoplasma genitalium* infection among women with clinically suspected pelvic inflammatory disease. *Sex Transm Infect* 2010;86:29–31.
21. Sweet RL. Treatment of acute pelvic inflammatory disease. *Infect Dis Obstet Gynecol* 2011;2011:561909.
22. Risser WL, Risser JM, Benjamins LJ, et al. Incidence of Fitz-Hugh-Curtis syndrome in adolescents who have pelvic inflammatory disease. *J Pediatr Adolesc Gynecol* 2007;20:179–180.
23. Kaul P, Stevens-Simon C, Saproo A, et al. Trends in illness severity and length of stay in inner-city adolescents hospitalized for pelvic inflammatory disease. *J Pediatr Adolesc Gynecol* 2008;21:289–293.
24. Mollen CJ, Pletcher JR, Bellah RD, et al. Prevalence of tubo-ovarian abscess in adolescents diagnosed with pelvic inflammatory disease in a pediatric emergency department. *Pediatr Emerg Care* 2006;22:621–625.
25. Demirtas O, Akman L, Demirtas GS, et al. The role of the serum inflammatory markers for predicting the tubo-ovarian abscess in acute pelvic inflammatory disease: a single-center 5-year experience. *Arch Gynecol Obstet* 2013;287:519–23.
26. Patrelli TS, Franchi L, Gizzo S, et al. Can the impact of pelvic inflammatory disease on fertility be prevented? Epidemiology, clinical features and surgical treatment: evolution over 8 years. *J Reprod Med* 2013;58:425–433.
27. Workowski KA, Bolan GA. Sexually Transmitted Diseases Guidelines, 2015. *MMWR Recomm Rep* 2015;64(RR-3):1–135.
28. Westrom L, Joesoef R, Reynolds G, et al. Pelvic inflammatory disease and fertility. A cohort study of 1,844 women with laparoscopically verified disease and 657 control women with normal laparoscopic results. *Sex Transm Dis* 1992;19:185–192.
29. Ness RB, Randall H, Richter HE, et al. Condom use and the risk of recurrent pelvic inflammatory disease, chronic pelvic pain, or infertility following an episode of pelvic inflammatory disease. *Am J Public Health* 2004;94:1327–1329.

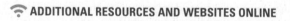 **ADDITIONAL RESOURCES AND WEBSITES ONLINE**

XIII

Syphilis

J. Dennis Fortenberry

Syphilis is an acute, localized sexually transmitted infection (STI) leading, if untreated, to systemic infection and chronic disease. Outbreaks among adolescents and young adults (AYAs) are common, often through connected social and sexual networks.[1] Syphilis is sometimes asymptomatic but often is associated with localized signs of primary infection such as an ulcer at the infection site, or evidence of disseminated secondary infection manifested by symptoms such as skin rash, lymphadenopathy, fever, or mucocutaneous lesions.

EPIDEMIOLOGY

1. Syphilis is caused by *Treponema pallidum*, a motile, spiral microorganism (spirochetes) 6 to 15 µm in length and about 0.20 µm in diameter.
2. Most infections are contracted by sexual contact, including kissing, penile-vaginal and penile-anal intercourse. Nonsexual transmission from direct contact with cutaneous or mucous membrane lesions is rare. Other transmission modes include maternal-fetal transplacental congenital infections, peripartum infection of newborns by contact with maternal genital lesions, and transfusion-related transmission. The estimated rate of transmission after sexual exposure to a person with primary or secondary syphilis is 30% or higher.
3. Syphilis in the US waxes and wanes in 7- to 10-year cycles. Rates of primary and secondary syphilis in the general population increased annually during 2001 to 2009, decreased in 2010, and increased between 2011 and 2013. In 2013, rates again increased (to 5.5 cases per 100,000 population), when 17,375 cases of primary and secondary syphilis were reported in the US. Of these, 900 (5.2%) were 15- to 19-year-olds and 3,642 (21%) were among 20- to 24-year-olds. In 2013, 23 cases of syphilis were reported among 10- to 14-year-olds.
4. Syphilis epidemiology demonstrates the extreme health disparities associated with many STIs.[2]
   a. Geographic disparity: Syphilis has substantial geographic concentration, with more than 50% of primary and secondary cases reported from 1% of the US counties. The southeastern part of the US bears a heavy burden of syphilis, with more than 40% of national cases of primary and secondary syphilis reported from this region.
   b. Racial disparity: Primary and secondary syphilis rates in 2013 were 16.8 per 100,000 among Black 15- to 19-year-olds, compared to 1.2 per 100,000 among White 15- to 19-year-olds. Comparable rates among 20- to 24-year-olds were 56.8 and 6.1 per 100,000 for Black and for White youth, respectively.
   c. Gender disparity: Men-to-women ratios of primary and secondary syphilis were 3.5 among 15- to 19-year-olds in 2013, compared to 7.4 among 20- to 24-year-olds. Recent increases in rates were among men (rising from 8.1 to 9.2 to 10.3 cases per 100,000 in 2011, 2012, and 2013, respectively), compared to relatively stable rates among women (about 0.9 cases per 100,000).
   d. Sex partner disparity: Men with men sex partners account for the majority of cases of primary and secondary syphilis in the US. Among heterosexual individuals, cases decreased during 2008 to 2011 (18.4% among women and 25.9% among men who have sex with women), but increased during 2011 to 2013 (2.9% among women and 14.4% among men who have sex with women). Among men who have sex with men, cases increased annually during 2007 to 2013 (75%).

PATHOGENESIS

T. pallidum produces an immediate localized inflammatory response, associated with regional lymphadenopathy. Antibody responses can be detected within a week of infection. A delayed hypersensitivity response clears most—but not all—organisms in local lesions within about 14 days.[3] Inflammation and local tissue necrosis cause the characteristic induration and ulcer formation of primary syphilis. Dissemination via blood and lymphatics occurs within a few days of infection. Dysregulation of the delayed hypersensitivity response is associated with gumma formation characteristic of late syphilis.[4]

CLINICAL MANIFESTATIONS

The clinical manifestations of syphilis depend on the time since infection and the specific body areas and organs infected. Five stages of syphilis are identified: primary, secondary, early latent, late latent, and late syphilis. Late syphilis (other than late congenital syphilis) is not seen in AYAs and is not additionally considered in this chapter. Neurosyphilis has various manifestations and occurs at any stage.[5]

Primary Syphilis

Syphilis should be considered for any ulcerating lesion of the genitals, cervix, anus, or lips/mouth, but lesions of fingers, arms, and breasts are more common than reported. Primary lesions appear after an incubation period of 9 to 90 days (average is 21 days). Characteristics of primary syphilis are:

1. Ulcer characteristics (Figs 59.1 to 59.3)
   a. Single lesions are 1 to 2 cm in size, but multiple lesions are common. Lesions may also appear as "kissing lesions," adjacent ulcers across a fold of skin.
   b. Ulcers are typically painless and described as having a punched out, clean appearance, with slightly elevated, firm margins. However, ulcer characteristics are an unreliable basis for the diagnosis of syphilis.[6]
2. Bilateral regional lymphadenopathy, with firm, nonsuppurative, usually nontender nodes.
3. Ulcers typically heal within 3 to 6 weeks.
4. Systemic symptoms such as fever, myalgia, or malaise are uncommon.

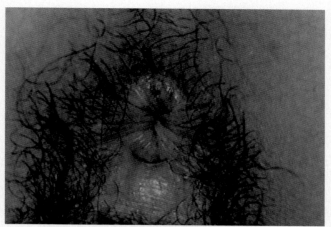

FIGURE 59.3 Primary syphilis: an ulcer at the anus, indicated by the arrow at 12 o'clock. (From Riddell R, Jain D. *Lewin, Weinstein and Riddell's gastrointestinal pathology and its clinical implications*. Philadelphia, PA: Wolters Kluwer, 2014).

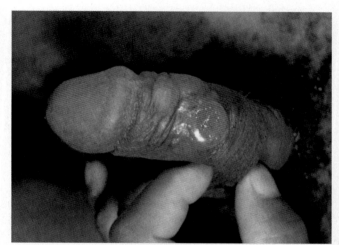

FIGURE 59.1 Primary syphilis: a "cleanly" bordered ulcer on the penil shaft. (From Lugo Somolinos A, McKinley-Grant L, Goldsmith LA, et al. *VisualDx: essential dermatology in pigmented skin*. Philadelphia, PA: Lippincott Williams &Wilkins, 2011.)

Secondary Syphilis

Secondary syphilis appears 6 to 8 weeks after infection and 4 to 10 weeks after the onset of the primary ulcer. *T. pallidum* can be identified in lesions and body fluids.[7] Signs and symptoms:

1. Rash (about 90% of individuals with secondary syphilis).
   a. Involves the trunk and extremities with predilection for palms and soles. Lesions on palms and soles may be scaly and hyperkeratotic (Fig. 59.4).
   b. Rashes are bilateral and symmetrical, and tend to follow the lines of cleavage.

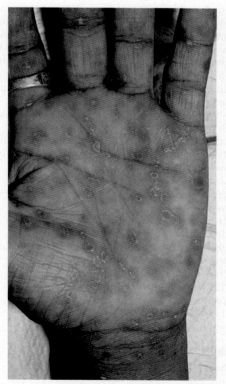

FIGURE 59.4 The rash of secondary syphilis has a predilection for palms and soles. Lesions on palms and soles may be scaly and hyperkeratotic. (From Rosdah CB, Kowalski MT. *Textbook of basic nursing*. 10th ed. Philadelphia, PA: Lippincott Williams & Wilkins, 2011.)

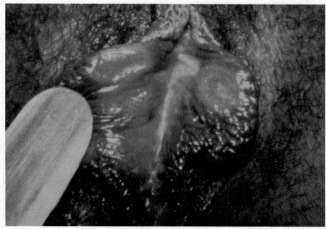

FIGURE 59.2 Primary syphilis: an ulcer on the left labium. (From Sweet RL, Gibbs RS. *Atlas of infectious diseases of the female genital tract*. Philadelphia, PA: Lippincott Williams & Wilkins, 2005.)

XIII

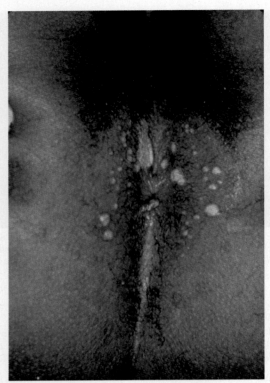

FIGURE 59.5 Condyloma lata. (From Goodheart HP. *Goodheart's same-site differential diagnosis: a rapid method of diagnosing and treating common skin disorders.* Philadelphia, PA: Lippincott Williams & Wilkins, 2010.)

   c. Sharply demarcated lesions, 0.5 to 2.0 cm in diameter, with a reddish-brown hue.

   d. Rash is most commonly macular, papular, or papulosquamous, but almost any type of rash is reported, including acneform lesions, herpetiform lesions, and lesions similar to psoriasis. Lesions in intertriginous areas may erode and fissure, especially in the nasolabial folds and near the corners of the mouth. In warm, moist areas, hypertrophic granulomatous lesions (condylomata lata) may occur (Fig. 59.5).

   e. Lesions are typically nonpruritic, but pruritus is sometimes reported.

   f. Rash lasts a few weeks to 12 months but resolves quickly with treatment.

2. General or regional lymphadenopathy (approximately 70%)
   a. Rubbery, nonpainful nodes, without suppuration
   b. Occasional hepatosplenomegaly

3. Flu-like syndrome (approximately 50%)
   a. Sore throat, fever, and malaise most common
   b. Headaches
   c. Lacrimation and nasal discharge
   d. Arthralgia and myalgia

4. Alopecia (uncommon): Moth-eaten—appearing alopecia of the scalp and eyebrows

5. Other rare manifestations
   a. Arthritis or bursitis
   b. Hepatitis
   c. Iritis and anterior uveitis
   d. Glomerulonephritis

Latent Syphilis

Latent syphilis is characterized by the following:

1. Absence of clinical signs and symptoms of syphilis
2. Positive serologic tests for syphilis, including both nontreponemal and treponemal tests.

Two stages of latent syphilis are differentiated to guide treatment. *Early latent syphilis* is defined as seroconversion (or four-fold or greater increase in a nontreponemal test) during the past 12 months, without clinical evidence of syphilis. For treatment purposes, early latent syphilis is grouped with primary and secondary syphilis. *Late latent syphilis* refers to seroconversion after 12 months, and requires a different treatment regimen. The term "latent syphilis of unknown duration" is used when the timing of seroconversion cannot be established.[8]

Neurosyphilis

Clinically significant neurosyphilis develops in up 20% of patients with untreated early syphilis, but abnormal cerebrospinal fluid (CSF) can be found in a much higher proportion of patients with early syphilis. Neurosyphilis in AYAs is usually asymptomatic but may manifest as acute meningitis. Meningovascular syphilis is rare.

1. Asymptomatic neurosyphilis: Characterized by abnormal CSF, including pleocytosis, elevated protein, and positive CSF-venereal diseases research laboratory (VDRL)
2. Acute syphilitic meningitis
   a. Usually occurs during secondary syphilis or the early latent period
   b. Common symptoms: Fever, headache, photophobia, and meningismus
   c. Less frequent symptoms: Confusion, delirium, and seizures
   d. Common findings include cranial nerve palsies (40%) and altered CSF (increased protein, lymphocytic pleocytosis, and lowered glucose)
3. Meningovascular syphilis
   a. Rare in AYAs (occurs 5 to 12 years after initial infection)
   b. Symptoms and signs result from an endarteritis producing local areas of infarction
   c. Symptoms: Headache, dizziness, mood changes, and memory loss
   d. Signs: Hemiparesis, hemiplegia, aphasia
   e. Parenchymal nervous system injury causing Argyll Robertson pupils (accommodation, but no response to light); posterior column spinal cord injury causing tabes dorsalis

Congenital Syphilis

AYAs with congenital syphilis bear the stigmata of early disease and may develop additional manifestations of syphilis.[9]

1. 1. Early congenital syphilis parallels secondary syphilis among adults and occurs before age two. The most common abnormalities include the following:
   a. Skeletal abnormalities, including osteochondritis (up to 90% of those affected)
   b. Hepatomegaly or splenomegaly (approximately 50%)
   c. Petechiae; hemolytic anemia and thrombocytopenia (35% to 40%)
   d. Skin lesions (approximately 40%)
   e. Persistent rhinitis (snuffles) (approximately 20%)
   f. Neurosyphilis (approximately 25%)
2. Late congenital syphilis corresponds to late syphilis in adults, and often presents during puberty. Most infections (60%) are latent, but new findings include the following:
   a. Abnormal faces, including saddle nose and frontal bossing (approximately 85%)
   b. Palatal deformity (approximately 75%)
   c. Dental deformities including Hutchinson incisors (approximately 55%)
   d. Interstitial keratitis (up to 50%)
   e. Symmetrical, painless swelling of knees (30% to 45%)
   f. Sensorineural 8th nerve deafness (3% to 4%)
   g. Neurosyphilis (up to 5%)

DIFFERENTIAL DIAGNOSIS

Primary Syphilis
Sexually Transmitted Genital Ulcer Diseases

The most common sexually transmitted genital ulcer is genital herpes. Fewer than 100 cases of chancroid were reported in the past 5 years in the US; ulcers due to lymphogranuloma venereum and granuloma inguinale are also rare.

1. Herpes simplex (see Chapter 60): Painful, multiple lesions beginning as vesicles on an erythematous base. Primary lesions may be extensive, and associated with tender adenopathy, and recurrent lesions are usually unilateral without significant adenopathy.
2. Chancroid: Painful lesions with a deep purulent base and often erythematous borders. Local lymph nodes are often fluctuant and tender.
3. Lymphogranuloma venereum: Nonindurated, herpetiform ulcer that heals rapidly. Many patients present with advanced disease, including fever and massive regional adenopathy.
4. Granuloma inguinale (donovanosis) (see Chapter 62): Nontender, fleshy, beefy-red, easily bleeding ulcers.

Nonsexually Transmitted Causes of Genital Ulcers
1. Traumatic lesions
2. Candida balanitis
3. Behçet syndrome

Secondary Syphilis
1. Psoriasis
2. Pityriasis rosea
3. Drug associated rash
4. Tinea versicolor
5. Alopecia areata
6. Lichen planus
7. Lupus erythematosus
8. Scabies
9. Pediculosis
10. Rosacea
11. Infectious mononucleosis
12. Condyloma acuminatum (the differentiation is to condyloma lata)

DIAGNOSIS

T. pallidum does not grow in artificial media. Syphilis serologic screening is routine during pregnancy and often done as part of evaluation for other STIs, including human immunodeficiency virus (HIV). Routine syphilis screening is recommended for youth with high-risk markers such as commercial sex work, injection drug use, and men with multiple same-sex partners; however, routine syphilis screening for AYAs is not recommended.

Laboratory Findings

Screening and diagnostic algorithms for syphilis have undergone substantial changes in recent years; clinicians are advised to review and understand the algorithm used in local laboratories.

Dark-Field Examination

The dark-field examination allows immediate diagnosis but requires specialized equipment and training. Technique is as follows:

1. Clean lesion with saline and gauze.
2. Abrade gently with dry gauze. Avoid inducing bleeding.
3. Squeeze lesion to express serous transudate.
4. Place a drop of transudate on a slide.
5. Place a drop of saline on transudate and cover with a coverslip.
6. Examine under dark-field microscope for typical motile, corkscrew-shaped organisms.
7. For internal lesions, a bacteriologic loop can be used to transfer the fluid to a slide.

Serological Tests

1. *Nontreponemal antibody tests* assess anticardiolipin antibodies formed to surface lipids on *T. pallidum*.
   a. Rapid plasma reagin (RPR) is visually assessed by agglutination.
   b. VDRL is assessed by flocculation seen by microscopy
   c. Nontreponemal tests are used for screening and to monitor response to treatment. Nontreponemal test titers correlate with disease activity and fall—usually to nondetectable levels—within 12 months of treatment. Peak titers are seen within 2 to 4 weeks of initial treatment, and subsequently decline. A four-fold change in titer, equivalent to a change of two dilutions (e.g., from 1:8 to 1:32 or 1:16 to 1:4), demonstrates a substantial change. RPR and VDRL are equally valid, but quantitative titers cannot be directly compared.
2. Treponemal antibody tests
   a. Fluorescent treponemal antibody-absorbed (FTA-ABS) is used to confirm a positive result from RPR or VDRL.
   b. *T. pallidum* particle agglutination (TP-PA) test is widely used as the treponemal test to confirm a positive nontreponemal test and to resolve discrepant results of reverse sequence syphilis screening algorithms (see 2e below and Fig. 59.6).
   c. Enzyme immunosorbent assay (EIA) and chemiluminescence immunoassay (CLIA) are treponemal tests, with high specificity but cannot be titered.
   d. Treponemal tests remain positive for life, limiting their usefulness in distinguishing new from previously treated infections.
   e. Advances in laboratory technology have led to reverse sequence syphilis screening algorithms (Fig. 59.6B).[10] This approach uses automated, high throughput EIA or CIA as the screening test, with confirmation by a nontreponemal test. Advantages include improved laboratory efficiency and increased detection of latent and late infections (although potentially with increased rates of false-positive tests).
3. Sensitivity
   a. The sensitivity of nontreponemal tests in primary syphilis depends on the duration of infection. With ulcer appearance, nontreponemal tests are positive in about 25% of persons. Positivity rates at 2 weeks, 3 weeks, and 4 weeks are 50%, 75%, and 100%, respectively.
   b. Treponemal tests are positive in 80% to 100% of primary syphilis. Sensitivity of nontreponemal and treponemal tests approaches 100% in secondary syphilis.
4. False-positive serology test results: Up to 40% of positive nontreponemal test results are false positive, as shown by a nonreactive treponemal test. Most false-positive nontreponemal test results show a low titer (dilution <1:8), and the probability of a false-positive finding decreases with increasing titer. The causes of false-positive test results include the following:
   a. Acute infection: Viral infections, chlamydial infections, Lyme disease, *Mycoplasma* infections, nonsyphilitic spirochetal infections, and various bacterial, fungal, and protozoal infections
   b. Autoimmune diseases
   c. Narcotic addiction
   d. Aging
   e. Hashimoto thyroiditis
   f. Sarcoidosis

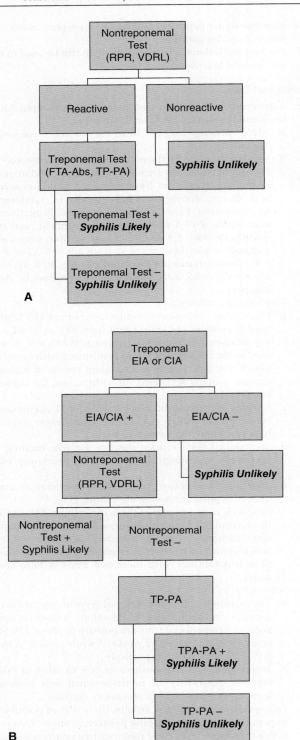

FIGURE 59.6 Traditional nontreponemal—treponemal sequence syphilis seroscreening algorithm (panel A) and reverse sequence syphilis screening algorithm (panel B).

g. Lymphoma
h. Leprosy
i. Cirrhosis of the liver
j. HIV infection: Can lead to unusually high, unusually low, or fluctuating titers
5. False-positive treponemal tests occur but most are reported as borderline and not positive.

Diagnosis by Stage
Primary Syphilis
1. Identification of spirochetes by dark-field examination of ulcer transudate.
2. A positive nontreponemal test result with a high titer (1:8 or higher) or rising titer (two or more than two dilutions) *and* a positive treponemal test result (e.g., FTA-ABS or TP-PA).

AYAs with a positive dark-field examination should be treated, as should those with a typical lesion and a positive serologic test result. If the initial serologic test result is negative, it should be repeated 1 week, 1 month, and 3 months later in suspected cases. A treponemal test should be used to confirm a positive nontreponemal test result.

Secondary Syphilis
1. Dark-field examination of material from lesions or lymph nodes
2. Serodiagnosis with combination of nontreponemal and treponemal tests

Treatment should be provided if the dark-field examination result is positive or for typical findings of secondary syphilis and a positive nontreponemal test that is confirmed with a treponemal test.

Early and Late Latent Syphilis
RPR/VDRL and a FTA-ABS/TP-PA (or other treponemal) test should be done. Treponemal tests are essential in latent and late syphilis because the nontreponemal tests are only approximately 70% sensitive in these states. Patients should be treated if the treponemal test result is positive and there is no documentation of appropriate prior treatment. A decision about a lumbar puncture in these instances should be done in consultation with an expert in this area.

Neurosyphilis
A positive CSF-VDRL is diagnostic of neurosyphilis, especially when accompanied by CSF pleocytosis. The CSF-VDRL cannot be replaced by other nontreponemal tests (such as the RPR) even if those tests are used to monitor serologic response to treatment.[11] A CSF FTA-ABS can be evaluated if the CSF-VDRL is negative, as neurosyphilis is highly unlikely with a negative CSF FTA-ABS.[12]

1. Central nervous system infection occurs in 30% to 40% of patients with primary or secondary syphilis, although not all develop symptomatic disease.
2. CSF examination is not routine in early syphilis without neurologic signs or symptoms.
3. Indications for CSF examination continue to be refined, but the following apply regardless of disease stage[13]:
   a. Neurologic or ophthalmologic signs or symptoms
   b. Treatment failure
   c. Serum nontreponemal test titer is greater than or equal to 1:32.
   d. Nonpenicillin therapy is planned.
   e. HIV infection

Syphilis in Pregnancy
Pregnant AYAs should be screened early in pregnancy. Seropositive patients are considered infected unless treatment is documented and serologic titers have appropriately declined. Screening should be repeated in the third trimester and again at delivery in areas or populations with a high prevalence of syphilis. Syphilis should be considered for pregnancy loss after 20 weeks' gestation.[14]

Syphilis and HIV
Ulcerative lesions increase the risk of HIV transmission. Treponemal and nontreponemal serologic tests for syphilis are accurate for most individuals with both syphilis and HIV infection. HIV-infected

individuals with neurologic symptoms or failure to respond to antibiotic treatment should be evaluated for neurosyphilis.

 THERAPY

Penicillin is the optimal antibiotic for syphilis treatment: the dosage and length depends on the syphilis stage. For individuals with a history of penicillin allergy, skin testing and desensitization, if indicated, are recommended. Few data are available on nonpenicillin regimens, especially among adolescents. Health care professionals should always review the Centers for Disease Control and Prevention STI guidelines available at http://www.cdc.gov/std/treatment/update.htm.

Primary and Secondary Syphilis

1. Benzathine penicillin G: The total recommended dose is a single injection of 2.4 million units intramuscularly (IM).
2. Penicillin-allergic nonpregnant patients:
   a. Doxycycline 100 mg orally two times a day for 14 days, or
   b. Tetracycline 500 mg orally four times a day for 14 days is recommended.
   c. Ceftriaxone is effective for treatment of early syphilis, but the optimal dose and duration have not been defined.
   d. Azithromycin 2 g as a single oral dose. However, treatment failure due to acquired azithromycin resistance of *T. pallidum* is reported. This treatment should be used only if other options are unavailable and careful follow-up is assured.
   e. Use of any alternative therapies in HIV-infected persons has been insufficiently studied.
   f. Patients who cannot tolerate an alternative therapy should be referred for penicillin desensitization.
   g. Pregnancy: Penicillin desensitization and penicillin treatment according to stage.
3. Other considerations
   a. Patients with syphilis should be tested for HIV. For high-risk patients or in high-prevalence areas, patients with primary syphilis should be retested for HIV after 3 months.
   b. Patients with signs or symptoms of neurologic or ophthalmic disease should be evaluated by CSF analysis or slit-lamp examination, respectively.
4. Follow-up
   a. Infected individuals should be reexamined clinically, and serologic test results should be rechecked at 3 and 6 months. Nontreponemal antibody titers should be used for follow-up. If signs or symptoms persist or nontreponemal antibody titers have not decreased four-fold by 6 months, the patient should have a CSF examination and HIV test and be re-treated. Most individuals with primary syphilis are seronegative by 3 to 12 months, and 75% to 95% of individuals with secondary syphilis are seronegative by 1 year. The drop in titers for primary and secondary syphilis applies only to first episodes of primary or secondary syphilis; those with reinfections have less predictable changes in antibody titers.
   b. Lack of four-fold decline of nontreponemal titers within 3 months of treatment indicates treatment failure. Re-treatment should include three weekly injections of benzathine penicillin G 2.4 million units IM unless neurosyphilis is identified.

Latent Syphilis

There are two regimens for nonpenicillin allergic patients with normal CSF:

1. Early latent syphilis: Benzathine penicillin G 2.4 million units IM in a single dose
2. Late latent syphilis or latent syphilis of unknown duration: Benzathine penicillin G 7.2 million units total, administered as three weekly doses of 2.4 million units IM each.

3. Penicillin-allergic patients: No data adequately document the efficacy of drugs other than penicillin for syphilis of more than 1 year's duration. CSF examinations should be performed before therapy with these regimens. Suggested regimens are doxycycline 100 mg orally two times a day or tetracycline 500 mg orally four times a day. Either is given for 14 days for individuals with early latent syphilis or 28 days for others. Patients with abnormal CSF examinations should be treated for neurosyphilis.
4. Follow-up
   a. Nontreponemal serologic titers should be assessed at 6, 12, and 24 months after treatment. If titers increase four-fold or initial high titers (1:32 or greater) fail to decrease four-fold (two dilutions) within 12 to 24 months, or if signs or symptoms of syphilis occur, the individual should be evaluated for neurosyphilis and re-treated appropriately.
   b. Approximately 75% of the patients with early latent disease become seronegative by 5 years; the remaining 25% have positive serology for life.

Neurosyphilis

1. Recommended regimen for neurosyphilis or ocular syphilis in individuals not allergic to penicillin: Aqueous crystalline penicillin G 18 to 24 million units daily administered as 3 to 4 million units intravenously (IV) every 4 hours for 10 to 14 days.
   a. Alternative regimen: Procaine penicillin G IM 2.4 million units daily, plus probenecid 500 mg orally four times a day, both for 10 to 14 days.
   b. Some experts add benzathine penicillin G 2.4 million units IM after completion of either of these two regimens.
2. Penicillin-allergic patients: Patients should be desensitized to penicillin, and treated with penicillin. No alternatives have been adequately evaluated. Some specialists recommend ceftriaxone 2 g daily IM or IV for 10 to 14 days.
3. Follow-up: If the initial CSF examination showed an increased cell count, the examination should be repeated every 6 months until the cell count is normal. If the count has not decreased at 6 months or is not normal by 2 years, re-treatment is recommended.

Syphilis in Pregnancy

Pregnant women should receive penicillin doses appropriate for the stage of syphilis. Penicillin is effective in preventing transmission to the fetus and in treating fetal infections. Some experts recommend additional therapy, such as a second dose of benzathine penicillin G 2.4 million units IM given 1 week after the first dose for women who have primary, secondary, or early latent syphilis. During the second half of pregnancy, syphilis treatment may be adjusted by sonographic fetal evaluation for congenital syphilis. Pregnant women with a history of an allergy to penicillin should be skin tested and either treated or desensitized.

Treatment of Sex Partners

1. Sex partners of persons with primary, secondary, or early latent syphilis within the preceding 90 days should be tested for syphilis but treated presumptively, even if seronegative. Treatment is the same as for primary syphilis. If exposure occurred more than 90 days before examination, the individual should be treated presumptively if serologic test results are not immediately available and follow-up is uncertain.
2. Partners should be notified and treated if the affected patient has syphilis of unknown duration and high nontreponemal serologic test titers (1:32 or greater).
3. Sex partners of patients with late syphilis should be evaluated both clinically and serologically for syphilis.
4. Identification of at-risk sex partners: Time periods used to identify partners at risk are as follows:

a. Three months plus duration of symptoms for primary syphilis
b. Six months plus duration of symptoms for secondary syphilis
c. One year for early latent syphilis

HIV-Infected Individuals

1. Penicillin regimens should be used whenever possible. Skin testing and desensitization can be used as appropriate.
2. Primary and secondary syphilis in HIV-infected patients: The Centers for Disease Control and Prevention recommends no change in therapy for early syphilis in HIV-infected patients. Some experts recommend adding multiple doses of benzathine penicillin G, similar to the dosages used to treat late syphilis.
   a. Because of the confusing CSF findings and difficulty in definitively diagnosing neurosyphilis, many authorities recommend CSF examination of all individuals who are HIV infected, with treatment altered accordingly.
   b. Follow-up: HIV-infected adolescents should have follow-up serologic testing at 3, 6, 9, 12, and 24 months. Those individuals with treatment failure should have a CSF examination and be re-treated similarly to those who are not HIV infected. If the CSF is normal, most experts would re-treat with benzathine penicillin G 7.2 million units as three weekly doses of 2.4 million units each.
3. Late latent syphilis
   a. Patients with HIV and latent syphilis should have a CSF examination.
   b. Treatment in those individuals with normal CSF should include benzathine penicillin G 7.2 million units (as three weekly doses of 2.4 million units each). Those with abnormal findings on CSF examination should be treated and managed as patients with neurosyphilis.

Jarisch–Herxheimer Reaction

Jarisch–Herxheimer reaction occurs within 2 hours of treatment in 50% of patients with primary syphilis, in 90% of those with secondary syphilis, and in 25% of those with early latent syphilis.[15] The reaction consists of the following:

1. Headache, fever, chills, myalgias
2. Elevated neutrophil count
3. Tachycardia

These symptoms may last up to 24 hours, and resolve with reassurance, rest, and antipyretics. The reaction can induce transient uterine contractions in pregnant women.

REFERENCES

1. Brewer TH, Schillinger J, Lewis FMT, et al. Infectious syphilis among adolescent and young adult men: implications for human immunodeficiency virus transmission and public health interventions. *Sex Transm Dis.* 2011;38:367–371.
2. Chesson HW, Kent CK, Owusu-Edusei K Jr, et al. Disparities in sexually transmitted disease rates across the "eight Americas". *Sex Transm Dis* 2012;39:458–464.
3. Lafond RE, Lukehart SA. Biological basis for syphilis. *Clin Microbiol Rev* 2006;19:29–49.
4. Carlson JA, Dabiri G, Cribier B, et al. The immunopathobiology of syphilis: the manifestations and course of syphilis are determined by the level of delayed-type hypersensitivity. *Am J Dermatopathol* 2011;33:433–460.
5. Ghanem KG. Neurosyphilis: a historical perspective and review. *CNS Neurosci Ther* 2010;16:e157–e168.
6. DiCarlo RP, Martin DH. The clinical diagnosis of genital ulcer disease in men. *Clin Infect Dis* 1997;25:292–298.
7. Mullooly C, Higgins SP. Secondary syphilis: the classical triad of skin rash, mucosal ulceration and lymphadenopathy. *Int J STD AIDS* 2010;21:537–545.
8. Shockman S, Buescher LS, Stone SP. Syphilis in the United States. *Clin Dermatol* 2014;32:213–218.
9. Chakraborty R, Luck S. Managing congenital syphilis again? The more things change. *Curr Opin Infect Dis* 2007;20:247–252.
10. Lipinsky D, Schreiber L, Kopel V, et al. Validation of reverse sequence screening for syphilis. *J Clin Microbiol* 2012;50:1501.
11. Marra CM, Tantalo LC, Maxwell CL, et al. The rapid plasma reagin test cannot replace the venereal disease research laboratory test for neurosyphilis diagnosis. *Sex Transm Dis* 2012;39:453–457.
12. Harding AS, Ghanem KG. The performance of cerebrospinal fluid treponemal-specific antibody tests in neurosyphilis: a systematic review. *Sex Transm Dis* 2012;39:291–297.
13. Ghanem KG, Moore RD, Rompalo AM, et al. Lumbar puncture in HIV-infected patients with syphilis and no neurologic symptoms. *Clin Infect Dis* 2009;48:816–821.
14. Gomez GB, Kamb ML, Newman LM, et al. Untreated maternal syphilis and adverse outcomes of pregnancy: a systematic review and meta-analysis. *Bull World Health Organ* 2013;91:217–226.
15. Myles TD, Elam G, Park-Hwang E, et al. The Jarisch-Herxheimer reaction and fetal monitoring changes in pregnant women treated for syphilis. *Obstet Gynecol* 1998;92:859–864.

📶 **ADDITIONAL RESOURCES AND WEBSITES ONLINE**

CHAPTER 60

Herpes Genitalis

Gale R. Burstein
Kimberly A. Workowski

Genital herpes is a chronic lifelong viral disease. Herpes genitalis lesions are caused by a large DNA virus, herpes simplex virus (HSV), with two serotypes, HSV type 1 (HSV-1) and HSV type 2 (HSV-2). Most cases of recurrent genital herpes are caused by HSV-2; however, HSV-1 is becoming more prominent as a cause of first-episode genital herpes, especially in young women and men who have sex with men (MSM).[1-3] These viruses have the ability to become latent and reactivate. Although among adolescents and young adults (AYAs) HSV-2 infection prevalence has not changed significantly over the last decade, HSV-1 seroprevalence has decreased, leaving young people more susceptible to HSV disease and incident HSV-1 infections at sexual debut.[3] Most HSV-1- and HSV-2-infected persons have not been diagnosed.[2,4] They may have mild or unrecognized infections but shed virus intermittently in the genital tract. Most genital herpes infections are transmitted by persons unaware that they have the infection or who are asymptomatic when transmission occurs.

EPIDEMIOLOGY

Prevalence[1] and Incidence

1. The National Health and Nutrition Examination Surveys (NHANES) conducted between 1999 and 2010 identified overall decreases in HSV-1 seroprevalence, especially among 14- to 19-year-olds, with no significant changes in HSV-2 seroprevalence.[3] As more youth lack HSV-1 antibodies at sexual debut, their susceptibility to genital HSV-1 increases.
   a. Among 14- to 19-year-olds, HSV-1 seroprevalence decreased by 23%, from 39% during 1999 to 2004, to 30% during 2005 to 2010, whereas HSV-2 seroprevalence did not change significantly (from 1.6% to 1.2%).
   b. Among 20- to 29-year-olds, HSV-1 seroprevalence decreased 9% over the 10-year period from 54% to 50%, whereas HSV-2 seroprevalence did not change significantly (from 11% to 10%).
2. HSV-1 and HSV-2 prevalence varies by age.[3]
   a. The prevalence of infection increases with age. In NHANES 2005 to 2010, approximately 30% of 14- to 19-year-olds and 50% of 20- to 29-year-olds were infected with HSV-1 and

1.2% of 14- to 19-year-olds and 9.9% of 20- to 29-year-olds were infected with HSV-2.[3]
3. Sociodemographic disparities exist with HSV-1 seroprevalence.[3,4]
   a. HSV-1 seroprevalence varies by race, gender, and income: Among 14- to 29-year-olds, estimated HSV-1 seroprevalence was higher among Mexican Americans and non-Hispanic Blacks compared to non-Hispanic Whites, females compared to males, and those with lower incomes.[3]
   b. Similar disparities exist with HSV-2 seroprevalence.[4]
4. HSV-1 incident infections are more than twice as common as HSV-2 infections.[2] Among healthy, HSV-1/2 seronegative females aged 18 to 30 years followed in an HSV vaccine trial for 20 months, the rate of new infections with HSV-1 (2.5/100 person years) was more than twice that of HSV-2 (1.1/100 person years), and HSV-1 infections in the genital area appeared three times more frequently than HSV-2 genital infections.[2]
   a. Among females 18 to 22 years, HSV-1 incident infections were most common (3.2/100 person years) and more than twice the rate of incident HSV-2 infections (1.3/100 person years).[2]

Recurrent Episodes

Persons with symptomatic first-episode genital HSV-2 infection frequently experience recurrent genital lesions; recurrences are less frequent after initial genital HSV-1 infection. However, intermittent shedding can occur with either strain, even in those without visible lesions. Therefore, identification of the type of infecting strain may have prognostic importance to the individual and may be useful in counseling.[5]

Transmission

1. Mode of transmission is through sexual contact, either genital–genital or oral–genital, and by mucosal contact with infected secretions.
2. Humans are the sole known reservoir of infection.
3. Risk of transmission
   a. Demographics: HSV-2 disproportionately affects Black Americans, particularly Black females, who reside in communities with a higher prevalence of HSV-2 infection, placing them at greater risk of infection. There are also additional biologic factors placing females at greater risk for HSV-2 than males.[4] The female genital tract has more exposed vascular, mucosal surface of the vagina and cervix compared to the male urethral meatus. Also, the female genital tract mucosa has more prolonged exposure to infected semen, which increases the probability of infection.

---

[1]The proportion of a population that is seropositive, i.e., has been exposed to HSV as evident by measurable antibodies. Type-specific serologic testing provides the best method to estimate HSV-1 and HSV-2 prevalence.

b. The decreasing seroprevalence of HSV-1 antibodies among AYAs results in increased susceptibility to incident genital HSV-1 infections.[3]

c. Although viral shedding is highest while genital lesions are present, most HSV-2 sexual transmission occurs on days when the source partner has no visible genital lesions.[2,5]

d. HSV-2 viral shedding rates are increased among persons with HIV infection.[6] HSV suppressive therapy in persons infected with HIV does not reduce the risk of HIV or HSV-2 transmission to susceptible sex partners.[7,8]

Infections by Serologic Type

1. HSV-1 infection typically manifests as oral–labial lesions, but the frequency of HSV-1 genital infections is increasing, especially among AYAs.[2,3] Genital recurrences and subclinical shedding are much less frequent than with genital HSV-2 infection.

2. HSV-2 infection typically manifests as anogenital lesions. Oral HSV-2 infection is uncommon.[2,9]

PATHOGENESIS

Virus particles can be shed in salivary, cervical, urogenital, and anorectal secretions of infected individuals. The virus gains entry into the body through mucosal surfaces or abraded skin and replicates in the epidermal and dermal cells of a susceptible host. After replication, the virus spreads through contiguous cells to mucocutaneous projections of sensory nerves.

After resolution of the primary disease, the virus becomes latent. Latency appears to be lifelong but is interrupted by periods of viral reactivation, leading to silent viral shedding or clinically apparent recurrences. Reactivation of latent virus leads to transport of viral genomes to the skin surface, where replication occurs in the dermis and epidermis. Reactivation can be triggered by a variety of stimuli, such as ultraviolet light, immunosuppression, fever, pneumococcal pneumonia, stress, and local trauma. Frequency and clinical severity of reactivation depend on factors such as the host immunological status and the severity and viral type of the primary infection.

CLINICAL MANIFESTATIONS

Definition of Terms

1. Primary infection: Genital herpes in a patient seronegative for antibody to either HSV-1 or HSV-2

2. First clinical episode: First clinical manifestations due to HSV-1 or HSV-2 infection. This term includes both nonprimary first episodes (i.e., positive serology), and primary infections.

3. Recurrent clinical episode: Recurrence of genital HSV lesions in a patient with a previously documented symptomatic genital herpes episode

4. Atypical clinical episode: Episode of clinical manifestations due to HSV-1 or HSV-2 infection that do not include *classic* genital lesions

Classic Primary Infection

1. Primary genital HSV infection involves both systemic and local symptoms.

2. Clinical manifestations begin approximately one week following initial infection.

3. Systemic symptoms occur over the first week of illness in more than half of infected individuals, which may include fever, headache, malaise, and myalgias.

4. Local symptoms may include painful lesions, dysuria, pruritus, vaginal, urethral, or rectal discharge, and tender inguinal adenopathy.

   a. Herpetic lesions can be extensive and can involve the vulva, perineum, vagina, perianal area, and cervix in females or, in males, large areas of the penis or anorectum. Lesions usually begin as small papules or vesicles on an erythematous base that rapidly spread over the genital area (Fig. 60.1).

   Multiple small vesicular/pustular lesions coalesce into large areas of ulceration. Pain and irritation from lesions usually peak between days 7 and 11 of disease and heal over the second week. Crusting and reepithelization occur in the penile and mons area, but crusting does not occur on mucosal surfaces. Scarring is uncommon. New crops of lesions may form during the primary outbreak between 4 and 10 days of disease in more than 75% of primary infections.[10] Lesions typically heal by the end of the third week of disease.

5. Central nervous system complaints, such as headache, stiff neck, and mild photophobia, may occur in the first week of illness.

6. Pharyngeal involvement is seen primarily with HSV-1.[2,9]

7. Median duration of viral shedding is 12 days.

8. Complications can include aseptic meningitis and other neurological complications (such as autonomic nervous system dysfunction and transverse myelitis), extragenital lesions (buttock, groin, or thigh areas), and disseminated disease.

First Clinical Episode

1. First episodes of genital herpes are more often associated with systemic symptoms and a prolonged duration of lesions and viral shedding, and are more likely to involve multiple genital and extragenital sites compared to recurrent episodes.

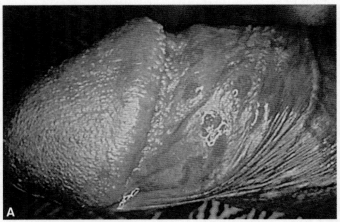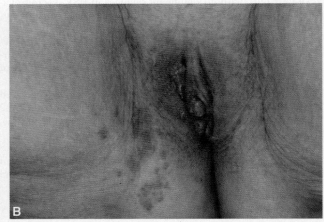

FIGURE 60.1 Genital herpes lesions **(A)** on the penis and **(B)** on the vulva. (**A** from Goodheart HP. *Goodheart's photoguide to common skin disorders: diagnosis and management.* 3rd ed. Philadelphia, PA: Lippincott Williams & Wilkins, 2009. B, © Dr. P. Marrazi/Photo Researchers, Inc.)

2. Most persons with their first clinical episode of symptomatic genital herpes have serologic evidence of prior HSV infection; that is, the first clinical episode is not a result of the primary infection.

3. Prior HSV-1 infection may diminish the severity of first genital HSV-2 episodes.

Recurrent Episodes

1. Clinical manifestations are localized to the genital region and are of mild to moderate severity compared to primary infection.

2. Duration: Usually ranges from 6 to 12 days

3. Prodromal symptoms: Variable presentation that can range from mild paresthesias to shooting pains in the buttocks, legs, or hips

4. Lesions in recurrent episodes occur on predominantly non-mucosal skin, are often unilateral with a much smaller area of involvement, and associated with fewer lesions compared to the primary infection (Figs. 60.2 and 60.3).

5. Clinical episodes can vary considerably in the severity and duration of disease between episodes in the same individual and among different individuals.

6. Symptoms tend to be more severe among females.

7. Duration: Lesions typically heal by the second week of disease.

8. Shedding: In untreated patients, the average duration of viral shedding is 4 days.

9. After the first year, genital recurrences tend to decrease in frequency.

Atypical Episodes

1. Atypical episodes may have manifestations of either a primary infection or a recurrent episode.

2. Episodes may present with genital pruritus, papules or fissures, dysuria, urethritis, or cervicitis.

🔵 DIFFERENTIAL DIAGNOSIS

Herpes genitalis lesions must be differentiated from early syphilis, chancroid, lymphogranuloma venereum, granuloma inguinale, excoriations, allergic and irritant contact dermatitis, intercourse-associated trauma, and genital lesions of Behçet syndrome.

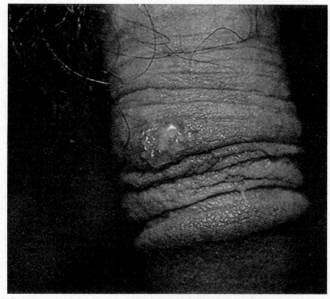

FIGURE 60.2 Recurrent genital herpes lesion on penis. (From *Lippincott's nursing advisor 2013*. Philadelphia: Lippincott Williams & Wilkins, 2013.)

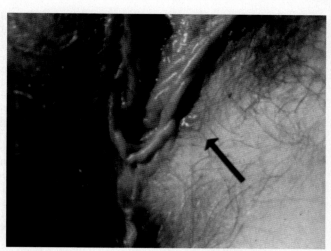

FIGURE 60.3 Recurrent genital herpes lesion on vulva. (From Nettina S. *The Lippincott manual of nursing practice*. 7th ed. Philadelphia, PA: Lippincott, Williams & Wilkins, 2001.)

🔵 DIAGNOSIS

Genital herpes is the most prevalent infectious cause of genital ulcers in the US. However, clinical diagnosis of genital herpes is both insensitive and nonspecific. The classic painful, multiple vesicular or ulcerative lesions are absent in many infected persons; a patient who presents with oral and/or genital sores may actually have a disease other than HSV. The clinical diagnosis of genital herpes should be confirmed by type-specific laboratory testing, since the prognosis and counseling depend on the type of genital herpes (HSV-1 or HSV-2).

Laboratory Evaluation

1. Virologic tests[5]: Cell culture and polymerase chain reaction (PCR) are the preferred HSV tests.[5] Viral culture sensitivity is low, especially for recurrent lesions, and declines rapidly as lesions begin to heal. Nucleic acid amplification tests, such as PCR for HSV DNA, are more sensitive and are increasingly available. Viral culture isolates and PCR amplicons should be typed to determine which HSV type is causing infection. Tzanck preparations and cervical Pap smears are insensitive and nonspecific diagnostic methods and should not be used.

2. Type-specific serologic tests: Both type-specific and type-common antibodies to HSV develop during the first several weeks following infection and persist indefinitely. Accurate type-specific HSV antibody assays must be based on the HSV-specific glycoprotein G2 for the diagnosis of HSV-2 infection and glycoprotein G1 for diagnosis of HSV-1 infection. Providers should specifically request type-specific gG-based assays when serology is performed.[5]

   a. Available tests: Currently, the US Food and Drug Administration-approved gG-based type-specific assays are laboratory-based and point-of-care tests that provide results for HSV-2 antibodies from capillary blood or serum.

   b. Sensitivity and specificity[5]: The sensitivities and specificities of these glycoprotein G type-specific tests for the detection of HSV-2 antibody vary. The most commonly used test, HerpeSelect HSV-2 ELISA, may be falsely positive at low index values (1.1 to 3.5).[11,12] Such low values should be confirmed with another test, such as Biokit or the Western blot. HerpeSelect HSV-2 Immunoblot should not be used for confirmation as it uses the same antigen as the HSV-2 ELISA. Repeat testing is also indicated if recent acquisition of genital herpes is suspected. The HerpeSelect HSV-1

XIII

ELISA is insensitive for detection of HSV-1 antibody. IgM HSV testing is not useful because it is not type specific and may be positive with recurrent HSV episodes.

c. Meaning of a positive test: Most persons with HSV-2 antibody by type-specific testing have anogenital HSV infection acquired during adolescence or adulthood, which may be asymptomatic. Positive HSV-1 antibody tests may indicate an acquired oral HSV infection in childhood. However, acquisition of genital HSV-1 is increasing, especially among AYAs, and genital infection can often be asymptomatic.[2] Therefore, it is impossible to determine if an asymptomatic person with a HSV-1 antibody positive test result has an anogenital, orolabial, or cutaneous site of infection. AYAs with HSV-1 infection remain at risk for HSV-2 acquisition.

d. Type-specific HSV-2 serologic assays may be useful in the following clinical situations:
   • Recurrent or atypical genital symptoms with negative HSV cultures
   • A clinical diagnosis of genital herpes without laboratory confirmation
   • A patient with a sex partner with genital herpes

HSV serologic testing should be considered for AYAs requesting an STI evaluation (especially for persons with multiple sexual partners), persons with HIV infection, and MSM at increased risk of HIV infection. HSV-1 or HSV-2 screening in the general population is not indicated.[5]

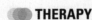 **THERAPY**

Principles of Genital Herpes Management

Counseling regarding the natural history of genital herpes, sexual and perinatal transmission, and methods to reduce transmission is integral to management. Antiviral chemotherapy offers clinical benefits to most persons with symptomatic infections or when used as daily suppressive therapy.[5]

Systemic antiviral drugs partially control the symptoms and signs of herpes episodes when used to treat first clinical episodes and recurrent episodes or when used as daily suppressive therapy. However, these drugs neither eradicate latent virus nor affect the risk, frequency, or severity of recurrences once the drug is discontinued. Randomized trials indicate that three antiviral medications provide clinical benefit for genital herpes—acyclovir, valacyclovir, and famciclovir.[5] Topical therapy with antivirals for genital HSV offers minimal clinical benefit and is not recommended.[5]

First Clinical Episode of Genital Herpes

Although AYAs with first-episode herpes may present with mild clinical manifestations, severe or prolonged symptoms can develop.

The Centers for Disease Control and Prevention (CDC)-recommended regimens for first clinical episodes include[5]:

Acyclovir 400 mg orally three times a day for 7 to 10 days, OR
Acyclovir 200 mg orally five times a day for 7 to 10 days, OR
Valacyclovir 1 g orally twice a day for 7 to 10 days, OR
Famciclovir 250 mg orally three times a day for 7 to 10 days
Treatment may be extended if healing is incomplete after 10 days of therapy.

Suppressive Therapy for Recurrent Genital Herpes

Suppressive therapy greatly reduces the frequency of genital herpes recurrences, even among those who have infrequent outbreaks, and decreases the risk for genital HSV transmission to susceptible partners.[13] Quality of life is often improved in patients with frequent recurrences who receive suppressive compared to episodic treatment. The frequency of recurrent outbreaks diminishes over time in many patients, and the patient's psychological adjustment to the disease may change. Therefore, the need to continue therapy should be discussed periodically during suppressive

treatment (e.g., once a year).[5] Ease of administration and cost also are important considerations for prolonged treatment.

The CDC-recommended regimens (www.cdc.gov/std/treatment) for suppressive therapy include:

Acyclovir 400 mg orally twice a day, OR
Valacyclovir 500 mg orally once a day*, OR
Valacyclovir 1 g orally once a day, OR
Famciclovir 250 mg orally twice a day.
*Valacyclovir 500 mg once a day might be less effective than other valacyclovir or acyclovir dosing regimens in persons who have very frequent recurrences (i.e., ≥10 episodes/year).

Episodic Therapy for Recurrent Genital Herpes

Effective episodic treatment of recurrent herpes requires therapy initiation within 1 day of lesion onset, or during the prodrome that precedes some outbreaks.[5] In those with known genital infection, a supply of drug or a prescription can be provided with instructions to self-initiate treatment immediately when symptoms begin.

The CDC-recommended regimens for episodic therapy include[5]:

Acyclovir 400 mg orally three times a day for 5 days, OR
Acyclovir 800 mg orally twice a day for 5 days, OR
Acyclovir 800 mg orally three times a day for 2 days, OR
Valacyclovir 500 mg orally twice a day for 3 days, OR
Valacyclovir 1 g orally once a day for 5 days, OR
Famciclovir 125 mg orally twice a day for 5 days, OR
Famciclovir 1,000 mg orally twice daily for 1 day, OR
Famciclovir 500 mg orally once followed by 250 mg twice daily for 2 days.

Management of Sex Partners

The sex partners of adolescents or young adults who have genital herpes likely benefit from evaluation and counseling. Symptomatic sex partners should be evaluated and treated in the same manner as persons who have genital lesions. Asymptomatic sex partners of patients who have genital herpes should be questioned concerning past genital lesions and offered HSV type-specific serologic testing.

PREVENTION COUNSELING

Below are counseling messages that should be provided to AYAs diagnosed with genital HSV.

1. HSV sexual transmission can occur during asymptomatic periods. Persons with active lesions or prodromal symptoms should abstain from intercourse with uninfected partners until the lesions are clearly healed.
2. Since viral shedding can occur in the absence of lesions, consistent and correct condom use should be recommended to any person who has had a genital herpes episode. Male latex condoms can reduce, but not eliminate, the risk of HSV.[14]
3. HSV-2 discordant couples should be encouraged to consider suppressive antiviral therapy as part of a strategy to prevent transmission, in addition to consistent condom use and avoidance of sexual activity during recurrences. These recommendations may also be given to symptomatic persons with multiple partners, to those who are HSV-2 seropositive without a history of genital herpes, and to MSM.
4. Many patients newly diagnosed with HSV develop psychological distress due to shame, stigma, and having to live with an incurable infection that could substantially interfere with future relationships. Providers can address these concerns by encouraging patients to recognize that herpes is a manageable condition by (1) giving information, (2) providing support resources, and (3) helping define treatment options.
5. Since a genital herpes diagnosis may affect perceptions about existing or future sexual relationships, it is important for patients to understand how to talk to sexual partners about STIs.

COMPLICATIONS

1. Significant psychological distress: Initially, denial, shock, fear, guilt, feelings of social isolation, and anger are common. Anxiety and depression also occur and may persist. Some persons have concerns about how herpes will impact their future sex life and relationships. There can be considerable embarrassment, shame, and stigma associated with a herpes diagnosis and this can substantially interfere with a patient's relationships.

2. Local complications: Secondary bacterial infection of lesions, phimosis (males) or labial adhesions (females), urinary retention, constipation, and impotence. Sacral radiculopathy can also occur, causing paresthesias in the lower extremities.

3. Proctitis can occur in persons who participate in receptive anal intercourse. Presenting complaints may include rectal bleeding, mucoid discharge, constipation, tenesmus, fever, and, occasionally, impotence.

4. Herpes keratitis is predominantly associated with HSV-1 infection.

5. Encephalitis is typically associated with oral HSV-1 infection and aseptic meningitis is typically associated with genital HSV-2 infection.

6. Most mothers of infants who acquire neonatal herpes lack histories of clinically evident genital herpes.

ACKNOWLEDGMENTS

We would like to acknowledge Elissa Meites for her assistance with references and editorial changes.

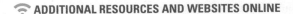 ADDITIONAL RESOURCES AND WEBSITES ONLINE

REFERENCES

1. Ryder N, Jin F, McNulty AM, et al. Increasing role of herpes simplex virus type 1 in first-episode anogenital herpes in heterosexual women and younger men who have sex with men, 1992–2006. *Sex Transm Infect* 2009;85:416–419.
2. Bernstein DI, Bellamy AR, Hook EW III, et al. Epidemiology, clinical presentation, and antibody response to primary infection with herpes simplex virus type 1 and type 2 in young women. *Clin Infect Dis* 2013;56:344–351.
3. Bradley H, Markowitz LE, Gibson T, et al. Seroprevalence of herpes simplex virus types 1 and 2—United States, 1999–2010. *J Infect Dis* 2014;209:325–333.
4. Xu F, Sternberg MR, Gottlieb SL, et al. Seroprevalence of herpes simplex virus type 2 among persons aged 14–49 Years—United States, 2005–2008. *MMWR* 2010;59:456–459. Available at www.cdc.gov/mmwr/preview/mmwrhtml/mm5915a3.htm. Accessed March 12, 2014.
5. Centers for Disease Control and Prevention. Sexually Transmitted Diseases Treatment Guidelines, 2015. *MMWR Recomm Rep* 2015;64(RR-3):27–32. Available at http://www.cdc.gov/std/tg2015/herpes.htm. Accessed June 20, 2015.
6. Tobian AA, Grabowski MK, Serwadda D, et al. Reactivation of herpes simplex virus type 2 after initiation of antiretroviral therapy. *J Infect Dis* 2013;208:839–846.
7. Mujugira A, Magaret AS, Celum C, et al. Daily acyclovir to decrease herpes simplex virus type 2 (HSV-2) transmission from HSV-2/HIV-1 coinfected persons: a randomized controlled trial. *J Infect Dis* 2013;208:1366–1374.
8. Celum C, Wald A, Lingappa JR, et al. Acyclovir and transmission of HIV-1 from person infected with HIV-1 and HSV-2. *N Engl J Med* 2010;362:427–439.
9. Wald A, Ericsson M, Krantz E, et al. Oral shedding of herpes simplex virus type 2. *Sex Transm Infect* 2004;80:272–276.
10. Corey L, Wald A. Genital herpes. In: Holmes KK, Sparling PF, Mardh PA, et al, eds. *Sexually transmitted diseases*. 4th ed. New York, NY: McGraw-Hill, 2008: 399–438.
11. Ngo TD, Laeyendecker O, Morrow RA, et al. Comparison of three commercial immunoassays for detection of herpes simplex virus type 2 antibodies in commercial sex workers in Yunnan Province, China. *Clin Vaccine Immunol* 2008;15:1301–1303.
12. Morrow RA, Friedrich D, Meier A, et al. Use of "biokit HSV-2 rapid assay" to improve the positive predictive value of Focus HerpeSelect HSV-2 ELISA. *BMC Infect Dis* 2005;5:84.
13. Corey L, Wald A, Patel R, et al. Once-daily valacyclovir to reduce the risk of transmission of genital herpes. *N Engl J Med* 2004;350:11–20.
14. Martin ET, Krantz E, Gottlieb SL, et al. A pooled analysis of the effect of condoms in preventing HSV-2 acquisition. *Arch Intern Med* 2009;169:1233–1240.

61 Human Papillomavirus Infection and Anogenital Warts

Shelly T. Ben-Harush Negari
Jessica A. Kahn

KEY WORDS

- Anogenital warts
- External genital warts
- Human papillomavirus
- Human papillomavirus vaccines
- Management
- Oral human papillomavirus
- Sexually transmitted infection
- Treatment

HUMAN PAPILLOMAVIRUS GENOTYPES AND CLINICAL SEQUELAE

Human papillomaviruses (HPVs) are small, nonenveloped, double-stranded DNA viruses of the Papillomaviridae family. More than 40 HPV types have been identified that infect the anogenital and oropharyngeal mucosa.[1] Genital HPV types are classified as low risk and high risk.[2] Low-risk types (e.g., HPV-6 and -11) may cause anogenital warts, mild vulvar intraepithelial neoplasia (VIN), vaginal intraepithelial neoplasia (VAIN), cervical intraepithelial neoplasia (CIN), penile intraepithelial neoplasia (PIN), and anal intraepithelial neoplasia (AIN). Vertical transmission of low-risk types from mother to child during delivery rarely may cause recurrent respiratory papillomatosis (RRP) in young children. High-risk types (e.g., HPV-16 and -18) may cause mild, moderate, or severe VIN, VAIN, CIN, PIN, and AIN; vulvar, vaginal, cervical, penile, and anal cancers; and oropharyngeal cancer.[3]

Epidemiology

Prevalence

At least 80% of sexually active adult men and women in the US have been exposed to genital HPV types at some point in their lives. The prevalence of HPV infection peaks during adolescence and young adulthood. In a nationally representative sample of US women, 20% of 14- to 17-year-olds, 38% of 18- to 21-year-olds, and 42% of 22- to 25-year-olds were positive for genital HPV.[4] Prevalence rates in men are similar to those in women. Cross-sectional prevalence rates for oral HPV range widely, from approximately 2% to 20% in studies of adolescents and young adults (AYAs).[5] The prevalence rate of symptomatic anogenital warts among US adults is estimated to be 1% to 5%, but rates up to 40% have been reported in patients presenting to sexually transmitted infection (STI) clinics. A population-based study in Sweden demonstrated that among 1,045,157 women, the crude incidence rate of condyloma was 528 per 100,000 person-years in unvaccinated individuals, and 138 per 100,000 person-years in fully vaccinated individuals.[6] The prevalence of RRP is approximately four cases per 100,000 in children.[7]

Transmission

In AYAs, HPV transmission occurs primarily through sexual contact, including genital–genital, oral–genital, and digital–genital contact. AYAs acquire HPV infection rapidly after sexual initiation, often within a few months.[8] Women who have sex only with women are also at risk for HPV infection and CIN.[9]

Risk Factors

Increased number of sexual partners, early age of sexual initiation, inconsistent condom use, cigarette smoking (also a cofactor in cervical carcinogenesis), immunosuppression, cervical ectopy, and history of genital warts and other STIs.

Pathophysiology and Natural History of HPV Infection

HPV initially infects the basal layer of epithelial cells through microabrasions in the skin or mucosa. Infected cells migrate to the suprabasal layers, where viral gene expression, viral replication, and particle formation occur. Although HPV infection is extremely common in AYAs, the vast majority of infections do not progress to anogenital warts, precancers, or cancer.[10]

Clinical Manifestations

Types of Anogenital Warts

1. Condylomata acuminata: Exophytic growths with a granular, irregular surface and finger-like projections. They usually have highly vascular cores that produce punctuated or loop-like patterns unless obscured by overlying keratinized surfaces (Figs. 61.1 and 61.2).
2. Papular warts: Smooth, skin-colored, well-circumscribed papules that are usually 1 to 4 mm in diameter and have a round, slightly hyperkeratotic or smooth surface (Fig. 61.3).
3. Keratotic warts: These have a thick, horny (crust-like) layer; they resemble common warts or seborrheic keratoses (Fig. 61.4).
4. Flat-topped macules: These are subclinical lesions that are difficult to detect without techniques such as treatment with a weak acetic acid solution.

Location

Typical sites for anogenital warts in women include the cervix, vagina, vulva, urethra, and anus. Typical sites in men include the inner surface of the prepuce, frenulum, corona, penile shaft, glans, scrotum, and anus. Condylomata can be multifocal or multicentric. Condylomata acuminata tend to occur on partially keratinized, non–hair-bearing ("moist") skin; keratotic and papular warts tend

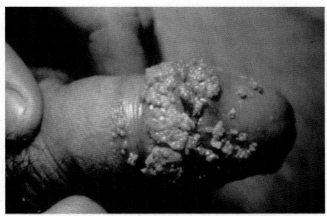

FIGURE 61.1 Condylomata acuminata (penis). (From Goodheart HP. *Goodheart's photoguide to common skin disorders: diagnosis and management.* 3rd ed. Philadelphia, PA: Lippincott Williams & Wilkins, 2009.)

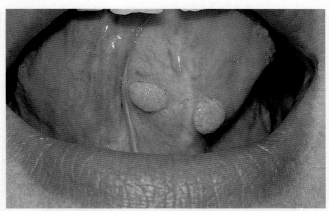

FIGURE 61.3 Papular warts (tongue). (From *Lippincott Williams & Wilkins' comprehensive dental assisting.* Philadelphia, PA: Lippincott Williams & Wilkins, 2011.)

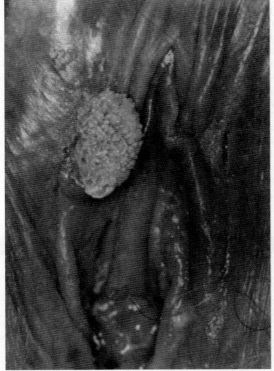

FIGURE 61.2 Condylomata acuminata (vaginal introitus). (From Wilkinson EJ, Stone IK. *Atlas of vulvar disease.* Baltimore, MD: Williams & Wilkins, 1994, Figure 17.9a.)

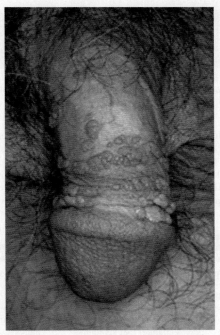

FIGURE 61.4 Keratotic warts (penis). (From Edwards L, Lynch PJ. *Genital dermatology atlas.* 2nd ed. Philadelphia, PA: Lippincott Williams & Wilkins, 2010.)

to occur on fully keratinized (hair-bearing or non–hair-bearing) skin; and flat-topped warts may occur on either skin surface.

Color
Pink, red, tan, brown, or gray.

Symptoms
Usually asymptomatic but may cause pruritus, burning, pain, urethral or vaginal discharge, urethral bleeding, or postcoital bleeding.

Exacerbating Factors
Pregnancy, skin moisture, and/or vaginal or urethral discharge.

Clinical Course
Lesions usually appear 2 to 3 months after infection, with a range of approximately 3 weeks to 8 months.[11] Warts may regress

spontaneously, persist, or increase in size or number. Over a period of months to years, most anogenital warts resolve.

Differential Diagnosis
The differential diagnosis for anogenital warts includes micropapillomatosis labialis of the labia minora, pearly penile papules, seborrheic keratosis, other benign genital lesions (skin tags, fibromas, lipomas, hidradenomas, and adenomas), condylomata lata (secondary syphilis) (see Fig. 61.5), molluscum contagiosum, granuloma inguinale, and high-grade intraepithelial lesions and cancer (Bowen disease, Bowenoid papulosis, dysplastic nevi, VIN, VAIN, PIN, AIN, and squamous cell carcinoma).

Diagnosis
Subclinical HPV Infection
HPV detection methods can be categorized generally as target amplification methods such as polymerase chain reaction, and signal amplification methods.[12] In the US, HPV DNA testing is generally

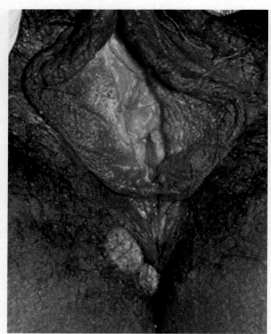

FIGURE 61.5 Condylomata lata (perineum). (From Edwards L, Lynch PJ. *Genital dermatology atlas.* 2nd ed. Philadelphia, PA: Lippincott Williams & Wilkins, 2010.)

recommended only in the context of cervical cancer screening for women ≥25 years of age to guide further management (i.e., reflex HPV testing for women with a cytologic test demonstrating atypical squamous cells of undetermined significance, and as a "cotesting" strategy with cytologic testing for women 30 to 65 years of age), as discussed in more detail in Chapter 50.[13]

Genital Warts

Genital warts can usually be diagnosed using direct visual inspection with a bright light and, if necessary, magnification.[14] A speculum examination is helpful in women with external genital warts to evaluate for vaginal and cervical warts. An otoscope and small spreader are helpful to inspect the male urinary meatus. Anoscopy should be considered for immunosuppressed men and women with recurrent perianal warts and a history of anoreceptive intercourse, and urethroscopy should be considered for men with gross hematuria or an altered urinary stream. Acetowhite testing, HPV DNA testing, and biopsy are not recommended routinely for diagnosis. However, patients with anogenital warts who are not responsive to therapy or have features suggestive of neoplasia (e.g., blue or black discoloration, induration, bleeding, ulceration, increased pigmentation, rapid growth, or fixation to underlying structures) should be referred to a specialist for further evaluation and possible biopsy.

Treatment

General Considerations

The goal of therapy is to eradicate or reduce the size of clinically apparent anogenital warts in order to ameliorate clinical symptoms or cosmetic concerns.[14,15] However, it is reasonable not to begin treatment unless the warts persist or enlarge because anogenital warts may resolve spontaneously and it is not clear whether treatment of anogenital warts alters the natural history of the infection or decreases future viral transmission. Treatment should be guided by the patient's preferences, extent and type of lesion, the provider's experience, and available resources.

Treatments for external genital warts are classified as patient-applied or clinician-applied. Patient-applied therapies require that the patient can adequately visualize the lesions to be treated and can adhere to the specified treatment schedule. There is no definitive evidence that any one treatment is more effective than another. Treatment strategies are presented in **Table 61.1**. If one treatment strategy fails, another may be tried. However, if anogenital warts

---

TABLE 61.1

Recommended Treatment Options for External Genital Warts

Treatment Option	Mechanism of Action	Instructions for Use	Advantages	Disadvantages
Patient-applied				
Imiquimod 3.75% or 5% cream	Topically active immune enhancer that stimulates production of interferon	The cream is provided in individual packets. Apply the 3.75% cream every night for up to 8 wk, or the 5% cream three times per week for up to 16 wk, until all lesions have disappeared. Both are left on overnight (6–10 h), then washed off with soap and water. Wash off before sexual intercourse.	May be applied at home. Can be applied to new warts as they appear	Local erythema, erosion, itching, and burning; rarely, may worsen autoimmune skin disorders. May weaken condoms/diaphragms. Takes up to 16 wk to treat. Safety during pregnancy has not been established.
Synecatechins 15% ointment (Polyphenon E)	Botanical quantified extract from green tea leaves consisting of more than 85% catechins—an active ingredient that exhibits specific antioxidant, antiviral, antitumor and, immunostimulatory properties	Apply 0.5-cm strand of ointment to each wart using a finger to ensure coverage with a thin layer of ointment until complete clearance of warts. Use three times daily for a maximum of 16 wk.	May be applied at home	May cause erythema, pruritus/burning, pain, ulceration, edema, induration, and vesicular rash. May weaken condoms/diaphragms. Sexual contact should be avoided while the ointment is on the skin. Not recommended for immunocompromised persons or those with clinical genital herpes. Safety during pregnancy is unknown.

(Continued)

TABLE 61.1

Recommended Treatment Options for External Genital Warts (*Continued*)

Treatment Option	Mechanism of Action	Instructions for Use	Advantages	Disadvantages
Podophyllotoxin/ podofilox 0.5% solution or gel	Antimitotic	Using a cotton swab for the solution or a finger for the gel, apply to genital warts twice daily for 3 d, followed by 4 d of no therapy. The cycle can be repeated up to four times if needed. Total wart area treated should not exceed 10 cm^2, and total volume of podofilox should not exceed 0.5 mL/d.	Widely available Inexpensive Easy to apply May be applied at home	May cause local erosion, burning, pain, and itching Not useful for cervical or mucosal lesions or extensive disease Safety during pregnancy has not been established
Clinician-applied				
Trichloroacetic acid (TCA) or bichloracetic acid (BCA) 80%–90%	Caustic agent—chemical coagulations of proteins	Provider first applies occlusive ointment to the healthy tissue surrounding lesion, or treats the area with a topical anesthetic (e.g., benzocaine topical solution). The back or front end of a cotton swab is used to apply the solution sparingly until the lesions blanch (frost). The solution should air-dry before the patient resumes a normal position. If necessary, sodium bicarbonate, soap, or talc may be applied to remove unreacted acid. Avoid contact with normal skin. Repeat weekly for up to 6 wk until warts have resolved.	Inexpensive Easy to apply Safe in pregnancy	Destroys normal tissue if overapplied
Cryotherapy with liquid nitrogen or cryoprobe	Thermal-induced cytolysis	Liquid nitrogen can be used to treat vaginal warts, but use of a cryoprobe is not recommended because of the risk of vaginal perforation or fistula formation. A cotton applicator designed for cryotherapy is placed in liquid nitrogen briefly and then quickly applied with gentle pressure for 2–3 sec to the wart to be treated as well as 2–3 mm of surrounding skin. The surface of the wart should briefly turn white and then return to its normal color. Process can be repeated every 1–2 wk.	Well tolerated Safe in pregnancy No anesthesia needed Minimal risk of scarring	May cause pain, necrosis, blistering Overapplication may lead to complications, while underapplication may lead to poor results
Surgical procedures		These procedures may include excision with a scalpel, curettage, or scissors; electrosurgery; and laser therapy.	Useful for extensive disease, intraurethral warts, or lesions resistant to other therapies Safe in pregnancy Rapid resolution of condylomata	Requires hospital setting, provider expertise, appropriate equipment, and anesthesia Expensive With surgical excision, scarring and bleeding are possible Laser is not readily available, and intact DNA may be liberated into the air with laser

persist, then patients should be referred to a specialist. The use of more than one treatment modality at the same time has not been shown to be effective and may increase the risk of side effects. Risk factors for long-term wart persistence include host immunosuppression, infection with a high-risk HPV type, and older patient age.[11] Partner evaluation is valuable if feasible, in that it provides an opportunity for the clinician to screen partners for anogenital warts and other STIs and to educate partners about HPV and genital warts.

Specific Treatment Recommendations and Considerations (www.cdc.gov/std/treatment)

- *Patient-applied treatments* for external genital warts (**Table 61.1**) include Imiquimod 3.75% or 5% cream, Podophyllotoxin/podofilox 0.5% solution or gel, and Synecatechins 15% ointment. If possible, the provider should apply the first treatment to demonstrate both the application technique and the warts to be treated.

- *Clinician-applied treatments for* external genital warts (**Table 61.1**) include bichloracetic acid (BCA) or trichloroacetic acid (TCA) 80% to 90% solution, cryotherapy with liquid nitrogen or cryoprobe, and surgical therapies including carbon dioxide laser therapy.
- *Treatment by location:* Patients with cervical warts may be treated with cryotherapy with liquid nitrogen or with TCA or BCA 80% to 90%, but should be managed with a specialist. Patients with vaginal warts may be treated using cryotherapy with liquid nitrogen (but not a cryoprobe due to a risk of perforation), TCA/BCA 80% to 90%, or surgical removal. Patients with urethral meatus warts may be treated using cryotherapy with liquid nitrogen or surgical removal. Intra-anal warts may be treated using cryotherapy with liquid nitrogen, TCA/BCA 80% to 90%, or surgical removal. They should be managed in consultation with a specialist. Finally, oral warts may be treated with cryotherapy or surgical removal.
- *Treatment in patients with special conditions:*
  a. Pregnancy: Several factors associated with pregnancy, such as hormonal factors and relative immunosuppression, may promote growth of anogenital warts. The only treatments recommended during pregnancy are BCA/TCA, cryotherapy, electrocautery, and surgical excision. Cesarean delivery is indicated for women with genital warts if the pelvic outlet is obstructed or if vaginal delivery would result in excessive bleeding; a cesarean delivery should not be performed solely to prevent transmission of HPV to the newborn.
  b. Immunosuppression: AYAs who are immunosuppressed due to HIV infection, organ transplantation, or other conditions may have more extensive genital warts, may not respond to treatment as well as immunocompetent adolescents, and may have more frequent recurrences. In addition, squamous cell carcinomas originating in or resembling genital warts occur more frequently among immunocompromised patients. Therefore, evaluation by a specialist should be considered.

Counseling

Clinicians should educate patients with anogenital warts about HPV infection, its transmission, and its clinical consequences. Key messages are as follows: Genital warts are caused by specific HPV types that are usually different from the types that cause cervical cancer; genital warts may recur after treatment; it is unclear whether treatment reduces transmission of HPV to partners; condom use may reduce transmission of HPV and acquisition of genital warts but is not fully protective against transmission of HPV; during treatment AYAs should avoid sexual activity; and HPV infection does not affect fertility. Clinicians should provide information about available treatment options for genital warts, their prognosis, and strategies to prevent HPV-related disease and other STIs (for example, abstinence, limiting number of sexual partners, avoiding tobacco, and using condoms consistently). It is not necessary to perform Pap testing more frequently in those with genital warts.

Clinicians should make sure that patients being treated for external genital warts can see their warts, especially those who are using patient-applied therapies. Patients should be advised to examine the areas being treated for signs of inflammation or infection (such as redness, swelling, or discharge) regularly and report these immediately to the clinician. General perineal care may promote healing, including sitz baths and keeping the area clean and dry. During treatment and after visible warts have resolved, follow-up visits are helpful to monitor for complications of therapy, educate AYAs about signs of recurrence, and reiterate prevention messages. The diagnosis of HPV infection or genital warts may cause anxiety, distress, and fear of social stigmatization in AYAs.[16] Clinicians should provide support and when necessary may refer patients to support groups or for individual counseling.

HPV Vaccines

Prophylactic HPV vaccines consist of virus-like particles, which are recombinant viral capsids that are identical to HPV virions morphologically, but do not contain viral DNA. Therefore, they cannot replicate and pose no infectious or oncogenic risk. They are highly effective in preventing infection with the HPV types targeted by the vaccines, and with precancers associated with those HPV types.[17-20] The three licensed vaccines are an HPV-16, 18 vaccine (HPV-2; Cervarix, GlaxoSmithKline), an HPV-6, 11, 16, 18 vaccine (HPV-4; Gardasil, Merck & Co., Inc.), and a recently approved HPV-6, 11, 16, 18, 31, 33, 45, 52, 58 vaccine (Gardasil 9; Merck and Co., Inc). Clinical trials, as well as post-marketing surveillance for the HPV-2 and HPV-4 vaccines, have demonstrated that they are safe and well tolerated. As more than 90% of genital warts are caused by HPV-6 and/or HPV-11, approximately 70% of cervical cancers are caused by HPV-16 and/or HPV-18, approximately 90% of cervical cancers are caused by the genotypes targeted by the HPV-9 vaccine, and approximately 90% of anal cancers are caused by HPV-16 and/or HPV-18, these vaccines are expected to have a significant public health impact. The Advisory Committee on Immunization Practices of the US Centers for Disease Control and Prevention recommends routine HPV vaccination on a schedule of 0, 1 to 2, and 6 months for all adolescents 11 to 12 years of age.[21,22] Either the HPV-2, HPV-4, or HPV-9 may be used for females, but only HPV-4 and HPV-9 may be used for males. The vaccine series may be started as early as age 9 years. Catch-up vaccination is recommended for girls and women 13 to 26 years of age (with either HPV-2, HPV-4, or HPV-9) and for boys and men 13 to 21 years of age (with HPV-4 or HPV-9) if not previously vaccinated. Vaccination with HPV-4 or HPV-9 is also recommended for men 22 to 26 years of age at high risk for HPV. HPV vaccines are not recommended for use in pregnant women. Vaccination is not contraindicated for those who have a history of sexual activity, anogenital warts, or HIV infection. If clinicians do not know which vaccine a patient received previously, does not have it available, or is in a setting transitioning to the HPV-9 vaccine, either the HPV-2, HPV-4, or HPV-9 vaccine may be used to continue or complete the series for females, and either the HPV-4 or HPV-9 vaccine may be used to continue or complete the series for males.

To maximize HPV vaccine uptake, clinicians should utilize key messages that drive parents' and AYAs' decisions about vaccination. These messages should include the following: the clinician strongly supports vaccination; HPV vaccines are safe, effective, and should prevent most HPV-associated anogenital cancers; HPV is very common and adolescents are often infected soon after sexual initiation; it is important to vaccinate girls and boys before they are exposed to HPV; and it is important to complete the vaccine series.[23-26] Clinicians can reassure parents that evidence has shown that vaccination does not lead to riskier sexual behaviors.[27] AYAs should understand that HPV vaccines do not prevent STIs other than HPV, and that Pap testing is still recommended after vaccination.

REFERENCES

1. de Villiers EM, Fauquet C, Broker TR, et al. Classification of papillomaviruses. *Virology* 2004;324:17–27.
2. Kahn JA. HPV vaccination for the prevention of cervical intraepithelial neoplasia. *N Engl J Med* 2009;361:271–278.
3. Munoz N, Castellsague X, Berrington de Gonzalez A, et al. Chapter 1: HPV in the etiology of human cancer. *Vaccine* 2006;24 (suppl 3):1–10.
4. Kahn JA, Lan D, Kahn RS. Sociodemographic factors associated with high-risk HPV infection. *Obstet Gynecol* 2007;110:87–95.
5. Kahn JA, Rudy B, Xu J et al. Behavioral, immunologic, and virologic correlates of oral human papillomavirus infection in HIV-infected adolescents. *Sex Transm Dis* 2015;42(5):246–252.
6. Herweijer E, Leval A, Ploner A et al. Association of varying number of doses of quadrivalent human papillomavirus vaccine with incidence of condyloma. *JAMA* 2014;311:597–603.
7. Larson DA, Derkay CS. Epidemiology of recurrent respiratory papillomatosis. *APMIS* 2010;118:450–454.
8. Winer RL, Feng Q, Hughes JP, et al. Risk of female human papillomavirus acquisition associated with first male sex partner. *J Infect Dis* 2008;197:279–282.
9. Marrazzo JM, Steine K, Koutsky LA. Genital human papillomavirus infection in women who have sex with women: a review. *Am J Obstet Gynecol* 2000;183:770–774.

10. Brown DR, Shew ML, Qadadri B. A longitudinal study of genital human papillomavirus infection in a cohort of closely followed adolescent women. *J Infect Dis* 2005;191:182–192.
11. Yanofsky VR, Patel RV, Goldenberg G. Genital warts: a comprehensive review. *J Clin Aesthet Dermatol* 2012;5:25–36.
12. Snijders PJ, Heideman DA, Meijer CJ. APMIS. Methods for HPV detection in exfoliated cell and tissue specimens. *APMIS* 2010;118:520–528.
13. Saslow D, Solomon D, Lawson HW. American Cancer Society, American Society for Colposcopy and Cervical Pathology, and American Society for Clinical Pathology screening guidelines for the prevention and early detection of cervical cancer. *J Low Genit Tract Dis* 2012;62:47–72.
14. Workowski KA, Bolan GA. Sexually Transmitted Diseases Treatment Guidelines, 2015. *MMWR Recomm Rep* 2015;64(RR3):1–137.
15. Tzellos TG1, Sardeli C, Lallas A, et al. Efficacy, safety and tolerability of green tea catechins in the treatment of external anogenital warts: a systematic review and meta-analysis. *J Eur Acad Dermatol Venereol* 2011;25:345–353.
16. Drolet M, Brisson M, Maunsell E, et al. The impact of anogenital warts on health related quality of life: a 6 month prospective study. *Sex Transm Dis* 2011;38:949–956.
17. Harper DM, Franco EL, Wheeler C, et al. Efficacy of a bivalent L1 virus-like particle vaccine in prevention of infection with human papillomavirus types 16 and 18 in young women: a randomised controlled trial. *Lancet* 2004;364:1757–1765.
18. Garland SM, Hernandez-Avila M, Wheeler CM, et al. Quadrivalent vaccine against human papillomavirus to prevent anogenital disease. *N Engl J Med* 2007;356:1928–1943.
19. Koutsky LA; FUTURE II Study Group. Quadrivalent vaccine against human papillomavirus to prevent high-grade cervical lesions. *N Engl J Med* 2007;356:1915–1927.
20. Villa LL, Costa RL, Petta CA et al. Prophylactic quadrivalent human papillomavirus (types 6, 11, 16, and 18) L1 virus-like particle vaccine in young women: a randomised double-blind placebo-controlled multicentre phase II efficacy trial. *Lancet Oncol* 2005;6:271–278.
21. Centers for Disease Control and Prevention (CDC). FDA licensure of quadrivalent human papillomavirus vaccine (HPV4, Gardasil) for use in males and guidance from the Advisory Committee on Immunization Practices (ACIP). *MMWR* 2010;59:630–632.
22. Centers for Disease Control and Prevention. FDA licensure of bivalent human papillomavirus vaccine (HPV2, Cervarix) for use in females and updated HPV vaccination recommendations from the Advisory Committee on Immunization Practices (ACIP). *MMWR* 2010;59:626–629.
23. Kahn JA, Rosenthal SL, Tissot AM, et al. Factors influencing pediatricians' intention to recommend HPV vaccines. *Ambul Pediatr* 2007;7:367–373.
24. Kahn JA, Cooper HP, Vadaprampil S, et al. HPV vaccine recommendations and agreement with mandated HPV vaccination for 11–12 year-old girls: a state-wide survey of Texas physicians. *Cancer Epidem Bio Prev* 2009;18:2325–2332.
25. Kahn JA, Ding L, Huang B, et al. Mothers' intention for their daughters and themselves to receive the human papillomavirus vaccine: a national study of nurses. *Pediatrics* 2009;123:1439–1445.
26. Griffioen AM, Glynn S, Mullins TK, et al. Perspectives on decision-making about HPV vaccination among 11–12 year old girls and their mothers. *Clin Pediatr* 2012;51:560–568.
27. Mayhew A, Mullins TLK, Ding L, et al. Risk perceptions and subsequent sexual behaviors after HPV vaccination in adolescents. *Pediatrics* 2014;133(3):404–411. doi:10.1542/peds.2013-2822.

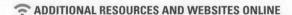 **ADDITIONAL RESOURCES AND WEBSITES ONLINE**

62

Other Sexually Transmitted Infections Including Genital Ulcers, Pediculosis, Scabies, and Molluscum

Wendi G. Ehrman
Mandakini Sadhir
M. Susan Jay

KEY WORDS

- Buboes
- Chancroid
- Genital ulcers
- Granuloma inguinale
- Lymphogranuloma venereum
- Molluscum
- Pubic lice
- Scabies

Chancroid, lymphogranuloma venereum (LGV), and granuloma inguinale constitute the classic minor ulcerative sexually transmitted infections (STIs) and should be considered in the differential diagnosis of genital ulcers (see **Table 62.1**). In the US, the most common causative agent of genital ulcers is the herpes simplex virus (HSV), followed by syphilis. Approximately 3% to 10% of these patients will have more than one infection. There is also an increased risk of human immunodeficiency virus (HIV) infection associated with these ulcerative infections.[1] Other potentially sexually transmissible minor infections include scabies, pediculosis, and molluscum contagiosum.

CHANCROID

Etiology

Chancroid is caused by the gram-negative facultative anaerobic coccobacillus, *Haemophilus ducreyi*.[2]

Epidemiology

This disease is uncommon in the US. According to Centers for Disease Control and Prevention (CDC), chancroid in the US has fallen dramatically from 4,212 cases in 1990 to only 10 cases in 2013.[3] While the reduction in cases is striking, the CDC is concerned that this may in part be related to the difficulty in culturing the causative agent. Worldwide, the highest prevalence of infection is in southern, central, and eastern Africa. In the US, 8 of the 10 cases were in the southern states of California (6), Texas (1), and Alabama (1); 6 cases were in males and 4 in females. Chancroid is a known risk factor for HIV and enhances disease transmission. Co-infection with syphilis or herpes simplex may also occur.[4]

Clinical Manifestations

The incubation period is generally 3 to 10 days. Classically, chancroid presents as a tender inflammatory papule on the genitalia that becomes pustular and then ulcerates in 1 to 2 days. The characteristic ulcer is painful, soft, friable, and nonindurated with ragged undermined margins, a granulomatous base, and a foul-smelling yellow or gray, necrotic purulent exudate (**Fig. 62.1**). Males may present with inguinal pain or ulcers located on the prepuce, coronal sulcus, or frenulum. In females, multiple lesions may be present on the vulva, clitoris, cervix, or perianal region. Females may be asymptomatic or present with dysuria, dyspareunia, vaginal discharge, pain with defecation, and rectal bleeding. Rarely, extragenital sites may be involved (breasts, thighs, fingers, and mouth[5]).

Painful unilateral inguinal lymphadenitis—known as a *bubo*—develops in as many as 50% of patients and may become suppurative, rupture, and ulcerate. Large inguinal abscesses can occur, leading to significant destruction of skin and soft tissue.[5]

Diagnosis

Probable diagnosis of chancroid can be made using CDC criteria (**Table 62.1**). Accuracy of clinical diagnosis ranges from 33% to 80%. Direct examination of Gram-stained ulcer material or aspirate from an infected lymph node (bubo) may show gram-negative coccobacilli arranged in parallel short chains described as "schools of fish." However, Gram stain has poor sensitivity and specificity and should not be used alone for diagnosis. Culture is the "gold standard" for diagnosis, with a sensitivity of 35% to 75% and specificity of 94% to 100%. Culture material may be obtained from genital ulcers or buboes, although intact buboes tend to be sterile. Laboratories should be notified in advance for receipt of the specimens.[5,6] Immunodiagnostic DNA probes and DNA amplification tests (multiplex polymerase chain reaction) can be performed by commercial laboratories that have developed their own polymerase chain reaction (PCR) test.

Treatment

Treatment is outlined in **Table 62.2**.

Other Management Considerations

Clinical improvement should be seen within 3 to 7 days. Failure to improve should raise the possibility of an incorrect diagnosis or co-infection with another STI such as HIV. Large ulcers may require more than 2 weeks to resolve; fluctuant lymphadenopathy heals even more slowly. Adenopathy may progress to fluctuation despite successful therapy and does not represent treatment failure.

LYMPHOGRANULOMA VENEREUM

Etiology

LGV is caused by the obligate intracellular organism *Chlamydia trachomatis*. Chlamydia has 18 serovars associated with disease; serovars L_1, L_2, and L_3 cause LGV. LGV strains can cause a systemic infection that, if untreated, can lead to colorectal fistulas and

TABLE 62.1

Differential Diagnosis of Genital Ulcers[1,7]

Infection	Clinical Manifestation	Diagnosis

Chancroid
Cause: *H. ducreyi*
	• Painful, shallow, friable, nonindurated genital ulcer with ragged undermined margins, granulomatous base, and foul-smelling yellow or gray, necrotic purulent exudate.
	• Painful inguinal adenopathy known as "buboes" present.
		• Culture of lesion (not widely available).
		• CDC criteria for "probable" diagnosis:
		  a. ≥1 painful genital ulcer(s)
		  b. No evidence of syphilis infection on dark-field examination or serologic test performed 7 days after onset of ulcer
		  c. Typical clinical presentation
		  d. Negative HSV test of ulcer

Lymphogranuloma venereum Cause: *C. trachomatis*	• Painful inguinal and/or femoral lymphadenopathy. "Groove" sign is pathognomonic. • Self-limited genital ulcer or papule at site of inoculation.	Genital lesion swab or lymph node aspirate tested using NAATs, immunofluorescence
Granuloma inguinale Cause: *K. granulomatis*	• Painless, slowly progressive ulcerative lesions on genitals or perineum; bleed easily on contact. • Regional lymphadenopathy uncommon.	Identification of Donovan bodies within histiocytes of granulation tissue smears or biopsy specimens
Syphilis Cause: *Treponema pallidum*	• Primary chancre: Painless ulcer with indurated hard raised border and "punched out" appearance. • Regional lymphadenopathy may occur.	• Screen: Nontreponemal tests (RPR, VDRL) • Confirm: Treponemal tests (FTA-ABS or TPPA) • Dark-field microscopy showing spirochetes
Genital Herpes Cause: HSV 1 and 2	• Painful vesicular lesions developing into ulcers. • Constitutional symptoms present in primary infection.	Viral culture or PCR for HSV DNA
Nonsexually transmitted genital ulcers	• Painful, well-demarcated ulcer. • Constitutional symptoms may be present if viral in etiology (CMV, EBV).	Negative for HSV or other STIs

RPR, Rapid plasma reagin; VDRL, venereal diseases research laboratory; FTA-ABS, Fluorescent treponemal antibody-absorbed; TPPA, *Treponema pallidum* particle agglutination; CMV, cytomegalovirus; EBV, Epstein–Barr virus.

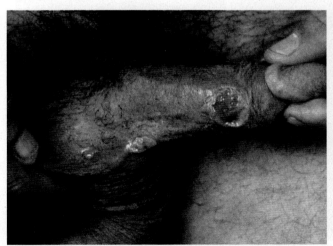

FIGURE 62.1 The lesions in chancroid are painful and more irregular than in syphilis. (From Craft N, Taylor E, Tumeh PC, et al. *VisualDx: essential adult dermatology.* Philadelphia, PA: Lippincott Williams & Wilkins, 2010.)

strictures and chronic pain.[6,7] These lesions can become superinfected with other STIs or pathogens.

Epidemiology

LGV is endemic in parts of Africa, India, South America, and the Caribbean. Outbreaks have been reported in Europe among HIV-positive MSM.[8]

Clinical Manifestations

The incubation period is 3 to 30 days (usually 7 to 12). Infection occurs in three stages:

a. *Primary stage:* The initial lesion begins as a small, painless papule or pustule at the site of inoculation that can erode into an asymptomatic herpetiform ulcer that often heals without scarring within a week. Lesions are typically found on the penis, urethral glans, and scrotum in men and on the vulva, vaginal wall, fourchette, and cervix in women. Rectal lesions occur in both sexes from receptive anal intercourse and can be associated with diarrhea, rectal discharge, and tenesmus. Mucopurulent cervicitis and urethritis may also occur. Women usually have primary involvement of the rectum, vagina, and cervix.

b. *Secondary or inguinal stage:* This stage typically occurs 2 to 6 weeks after the appearance of the primary lesion and involves painful inflammation of the inguinal and femoral lymph nodes. Inguinal adenopathy is unilateral in 70% of cases and is more common in males (Fig. 62.2). The "groove" sign is the result of enlarged inguinal nodes above Poupart's ligament and the femoral nodes below it and is considered "pathognomonic" for LGV (Fig. 62.3). Nodes can become matted and fluctuant and produce the characteristic bubo.[7] Buboes may rupture in one-third of patients or develop into hard, nonsuppurative masses. Most buboes eventually heal, but some will form sinus tracts. Bubonic relapse occurs in 20% of untreated cases. Constitutional symptoms may occur with the inguinal buboes and be associated with systemic spread of chlamydia, leading to arthritis, hepatitis, and pneumonitis.

XIII

TABLE 62.2

Treatment of Chancroid[5,18]

CDC Recommended Treatments	Other Management Considerations	Follow-Up
Azithromycin 1 g orally in a single dose or Ceftriaxone 250 mg IM in a single dose or Ciprofloxacin 500 mg orally twice daily × 3 d or Erythromycin base 500 mg orally 3 times daily × 7 d	**HIV-positive patients:** May require longer or repeated treatment due to treatment failures and slow healing. Use single-dose therapies only when close follow-up assured. **Pregnancy/lactation:** Ciprofloxacin contraindicated **Uncircumcised males:** Higher treatment failure rates and slower healing especially if ulcers under foreskin **Sex partners:** Examine and treat sex partners who had sexual contact with patient in the 10 days preceding the patient's onset of symptoms	Within 3–7 d of start of therapy Weekly follow-up until resolution of lesions and symptoms Test for HIV at time of diagnosis and 3 mo later along with syphilis if initial test negative

Buboes (fluctuant adenopathy): Treat by aspiration for symptomatic relief and to prevent rupture or by incision and drainage with wound packing (more definitive). Clinical resolution of fluctuant lymphadenopathy is slower than that of ulcers.

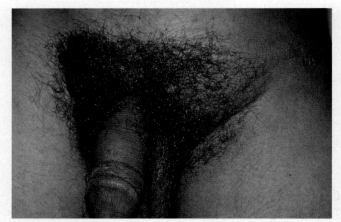

FIGURE 62.2 Lymphogranuloma venereum. Painful inguinal lymphadenopathy in a man infected with *C. trachomatis*. (Image from Rubin E, Farber JL. *Pathology*. 3rd ed. Philadelphia, PA: Lippincott Williams & Wilkins, 1999.)

c. *Tertiary or genito-anorectal syndrome (uncommon):* This stage occurs more often in women who were asymptomatic during previous stages and in men who have receptive anal intercourse.[9] Patients initially develop symptoms of proctocolitis (anal pruritus, rectal discharge, rectal pain, tenesmus, and fever). Subsequent manifestations include perirectal abscesses, rectovaginal and anorectal fistulas, rectal strictures, and rectal stenosis. Chronic untreated LGV can lead to repetitive scarring and fistulous tract formation in the genital region.

Diagnosis

Diagnosis of LGV is usually based on clinical findings. Nucleic acid amplification tests (NAATs) are the most sensitive tests for diagnosing chlamydia,[6] but do not differentiate between LGV and non-LGV serovars. If the NAAT is positive, specimens may need to be sent to a reference lab for specific genotyping. Chlamydia culture has a low recovery rate and is not specific for LGV. Other tests include complement fixation and microimmunofluorescence tests. The microimmunofluorescence test is more sensitive and specific than complement fixation. Immunofluorescence techniques are usually applied to lymph node aspirates and may not be useful in diagnosing LGV proctitis. A single complement fixation titer of >1:64 along with clinical correlation is consistent with a diagnosis of LGV infection.

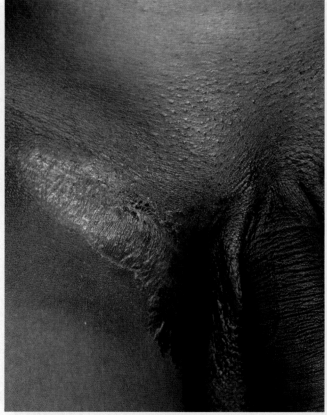

FIGURE 62.3 Lymphogranuloma venereum with groove sign of swelling above and below the inguinal fold. (From Lugo-Somolinos A, McKinley-Grant L, Goldsmith LA, et al. *VisualDx: essential dermatology in pigmented skin*. Philadelphia, PA: Lippincott Williams & Wilkins, 2011.)

Antibody titers do not correlate with disease severity. A high titer (typically >1:128) is consistent with a diagnosis of LGV.[6]

Treatment

Due to the limitations of diagnostic testing for LGV, patients with a clinical syndrome consistent with LGV should be treated presumptively for LGV (see **Table 62.3**).

TABLE 62.3			
Treatment of LGV[6,19]			
CDC Recommended Treatment	**Alternative Treatments**	**Other Management Considerations**	**Follow-Up**
Doxycycline 100 mg orally twice daily × 21 d	Erythromycin base 500 mg orally four times a day for 21 d	**HIV-positive patients:** May require prolonged treatment	Monitor until signs and symptoms resolve
		Pregnancy/lactation: Use erythromycin first line, azithromycin may be used as an alternative although safety and efficacy data lacking	Test for otyhers STIs, especially HIV, gonorrhea, and syphilis
		Sexual Contacts: Examine, test, and treat contacts within 60 d prior to onset of symptoms. For asymptomatic contacts use, azithromycin 1 g single dose or doxycycline 100 mg orally twice daily × 7 d	

Buboes (fluctuant adenopathy): May require aspiration or incision and drainage (abscess) for prevention of ulcer formation or relief of pain. Formation of Anorectal fistulas and sinuses may require surgical intervention.

GRANULOMA INGUINALE

Etiology

Granuloma inguinale, or *Donovanosis*, is caused by *Klebsiella granulomatis*, an intracellular gram-negative bacillus.[2]

Epidemiology

Granuloma inguinale is considered endemic in Papua, New Guinea, southeast India, South Africa, central Australia, Brazil, and the Caribbean. It is extremely rare in the US and Western Europe.[6,7] It is transmitted primarily through sexual contact; autoinoculation can also lead to spread of the disease.

Clinical Manifestations

Infection can result in granulomatous and destructive ulcers on the genital, inguinal, and perineal skin and should be included in the differential diagnosis of chronic progressive genital ulcers. Lesions are typically localized without accompanying constitutional symptoms. The genital area is involved in 90% of cases and the inguinal area in the remainder. Extragenital lesions occur in 6% of cases secondary to autoinoculation. Lesions are more common in uncircumcised men with poor genital hygiene, and occur on the coronal sulcus, prepuce, frenulum, glans penis, and anus. In women, the labia minora and fourchette are commonly affected. Infection of the cervix and upper genital tract can mimic cervical cancer. The ulcerovegetative or ulcerogranulomatous form is the most common clinical presentation.[7] It produces large, extensive, nonindurated ulcerations with beefy-red, highly vascular, and friable granulation tissue (Fig. 62.4). True inguinal lymphadenopathy does not occur with granuloma inguinale unless bacterial superinfection develops. However, subcutaneous granulomas near the inguinal nodes (pseudobuboes) can result in inguinal enlargement.

Diagnosis

Tissue smears or crush biopsies of the lesions are used to diagnose granuloma inguinale. Tissue smears are obtained by firmly rolling a cotton swab across the base of a nonbleeding ulcer and then across a slide. "Crush biopsies" involve removing tissue from the advancing surface of the ulcer and "crushing" or smearing the specimen between two slides. Giemsa or Wright's stain is used to identify the dark-staining, safety pin–shaped intracytoplasmic inclusion bodies within large mononuclear cells or histiocytes known as *Donovan bodies*.[7]

Treatment

Treatment is outlined in **Table 62.4.**

PEDICULOSIS AND SCABIES

Scabies and pediculosis are ubiquitous and highly contagious parasitic skin infections that occur both in individuals and in clusters of

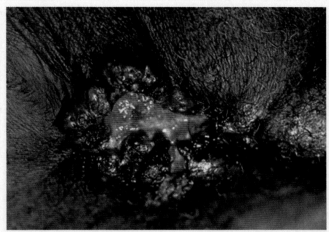

FIGURE 62.4 This perianal ulceration with heaped-up borders is typical of granuloma inguinale (Donovanosis). (Courtesy of Jack Mosley. In: Edwards L, Lynch PJ, eds. *Genital dermatology atlas.* 2nd ed. Philadelphia, PA: Lippincott Williams & Wilkins, 2010.)

individuals such as school children, homeless people, hospital staff, and immunocompromised individuals.

Pediculosis Pubis

Etiology

Pediculosis pubis is caused by the pubic or crab louse, *Pthirus pubis,* an obligate human parasite (Fig. 62.5).

Epidemiology

1. Transmission: Infestations are most common among adolescents and young adults (AYAs). Transmission occurs as a result of close bodily contact, chiefly through sexual contact. Condoms do not prevent transmission, and infestations frequently coexist with other STIs.[5] Pubic lice can be transmitted by infected clothing, towels, and bedding. There is no current evidence linking ectoparasites to transmission of HIV.
2. Life cycle: The parasite spends its life on skin and feeds on blood. It dies approximately 24 hours after being off its human host, but lower environmental temperatures can prolong survival. Female lice lay eggs that are cemented to hair shafts as nits. After 6 to 10 days, nits hatch into nymphs that mature into adult lice within 10 to 14 days. Adult lice live approximately 1 month.

Clinical Manifestations

Symptoms occur 2 or more weeks after contact and occur more rapidly with subsequent infections. Once symptoms are present,

XIII

TABLE 62.4

Treatment of Granuloma Inguinale[6,20,21]

CDC Recommended Treatment	Alternative Treatments	Other Management Considerations	Follow-Up
Azithromycin 1 g orally once per week or 500 mg daily for at least 3 weeks and until all lesions have completely healed[a]	Use all medications below for at least 3 wk and until all lesions healed Doxycycline 100 mg orally twice a day for at least 3 weeks and until all lesions have completely healed[a] or Ciprofloxacin 750 mg orally twice daily[a] or Erythromycin base 500 mg orally 4 times daily[a] or Trimethoprim-sulfamethoxazole one double-strength (160 mg/800 mg) tablet orally twice daily[a]	**HIV positive:** Consider addition of an aminoglycoside **Pregnancy/lactation:** Erythromycin with consideration of additional aminoglycoside such as gentamicin or Azithromycin[21] **Sexual contacts:** Examine and offer treatment to all contacts exposed 60 d prior to the onset of symptoms in the infected partner or treat all who are symptomatic[b]	Follow until resolution of all lesions Test for other STIs, including gonorrhea, chlamydia, herpes, syphilis, HIV, and hepatitis B

[a]The addition of an aminoglycoside (e.g., gentamicin 1 mg/kg IV every 8 h) to these regimens can be considered if improvement is not evident within the first few days of therapy.
[b]Value of treatment of an asymptomatic contact is unknown.

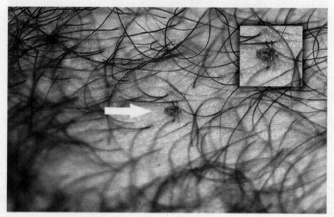

FIGURE 62.5 Pubic lice. (Reproduced with permission from Goodheart HG. *A Photoguide to common skin disorders: diagnosis and management.* 3rd ed. Philadelphia, PA: Lippincott Williams & Wilkins, 2009.)

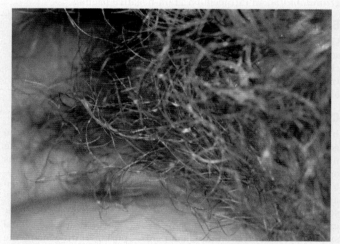

FIGURE 62.6 Multiple nits on pubic hairs suggestive of pubic lice infestation. (From Craft N, Taylor E, Tumeh PC, et al. *VisualDx: essential adult dermatology.* Philadelphia, PA: Lippincott Williams & Wilkins, 2010.)

the infection is usually well established. Common areas of infection include hair on the chest, axilla, abdomen, thighs, genitals, and occasionally the male beard. Pruritus, the main symptom, is probably a hypersensitivity reaction to the louse bite. Small blue spots known as maculae caeruleae may appear on the thighs and abdomen after prolonged infestations and represent feeding sites of the louse.

Diagnosis

Diagnosis of pubic lice is made by direct visualization of lice and/or nits (eggs) on the hair shafts (Fig. 62.6). Lice appear as tiny, tan to grayish-white oval insects. Nits can be seen as small yellowish-white, glistening oval kernels attached to hair shafts.

Treatment

Pubic lice do not transmit systemic disease. Treatment is for symptomatic relief and prevention of reinfestation and transmission. Topical treatments are more effective when applied to dry hair. Embryos may survive initial treatment, requiring a second treatment in 7 to 10 days (**Table 62.5**).

Additional Management Considerations[10]

1. Clothing or bed linens worn or used within 2 days of diagnosis should be machine washed at 130 to 140°F and machine dried using the hot cycle for at least 20 minutes, or dry cleaned.

Clothing that cannot be decontaminated as above should be bagged for at least 72 hours (preferentially for 2 weeks) to allow newly hatched lice to die. Fumigation is not necessary.
2. Residual nits should be removed with a fine comb. A solution of vinegar and water can be used to loosen them.
3. All sexual contacts within the past month should be treated and sexual contact avoided until both patient and partner(s) are reevaluated for persistent infection.
4. *HIV infection:* treat the same as for noninfected AYAs.
5. Pediculosis of eyelashes: Apply occlusive ophthalmic ointment to the eyelid margins two times a day for 10 days to smother lice and nits.

Scabies

Etiology

Scabies is a highly contagious, ectoparasitic infection caused by *Sarcoptes scabiei* var *hominis*, a small mite; it is host specific to humans.

Epidemiology

1. Transmission: The mite is transmitted by prolonged (10 to 20 minute) skin-to-skin contact.[11] Sexual transmission is common, as is nonsexual spread in family groups. Transmission

TABLE 62.5

Treatment of Pediculosis[6,10]

Drug	Application Instructions/Dosing	Warnings/Precaution	Other
CDC Recommended Regimens			
Permethrin 1% cream rinse	Apply to affected areas and wash off after 10 min Avoid eyes	Pruritus, erythema, burning, and stinging	Can be used in pregnancy
Pyrethrins with piperonyl butoxide (RID)	Apply to affected areas and wash off after 10 min Avoid eyes	Pruritus, burning, and stinging	Can be used in pregnancy
CDC Alternative Regimens			
Malathion 0.5% lotion	Apply to affected areas for 8–12 h and wash off	Bad odor, potentially flammable, toxic if ingested, avoid eyes	FDA approved *only* for treatment of *HEAD* lice
Ivermectin	250 µg/kg orally, repeat in 2 wk	Human data suggest low risk in pregnancy and probably compatible with breastfeeding Inadequate safety data on use in children <15 kg Potential for neurotoxicity, useful in multiple parasitic infections, avoid eyes	Not FDA approved treatment

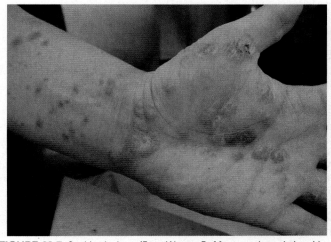

FIGURE 62.7 Scabies lesions. (From Werner R. *Massage therapist's guide to pathology.* 5th ed. Philadelphia: Lippincott Williams & Wilkins, 2012.)

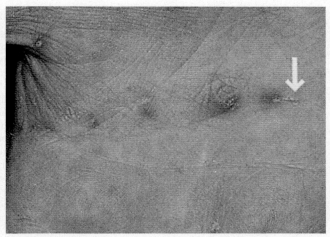

FIGURE 62.8 Burrow of scabies—a person with scabies has intense itching. Skin lesions include small papules, pustules, lichenified areas, and excoriations. With a magnifying lens, look for the burrow of the mite that causes it. A burrow is a minute, slightly raised tunnel in the epidermis and is commonly found on the finger webs and on the sides of the fingers. It looks like a short (5 to 15 mm), linear or curved, gray line and may end in a tiny vesicle. (From Goodheart HP. *A photoguide of common skin disorders: diagnosis and management.* Philadelphia, PA: Lippincott Williams & Wilkins, 1999.)

can occur before the patient is symptomatic and throughout the infestation as long as it remains untreated. Scabies is frequently found in institutional settings.

2. Life cycle: Female mites burrow into the epidermal layer of the skin laying 2 to 4 eggs per day for 4 to 5 weeks. The adult female then dies within the burrow. After 3 to 5 days the eggs hatch, and the larvae return to the skin surface to mature in 10 to 17 days. Only 10% of eggs become adults.[12] Away from the host, human mites have been shown to survive up to 72 hours.

Clinical Manifestations

Symptoms occur 3 to 6 weeks after first exposure and 1 to 4 days after reexposure, resulting in an intensely pruritic, papular eruption associated with eczematous lesions and areas of excoriation (Fig. 62.7).[11] Pruritus is often worse at night or after a hot bath and is caused by a cell-mediated immune reaction to the mite and its by-products. Burrows (Fig. 62.8), if seen, appear as short wavy lines a few millimeters to 1 cm in length. Skin lesions are typically seen between finger webs, on the flexor surfaces of the wrists, in the axillary folds, and on the nipples, waist, umbilicus, buttocks,

thighs, knees, ankles, and genital areas. Scabies usually spares the face, neck, and scalp except in children.

Crusted or Norwegian scabies is a rare and aggressive form of scabies found in immunodeficient, debilitated, or malnourished patients. It is characterized by a hyperinfestation of the mite with a concomitant inflammatory and hyperkeratotic reaction. The thick, crusted scales are highly contagious. Treatment failures occur frequently, and septicemia is a common complication.

Scabies infections can become secondarily infected.[11] In countries where scabies is seen in large numbers, there has been an association with poststreptococcal glomerulonephritis and chronic kidney disease as well as rheumatic fever and heart disease.[13]

Diagnosis

1. Diagnosis is usually made on the basis of the distribution of lesions and a history of intense itching and similar symptoms

XIII

TABLE 62.6

Treatment of Scabies[6,15,24,26]

Medication	Application/Dosing	Warnings/Precautions	Other
CDC Recommended Regimens			
Permethrin cream 5%	Apply neck down and wash off after 8–14 h, including fingernails and skin folds Can apply at bedtime and wash off in a.m.	Pruritus Erythema Burning, and stinging	FDA approved for use in pregnant and lactating women and children ≥2 years of age
Ivermectin	200 µg/kg orally, repeat in 2 wk	Not for use with crusted scabies	Not FDA approved, safety not established in pregnant or lactating women Consider for use in epidemics
CDC Alternative Regimens			
Lindane 1% (infants and young children aged <10 years should not be treated with lindane)	Apply 1 oz of lotion or 30 g of cream in thin layer from neck down and wash off after 8 h, including web spaces and beneath nails	Neurotoxic Reports of aplastic anemia Do not apply after bathing due to absorption, do not use with extensive dermatitis, seizure disorders, or in pregnant or lactating women	Resistance has been reported Only use when recommended treatments fail or are not tolerated

in family members or sexual partners. Definitive diagnosis requires microscopic identification of mites, eggs, or feces from skin scrapings of papules or burrows. Burrows are virtually pathognomonic for human scabies, but are often difficult to demonstrate.

2. Isolation of mite: Best results are obtained using a no.15 scalpel blade to scrape the leading edge of an intact burrow or affected areas under the fingernails. Visibility of burrows can be enhanced by applying mineral or immersion oil, saline, or ink to the skin. Scrapings are examined under oil or saline on low power for the presence of eggs, feces, or mites. Alternately, punch or shave biopsies of inflamed lesions can be used with varying results. In resource-poor areas, handheld dermatoscopes and adhesive tape (placed over lesions, pulled off rapidly, and transferred to a slide) have been used to identify mites and burrows.[14,15]

Treatment

Treatment is outlined in **Table 62.6.**

Additional Management Considerations[5,6,12,25]

1. Environmental control: Bedding and clothing worn during the 4 days preceding treatment should be machine washed, dried using the hot cycle, dry cleaned, or set aside in a sealed plastic bag for at least 72 hours. Fumigation is not necessary.

2. Follow-up: Pruritus may persist for up to 2 weeks after treatment. Symptoms persisting longer may be due to medication resistance, incorrect scabicidal application, poor skin penetration in crusted scabies, reinfection, or other allergies. Consideration can be given to re-treatment with a different regimen after 1 to 2 weeks, although some specialists recommend this only with confirmation of live mites.

3. Sex partners as well as close personal and household contacts from within the previous month should be treated.

4. *HIV infection*: Treat the same as HIV-negative individuals. However HIV-positive individuals are at increased risk for crusted scabies, which should be managed in consultation with a specialist.

5. *Crusted scabies:* It may require combined treatment with ivermectin and topical scabicides and keratolytic therapy or multiple doses of ivermectin, see Ref. 6 for details.

MOLLUSCUM CONTAGIOSUM

Etiology

Molluscum contagiosum is caused by a large double-stranded DNA virus of the genus *Molluscipoxvirus* in the family *Poxviridae*.

Epidemiology

Humans appear to be the only known host. Transmission occurs by direct person-to-person contact, fomites, or autoinoculation. Sexual contact is the most common form of transmission in AYAs. Activities such as swimming may be associated with disease spread through use of contaminated fomites. Individuals with atopic dermatitis may be at increased risk for infection.[16,27,28]

Clinical Manifestations

The incubation period varies from 2 weeks to 6 months. Lesions commonly occur on the face, trunk, and extremities. In sexually active AYAs, the lesions are commonly seen on the genitals, abdomen, and inner thighs. These may be more widespread in immunocompromised individuals.[2] Lesions present as smooth, firm, dome-shaped, flesh-colored, and semi-translucent papules with central umbilication (Fig. 62.9). Immunocompetent hosts typically have less than 20 lesions that are 2 mm to 5 mm in diameter. HIV-positive and immunocompromised patients may develop hundreds of lesions that may occur in clusters (Fig. 62.10) or can present with "giant molluscum" up to 15 mm in diameter that are difficult to eradicate and are easily spread. Most lesions are asymptomatic; however, 10% of patients may have an encircling eczematoid reaction.[2]

Diagnosis

The clinical appearance of the lesion is usually diagnostic. Wright or Giemsa staining of the caseous material within the core demonstrates intracytoplasmic inclusion bodies known as molluscum bodies.

Treatment

Molluscum contagiosum has a self-limiting course in immunocompetent individuals. Lesions usually resolve in 2 to 6 months, but untreated infections may last for 12 months and even up to 4 years.

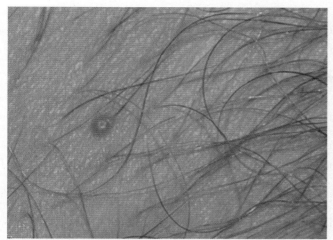

FIGURE 62.9 This skin-colored, shiny papule with a central dell is typical of molluscum contagiosum. (From Edwards L, Lynch PJ. *Genital dermatology atlas*. 2nd ed. Philadelphia, PA: Lippincott Williams & Wilkins, 2010.)

Treatment may be indicated to prevent spread of disease via auto-inoculation and further transmission in sexually active individuals. Immunocompromised individuals are also at greater risk of secondary inflammation and bacterial infection. Currently, no evidence-based recommendations exist for the treatment of molluscum.[17] Various treatment options are described in **Table 62.7**.

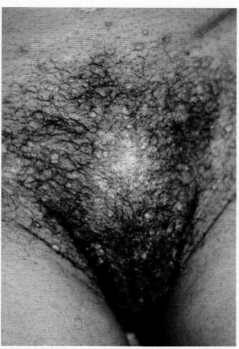

FIGURE 62.10 Molluscum contagiosum in an HIV-positive female: typical umbilicated papules are shown. (From Kroumpouzos G. Text atlas of obstetric dermatology. Philadelphia, PA: Lippincott Williams & Wilkins, 2013.)

TABLE 62.7

Treatment of Molluscum Contagiosum[16,22]

	Method	Side Effects	Comments
Mechanical			
Curettage/needle extraction	Lesions scraped away after using topical anesthetic	Pain, bleeding, scarring	• Works best when there are few lesions • Safe in pregnancy
Cryotherapy	Liquid N_2 applied for 10–20 sec in 2 freeze-thaw cycles. Repeat in 1 wk as needed	Pain, blistering, scarring, hyper- or hypopigmentation	• Effective and preferred for large single or few lesions
Pulse dye laser (585 nm)	Single pulse to each lesion after topical anesthetic. May repeat in 2–3 wk if needed	Minimal pain, transient hyperpigmentation	Option for recalcitrant lesions
Chemical			
Trichloroacetic acid (TCA) (100%)	Applied to the lesion(s) once weekly for 4–6 wk	Mild pain, irritation, and scarring	• Safe in pregnancy • Can be used in recalcitrant lesions
Cantharidin (0.7%)	Applied sparingly to lesions and washed off in 4 h (2–6 h). May be repeated in 2–4 wk	Pain, blistering	• Not FDA approved. • Not recommended for use on face or genitalia
Podophyllotoxin (0.5%)	Apply twice daily for 3 d, wait 4 d, and repeat weekly up to 4 wk	Erythema, pruritus, irritation, inflammation	
Retin A (0.025%, 0.05%, or 0.1%)	Apply 1–2 times daily for 4 wk	Mild erythema, irritation	• Data limited to case reports • Not for use in pregnancy
Potassium hydroxide aqueous solution (5%–10%)[17]	Applied with a cotton swab twice daily until lesions cleared	Erythema, stinging, hyper- or hypopigmentation	
Salicylic acid gel (12%)	Apply to each lesion 1–2 times a week until cleared	Stinging	
Immunomodulators			
Topical 5% imiquimod	Applied 3 times/wk for 8 h (overnight), washed off in a.m. Used for 4–12 wk	Erythema, itching, burning sensation, mild pain	Not FDA approved for this use. Not for use in pregnancy
Intralesional Candida antigen injection[23]	0.3 mL injected directly into lesion with a 1 mL syringe and 30 G needle	Pain	Single study reported with 93% response rate

XIII

HIV-Positive/Immunosuppressed Patients

Molluscum contagiosum is considered an opportunistic infection in HIV disease and as a marker for advanced infection. HIV-infected individuals have high treatment failure rates with almost all standard therapies. The antiviral agent cidofovir used topically or systemically has been shown to be beneficial. Other experimental treatments using photodynamic, electron beam, and contact immunotherapy with diphencyprone have shown some improvement in HIV-positive patients. Interferon α has been used with success in immunocompromised individuals.[16]

⬤ FOLLOW-UP

Patients should watch for the development of new lesions after several weeks that may have been incubating at the time of the initial treatment. Patients should refrain from sharing clothing or towels with others. Lesions should be kept clean and covered with clothing or watertight bandages, especially before participating in contact sports or sharing equipment (swimming pools).

REFERENCES

1. Wu JJ, Huang DB, Pang KR, et al. Selected sexually transmitted diseases and their relationship to HIV. *Clin Dermatol* 2004;22:499.
2. American Academy of Pediatrics. Committee on Infectious Diseases. *Red book: report of the committee on infectious diseases*. Elk Grove Village, IL: American Academy of Pediatrics, 2012.
3. Centers for Disease Control and Prevention (U.S.), National Center for HIV/AIDS, Viral Hepatitis, STD, and TB Prevention (U.S.), Division of STD Prevention. *Sexually transmitted disease surveillance 2012*. Atlanta, GA: U.S. Department of Health and Human Services, Centers for Disease Control and Prevention, National Center for HIV/AIDS, Viral Hepatitis, STD, and TB Prevention, Division of STD Prevention, 2014:80. Available at http://www.cdc.gov/std/stats12/Surv2012.pdf. Accessed February 02, 2014.
4. Mookerjee AL, Newell GC. Chancroid. In: Lebwohl M, Heymann WR, Berth-Jones J, et al. eds. *Treatment of skin disease: comprehensive therapeutic strategies*. 4th ed. Oxford: Saunders, 2014:133–134.
5. Holmes KK. *Sexually transmitted diseases*. 4th ed. New York, NY: McGraw-Hill Medical, 2008:2166.
6. Workowski KA, Bolan GA. Sexually Transmitted Diseases Guidelines, 2015. *MMWR Recomm Rep* 2015;64(RR-3):1–137.
7. Edwards L, Lynch PJ, Neill SM. *Genital dermatology atlas*. 2nd ed. Philadelphia, PA: Lippincott Williams & Wilkins, 2011:336.
8. Blank S, Schillinger JA, Harbatkin D. Lymphogranuloma venereum in the industrialised world. *Lancet* 2005;365(9471):1607–1608.
9. Weir E. Lymphogranuloma venereum in the differential diagnosis of proctitis. *CMAJ* 2005;172:185.
10. http://www.cdc.gov/parasites/lice/pubic/health_professionals/index.html. Accessed January 01, 2014.
11. Hay RJ, Steer AC, Engelman D, et al. Scabies in the developing world—its prevalence, complications, and management. *Clin Microbiol Infect* 2012;18(4):313–323.
12. http://www.cdc.gov/parasites/scabies/biology.html. Accessed February 02, 2014.
13. Chung SD, Wang KH, Huang CC, et al. Scabies increased the risk of chronic kidney disease: A 5-year follow-up study. *J Eur Acad Dermatol Venereol* 2014;28(3):286–292.
14. Walter B, Heukelbach J, Fengler G, et al. Comparison of dermoscopy, skin scraping, and the adhesive tape test for the diagnosis of scabies in a resource-poor setting. *Arch Dermatol* 2011;147(4):468–473.
15. Dupuy A, Dehen L, Bourrat E, et al. Accuracy of standard dermoscopy for diagnosing scabies. *J Am Acad Dermatol* 2007;56(1):53–62.
16. van der Wouden JC, van der Sande R, van Suijlekom-Smit LW, et al. Interventions for cutaneous molluscum contagiosum. *Cochrane Database Syst Rev* 2009;(4):CD004767. doi(4):CD004767.
17. Short KA, Fuller LC, Higgins EM. Double-blind, randomized, placebo-controlled trial of the use of topical 10% potassium hydroxide solution in the treatment of molluscum contagiosum. *Pediatr Dermatol* 2006;23(3):279–281.
18. Kemp M, Christensen JJ, Lautenschlager S, et al. European guideline for the management of chancroid, 2011. *Int J STD AIDS* 2011;22(5):241–244.
19. Pereira FA. Lymphogranuloma venereum. In: Lebwohl M, Heymann WR, Berth-Jones J, et al., eds. *Treatment of skin disease: comprehensive therapeutic strategies*. 4th ed. Oxford: Saunders, 2014:428–429.
20. Guidry JA, Rosen T. Granuloma inguinale. In: Lebwohl M, Heymann WR, Berth-Jones J, et al., eds. *Treatment of skin disease: comprehensive therapeutic strategies*. 4th ed. Oxford: Saunders, 2014:286–287.
21. O'Farrell N. Moi H. IUSTI/WHO European STD guidelines Editorial Board. European guideline for the management of donovanosis, 2010. *Int J STD AIDS* 2010;21(9):609–610.
22. Enns LL, Evans MS. Intralesional immunotherapy with candida antigen for the treatment of molluscum contagiosum in children. *Pediatr Dermatol* 2011;28(3):254–258.
23. Rome E. Other sexually-transmitted diseases. In: Hillard PA, ed. *Practical pediatric and adolescent gynecology*. Chichester, West Sussex: Wiley-Blackwell, 2013:318–324.
24. Leone PA. Scabies and pediculosis pubis: An update of treatment regimens and general review. *Clin Infect Dis* 2007;44 (suppl 3):S153–S159.
25. Chosidow O. Clinical practices. Scabies. *N Engl J Med* 2006;354(16):1718–1727.
26. Strong M, Johnstone P. Cochrane review: interventions for treating scabies. *Evid-Based Child Health* 2011;6(6):1790–1862.
27. Chen X, Anstey AV, Bugert JJ. Molluscum contagiosum virus infection. *Lancet Infect Dis* 2013;13(10):877–888.
28. Olsen JR, Gallacher J, Piguet V, et al. Epidemiology of Molluscum contagiosum in children: a systematic review. *Fam Pract* 2014;31(2):130–136.

📶 ADDITIONAL RESOURCES AND WEBSITES ONLINE

PART XIV

Substance use and Abuse

CHAPTER 63

Adolescent and Young Adult Substance Use and Abuse

Leslie R. Walker
Erin N. Harrop

KEY WORDS

- Addiction
- Adolescent brain development
- Adolescent research
- Alcohol
- Drug dependence
- Drug use
- Drug use prevention
- Generational forgetting
- Marijuana
- Risk and protective factors

Adolescent and young adult (AYA) use of alcohol, marijuana, tobacco, and other illicit drugs (AMTOD) is a major public health problem. The last decade has brought a new complexity to drug use in the US with legalization of marijuana for medicinal and/or recreational purposes in a growing number of states. The continued use of prescription and synthetic drugs for recreational purposes continues to be a national concern. In the short term, drug use is associated with significant morbidity and mortality in the AYA population. In the long term, much of the adult morbidity and mortality attributed to AMTOD use can be traced to behaviors that began during adolescence. Alcohol, tobacco, and marijuana are the three drugs most abused by the AYA age-groups. Other drugs wax and wane in popularity and their use, following a predictable pattern. A phenomenon called generational forgetting contributes to the popularity of a particular drug over time. Generational forgetting occurs in the absence of knowledge; otherwise, Drug "X" is perceived as safer than other drugs, and its use increases. As use increases, the drug's negative effects become more widely known, and use of Drug "X" is perceived as increasingly risky. This increased perception of risk causes the popularity of Drug "X" to wane, leading to Drug X's replacement by a different drug that is perceived as being of lower risk. Decades later, when the risk of Drug "X" is no longer common knowledge, it again becomes popular.

Advances in neuroimaging techniques and research using animal models of human puberty have elucidated the unique vulnerability of the still-developing AYA brain to the effects of alcohol and other drugs; many observed neural changes in response to drug use might be permanent.[1,2] Ongoing research into the brain's reward circuitry (e.g., the ventral tegmental area, the prefrontal cortex, and the nucleus accumbens) continues to demonstrate that in the brain, drugs of abuse share common pathways and exert their effects through similar mechanisms. For example, the active ingredient in marijuana, Δ^9-tetrahydrocannabinol, stimulates the same µ1 opioid receptor as does heroin. Similarly, when rats previously exposed on a chronic basis to a cannabinoid agonist are given a cannabinoid antagonist to produce an acute withdrawal state, they secrete elevated amounts of corticotropin-releasing factor. This same pattern is seen in withdrawal from other drugs of abuse. Given this growing body of research, drug addiction is best viewed as a chronic disease, with relapses being common. However, recent data indicate that treatment of AYAs with drug use disorders is effective.

EPIDEMIOLOGY

Middle and High School Youth

The best data on adolescent substance abuse come from the *Monitoring the Future (MTF) study*, conducted by the Institute for Social Research at the University of Michigan (www.monitoringthefuture.org). This school-based study began in 1975, and currently surveys a nationally representative sample of 8th, 10th, and 12th graders. The sample in 2014 consists of 41,600 youth in 377 secondary schools nationwide. Because the anonymous surveys are conducted in schools, MTF data do not reflect drug use by out-of-school youth (including youth who dropout, are homeless, or incarcerated), whose use is typically higher. Declining use of a number of licit and illicit substances is a main finding in 2014. The annual prevalence of drug use declined for 28 of the 34 drug outcomes reported for the combined pool of 8th, 10th, and 12th graders. The most important findings from the 2014 MTF survey are discussed in the following section. Overall trends in drug use among 8th, 10th, and 12th graders have fluctuated since 1975, with peak use in 1981 when 66% of MTF adolescents reported use of an illicit drug in their lifetime. After reaching a low of 29.8% in 1992, lifetime drug use then increased to a peak level of 43.3% in 1997; it then decreased again to a low of 32.6% in 2008. Lifetime illicit drug use then increased steadily to 36.0% in 2013, but then decreased slightly to 34.9% in 2014. The major cause of this decline was a drop in marijuana use. One of the more concerning trends has been in the change of perception of risk of substances in the MTF samples. Along with the increase in use over the last few years, there has been a decline in perceived risk, which can foreshadow future increases in drug use in this cohort. The MTF survey categorizes use across a continuum by asking about lifetime use (ever used), annual use (any use in the last year), 30-day use (a measure of regular use), and daily use. The data are then able to give an estimate of chronicity of use for 8th, 10th, and 12th graders. Figure 63.1 shows trends in lifetime use of various drugs; Table 63.1 shows prevalence of lifetime, annual, past 30 day, and daily use of various drugs for 8th, 10th and 12th graders in 2012.

Some of the most notable findings across all three grades were slight decreases in lifetime and annual illicit drug use and the prevalence of alcohol and marijuana use. Both alcohol and marijuana are illicit for this age-group. It is also important to note that for all other measured reports of illicit drug use, the overall combined use rates are much more consistent than is the rate of use of a particular drug by year or decade. This again illustrates generational

TABLE 63.1

Prevalence of Use of Various Drugs for 8th, 10th, and 12th Graders, 2012

	Lifetime			Annual			Past 30 days			Daily		
	8th	10th	12th	8th	10th	12th	8th	10th	12th	8th	10th	12th
Approximate weighted N =	15,100	15,000	13,700	15,100	15,000	13,700	15,100	15,000	13,700	15,100	15,000	13,700
Any Illicit Drug	18.5	36.8	49.1	13.4	30.1	39.7	7.7	18.5	25.2	-	-	-
Any Illicit Drug other than Marijuana	8.7	14.9	24.1	5.5	10.8	17.0	2.5	5.0	8.4	-	-	-
Any Illicit Drug Including Inhalants	25.1	40.0	50.3	17.0	31.5	40.2	9.5	19.3	25.2	-	-	-
Marijuana/Hashish	15.2	33.5	45.2	11.4	28.0	36.4	6.5	17.0	22.9	1.1	3.5	6.5
Synthetic Marijuana	-	-	-	4.4	8.8	11.3	-	-	-	-	-	-
Inhalants	11.8	9.9	7.9	6.2	4.1	2.9	2.7	1.4	0.9	-	-	0.1
Hallucinogens	2.8	5.2	7.5	1.5	3.5	4.8	0.6	1.2	1.5	-	-	0.1
Hallucinogens, Adjusted	-	-	7.9	-	-	-	-	-	1.8	-	-	-
LSD	1.3	2.5	3.8	0.8	1.7	2.4	0.3	0.5	0.8	-	-	0.1
Hallucinogens other than LSD	2.3	4.5	6.6	1.3	3.0	4.0	0.5	0.9	1.3	-	-	0.1
PCP	-	-	1.6	-	-	0.9	-	-	0.5	-	-	0.1
Ecstasy (MDMA)	2.0	5.0	7.2	1.1	3.0	3.8	0.5	1.0	0.9	-	-	0.1
Salvia	-	-	-	1.4	2.5	4.4	-	-	-	-	-	-
Cocaine	1.9	3.3	4.9	1.2	2.0	2.7	0.5	0.8	1.1	-	-	0.1
Crack	1.0	1.4	2.1	0.6	0.8	1.2	0.3	0.4	0.5	-	-	0.1
Other Cocaine	1.6	3.0	4.4	1.0	1.8	2.4	0.3	0.7	1.0	-	-	0.1
Heroin												
Any Use	0.8	1.1	1.1	0.5	0.6	0.6	0.2	0.4	0.3	-	-	0.1
With A Needle	0.6	0.7	0.7	0.4	0.4	0.4	0.2	0.2	0.3	-	-	0.1
Without A needle	0.5	0.8	0.8	0.3	0.4	0.4	0.1	0.2	0.2	-	-	0.1
Narcotics other than Heroin	-	-	12.2	-	-	7.9	-	-	3.0	-	-	0.2
OxyContin	-	-	-	1.6	3.0	4.3	-	-	-	-	-	-
Vicodin	-	-	-	1.3	4.4	7.5	-	-	-	-	-	-
Amphetamines	4.5	8.9	12.0	2.9	6.5	7.9	1.3	2.8	3.3	-	-	0.3
Ritalin	-	-	-	0.7	1.9	2.6	-	-	-	-	-	-
Adderall	-	-	-	1.7	4.5	7.6	-	-	-	-	-	-
Methamphetamine	1.3	1.8	1.7	1.0	1.0	1.1	0.5	0.6	0.5	-	-	-
Crystal Methamphetamine (Ice)	-	-	1.7	-	-	0.8	-	-	0.4	-	-	0.2
Bath Salts (Synthetic Stimulants)	-	-	-	0.8	0.6	1.3	-	-	-	-	-	-
Seductive (Barbiturates)	-	-	6.9	-	-	4.5	-	-	2.0	-	-	0.1
Seductive, Adjusted	-	-	7.2	-	-	4.5	-	-	2.1	-	-	0.3
Methaqualone	-	-	0.8	-	-	0.4	-	-	0.3	-	-	0.3

TABLE 63.1

Prevalence of Use of Various Drugs for 8th, 10th, and 12th Graders, 2012 (Continued)

	Lifetime			Annual			Past 30 days			Daily		
	8th	10th	12th	8th	10th	12th	8th	10th	12th	8th	10th	12th
Approximate weighted N =	15,100	15,000	13,700	15,100	15,000	13,700	15,100	15,000	13,700	15,100	15,000	13,700
Tranquilizers	3.0	6.3	8.5	1.8	4.3	5.3	0.8	1.7	2.1	-	-	0.1
Any Prescription Drug	-	-	21.2	-	-	14.8	-	-	-	-	-	-
Over-the-Counter Cough/Cold Medication	-	-	-	3.0	4.7	5.6	-	-	-	-	-	-
Rohpnol	1.0	0.8	-	0.4	0.5	1.5	0.1	0.2	-	-	-	-
GHB	-	-	-	-	-	1.4	-	-	-	-	-	-
Ketamine	-	-	-	-	-	-	-	-	-	-	-	-
Alcohol												
Any Use	29.5	54.0	69.4	23.6	48.5	63.5	11.0	27.6	41.5	0.3	0.1	2.5
Been Drunk	12.8	34.5	54.2	8.5	28.2	45.0	3.4	14.5	28.1	0.1	0.4	1.5
Flavored Alcoholic Beverages	23.5	46.7	60.5	17.0	37.8	45.0	3.5	14.5	28.1	0.1	0.4	1.5
Alcoholic Beverages Containing Caffeine	-	-	-	10.9	19.7	25.4	-	-	-	-	-	-
5+ Drinks in a Row in Last 2 wk	-	-	-	-	-	-	-	-	-	5.1	15.5	23.7
Cigarettes												
Any Use	15.5	27.7	39.5	-	-	-	4.9	10.8	17.1	1.9	5.0	9.3
1/2 Pack+/Day	-	-	-	-	-	-	-	-	-	0.6	1.5	4.0
Kreteks	-	-	-	-	-	3.0	-	-	-	-	-	-
Tobacco using a Hookah	-	-	-	-	-	18.3	-	-	-	-	-	-
Small Cigars	-	-	-	1.0	1.6	1.6	-	-	-	-	-	-
Dissolvable Tobacco Products	-	-	-	2.4	6.9	7.9	-	-	-	-	-	-
Snuff	8.1	15.4	17.4	-	-	-	2.8	6.4	7.9	-	-	-
Smokeless Tobacco	1.2	1.3	1.8	0.6	0.8	1.3	0.3	0.4	0.9	-	-	-

Trends in annual prevalence of an illicit drug use index for 8th, 10th, and 12th graders. (From Johnston LD, O'Malley PM, Bachman JG, et al. *Monitoring the Future national survey results on drug use, 1975–2012: Volume I, Secondary school students.* Ann Arbor: Institute for Social Research, The University of Michigan, 2013. Available at http://www.monitoringthefuture.org/pubs/monographs/mtf-vol1_2012.pdf. Accessed February 3, 2014.)

forgetting and the perceived risk of particular drugs waxing and waning over time. However, it also illustrates that the number of youth interested in other illicit drugs remains relatively stable over time (see Fig. 63.1).

Other surveys that track adolescent substance abuse to varying degrees are the *Youth Risk Behavior Surveillance System (YRBSS)*, also administered in schools, (www.cdc.gov/Healthy Youth/yrbs/index.htm) and the *National Survey on Drug Use and Health (NSDUH)* (www.oas.samhsa.gov/nhsda.htm). The latter survey, administered in the home, includes out-of-school youth, but may result in underreporting if parents are present. Drug use estimates from the MTF surveys consistently yield higher estimates than the NSDUH (see Fig. 63.2).

Alcohol

Alcohol continues to be the drug most abused by adolescents. In 2014, the MTF study reported a continued decline in use since 1975, with approximately 20.8% of 8th graders, 44% of 10th graders, and 60.2% of 12th graders reporting use in the last year. Binge drinking (defined as five or more drinks in a row over a 2-hour period) was also at historic lows in 2014, reported by 4.1% of 8th graders, 12.6% of 10th graders, and 19.4% of 12th graders. There are only small differences between 8th and 10th grade female use compared to male use. By the 12th grade, males consume significantly more alcohol and report significantly more binge drinking episodes than females.

The *European School Survey Project on Alcohol and Other Drugs (ESPAD)*, published in 2012, reported data collected in 2011

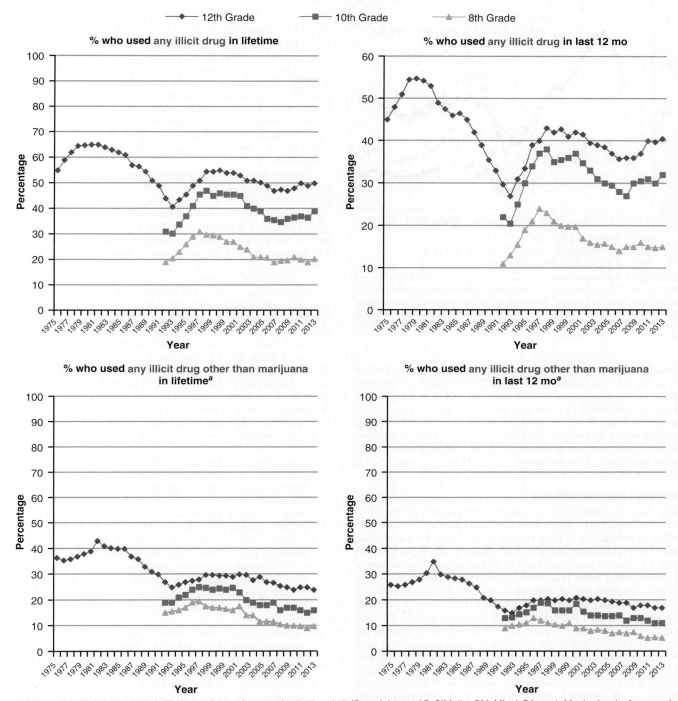

FIGURE 63.1 Any illicit drug: trends in lifetime and annual use grades 8, 10, and 12. (From Johnston LD, O'Malley PM, Miech RA, et al. *Monitoring the future national results on drug use: 1975–2014: overview, key findings on adolescent drug use.* Ann Arbor: Institute for Social Research, the University of Michigan, 2015. Available at http://www.monitoringthefuture.org/. Accessed February 20, 2015.
[a]In 2001, a revised set of questions on other hallucinogen use and tranquilizer use were introduced. In 2013, a revised set of questions on amphetamine use was introduced. Data for any illicit drug other than marijuana were affected by these changes.

on substance use in 36 European countries and regions among 15- to 16-year-old students (mean age 15.8 years old). This study permitted the comparison of alcohol use between the US, where the legal age for alcohol consumption is 21 years, and European countries, most of which have legal drinking ages below 21 years. In comparing binge drinking (five or more drinks in a row), the 2011 ESPAD data indicated that on average 38% of students in European countries reported binge drinking compared to 15% in the US. Concerning report of drunkenness, 41% of students in France, 50% of students in the United Kingdom, and 28% of students in the US reported they had

been drunk in the last year. These differences underscore that increased restrictions on underage drinking in the US have resulted in lower levels of reported alcohol use compared to countries with less restrictive policies.

Marijuana

Marijuana use is undergoing change nationally, with over 21 states legalizing the use of marijuana for medicinal purposes and two states (Washington and Colorado) additionally legalizing recreational use in 2013. These changes have coincided with a significant decrease in

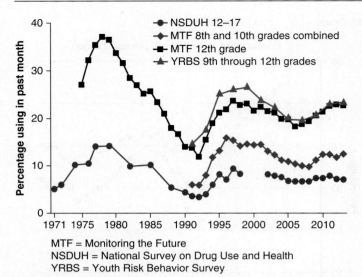

MTF = Monitoring the Future
NSDUH = National Survey on Drug Use and Health
YRBS = Youth Risk Behavior Survey

FIGURE 63.2 Past month marijuana use among youths in NSDUH, MTF, and YRBS: 1971 to 2013 substance abuse and mental health services Administration. (Results from the *2013 National Survey on Drug Use and Health: summary of National Findings*. NSDUH Series H—48, HHS Publication No. (SMA) 14-4863. Rockville, MD: Substance Abuse and Mental Health Services Administration, 2014.

adolescents' perceived risk of use, which is reflected in both the MTF and YRBSS surveys. Currently marijuana, both inhaled and ingested, is illegal for recreational use in every state under the age of 21; medicinal use age limits vary by state. Well before changes in state laws regarding this drug, the MTF showed that marijuana is the second most used drug during adolescence. Since 2010, there has been a significant increase in daily use in all grades. In 2014, the MTF study reported the lifetime prevalence of marijuana use was 15.6% in 8th grade, 33.7% in 10th grade, and 44,4% in 12th grade.

Prescription Medication Misuse

Taken together, misuse of prescription medications is the third most common form of drug use in adolescence, with 19.9% of 12th graders reporting use of prescription medications for nonmedical purposes. Prescription misuse encompasses using medications without a prescription, in addition to using a prescription in a manner inconsistent with prescriber instructions. This typically includes nonmedical use of pain relievers, stimulants, tranquilizers, and sedatives. According to the 2013 NSDUH, 17.4% of 17-year-olds surveyed had abused prescription pain relievers, with 11.2% using them in the last year and 4.3% in the last month. The largest group of new drug users was those who began using prescription pain relievers without a prescription. According to the *2012 Partnership for a Drug Free America Tracking Survey*, 16% of teenagers have used hydrocodone (Vicodin) or oxycodone (OxyContin) and 13% have used methylphenidate (Ritalin) or dextroamphetamine (Adderall) without a prescription. Approximately 43% of teens in this survey indicated that these drugs were easier to get than illegal drugs, and 56% reported that they were easy to get from their parents' medicine cabinets.

Young Adults

Young adult (aged 18 to 25 years—26th birthday) substance use trajectories after high school can include continued abstinence, initiation, or a decrease, increase, or maintenance of past levels of use. Data for young adults do not have uniform age brackets, with some studies including 19- to 24-year-olds and others using 18- to 25–year-olds. Nonetheless, these data show concerning trends in young adult use in the US. In describing this age-group, overall use of AMTOD is higher than among adolescents and older adults. For those over age 21 who can legally purchase alcohol (and perhaps marijuana, depending on the state), controls for

use no longer exist. However, even for those between the ages of 18 and 21 (who cannot purchase alcohol legally in the US), the vast majority have used alcohol. In the 2013 NSDUH data, approximately 83.8% of 18- to 25-year-olds reported lifetime use of alcohol, with 59.6% reporting consumption of alcohol in the last 30 days. Marijuana use is also higher in the 18 to 25 age range, with 51.9% reporting lifetime use and 19.1% reporting use in the last 30 days. Females report significantly less illicit drug use than males; however, female use has been increasing. Asian and African American young adults report lower levels of drug use compared to White and Latino young adults, similar to patterns among adolescents.

Tobacco use is less prevalent in full-time college students compared to all other young adults. In the 2013 NSDUH, 21.0% of college students reported cigarette use, compared to 34.4% of 18- to 22-year-olds who were not full-time college students. E-cigarettes, vaporizers, and flavored cigarettes are becoming more popular in this age-group as well as among younger adolescents, and it will be important to observe future tobacco and nicotine use as a result.

A longitudinal comparison of substance use rates among those in college versus those not in college (with 12th graders as a comparison) can be seen in MTF data from 1980 to 2013. In general, rates of drug use reported by young adults and 12th graders over that 30-year period are quite similar (including 2013) and are reported at higher rates than in the NSDUH (see Fig. 63.3).

Use of illicit drugs in the last 12 months among college students and young adults in general reached a low point in 1991 and then began to trend upward, peaking in 2001. Since then, rates of illicit drug use (except marijuana) have decreased. After alcohol, marijuana is the drug most often used by both college and noncollege students. Other notable findings regarding drug use in the last 12 months among young adults are as follows:

1. 3,4-Methylenedioxy-N-methylamphetamine (MDMA). MDMA ("ecstasy") use grew rapidly in popularity among college students, with peak use occurring in 2001 and declining rapidly after that.
2. Amphetamines. The recent MTF survey asked about the use of amphetamines, particularly Adderall, and found that 10.6% of college students compared to 7.8% of young adults in general reported using. This nonprescribed use may be due to a desire to increase academic performance or increase alertness. Several recent studies have linked amphetamine prescription misuse with unhealthy weight loss, increased anxiety and impulsivity, increased use of other substances, and other psychiatric issues.[3,4]
3. Cocaine. Cocaine use reached a nadir in 1994. Among college students, rates of use plateaued from 2000 to 2002 and then increased in 2003 and 2004 with a continued decrease since that time. Among young adults in general, rates of use increased through 2004 and then decreased after a period of plateau.
4. Synthetic drugs. In 2011, a question about synthetic marijuana use was added to the MTF study; synthetic marijuana was noted to be the second most abused drug after marijuana. Bath salts were added to MTF in 2012. It is important to monitor new trends and synthetic products that come on the market. Generational forgetting will make it likely that these will wax and wane in popularity.
5. Prescription pain relievers. In 2006, approximately 7.6% of college students and 9.1% of young adults in general reported nonmedical use of hydrocodone in the last 12 months. Since that time, OxyContin also became popular, with current combined annual use of 5.0% in college students compared to 8.6% use in young adults in general in 2012. Generally, there appear to be two main types of pain reliever misuse: self-treatment (of unmanaged pain or underlying psychiatric issues) and recreational use[4]. While recreational use is more indicative of other risky behaviors, increases in the misuse of pain relievers are

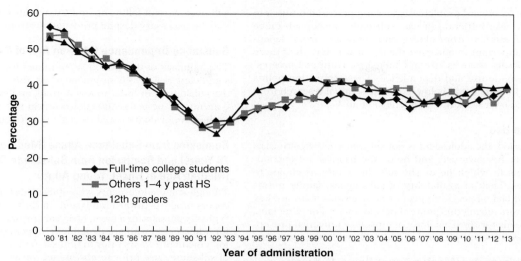

FIGURE 63.3 Trends in annual prevalence college students vs others any illicit drug use (twelfth graders included for comparison). (From Johnston LD, O'Malley PM, Bachman JG, et al. *Monitoring the future national survey results on drug use, 1975–2013*. Vol 2. College students and adults ages 19–55. Ann Arbor: Institute for Social Research, the University of Michigan, 2014.) HS = High school.

linked to increased heroin use and increased mortality according to the Centers for Disease Control and Prevention.

LONG-TERM OUTCOMES OF DRUG USE

Over the last 10 years, advances in neuroimaging technology and longitudinal studies provide evidence that use of drugs, especially if initiated in early to mid-adolescence, is associated with significant long-term consequences. Below the cognitive effects of marijuana use are examined:

1. A longitudinal study from New Zealand, which followed toddlers into middle adulthood, showed that permanent cognitive impairment and loss of intelligence quotient (IQ) could occur in persistent marijuana users.[5]
2. Another longitudinal birth cohort study from New Zealand demonstrated that cannabis use (especially by age 14 to 15) was significantly related to depression, suicidal ideation and attempts, and participation in violent crimes at 21 years.[6]
3. The research examining the correlation between schizophrenia and marijuana use continues to grow. Smith et al.[7] found that the younger a person begins to use marijuana heavily and consistently, the more brain abnormalities are seen. Furthermore, those abnormalities resemble the same abnormalities seen in schizophrenia. Another study, controlling for childhood psychotic symptoms and other drug use, found that those who smoked marijuana by age 15 were 7.2 times more likely to develop psychotic symptoms at age 26 than controls.[8]

ADOLESCENT BRAIN DEVELOPMENT AND SUSCEPTIBILITY TO DRUG USE AND DRUG-ASSOCIATED BRAIN DAMAGE

Use of sophisticated neuroimaging techniques demonstrates that adolescence is a period of significant brain development particularly in regards to learning and reward systems.[9] In a longitudinal study of 145 healthy children (56 females, age range 4.2 to 21.6 years), Giedd et al.[10] noted that the dorsal lateral prefrontal cortex, which is responsible for controlling impulses, did not reach maturity until the early 20s. Observed changes in the frontal cortex are consistent with neuropsychological studies that show that frontal lobes are involved with emotional regulation, planning, organizing, and response inhibition (the latter three constituting "executive functioning"). Such brain development

may contribute to the increase in risk-taking behaviors experienced by adolescents, particularly in regards to substance use.

Studies in rats show that mesolimbic dopamine (DA) synthesis in the nucleus accumbens is lower in preadolescent than adolescent rats, which in turn are lower than in adult rats. Dopaminergic and noradrenergic systems show large increases in neurotransmitter levels and activity during adolescence, and the hippocampus increases significantly in size. The hippocampus is intricately involved with new memory formation, a critical process in learning. This development in the reward circuitry and memory systems may contribute to the findings that adolescents may be at increased risk for substance dependence due to brain development.[11]

In addition to adolescents being uniquely susceptible to substance use due to developmental changes, adolescents may also face increased consequences with substance use. One recent study revealed that the brains of adolescents who were heavy drinkers for at least 1 year (<20 drinks/month) showed significantly decreased gray matter and functioning.[12] Brown, Tapert, Granholm, and Delis[13] found that alcohol-dependent adolescents showed distinct deficits when retrieving verbal and nonverbal information compared to healthy peers. Given the significant brain changes that occur during adolescence, including frontal lobe changes linked to impulse control and decision making, and the areas involved in the brain's reward circuitry, it is not surprising that adolescents may be uniquely susceptible to the harmful effects of drug use, including dependence or addiction.

PROGRESSION OF SUBSTANCE USE

It is clinically useful to conceptualize AYA substance abuse as occurring across a continuum. Diagnostic criteria for substance use disorders in the fifth edition of the *Diagnostic and Statistical Manual of Mental Disorders (DSM-5)* involve classifying problematic use as "mild," "moderate," and "severe," with individuals moving back and forth through this continuum. Individuals are considered in "early remission" once abstinence is achieved for 3 to 12 months and considered in "sustained remission" when continuous abstinence is maintained for 1 year. However, along the spectrum, relapses can be frequent, cycling the individual back to earlier points in use patterns.

It is useful to consider the various transition points that occur in substance use behaviors for AYAs. The National Institutes of Health currently recognizes six distinct transition points that

XIV

mark progression toward problematic use and potential remission: opportunity to use, initiation of use, substance abuse, substance dependence, remission from abuse, and remission from dependence.[14] It is important to note that the age at which each of these transitions initially occur is strongly linked to continued progression to problematic use and dependence. These transition points are described in more detail below, adapting seminal research from MacDonald and later work by Swendenson et al.[14]

No Substance Use

During this period, the adolescent is not subject to any health risks posed by his or her own use, and he or she has not yet encountered situations in which he or she has the ability or choice to use substances. Lack of availability of substances, family norms of nonuse, and lack of access to peers who use substances are key protective factors during this point of development. For clinicians, the primary focus for these adolescents involves universal prevention techniques aimed at preventing and delaying initiation of use.

First Opportunity to Use (Median Age of Onset, 16 Years)

At this point, the adolescent is still not subject to any health risks posed by their own use. However, the adolescent is subject to risks from use of substances by friends (e.g., riding with an impaired driver, sexual assault in association with substances, being in a fight with an intoxicated individual). For clinicians, the primary focus is on safety, praising and normalizing abstinence, and prevention of initiation (refusal skills).

Initiation of Use (Median Age of Onset, 17 Years)

The age of substance use initiation has been linked to the development of substance use problems later in life.[15] Following initiation of use of one drug, adolescents may try various other drugs, typically out of curiosity or to fit in with friends. The most commonly used drugs at this point are alcohol, marijuana, and tobacco. Once adolescents initiate substance use, they place themselves at risk for the health risks associated with this use. Even a single episode or very sporadic use can involve significant risk—even death—depending on the circumstances of use and the substances used. Some adolescents may cease using substances for a time, having found the experience unpleasant. Other adolescents will continue to experiment with substances, trying different types of substances with increasing frequency. Use typically occurs in social settings, and positive or pleasurable experiences generally outweigh negative consequences, though this may change as use continues to increase. For clinicians, the primary focus (using motivational interviewing (MI) techniques) should be on reviewing risks of substance use, assessing the adolescent for risk factors associated with use progression, safety, encouraging and normalizing abstinence, and practicing refusal skills.[16]

Drug Abuse (Median Age of Onset, 18 Years)

At this point, adolescents will actively seek out substances and begin to organize their lives around assuring a supply. They will actively seek out settings where substances are likely to be and avoid ones where substance use is unlikely. They may buy or perhaps sell substances to assure a supply. The types of substances used continue to expand. The social network will largely consist of using peers. Nonusing friends may become less desirable and distant. Behavioral changes may become apparent. The hallmark of this point in substance use progression is the increasing amount of negative consequences associated with substance use. In addition, the adolescent will need to be increasingly vigilant to hide substance use. Often, individuals who progress to substance abuse continue on to dependence; this transition typically takes less than 1 year. For clinicians, the focus should be on MI, reviewing risks, safety, assessing increasing problems, and increasing adolescent ambivalence about use and promoting change behaviors.[16] Adolescents at this stage

will need careful follow-up and treatment. Involvement of parents may be necessary despite protestations from the adolescent.

Substance Dependence (Median Age of Onset, 19 Years)

The hallmark of this period is continued use despite experiencing significant negative consequences. At this point, AYAs will often use substances in order to feel normal, and negative consequences continue to increase. Any adolescent in this stage requires a comprehensive evaluation and intensive treatment.

Remission from Substance Abuse (Median Age of Onset, 26 Years) and Remission from Substance Dependence (Median Age of Onset, Young Adult)

Though some adolescents who abuse substances continue to use, others progress toward remission. In these cases, substance abuse typically persists for a mean of 5 years prior to remission. Similarly, for adolescents who are dependent, dependence typically persists for a mean of 7 years prior to remission of use. In each case, length of substance use prior to abstinence varies greatly based on type of substance and history of substance use. For clinicians, the focus should be on involving the adolescents in evidence-based treatments of substance use disorders, such as cognitive-behavioral therapy, contingency management, motivational enhancement therapy, 12-step facilitation therapy, functional family therapy, and multisystemic therapy.

PREVENTION

Risk and Protective Factors for Substance Use

Research on the prevention of substance use in AYAs has made significant strides in the past three decades. Prevention science is based on risk and protective factors. *Risk factors* include individual, family, peer, school, and community characteristics (both malleable and unchanging) that precede problem behaviors (e.g., substance abuse) and contribute to an individual's likelihood of developing problems. At the same time, *protective factors* buffer individuals from the effects of these risks, decreasing an individual's likelihood of developing problems. Substance use prevention is based on the premise that substance use may be prevented by reducing an individual's malleable risk factors and reinforcing an individual's protective factors. Ultimately, adolescent substance use is a complex phenomenon; no single risk factor predicts with certainty that an adolescent will use substances or develop a substance abuse problem, nor does the presence of a single protective factor offer reassurance that no use will occur. Rather, substance use or nonuse results from a combination of these factors.

A small list of risk factors has consistently emerged as significantly contributing to substance use. Interestingly, many of these risk factors overlap with risk factors for other problematic behaviors, such as delinquency, teen pregnancy, school dropout, and violence. This convergence of risk factors suggests that adolescents who are at greater risk for substance use may also be at risk for developing other problems. **Table 63.2** lists the risk factors identified by the *Substance Abuse and Mental Health Services Administration (SAMHSA)*. To summarize, the more that various substances are readily available and that use of these substances is visible and perceived to be safe and accepted within communities, the more likely AYAs are to use substances.

Additionally, at a population level, perception of the risks of substance use is linked to the prevalence of use. For example, according to the MTF study, over the last 30 years, the prevalence of marijuana use rose and fell according to risk perception. The percentage of 12th graders who perceived "great risk" in regular marijuana use reached a nadir (approximately 35%) in 1979. In that same year, reported use of marijuana in the past year by 12th graders peaked at approximately 50%. Perceived risk then began to rise, peaking in 1992. Not surprisingly, use fell to its lowest level at

TABLE 63.2

Risk Factors	Adolescent Problem Behaviors				
Community	**Substane Abuse**	**Delinquency**	**Teen Pregnany**	**School Dropout**	**Violence**
Availability of drugs					•
Availability of firearms					•
Community laws and norms favorable toward drug use, firearms, and crime	•	•			•
Media portrayals of violence					•
Transitions and mobility	•	•		•	
Low neighborhood attachment and community disorganization	•	•			•
Extreme economic deprivation	•	•	•	•	•
Family					
Family history of the problem behavior	•	•	•	•	•
Family management problems	•	•	•	•	•
Family conflict	•	•		•	•
Favorable parental attitudes and involvement in the problem behavior	•	•			•
School					
Academic failure beginning in late elementary school	•	•	•	•	•
Lack of commitment to school	•	•	•		•
Peer and Individual				•	
Early and persistent antisocial behavior	•	•	•	•	•
Rebelliousness	•	•			
Friends who engage in the problem behavior	•	•	•	•	•
Gang involvement	•	•			•
Favorable attitudes toward problem behavior	•	•	•	•	
Early initiation of the problem behavior	•	•			•
Constitutional factors	•	•			•

From Adolescent Problem Behaviors. Social Development Research Group. (n.d.). *Communities that care: social development strategy chart & risk factor checklist.* Available at http://www.sdrg.org/ctcresource/Community%20Building%20and%20Foundational%20Material/Building_Protection_Social_Dev_Strategy_Chart.pdf. Accessed January 13, 2014.

the same time. Following that, perceived risk then began to fade, and use began to rise. Perception of risk not only differs by historical time point, but also by age. According to research done by SAMSHA, young adults aged 18 to 25 years have the highest rates of marijuana use and the lowest perception of risk, compared to any other age-group.

While adolescents are exposed to multiple risk factors, they typically have some protective factors in place. Protective factors for substance use are broadly conceptualized as centered around two concepts: strong social bonding and clear standards for behavior. Generally, the more bonded adolescents are to their family, prosocial peers, school, and community, the more likely adolescents are to abide by the behavioral standards of their family and community. By offering opportunities for prosocial involvement and rewarding prosocial participation, parents, educators, and community members can increase the bonding young people experience in their families, schools, and communities. A recent study on emerging adults transitioning from high school to college found that having prosocial peers who did not frequently use substances protected young adults from experiencing increasing alcohol and marijuana use rates with their transition to college.[17] Similarly, young adults who reported higher rates of parental monitoring while in high school reported less heavy drinking and marijuana use when they transitioned to college.[17]

XIV

TABLE 63.3
Protective Factors for Preventing Drug Use

Domain	Protective Factors
Individual	High intelligence Achievement oriented Positive self-esteem Optimistic view of future Good coping skills Prosocial orientation High religiosity
Family	Clear messages about no use Parents model appropriate alcohol/drug use Strong family–youth attachment Moderate to high levels of parental monitoring Supportive parents
Peers	Peers do not use drugs Peers have prosocial/conventional values
Schools	Offer opportunities for success and involvement Students feel connected to school School personnel perceived as fair and caring
Community	Recreational activities offered Strong community institutions Media realistically portrays harms associated with drug use Counter marketing media

Additional protective factors include social skills, refusal skills, belief in the moral order, and religiosity.[18] **Table 63.3** shows primary protective factors. Prevention programs are most effective if they specifically target malleable risk factors within communities, while simultaneously, bolstering the protective factors in young people's lives.

One major protective factor associated with drug use is race/ethnicity. Since 1975, African American 12th graders have consistently had lower rates of illicit drug use than White adolescents, with Hispanic adolescents having rates in-between those of African Americans and Whites. African American 8th and 10th graders also have lower rates of illicit drug use than their White classmates although the differences are less pronounced than among 12th graders. In 2004, Hispanic 8th and 10th graders had higher rates of drug use than did Whites.

Prevention Interventions

Early efforts at substance use prevention focused on providing knowledge of the harmful effects of substance use. Evaluation of these programs failed to show an effect; some studies showed an increase in use following the programs. Other unsuccessful efforts relied on the use of authority figures (e.g., police) to deliver anti-drug messages. Beginning in the 1980s, prevention efforts became more sophisticated, recognizing the multiple risk factors of drug use. Today prevention programs focus on reducing community, school, family, or individual risk factors.

Community or structural prevention interventions typically intercede at county or state levels and often involve policy and media work. These interventions include increased taxes on alcohol and tobacco, the minimum legal drinking age, and graduated licensing policies. Increasing taxes on alcohol is linked to lowered mortality rates, fewer traffic crash fatalities, and lower rates of sexually transmitted infections, violence, and crime. Similarly, increasing the minimum drinking age is linked to decreased rates of drinking in AYAs and to decreased mortality rates in vehicular crashes. Additional structural

prevention programs involve media campaigns, which can increase health behaviors when targeted and well executed.

Family-based prevention programs typically target parent and child interactions and span child development. Early interventions, such as the Nurse Family Partnership, focus on prenatal health up to 2 years, and increasing parenting skills for low-income, single, first-time mothers. Though this intervention occurs early in a child's life, it has been linked with reduced substance use when the children reach the age of 15.[19] Other interventions include the Strengthening Families and Guiding Good Choices programs, for parents and early adolescents aged 10 to 14 years. These programs involve five to seven parent-training sessions that focus on family management skills, conflict resolution, refusal skills, and parent–child bonding. Both programs have been shown to reduce substance initiation and substance use years after participation.[20]

Most school interventions are delivered in primary and secondary education settings, and they target school risk factors by teaching skills to students and bolstering teacher instructional and management skills.[21] Programs, such as the Seattle Social Development Project, increase teachers' skills by promoting interactive styles, cooperative learning strategies, and proactive classroom management. This program also facilitates parent classes to equip parents with skills to help their children succeed in an academic environment. This program showed a decrease in substance use, criminal activity, and mental health problems at 21 years.[22]

In addition to these programs, some prevention interventions focus on peer and individual risk factors. These interventions typically occur in school-based settings or involve community agencies. Life Skills Training is a 3-year prevention curriculum designed for implementation in middle school. The modules focus on decision making, goal setting, anger management, communication, stress reduction, media, peer pressure, and consequences of drug use.[21] Three years after receiving these classes, students had reduced substance use compared to controls, including cigarette smoking, binge drinking, and illicit drug use.[23] For a more comprehensive review of drug prevention programs, see the review by Catalano et al.[21]

ACKNOWLEDGMENT

This chapter is based on Chapter 68 from the 5th edition, Adolescent Health Care: A Practical Guide, authored by Alain Joffe and Robert E. Morris.

REFERENCES

1. Volkow ND, Baler RD. Addiction science: uncovering neurobiological complexity. *Neuropharmacology* 2014;76:235–249.
2. Casey BJ, Jones RM, Hare TA. The adolescent brain. *Ann N Y Acad Sci* 2008;1124:111–126.
3. Jeffers A, Benotsch EG, Koester S. Misuse of prescription stimulants for weight loss, psychosocial variables, and eating disordered behaviors. *Appetite* 2013;65:8–13.
4. Zullig KJ, Divin AL. The association between non-medical prescription drug use, depressive symptoms, and suicidality among college students. *Addict Behav* 2012;37(8):890–899.
5. Meier MH, Capsi A, Ambler A, et al. Persistent cannabis users show neuropsychological decline from childhood to midlife. *Proc Natl Acad Sci U S A* 2012;109(40): E2657–E2664.
6. Fergusson DM, Horwood LJ, Swain-Campbell N. Cannabis use and psychosocial adjustments in adolescence and young adulthood. *Addiction* 2002;97:1123.
7. Smith MJ, Cobia DJ, Wang L, et al. Cannabis-related working memory deficits and associated subcortical morphological differences in healthy individuals and schizophrenia subjects. *Schizophr Bull* 2014;40(2):287–299. doi:10.1093/schbul/sbt176.
8. Arseneault L, Cannon M, Poulton R, et al. Cannabis use in adolescence and risk for adult psychosis: longitudinal prospective study. *BMJ* 2002;325:1212.
9. Sowell ER, Thompson PM, Holmes CJ, et al. In vivo evidence for post-adolescent brain maturation in frontal and striatal regions. *Nat Neurosci* 1999;2:859.
10. Giedd JN. Structural magnetic resonance imaging of the adolescent brain. *Ann N Y Acad Sci* 2004;1021:77–85.
11. Casey BJ, Jones RM. Neurobiology of the adolescent brain and behavior: implications for substance use disorders. *J Am Acad Child Adolesc Psychiatry* 2010;49(12):1189–1201.
12. Squeglia LM, Jacobus J, Tapert SF. The influence of substance use on adolescent brain development. *Clin EEG and Neurosci* 2009;40(1):31–38.
13. Brown SA, Tapert SF, Granholm E, et al. Neurocognitive functioning of adolescents: effects of protracted alcohol use. *Alcohol Clin Exp Res* 2000;24(2):164–171.
14. Swendsen J, Anthony JC, Conway KP, et al. Improving targets for the prevention of drug use disorders: sociodemographic predictors of transitions across

drug use stages in the national comorbidity survey replication. *Prev Med* 2010;47(6):629–634.

15. McGue M, Iacono WG. The adolescent origins of substance use disorders. *Int J Methods Psychiatr Res* 2008;17(S1):S30–S38.
16. Jensen CD, Cushing CC, Aylward BS, et al. Effectiveness of motivational interviewing interventions for adolescent substance use behavior change: a meta-analytic review. *J Consult Clin Psychol* 2011;79(4):433.
17. White HR, McMorris BJ, Catalano RF, et al. Increases in alcohol and marijuana use during the transition out of high school into emerging adulthood: the effects of leaving home, going to college, and high school protective factors. *J Stud Alcohol* 2006;67(6):810–822.
18. Beyers JM, Toumbourou JW, Catalano RF, et al. A cross-national comparison of risk and protective factors for adolescent substance use: the United States and Australia. *J Adolesc Health* 2004;35(1);3–16.
19. Olds D L. The nurse–family partnership: an evidence-based preventive intervention. *Infant Ment Health J* 2006,27(1):5–25.
20. Robertson EB, David SL, Rao SA. *Preventing drug use among children and adolescents: a research-based guide for parents, educators, and community leaders* (No. 4). 2003; Bethesda, MD: Diane Publishing.
21. Catalano RF, Fagan AA, Gavin LE, et al. Worldwide application of prevention science in adolescent health. *The Lancet* 2012;379(9826):1653–1664.
22. Hawkins JD, Kosterman R, Catalano RF, et al. Promoting positive adult functioning through social development intervention in childhood: long-term effects from the Seattle Social Development Project. *Arch Pediatr Adolesc Med* 2005;159: 25–31.
23. Botvin GJ, Kantor LW. Preventing alcohol and tobacco use through life skills training. *Alcohol Res Health* 2000;24:250.

ADDITIONAL RESOURCES AND WEBSITES ONLINE

Alcohol

Rachel Gonzales-Castaneda
Martin M. Anderson

KEY WORDS

- Alcohol
- Alcoholism
- Alcohol intoxication
- Alcohol treatment
- Alcohol use
- Binge drinking
- Screening and brief intervention
- Underage drinking

Alcohol is the most widely used substance in the US. It is readily available and inexpensive. Alcohol is a central nervous system (CNS) depressant that has the ability to increase brain activity in areas that produce endorphins and in those that activate the dopaminergic reward system. In terms of physiology and metabolism, alcohol is a nonionized lipid soluble compound that is completely miscible in water. It is rapidly absorbed from the gastrointestinal tract and is distributed throughout the total body water. It easily penetrates the CNS because of its lipid solubility. Alcohol intoxication by legal definition is a blood alcohol concentration (BAC) of 0.08 g/dL or greater.[1] Physiologically, alcohol intoxication depresses the CNS so that mood, physical, and mental abilities are noticeably changed. Factors that affect alcohol intoxication include body weight/body type, functional tolerance, medication use, illness, and food consumption, as well as the rate of consumption and strength of drink. Given differences in alcohol metabolism by body weight, type, and physiologic mechanisms, alcohol dose in terms of BAC levels will have different intoxication effects on the body (Table 64.1).

The principal ingredient of all alcoholic beverages is ethanol. A standard drink in the US contains approximately 14 g of "pure" ethanol; however, levels of alcohol vary by type of alcoholic beverage.[1] For instance, a standard drink of beer constitutes 12 oz (which contains about 5% alcohol), whereas wine is 5 oz (containing about 12% alcohol), and distilled spirits is 1.5 oz (including about 40% alcohol). Hence, alcohol content for beers, wines, and distilled spirits vary and contain between 3% and 20% alcohol.

EPIDEMIOLOGY OF ALCOHOL USE AMONG ADOLESCENTS AND YOUNG ADULTS

The following highlights the epidemiologic data of alcohol use among adolescents and young adults (AYAs) separately, using standard national survey sources.

Adolescents

Youth Risk Behavior Survey (2013)

The Centers for Disease Control and Prevention's (CDC's) Youth Risk Behavior Survey (YRBS) reveals the following trends in alcohol use among high school–aged adolescents in the US.[2]

- *Incidence*: 18.6% of high school youth in the US reported that they drank alcohol before the age of 13 years (for the first time, other than a few sips).
- *Lifetime prevalence*: 66.2% reported that they ever had at least one drink of alcohol (on at least one day during their life).
- *Current prevalence*: 34.9% reported that they currently drank alcohol (had at least one drink of alcohol on at least 1 day during the past 30 days).
- *Binge drinking*: Binge drinking is defined as excessive alcohol intake within a 2-hour period such that BAC levels reach 0.08 g/dL (the legal limit of intoxication) or more. This typically happens when males consume five drinks or more and when women drink four drinks or more, within a 2-hour period.[1] Research suggests that for 9- to 13-year-old children and girls aged 14 to 17 years, binge drinking should be defined as three or more drinks. For boys, binge drinking should be defined as four drinks or more for those aged 14 or 15 years and five or more drinks for those aged 16 or 17 years. These figures are based on the number of drinks required to reach a BAC of 0.08 g/dL.[1] Data suggest that 20.8% of adolescents reported that they had five or more drinks of alcohol in a row (within a couple of hours on at least 1 day in the past month).

Monitoring The Future (MTF): Data from the 2014 MTF survey reveal lifetime, current, and binge drinking trends across 8th, 10th, and 12th grade levels[3]:

- *Lifetime prevalence*: The prevalence of lifetime alcohol use for 8th, 10th, and 12th graders combined in 2014 was 40.7%. The percentage reporting ever being drunk in one's lifetime across all three grade levels was 23.6%.
- *Current prevalence*: Current alcohol use (drinking in the 30-day period prior to the survey) was 9% for 8th graders, 24% for 10th graders, and 37% for 12th graders. Overall, the current prevalence in the past month across the three grades combined in 2014 was 22.6%.
- *Binge drinking*: The proportion of binge drinking (i.e., having five or more drinks in a row at least once in the prior 2 weeks) for 8th, 10th, and 12th graders was 5.1%, 13.7%, and 22.1%, respectively. Overall, the current prevalence of binge drinking during the past month across the three grades combined was 11.7%.

National Survey on Drug Use and Health (NSDUH): Data from the NSDUH (2014) survey also provide current, binge, and heavy alcohol use among adolescents in the US.[4] The NSDUH defines current (past month) use as at least one drink in the past 30 days; binge use as five or more drinks on the same occasion (i.e., at the same time or within a couple of hours of

TABLE 64.1

Effects of Alcohol Consumption in the Nontolerant Individual

Blood Alcohol Level (g/dL)	Effects
0.02	Reached after approximately one drink; light or moderate drinkers feel some effect—warmth and relaxation
0.04	Most people feel relaxed, talkative, and happy; skin may become flushed
0.05	First sizable changes begin to occur; light-headedness, giddiness, lowered inhibitions, and less control of thoughts may be experienced; both restraint and judgment are lowered; coordination may be slightly altered
0.06	Judgment is somewhat impaired; ability to make rational decisions about personal capabilities is affected (such as being able to drive)
0.08	Definite impairment of muscle coordination and slower reaction time occurs; driving ability becomes suspect; sensory feelings of numbness of the cheeks and lips occur; hands, arms, and legs may tingle and then feel numb (this constitutes legal impairment in Canada and in some US states, e.g., California)
0.10	Clumsiness; speech may become fuzzy; clear deterioration of reaction time and muscle control (this level previously constituted drunkenness in most US states)
0.15	Definite impairment of balance and movement
0.20	Motor and emotional control centers are measurably affected; slurred speech, staggering, loss of balance, and double vision can all be present
0.30	Lack of understanding of what is seen or heard occurs; individuals are confused or stuporous and may lose consciousness
0.40	Usually unconscious; the skin becomes clammy
0.45	Respiration slows and may stop altogether
0.50	Death occurs

From Morrison SF, Rogers PD, Thomas MH. Alcohol and adolescents. *Pediatr Clin North Am* 1995;42:371–387.

each other) on at least 1 day in the past 30 days; and heavy use as five or more drinks on the same occasion on each of 5 or more days in the past 30 days:

- *Current use:* Of the approximately 24.3 million adolescents in the US, 16.6% had used alcohol in the past month (10.3% to the point of intoxication), with 8.0% meeting criteria for substance abuse/dependence in the past year.[3] Data also show that rates of current alcohol use were lowest for youth aged 12 or 13 (2.1%) and increased with age (9.5% for 14- to 15-year-olds and 22.7% for 16- to 17-year-olds).
- *Binge drinking:* Rates of binge alcohol use followed trends similar to current use, with rates lowest for 12- to 13-year-olds (0.8%) and increasing to 4.5% for 14- to 15-year-olds and 13.1% for 16- to 17-year-olds.
- *Heavy drinking:* Heavy alcohol use rates for adolescents aged 12 to 13 and 14 to 15 were less than 1% (0.1% and 0.7%, respectively) and up to 3% for 16- to 17-year-olds.

Young Adults and College Students

MTF: Prevalence of various measures of alcohol use among young adults and college students in the 2014 MTF survey[5] is as follows:

- *Lifetime prevalence:* Lifetime prevalence of alcohol use for young adults in 2014 increased with age: 72.1% for 19- to 20-year-olds; 85.2% for 21- to 22-year-olds; 88.8% for 23- to 24-year-olds; and 91.1% for 25- to 26-year-olds.
- *Annual prevalence:* The annual prevalence of alcohol use for young adults followed a pattern comparable to those of lifetime rates in 2014: 68.4% for 19- to 20-year-olds; 82.8% for 21- to 22-year-olds; 84.7% for 23- to 24-year-olds; and 87.9% for 25- to 26-year-olds.
- *Current use:* The current rates of alcohol use (past 30 day use) for young adults also escalated with increasing age: 51.5% for 19- to 20-year-olds; 70.5% for 21- to 22-year-olds; 72.7% for 23- to 24-year-olds; and 75.9% for 25- to 26-year-olds.
- *Binge drinking:* The proportion of young adults who reported binge drinking (i.e., having five or more drinks in a row at least once in the prior 2 weeks) was lower for 19- to 20-year-olds (27.2%) compared to 21- to 22-year-olds, 23- to 24-year-olds, and 25 to 26-year-olds (40%, 38%, and 37%, respectively).

National Survey on Drug Use and Health: Trends in alcohol use among young adults in the US from the NSDUH data are summarized below.[6]

- *Current use:* Rate of current alcohol use in 2013 among young adults aged 18 to 25 was 59.6%.
- *Binge drinking:* Rates of binge drinking among young adults ranged from 29.1% among 18- to 20-year-olds to 43.3% for those aged 21 to 25. Figure 64.1 shows that young adults aged 18 to 25 have the highest prevalence of binge drinking in the US (estimated at 37.9%).
- *Heavy drinking:* Rates of heavy alcohol use in 2013 were 8.5% for young adults aged 18 to 20, peaking at 13.1% for those aged 21 to 25. As a whole, heavy alcohol use was reported by 11.3% of young adults aged 18 to 25 years.

American College Health Association

- According to 2013 data from the **American College Health Association's National College Health** Assessment (NCHA) survey,[6] the proportion of young adult college students who reported any alcohol use within the last 30 days was 66.8% (67.0% for females and 66.8% for males).

Sociodemographic Trends of Alcohol Use among Youth
Gender and Race

Lifetime Prevalence: The **2013 YRBS data**[2] show that the prevalence of lifetime alcohol use for females is higher than for males (67.9% versus 64.4%, respectively). Lifetime prevalence of alcohol use was highest among Hispanic/Latino adolescents (72.4%), followed by non-Latino Whites (65.9%) and Blacks (63.4%).

Current Use: Current use of alcohol was slightly higher for female than male adolescents (35.5% versus 34.4%, respectively). Current alcohol use rates in 2013 were higher among Hispanic (37.5%) and non-Latino White (36.3%) compared to Black (29.6%) youth. Data also reveal that alcohol use in the past month was higher among Hispanic female (39.7%) than Black female (31.3%) students and higher among non-Latino White (36.9%) and Hispanic male (35.2%) students than Black male (27.7%) students.

Binge Drinking: According to the **YRBS (2013),** binge drinking was higher for male than female adolescents (22.0% versus 19.6%, respectively). Binge drinking was highest among Hispanic/Latino youth (22.6%), followed by non-Latino White (23.2%) and Black students (12.4%). Data for young adult college students from the MTF (2014) suggest that since 2005 there has been considerable similarity in daily alcohol use patterns among males and females,

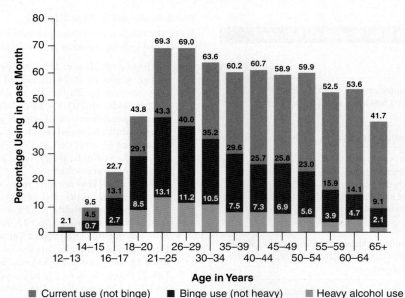

FIGURE 64.1 Percentage of current, binge, and heavy drinking by age-groups in the US. Results from the 2013 National Survey on Drug Use and Health: Summary and National Findings.

with the exception of the 19- to 22-year-old age-group. Specifically, males in this age-group have higher rates of daily drinking than their female age counterparts (5.6% for males versus 2.4% for females).

Puberty

Pubertal timing has been identified as a potential factor in understanding alcohol use among youth. Girls who become physically mature earlier than their same-aged peers are at risk for greater alcohol use than girls who mature on time or are late developing.[7] The situation for boys is less clear, but there is some evidence that early development may also be linked to increased levels of alcohol consumption among boys.

Consequences of Alcohol Use among Youth

The costs of problematic alcohol consumption in the US are substantial. In 2006, costs of alcohol use were estimated at $224 billion from losses in productivity, health care costs, crime, and other expenses,[8] with 11% of the costs ($24.6 billion) attributed to underage drinking. Alcohol use among young adults has been related to multiple adverse consequences, affecting individuals, families, communities, and society at large. Mortality tied to alcohol consumption in the US accounts for approximately 88,000 deaths per year, with young people less than 21 years of age accounting for more than 4,300 of those deaths.[9] Specific factors associated with alcohol mortality and injuries include engaging in high-risk behaviors, driving under the influence, unsafe sexual practices, and criminal behaviors.

Drinking and Driving

According to the 2013 YRBS survey,[2] 10% of high school–aged youth reported that they "drove after drinking alcohol," while 21.9% reported riding "with a driver who had been drinking alcohol." Motor vehicle accidents caused by driving under the influence of alcohol are among the leading causes of injuries for those younger than 21 years old. According to the most recent NCHA data,[6] 2.2% of college students reported driving after having five or more drinks in the last 30 days and 21.2% of college students reported driving after having any alcohol in the last 30 days. According to the US Department of Health and Human Services, an estimated 5.8% of youth between 16 and 17 and 15.1% of youth 18 to 20 reported

driving under the influence of alcohol in 2010. The US Department of Transportation found that a total of 3,115 youth between 13 and 19 died in motor vehicle crashes that year related to alcohol (with 2 out of 3 fatalities being identified as male). Overall, national risk estimates for being seriously injured (including death) while driving under the influence of alcohol are significantly higher among 16- to 20-year-olds[10] compared to other youth groups reported. Approximately 5,244 (66%) of traffic deaths among persons aged 16 to 20 years were alcohol related. In 2010, there were roughly 189,000 emergency department visits by youth under age 21 for injuries and other conditions associated with alcohol consumption, such as DUIs, violence, and other unintentional injuries, such as falls, drownings, etc.[10] According to the NSDUH (2013), roughly 1 in 9 persons aged 12 or older (10.9%) drove under the influence of alcohol at least once in the past year.[5] Figure 64.2 shows the prevalence of driving under the influence for young persons in the US.[11] As shown, young people aged 21 to 25 have the second highest rate (19.7%) of driving under the influence of alcohol among persons aged 16 or older.[11]

In 2008, more than 100 US college presidents and other higher education officials signed onto the Amethyst Initiative, which calls for a reexamination of the minimum legal drinking age in the US. The current age limit of 21 years in the US is higher than in Canada (18 or 19, depending on the province), Mexico (approximately 18), and most western European countries (typically 16 or 18). The thrust of their argument is that the US minimum legal drinking age policy results in more dangerous drinking than would occur if the legal drinking age were lower and youth were able to learn responsible drinking earlier. However, when examining epidemiologic and morbidity data over the past three decades, from sources such as the US Fatality Analysis Reporting System, MTF surveys, and Vital Statistics Data, lowering the drinking age (from 21 to 18) would result in the following among 18- to 20-year-olds: (1) a 17% increase in nighttime fatal crashes (those most likely to involve alcohol)—the highest percentage of any age-group and (2) a 10% increase in suicides, past-month drinking, and heavy episodic ("binge") drinking.[12–14]

Drinking and High-Risk Behaviors

Alcohol use is linked to a number of risky behaviors. According to data from the NCHA survey,[6] college students who drank alcohol

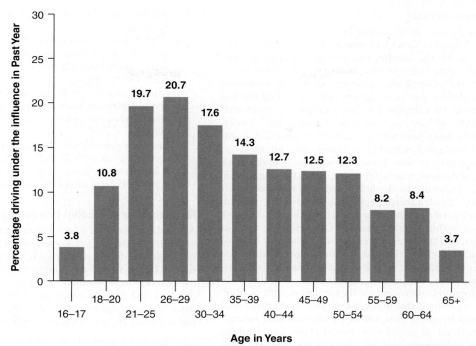

FIGURE 64.2 Percentage of individuals driving under the influence in the US by age-groups. Results from the 2010 National Survey on Drug Use and Health: Summary of National Findings.

reported experiencing the following problems in the last 12 months when drinking alcohol:

- Did something you later regretted (36.5%)
- Forgot where you were or what you did (32.3%)
- Got in trouble with the police (3.0%)
- Someone had sex with me without my consent (2.1%)
- Had sex with someone without their consent (0.6%)
- Had unprotected sex (20.4%)
- Physically injured yourself (14.9%)
- Physically injured another person (1.8%)
- Seriously considered suicide (2.5%)
- Reported one or more of the above (53.4%)

Data from the **2013 YBRS** also show the co-occurrence of drinking and high-risk sexual behaviors among youth, as 22.4% of high school adolescents in the US reported drinking alcohol or using drugs before their last sexual intercourse.[2]

Drinking and Disordered Eating/Energy Drinks

In a study of 697 college students, almost one-quarter of "current drinkers" reported mixing alcohol with energy drinks. Although there is still limited research regarding the growing use of mixing alcohol with energy drinks among youth, some reports have associated such growing use to increased marketing tactics from the alcohol industry and increased availability of such drinks in bars and clubs as "mixers."[15] These students were at increased risk for alcohol-related consequences, even after adjusting for the amount of alcohol consumed. Use of energy drinks alone is associated with a higher rate of sensation seeking, depression, and substance use in high school students. "Drunkorexia" is a term coined to describe college students' purposefully decreasing caloric intake, increasing exercise, and/or drinking until vomiting occurs (purging) to offset the excess calories consumed from drinking alcohol.[16]

Risk Factors for Alcohol Use among AYAs

There are many factors that contribute to alcohol initiation, use, and alcohol-related problem behaviors among AYAs. Many of these factors are similar to the ones for substance abuse in general, outlined in Chapter 63.

Parental Alcoholism

Various research studies have suggested that children of alcoholics are more susceptible to alcohol use disorders (AUDs) than those without a family history of alcoholism. Studies of twins and adopted children, for example, indicate that alcohol initiation arises from genetic, shared, and nonshared environmental contributions, since offspring of alcoholics are significantly more likely to develop alcoholism as compared to children of nonalcoholics.[17] Research has shown that parents who have heavy drinking episodes and who meet alcohol-dependence criteria are twice as likely as abstainers to have children with heavy drinking episodes (20% and 10% versus 10% and 5%, respectively). Moreover, studies have found that children of alcoholics are 4 to 10 times more likely to have alcohol use problems (abuse/dependence) than children whose parents were not alcoholic.[17]

Parental Drinking Standards

Problem alcohol use can be shaped by environmental exposure in the home through socialization patterns of parents.[18] Parents who provide structure around drinking (i.e., rules and communication) foster better regulatory skills in their children, including increased self-control and less risk for alcohol use problem behaviors.[18] Youth perceptions of parental approval of alcohol use and parents' use of alcohol have been identified as risk factors for youth initiation of drinking behaviors. Studies have shown, for instance, that if parents are perceived as being permissive toward drinking, youth are at higher risk of early initiation.[18] Early initiation or early onset of alcohol use (before age 14) has been identified as a risk factor for the later development of alcohol-related problems and disorders in adulthood. For example, studies have found that youth who started drinking before 13 years are nine times more likely to engage in problem drinking, such as binge drinking, than youth who initiated drinking later.[19] Moreover, the risk for lifetime alcohol dependence was 40% for individuals who started drinking at 14 compared to only 10% for those who started drinking after age 21.[20]

Media/Advertising of Alcohol

Media influences on the use of alcohol by young people are substantial. Research studies have demonstrated the extensive marketing efforts used by the alcohol industry to promote alcohol products to youth, including advertisements and depictions in entertainment outlets.[21] The alcohol industry spends an estimated 15 to 20 million dollars per year aggressively marketing alcohol to youth, conveying that drinking is fun and an important part of achieving social, athletic, and even sexual success.[21] Underage youth saw 45% more beer and ale, 12% more distilled spirit, and 65% more low-alcohol refresher beverage ads (for alcopops or lemonades, iced teas, or fruit-flavored beverages containing alcohol) as well as 69% more wine advertising than did people aged 21 years or older. Exposure to alcohol advertising was greater for girls than for boys.[22] Such advertising has been a powerful medium for setting and reinforcing existing prosocial trends and attitudes about alcohol use within youth culture.[23] Other media, such as television, movies, and the Internet, are known to be very influential in promoting alcohol use through attractive portrayals of use without mention of associated negative consequences. Considerable research has shown that media exposure increases the probability that children and adolescents will experiment with alcohol. Teunissen et al. examined the influence of pro- and antialcohol messages delivered by peers to youth in an Internet chat room.[23] When peers identified as popular delivered these pro-drinking messages, youths' willingness to drink changed accordingly. Similarly, Litt and Stock reported that youth had greater willingness to drink alcohol after viewing experimenter-generated Facebook pages portraying alcohol use as normative among older peers.[24] Smith and Foxcroft reviewed prospective cohort studies involving more than 13,000 youth aged 10 to 26 years and found that baseline nondrinkers who reported greater exposure to alcohol content online were more likely to become drinkers at follow-up.[25]

Alcohol Industry Developments and Social Norms

Increasingly, the alcohol industry has used various strategies to promote the use of alcohol within American culture, especially among youth.[25] For instance, flavored alcohol beverages (alcopops) (e.g., Mike's hard lemonade)—which mask the taste of alcohol—have become popular among young people. Developmentally, this is concerning since it can create social norms that drinking is a standard and accepted practice in the community (part of the culture), which can have a strong influence over youth behavior, especially the early initiation of alcohol use and progression from use to abuse/dependence.[24]

Societal Provision of Alcohol

In the US, the minimum alcohol drinking age is set at 21. Even so, research shows that patterns of drinking behavior are a major concern among 21- to 24-year-olds, especially college students, and national data reflect that many students come to college with already established drinking habits, as highlighted above.[3,5] Furthermore, studies have documented that drinking during college is a ritual that students often feel is an integral part of their higher education experience.[26] Surveys of college students reveal that about two out of three students who drink do so to the point of intoxication, typically on multiple occasions.[27] Alcohol drinking is related to several consequences, including injury/death, assault and sexual risk behaviors, and academic problems.[28] According to the National Institute on Alcohol Abuse and Alcoholism (NIAAA) (http://pubs.niaaa.nih.gov/publications/CollegeFactSheet/Collegefactsheet.pdf), each year among college students aged 18 to 24, an estimated:

- 1,825 die from alcohol-related unintentional injuries, including motor vehicle crashes.
- 599,000 are unintentionally injured under the influence of alcohol.
- 696,000 are assaulted by another student who has been drinking.
- 97,000 are victims of alcohol-related sexual assault or date rape.
- 400,000 have unprotected sex, and more than 100,000 students report having been too intoxicated to know if they consented to having sex.
- One-quarter report having academic consequences because of their drinking, including missing class, falling behind, doing poorly on examinations or papers, and receiving lower grades overall.
- Nineteen percent met the criteria for alcohol abuse or dependence, but only 5% of these students sought treatment for alcohol problems in the year preceding the survey.
- 3,360,000 drive under the influence of alcohol.

Neurotoxicity of Alcohol Use among Youth

Alcohol is considered a neurotoxin. Its full effects on the developing youth brain are not yet known (for a more detailed discussion of brain growth during adolescence and young adulthood, see Chapter 2). This dynamic developing brain is potentially susceptible to damage due to problematic alcohol consumption, especially binge drinking and heavy alcohol use patterns among young people. To date, research demonstrates the following neurologic, structural, and cognitive effects on the developing brain system among youth[28]:

- Youth are relatively resistant to the sedative effects of alcohol. They show less ataxia, social impairment, and fewer acute withdrawal effects than adults. They are more sensitive, however, to the social facilitation that may serve to encourage alcohol consumption.
- Imaging studies of youth with significant alcohol use show a reduced hippocampal volume and abnormalities of the corpus callosum, as well as subtle white matter microstructure abnormalities, particularly in the splenium of the corpus callosum.
- Functional magnetic resonance imaging shows decreased functional activity of the frontal and parietal areas of the right hemisphere, areas responsible for spatial memory.
- Studies show a disruption in learning and memory, especially memory retrieval, and in visual spatial functioning.
- Neurocognitive testing of alcohol abusers shows decreased visuospatial motor speed, decreased reading recognition, total reading, and spelling subtests on IQ testing.
- Increased consumption is associated with decreased memory, abstract thought, and language.
- Youth with more than 100 lifetime drinking episodes showed decreased verbal and nonverbal retention when compared to nondrinking controls.
- Withdrawal from alcohol also has neurocognitive effects. An increased number of withdrawal episodes are associated with greater decrease in visuospatial function with poor retrieval of verbal and nonverbal information.
- Alcohol use is also known to disrupt the sleep–wake cycle, resulting in increased sleep latency and increased daytime sleepiness.

AUDs among Youth

In the *Diagnostic and Statistical Manual for Mental Disorders (DSM-5)*, alcohol abuse and alcohol dependence are now combined into a single entity, Alcohol Use Disorders. According to the *DSM-5* (**Table 64.2**), anyone meeting any two of the 11 diagnostic criteria for abuse and dependence during the same 12-month period would receive a diagnosis of AUD. AUDs are now characterized as mild, moderate, and severe, depending on the number of criteria met.[29]

Approximately 855,000 adolescents (aged 12 to 17) in the US in 2012 were estimated to have an AUD. In 2013, among young adults aged 18 to 25, 13% were estimated to have past-year alcohol dependence or abuse (http://www.samhsa.gov/data/sites/default/files/National_BHBarometer_2014/National_BHBarometer_2014.pdf).

TABLE 64.2

DSM-5 Criteria for Diagnosis of Alcohol Use Disorder

Alcohol Use Disorder DSM-5[a]

Alcohol is often taken in larger amounts or over a longer period than was intended

There is a persistent desire or unsuccessful efforts to cut down or control alcohol use

A great deal of time is spent in activities necessary to obtain alcohol, use alcohol, or recover from its effects

Craving, or a strong desire or urge to use alcohol

Recurrent alcohol use resulting in a failure to fulfill major role obligations at work, school, or home

Continued alcohol use despite having persistent or recurrent social or interpersonal problems caused or exacerbated by the effects of alcohol

Important social, occupational, or recreational activities are given up or reduced because of alcohol use

Recurrent alcohol use in situations in which it is physically hazardous

Alcohol use is continued despite knowledge of having a persistent or recurrent physical or psychological problem that is likely to have been caused or exacerbated by alcohol

Tolerance, as defined by either of the following:
  a. A need for markedly increased amounts of alcohol to achieve intoxication or desired effect
  b. A markedly diminished effect with continued use of the same amount of alcohol

Withdrawal, as manifested by either of the following:
  a. The characteristic withdrawal syndrome for alcohol (see criteria A and B below)[b]
  b. Alcohol (or a closely related substance, such as a benzodiazepine) is taken to relieve or avoid withdrawal symptoms.

[a] The presence of at least 2 of these symptoms indicates an **Alcohol Use Disorder (AUD)**.
The severity of the AUD is defined as:
Mild: The presence of 2–3 symptoms
Moderate: The presence of 4–5 symptoms
Severe: The presence of 6 or more symptoms

[b] **Alcohol withdrawal-Criteria A and B**
A. Cessation of (or reduction in) alcohol use that has been heavy and prolonged
B. Two (or more) of the following, developing within several hours to a few days after Criterion A:
  (1) Autonomic hyperactivity (e.g., sweating or pulse rate greater than 100)
  (2) Increased hand tremor
  (3) Insomnia
  (4) Nausea or vomiting
  (5) Transient visual, tactile, or auditory hallucinations or illusions
  (6) Psychomotor agitation
  (7) Anxiety
  (8) Grand mal seizures

Adapted from NIH Publication No. 13-7999, 2013. Available at http://pubs.niaaa.nih.gov/publications/dsmfactsheet/dsmfact.htm. Accessed July 4,2015.

Although problematic in nature, research shows that most people with an AUD do not receive treatment. In 2012, for instance, only 1.4 million people received treatment for an AUD at a specialized facility (8.4% of population in need).[30]

Screening and Treatment Approaches for AUD among Youth

The American Medical Association's Guidelines for Adolescent Preventive Services, Bright Futures, and the American Academy of Pediatrics Policy Statement on Substance Abuse all recommend that every adolescent be screened for alcohol, tobacco, and other drug abuse (ATODA) as part of routine care. The US Preventive Services Task Force recommends screening everyone aged 18 years and older for alcohol misuse (Grade B recommendation), but concludes there is not sufficient evidence to make recommendations for or against screening youth less than 18 (Grade I recommendation). The NIAAA recommends screening all 9- to 18-year-olds using two questions: one about their friends' drinking and one about their own drinking. The questions vary by age. For example, if in middle school (aged 11 to 14), youth are asked first about friends' use ("Do you have any friends who drank beer, wine, or any drink containing alcohol in the past year?") followed by personal use questions ("How about you—in the past year, on how many days have you had more than a few sips of beer, wine, or any drink containing alcohol?"). However, high school youth (aged 14 to 18) should first be questioned about personal use ("In the past year, on how many days have you had more than a few sips of beer, wine, or any drink containing alcohol?") followed by friends' use ("If your friends drink, how many drinks do they usually drink on an occasion?") (http://pubs.niaaa.nih.gov/publications/Practitioner/YouthGuide/YouthGuideAlgorithm.pdf.).[31]

Currently, screening, brief intervention, and referral to treatment, referred to as "SBIRT," has been nationally recognized as an evidence-based approach to prevent/reduce substance use, by identifying substance use "risk" and following with a tailored intervention/treatment response.[28] To date, SBIRT efforts have been effective in both identifying and reducing substance use risk in a wide array of settings, including emergency departments, primary care offices, dental settings, and mental health agencies. Most of these efforts have primarily targeted adults, with fewer efforts among youth populations. Given the call to meet national goals of "reducing the rate of youth substance use over the next 5 years by 15%" as put forth by the National Drug Prevention Alliance, efforts are needed to better identify and address substance use–related behaviors among youth. Studies have identified as much as a $4 cost savings in treatment for every $1 spent on SBIRT. There is a broad base of evidence to support the effectiveness of SBIRT for alcohol use in the population over age 18.[32]

There are several widely available screening instruments to guide professionals in identifying individuals with alcohol problems. Screening tools can be administered by the professional as part of the general health interview or while performing related clinical or diagnostic screening (i.e., physical examinations). To be practical, screening tools must be easy to administer, score, and remember. Simple "yes" or "no" questions that lend themselves to mnemonic acronyms are ideal. The screening tools specific to youth that have been widely used and recommended are described below.[32]

Alcohol Use Disorders Identification Test (AUDIT) was developed by the World Health Organization (WHO) as a simple way to screen and identify people who are at risk of developing alcohol problems (see http://www.talkingalcohol.com/files/pdfs/WHO_audit.pdf). The AUDIT screening test has 10 multiple choice questions that focus on identifying the preliminary signs of hazardous drinking and mild dependence experienced within the last year (including questions on quantity and frequency of alcohol consumption, drinking behavior, and alcohol-related problems or reactions to problems). It is one of the most accurate alcohol screening tests available, rated 92% effective in detecting hazardous or harmful drinking. The test was modified into the AUDIT-C, which contains a simple three-question screen for hazardous or harmful drinking that can stand alone or be incorporated into general health assessments (see http://www.integration.samhsa.gov/images/res/tool_auditc.pdf).

The *CRAFFT* is also a validated, behavioral health screening tool. It consists of six items that are meant to assess whether a more in-depth conversation about the context and frequency of use and other risks and consequences of alcohol and other drug use is warranted. CRAFFT is a mnemonic acronym of the first letters of key words in the six screening questions, and the questions should be asked exactly as written (see below). Before being asked the CRAFFT questions, the young person is asked to answer the following three questions: "During the past 12 months, did you (1) drink any alcohol (more than a few sips)? (2) smoke any marijuana or hashish? (3) use anything else to get high? ("Anything else" includes illegal drugs, over-the-counter and prescription drugs, and things that you sniff or "huff"). If they respond "no" to all three questions, they just answer the CAR question (see below), whereas if they answer "yes" to any one of the three, they get all six CRAFFT questions.

C: Have you ever ridden in a CAR driven by someone (including yourself) who was "high" or had been using alcohol or drugs?
R: Do you ever use alcohol or drugs to RELAX, feel better about yourself, or fit in?
A: Do you ever use alcohol or drugs while you are by yourself, or ALONE?
F: Do you ever FORGET things you did while using alcohol or drugs?
F: Do your family or FRIENDS ever tell you that you should cut down on your drinking or drug use?
T: Have you ever gotten into TROUBLE while you were using alcohol or drugs?

Each "Yes" response to the CRAFFT questions is scored as one point. Youth who report no use of alcohol or drugs and have a CRAFFT score of 0 receive praise and encouragement. Those who report any use of alcohol or drugs receive a CRAFFT score of 1 and are encouraged to stop, and receive brief advice regarding the adverse health effects of substance use. A score of 2 or greater is a "positive" screen and indicates that the adolescent or young adult is at high risk for having an alcohol or drug-related disorder and requires further assessment.

The *CAGE* is a commonly used screening tool for alcohol use. Like the CRAFFT, the CAGE is an acronym formed from the italicized letters in the questionnaire (cut-annoyed-guilty-eye), which includes the following questions for identifying problems with alcohol:

Have you ever felt you should *C*ut down on your drinking?
Have people *A*nnoyed you by criticizing your drinking?
Have you ever felt bad or *G*uilty about your drinking?
Have you ever had a drink first thing in the morning to steady your nerves or to get rid of a hangover (*E*ye opener)?

Drug abuse screen test (DAST-10) is an adapted version of the *DAST* 28-item instrument that takes less than 8 minutes to complete. The *DAST-10* was designed to provide a brief instrument for clinical screening and treatment evaluation and can be used with older youth (see http://smchealth.org/sites/default/files/docs/13095 87937DRUGUSEQUESTIONNAIRE.pdf).

Alcohol, smoking, and substance involvement screening test (ASSIST) is another standardized, scripted screening tool developed by the WHO (see http://www.who.int/substance_abuse/activities/assist_test/en/). The ASSIST has gained much prominence by the Substance Abuse Mental Health Services Administration (SAMHSA) as it has been studied cross-culturally in eight countries. This interview-guided screening tool provides a detailed assessment of both alcohol and illicit drug use (including hazardous, harmful, or dependent use). Originally developed for use in primary care settings, it has been increasingly applied in other settings, including trauma centers, mental health settings, and college health centers.

The NIAAA developed a program for screening youth aged 9 to 18 years, described in its Alcohol Screening and Brief Intervention Guide for Youth, which can be downloaded at: http://pubs.niaaa.nih.gov/publications/Practitioner/YouthGuide/YouthGuideOrderForm.htm. Briefly, it consists of two questions that ask about friends' and the patient's number of drinks over the past year.

Depending on their answers and age, individuals are assigned to low-, moderate-, or high-risk categories and potential brief interventions are discussed.

Treatment for AUDs is a growing field. There has been substantial progress in research on behavioral treatments for adults aged 18 years and older with AUDs.[27] To date, evidence-based treatments for reducing alcohol problems include motivational enhancement therapy, cognitive behavioral therapy, behavioral couples therapy, brief interventions, twelve-step facilitation therapy, and the community reinforcement approach. Overall, treatment requires that young people (both AYAs) learn substitute activities that provide pleasures and rewards to replace the "highs" of drug use. These activities should be realistic and attainable, as well as facilitate the development of a healthy support system, such as sober peer-support systems (e.g., Alcoholics Anonymous), that are essential for recovery. Treatments that include family components have also shown to be effective with younger-aged youth, since the abuse of alcohol by one member of the family system affects other members. Family members are encouraged to attend Al-Anon or Alateen, which are 12-step self-help groups for family members.

REFERENCES

1. Donovan JE. Estimated blood alcohol concentrations for child and adolescent drinking and their implications for screening instruments. *Pediatrics* 2009;123(6):e975–e981.
2. Kann L, Kinchen S, Shanklin, SL, et al. Youth Risk Behavior Surveillance—United States, 2013. *MMWR* 2014;63 (SS-4):17–19.
3. Johnston LD, O'Malley PM, Miech RA, et al. *Monitoring the future national survey results on drug use: 1975–2014: overview, key findings on adolescent drug use.* Ann Arbor: Institute for Social Research, the University of Michigan, 2015.
4. Substance Abuse and Mental Health Services Administration. *Results from the 2013 National Survey on Drug Use and Health: Summary of National Findings.* NSDUH Series H-48, HHS Publication No. (SMA) 14-4863. Rockville, MD: Substance Abuse and Mental Health Services Administration, 2014. Available at http://store.samhsa.gov/
5. Johnston LD, O'Malley PM, Bachman JG, et al. *Monitoring the future national survey results on drug use, 1975–2013. Vol 2. College students and adults ages 19–55.* Ann Arbor: Institute for Social Research, the University of Michigan, 2014.
6. American College Health Association. *American College Health Association-National College Health Assessment II: Reference Group Executive Summary Spring 2014.* Hanover, MD: American College Health Association, 2014.
7. Singer M. Toward a bio-cultural and political economic integration of alcohol, tobacco and drug studies in the coming century. *Soc Sci Med* 2001;53(2):199–213.
8. Bouchery EE, Harwood HJ, Sacks JJ, et al. Economic costs of excessive alcohol consumption in the United States, 2006. *Am J Prev Med* 2011;41:516–24.
9. Substance Abuse and Mental Health Services Administration, Center for Behavioral Health Statistics and Quality. *The DAWN report: highlights of the 2010 Drug Abuse Warning Network (DAWN) findings on drug-related emergency department visits.* Rockville, MD, 2012.
10. National Highway Traffic Safety Administration. *Traffic safety facts: 2011 data: young drivers (DOT HS 811-744).* Washington, DC: 2013. Available at http://www-nrd.nhtsa.dot.gov/Pubs/811744.pdf
11. Neinstein LS. *The new adolescents: an analysis of health status.* 2013. Available at http://www.usc.edu/student-affairs/Health_Center/thenewadolescents/doc/TheNewAdolescents_Final_Locked.pdf
12. National Highway Traffic Safety Administration. *U.S. fatality analysis reporting system.* Available at http://www-fars.nhtsa.dot.gov Alcoholism. (2011). Unpublished analysis of 2000–2009 data from the National Survey on Drug Use and Health (NSDUH), an annual nationwide survey sponsored by the Substance Abuse and Mental Health Services Administration. 2013.
13. Murphy SL, Xu JQ, Kochanek KD. Deaths: final data for 2010. *Natl Vital Stat Rep* 2013;61(4).
14. Carpenter C, Dobkin C. The minimum legal drinking age and public health. *J Econ Perspect* 2011;25(2):133–156.
15. O'Brien MC, McCoy TP, Rhodes SD, et al. Caffeinated cocktails: energy drink consumption, high-risk drinking, and alcohol-related consequences among college students. *Acad Emerg Med* 2008;15(5):453–460.
16. Barry AE, Piazza-Gardner AK. Drunkorexia: understanding the co-occurrence of alcohol consumption and eating/exercise weight management behaviors. *J Am Coll Health* 2012;60(3):236–243.
17. National Institute on Alcohol Abuse and Alcoholism, U.S. Department of Health and Human Services. Alcohol and development in youth—a multidisciplinary overview. Genetics, pharmacokinetics, and neurobiology of adolescent alcohol use. *Alcohol Res Health* 2004/05c;28(3):133.
18. Koning IM, Van den Eijnden RJJM, Engels, RCME, et al. Why target early adolescents and parents in alcohol prevention? The mediating effects of self-control, rules and attitudes about alcohol use. *Addiction* 2011;106:538–546.
19. Foxcroft DR, Tsertsvadze A. Universal alcohol misuse prevention programmes for children and adolescents: Cochrane systematic reviews. *Perspect Public Health* 2012; 132:128–134.
20. Spoth R, Trudeau L, Guyll M, et al. Universal intervention effects on substance use among young adults mediated by delayed adolescent substance initiation. *J Consult Clin Psychol* 2009;77:620–632.

21. American Academy of Pediatrics, Committee on Communications. Children, adolescents, and advertising [published correction appears in Pediatrics. 2007; 119(2): 424]. *Pediatrics* 2006;118(6):2563–2569.

22. Jernigan DH, Ostroff J, Ross C, et al. Sex differences in adolescent exposure to alcohol advertising in magazines. *Arch Pediatr Adolesc Med* 2004;158(7):629–634.

23. Teunissen HA, Spijkerman R, Prinstein MJ, et al. Adolescents' conformity to their peers' proalcohol and anti-alcohol norms: the power of popularity. *Alcohol Clin Exp Res* 2012;36:1257–1267.

24. Litt DM, Stock ML. Adolescent alcohol-related risk cognitions: the roles of social norms and social networking sites. *Psychol Addict Behav* 2011;25:708–713.

25. Smith LA, Foxcroft DR. The effect of alcohol advertising, marketing and portrayal on drinking behaviour in young people: systematic review of prospective cohort studies. *BMC Public Health* 2009;9:51.

26. Presley CA, Meilman PW, Cashin JR. *Alcohol and drugs on American college campuses: use, consequences, and perceptions of the campus environment.* Vol. IV: 1992–1994. Carbondale, IL: Core Institute, Southern Illinois University, 1996.

27. Engs, RC, Diebold, BA, Hansen DJ. The drinking patterns and problems of a national sample of college students, 1994. *J Alcohol Drug Educ* 1996;41(3):13–33.

28. National Institute on Alcohol Abuse and Alcoholism, U.S. Department of Health and Human Services. *Underage drinking.* Available at http://www.niaaa.nih.gov/alcohol-health/special-populations-co-occurring-disorders/underage-drinking

29. National Institute on Alcohol Abuse and Alcoholism, U.S. Department of Health and Human Services. *Alcohol use disorder: a comparison between DSM–IV and DSM–5.* NIH publication No. 13-7999. November 2013. Available at http://pubs.niaaa.nih.gov/publications/dsmfactsheet/dsmfact.htm

30. NIAAA. National Institute on Alcohol Abuse and Alcoholism, U.S. Department of Health and Human Services. *Alcohol use disorder.* Available at http://www.niaaa.nih.gov/alcohol-health/overview-alcohol-consumption/alcohol-use-disorders

31. American Academy of Pediatrics Committee on Substance Abuse. Substance use screening, brief intervention, and referral to treatment for pediatricians. [Electronic version]. *Pediatrics* 2011;128:e1330. Available at http://pubs.niaaa.nih.gov/publications/Practitioner/YouthGuide/YouthGuideAlgorithm.pdf

32. Young MM, Stevens A, Porath-Waller A, et al. Effectiveness of brief interventions as part of the screening, brief intervention and referral to treatment (SBIRT) model for reducing the non-medical use of psychoactive substances: a systematic review protocol. *Syst Rev* 2012;1:22.

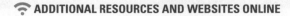 **ADDITIONAL RESOURCES AND WEBSITES ONLINE**

Tobacco

Mark L. Rubinstein
Judith J. Prochaska

KEY WORDS

- Addiction
- Cessation
- Cigarettes
- e-Cigarettes
- Nicotine
- Smoking
- Tobacco

"Tobacco use is a pediatric epidemic, around the world as well as in the United States."

Regina Benjamin, M.D., M.B.A. Surgeon General 2012[1]

More than 80% of all cigarette smokers start before the age of 18, and the majority of these will be addicted by young adulthood. Great strides have been made in limiting environmental exposure to tobacco smoke and banning direct marketing and sales of cigarettes to youth, resulting in a decline in adolescent and young adult (AYA) cigarette use in the US. However, challenging these public health efforts is the evolving tobacco market, with greater promotion of cigarillos (mini-cigars distinguishable from cigarettes only by their tobacco leaf rolling paper) and electronic or e-cigarettes (battery powered devices that generate an aerosol for inhalation typically containing nicotine). Both cigarillos and e-cigarettes are available for single purchase in a variety of child-friendly candy-flavorings (e.g., chocolate, bubble gum, cotton candy), and alterable for smoking other substances (e.g., marijuana). Use of cigarillos and e-cigarettes is on the rise among AYAs in some areas, generating concern that these products may represent a new gateway into tobacco smoking. The role of health care providers in immunizing their young patients from initiation of smoking and assisting those patients or the parents of their patients who already smoke to stop is critical.

PREVALENCE

Use among Adolescents

Tobacco use by adolescents remains a serious public health problem with roughly 1,000 American teenagers becoming regular smokers each day. In the 2014 Monitoring the Future (MTF) study of adolescents, there were two major findings:

- Cigarette smoking continues to decline and is now at the lowest levels recorded in the history of the survey.
- e-Cigarettes: This new product has made significant inroads among adolescents. Its prevalence among adolescents is now higher than the prevalence of tobacco cigarette smoking.

Past-month smoking among youth younger than 18 years declined from a peak of 36% in 1996 to 1997 to 18% in 2011 (Fig. 65.1). In the 2014 MTF survey (www.monitoringthefuture.org), 30-day prevalence of cigarette use reached a peak in 1996 in grades 8 and 10. Between 1996 and 2014, "current smoking" fell dramatically in these grades (by 81% and 77%, respectively). This decline slowed in recent years, and in 2010 there was a suggestion of a slight increase in smoking rates among 8th and 10th graders. However, use in these grades declined further between 2011 through 2014. Among 12th graders, peak use occurred in 1997 at 37%, and declined more modestly since then to 14% in 2014 (a 63% decline). In the 2014 survey, 4% of 8th graders, 7.2% of 10th graders, and 13.6% of 12th graders reported smoking one or more cigarettes during the previous 30 days. Declines in "daily smoking" are seen across all grades (currently 1% of 8th graders, 3.4% of 10th graders, and 5.8% of 12th graders).

Gender and Race

In the 2014 MTF study, there was more use among 12th grade males (15%) than females (12%) and among non-Hispanic Whites (18%) compared to Hispanics (11%) and Blacks (9%).

Smokeless Tobacco

Use of smokeless tobacco also has declined, with current rates for 30-day use in the 2014 MTF survey being 3% among 8th graders, 5.3% among 10th graders, and 8.4% among 12th graders.

Other Studies

The same trends in the prevalence of smoking among youth have been observed in the Centers for Disease Control and Prevention's (CDC's) biannual school-based Youth Risk Behavior Surveillance System (YRBSS; www.cdc.gov/HealthyYouth/yrbs) and the Substance Abuse and Mental Health Services Association (SAMHSA) non-school-based sample of adolescents in the biannual National Survey on Drug Use and Health (NSDUH; http://oas.samhsa.gov/nsduh.htm). While cigarette use has declined, there has been a significant increase in cigar use among Blacks adolescents, from 7% in 2009 to 12% in 2011.[2]

Tobacco Use among College Students and Young Adults

Young adults aged 18 to 24 have the highest prevalence of smoking and use of noncigarette, nicotine-containing tobacco products than any other age–group.[3] For both male and female college students, cigarettes remain the most commonly used tobacco product. Smokeless tobacco, traditional cigars, and pipes are less common, while flavored cigarillos, hookah (water pipe), and e-cigarettes are gaining in popularity. According to the 2013 National Health Interview Survey, among young adults aged 18 to 24, 23% of men and 17% of women are current smokers.[4] The 2013 MTF survey (Table 65.1) yielded similar results among young adults aged 19 to 28, with 20% reporting current smoking.[5] Whites have the highest use of tobacco products, followed by Hispanics, Asians, and Blacks.[4]

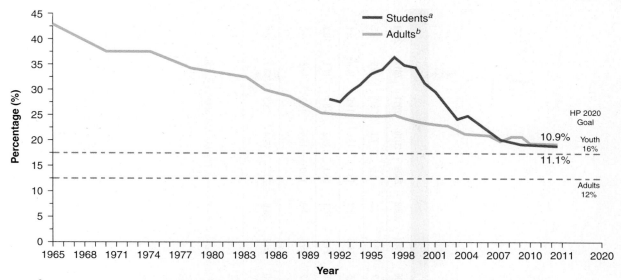

[a]Percentage of high school students who smoked cigarettes on 1 or more of the 30 d preceding the survey (Youth Risk Behavior Survey, 1991–2011).

[b]Percentage of adults who are current cigarette smokers (National Health Interview Survey, 1965–2011).

FIGURE 65.1 Trends in current cigarette smoking among high school students and adults, in the US, 1965 to 2011. (From the Centers for Disease Control and Prevention. Updated November 2013. Available at http://www.cdc.gov/tobacco/data_statistics/tables/trends/cig_smoking/)

College students who use tobacco are more likely to be single, White, and engaged in other risky behaviors involving substance use and sexual activity. Based on the Surgeon General report from 2012, of every three young smokers (i.e., AYAs), one will quit and one will die from tobacco-related causes.[1] The tobacco industry has overtly and heavily targeted young adult smokers, sponsoring events in bars and clubs, musical events, and movies popular with young adults.

FACTORS ASSOCIATED WITH YOUTH TOBACCO USE

Factors related to smoking initiation for boys and girls include low educational aspirations or attainment; low self-esteem or ongoing stress or depression; risk-taking; minimizing perceived hazards of smoking; and favorable attitudes toward smoking or smokers. Other variables associated with adolescent smoking include peer, parental, and sibling smoking; perceived parental or peer support for smoking; lower socioeconomic status or parental educational attainment; a history of abuse; exposure to tobacco advertising on the Internet or in the movies; and accessibility, availability, and price of tobacco products.[1,6] There are also gender-specific factors associated with smoking. For example, girls are more likely to smoke cigarettes for weight control, while teenage boys may smoke for a sense of adventure or daring.[6] Youth who identify as gay, lesbian, or bisexual smoke at rates far greater than those of their straight counterparts.[7]

NICOTINE ADDICTION AND HEALTH CONSEQUENCES

Addiction

Nicotine is one of the most addictive substances known. Tobacco use by adolescents, which may have started primarily for psychosocial reasons, can become a serious drug addiction. Preteens and early adolescents may believe that there are benefits to smoking and underestimate the addictive nature of cigarettes. Yet, initial symptoms of nicotine dependence occur in some teens, within days to weeks of onset of use.

Modes of Action

Nicotine seems to function as a positive reinforcer through its actions on nicotinic acetylcholine receptors in the mesocorticolimbic dopamine pathway. Stimulation of brain dopamine systems is of great importance for the rewarding and dependence-producing properties of nicotine.[8] Abstinence from nicotine is associated with depletion of dopamine and other neurotransmitters, which may cause numerous withdrawal symptoms, including anxiety, irritability, and cravings.[9] There are likely genetic factors (e.g., genetic variants in the CYP2A6 gene that influence the rate at which a smoker clears nicotine) in an individual's susceptibility to tobacco addiction as well as to response to the various pharmacologic treatments.[10] This is an active area of ongoing research.

Pharmacology

- Each cigarette delivers 1 to 2 mg of nicotine to the smoker.
- Each dose of the drug acts on the user within seconds of being inhaled.

Plasma concentrations of nicotine decline in a biphasic manner. Typically, the initial half-life is 2 to 3 minutes, and the terminal half-life is 30 to 120 minutes. Most nicotine is metabolized in the liver to cotinine. Cotinine has a plasma half-life that varies from approximately 16 to 20 hours. Nicotine and its metabolites are excreted by the kidneys; approximately 10% to 20% of the nicotine is eliminated unchanged in the urine.[11]

Effects of Other Compounds in Cigarettes

In addition to nicotine, cigarettes contain tar—a toxic compound. Cigarettes usually contain thousands of other chemicals, many poisonous and cancer causing, including arsenic, ammonia, benzene, cadmium, carbon monoxide, cyanide, formaldehyde, lead, nitrosamines, polonium, and polynuclear aromatic hydrocarbons.

Systemic Effects of Tobacco

The 2014 US Surgeon General's report updated the list of diseases related to tobacco use and concluded that unless use rates decline, smoking will result in the premature death of 1 of every 13 or 5.6 million US children alive today. The 2014 report concluded that

XIV

TABLE 65.1

Trends in 30-Day Prevalence[a] of Use[b] of Cigarettes for 8th, 10th, and 12th Graders, College Students, and Young Adults (Aged 19–28)

	1991	1992	1993	1994	1995	1996	1997	1998	1999	2000	2001	2002	2003	2004	2005	2006	2007	2008	2009	2010	2011	2012	2013
8th Grade	14.3	15.5	16.7	18.6	19.1	21.0	19.4	19.1	17.5	14.6	12.2	10.7	10.2	9.2	9.3	8.7	7.1	6.8	6.5	7.1	6.1	4.9	4.5
10th Grade	20.8	21.5	24.7	25.4	27.9	30.4	29.8	27.6	25.7	23.9	21.3	17.7	16.7	16.0	14.9	14.5	14.0	12.3	13.1	13.6	11.8	10.8	9.1
12th Grade	28.3	27.8	29.9	31.2	33.5	34.0	36.5	35.1	34.6	31.4	29.5	26.7	24.4	25.0	23.2	21.6	21.6	20.4	20.1	19.2	18.7	17.1	16.3
College Students	23.2	23.5	24.5	23.5	26.8	27.9	28.3	30.0	30.6	28.2	25.7	26.7	22.5	24.3	23.8	19.2	19.9	17.9	17.9	16.4	15.2	12.5	14.0
Young Adults	28.2	28.3	28.0	28.0	29.2	30.1	29.9	30.9	30.3	30.1	30.2	29.2	28.4	29.2	28.6	27.0	26.2	24.6	23.3	22.4	21.3	19.7	20.0

[a]Numbers are percentages.
[b]Refers to any use.
From Johnston LD, O'Malley PM, Miech RA, et al. *Monitoring the future national results on drug use: 1975–2014: overview, key findings on adolescent drug use.* Ann Arbor: Institute for Social Research, The University of Michigan, 2015.
Available at http://monitoringthefuture.org//pubs/monographs/mtf-vol2_2013.pdf; Table 2.3.

smoking is even more dangerous than previously thought. Use of tobacco products can adversely affect virtually every organ system in the body (http://www.surgeongeneral.gov/library/reports/50-years-of-progress/). Some of these adverse effects include the following:

- Cardiovascular disease—coronary heart disease, stroke, atherosclerotic peripheral vascular disease, aortic aneurysm, early abdominal aortic atherosclerosis in young adults
- Cancers—oropharynx, larynx, esophagus, trachea, bronchus, lung, stomach, pancreas, kidney and ureter, bladder, acute myeloid leukemia, colorectal
- Diminished bone density and hip fractures
- Pulmonary effects—chronic obstructive pulmonary disease and worsening asthma
- Gastrointestinal effects—gastroesophageal reflux and peptic ulcer disease
- Cataracts, blindness, and age-related macular degeneration
- Premature wrinkling of the skin
- Periodontitis
- Weakening effect on immune system
- Reproductive effects and adverse pregnancy outcomes in women—reduced fertility, ectopic pregnancy, spontaneous abortion, cancer of the cervix, and low birth weight babies
- Erectile dysfunction (impotence) in men

Smokeless Tobacco

Smokeless tobacco is classified as either chewing or dipping (also known as snuff) tobacco. Chewing tobacco, including loose leaf, plug, and twist, is chewed or held in the cheek or lower lip. Snuff, further categorized as moist or dry, has a much finer consistency than chewing tobacco and is held in place in the mouth without chewing. In addition to suffering from many of the same systemic adverse effects as smokers due to tars and tobacco additives, smokeless tobacco users have higher rates of oral, prostate, pancreatic, and cervical cancers compared with nonsmokers. Smokeless tobacco use is associated with numerous dental, periodontal, and oral soft tissue problems, including gingival recession, periodontal attachment loss, tooth staining, halitosis, and leukoplakia.[12]

Another smokeless tobacco product, with growing use in the US since its entry as a product in 2011, is snus. Snus originated in Sweden from a variant of dry snuff. Portion snus, the original and most common form, comes in small teabag-like sachets that are placed under the upper lip, delivering nicotine for an extended period of time without the need for spitting. Snus is viewed as an alternative to smoking, chewing, or dipping tobacco, with evidence of lower harm, although pancreatic cancer rates appear higher than nonusers.[13]

e-Cigarettes

e-Cigarettes are battery-operated devices that generate an aerosol for inhalation typically containing nicotine. Although there remains controversy, some propose that e-cigarettes are a safer alternative or form of harm reduction for current smokers since these products are not thought to contain many of the harmful elements found in traditional cigarettes. The safety of these devices, however, has not been fully established by a reputable national regulatory body, and the two randomized trials published to date do not indicate efficacy for aiding with quitting of conventional cigarettes. Although the US Food and Drug Administration (US FDA) proposed a ban on the sale to minors, with the liquid nicotine available in youth-friendly flavors (Figs. 65.2 and 65.3) and widespread marketing of e-cigarettes including on television and social media sites (see http://tobacco.stanford.edu/tobacco_main/ecigs.php), there is also concern that these products may be a gateway for youth to traditional cigarette smoking. In 2014, more teens reported using e-cigarettes than traditional cigarettes (ww.monitoringthefuture.org), and dual use of e-cigarettes and conventional cigarettes is also common.[14]

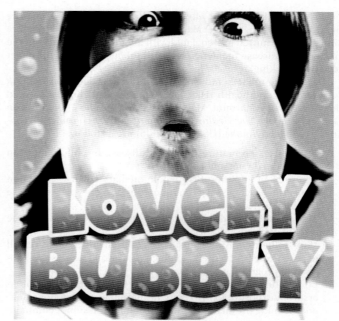

FIGURE 65.2 Youth-friendly e-cigarette flavor: bubble gum. (From Stanford School of Medicine. *Stanford research into the impact of tobacco advertising.* Available at http://tobacco.stanford.edu/tobacco_main/ecigs.php)

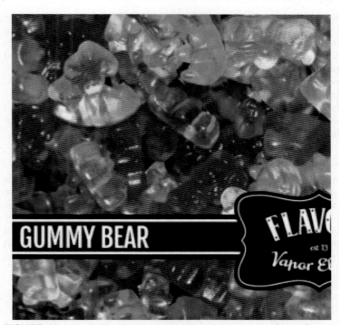

FIGURE 65.3 Youth-friendly e-cigarette flavor: gummy bear. (From Stanford School of Medicine. *Stanford research into the impact of tobacco advertising.* Available at http://tobacco.stanford.edu/tobacco_main/ecigs.php)

Secondhand Smoke

Secondhand smoke (SHS) is a mixture of *sidestream smoke,* which comes from the lit end of a combusted tobacco product, and *mainstream smoke,* which is exhaled by a smoker. Because the cigarette is burning at a lower temperature when it is not being smoked, the combustion is less complete and the smoke is richer in toxic chemicals than the mainstream smoke that the smoker inhales. Relative to mainstream smoke, sidestream smoke also has smaller particles, which more easily make their way into the lungs and the body's cells. Even though nonsmokers receive a much lower total dose of these chemicals (because the smoke is diluted in the air before nonsmokers inhale it), the effects on blood vessels, blood, and the heart are surprisingly large. Marriage to a smoker or working where smoking is permitted is associated with about a 30% increase in the risk of heart disease incidence or death (about one-third the effect of active smoking).

Despite the tobacco industry's efforts to cast doubt on the link between SHS and health risks, few scientists and clinicians would deny that SHS is harmful. Major conclusions of the 2006 Surgeon General's report *The Health Consequences of Involuntary Exposure to Tobacco Smoke* (USDHHS, 2006) are as follows:

1. SHS causes premature death and disease in children and in adults who do not smoke.
2. Exposure of adults to SHS has immediate adverse effects on the cardiovascular system and causes coronary heart disease and lung cancer.
3. The scientific evidence indicates that there is no risk-free level of exposure to SHS.
4. Many millions of Americans, both children and adults, are still exposed to SHS in their homes and workplaces despite substantial progress in tobacco control.
5. Eliminating smoking in indoor spaces fully protects nonsmokers from exposure to SHS. Separating smokers from nonsmokers, cleaning the air, and ventilating buildings cannot eliminate exposures of nonsmokers to SHS.

⬤ PREVENTION AND TREATMENT

Research has demonstrated that *brief clinician interventions* (<5 minutes) can have a significant impact for treating tobacco dependence.[15] It is feasible for busy practitioners to address tobacco use in a meaningful way in a short period of time. Given the medical problems associated with SHS and that parents are one of the most important role models for children and adolescents, clinicians must also provide tobacco cessation referrals and/or interventions for the family. AYAs are far more likely to start smoking and less likely to quit if their parents, siblings, or partners smoke. Therefore, siblings, parents, and partners need to be encouraged to quit too.

Clinical Interventions for Tobacco Prevention and Treatment

Anticipatory guidance should always include tobacco-use counseling. Tobacco exposure may start in utero, and first cigarette use may occur in the early school-age years; hence, clinical attention to tobacco starts with the prenatal visit and continues throughout childhood, adolescence, and into young adulthood. More than 70% of smokers visit a physician each year and thus this is an ideal time for intervention.[15,16] The National Cancer Institute created

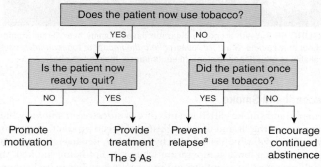

*a*Relapse prevention interventions not necessary if patient has not used tobacco for many years and is not at risk for reinitiation.

FIGURE 65.4 Tailoring assistance to readiness to quit. (From Fiore MC, Jaen CR, Baker TB, et al. *Treating tobacco use and dependence: 2008 update. Clinical practice guideline*. Rockville, MD: US Department of Health and Human Services. Public Health Service, 2008.)

the 5-A framework to Ask, Advise, Assess, Assist, and Arrange Follow-up, summarized in Figure 65.4 and discussed below:

1. Ask all patients at each visit systematically about all forms of tobacco and nicotine use (including cigars, mini-cigars, and e-cigarettes) and exposure to SHS. A simple and effective way to operationalize this is to add a question about tobacco exposure to the electronic health record or intake assessment. Including assessment of tobacco as a vital sign gives a simple and effective patient-centered, pro-health message at the beginning of the visit, prompts the health care provider to discuss the issue, and helps increase the chances of patients quitting or never using tobacco in the first place. Smoking status can change quickly in teenagers and young adults, and a previous nonsmoker may be smoking by the time of the next visit—or a regular smoker who did not wish to quit in the past may now wish to quit smoking.[16] Because AYAs often come in only sporadically for health care, the tobacco issue should be raised at every office visit, regardless of the chief complaint. Assessment of tobacco use among youth also has relevance for detection of other risk behaviors and substances used, given the high rates of co-occurrence. Other substances can be a trigger for tobacco use and vice versa, warranting consideration and clinical attention.

2. Strongly advise all nonsmokers not to start and all smokers to quit. The clinician's message should be varied according to the smoking status, age, and developmental stage of the patient. Advice that is clear and personally relevant is most effective. Physicians are looked upon as authoritative figures, even by teens, and giving a consistent cessation message is important. With never smokers, nonsmoking should be praised and the behavior normalized, as youth may overestimate the likelihood of their peers smoking. Urge continuation of nonsmoking: "Keep making smart choices."

   For someone who is considering smoking and who lives in an environment with exposure to smokers (e.g., parents, siblings, friends who smoke), offer praise for nonsmoking to date, encourage healthy alternatives to smoking (e.g., physical activity, involvement in school clubs), and role-play methods to gracefully bow out of smoking with peers. For example, the teen may refuse opportunities to smoke by saying, "No thanks, one of my relatives died of lung cancer" or "I don't want to smell like an ashtray." For someone who is experimenting or regularly using tobacco, immediate quitting should be encouraged.

3. Assess patients' willingness to make a quit attempt so that you can tailor your counseling strategy. Have they tried to quit in the past year? Are they intending to quit in the near future (i.e., next 6 months), and if so, are they interested in quitting in the next month? Patients who are uninterested in quitting (called "precontemplators") may be in that stage for any number of reasons—lack of knowledge of the health effects (though less likely these days); low confidence in their perceived ability to quit (called self-efficacy); lack of nonsmoking friends or role models; stress or high levels of nicotine addiction and withdrawal; or more globally, the good things they get from smoking (the pros) outweigh the cons of smoking. Patients who are interested in quitting, but not immediately, are called "contemplators." These individuals typically are aware that smoking is a problem for them and they want to quit, but they also perceive a number of barriers in the way such as concerns around withdrawal, weight gain, stress, and mood. With support and problem solving around the barriers to quitting, patients may increase in motivation and move into the preparation stage, with intention to quit in the next 30 days.

4. Assist the patient in stopping smoking, tailoring your strategy to their readiness to quit.
   a. Assisting patients not ready to quit (precontemplators and contemplators): A quick and easy method to encourage

patients to generate their own reasons for quitting is the following technique from motivational interviewing. Ask, "On a scale from 1 to 10, how important is it for you right now to quit smoking?" With the value they report, ask "Why is it an X (e.g., 2) and not a 1?" This question gets the patient to identify the factors important to them (e.g., cost, smell of smoke). Next ask, "On a scale from 1 to 10, how confident are you that you could quit right now and not go back to smoking?" Then ask, "What would it take to get your confidence to a 10?" The answer to this question gets at the barriers to change that the patient anticipates and helps for strategizing ways to overcome them. Instead of lecturing patients about how bad tobacco is for their health (which most patients know), asking these two questions effectively encourages patients to self-identify their own benefits and barriers to quitting. The interaction, though brief, sets up for a collaborative process with quitting smoking.

b. Assisting patients ready to quit (those in preparation): *Setting a quit date* is an important and effective first step in smoking cessation. Once the quit date has been selected (usually 2 to 4 weeks away), the patient can prepare to become a nonsmoker. Preparation to quit smoking has physical, psychological, and emotional components. For example, in getting ready to quit (before the quit date), the patient should *keep a journal* noting when and why and how much he or she smokes, as well as any routine activities in which smoking plays a part, such as drinking coffee or alcohol. The patient can attempt to *change smoking routines* by keeping cigarettes in a different place, smoking with the other hand, or smoking only in self-designated areas. The patient should occasionally *chew gum or drink a glass of water* instead of smoking a cigarette; he or she will notice that the smoking craving usually subsides within a few minutes. Gum, hard candy, sunflower seeds, carrot sticks, or toothpicks can be carried around and used as cigarette substitutes. By the quit date, the patient's *environment should be rid of cigarette cues*. For example, clothes, the living space, and the inside of the car should all be cleaned to get rid of the tobacco smell. Ashtrays and all cigarettes should be disposed of. The patient should make it a point to find nonsmoking spaces to be in and to stay away from places where smoking occurs. Patients need to think of themselves as nonsmokers, and they should literally say to themselves that being a nonsmoker is important. When the going gets tough, patients need to remember the benefits of nonsmoking! Writing down the benefits on a 3 × 5 card for looking at in tempting situations may be helpful. To maintain the quit effort, patients need to know that withdrawal symptoms are common but transient and that pharmacotherapy is available if necessary. *Exercise*, including walking or riding a bicycle, can help attenuate withdrawal symptoms. For reinforcement and reward, suggest that the patient start a *money jar* with the money saved from not buying cigarettes. This will add up quickly; will provide a visual of the money saved; and can be used on alternative reinforcers such as new music, going to the movies, or new apps. Support from clinicians has been shown to lead to more successful quit attempts. For additional support, the patient should be encouraged to call the toll-free smokers' quit line (1-800-QUIT-NOW) and sign up with the National Cancer Institute's SmokeFree Teen website and texting support (http://teen.smokefree.gov/).

Concerns about postcessation weight gain can be an impediment to quitting smoking, particularly among girls. Weight gain after cessation varies greatly and in adults is more common among women, African Americans, heavier smokers, and adults under 55 years of age. Strict dieting may reduce success with quitting smoking, and patients should instead be encouraged to engage in physical activity (e.g., walking, biking), eat a healthy diet with planned meals and high-fiber foods, increase water intake, chew sugarless gum, and select nonfood rewards.

While cessation pharmacotherapy—including nicotine replacement products (patch, gum, lozenge, inhaler, or nasal spray), bupropion (Zyban), and varenicline (Chantix)—is recommended for smokers 18 years of age and older interested in quitting, to date, the few that have been tested in adolescents have demonstrated only limited success and are not FDA approved for use with youth.[17–19] For young adult smokers and possibly for adolescent smokers with usage patterns closer to that of adults (i.e., >5 to 10 cigarettes/day), clinicians may consider prescribing a cessation medication. (Prescribing instructions for these medications can be found in **Table 65.2**.) Note that nicotine patches, gum, and lozenges are available over the counter for smokers 18 years of age and older, but available only by prescription for youth under age 18. Both bupropion and varenicline have boxed warnings for risk of serious neuropsychiatric symptoms.

5. *Arrange* follow-up. Cessation rates have been shown to significantly improve with regular follow-up. For example, a call, email, or text to patients on their quit date to congratulate their effort, followed by in-person visits every 1 or 2 weeks during the first 3 months of the quit attempt—the time of greatest relapse. Clinician contacts can be augmented or replaced by follow-up arranged via the state's tobacco quit line, a local group, or emerging social media cessation support. If a patient is able to quit for 3 straight months, he or she is more likely to successfully quit for good.

Most smokers try to quit many times before ultimately quitting for good. Patients should be advised that it is a learning process and that the longer they can remain tobacco-free with each attempt, the more likely they are to quit for good. Irritability, dysphoric mood, and sleep disturbance may occur during a quit attempt, and the patient should be asked about mood changes.[20] For smokers with numerous unsuccessful quit attempts, referral to an evidence-based cessation group may be helpful. One particular program approved by the CDC and with demonstrated success is the school-based Not On Tobacco (NOT) program (http://www.cdc.gov/prc/pdf/not-on-tobacco-smoking-cessation.pdf). Developed by the American Lung Association, NOT is one of the most popular and efficacious, teen-specific smoking cessation programs.[21] More behavioral therapies shown to be efficacious for AYAs are listed in the 2012 Public Health Service (PHS) guidelines.[1] In addition, 12-step programs, such as Nicotine Anonymous, also exist, though they have not been researched for effectiveness with quitting smoking in young adults or adolescents.

OFFICE PRACTICES

Office practices should attend to tobacco to ensure systematic, and time efficient, assessment, treatment, and referrals.

1. *Select a smoking cessation coordinator*: Office practices will benefit from having a point person to maintain attention to tobacco treatment in the clinic, including periodic staff inservices and news alerts, inclusion of smoking status in intake forms and online medical records, and signage (posters in the waiting area and/or visit rooms, quit line cards, and brochures). If the clinic or medical center is not yet smoke-free, that should be an immediate goal to coordinate a date and plan.

TABLE 65.2

FDA-Approved Medications for Smoking Cessation

	Nicotine Replacement Therapy (NRT) Formulations					Buproprion SR	Varenicline
	Gum	Lozenge	Transdermal Patch	Nasal Spray	Oral Inhaler[2]		
Production	Nicorette[1], Generic OTC 2 mg, 4 mg original, cinnamon, fruit, mint, orange	Nicorette Lozenge,[1] Nicorette Mini Lozenge,[1] Generic OTC 2 mg, 4 mg cherry, mint	NicoDerm CQ[1], Generic OTC (NicoDerm CQ, generic) Rx (generic) 7 mg, 14 mg, 21 mg (24-hour release)	Nicotrol NS[2] Rx Metered spray 0.5 mg nicotine in 50 mcL aqueous nicotine solution	Nicotrol Inhaler[2] Rx 10 mg cartridge delivers 4 mg inhaled nicotine vapor	Zyban[1], Generic Rx 150 mg sustained-release tablet	Chantix[2] Rx 0.5 mg, 1 mg tablet
Precautions	• Recent (≤ 2 weeks) myocardial infarction • Serious underlying arrhythmias • Serious or worsening angina pectoris • Temporomandibular joint disease • Pregnancy[3] and breastfeeding • Adolescents (<18 years)	• Recent (≤ 2 weeks) myocardial infarction • Serious underlying arrhythmias • Serious or worsening angina pectoris • Pregnancy[3] and breastfeeding • Adolescents (<18 years)	• Recent (≤ 2 weeks) myocardial infarction • Serious underlying arrhythmias • Serious or worsening angina pectoris • Pregnancy[3] (Rx formulations, category D) and breastfeeding • Adolescents (<18 years)	• Recent (≤ 2 weeks) myocardial infarction • Serious underlying arrhythmias • Serious or worsening angina pectoris • Underlying chronic nasal disorders (rhinitis, nasal polyps, sinusitis) • Severe reactive airway disease • Pregnancy[3] (category D) and breastfeeding • Adolescents (<18 years)	• Recent (≤ 2 weeks) myocardial infarction • Serious underlying arrhythmias • Serious or worsening angina pectoris • Bronchospastic disease • Pregnancy[3] (category D) and breastfeeding • Adolescents (<18 years)	• Concomitant therapy with medications or medical conditions known to lower the seizure threshold • Severe hepatic cirrhosis • Pregnancy[3] (category C) and breastfeeding • Adolescents (<18 years) • BLACK-BOXED WARNING for neuropsychiatric symptoms[4] **Contraindications:** • Seizure disorder • Concomitant bupropion (e.g., Wellbutrin) therapy • Current or prior diagnosis of bulimia or anorexia nervosa • Simultaneous abrupt discontinuation of alcohol or sedatives/benzodiazepines • MAO inhibitor therapy in previous 14 days	• Severe renal impairment (dosage adjustment is necessary) • Pregnancy[3] (category C) and breastfeeding • Adolescents (<18 years) • BLACK-BOXED WARNING for neuropsychiatric symptoms[4]

Dosing	*1st cigarette ≤30 minutes after waking:* 4 mg
	1st cigarette >30 minutes after waking: 2 mg
	Weeks 1–6:
	  1 piece q 1–2 hours
	Weeks 7–9:
	  1 piece q 2–4 hours
	Weeks 10–12:
	  1 piece q 4–8 hours
	• Maximum, 24 pieces/day
	• Chew each piece slowly
		1st cigarette ≤ 30 minutes after waking: 4 mg
		1st cigarette >30 minutes after waking: 2 mg
		Weeks 1–6:
		  1 lozenge q 1–2 hours
		Weeks 7–9:
		  1 lozenge q 2–4 hours
		Weeks 10–12:
		  1 lozenge q 4–8 hours
		• Maximum, 20 lozenges/day
			> 10 cigarettes/day:
			  21 mg/day × 4 weeks (generic)
			  6 weeks (NicoDerm CQ)
			  14 mg/day × 2 weeks
			  7 mg/day × 2 weeks
			≤10 cigarettes/day:
			  14 mg/day × 6 weeks
			  7 mg/day × 2 weeks
			• May wear patch for 16 hours if patient experiences sleep disturbances (remove at bedtime)
				1–2 doses/hour (8–40 doses/day)
				One dose = 2 sprays (one in **each** nostril; each spray delivers 0.5 mg of nicotine to the nasal mucosa
				• Maximum
				  – 5 doses/hour or
				  – 40 doses/day
				• For best results, initially use at least 8 doses/day
					6–16 cartridges/day
					Individualize dosing; initially use 1 cartridge q 1–2 hours
					• Best effects with continuous puffing for 20 minutes
					• Initially use at least 6 cartridges/day
					• Nicotine in cartridge is depleted after 20 minutes of active puffing
						150 mg po q AM × 3 days, then 150 mg po bid
						• Do not exceed 300 mg/day
						• Begin therapy 1–2 weeks **prior** to quit date
						• Allow at least 8 hours between doses
						• Avoid bedtime dosing to minimize insomnia
						• Dose tapering is not necessary
						• Duration: 7–12 weeks, with maintenance up to 6 months in selected patients
							Days 1–3:
							  0.5 mg po q AM
							Days 4–7:
							  0.5 mg po bid
							Weeks 2–12:
							  1 mg po bid
							• Begin therapy 1 week prior to quit date; alternatively, the patient can begin therapy and then quit smoking between days 8–35 of treatment

	• Park between cheek and gum when peppery or tingling sensation appears (~15–30 chews) • Resume chewing when tingle fades • Repeat chew/park steps until most of the nicotine is gone (tingle does not return; generally 30 min) • Park in different areas of mouth • No food or beverages 15 minutes before or during use • Duration: up to 12 weeks	• Allow to dissolve slowly (20–30 minutes for standard; 10 minutes for mini) • Nicotine release may cause a warm, tingling sensation • Do not chew or swallow • Occasionally rotate to different areas of the mouth • No food or beverages 15 minutes before or during use • Duration: up to 12 weeks	• Do not sniff, swallow, or inhale through the nose as the spray is being administered • Duration: 8–10 weeks	• Inhale into back of throat or puff in short breaths • Do NOT inhale into the lungs (like a cigarette) but "puff" as if lighting a pipe • Open cartridge retains potency for 24 hours • No food or beverages 15 minutes before or during use • Duration: 3–6 months			• Take dose after eating and with a full glass of water • Dose tapering is not necessary • Dosing adjustment is necessary for patients with severe renal impairment • Duration: 12 weeks; an additional 12-week course may be used in selected patients
Adverse Effects	• Mouth/jaw soreness • Hiccups • Dyspepsia • Hypersalivation • Effects associated with incorrect chewing technique: – Lightheadedness – Nausea/vomiting – Throat and mouth irritation	• Nausea • Hiccups • Cough • Heartburn • Headache • Flatulence • Insomnia	• Nasal and/or throat irritation (hot, peppery, or burning sensation) • Rhinitis • Tearing • Sneezing • Cough • Headache	• Mouth and/or throat irritation • Cough • Headache • Rhinitis • Dyspepsia • Hiccups	• Local skin reactions (erythema, pruritus, burning) • Headache • Sleep disturbances (insomnia, abnormal/vivid dreams); associated with nocturnal nicotine absorption	• Insomnia • Dry mouth • Nervousness/difficulty concentrating • Rash • Constipation • Seizures (risk is 0.1%) • Neuropsychiatric symptoms (rare; see PRECAUTIONS)	• Nausea • Sleep disturbances (insomnia, abnormal/vivid dreams) • Constipation • Flatulence • Vomiting • Neuropsychiatric symptoms (rare; see PRECAUTIONS)
Advantages	• Might satisfy oral cravings • Might delay weight gain • Easy to use and conceal • Patients can titrate therapy to manage withdrawal symptoms • Variety of flavors are available	• Might satisfy oral cravings • Might delay weight gain • Easy to use and conceal • Patients can titrate therapy to manage withdrawal symptoms • Variety of flavors are available	• Patients can titrate therapy to rapidly manage withdrawal symptoms	• Patients can titrate therapy to manage withdrawal symptoms • Mimics hand-to-mouth ritual of smoking (could also be perceived as a disadvantage)	• Provides consistent nicotine levels over 24 hours • Easy to use and conceal • Once daily dosing associated with fewer compliance problems • FDA-approved for use in combination with bupropion SR	• Easy to use; oral formulation might be associated with fewer compliance problems • Might delay weight gain • Can be used safely with NRT; FDA-approved for use in combination with nicotine transdermal patch • Might be beneficial in patients with depression	• Easy to use; oral formulation might be associated with fewer compliance problems • Offers a new mechanism of action for patients who have failed other agents

(Continued)

XIV

TABLE 65.2

FDA-Approved Medications for Smoking Cessation (Continued)

Disadvantages	• Need for frequent dosing can compromise compliance • Might be problematic for patients with significant dental work • Gastrointestinal side effects (nausea, hiccups, heartburn) might be bothersome • Patients must use proper chewing technique to minimize adverse effects • Gum chewing may not be socially acceptable	• Patients cannot titrate the dose to acutely manage withdrawal symptoms • Allergic reactions to adhesive might occur • Patients with dermatologic conditions should not use the patch	• Need for frequent dosing can compromise compliance • Nasal/throat irritation may be bothersome • Patients must wait 5 minutes before driving or operating heavy machinery • Patients with chronic nasal disorders or severe reactive airway disease should not use the spray	• Need for frequent dosing can compromise compliance • Initial throat or mouth irritation can be bothersome • Cartridges should not be stored in very warm conditions or used in very cold conditions • Patients with underlying bronchospastic disease must use with caution	• Seizure risk is increased • Several contraindications and precautions preclude use in some patients (see Precautions) • Patients should be monitored for potential neuropsychiatric symptoms[4] (see Precautions)	• May induce nausea in up to one third of patients • Patients should be monitored for potential neuropsychiatric symptoms[4] (see Precautions)
Cost/day[5]	2 mg or 4 mg: $1.90–$5.48 (9 pieces)	2 mg or 4 mg: $3.05–$4.10 (9 pieces)	$1.52–$3.40 (1 patch)	$4.32 (8 doses)	$7.74 (6 cartridges)	$2.54–$6.22 (2 tablets)	$6.54 (2 tablets)

[1]Marketed by GlaxoSmithKline.

[2]Marketed by Pfizer.

[3]The US Clinical Practice Guideline states that pregnant smokers should be encouraged to quit without medication based on insufficient evidence of effectiveness and theoretical concerns with safety. Pregnant smokers should be offered behavioral counseling interventions that exceed minimal advice to quit.

[4]In July 2009, the FDA mandated that the prescribing information for all bupropion- and varenicline-containing products include a black-boxed warning highlighting the risk of serious neuropsychiatric symptoms, including changes in behavior, hostility, agitation, depressed mood, suicidal thoughts and behavior, and attempted suicide. Clinicians *should advise patients to stop taking varenicline or bupropion SR and contact a healthcare provider immediately if they experience agitation, depressed mood, and any changes in behavior that are not typical of nicotine withdrawal, or if they experience suicidal thoughts or behavior. If treatment is stopped due to neuropsychiatric symptoms, patients should be monitored until the symptoms resolve.*

[5]Wholesale acquisition cost from Red Book Online. Thomson Reuters, July 2013

Abbreviations: MAO, monoamine oxidase; NRT, nicotine replacement therapy; OTC, over-the-counter (non-prescription product); Rx, prescription product.

For complete prescribing information, please refer to the manufacturers' package inserts.

Copyright © 1999–2014 The Regents of the University of California. All rights reserved. Updated July 7, 2013

2. *Post tobacco prevention and treatment posters in the office area*: In your waiting and examination rooms, prominently display tobacco cessation materials, such as posters and cards from the state tobacco quit line.
3. *Eliminate all tobacco advertising from the waiting room,* either by not subscribing to magazines that carry tobacco advertisements (e.g., Rolling Stone) or by having the office smoking coordinator write over cigarette ads or place stickers with slogans such as, "Don't fall for this" or "This is a rip-off."
4. *Have the office recognize and celebrate the "Great American Smoke-out,"* which is always the Thursday before Thanksgiving, and *"World No-Tobacco Day,"* which is always May 31. These are particularly high-profile public events to encourage smoking cessation.

HEDIS (Health Plan Employer Data and Information Set) Standards and Billing Issues

Smoking prevention and cessation counseling is considered a standard of care, and formal ratings of health plans and individual physicians commonly include these efforts. The National Committee on Quality Assurance (NCQA; www.ncqa.org) issues annual reports on the state of health care quality. Concerning billing issues for follow-up, if smoking cessation per se is not covered, there is almost always a related medical issue that may be billed, such as asthma, bronchitis, cough, pharyngitis, or an upper respiratory infection.

Educational Materials

Educational materials for AYAs, parents, and physicians are available from a variety of sources either free or for nominal fees. The CDC's Office on Smoking and Health (www.cdc.gov/tobacco) summarizes national trends in youth smoking and provides educational materials, posters, hypertext links, and other information. RxforChange is a turnkey interdisciplinary medical education tobacco treatment curriculum available at no-cost online with patient materials (http://rxforchange.ucsf.edu). Local chapters of the American Cancer Society (www.cancer.org) and the American Lung Association (www.lung.org/stop-smoking/), the American Academy of Pediatrics (www.aap.org), the National Cancer Institute (www.teen.smokfree.gov), and the Agency for Health Care Research and Quality (www.ahcpr.gov) provide tobacco treatment materials and trainings for physicians and patients.

ADVOCACY ISSUES

The most successful tobacco control efforts involve a number of concerted actions. These include the following:

- Increasing the cost of tobacco products through higher taxes on the products
- Banning advertising of tobacco products in youth-oriented media and youth-frequented activities such as sporting events
- Enforcing laws that ban adolescents less than 18 years old from buying nicotine-containing products
- Banning cigarette-vending machines
- Promoting adoption of clean indoor air laws and smoke-free facilities such as schools, day care centers, office buildings, restaurants, and bars

Organizations such as Action on Smoking and Health (http://www.ash.org), Americans for Nonsmokers' Rights (www.no-smoke.org), and the Campaign for Tobacco-Free Kids (www.tobaccofreekids.org) advocate for public policies that prevent kids from smoking, help smokers quit, and protect all from SHS exposure. The sites have many useful fact sheets, educational materials, and up-to-date information. The American Legacy Foundation (www.americanlegacy.org) was founded as part of the master settlement agreement between the states and tobacco industry, and its counter-advertising Truth campaign in particular involved youth in its tobacco control activities. The University of California, San Francisco, provides online access to the Tobacco Control Archives Print Collection, tobacco industry Web sites and documents, state-by-state reports on tobacco industry activities, the "Cigarette Papers," and information on smoking in the movies.

RESEARCH ISSUES

A number of questions concerning tobacco use prevention and cessation in AYAs are being actively investigated in the research setting, including the following:

1. What defines nicotine addiction in adolescents, and how is it similar/different from that in adults?
2. What are the best methods, and in which settings are programs and clinicians best able to help prevent and treat tobacco use in the AYA population?
3. Is there a role for pharmacologic aids for smoking cessation in adolescents?
4. What role will e-cigarettes play in the future landscape of tobacco use? Are e-cigarettes a useful form of harm reduction or are they a gateway into tobacco smoking for AYAs?

SUMMARY

Tobacco prevention and cessation counseling is one of the most important steps health care provider can take to improve the short-term and long-term health of patients and their parents. Smoking is a very serious disease with potentially lifelong and life-shortening consequences. Practitioners are in a unique position to help prevent smoking onset or intervene early to stop smoking by adolescents. The landscape, however, is evolving, and the emerging products, their health effects, and likelihood for addiction warrant continued attention.

ACKNOWLEDGMENT

The authors wish to acknowledge Dr. Seth D. Ammerman for his contributions to previous versions of this chapter.

REFERENCES

1. US Department of Health and Human Services. *Preventing tobacco use among youth and young adults: a report of the surgeon general.* Atlanta: U.S. Department of Health and Human Services, Centers for Disease Control and Prevention, National Center for Chronic Disease Prevention and Health Promotion, Office on Smoking and Health, 2012.
2. Centers for Disease Control and Prevention. Tobacco product use among middle and high school students—United States, 2011 and 2012. *MMWR* 2013;62(45):893–897.
3. Kasza KA, Bansal-Travers M, O'Connor RJ, et al. Cigarette smokers' use of unconventional tobacco products and associations with quitting activity: findings from the ITC-4, U.S. cohort. *Nicotine Tob Res* 2014;16(6):672–681.
4. Centers for Disease Control and Prevention. Vital signs: current cigarette smoking among adults aged >or=18 years—United States, 2009. *MMWR* 2010;59(35):1135–1140.
5. Johnston LD, O'Malley PM, Bachman JG, et al. *Monitoring the Future national survey results on drug use, 1975–2013.* Vol 2. College students and adults ages 19–55. Ann Arbor: Institute for Social Research, The University of Michigan, 2014.
6. Abroms L, Simons-Morton B, Haynie DL, et al. Psychosocial predictors of smoking trajectories during middle and high school. *Addiction* 2005;100(6):852–861.
7. Remafedi G, Carol H. Preventing tobacco use among lesbian, gay, bisexual, and transgender youths. *Nicotine Tob Res* 2005;7(2):249–256.
8. Benowitz NL. Neurobiology of nicotine addiction: implications for smoking cessation treatment. *Am J Med* 2008;121(4, suppl 1):S3–S10.
9. Benowitz NL. Nicotine addiction. *N Engl J Med* 2010;362(24):2295–2303.
10. Rubinstein ML, Shiffman S, Moscicki AB, et al. Nicotine metabolism and addiction among adolescent smokers. *Addiction* 2013;108(2):406–412.
11. Benowitz NL. Clinical pharmacology of nicotine: implications for understanding, preventing, and treating tobacco addiction. *Clin Pharmacol Ther* 2008;83(4):531–541.
12. Smokeless tobacco and some tobacco-specific N-nitrosamines. *IARC Monogr Eval Carcinog Risks Hum* 2007;89:1–592.
13. Boffetta P, Hecht S, Gray N, et al. Smokeless tobacco and cancer. *Lancet Oncol* 2008;9(7):667–675.

14. Centers for Disease Control and Prevention. Notes from the field: electronic cigarette use among middle and high school students—United States, 2011–2012. *MMWR* 2013;62(35):729–730.
15. Fiore M, Jaén C, Baker T. *Treating tobacco use and dependence: 2008 Update*. 2008. Available at http://www.ahrq.gov/path/tobacco.htm-Clinic. Accessed April 8, 2008.
16. Milton M, Maule C, Yee S, et al. *Youth tobacco cessation: a Guide for Making Informed Decisions*. Atlanta: U.S. Department of Health and Human Services, 2004.
17. Rubinstein ML, Benowitz NL, Auerback GM, et al. A randomized trial of nicotine nasal spray in adolescent smokers. *Pediatrics* 2008;122(3):e595–e600.
18. Moolchan ET, Robinson ML, Ernst M, et al. Safety and efficacy of the nicotine patch and gum for the treatment of adolescent tobacco addiction. *Pediatrics* 2005; 115(4):e407–e414.
19. Bailey SR, Crew EE, Riske EC, et al. Efficacy and tolerability of pharmacotherapies to aid smoking cessation in adolescents. *Paediatr Drugs* 2012;14(2):91–108.
20. Killen JD, Robinson TN, Ammerman S, et al. Major depression among adolescent smokers undergoing treatment for nicotine dependence. *Addict Behav* 2004;29(8):1517–1526.
21. Dino G, Horn K, Goldcamp J, et al. A 2-year efficacy study of not on tobacco in Florida: an overview of program successes in changing teen smoking behavior. *Prev Med* 2001;33(6):600–605.

🛜 ADDITIONAL RESOURCES AND WEBSITES ONLINE

CHAPTER 66

Marijuana

Kevin M. Gray
Amanda P. Roper

KEY WORDS

- Cannabis
- Cannabis use disorders
- Cognitive behavioral therapy
- Endocannabinoid system
- Family-based therapies
- Hashish
- Intoxication
- Marijuana
- Motivational enhancement therapy
- Synthetic cannabinoids (cannabimimetics)
- Δ^9-tetrahydrocannabinol (THC)
- Withdrawal

Marijuana is the most commonly used illicit substance among adolescents and young adults (AYAs) in the US and the world. Its psychoactive and pharmacologic effects are well characterized, but variations in potency and composition, as well as many other individual and environmental variables, may influence these effects. Young people appear to be particularly prone to adverse effects of chronic marijuana use, most notably including cannabis use disorders and cognitive impairments. Additionally, adolescent marijuana use is associated with adverse psychiatric and psychosocial outcomes. An expanding evidence base is available to guide efficacious treatments for adolescents with problematic marijuana use. The majority of evidence supports motivational enhancement, cognitive behavioral, and family therapies, while new findings suggest that contingency management as well as the pharmacotherapy *N*-acetylcysteine may enhance abstinence outcomes. More work is needed to optimize strategies to prevent and treat cannabis use disorders in young people, especially in an evolving public policy setting in which adolescents may be more prone to view marijuana favorably and initiate use.

PREVALENCE, EPIDEMIOLOGY, AND POLICY CONSIDERATIONS

Marijuana is the most commonly used illicit substance in the US and the world. Onset of use typically occurs in adolescence, and the peak prevalence of use is among young adults. Recent trends among young people suggest that perceptions of marijuana-associated risks are decreasing, though rates of use may be stabilizing or even slightly decreasing after prior notable increases.[1] Youth are more vulnerable than adults to adverse consequences of marijuana use, and more likely to develop cannabis use disorders.[2] Marijuana is the most common primary substance of use among AYAs entering substance use treatment.[3] Recent key prevalence findings are outlined below.

Adolescents

1. *Monitoring the Future (MTF) 2014:* Past-year use of marijuana was 11.7%, 27.3%, and 35.1% in 8th, 10th, and 12th graders, respectively. Lifetime (ever) use was 15.6%, 33.7%, and 44.1%, respectively, by grade, while past-month use was 6.5%, 16.6%, and 21.2% and daily use was 1.0%, 3.4%, and 5.8% by grade (www.monitoringthefuture.org).

2. *Youth Risk Behavior Survey (YRBS):* In the 2013 YRBS survey, 40.7% of 9th to 12th graders have ever used marijuana, with a prevalence of 39.2% in females and 42.1% in males. The proportion reporting ever use of marijuana was 36.7%, 46.8%, and 48.8% in White, Black, and Hispanic students, respectively, and by grade, 30.1%, 39.1%, 46.4%, and 48.6% for 9th through 12th grades, respectively. (http://www.cdc.gov/HealthyYouth/yrbs/index.htm)

3. *National Survey on Drug Use and Health (NSDUH):* In the 2013 NSDUH study among 12- to 17-year-olds, the prevalence of use in past month was 7.9% in 2011, 7.2% in 2012, and 7.1% in 2013 (http://www.samhsa.gov/data/sites/default/files/NSDUHresultsPDFWHTML2013/Web/NSDUHresults2013.pdf).

Young Adults and College Students

1. MTF 2013: Since 2000, the annual prevalence of marijuana use among college students reached a recent peak prevalence of 36% in 2001, declined to 30% in 2006, and then increased to 36% in 2013. Noncollege young adult peers showed comparable changes over the same time interval. The annual prevalence rates for both groups were comparable across this interval (www.monitoringthefuture.org).

2. National College Health Assessment (NCHA) 2014: Among this national survey of college students, 61% have never used marijuana, 20.7% used but not in last 30 days, and 18.3% used in the past month, with 2.6% reporting daily use (www.acha-ncha.org).

While the US Drug Enforcement Agency classifies marijuana as a schedule I drug (high potential for abuse, no currently accepted medical use in the US, and no accepted safety for use under supervision by a physician), several states have proceeded with policy changes to legalize/decriminalize marijuana for medical and/or recreational purposes. These changes may potentially present unintended downstream effects relevant to youth,[4–6] though more work is needed to clarify these issues.[7,8]

PREPARATION AND USE

Human use of marijuana, derived from the plant *Cannabis sativa*, dates back to at least 2700 BC. The main psychoactive component of marijuana is Δ^9-tetrahydrocannabinol (THC), which is present in varying concentrations across parts of the plant. Marijuana is composed of the dried seeds, stems, leaves, and flowering top of the plant. This preparation typically contains 0.5% to 5% THC, while hashish, a dried cannabis resin, contains 2% to 20% THC and an oil-based hashish extract contains 15% to 50% THC.[9] With advances in cultivation and preparation, the THC concentration in marijuana has increased significantly in recent decades.[10]

Marijuana may be smoked, vaporized/inhaled, or ingested. Smoking is the most common method of administration, and this results in the most rapid delivery of THC to the brain. A marijuana "joint" is composed of dried cannabis rolled into cigarette paper, whereas a "blunt" is a larger portion rolled into a hollowed/emptied cigar. Some users combine tobacco with marijuana when smoking joints or blunts. Marijuana is also often smoked in a pipe, also called a "bowl," or a water pipe, known as a "bong." Individuals seeking a higher THC concentration often smoke hashish using similar methods. Marijuana is commonly ingested in the form of brownies or other food products, though this leads to slower absorption and more delayed/gradual psychoactive effects than smoking/inhaling. Given the variety of products/routes of administration, the broad range of THC concentrations, and the frequency of sharing with a group, standardized quantification of marijuana use is considerably more challenging than for many other substances (e.g., cigarettes, alcohol).

Slang terms for marijuana and its various preparations are too numerous and geographically variable for an exhaustive review in this chapter, though "weed," "pot," "bud," "grass," "herb," "dope," and "Mary Jane" are particularly common. Slang terms reflecting potency often range from "schwag" (low potency) to "kine bud" (high potency). Recent preparations of highly concentrated cannabis may be referred to as "dabs," "wax," or "shatter."

PHARMACOLOGY AND NEUROBIOLOGY

Marijuana is composed of at least 60 distinct cannabinoid compounds and about 500 total chemical constituents. The relative concentrations and potencies of these ingredients vary significantly across strains and preparations. Cannabinoids exert their effects via binding to cannabinoid receptors, which are widely dispersed in the central and peripheral nervous system. To date, two cannabinoid receptors, CB_1 and CB_2, have been well characterized, and they, along with endocannabinoids (including anandamide and 2-arachidonoylglycerol), comprise the endocannabinoid system, which plays a modulatory role in a number of physiologic processes. While our understanding of the endocannabinoid system is likely in its infancy, it is known to be involved in cognition, memory, mood, appetite, immune function, motor coordination, and pain sensation.

THC, the primary psychoactive component of marijuana, binds to CB_1 and CB_2 receptors. Its potency, when delivered via smoked marijuana, is far greater than the analogous endocannabinoids. Activation of CB_1 receptors in the brain leads to downstream effects on several neurotransmitters, including dopamine, conveying marijuana's psychoactive and reinforcing effects.

THC is highly lipophilic and is rapidly distributed into tissues. While smoked marijuana leads to rapid uptake of THC into the central nervous system, most of the THC administered remains in the periphery. THC is primarily metabolized by the liver, and a number of active and inactive metabolites have been identified. The rate of excretion of THC is slowed by its propensity to deposit in lipid-rich tissues. THC metabolites are typically detectable in urine for 1 to 3 days after acute use, and may remain detectable for weeks in chronic/heavy users.[11]

Among other cannabinoids in marijuana is cannabidiol, which is now the subject of significant interest for potential therapeutic (e.g., anticonvulsant, anxiolytic, and antipsychotic) effects. Strains of marijuana with higher ratios of cannabidiol to THC appear to be associated with reduced likelihood of memory impairment and psychotomimetic effects. However, many strains have been developed with particularly low ratios of cannabidiol to THC, given many users' preference for stronger psychoactive effects associated with high-dose THC.

Behavioral and Physiologic Effects
Acute Effects

Immediate/short-term effects of marijuana vary significantly based on its potency/constituency, the user's expectations, the setting of use, the user's marijuana naivety versus experience, the amount used, and the route of administration. Psychoactive and physiologic effects are detectable within 30 minutes of smoking/inhalation and typically last for 2 to 3 hours, whereas effects of marijuana ingestion are detectable within 90 minutes and last 6 or more hours. Marijuana is most often used recreationally to achieve a mild euphoria or "high," to experience pleasant distortions of ordinary experiences, and to facilitate social interactions. Naïve users are more likely to report adverse acute experiences, including anxiety/panic as well as psychotic symptoms.

Acute physiologic experiences include increased heart rate, orthostatic hypotension, and supine hypertension. Users frequently experience injected and/or erythematous sclera and conjunctiva, dry mouth, and varying degrees of cognitive impairment and processing difficulties. Among associated risks with processing/cognitive difficulties is impaired driving. While overall effects on driving performance appear more modest than those associated with alcohol intoxication, epidemiologic and experimental studies have demonstrated that marijuana use does substantially increase the risk of motor vehicle accidents.[12]

As users recover from marijuana's acute intoxicating effects, they may experience increased appetite ("munchies") as well as sedation.

Chronic Effects (see also Chapter 63)

Repeated use of marijuana over time is associated with a number of adverse outcomes, particularly among young people. Significant among these is development of a maladaptive pattern involving continued marijuana use despite associated impairment and adverse consequences. Prior editions of the *Diagnostic and Statistical Manual of Mental Disorders (DSM)* included the diagnosis of cannabis abuse and cannabis dependence, whereas the current edition *(DSM-5)* utilizes the term "cannabis use disorder," with three levels of severity.[13] One in 6 adolescent marijuana users, compared to only 1 in 11 adult users, develop a use pattern consistent with cannabis dependence.[14] The 2012 NSDUH indicates that, in the US population, 3.2% of adolescents aged 12 to 17 and 5.7% of young adults aged 18 to 25 meet criteria for cannabis use disorder.[3] Tolerance to marijuana's effects occurs over repeated use, and a marijuana withdrawal syndrome has been well characterized and observed in adults and adolescents.[15,16]

Parsing the causality and directionality of associations between marijuana use and general health, psychiatric, and psychosocial outcomes is challenging, given the myriad potentially confounding factors (e.g., shared associations) and variations in use (e.g., age of onset, frequency/dosing). Epidemiologists approach these challenges via analysis within large-scale prospective population studies with detailed assessments occurring at multiple time points from childhood to adulthood, controlling for potential confounders. These studies are complemented by highly controlled experimental studies with comparisons between marijuana users and control groups.

Given the central role of educational attainment in AYA development, marijuana's effects on cognition are particularly relevant in this age-group. The issue is complicated by potential distinctions between marijuana intoxication effects, residual effects after resolution of intoxication, and long-term effects even after THC and its metabolites have been fully excreted. Marijuana use is most consistently associated with impairments in attention, declarative memory, and cognitive control.[17] In general, impairment is dependent on the dose and chronicity of use, and is more severe with earlier initiation of use (i.e., in early adolescence). While cognitive improvements in a number of domains have been noted with sustained abstinence, recent evidence suggests that significant impairment may persist long-term, reflecting a potentially lasting neurotoxic effect of adolescent-onset cannabis use.[18]

A confluence of evidence demonstrates that adolescent-onset marijuana use conveys a dose-dependent increased risk of developing a psychotic disorder.[19] While the underlying mechanism remains unclear, it has been posited that repeated exogenous cannabinoid administration disrupts a protective developmental role of the endocannabinoid system in adolescents genetically vulnerable to developing psychosis.[20] The association between adolescent marijuana use and psychotic disorders is sufficiently compelling to warn young people, particularly those with a family history of psychosis, of this risk. The association between adolescent marijuana use and other psychiatric disorders is less clear. In general, marijuana use is associated with a worsened course of co-occurring psychiatric illnesses, including affective disorders such as major depression and bipolar disorder. Some studies have shown an increased risk of subsequent depression and suicidality in early-onset adolescent marijuana users, but the association may be accounted for by confounding factors.[19] Several studies have shown that substance use, including marijuana use, is more common among adolescents with attention deficit hyperactivity disorder, but this may be due to a shared association with disruptive behaviors, such as oppositional defiant disorder and conduct disorder.

Adolescent marijuana use is associated with a number of adverse psychosocial outcomes, including impaired school performance, school dropout, unemployment, impaired interpersonal relationships, and life dissatisfaction, though these associations are likely multidetermined.[21–23] Preexisting risk, negative peer affiliation, and adverse effects of marijuana on cognition are all potential contributors. Adolescent marijuana users are more likely than nonusers to use other illicit substances, but this may reflect increased access to other substances and/or shared risk for use of multiple substances, rather than the long-hypothesized "gateway" effect.

Frequent marijuana smokers are more prone than nonusers to chronic bronchitis and impaired respiratory function, and these associations appear to be independent of cigarette smoking, which often co-occurs among marijuana users. Smoked marijuana contains several known carcinogens, some of which are also present in cigarette smoke. It is thus believed that chronic marijuana smoking may increase the risk for respiratory cancers, but a clear causal relationship has not been established.[24]

SYNTHETIC CANNABINOIDS

Synthetic cannabinoids (cannabimimetics) are compounds with chemical structures similar to THC and other naturally occurring cannabinoids, developed by scientists investigating the endocannabinoid system and potential avenues for treatments.[25] Scientific publication of methods to develop these compounds has unwittingly led to their manufacture and distribution as "marijuana substitutes" by underground laboratories. These compounds are typically sold in convenience stores, in "head shops," and online, and contain various synthetic cannabinoid constituents sprayed onto dried herbs. Common brand names include "K2" and "Spice." While the packaging indicates that these products are "not for human consumption," ostensibly to avoid Food and Drug Administration scrutiny, they are generally prepared and used similarly to marijuana. The appeal of these products is two-fold: (1) users may be attracted to their novelty and the opportunity for a new/distinct "high," and (2) users may wish to avoid detection of marijuana use by routine urine drug testing. Given the lack of product/quality control, the constituency and potency of these products may be highly variable and unpredictable. Several case reports and series suggest that many young people using these compounds experience significant adverse effects, including anxiety, agitation, paranoia,

hallucinations, tachycardia, nausea and vomiting, and diaphoresis.[26] Legislative bans initially targeted specific compounds, but manufacturers responded by utilizing alternative cannabimimetics. As a result, subsequent efforts to restrict or prohibit their manufacture and distribution have targeted these compounds as a class.

ASSESSMENT, MANAGEMENT, AND TREATMENT

Clinical assessment of marijuana use may include clinical interview for symptoms of *DSM-5* cannabis use disorder, physical examination for signs of intoxication (see **Acute Effects**) or withdrawal, and toxicology testing for marijuana metabolites. Urine testing is the most commonly available method, though in chronic, frequent, heavy users, urine cannabinoid tests may remain "positive" even after 1 to 3 weeks of abstinence.

Supportive care may be provided in the event of acute marijuana intoxication. Observation is often indicated to evaluate the acuity versus chronicity of adverse effects such as anxiety/panic and psychosis. In some cases, psychosis may be restricted to the intoxication event, but in other cases marijuana use, particularly in youth, may "unmask" or hasten the onset of a psychotic disorder in a vulnerable individual.

Marijuana withdrawal is common in chronic, daily users, and symptoms are similar in severity to those of nicotine withdrawal. Specific symptoms vary by individual, but often include increased anger/aggression, anxiety, depressed mood, irritability, restlessness, sleep difficulty and vivid/unusual dreams, decreased appetite, and weight loss.[15] Symptoms typically occur within 1 day of cessation, peak within 1 week, and last up to 2 weeks. Sleep difficulties may persist longer than other symptoms. Investigation of medications targeting marijuana withdrawal in adults is underway, but at present no specific pharmacotherapies are indicated. Withdrawal is often markedly unpleasant and is a clear factor associated with continued use and relapse in chronic users. Developing cognitive and behavioral skills to manage withdrawal symptoms and avoid using/relapsing is an important component of psychosocial marijuana cessation treatment.

An expanding evidence base is available to guide treatment of young people with substance use disorders in general, and cannabis use disorder in particular. The majority of evidence involves the use of individual- or group-delivered motivational enhancement therapy and cognitive behavioral therapy and/or family-based therapies.[27,28] While these treatments are often associated with reduced marijuana use and marijuana-associated adverse outcomes, few treatments have reliably yielded sustained abstinence outcomes. Recent developments indicate that additional modalities may augment other treatments to enhance outcomes. One is contingency management, in which rewards are provided based on substance abstinence (e.g., gift cards contingent upon "clean" urine cannabinoid tests).[29] This may be a key component of treatment for youth who are poorly motivated for cessation and only reluctantly engaged in treatment. Another recent development is evidence that the glutamate-modulating medication *N*-acetylcysteine is an efficacious pharmacotherapy to augment behavioral marijuana cessation treatment in adolescents.[30]

REFERENCES

1. Johnston LD, O'Malley PM, Miech RA, et al. *Monitoring the future national results on drug use*: 1975–2014: overview, key findings on adolescent drug use. Ann Arbor: Institute for Social Research, The University of Michigan, 2015.
2. Chen CY, Anthony JC. Possible age-associated bias in reporting of clinical features of drug dependence: epidemiological evidence on adolescent-onset marijuana use. *Addiction* 2003;98:71–82.
3. Substance Abuse and Mental Health Services Administration. *Results from the 2012 National Survey on Drug Use and Health: Summary of National Findings.* NSDUH Series H-46, HHS Publication No. (SMA) 13-4795. Rockville, MD: Substance Abuse and Mental Health Services Administration, 2013.
4. Joffe A, Yancy WS. Legalization of marijuana: potential impact on youth. *Pediatrics* 2004;113:e632–e638.
5. Salomonsen-Sautel S, Sakai JT, Thurstone C, et al. Medical marijuana use among adolescents in substance abuse treatment. *J Am Acad Child Adolesc Psychiatry* 2012;51:694–702.

6. Wang GS, Roosevelt G, Le Lait MC, et al. Association of unintentional pediatric exposures with decriminalization of marijuana in the United States. *Ann Emerg Med* 2014;63(6):684–689. doi:10.1016/j.annemergmed.2014.01.017

7. Wall MM, Poh E, Cerdá M, et al. Adolescent marijuana use from 2002–2008: higher in states with medical marijuana laws, cause still unclear. *Ann Epidemiol* 2011;21:714–716.

8. Lynne-Landsman SD, Livingston MD, Wagenaar AC. Effects of state medical marijuana laws on adolescent marijuana use. *Am J Public Health* 2013;103:1500–1506.

9. United Nations Office on Drugs and Crime. *World drug report 2006.* Vol. 1: analysis. Vienna: United Nations Office on Drugs and Crime, 2006.

10. Mehmedic Z, Chandra S, Slade D, et al. Potency trends of Δ9-THC and other cannabinoids in confiscated cannabis preparations from 1993 to 2008. *J Forensic Sci* 2010;55:1209–1217.

11. Huestis MA. Pharmacokinetics and metabolism of the plant cannabinoids, Δ9-tetrahydrocannbinol, cannabidiol and cannabinol. *Handb Exp Pharmacol* 2005;168:657–690.

12. Hartman RL, Huestis MA. Cannabis effects on driving skills. *Clin Chem* 2013;59:478–492.

13. American Psychiatric Association. *Diagnostic and statistical manual of mental disorders.* 5th ed. Arlington, VA: American Psychiatric Publishing, 2013.

14. Anthony J, Warner LA, Kessler RC. Comparative epidemiology of dependence on tobacco, alcohol, controlled substances, and inhalants: basic findings from the National Comorbidity Survey. *Exp Clin Psychopharmacol* 1994;2:244–268.

15. Budney AJ, Hughes JR, Moore BA, et al. Review of the validity and significance of cannabis withdrawal syndrome. *Am J Psychiatry* 2004;161:1967–1977.

16. Preuss UW, Watzke AB, Zimmerman J, et al. Cannabis withdrawal severity and short-term course among cannabis-dependent adolescent and young adult inpatients. *Drug Alcohol Depend* 2010;106:133–141.

17. Randolph K, Rurull P, Margolis A, et al. Cannabis and cognitive systems in adolescents. *Adolesc Psychiatry* 2013;3:135–147.

18. Meier MH, Caspi A, Ambler A, et al. Persistent cannabis users show neuropsychological decline from childhood to midlife. *Proc Natl Acad Sci U S A* 2012;109:E2657–E2664.

19. Moore TH, Zammit S, Lingford-Hughes A, et al. Cannabis use and risk of psychotic or affective mental health outcomes: a systematic review. *Lancet* 2007;370:319–328.

20. Rubino T, Parolaro D. Cannabis abuse in adolescence and the risk of psychosis: a brief review of the preclinical evidence. *Prog Neuropsychopharmacol Biol Psychiatry* 2014;52:41–44. doi: 10.1016/j.pnpbp.2013.07.020

21. Lynskey MT, Hall WD. The effects of adolescent cannabis use on educational attainment. *Addiction* 2000;96:433–443.

22. Fergusson DM, Horwood LJ, Swain-Campbell N. Cannabis use and psychosocial adjustment in adolescence and young adulthood. *Addiction* 2002;97:1123–1135.

23. Fergusson DM, Boden JM. Cannabis use and later life outcomes. *Addiction* 2008;103:969–976.

24. Hall W, Degenhardt L. Adverse health effects of non-medical cannabis use. *Lancet* 2009;374:1383–1391.

25. ElSohly MA, Gul W, Wanas AS, et al. Synthetic cannabinoids: analysis and metabolites. *Life Sci* 2014;97:78–90.

26. Brewer TL, Collins M. A review of clinical manifestations in adolescent and young adults after use of synthetic cannabinoids. *J Spec Pediatr Nurs* 2014;19(2):119–126. doi: 10.1111/jspn.12057

27. Waldron HB, Turner CW. Evidence-based psychosocial treatments for adolescent substance abuse. *J Clin Child Adolesc Psychol* 2008;37:238–261.

28. Tanner-Smith EE, Wilson SJ, Lipsey MW. The comparative effectiveness of outpatient treatment for adolescent substance abuse: a meta-analysis. *J Subst Abuse Treat* 2013;44:145–158.

29. Stanger C, Budney AJ, Kamon JL, et al. A randomized trial of contingency management for adolescent marijuana abuse and dependence. *Drug Alcohol Depend* 2009;105:240–247.

30. Gray KM, Carpenter MJ, Baker NL, et al. A double-blind randomized controlled trial of N-acetylcysteine in cannabis-dependent adolescents. *Am J Psychiatry* 2012;169:805–812.

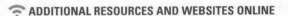

ADDITIONAL RESOURCES AND WEBSITES ONLINE

CHAPTER

67

Psychoactive Substances of Abuse

Diana Deister
Alan D. Woolf
Sharon Levy

KEY WORDS

- Barbiturate
- Benzodiazepine
- Cathinone ("bath salts" or "plant food")
- Cocaine
- D-Lysergic acid diethylamide tartrate (LSD)
- Inhalant
- Methamphetamine
- Methylene dioxymethamphetamine (MDMA)
- Opioid
- Phencyclidine (PCP)

Misuse of drugs, chemicals, plants and herbs, mushrooms, and other agents continues to be a major cause of mortality and morbidity for adolescents and young adults (AYAs). All psychoactive substances can have toxic effects, and use may result in overdose, serious injury, or death. Chronic drug use results in long-term neurologic and other health consequences and is associated with infections (i.e., hepatitis C and sexually transmitted infections), mental health disorders, increased rates of suicide, poor functional outcomes, and underachievement. In this chapter, we review the clinical toxicology and management of the effects of psychoactive substances of abuse other than alcohol, tobacco, and marijuana. AYAs may use several drugs and chemicals concurrently, so that the consequent toxic effects may not be those classically associated with one class of substances.

 COCAINE

Prevalence/Epidemiology

In 2013, 1 in 500 adolescents aged 12 to 17 were current cocaine users; the rate climbs to 1 in 90 for YAs aged 18 to 26.[1] Lifetime use of cocaine among US high school students has declined notably since the height of the "crack cocaine" epidemic in the mid-1980s; in 2014, 2.6% of high school seniors reported lifetime use of cocaine, the lowest rate since this data has been collected.[2] Recent cocaine initiates in 2013 were mostly (81.9%) over age 18.[1]

Medical Use

Cocaine is used medically to provide local anesthesia and hemostasis (via vasoconstriction) in surgery. It is often used topically in otolaryngological, plastic surgical, and emergency medical procedures.

Preparation and Dose

Cocaine (benzoylmethylecgonine) is a stimulant made from an alkaloid contained in the leaves of the coca bush, first used by the Inca people 3,000 years ago. The cocaine commonly available is actually the hydrochloride salt, which is 89% cocaine by weight. Most cocaine is "cut" by adding an inexpensive substance with similar appearance, leading to significant variability in concentration and potency, which can result in accidental overdose. Nasal insufflation is the most common route of exposure, giving a "high" that lasts 60 to 90 minutes. Cocaine hydrochloride easily dissolves in water for injection, resulting in a faster onset but shorter duration of the high.

"Crack" is cocaine hydrochloride that has been converted to a freebase by extraction (without purification) with the use of baking soda, heat, and water. It is usually smoked with marijuana, in a tobacco cigarette or cigar, or in a crack pipe resulting in a "high" that lasts about 20 minutes. Crack cocaine can also be injected.

Physiology and Metabolism

Cocaine has many potent pharmacological actions. It is a *stimulant* of the central and peripheral nervous systems; it has *local anesthetic* activity, and it is a *vasoconstrictor*.

Cocaine has three different effects on the central nervous system (CNS):

1. Stimulation of D1 and D2 presynaptic dopamine receptors, causing the release of dopamine (primarily), serotonin, and norepinephrine into the synaptic cleft
2. Blockade of neurotransmitter reuptake, causing synaptic entrapment and leaving an excess of neurotransmitters in the synapse
3. Increase in the sensitivity of the postsynaptic receptor sites

The dopamine reuptake transporter controls the level of the neurotransmitter in the synapse by carrying dopamine back into nerve terminals. Because cocaine effectively blocks this transporter, dopamine levels remain high in the synapse, affecting adjacent neurons and perpetuating the classic "high" associated with the drug. Depletion eventually occurs as enzymes break down entrapped neurotransmitters. This leaves the user dysphoric, with feelings of irritability, restlessness, and depression when the transporter resumes normal function. The "low" can be so intense that it leads to craving and repeated use to overcome the dysphoria. The study of the neurochemical pathways underlying these neuroadaptations is facilitating new approaches to treatment, such as N-methyl-D-aspartate (NMDA) receptor antagonists that block both dopaminergic and reinforcing effects.

Cocaine also blocks neuronal reuptake of norepinephrine and stimulates release of epinephrine, leading to what has been described as an "adrenergic storm" stimulating the neurological, respiratory, and cardiovascular systems. Cocaine is similar

551

to methamphetamine in that both drugs achieve their reinforcing effects via profound stimulation of the mesolimbic/mesocortical dopaminergic neuronal system, which consists of the ventral tegmental area, nucleus accumbens, ventral pallidum, and medial prefrontal cortex. Repeated exposure results in either sensitization (mediated by the D1 and D2 dopamine receptors) or tolerance depending on dose and pattern of use, and causes "neuroadaptation" or progressively decreasing sensitivity of neurons, a process that explains many aspects of addiction.

Cocaine is metabolized enzymatically by hepatic esterases, and, to a lesser degree, by plasma cholinesterase to the metabolite ecgonine methylester, which is hydrolyzed nonenzymatically to form benzoylecgonine. Between 5% and 10% of cocaine is metabolized by cytochrome p450–mediated N-demethylation into norcocaine, an active metabolite with greater vasoconstrictive and neurological activity than cocaine. Progesterone increases hepatic-N-demethylation, resulting in increased formation of norcocaine, potentially increasing toxic effects in women. Increased cocaine levels occur under conditions of decreased hepatic perfusion, such as hypotension or low cardiac output. Patients with genotype-mediated, reduced enzyme activity will have decreased metabolism by plasma cholinesterase. These patients may have extreme reactions, and sudden death can occur after seemingly small doses of cocaine (Table 67.1).

Effects of Intoxication

Signs of cocaine intoxication include hyper-alert state, increased talking, restlessness, elevated temperature, tachycardia, hypertension, anorexia, nausea, vomiting, dry mouth, dilated pupils, sweating, dizziness, tremors, hyperactive reflexes.

Adverse Effects

1. Psychiatric/neurologic: toxic psychosis, hallucinations, delirium, formication (sense of bugs crawling on the skin), body image changes, agitation, anxiety, irritability, seizures, paresthesias, hyperactive reflexes, tremor, pinprick analgesia, facial grimaces, headache, cerebral hemorrhage, cerebral infarctions, cerebral vasculitis, coma
2. Skin: excoriations, rashes, secondary skin infections (Fig. 67.1)
3. Cardiovascular: *Acute*: vasoconstriction, increased myocardial oxygen demand, tachycardia, angina, arrhythmias, chest pain, aortic dissection, hypertension, stroke, myocardial infarction, and cardiovascular collapse. Dysrhythmias and conduction disturbances range from sinus tachycardia or bradycardia to bundle branch block or a Brugada pattern, to complete heart block, idioventricular rhythms, Torsades de pointes, ventricular tachycardia or fibrillation, or sudden asystole. Cocaine and metabolites (benzoylocogenine and cocaethylene) contribute to Von Willebrand Factor (VWF) release by endothelium,[3] which may explain increased thrombosis. *Chronic*: accelerated atherosclerosis and thrombosis, endocarditis, myocarditis, cardiomyopathy, coronary artery aneurysms, bacterial endocarditis
4. Gastrointestinal: acute ischemia, gastro-pyloric ulcers, perforation of the small and large bowel, colitis, hepatocellular necrosis
5. Respiratory: *Acute*: pneumothorax, pneumomediastinum, pneumopericardium, pulmonary edema, "crack lung," pulmonary hemorrhage, tracheobronchitis, and respiratory failure. *Chronic*: interstitial lung damage
6. Musculoskeletal: up to a quarter of emergency department patients with cocaine-related problems have rhabdomyolysis, which may lead to acute renal failure, disseminated intravascular coagulation, and multiorgan failure.
7. Obstetric: low birth weight, prematurity, microcephaly, placental abruption
8. Adulterant-related reactions: Levamisole, a veterinary antihelminthic agent, appeared in 69% of cocaine samples entering the US (based on 2009 Drug Enforcement Administration (DEA) estimates), and composed about 10% of each sample. Complications often seen with Levamisole are neutropenia, agranulocytosis, arthralgias, retiform purpura, and skin necrosis.[3] Adulterants also include caffeine, acetaminophen, heroin, phenacetin, and many others.

Acute Overdose and Treatment

Cocaine is a short-acting drug, and treatment of cocaine overdose is similar to that for other cardiovascular and respiratory emergencies. The pathogenesis of cardiovascular complications is multifactorial and may be due not only to sympathomimetic effects but also to cocaine's direct effects on multiple cellular targets such as cardiac potassium and calcium channels.

Initial Management

The primary response is to support respiratory and cardiovascular functions, monitor vital signs and cardiac rhythm, and establish intravenous (IV) access. Screening of both urine and blood for drugs and other substances of abuse should be done to confirm cocaine use and to check for other substances. Electrocardiographic (ECG) monitoring, cardiac isoenzymes, and a chest x-ray are other useful studies in cocaine poisoning. Blood creatine kinase, urinalysis, and renal function tests may be necessary in patients suspected of having significant rhabdomyolysis.

Removal of Residual Cocaine

All residual cocaine should be removed from the patient's nostrils. If ingestions are suspected, or if the patient is a "body packer" or "stuffer" (see below), then activated charcoal should be administered orally or by gastric tube. If the patient presents with altered mental status, check for and treat hypoglycemia. Hyperthermia is life threatening and can be treated with antipyretics, a cooling blanket, and iced saline lavage. Muscle paralysis with a nondepolarizing agent may be necessary to reduce muscle contractions contributing to the hyperthermia. Seizures can be treated with benzodiazepines or other standard anticonvulsants. Ventricular dysrhythmias may require an antiarrhythmic agent such as lidocaine, whereas supraventricular arrhythmias may respond to therapy with calcium-channel blockers. Cardioversion may be necessary in some patients. Persistent dysrhythmias have been treated successfully in some cases with IV lipid emulsion, but its role in the routine management of patients remains unproven.[4] Cocaine-associated chest pain should be treated with nitroglycerin, calcium-channel blockers, and aspirin. β-Blockers should be avoided unless combined with α blockade. Thrombolysis should be considered if the symptoms and signs of toxicity, an ECG, and cardiac enzymes are consistent with acute myocardial infarction. Additionally, according to recent research, medications that disrupt platelet–VWF interactions may be indicated for prevention or management of thrombotic events.[5] Hypertensive crisis can precipitate cerebrovascular hemorrhage and must be treated emergently. Blood pressure elevations may be the result of direct CNS stimulation (treated with benzodiazepines), or peripheral α agonist effects (treated with either vasodilators (e.g., nifedipine, nitroglycerin, nitroprusside) or an α-adrenergic antagonist such as phentolamine). Agitation and psychosis may be treated with haloperidol or droperidol with consideration given to QTc prolongation from these medications and cocaine itself. To avoid further agitating acutely intoxicated patients, extraneous stimuli should be reduced. They should be approached in a subdued manner, with soft voice and slow movements. To achieve safe yet effective tranquilization in adults with agitated psychosis, the combination of intramuscular (IM) haloperidol 5 mg plus lorazepam 2 mg IM is generally well tolerated. Younger or smaller adolescents may warrant a dose reduction. Chlorpromazine should be avoided because of the possibility of a severe drop in blood pressure, provocation of arrhythmias or seizures, or anticholinergic crisis.

TABLE 67.1

Physiology and Metabolism of Common Drugs of Abuse

Receptors	Pharmacodynamics	Distribution	Metabolism
Cocaine			
D1 and D2 dopamine receptors	Release of dopamine, epinephrine, norepinephrine, and serotonin Blockade of neurotransmitter reuptake Increase sensitivity of postsynaptic receptor sites	Plasma and extracellular fluid	Hepatic esterases (80%) and plasma cholinesterase to form ecgonine methylester, then hydrolysis to benzoylecgonine Hepatic-*N*-demethylation to form norcocaine Excretion primarily in urine
Methamphetamine			
Serotonin binding sites and monoaminergic reuptake sites	Release of neurotransmitters from the presynaptic neurons Direct stimulation of postsynaptic catecholamine receptors Reuptake blockade Mild monoamine oxidase inhibitor	Crosses into the CNS with CSF levels approximately 80% of plasma levels	Little metabolism Renal excretion, enhanced in acidic urine
MDMA			
Serotonin 5HT2 receptors Central and peripheral catecholamine receptors	Release of serotonin into the synapse Release of endogenous catecholamines Inhibition of serotonin reuptake Depletion of serotonin stores occurs with repeated dosing, after which no further effect is achieved by taking more drug	Few pharmacologic studies have been performed in humans Peak concentrations at 2 h, half-life 8–9 h	Metabolized via cytochrome p450 isoenzyme CYP2D6 into 3,4-methylenedioxyamphetamine (MDA) 75% excreted in the urine as parent compound
Opioids			
Mu, kappa, and delta opioid receptors (primarily mu)	Stimulation of opioid receptors produces euphoria, pain relief, and other effects	Morphine—low lipid solubility, crosses blood–brain barrier slowly Heroin—high lipid solubility, crosses blood–brain barrier quickly and then is metabolized, creating a "morphine rush"	Metabolized by the liver (N-demethylation, N-dealkylation, O-dealkylation, conjugation, and hydrolysis) Primarily excreted in the urine (90%)
Barbiturates			
GABA-A agonists	Enhance GABA binding Open the chloride ion channel of the GABA receptor	Barbiturates bind to plasma proteins in varying amounts (50%–97%), and cross into the cerebrospinal fluid and the placenta to varying degrees	Metabolized in the liver, may enhance metabolism of other compounds Excreted by the kidney
Benzodiazepines			
GABA-A receptor agonists	Enhance the binding of GABA to the GABA receptor	Protein bound Cross into the CNS based on their solubility and lipophilicity	Metabolized in the liver Many active metabolites, which account for wide variation of half-lives
LSD			
Nonspecific intracellular binding throughout the CNS	Inhibition of serotonin release, resulting in: Increased firing of sensory neurons Nonspecific stress response	Primarily protein bound	Metabolized in the liver to multiple compounds; excreted by the kidney over hours (LSD) to days (metabolites).
Phencyclidine (PCP)			
Glutamate-NMDA receptors	Increases the production of dopamine Inhibits dopamine reuptake	Metabolites are fat soluble, though not physiologically active	Metabolized by the liver to monopiperidine conjugate pH-dependent urinary excretion

XIV

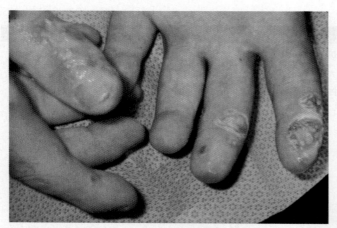

FIGURE 67.1 Crack pipe smoker's callus. (From Berg D, Worzala K. *Atlas of adult physical diagnosis*. Philadelphia, PA: Lippincott Williams & Wilkins, 2006.)

Flumazenil should be avoided as it may unmask seizure activity. Physical restraints should be avoided or discontinued as soon as possible due to increased risk of hyperthermia, lactic acidosis, and rhabdomyolysis.

Body Stuffer Syndrome

Body stuffers hastily swallow bags of drugs while running from law enforcement officials, whereas body packers carefully seal and swallow latex gloves or condoms filled with drugs prior to border crossings, with the intent to retrieve them later. Both are at risk of drug overdose if bags leak or break ("body stuffer syndrome"), with body stuffers at greater risk. Abdominal computed tomography may be necessary to rule out residual packets prior to hospital discharge. As many as 10% of body stuffers treated with whole bowel irrigation to facilitate evacuation of bags had remaining packets after two packet-free stools; these were largely undetectable on abdominal x-ray.[6]

Chronic Use

Cocaine is irritating to the mucosa, skin, and airways, and chronic use is associated with erosion of dental enamel, gingival ulceration, keratitis, chronic rhinitis, perforated nasal septum, midline granuloma, altered olfaction, optic neuropathy, osteolytic sinusitis, rashes, burns, and local skin necrosis. People addicted to cocaine also frequently experience anorexia, weight loss, sexual dysfunction, and elevated blood prolactin levels. Cognitively, cocaine can enhance some functions in acute use, similar to methylphenidate or amphetamines; however, chronic use leads to diminished abilities in most cognitive domains, possibly due to increased atherosclerosis of brain vasculature caused by cocaine use.

Tolerance and Withdrawal

Because of cocaine's powerful euphoric effects and short half-life, repeated use leads to rapid development of tolerance; addicts can progress from small doses to large daily quantities within weeks or months. No tolerance develops to the cardiovascular side effects. Symptoms of cocaine abstinence or withdrawal include depression, anhedonia, irritability, aches and pains, restless but protracted sleep, tremors, nausea, weakness, intense cravings for more cocaine, slow comprehension, suicidal ideation, lethargy, and hunger. There is currently no widely accepted treatment of cocaine withdrawal, and relapse rates are very high. Recent research on nonpharmacologic treatment for cocaine dependence shows that contingency management therapy—a well-established and effective treatment for adult cocaine users that consists of providing rewards for desired behaviors like clean urine tests or attending doctor's appointments—improves outcomes in adolescents when added to standard care.[7]

Cocaethylene

When alcohol is used with cocaine, a third substance, cocaethylene, is formed in the liver. The half-life of cocaethylene is 2 hours, compared with 38 minutes for cocaine. Cocaethylene is able to block dopamine reuptake, thereby extending the period of intoxication and toxicity. When alcohol and cocaine are used together, risk of sudden cardiac death or seizures is much higher. Chronically, neurobehavioral performance suffers even after periods of abstinence.

AMPHETAMINE (AMPHETAMINE, METHAMPHETAMINE, METHYLPHENIDATE, KHAT)

Prevalence/Epidemiology

In 2013, 0.5% of Americans aged 12 or older had used stimulants nonmedically in the last 30 days.[1] "Nonmedical" use of prescription amphetamines is increasingly common among youth, and ranges from taking someone else's prescription while studying to clear abuse and "getting high." The average age of first-time users of methamphetamine was 18.9 years in 2013,[1] indicating that prevention efforts must be made in early to mid-high school. From 2005 to 2010, emergency department visits in the US due to prescription stimulant use increased nearly three-fold, driven by dramatic increases in adult age-groups (especially for 18- to 25-year-olds) for both nonmedical use and adverse reactions, with no change in rates for adolescents. This may be due in part to greater cardiovascular risk at older ages.[8]

Medical Use

Amphetamines are used to treat attention-deficit/hyperactivity disorder and narcolepsy, and as a weight loss aid. Despite its potential for misuse, appropriate stimulant treatment does not appear to increase the risk of developing a substance use disorder (SUD). Longer-acting medications may have lower addiction potential than short-acting ones; once-daily dosing also facilitates easier supervision and pill counts by parents.

Preparation and Dose

The term "amphetamine" refers to a class of drugs containing an amphetamine base, available either in prescription form (such as amphetamine, dextroamphetamine, lisdexamfetamine), or illicitly manufactured (mainly in the form of methamphetamine). Amphetamines are CNS stimulants. Methamphetamine has a stronger effect on the CNS than other forms of amphetamine. Methylphenidate (and its enantiomer dexmethylphenidate) is a non-amphetamine stimulant with similar actions available in prescription form.

Amphetamine and methamphetamine differ structurally by the addition of one methyl group. Methamphetamine can be easily produced in clandestine "labs," beginning with ephedrine or pseudoephedrine found in over-the-counter medications, though availability of these precursors was limited by US federal law in 2005. Synthesis involves heating volatile solvents, which may often lead to explosions and fires. Meth labs are considered to be toxic waste sites that may be explosive; in the US, most are in residential areas, putting local residents at risk both during and after production. Illicitly synthesized methamphetamine may be contaminated by organic or inorganic impurities such as heavy metals (e.g., lead, mercury), solvents, and carcinogens. In recent years, the inexpensive and portable "shake and bake" method of methamphetamine production, which requires no lab equipment but can still be explosive, has gained popularity, leading to injuries, burns, and death.

The D-isomer (D-methamphetamine) is cortically more active than the L-isomer (the active ingredient in Vicks Inhaler). Water-soluble methamphetamine HCl is much more versatile than the hydrochloride salt of cocaine. It has high bioavailability in the salt form by any route of administration, such as snorting, smoking, ingesting by mouth, or passing across other mucous membranes such as the vaginal mucosa. "Ice" consists of pure crystals of D-methamphetamine.

Street methamphetamine may be mixed with many drugs, including cocaine. Studies show that 8% to 20% of street-available stimulants contain both drugs. Look-alikes containing combinations of caffeine, ephedrine, and phenylpropanolamine are particularly dangerous. A much larger dose of this combination is necessary to achieve the same level of cortical stimulation achieved with amphetamines. This combination also has greater cardiovascular stimulation, so abuse of look-alikes puts the user at great risk for stroke, myocardial infarction, or hypertensive crisis.

Prescription amphetamines are typically ingested orally or via nasal insufflation; illicit methamphetamine is usually smoked. Either preparation may be ground up, heated, and injected intravenously. Smoking methamphetamine may be more potent and addictive than snorting or ingesting it; smoking produces higher concentrations of drug in the brain for a shorter period.

Physiology and Metabolism

Amphetamines are CNS stimulants that work as sympathomimetic drugs. Amphetamines release neurotransmitters from presynaptic neurons, stimulate postsynaptic catecholamine receptors, prevent reuptake of neurotransmitters (dopamine, serotonin, and norepinephrine), and mildly inhibit the enzyme monoamine oxidase. Stimulation of the nucleus accumbens causes the experience of pleasure. Stimulation of the basal ganglia causes repetitive movements that may be seen in patients with amphetamine addiction. Increased serotonin levels are associated with changes in sleep and appetite patterns, increased body temperature, mood changes, aggressiveness, and psychosis.

Effects of Intoxication

As with cocaine, users experience increased energy, psychological euphoria, and physical well-being, but effects last much longer (12 hours versus 1 hour for cocaine).

Symptoms of amphetamine intoxication include hyperalertness, anxiety, confusion, irritability, aggression, delirium, dry mouth, tachycardia, hypertension, tachypnea, jaw clenching, bruxism (teeth grinding), reduced appetite, sweating, and psychosis. Amphetamine related deaths may arise from direct physiologic effects (myocardial infarction, cerebrovascular complications, seizures, maternal-fetal and infant exposures) or mental and behavioral impairments (assaults, suicides, homicides, accidents, driving impairment).

Adverse Effects

1. Psychiatric/Neurological: aggressiveness, confusion, delirium, psychosis, post-use dysphoria, seizures, choreoathetoid movements, cerebrovascular accidents, cerebral edema, cerebral vasculitis, hyperthermia
2. Cardiovascular: tachycardia, hypertension, atrial and ventricular arrhythmias, myocardial infarction, cardiac ischemia, coronary artery vasospasm, necrotizing angiitis, arterial aneurysms, aortic dissections. Li et al.[9] demonstrated in rats that cardiovascular collapse occurs due to concentration of methamphetamine in the brain stem nuclei responsible for regulation of respiration and circulation, leading to cell death by oxidative damage.
3. Gastrointestinal: ulcers, ischemic colitis, hepatocellular damage
4. Musculoskeletal: muscle contractions, tremors, rhabdomyolysis
5. Respiratory: pneumomediastinum, pneumothorax, pneumopericardium; acute noncardiogenic pulmonary edema, pulmonary hypertension
6. Renal: acute tubular necrosis, acute renal failure due to rhabdomyolysis
7. Dental: chronic gingivitis, numerous dental caries, severe dental abscesses and necrosis (known colloquially as "meth mouth") (Fig. 67.2)

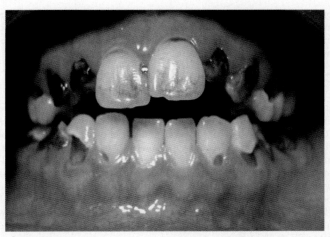

FIGURE 67.2 Dental changes such as blackened, stained, rotting teeth and tooth loss, referred to collectively as "meth mouth," are the result of abusing methamphetamine. (Photo by Dozenist, University of Tennessee Health Science Center, College of Dentistry, Memphis, Tennessee. In: Timby BK, Smith NE, eds. *Introductory medical-surgical nursing.* 11th ed. Philadelphia, PA: Lippincott Williams & Wilkins, 2013.)

Overdose and Emergency Treatment

Complications of amphetamine overdose resemble those of cocaine, although amphetamines do not affect nerve conduction as cocaine does. As with cocaine, emergency treatment is directed toward cardiovascular and respiratory stabilization and control of seizures. Agitation on presentation (39%), suicidal ideation (31%), and suicide attempt (21%) are commonly seen in methamphetamine poisonings in teens (age 11 to 18); suicidality was significantly higher than a control cohort, indicating the need for assessment for suicidal ideation after stabilization.[10] Patients who present to emergency departments for acute intoxication may require pharmacological intervention for agitation; multiple trials have shown effectiveness of antipsychotics (haloperidol, droperidol, risperidone, aripiprazole, quetiapine) and/or benzodiazepines (diazepam, lorazepam), though haloperidol should be used with caution as coadministration of methamphetamine and haloperidol caused excitotoxicity and cell death in the substantia nigra pars reticula in a rat model.[11] Avoid chlorpromazine (Thorazine), which can cause hypotension, anticholinergic crisis, or seizures.

Chronic Use

Chronic use of amphetamines can produce severe psychiatric as well as physical problems, including loss of executive function, delusions, hallucinations, long-term personality changes, and formication, leading individuals to tear and damage their skin. Choreoathetoid movements and other movement disorders are common and may persist after cessation of drug use. Chronic use of amphetamines or cocaine is associated with loss of gray matter volume in the frontal cortex.

Tolerance and Withdrawal

Tolerance to methamphetamine causes users to frequently escalate dose or change the route of administration to maintain the desired effect. Symptoms of withdrawal include irritability, agitation, depression, fatigue, sleep problems, increased appetite, headaches, and drug cravings; these symptoms may begin as soon as the high ends, can last up to 7 to 10 days, and are treated supportively.

STP

STP (2,5-dimethoxy-4-methylamphetamine, also known as DOM or the "serenity-tranquility-peace pill"), is a substituted amphetamine with selective serotonin (5-HT$_{2A}$, 5-HT$_{2B}$, and 5-HT$_{2C}$) partial agonist properties. Its powerful psychedelic, hallucinogenic properties are mediated by its 5-HT$_{2A}$ agonist activity. Its effects are also similar to those of other hallucinogenic drugs, with the exception that with STP the incidence of unpleasant sensations is increased, and the effects seem to last longer, up to 72 hours.

Cathinone (Khat) and Cathine, "Bath Salts," "Plant Food"

Cathinone is chemically similar to D-amphetamine, and cathine (D-norisoephedrine) is a form of cathinone with less psychoactive effect. These compounds are the active ingredients in khat leaves (*Catha edulis*), which are used as a tea or chewed for their euphoriant and stimulant effects by persons in Africa, the Middle East, and corresponding immigrant and refugee communities in developed nations. Outside of the US, khat is used within cultural norms with little evidence of abuse. Recently, synthetic cathinones have been marketed with names such as "bath salts" and "plant food." "Bath salt" use rates have been tracked since 2012 and remain low for high school students (about 1%) and lower for young adults aged 19 to 28 (0.4%).[2,12]

The most common synthetic compounds are 3,4-methylenedioxypyrovalerone, mephedrone, and methylone. While classified by the DEA as schedule I drugs, many chemical variants with similar properties are still legally marketed. These drugs are inexpensive to manufacture and easy to market on store shelves (in volumes of 200 mg to 10 g) and are often labeled as "not for human consumption." They are typically available as white or yellow powders (or rarely in pill form) and can either be ingested orally or through nasal insufflation. Banning the entire category is not feasible because other members are used medically as antidepressants or anorexiants.[13]

Effects of intoxication are similar to those for cocaine, methamphetamine, and methylene dioxymethamphetamine (MDMA); adverse reactions may be severe, including excited delirium and psychosis. Khat-induced psychosis most commonly occurs in the context of nonculturally sanctioned polydrug abuse. Khat and synthetic cathinones have been associated with multisystem organ failure: cardiac, gastrointestinal, neurologic, and psychiatric.[14]

⬤ ECSTASY/MDMA/MOLLY (METHYLENE DIOXYMETHAMPHETAMINE)

Prevalence/Epidemiology

According to the 2013 National Survey on Drug Use and Health, lifetime prevalence rates for MDMA use for teens aged 12 to 17 years and young adults aged 18 to 25 years were 1.5% and 12.8%, respectively.[1] Recently, MDMA has been rebranded as "Molly" (short for molecule) and advertised as "purer" and therefore "safer" than Ecstasy, although both are of highly variable content (varying from 0% to 100% MDMA).

Medical Use

MDMA was first patented in 1912 as an appetite suppressant; however, it was never manufactured or sold commercially and it has no current medical uses. MDMA continues to be studied as an adjunct to psychotherapy for conditions such as posttraumatic stress disorder (PTSD), with unconvincing results.

Preparation and Dose

The majority of pharmaceutical-grade MDMA tablets are now produced in Europe and smuggled into the US. The drug is sold as a tablet or capsule, often with a symbol printed on it. Tablets sold as MDMA may actually contain MDA, MDEA, or something entirely unrelated to the drug, such as LSD, caffeine, pseudoephedrine, or dextromethorphan. Orally ingested doses take approximately 30 to 60 minutes for onset of effect and the duration of action is 3 to 6 hours. Many users begin with a low dose (40 to 70 mg) and gradually add more pills until they experience the desired effect at a common dosage range of 75 to 125 mg, a practice known as "rolling." MDMA can be snorted, smoked, or injected, but is usually taken orally.

Physiology and Metabolism

MDMA binds to the serotonin transporter in vesicles and the plasma membrane and stimulates release of serotonin into the synapse where excess serotonin binding to postsynaptic receptors results in its effects. Serotonin has a variety of neurotransmitter actions, including control of wakefulness, appetite and satiety, regulation of mood and emotional states, and thermoregulation and circadian rhythms. Serotonin also causes release of oxytocin and vasopressin, both of which have roles in sexual arousal as well as such emotions as love and trust. Serotonin is largely broken down in the synapse by monoamine oxidase; repeated use of MDMA causes serotonin depletion, after which further doses have little or no effect. Single doses of MDMA have caused nerve damage in animal studies.

Effects of Intoxication

MDMA has both stimulant and hallucinogenic effects. Users describe feelings of enhanced well-being and introspection, empathy, love, affection, and increased energy.

Adverse Effects

1. Psychiatric/neurologic: confusion, depression, fatigue, sleep problems, anxiety, seizures, paranoia, spasms, bruxism, hyperthermia, sweating, syndrome of inappropriate antidiuretic hormone (SIADH), blurred vision, faintness, chills, excessive sweating, hyponatremia, hyponatremic dehydration, serotonin syndrome (with repeated dosing, or when taken with selective serotonin reuptake inhibitors [SSRIs])
2. Musculoskeletal: muscle rigidity, rhabdomyolysis
3. Cardiovascular: tachycardia, hypertension, arrhythmias, cardiovascular failure, asystole
4. Gastrointestinal: nausea, severe hepatic damage requiring transplantation.[8] MDMA enhances hepatic damage of alcohol by inhibiting aldehyde dehydrogenase 2, resulting in accumulation of toxic acetaldehyde (similarly to disulfiram).[15]
5. Developmental: infants of mothers who used MDMA regularly during the first trimester showed gross psychomotor retardation both at 4 and 12 months of age.[16]

Overdose and Emergency Treatment

The most common reaction to MDMA overdose is a syndrome of altered mental status, tachycardia, tachypnea, flushed appearance, profuse sweating, and hyperthermia; this syndrome is similar to the sympathomimetic effects of acute amphetamine overdose. MDMA should be suspected if a routine urine screen for amphetamines is negative. Serious complications such as delirium, seizures, and profound coma are more frequent with the combination of MDMA and other substances. AYAs who present late at night on weekends and have clinical manifestations of sympathetic overactivity and increased temperature ("Saturday night fever") should be suspected of using stimulants, and MDMA in particular. Patients chronically taking serotonin reuptake inhibitors or MAO inhibitors for depression risk fatal drug interactions when they ingest MDMA.

Treatment of toxic ingestions of MDMA is supportive, including support of airway, breathing, and circulation; assessment and treatment of cardiac arrhythmias; and monitoring of vital signs and level of consciousness. Close monitoring of serum electrolytes and fluid balance is required to detect the SIADH and/or water loading-induced hyponatremia. Hyperthermia should be treated with cooling blankets and IV fluids; muscle relaxants, anticonvulsants, and sedatives may be indicated. MDMA can be lethal due to hyperthermia, disseminated intravascular coagulation, rhabdomyolysis, renal failure, cardiac arrhythmias and sudden asystole, hyponatremia, seizures, serotonin syndrome, hepatic failure, cerebral infarction, and cerebral hemorrhage.

Chronic Use

Chronic MDMA use is associated with long-term cognitive impairments in retrospective memory, prospective memory, higher cognition, problem solving, and social intelligence.[17] Impairments in sleep, vision, and cortisol metabolism (with cortisol levels 800% above baseline during MDMA use) have been well documented. Long-lasting impairment of the 5-hydroxytryptamine (5-HT) system has been found in past users of MDMA, which may be more prominent in females and may be reversible in some patients. In rats, use of caffeine with MDMA or MDA enhances hyperthermic effects acutely and serotonergic loss in the long term.[18]

Withdrawal Syndrome

MDMA withdrawal is similar to that for other stimulants. The most common symptoms include depression, anxiety, panic attacks, sleeplessness, paranoia, and delusions. Treatment is supportive. The role of psychopharmacological management is uncertain, as an animal model found decreased fluoxetine antidepressant effects following prior exposure to MDMA, possibly due to damage to serotonergic systems.[19]

OPIODS (OPIUM, HEROIN, MEPERIDINE, OXYCONTIN, OXYCODONE, FENTANYL, SUFENTANYL, DESOMORPHINE)

Opioids, especially the potent oral analgesics such as hydrocodone (Vicodin) and oxycodone (OxyContin) and oxycodone+ acetaminophen (Percocet), continue to be attractive to AYAs, with 9.5% of high school seniors and 11% to 28% of 18- to 26-year-olds reporting lifetime use of "narcotics other than heroin … on your own—that is, without a doctor telling you to take them."[2,12]

Motive for misuse of prescription pain killers has significant implications. McCabe et al reported that the majority of adolescents misusing pain medication were seeking pain relief. Unfortunately, if other motives were also present (such as using to get "high"), chances were increased for having a SUD.[20] Annual prevalence rates of heroin use by AYAs remain less than 1%.[2,12]

Medical Use

Opioids are potent antitussives, antidiarrheals, and extremely potent pain relievers. Newer oral medications with extended half-lives are a tremendous asset in the field of pain management, but also come with the significant risk of addiction, particularly if use results in euphoria. Synthetic narcotics such as fentanyl, which is 80 times more potent than morphine, pose an increased danger of death by overdose.

Preparation and Dose

Opium has been used for centuries. The term *opioid* refers to all drugs, natural and synthetic, that bind to opioid receptors. Naturally occurring opiates (morphine, codeine, and heroin) are prepared from the opium poppy, *Papaver somniferum*. Synthetic opioid pain relievers such as oxycodone, hydrocodone, and oxymorphone are pharmaceutical products that are diverted and sold illegally. Many AYAs believe that these products are safer than illicit drugs.

Illicit synthetic opioids such as desomorphine ("krocodil") also are highly potent and may be attractive to individuals who have developed tolerance to other opioids. Use of krocodil, which is easily synthesized from codeine and household chemicals (similarly to meth), was a large public health problem in Russia and the Ukraine, where codeine was available without prescription until 2012, and now has spread to other countries throughout Europe. Fast onset and short duration of action make this drug highly addictive. Toxicity from impurities in the production process leads to significant tissue damage and often death in a relatively short time.

Routes of Administration

Opioids can be ingested, insufflated nasally, smoked, or injected intravenously or subcutaneously. Most AYAs first use prescription pain medications either orally or by nasal insufflation ("snorting"). "Long-acting" formulations can be crushed, making the entire dose available at once. Because of the rapid development of tolerance, many individuals with opioid dependence cannot keep up with the higher cost of prescribed opioids, and switch to less-expensive heroin.

Heroin, or diacetylmorphine, is a semisynthetic drug that quickly crosses the blood–brain barrier and is metabolized to morphine. It is produced illicitly and commonly mixed with sugar, talcum powder, Epsom salt, or quinine. The relatively pure heroin available today can be smoked, insufflated nasally, injected intravenously, or rarely injected subcutaneously ("skin popping"). The ability to use heroin without needles has lowered the barriers to initiation for many youth. The duration of the effects of intravenously injected heroin is 3 to 6 hours; addicted individuals often need to use heroin 2 to 4 times a day to avoid withdrawal.

Physiology and Metabolism

There are four opioid receptors in humans. Mu, kappa, and delta (subclasses: mu 1 and 2, delta 1 and 2, and kappa 1, 2, and 3) are G-protein–coupled receptors, but they also activate other biochemical pathways such as the arrestin pathway; a fourth receptor, sigma, is in a unique class. Mu is the major opioid receptor in the brain and is responsible for the majority of neurological effects, including euphoria and pain relief. The kappa receptor is found primarily in the brain stem and spinal cord and contributes to pain relief and sedation. Delta receptors are located in the limbic system and are believed to be responsible for affective and emotional changes associated with opioid use.[13] Sigma-1 receptors bind inactive opioids and modulate action of mu, kappa, and delta receptors; their contributions to plasticity, reinforcement, and addiction are still being explored. They also bind cocaine, methamphetamine, and dextromethorphan and mediate some effects of these drugs as well.[21]

Naloxone (Narcan) is a synthetic opioid antagonist that binds to mu, kappa, and delta opioid receptors with greater affinity than other opioids, and is used to treat opioid overdose,[13] resulting in reversal of effect and sudden withdrawal. Buprenorphine is a new synthetic opioid partial agonist that has been approved for use as therapy for opioid addiction. It has intermediate avidity for the opioid receptor, between that of naloxone and other opioids.

Effects of Intoxication

Opioids produce analgesia, and, in high doses, euphoria. Symptoms of intoxication include anxiety, slow comprehension, euphoria, floating feeling, flushing, hypotonia, pinpoint pupils, skin picking, sleepiness, poor appetite, and constipation. The analgesia produced by opioids dissociates the perception of pain from the emotional response and is often described as "I feel it, but it doesn't hurt."

Adverse Effects

1. Psychiatric/neurologic: sedation, apathy, dysphoria, psychomotor agitation or retardation, impaired judgment, delirium, stupor, diminished reflexes, miosis, pinprick analgesia, ataxia, hypothermia, hypotonia, coma
2. Cardiovascular: circulatory collapse, hypotension, hypothermia, thrombosis, phlebitis, and endocarditis
3. Respiratory: blocked cough reflex, bradypnea, respiratory failure, pulmonary edema
4. Gastrointestinal: constipation
5. Skin: rashes, allergic reactions, secondary bacterial infections, abscesses, cellulitis
6. Obstetric: low birth weight, neonatal withdrawal, and respiratory compromise

XIV

Overdose and Emergency Treatment

Opioid overdose results in coma, respiratory depression or failure, and circulatory collapse. Treatment begins with support of respiratory and circulatory function, protection of the airway to prevent aspiration, and treatment of hypoglycemia if present. Patients should receive naloxone (0.4- 2 mg) intravenously every 2-3 minutes until a response occurs or up to a maximum dose of 10 mg. Naloxone has a short duration of action compared to most opioid agonists, and must be repeated every 20 to 60 minutes or given by IV infusion, to cover the patient for the duration of the overdose. Close observation for reemergence of sedation and respiratory failure is necessary. Naloxone does not reverse hypotension caused by opiate-induced histamine release. Nasal naloxone has been successfully deployed in community health programs for administration by friends and family members of patients with opioid addiction while waiting for EMS to arrive, significantly reducing rates of opioid overdose deaths.[22]

Chronic Use

Problems related to chronic use of opioids are primarily due to impurities, complications of injection or insufflation, and behaviors associated with addiction, such as prostitution, lying, and stealing. Frequent complications include:

1. Skin: abscesses and cellulitis
2. Vascular: arteritis and thrombosis of the pulmonary vessels
3. Infectious: lung abscesses with resulting pulmonary fibrosis and pulmonary hypertension; endocarditis and secondary septic emboli; osteomyelitis, septic arthritis, tetanus, HIV and hepatitis C from injecting infectious organisms directly into a vein
4. Liver and kidney: hepatitis and glomerulonephritis from injecting foreign material (talc, sugar) into a vein
5. Respiratory: recurrent aspiration pneumonia from respiratory suppression and blocking of the cough reflex, pulmonary edema, and arrhythmias caused by quinine
6. Myositis ossificans: extraosseous metaplasia of muscle caused by needle manipulation

Tolerance and Withdrawal

Tolerance, dependence, and addiction occur very quickly, and patients must constantly increase dose and frequency to avoid withdrawal symptoms. Opioid withdrawal presents with flu-like symptoms, which can be extremely unpleasant, but are generally not life threatening in otherwise healthy individuals. Symptoms include anxiety, irritability, yawning, restlessness, sleep disturbances, muscle aches, chills and sweating, piloerection, hyperthermia, lacrimation and nasal secretions, abdominal cramps with vomiting and diarrhea, paresthesias, tremors, mydriasis, hypertension, and tachycardia. The Clinical Opiate Withdrawal Scale,[23] http://www.naabt.org/documents/cows_induction_flow_sheet.pdf, was developed to quantify the symptoms of opioid withdrawal and may be useful clinically during buprenorphine induction. Induction should only be started once a sufficient number of opioid receptors are available (either after all withdrawal symptoms have subsided, or during significant symptoms of withdrawal), in order to avoid precipitating the rapid withdrawal that occurs when the partial opioid agonist (buprenorphine) replaces a full agonist (heroin, hydrocodone, etc.) on the receptor.

Treatment for opioid withdrawal is supportive, and includes symptomatic treatment of aches and pains with nonsteroidal anti-inflammatory medications, abdominal cramping with dicyclomine (Bentyl), and reassurance. The α-2 adrenergic agonists clonidine and lofexidine improve tolerability of opioid withdrawal; it can also be managed with buprenorphine.

Medical Management of Opioid Addiction

Opioid dependence, regardless of the specific preparation chosen or route of administration, creates intense addictive disease and carries a guarded prognosis. However, newer medications have been shown to reduce relapse rates substantially, particularly when combined with supportive counseling. Methadone and buprenorphine have both been shown to reduce relapse rates in patients seeking treatment. Naltrexone, administered orally or as a monthly injection, improves sobriety outcomes in both opioid and alcohol use disorders.[24]

NON-NARCOTIC CNS DEPRESSANTS

CNS depressants include barbiturates, benzodiazepines, γ-hydroxyl butyrate (GHB), flunitrazepam (Rohypnol), major tranquilizers (phenothiazines), and carbamates such as meprobamate (Equanil and Miltown). Physical symptoms of sedative-hypnotic intoxication include slurred speech, incoordination, unsteady gait, nystagmus, decreased reflexes, impaired attention or memory, and stupor or coma. Psychiatric symptoms of intoxication include inappropriate behavior, mood lability, impaired judgment, and impaired social and occupational functioning.

Barbiturates

Prevalence/Epidemiology

Nonmedical use of barbiturate tranquilizers continues to be a problem among AYAs. The Monitoring the Future study recorded the rate of lifetime use of sedatives/barbiturates among high school seniors to be 6.8%; use increases until age 25 to 26 with rates of 13% to 16%.[2,12]

Medical Uses

Barbiturates are sedative/hypnotic drugs derived from barbituric acid, and are used as sleep aides, for sedative-hypnotic anesthesia, as anticonvulsants, for reduction of intracranial pressure and cerebral ischemia after head trauma, for post-stroke management, and for pre-induction of anesthesia. Their medical use has decreased over the past decades as they have been replaced by benzodiazepines for several indications due to less respiratory depression and higher therapeutic index (the ratio between effective dose and overdose).

Preparation and Dose

About 12 types of barbiturates are used medically in the US. The most frequently abused barbiturates are secobarbital, pentobarbital, and amobarbital. Many of the illicit pills are made in Mexico and contain varying amounts of secobarbital. Duration of action of barbiturates may vary from minutes to days. Approximately 75% of phenobarbital is hydroxylated in the liver and 25% is excreted unchanged in urine, whereas secobarbital and butabarbital undergo 99% hepatic metabolism. Barbiturates are usually taken orally, although some users inject them intravenously.

Physiology and Metabolism

Barbiturates are GABA (γ-aminobutyric acid) A receptor agonists. GABA is the main inhibitory neurotransmitter of the CNS. Barbiturates bind to a unique location on the GABA receptor (separate from the GABA, benzodiazepine, and the endogenous neuroactive steroid binding sites). Once bound, barbiturates have three effects. First, they enhance binding of GABA *and* benzodiazepines to their unique sites. Second, they open the chloride ion channel of the GABA receptor even in the absence of GABA. Third, they increase the duration of channel opening. Increased chloride conductance reduces neuron firing, thus the antiseizure effects. Together, these effects make barbiturates potent drugs with a narrow window of safety. By enhancing GABA actions, barbiturates can produce all degrees of CNS depression. The mesencephalic reticular activating system, which contributes to homeostasis, is particularly sensitive to barbiturates.

Barbiturates are metabolized by the liver and enhance liver metabolism, shortening the half-life of other drugs (e.g., anticoagulants, corticosteroids, phenothiazines, oral contraceptives), reducing their clinical effectiveness. They can increase the CNS depressant effects of meperidine by increasing its active metabolites.

Effects of Intoxication

Barbiturates are CNS depressants: low doses result in mild sedation; higher doses result in hypnosis; and still higher doses result in anesthesia and death. Symptoms of intoxication include sleepiness, yawning, slowed comprehension, slurred speech, lateral nystagmus, anorexia, dizziness, and orthostatic hypotension. Allergic reactions including bronchospasm, urticaria, dermatitis, fever, and angioedema can occur. When barbiturates are used in combination with other depressants such as alcohol, benzodiazepines, or opioids, the effects of both are potentiated and lethal overdoses can occur more easily.

Adverse Effects

1. Psychiatric/Neurological: fatigue, euphoria or depressed mood, irritability, violent behavior, toxic psychosis, ataxia, slowed comprehension, diplopia, dizziness, dysmetria, hypotonia, poor memory, lateral nystagmus, and slowed speech
2. Skin: Cutaneous lesions, urticarial rashes, and bullae
3. Respiratory: respiratory depression, acidosis, respiratory failure

Overdose and Emergency Treatment

Signs and symptoms of barbiturate overdose include miosis, hypotension, hypothermia, respiratory depression, and decreased gastrointestinal motility. Coma, shock, and death are possible. The presentation is indistinguishable from opiate or other sedative overdose on clinical examination. Urine toxicology can be helpful for diagnosis, but quantitative levels are not predictive of the clinical course. Ingestion of more than 3 g or a blood level of more than 2 mg/dL is the lethal dose for short-acting barbiturates; ingestion of more than 6 to 9 g or a blood level greater than 11 to 12 mg/dL is the lethal dose for long-acting barbiturates. Treatment of barbiturate overdose is primarily supportive, and aimed at supporting airway, breathing, and circulation. Unabsorbed barbiturate should be removed by gastric lavage followed by activated charcoal. In severe, life-threatening barbiturate poisoning, extracorporeal methods of drug removal, such as hemodialysis, might be considered. CNS stimulants should be avoided.

Tolerance and Withdrawal

If dependence is suspected, detoxification must be done under close medical supervision, as withdrawal can be life threatening. Withdrawal symptoms include anxiety, delirium, hallucinations, irritability, sleep disturbance, seizures, headaches, weakness, hyperactive reflexes, tremor, abdominal cramps, flushing, nausea, sweating, and increased temperature. Orthostatic hypotension may also occur, in contrast to benzodiazepine withdrawal, which typically presents with hypertension. Barbiturate withdrawal is treated with replacement by phenobarbital followed by a slow taper until the patient is drug free.

Benzodiazepines
Prevalence/Epidemiology

Nonmedical use of benzodiazepines by AYAs has declined since a peak in 2002. In 2014, annual nonmedical use rates were 1.7%, 3.9%, and 4.7% for 8th, 10th, and 12th graders; rates for college students and young adults (2013) were 4.4% and 5.4%, respectively.[2,12]

Medical Use

Medical use of benzodiazepines became widespread in the 1970s, and this class of drugs continues to be used clinically as

TABLE 67.2

Major Pharmacological Actions of Various Benzodiazepines

Benzodiazepine	Major Pharmacological Action
Diazepam, chlordiazepoxide, oxazepam, chlorazepate, lorazepam, prazepam, alprazolam, halazepam	Anxiolytic
Flurazepam, temazepam, flunitrazepam, triazolam, midazolam	Sedative-hypnotic
Diazepam, clonazepam	Anticonvulsant
Diazepam	Muscle relaxant

anxiolytic, hypnotic, anticonvulsant, and antispasmodic medications (Table 67.2). Benzodiazepines are also used to treat alcohol withdrawal and catatonia. Initially, benzodiazepines were thought to be free of negative consequences, but it is now known that they carry the risk of dependence, withdrawal, and negative side effects.

Preparation and Dose

Benzodiazepines are readily available on the street in the US, and may be obtained by diverting legitimate prescriptions or by theft from pharmaceutical supplies. Abuse of benzodiazepines generally occurs within the context of another substance abuse disorder as they are often used to augment the effects of or prevent withdrawal from another drug. However, benzodiazepines are the drug of choice for a small proportion of adolescents with substance abuse problems and severe sedative/hypnotic use disorder has been described.

Benzodiazepines are most often taken orally, though some users may snort or inject them intravenously. Regardless of route of administration, those that cross the blood–brain barrier more quickly have a higher abuse potential than those that cross more slowly.

Physiology and Metabolism

Benzodiazepines bind to a unique site on the GABA-A receptor and enhance the inhibitory effects of GABA. Like barbiturates, benzodiazepines enhance the binding of GABA to its receptor. They also increase the frequency of channel opening. Unlike barbiturates, however, benzodiazepines do not open the chloride ion channel of the GABA receptor in the absence of GABA. This makes benzodiazepines relatively milder in effect and safer to use than barbiturates. However, in combination, benzodiazepines and barbiturates synergistically enhance channel opening (by increasing both frequency and duration of opening), and are thus a dangerous combination. GABA-A receptors have five subunits, all of which have multiple variants; different channel subtypes are expressed in varying neuronal populations and likely account for specific effects of individual benzodiazepines.

The liver metabolizes benzodiazepines. The duration of the clinical effect is often determined by the half-life of active metabolites, and they are often classified this way. Long-acting drugs are diazepam, chlordiazepoxide, clonazepam, flurazepam, and clorazepate. Diazepam is highly lipophilic and has rapid absorption after ingestion, with an elimination half-life ranging from 18 to 100 hours. It is metabolized in the liver via a two-phase process of demethylation involving the cytochrome p450 system, followed by glucuronidation. Shorter-acting benzodiazepines include oxazepam and lorazepam, which are metabolized directly in the liver by single-step glucuronidation and have elimination half-lives of about 6 hours. Ultra-short–acting agents include triazolam, temazepam, and midazolam. Benzodiazepines can cross the placenta and are excreted in breast milk.

Benzodiazepines and their metabolites may accumulate in the body, resulting in a delayed appearance of adverse reactions and continued clinical effects beyond discontinuation of the drug. Unlike the barbiturates, benzodiazepines do not induce the metabolism of other drugs.

Effects of Intoxication

Benzodiazepines are CNS depressants. They produce drowsiness, dizziness, weakness, sedation, and a sense of calmness.

Adverse Effects

1. Psychiatric/Neurologic: disinhibition, paradoxical aggression, anxiety, delirium, agitation, visual hallucinations, ataxia, memory loss, impaired psychomotor function. These effects are prominent with the "date rape" drug flunitrazepam (Rohypnol).
2. Cardiovascular: mild hypotension.

Overdose and Emergency Treatment

Benzodiazepine overdose typically presents with dizziness, confusion, drowsiness or unresponsiveness, and blurred vision. Some patients may present with anxiety and agitation. Physical exam signs include nystagmus, slurred speech, ataxia, weakness or hypotonia, hypotension, and respiratory depression. Treatment for benzodiazepine overdose is primarily supportive, including securing the airway, and cardiovascular and respiratory stabilization. Flumazenil is a benzodiazepine receptor antagonist/partial agonist capable of reversing the sedative effects of benzodiazepines. To treat coma from severe benzodiazepine overdose, flumazenil is given in incremental doses over a few minutes. If a clinical effect is not seen after five spaced doses have been given, it is unlikely that higher doses will be helpful. Similar to naloxone for opiate overdose, flumazenil has a shorter action than many benzodiazepines and may require repeated doses to prevent return of symptoms.

Flumazenil is contraindicated in mixed overdoses involving seizure-causing agents, because it can counteract anticonvulsant protection conferred by benzodiazepines. It is also relatively contraindicated in individuals who are physically dependent on benzodiazepines because it can precipitate a full-blown benzodiazepine withdrawal state (agitation, tremor, flushing). Like the opiate partial agonist buprenorphine, flumazenil can relieve withdrawal symptoms when receptors are unoccupied.

Chronic Use, Tolerance, and Withdrawal

Benzodiazepines have a high abuse and dependence potential. Care should be used in prescribing benzodiazepines for the management of sleep disturbances or anxiety in any patient who has been diagnosed with drug problems, or who takes barbiturates for other conditions such as migraine. Benzodiazepines are relatively contraindicated in adolescents with alcohol or opioid use disorders, or who are taking methadone or buprenorphine for treatment of an opioid use disorder.

If benzodiazepine dependence is suspected, withdrawal must be carefully supervised. Patients who abruptly stop taking benzodiazepines can develop life-threatening, protracted seizures (delirium tremens when it occurs with altered sensorium). Patients with a prior seizure history are at much greater risk and will more likely need inpatient detoxification. Other symptoms of benzodiazepine withdrawal include anxiety, agitation, confusion, sleep disturbance, and flu-like symptoms, including fatigue, headache, muscle pain and weakness, sweating, chills, nausea, vomiting, and diarrhea.

There is an extensive literature on benzodiazepine detoxification. It may be done in an inpatient or outpatient setting, by using a benzodiazepine taper and/or benzodiazepine symptom- triggered protocol (for inpatients); by using anticonvulsants (carbamazepine) with baclofen augmentation; or by using a combination of low-dose flumazenil coupled with clonazepam replacement[25]

γ-Hydroxybutyrate (Precursors: 1,4 Butane-Diol, Butyrolactone, γ-Valerolactone)

GHB is a CNS depressant that acts through a metabolite of the inhibitory neurotransmitter GABA and can function as a neurotransmitter itself. GHB triggers the release of an opiate-like substance and can mediate sleep cycles, temperature regulation, memory, and emotional control. In some countries, GHB is used as an anesthetic and to treat narcolepsy. It is available as a liquid or powder and is rapidly absorbed after oral ingestion. Precursors of GHB, such as 1,4 butanediol and butyrolactone, may have sedative effects that are delayed by several hours, until their metabolism is complete.

GHB stimulates protein synthesis, so is used by body builders to increase lean body mass. It is used as a euphoriant by people attending raves. It is also considered to be a "date rape" drug because it has been used to incapacitate victims and is difficult to detect.

Adverse effects include bradycardia, increased or decreased blood pressure, respiratory depression or failure with acidosis, vomiting, and mild hyperglycemia. Neurological effects include hypothermia, dizziness, weakness, ataxia, vertigo, nystagmus, short-term amnesia, coma, tonic–clonic seizures, and myoclonus. Confusion, sedation, aggression, impaired judgment, and hallucinations may lead to accidental injury.

Heavy doses can induce coma and respiratory depression, which are exacerbated by the use of alcohol. There is no antidote for GHB overdose; the treatment is supportive care. Withdrawal effects include insomnia, anxiety, tremors, and sweating, and are potentially life threatening. Decision rules about when to recommend inpatient detoxification have been proposed.[26]

Phencyclidine

Prevalence/Epidemiology

The use of phencyclidine (PCP) has steadily declined from the 1970s. In 2013 to 2014, 0.8% of high school seniors and 0.2% of YA reported using PCP within the previous 12 months.[2,12]

Medical Use, Preparation, and Dose

PCP is an arylamine (1-[1-phenyl{cyclohexyl}piperidine]) introduced in the 1950s as a general anesthetic. Due to adverse effects such as excessive agitation, excitement, and disorientation during surgical recovery, it was discontinued as a medicine for human use in 1965. PCP may be packaged as a liquid, powder, tablet, leaf mixture, or rock crystal. It can be used intravenously, intramuscularly, or orally, or it can be snorted or smoked.

Physiology and Metabolism

The hydrogen chloride salt of PCP is structurally related to ketamine. It is a dissociative anesthetic with analgesic, stimulant, depressant, and hallucinogenic properties whose pharmacology is complex and not fully understood. Its major psychiatric effects are thought to be the result of binding to glutamatergic NMDA receptors leading to increased production of dopamine and inhibition of its reuptake. PCP is rapidly inactivated by hepatic metabolism and is excreted in the urine as monopiperidine conjugate. Because PCP is fat soluble, it easily crosses the blood brain barrier and may remain in the body for prolonged periods, with a half-life of 3 days. Its urinary excretion is highly dependent on urine pH, with significantly higher excretion rates at an acidic pH. However, the urine should not be acidified in case of overdose as this can worsen the patient's clinical status and promote renal injury from myoglobinuria.[27]

Effects of Intoxication

The clinical symptoms of PCP use vary with the dose, route of administration, and experience of the user (inexperienced users have more side effects). IV, IM, and oral routes of administration are more difficult to regulate than the smoking of PCP. PCP usually induces one of several clinical states (**Table 67.3**).

TABLE 67.3
PCP-Induced Intoxication States

Acute intoxication	Delusion, disinhibition, dissociation ("out of body" experience)
Acute or prolonged delirium	Disorientation, clouded consciousness, and abnormal cognition
Schizophreniform psychosis	Hallucinations, thought disorder, and delusions
Mania	Hallucinations, elevated mood, elevated self-attitude, feelings of omnipotence
Depressive reactions	Dysphoria, social withdrawal, paranoia, isolation

TABLE 67.4
Adverse Effects of PCP by Dose

Low dose (<5 mg)

Physical: horizontal and vertical nystagmus, blank stare, ataxia, hypertension, increased deep tendon reflexes, decreased proprioception and sensation, miosis or midposition reactive pupils, diaphoresis, flushing

Cognitive and behavioral: disorganized thought processes, distortion of body image and of objects, amnesia, agitated or combative behavior, unresponsiveness, disinhibition of underlying psychopathology, schizophrenic reactions, catalepsy, catatonia, illusions, anxiety, and excitement

Moderate dose (5–10 mg)

Physical: vertical and horizontal nystagmus, hypertension, myoclonus, midposition pupil size, dysarthria, diaphoresis, fever, hypersalivation

Cognitive and behavioral: amnesia, mutism, anxiety, excitement, delusions, stupor or extreme agitation, violent or psychotic behavior

High dose (>10 mg)

Physical: eyes that may remain open during coma, hypertension, arrhythmias, increased deep tendon reflexes, muscle rigidity, decerebrate posturing, convulsions, spontaneous nystagmus, miosis, decreased urine output, dysarthria, diaphoresis and flushing, fever

Cognitive and behavioral: unresponsive, immobile state, amnesia, mutism

Extremely high dose (>500 mg)

Physical: prolonged coma, rigidity, extensor (decerebrate) posturing, seizures, hypoventilation, hypertension or hypotension

Cognitive and behavioral: prolonged and fluctuating confusional state after recovery from coma

PCP causes a characteristic vertical nystagmus, and may also cause horizontal or rotatory nystagmus. PCP use should be suspected in all AYAs with a distorted thought process, especially when there is evidence of analgesia or nystagmus. Any individual with open-eye coma, horizontal and vertical nystagmus, hypertension, and rigidity should be considered to have taken PCP. PCP is best detected in the urine but, unfortunately, several other drugs such as tramadol and dextromethorphan may cause a false-positive PCP screen. Confirmatory testing is critical. A serum concentration of 25 to 100 ng/mL may be found in patients who are in an acute state of confusion; higher levels may be found in comatose patients.

Adverse Effects

Adverse effects associated with PCP use are dose related (see Table 67.4).

Overdose and Emergency Treatment

PCP use may result in generalized motor seizures either early in the course of intoxication or delayed in appearance. Death can occur from injuries sustained during periods of analgesia and aggression or as a result of convulsions and/or cerebral hemorrhage.

Reduction of Stimuli: When treating patients with PCP overdose, health care providers must use extreme caution. Patients are unpredictable and often have little awareness of the consequences of their behavior. Reducing the levels of light, sound, and other external stimuli can rapidly bring down a PCP user; if possible, patients should not be touched or cornered or engaged in conversation. In an emergency, covering the intoxicated patient with a blanket may be helpful. All hazards should be removed from the environment. Restraints are not recommended; they may cause the patient to harm himself or herself in an attempt to escape and can increase the risk of rhabdomyolysis if the patient continues to struggle.

Supportive Care: Treatment for PCP overdose is largely supportive. In addition to basic cardiopulmonary resuscitation, it is essential to check for signs of head, neck, back, and internal injuries, which can occur from trauma while the patient is under the behavioral effects of the drug. Because PCP travels through enterohepatic circulation, repeated doses of activated charcoal may be beneficial regardless of how PCP was used.[27]

Medications: Medication use is relatively contraindicated, but, if necessary, IV diazepam or lorazepam can be used to treat seizures. PCP-induced dystonia does not respond to diphenhydramine.[26] Severe agitation and psychosis caused by PCP can be treated with haloperidol.

Recovery: Recovery usually occurs within 24 hours but, depending on the dose, can take days. During the recovery phase, a user of PCP may require short-term inpatient psychiatric care to deal with paranoia, regressive behavior, and a slow phase of reintegration. With higher doses the coma can last 5 to 6 days and can be followed by a prolonged recovery period marked by behavioral disorders. Cognitive, memory, and speech disorders may last up to one year after the last use of PCP. Flashbacks may occur, as with LSD.

Ketamine

Ketamine ("Special K") is an arylcycloalkylamine chemical congener of PCP; it is similar to PCP pharmacologically. It is a rapid-acting dissociative anesthetic that combines sedative-hypnotic, analgesic, and amnesic effects with the maintenance of pharyngeal reflexes and respiratory function at normal doses. Like PCP, ketamine is an NMDA receptor antagonist and is used as a human and veterinary anesthetic. Like PCP-induced anesthesia, it occasionally produces unpleasant reactions, anxiety, dysphoria, and hallucinations. Due to reports that ketamine can alleviate refractory depression, it has been studied for this use, although barriers to safe use are sizeable. Users are attracted to the "dreamy" state of mild hallucinations and "out of body" experiences induced by light ketamine anesthesia. Adverse effects include a cataleptic state, with nystagmus, excessive salivation, involuntary tongue and limb movements, and hypertonus. Laryngospasm, seizures, apnea, and respiratory arrest have all been reported on rare occasions with ketamine-induced anesthesia. Accidents are often of greater threat to the individual than the drug's toxicity. Ketamine can be used as an alternative to cocaine, and it is often snorted. The drug is also often sold in tablets, and users may take ketamine thinking they are using MDMA. Ketamine overdose treatment is supportive, with attention to neurological, cardiovascular, and respiratory monitoring; ventilatory support may be necessary. Treatment of agitation related to an emergence reaction entails dim lighting, reduction of extraneous external stimuli, and administration of a benzodiazepine. For idiosyncratic dystonic reactions, IV diphenhydramine may be of benefit.

Baclofen and Muscle Relaxants

Abuse of prescription drugs such as muscle relaxants has become more common among adolescents. Muscle relaxants are diverse in chemical structure and actions; they include such drugs as baclofen, meprobamate, orphenadrine, and methocarbamol. Baclofen (Lioresal) is chemically related to the inhibitory neurotransmitter, GABA, and can induce drowsiness, coma, muscle flaccidity, cardiac dysrhythmias, and respiratory depression or sudden respiratory arrest. Treatment of patients who overdose on muscle relaxants includes oral decontamination with activated charcoal, close monitoring of neurological and cardiovascular status, and supportive care. Intubation and mechanical ventilation may be necessary in cases of severe poisoning.

INHALANTS

Prevalence/Epidemiology

Based on the National Survey on Drug Use and Health, 0.5% of youth aged 12 to 17 had used inhalants within the past 30 days.[1] Data were not collected below age 12, so that very early use is not accounted for in this sample; however, inhalants are most frequently used by younger children (ages 8 to 12) and prevalence of use decreases with age. Only 0.5% of college students and young adults aged 19 to 28 reported past-year use of inhalants in 2013.[12] "Fad" use of inhalants is also common, such that misuse of a specific product may gain short-term popularity in a particular school or town based on word-of-mouth reports among teens.

Preparation

Inhalants are especially attractive to younger adolescents because of their rapid onset of action, low cost, and easy availability. They are typically used by inhaling from a plastic bag containing the substance ("bagging") or by inhaling through a cloth saturated with the substance ("huffing"). The initial effect is stimulation and excitation, which then progresses to a depressant effect on the CNS. Of the myriad products and substances abused, toluene is the most common and is found in spray paint, airplane glues, rubber cement, cleaning fluids, permanent markers, and lacquer thinner (Table 67.5).

Circumstances of Abuse

Inhalants are inexpensive, legal products that do not arouse suspicion in most homes (Table 67.5). Inhalant abuse should be asked about directly if parents report finding fluid-saturated clothes, empty spray paint cans or plastic bags, or unusual chemicals in a bedroom or among personal items where they would not usually be stored. Users may have a distinctive chemical odor to their breath, hair, or clothing, and may appear disheveled.

Physiology and Metabolism

Inhalants are lipophilic, and their effects are felt within minutes of inhalation due to rapid absorption into the blood and then the brain. Their pharmacology often involves anesthetic effects at the cellular level. Peak effects occur within minutes and excretion is rapid, such that the course of intoxication after one huffing event may last only 15 to 30 minutes.

Effects of Intoxication

Inhalant use results in euphoria, decreased inhibition, and decreased judgment. Symptoms of inhalant use include heavy-lidded glazed eyes, slowed reflexes, slurred speech, lacrimation, rhinorrhea, salivation, and irritation of the mucus membranes. Anesthesia is common with drowsiness, stupor, or even obtundation, accompanied by respiratory depression. Users report spinning or floating sensations, exhilaration, and mild delirium.

Adverse Effects

Common adverse effects associated with inhalant abuse include gastrointestinal complaints such as anorexia, vomiting, and abdominal pain associated with gastritis. Neurological effects accompanying inhalant abuse include sleepiness, headaches, dizziness, ataxia, incoordination, and diplopia. Defatting properties of solvents may lead to perinasal and perioral skin rashes and nosebleeds. Respiratory irritation may cause a chronic dry cough, new-onset wheezing, and shortness of breath.

Overdose of inhalants can result in life-threatening complications, such as seizures, loss of consciousness, arrhythmias, respiratory failure, or cardiopulmonary arrest (Table 67.6). Death can occur, either directly from respiratory or cardiac toxicity or as a result of trauma from risk-taking behaviors and poor judgment. The "sudden sniffing death syndrome" occurs when halogenated hydrocarbons are inhaled, directly sensitizing the His bundle and cardiac electrical system. The patient, in an excited state, then starts running or dancing and has an adrenergic surge, provoking a fatal arrhythmia.

Chronic Use

Inhalant abuse is notable for escalation in the frequency of use and in binge behaviors, due to the short duration of the "high." Chronic effects of inhalant abuse are characterized by irreversible damage to target organs such as the brain, kidneys, heart, or liver. Fatty brain tissues such as myelin, axons, and neuronal cell bodies are damaged or destroyed, and often there is diffuse cerebral atrophy; the developing brain is more susceptible to damage than adult brains. In addition to cognitive decline, chronic inhalant users are more likely to attempt or complete suicide, have mood or anxiety disorders, and have other SUDs.[28] Although tolerance to inhalants may develop, withdrawal symptoms do not usually occur.

Diagnosis

Many inhalants are so quickly metabolized and/or excreted that they cannot be detected by the time the patient arrives in the emergency department. Standard toxicological screening tests of the blood or urine do not include such chemicals as hydrocarbons

TABLE 67.5		
Classes of Inhalants, Chemical Examples, and Toxicity		
Class of Inhalant	**Product/Chemical Examples**	**Toxicity**
Volatile Products	Glues, Gasoline, Spray Paints, Butane, Paint Thinner	Cardiac Arrhythmias, Respiratory Failure, Coma, Pneumothorax
Gases	Nitrous Oxide	Simple Asphyxia
Anesthetics	Ether	Coma, Respiratory Failure
Nitrates	Amyl Nitrate, Butyl Nitrate	Cardiovascular Failure, Coma, Methemoglobin

TABLE 67.6	
Agent-Specific Toxicities of Inhalant Chemicals	
Inhalant Chemical	**Agent-Specific Toxicity**
Toluene	Renal Damage, Embryopathy
Amyl and Butyl Nitrites	Methemoglobinemia, Hypotension
Gasoline	Lead poisoning, Benzene-induced Leukemia
Carbon Tetrachloride, Trichloroethylene	Hepatitis, Cirrhosis
Nitrous Oxide	Vitamin B_{12} Deficiency
Methylene Chloride (paint thinner)	Carbon Monoxide Poisoning

or nitrites. However, some products, such as paint thinners or glue, may leave chemical signatures behind. For example, heavy toluene exposure can be detected by elevated urinary hippuric acid levels.

Treatment

Treatment is supportive, and is aimed at control of arrhythmias, and respiratory and circulatory support. Epinephrine should be avoided since it may provoke cardiac irritability in those patients who have inhaled halogenated hydrocarbons. Intubation and mechanical ventilation may be necessary in severely affected patients who present with respiratory depression and blood gas evidence of hypoxia, hypercarbia, and respiratory acidosis.

Nitrous Oxide

Also known as laughing gas, nitrous oxide (N_2O) has long been abused by health care personnel. More recently, there has been a resurgence of interest in the AYA population. It is most commonly sold in small balloons or inhaled from whipped-cream cans ("whippets"), in which it is used as a propellant. Occasionally, individual users gain access to a tank of nitrous oxide. Deaths have occurred after prolonged inhalation of 100% N_2O in a closed space due to displacement of oxygen in the blood with subsequent suffocation. N_2O is known to deplete vitamin B-12, and many patients who present with psychiatric symptoms following exposure also have B-12 deficiency.[29]

Nitrites

Amyl, butyl, and isobutyl nitrites are examples of nitrites. Known as "poppers," they are volatile liquids abused for their vasodilatory action, enhancement of sexual pleasure, and subjective feeling of light-headedness (known as the "rush"). Amyl nitrite requires a prescription and is currently indicated in cyanide poisoning as the first step in a three-step antidote kit. Butyl and isobutyl nitrite are available over the counter in "head shops" as a room deodorizer, cologne, or liquid incense. Individuals abusing nitrites rarely seek medical attention for complications of abuse. The most common side effects are a result of smooth muscle relaxation: severe headache, dizziness, orthostatic hypotension, and occasionally syncope. Nitrites can cause methemoglobin formation, although clinically significant methemoglobinemia is extremely rare as a complication of nitrite abuse. Frequent abusers may have crusty yellow skin lesions on the face that can be misdiagnosed as impetigo or seborrheic dermatitis.[30]

HALLUCINOGENS

The hallucinogen class of drugs includes LSD (D-lysergic acid diethylamide tartrate), PCP, psilocybin, peyote, mescaline, dimethyltryptamine (DMT), morning glory seeds, Jimson weed, dextromethorphan, MDMA, MDA, and MDEA, and salvia. The term *hallucinogen* ("producer of hallucinations") is actually a misnomer, because prototypical hallucinogens such as LSD, mescaline, and psilocybin at typical dosage levels do not cause hallucinations (sensory perception changes without a corresponding environmental stimulus) but rather illusions (perceptual distortion of a real environmental stimulus). Hallucinogen-persisting perception disorder (HPPD), long-term recurrence of fleeting distortions and illusions, or "flashbacks" is not uncommon; lamotrigine was reported to improve symptoms of one patient who had HPPD for over a decade after stopping hallucinogen use.[31]

Past-month use of hallucinogens was 1.8% in young adults aged 18 to 25, 1.3% in 16- to 17-year-olds, 0.4% in 14- to 15-year-olds, and 0.1% in 12- to 13-year-olds in 2013, based on the National Survey on Drug Use and Health.[1]

Types of Hallucinogens

Table **67.7** contains the subgrouping of hallucinogens based on distinctive psychoactive effects and structure–activity relationship similarities.

TABLE 67.7

Types of Hallucinogens and the Psychoactive Effects They Produce

Category	Psychoactive Effect	Examples
Psychedelics	Prominent hallucinations and synesthesias with mild distortion of time and reality, impaired attention/concentration, mild disruption in ego structure	• Indolealkylamines: LSD, psilocybin, DMT • Phenlyalkylamines: mescaline
Enactogens	Structural similarities to psychedelics (mescaline) and amphetamines; unique psychoactive characteristics include improved communication, empathy with others, and positive mood enhancement	MDMA, MDA, MDEA
Dissociative anesthetics	Causes anesthesia, emergence reactions, and "out of body" experiences	PCP, Ketamine

D-Lysergic Acid Diethylamide

In the 1950s, LSD was marketed for the treatment of mental illness. The military also had interest in developing the drug as an agent for "mind control." By the mid-1960s no significant medical benefits of the drug had been found, and development stopped. LSD became illegal in the US in 1968.

Prevalence/Epidemiology

LSD abuse peaked in the 1960s, then fell until regaining popularity in the 1990s. In 1997, the lifetime use rate of LSD among high school seniors was 13.6% and surpassed the rate of 11.3% recorded in 1975. Since that time its popularity has waned, hovering between 3% and 4% in the decade 2003 to 2013.[2] The rate of LSD use among young adults (19 to 28) is higher: it peaked at 16.4% in 2000, and its popularity has declined, with 6.3% endorsing lifetime use in 2013.[12]

Preparation and Dose

Because the production of LSD from an alkaloid found in rye ergot fungus (e.g., *Claviceps purpurea*) is difficult, much of the LSD sold on the street is either adulterated or contains no LSD.

LSD is extremely potent, with doses measured in micrograms. Low doses of LSD (50 to 75 μg) produce euphoria while higher doses result in typical LSD illusions or "trips." The current average dose of 20 to 80 μg is an order of magnitude lower than the 1960s doses of up to 500 μg. There is clearly a disregard for, and underestimation of, the dangers of LSD due to less frequent aversive effects with lower doses. Even at lower doses, users remain at risk for chronic psychiatric problems, acute physical trauma, and other consequences of risk-taking behaviors that might occur under the influence of the drug.

LSD is commonly distributed as a soluble, colorless powder or liquid, sold as colored cylindrical tablets or gelatin squares, or applied to small pieces of paper. These preparations, known as "microdots," "windowpanes," or "blotters," are placed on the oral mucosa for absorption. LSD is also sold as colorful decals or stickers, some with cartoon characters, which may be appealing to young children. LSD can also be mixed with foods or liquids for oral consumption, or delivered in eye drops; it cannot be smoked as it is destroyed by heat.

Physiology and Metabolism

LSD is rapidly absorbed, binds to receptors throughout the CNS, and has onset of action in 30 to 40 minutes and a half-life of about

XIX

3 hours. The neurologic effects of LSD are not fully understood. LSD is similar in chemical structure to the serotonin molecule. It has inhibitory effects through binding to serotonin 5-HT1 receptors, and stimulatory effects through serotonin 5-HT2A receptors. The latter results in glutamate release, alterations in cortical function, and likely the hallucinogen effects.[32]

Effects of Intoxication

LSD intoxication results in euphoria and sensory illusions that may give rise to hallucinations. The sense of being an observer (depersonalization, loss of body image) is frequently reported and distinguishes LSD psychosis from schizophrenia. "Mystical experiences" are also reported. Synesthesias (i.e., the perception of one sensory experience as another, such as seeing colored waves in the air emanating from music), "trails" (visual after-images), and loss of time sense are hallmarks of LSD use.

Adverse Effects

1. Psychiatric/Neurologic: visual and auditory hallucinations, synesthesias, depersonalization, loss of sense of time, loss of ego boundaries, impairment of attention, motivation and concentration, anxiety, depression, paranoia, confusion, flashbacks, flushing, hyperthermia, piloerection, dizziness, paresthesia, dilated pupils, photophobia, blurred vision, conjunctival injection, lacrimation, hyperactive reflexes, ataxia and tremor, loss of muscle coordination and pain perception, restlessness, and sleep disturbances
2. Cardiovascular: hypertension and tachycardia
3. Gastrointestinal: anorexia, nausea, dry mouth

Overdose and Emergency Treatment

LSD overdose may result in grand mal seizures, circulatory collapse, coagulopathies, and coma. Some LSD users experience "bad trips," which terrify the user and may produce a sense of panic, fragmentation, fear of "going crazy," or fear of being intoxicated forever. LSD can be readily detected in urine by thin layer chromatography or other analytical techniques.

Treatment is supportive. Physical restraints and emergency medications are discouraged. Important components of treatment include providing a peaceful, calm environment (darkened lights, few extraneous stimuli), and reassurance that unusual sensations will cease when the drug wears off. Health care providers should avoid discussing the reasons for use of the drug or personal problems during a "bad trip." Frequent cycling between lucidity and periods of intense reactions to the drug occur early during intoxication and slow down over time.

History of hallucinogen use is often unreliable; adulteration and misrepresentation of the substances are common. In the case of a patient with clouded sensorium and fever, even with a history of ingestion of LSD, the differential diagnosis must include CNS infection, endocrine disorder, drug or alcohol withdrawal syndrome, and ingestion of a different toxin.

Chronic Use

Chronic adverse effects may include psychosis, depression, and personality changes. The use of a hallucinogen should be considered in the differential diagnosis of an adolescent who presents with new-onset psychosis.

Tolerance and Withdrawal

Tolerance to LSD develops rapidly but is short-lived. Some daily users of LSD describe the practice of "doubling up" (doubling the previous day's dose when using on consecutive days) to counteract tolerance. No withdrawal syndrome is described.

Dextromethorphan

Dextromethorphan, the dextro isomer of the codeine analog, levorphanol, has a chemical structure resembling a synthetic opiate, but lacks an opiate's potent analgesic and sedative properties.

It does not bind to the mu opioid receptor, but does bind to the opioid sigma receptor. The drug's prominent antitussive properties make it a common ingredient in nonprescription cough and cold syrups, with maximum daily doses ranging from 30 mg for children to 120 mg for adults.

To experience euphoria, users may drink 8 to 16 oz or more of dextromethorphan-containing cough syrup. The volume of cough syrup required to get "high" has led adolescents to order the pure, highly concentrated powder from Internet sources, or to purchase high-concentration dextromethorphan-containing tablets such as Coricidin products.[33]

Physiology and Metabolism

Dextromethorphan binds to opioid sigma receptors, which may account for some of its sedative and psychomimetic properties. The drug is metabolized by *CYP2D6* via O-demethylation to an active metabolite, dextrorphan, which interacts with the PCP and ketamine receptor in the NMDA neurotransmitter complex. Antagonism of NMDA receptors may be responsible for some of the adrenergic effects (e.g., hypertension, tachycardia, diaphoresis) seen clinically with large doses of dextromethorphan due to inhibition of catecholamine reuptake. The drug undergoes secondary conjugation in the liver to inactive glucuronide and sulfate esters, and has an elimination half-life of about 3.3 hours. Quinidine inhibition of *CYP2D6* and the conversion to dextrorphan alter the psychoactive properties of dextromethorphan ingestion, with a reduction in euphoria and an increase in unpleasant effects.[34]

Intoxication

Dextromethorphan can induce euphoria and produce dissociative effects. The actions of dextrorphan may explain dextromethorphan's PCP-like symptoms in overdose. It can produce stupor, somnolence and ataxia, coma, slurred speech, hallucinations, toxic psychosis, dysphoria, nystagmus, dystonia, tachycardia, and elevated blood pressure. Dextromethorphan also blocks presynaptic serotonin reuptake and has dopaminergic properties. Dextromethorphan interacts with other drugs that are substrates or inhibitors of *CYP2D6*, including SSRIs, MAO inhibitors, neuroleptics, and tricyclic antidepressants, to produce movement disorders, serotonin syndrome, or neuroleptic malignant syndrome.

Diagnosis and Treatment

Dextromethorphan is not detected by opiate or opioid panels on toxicologic screens. However, depending on concentration, the test for PCP may be weakly positive in some cases of dextromethorphan poisoning. Generally, patients with dextromethorphan poisoning will recover with supportive care. If they present to the emergency department early enough after ingestion, oral activated charcoal may be indicated. Health care providers should note that dextromethorphan poisonings often involve con- comitant intoxications with other ingredients in nonprescription medications such as acetaminophen, antihistamines, pseudoephedrine, and guaifenesin. Since dextromethorphan is formulated as a hydrobromide salt, an overdose with the drug can also produce toxic effects, such as somnolence, related to bromide poisoning.

Psilocybin

Mushrooms containing psilocybin and psilocin produce effects similar to those of the other hallucinogens. Users reportedly experience euphoria, prominent visual and auditory hallucinations, and synesthesias (i.e., perceptual distortions resulting in an apparent ability to visualize sounds or hear colors). The mushrooms are ingested orally, and the onset of effects occurs in 20 to 40 minutes. The effects peak at 90 minutes and usually abate within 5 or 6 hours. Hallucinogenic effects occur at doses above 15 mg of orally ingested psilocybin, and are mediated primarily by the 5-HT 2A/C receptor. Since many other species can be confused with true *psilocybe* mushrooms, ingestion of misidentified, toxic non-*psilocybe* species can pose a special danger to users.

Jimson Weed

Jimson weed (*Datura stramonium*) is an annual plant found growing wild in parts of North America and the West Indies. The plant has strong anticholinergic and mildly hallucinogenic properties. Users eat or make tea from the seeds, or smoke cigarettes made from Jimson weed.

Peyote and Mescaline

Peyote is a cactus (*Lophophora*) that grows in the southwestern United States and in Mexico; mescaline is a psychedelic alkaloid found in peyote. Because the cactus is hard to find, most drugs sold as "mescaline" capsules contain no mescaline, but rather LSD, PCP, both LSD and PCP, or something else. Peyote is sold either as buttons derived from the cactus or as capsules containing ground peyote. The usual dose ranges from 100 to 500 mg.

Mescaline has its onset of action within 30 minutes to 2 hours after ingestion, and the effects last for 6 to 12 hours. The mescaline high is less intense and less disorienting than LSD and tends to intensify body sense. Mescaline use is frequently accompanied by unpleasant side effects such as nausea and vomiting. Bad trips are less severe and less frequent with mescaline than with LSD.

Dimethyltryptamine

DMT is a natural constituent of the seeds of several plants found in the West Indies and South America. DMT is usually prepared as an orange liquid in which either tobacco, marijuana, or parsley is soaked and then smoked; it is inactive orally. This drug has effects similar to those of other hallucinogens, except that the "trip" is short, lasting only 1 to 3 hours, which leads to its street name of "businessman's special" or "businessman's lunch."

Morning Glory Seeds

The seeds of some members of the bindweed family, including the morning glory (*Rivea corymbosa* and *Ipomoea*), have been used for centuries for their hallucinogenic effects. Morning glory seeds are legally available on seed racks, but, to prevent spoilage, seeds intended for planting are usually coated with dangerous chemicals such as methyl mercury. The effects of morning glory seeds are similar to those of LSD; however, there is an increase in side effects such as nausea, dizziness, and diarrhea, and there is an extremely bitter taste.

Nutmeg

Nutmeg (*Myristica fragrans*) abuse requires the ingestion of large quantities of freshly ground seeds. Nutmeg includes the active chemical, myristicin, a mild MAO inhibitor and psychoactive agent. Effects include delirium, hallucinations, and euphoria, with onset within 30 minutes or so, and effects that can last as long as 24 hours. The predominant effects of nutmeg overdose are anticholinergic mydriasis, dry mouth, tachycardia, dizziness, headache, and repeated vomiting. Patients may experience anxiety reactions with agitation and restlessness, can experience seizures, or develop allergic reactions and rashes.

Salvia

Salvia divinorum is a plant that grows wild in Mexico and produces the psychedelic drug Salvinorin A. Leaves may be chewed and swallowed, smoked, or extracted in various ways. Hallucinogenic "trips" are short (1 to 2 hours for oral ingestion, and a few minutes when smoked). It is not a federally controlled substance, but restrictions have been enacted by some localities.

⬤ ANABOLIC STEROIDS

Anabolic steroids are synthetic derivatives of testosterone. Abusers of this class of drug exhibit tolerance, withdrawal, and psychological dependence. Treatment may require detoxification and a rehabilitation phase comparable to traditional drug treatment.

The numerous agents fit into two basic categories: the oral agents are 17α-methyl derivatives of testosterone, and the injectable agents are esters of testosterone and 19-nortestosterone. Many abusers use 10 times the usual therapeutic dose and use combinations of oral and injectable agents concurrently in 6- to 12-week cycles ("stacking").

Prevalence and Epidemiology

In the 2013 Youth Risk Behavior Survey, 4.0% of high school males and 2.2% of females reported ever having used steroids illegally.[35] In the young adult group (aged 18 to 26), annual prevalence of steroid use was 0.4% to 1.5% in 2013.[12]

Adverse Effects

1. Psychiatric: psychosis, mania, mood swings, hyper-aggressive behavior, violence, neurotoxicity, and body dysmorphia. Withdrawal may be associated with depression.
2. Cardiovascular: decreased high-density lipoprotein cholesterol, hypertension, ventricular remodeling, myocardial ischemia, sudden death
3. Endocrine: premature epiphyseal closure and shortened stature, female virilization and hypogonadism, testicular atrophy, reduced libido, infertility
4. Other: acne, hemolysis, enlarged prostate gland, hepatocellular carcinoma with chronic use.[36]

Treatment of Withdrawal or Dependence

Patients exhibiting psychotic behavior or severe depression require inpatient care. For the patient meeting DSM-5 criteria for a SUD, a traditional drug treatment approach is indicated.

REFERENCES

1. Substance Abuse and Mental Health Services Administration. *Results from the 2013 NSDUH: summary of national findings. NSDUH series H-48 [Internet].* HHS Public. Rockville, MD: Substance Abuse and Mental Health Services Administration, 2014:14–4863. Available at http://www.samhsa.gov/data/NSDUH/2013SummNatFindDetTables/NationalFindings/NSDUHresults2013.htm
2. Johnston LD, O'Malley PM, Miech RA, et al. *Monitoring the future national survey results on drug use: 1975–2014. Overview, key findings on adolescent drug use [Internet].* Ann Arbor, 2015. Available at http://monitoringthefuture.org/pubs/monographs/mtf-overview2014.pdf
3. Lee KC, Ladizinski B, Federman DG. Complications associated with use of levamisole-contaminated cocaine: an emerging public health challenge. *Mayo Clin Proc* 2012;87(6):581–586.
4. Arora NP, Berk WA, Aaron CK, et al. Usefulness of intravenous lipid emulsion for cardiac toxicity from cocaine overdose. *Am J Cardiol* 2013;111(3):445–447.
5. Hobbs WE, Moore EE, Penkala RA, et al. Cocaine and specific cocaine metabolites induce von willebrand factor release from endothelial cells in a tissue-specific manner. *Arterioscler Thromb Vasc Biol* 2013;33(6):1230–1237.
6. Rousset P, Chaillot PF, Audureau E, et al. Detection of residual packets in cocaine body packers: low accuracy of abdominal radiography—A prospective study. *Eur Radiol* 2013;23(8):2146–2155.
7. Lott DC, Jencius S. Effectiveness of very low-cost contingency management in a community adolescent treatment program. *Drug Alcohol Depend* [Internet]. 2009;102(1/3):162–165. Available at: http://www.sciencedirect.com/science/article/B6T63-4VPV8R5-2/2/0df6e310b2425c89391d738887e98e32
8. Caballero F, Lopez-Navidad A, Cotorruelo J, et al. Ecstasy-induced brain death and acute hepatocellular failure: multiorgan donor and liver transplantation. *Transplantation* 2002;74(4):532–537.
9. Li FCH, Yen JC, Chan SHH, et al. Bioenergetics failure and oxidative stress in brain stem mediates cardiovascular collapse associated with fatal methamphetamine intoxication. *PLoS One* 2012;7(1).
10. Auten JD, Matteucci MJ, Gaspary MJ, et al. Psychiatric implications of adolescent methamphetamine exposures. *Pediatr Emerg Care.* 2012;28(1):26–29.
11. Hatzipetros T, Raudensky JG, Soghomonian J-J, et al. Haloperidol treatment after high-dose methamphetamine administration is excitotoxic to GABA cells in the substantia nigra pars reticulata. *J Neurosci* 2007;27(22):5895–5902.
12. Johnston LD, O'Malley PM, Bachman JG, et al. *Monitoring the future national survey results on drug use, 1975–2013: Vol 2, College students and adults ages 19–55 [Internet].* Ann Arbor, MI, 2014. Available at http://monitoringthefuture.org//pubs/monographs/mtf-vol2_2013.pdf
13. Pasternak GW, Pan Y-X. Mu opioids and their receptors: evolution of a concept. *Pharmacol Rev* [Internet] 2013;65(4):1257–317. Available at http://www.ncbi.nlm.nih.gov/pubmed/24076545
14. Valente MJ, Guedes De Pinho P, De Lourdes Bastos M, et al. Khat and synthetic cathinones: a review. *Arch Toxicol* 2014;15–45.
15. Upreti VV, Eddington ND, Moon KH, et al. Drug interaction between ethanol and 3,4-methylenedioxymethamphetamine ("ecstasy"). *Toxicol Lett* 2009; 188(2):167–172.

XIV

16. Singer LT, Moore DG, Min MO, et al. One-year outcomes of prenatal exposure to MDMA and other recreational drugs. *Pediatrics* 2012;407–413.

17. Parrott AC. Human psychobiology of MDMA or "Ecstasy": an overview of 25 years of empirical research. *Hum Psychopharmacol* 2013;28(4):289–307.

18. McNamara R, Kerans A, O'Neill B, Harkin A. Caffeine promotes hyperthermia and serotonergic loss following co-administration of the substituted amphetamines, MDMA ("Ecstasy") and MDA ("Love"). *Neuropharmacology* 2006;50(1):69–80.

19. Durkin S, Prendergast A, Harkin A. Reduced efficacy of fluoxetine following MDMA ("Ecstasy")-induced serotonin loss in rats. *Prog Neuro-Psychopharmacol Biol Psychiatry* 2008;32(8):1894–901.

20. McCabe SE, West BT, Boyd CJ. Motives for medical misuse of prescription opioids among adolescents. *J Pain* 2013;14(10):1208–1216.

21. Maurice T, Su TP. The pharmacology of sigma-1 receptors. *Pharmacol Ther* 2009;195–206.

22. Walley AY, Xuan Z, Hackman HH, et al. Opioid overdose rates and implementation of overdose education and nasal naloxone distribution in Massachusetts: interrupted time series analysis. *BMJ* [Internet]. 2013;346:f174. Available at http://www.ncbi.nlm.nih.gov/pubmed/23372174

23. Tompkins DA, Bigelow GE, Harrison JA, et al. Concurrent validation of the Clinical Opiate Withdrawal Scale (COWS) and single-item indices against the Clinical Institute Narcotic Assessment (CINA) opioid withdrawal instrument. *Drug Alcohol Depend* 2009;105(1/2):154–159.

24. Syed YY, Keating GM. Extended-release intramuscular naltrexone (VIVITROL®): a review of its use in the prevention of relapse to opioid dependence in detoxified patients. *CNS Drugs* 2013;27(10):851–861.

25. Hood SD, Norman A, Hince DA, et al. Benzodiazepine dependence and its treatment with low dose flumazenil. *Br J Clin Pharmacol* 2014;77(2):285–294.

26. Kamal RM, van Iwaarden S, Dijkstra BAG, et al. Decision rules for GHB (gamma-hydroxybutyric acid) detoxification: A vignette study. *Drug Alcohol Depend* 2014;135(1):146–151.

27. Piecuch S, Thomas U, Shah BR. Acute dystonic reactions that fail to respond to diphenhydramine: think of PCP. *J Emerg Med* [Internet] 1999;17(3):527. Available at http://www.sciencedirect.com/science/article/pii/S0736467999000335

28. Howard MO, Bowen SE, Garland EL, et al. Inhalant use and inhalant use disorders in the United States. *Addict Sci Clin Pract* [Internet] 2011;6(1):18–31. Available at http://www.pubmedcentral.nih.gov/articlerender.fcgi?artid=3188822&tool=pmc entrez&rendertype=abstract

29. Céline C, Gunter H, Kurt A. Laughing gas abuse is no joke. An overview of the implications for psychiatric practice. *Clin Neurol Neurosurg* 2013;115(7):859–862.

30. Romanelli F, Smith KM, Thornton AC, et al. Poppers: epidemiology and clinical management of inhaled nitrite abuse. *Pharmacotherapy* 2004;24(1):69–78.

31. Hermle L, Simon M, Ruchsow M, et al. Hallucinogen-persisting perception disorder. *Ther Adv Psychopharmacol* 2012;2(5):199–205.

32. Passie T, Halpern JH, Stichtenoth DO, et al. The pharmacology of lysergic acid diethylamide: a review. *CNS Neurosci Ther* 2008;14(4):295–314.

33. Kirages TJ, Sulé HP, Mycyk MB. Severe manifestations of coricidin intoxication. *Am J Emerg Med* 2003;21(6):473–475.

34. Zawertailo LA, Tyndale RF, Busto U, et al. Effect of metabolic blockade on the psychoactive effects of dextromethorphan. *Hum Psychopharmacol* 2010;25(1):71–79.

35. Kann L, Kinchen S, Shanklin SL, et al. Youth Risk Behavior Surveillance—United States, 2013. *MMWR Surveill Summ* [Internet] 2014;63(4):17–20. Available at http://www.cdc.gov/mmwr/preview/mmwrhtml/ss6304a1.htm?s_cid=ss6304a1_w

36. Pope HG, Wood RI, Rogol A, et al. Adverse health consequences of performance-enhancing drugs: an endocrine society scientific statement. *Endocrine Rev* 2014;35(3):341–375.

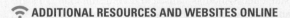 **ADDITIONAL RESOURCES AND WEBSITES ONLINE**

68

Approaches to Adolescent and Young Adult Substance Use

Sharon Levy
Elissa R. Weitzman

KEY WORDS

- Brief intervention
- Confidentiality
- Drug testing
- Screening
- Substance use disorders

THE ROLE OF THE PRIMARY CARE PROVIDER

Despite declines over the past decade, alcohol and drug exposure remain common among adolescents and young adults (AYAs) in the US. By high school graduation, approximately 7 of 10 American students have tried alcohol, more than half of students have tried an illicit drug, and approximately one-fourth have tried an illicit drug other than marijuana. One-fourth of students try an illicit substance by the end of 8th grade.[1] Alcohol and drug use are related to the four leading causes of death in the adolescent age-group and therefore present a major public health problem. In addition, the likelihood of developing addiction is inversely correlated with age of initiation.[2]

Clinicians who provide primary care to youth are on the "front-lines"; they are ideally positioned to provide primary and secondary prevention to those who have not initiated nor developed a substance use disorder (SUD) and early intervention to those who have developed a mild or moderate SUD. They may also leverage their position as a knowledgeable professional to assist AYAs who have developed a SUD in engaging in appropriate treatment. The Substance Abuse and Mental Health Services Administration (SAMHSA) has coined the term "SBIRT," which refers to the clinical framework of Screening, Brief Intervention, and Referral to Treatment. While a recent review by the US Preventive Services Task Force found that to date, there is insufficient evidence to evaluate the efficacy of brief interventions for substance use with adolescents in primary care,[3] emerging research is promising, and SBIRT is low cost and not associated with known harms. The findings for adults 18 and older are different. The Brief Intervention approach is effective for reducing "risky" alcohol use in adults but the evidence also suggests this approach is not effective for reducing illicit drug use in adult patients. Notably, there are also no competing approaches to address substance use, a known health risk factor for AYAs, within primary care. Therefore, the American Academy of Pediatrics (AAP) and other professional organizations recommend annual confidential screening and brief intervention as part of routine health maintenance for AYAs. Beyond SBIRT, clinicians should be prepared to assess AYAs who present with concerns stemming from substance use. Drug testing may be helpful as part of an assessment or for monitoring, and clinicians should be prepared to use this procedure. Clinicians should be familiar with varying levels of treatment for SUDs and aware of local resources.

CONFIDENTIALITY

Regardless of the format used to assess drug and alcohol use, questions about these behaviors and other sensitive health topics should always be asked in private, without a parent or guardian present. Before beginning a discussion about alcohol and drugs, we recommend that clinicians review their guidelines regarding confidentiality with AYA patients, and, when present, with parents. In general, adolescents should be afforded confidentiality unless their behavior poses an acute safety concern to themselves or others. Determining whether a specific behavior presents a safety concern is a matter of clinical judgment; the patient's age, other diagnoses, and social situation should be taken into account. Occasional use of alcohol or marijuana can usually be kept confidential. In all cases, adolescents should be assured that if confidentiality is to be broken, the health care provider and patient will review what will be said before speaking with parents, and only diagnostic and planning information will be shared; specific details generally need not be disclosed. For young adults over age 18, their medical information must remain confidential unless they have signed a release of information for a clinician to communicate with a parent. Regardless of a patient's age, it is good clinical practice to ask patients with SUDs what parents already know regarding their substance use whenever parents play a supportive role (i.e., in the case of a young adult who lives at home or is supported at school by parents). In many situations, parents are already aware of adolescents' high-risk behaviors by the time they reach a level that requires breach of confidentiality, though parents may underestimate frequency or severity. Young adults whose parents are aware of the substance use problem can be encouraged to include them in treatment planning, though ultimately information should not be shared without a specific signed consent. When parents are involved, the discussion can focus on treatment recommendations. Adolescents who report a behavior to their physician, such as intravenous drug use, may be asking for help. In these cases, we recommend evaluating for possible abuse and/or neglect before speaking with parents and managing accordingly.

In all 50 states, 18 years is the age of majority at which a young person is officially recognized as an adult. While this age is a landmark, for many American youth the 18th birthday signifies the beginning of a transition to adulthood, with a continued tapering of reliance on parents, rather than full independence. Many individuals continue to live at home with parents or are supported by parents while they continue their education. In accordance with these current cultural standards, imaging studies have found that the brain, and in particular the frontal lobes to which "executive functioning" is attributed, continue to mature well into the mid-third decade of life.[4] We recommend that clinicians treat the period of "young adulthood" as a transition period—both respecting the growing need for independence as well as the continued benefit of parental involvement in most cases. The approaches and recommendations in this chapter vary only minimally when working with adolescents or young adults, though one important change is that young adults over the age of 18 must formally give consent to include parents in their treatment.

SCREENING

All AYAs are at risk of exposure to alcohol and drugs. Therefore, every AYA should be screened regardless of race, ethnicity, socioeconomic status, religion, or gender. The National Institute on Alcohol Abuse and Alcoholism (NIAAA) recommends screening for alcohol use in children as young as 9 years of age, or the first time that the child is interviewed privately.[5] The AAP recommends screening for drug use beginning at age 12.[6]

Screens may be self-administered electronically, in a paper-and pencil format, by a clinical assistant or by a clinician; research suggests that all of these methods yield reliable results. A number of screens have been validated to determine likelihood of an alcohol or SUD (see **Table 68.1** for validated screening and assessment tools and **Table 68.2** for DSM-5 criteria for a SUD). The NIAAA youth alcohol screening tool is particularly notable because it is very brief (two questions), empirically derived, and recommended for children starting at age nine. The two screening questions provide information about (1) current risk of an alcohol use disorder (frequency of past year drinking) and

TABLE 68.1
Substance Abuse Screening and Assessment Tools Validated for Use with AYAs

Brief Screens

S2BI	• 2 question frequency screen • Screens for tobacco, alcohol, marijuana, and other illicit drug use • Discriminates between no use, no SUD, moderate SUD, and severe SUD, based on DSM-5 diagnoses
BSTAD	• Brief Screener for Tobacco, Alcohol, and Other Drugs • Identifies problematic tobacco, alcohol, and marijuana use in pediatric settings
NIAAA Youth Alcohol Screen	• 2 question screen • Screens for friends' use and own use
DAST-A[31]	• 27 questions • Queries adolescents about any adverse consequences they may have experienced secondary to drug use

Brief Assessments

CRAFFT	• Car, Relax, Alone, Friends/Family, Forget, Trouble • The CRAFFT is a good tool for quickly identifying problems associated with substance use • Not a diagnostic tool
GAIN	• Global Appraisal of Individual Needs • Assesses for both SUDs and mental health disorders
AUDIT	• Alcohol Use Disorders Identification Test • Assesses risky drinking • Not a diagnostic tool
DAST AND DAST 10	• Provides a quantitative score for problems related to drug misuse in adults • DAST-10 has been evaluated in college students[32]

TABLE 68.2
DSM-5 SUD Criteria

A problematic pattern of substance use leading to clinically significant impairment or distress, as manifested by at least two of the following, occurring within a 12-month period.

1. Taking the substance in larger amounts or for longer than you meant to
2. Wanting to cut down or stop using the substance but not managing to
3. Spending a lot of time getting, using, or recovering from use of the substance
4. Cravings and urges to use the substance
5. Not managing to do what you should at work, home, or school, because of substance use
6. Continuing to use, even when it causes problems in relationships
7. Giving up important social, occupational, or recreational activities because of substance use
8. Using substances again and again, even when it puts you in danger
9. Continuing to use, even when you know you have a physical or psychological problem that could have been caused or made worse by the substance
10. Needing more of the substance to get the effect you want (tolerance)
11. Development of withdrawal symptoms, which can be relieved by taking more of the substance

(2) future risk of an alcohol use disorder (friends' drinking). Alcohol-only screening may be particularly useful with younger children, when time is very limited or when alcohol use is a particular concern. The NIAAA published accompanying resource material and a web-based training course to guide clinicians in using this tool (**Table 68.1**).

Recently, the National Institute on Drug Abuse funded the development of brief adolescent substance use screening tools that are compatible with electronic health records, which resulted in the development of two new tools: Brief Screener for Tobacco, Alcohol and other Drugs (BSTAD)[7] and "Screening to Brief Intervention" (S2BI).[8] Both have been validated for ages 12 to 18. The BSTAD tool is built upon the NIAAA screening tool with added questions for tobacco and "drugs." The optimal cut points for identifying a SUD were ≥6 days of tobacco use (sensitivity = 0.95; specificity = 0.97); ≥2 days of alcohol use in the past year (sensitivity = 0.96; specificity = 0.85); and ≥2 days of marijuana use (sensitivity = 0.80; specificity = 0.93).[7] The S2BI uses a comprehensive stem question to assess the frequency of past-year use (none, once or twice, monthly, weekly or more) for tobacco, alcohol, marijuana, and five other classes of substances commonly used by adolescents. In the initial validation study, this tool had high sensitivity and specificity for discriminating between clinically relevant risk categories of adolescent substance use: no use; substance use without a SUD, which correlated to a response of "once or twice:" mild or moderate SUD, which correlated to a response of "monthly:" and severe SUD, which correlated to a response of "weekly or more."[9] The ability to detect adolescents who already have developed a severe SUD (addiction) is important: SAMHSA estimates that less than 10% of teens in need of specialty substance use treatment receive it and the majority who do are referred from the justice system.[10,11] The primary care arena has been notably poor in identifying teens with severe SUDs and connecting this vulnerable group with treatment. Indeed, clinical impressions alone, even those of experienced physicians, significantly underestimate the severity of an adolescent's substance-related problems.[12] It is therefore imperative that screening be done with a validated tool.

BSTAD and S2BI have been validated for ages 12 to 18. As young adults typically have patterns of substance use consumption much more similar to adolescents than older adults, these two tools likely would be the "off-label" tool of choice for this group as well. In addition to the very brief screening adolescent-specific screening tools, the AUDIT and DAST[13] can be used both with adolescents and also with college students and young adults.

AYAs WITH CHRONIC MEDICAL CONDITIONS

In the US, one in four AYAs has a chronic medical condition such as diabetes, asthma, or arthritis that requires long-term follow-up by a regular care team.[14] AYAs or youth with chronic medical conditions (YCMC) are heterogeneous in terms of specific diagnoses, disease management, and treatment regimens. However, they share a number of attributes that may interact negatively with substance use, including the need to follow a medication regimen, participate in regular clinical monitoring, self-monitor/manage their condition, and manage sleep, diet/meals, and activity levels. Adverse effects of substance use on these issues and attendant risks for poor health outcomes are vital topics to discuss and may be anchor points for screening and brief intervention. Frequent interactions with a clinical care team to address underlying health issues may provide physicians with opportunities for SBIRT, leveraging the strong patient–provider bonds established by long-term clinical management of pediatric onset chronic illness.

Tailoring Screening Tools for YCMC

Current existing screening tools have been developed using data derived from healthy youth. Screens may underestimate risks to YCMC from substance use if algorithms for assigning risk and guidelines for advising youth do not take into consideration special risks facing chronically ill adolescents from substance use. To the extent that screens underestimate risks from substance use, physicians may miss important opportunities for giving relevant medical advice and promoting intervention or treatment when warranted. Since there are no validated screening tools for use with YCMC, we recommend the use of existing tools coupled with probes to elicit reports of specific problems that these youth might encounter—such as substance use causing deterioration in an underlying condition or interfering with medications or self-care.

Salient Points for Brief Interventions

Like their peers, YCMC are vulnerable to acute and long-term consequences of substance use.[15] For chronically ill youth, however, substance use may amplify risks for treatment nonadherence and medical complications. By preventing or reducing substance use, screening and brief intervention may also reduce other risky behaviors, leading to better long-term medical outcomes. As a group, YCMC are taught from diagnosis about the importance of medication adherence, self-care/monitoring, healthy sleep, and diet patterns to avoid *salient near-term health problems*. Immediacy of substance use–related risk creates an opportunity to engage this population using the motivational interviewing paradigm, eliciting from them areas of ambivalence, motivators, and behavioral goals.

Follow-up and Coordination with Specialty Care

While the primary care physician can advance SBIRT within her/his practice, many YCMC use a specialty care setting as their medical home. The specialty care infrastructure and multidisciplinary team approach *could* be used to facilitate follow-up, internal referral to the team mental health specialist, and/or referral to an addiction specialist if needed. Improved tools, better integration of services, and more behavioral health services promised by current health care reform efforts may help to improve the situation.

BRIEF INTERVENTION

Most AYAs who use alcohol and drugs can be managed effectively in the primary care setting, and even patients who will ultimately require referral to an addiction or mental health specialist may receive direct benefit, or be more likely to accept treatment recommendations after a brief office intervention.[16] Brief interventions by health care providers, ranging in intensity from a few seconds up to several hours, can significantly reduce drug and alcohol use. In this chapter, we define *brief advice* as an intervention lasting seconds to minutes in which the health care provider gives general information to discourage substance use to a patient and *brief motivational intervention* as a very brief counseling session focused on details specific to the patient's substance use.

No Past-Year Substance Use

Positive reinforcement from a physician for abstaining from substance use can reduce the odds of initiating alcohol use within 12 months after a primary care appointment.[17] This very "brief intervention" may be one of the most under used, effective prevention strategies. If appropriate, statements can emphasize and praise the patient's decision not to use substances. While there is no evidence that screening older children or teens for substance use results in *increased* use, the NIAAA recommends including a statement about behavioral norms to avert any suggestion that screening implies that drinking is common among peers, especially for younger teens. An example is "*I am really glad that you have never had a drink with alcohol in it and I recommend that you keep it up. Alcohol use is dangerous for kids. Most kids your age don't drink, and those who do often end up having problems.*"

No SUD

Regardless of the screening tool selected, adolescents in the "lower risk" category are unlikely to have had problems associated with their use or a SUD. Nonetheless, even occasional use puts adolescents at risk of consequences such as injuries, fights, and unprotected sex. The AAP recommends that adolescents receive general advice to avoid all alcohol and drug use.[18] In one small study, brief health advice from a physician increased the percentage of low-risk adolescents who reported "no alcohol use," 3 and 12 months after their appointment.[17] We recommend clear advice not to use substances, such as "*As a clinician, I recommend that you don't drink at all. Alcohol use can interfere with your memory and learning.*" Knowledge of the patient can help the health care provider select the most relevant piece of information to share. We also recommend a strengths-based approach in which the clinician emphasizes skills, talents, and abilities, such as "*You are such a good student, I wouldn't want to see anything interfere with your education.*" While alcohol use is legal for young adults over age 21, heavy episodic ("binge") drinking remains common in young adulthood and is associated with a wide variety of health risks (see Chapter 64); thus, we recommend that brief advice include the health risks associated with this pattern of drinking.

Mild or Moderate SUD

AYAs with a mild or moderate SUD have already begun experiencing problems associated with their use of substances, and may respond to a "brief motivational intervention." Brief motivational interventions are based on motivational interviewing—a counseling technique that uses a nonjudgmental, empathetic, clinician-guided exploration of a behavior, identifies ambivalence, and works toward resolving ambivalence through behavior change.

Effectiveness

Brief motivational interventions reduce "unhealthy" drinking by adults.[19] Work with adolescents has found that brief motivational interventions decreased tobacco initiation and increased quit attempts,[20] decreased intentions to use substances in high-risk teens,[16] reduced marijuana use among "problem" marijuana smokers in the emergency department,[21] and improved engagement in SUD treatment among adolescents presenting to an emergency department.[22] Compared to feedback and advice, motivational interventions resulted in greater reductions of alcohol use among "problem" drinkers.[23]

Method

The crux of brief motivational interventions involves quickly identifying problems experienced by the patient, briefly exploring

XIV

them and leveraging attendant ambivalence expressed into a commitment for behavior change. Common problems experienced by AYAs with mild to moderate alcohol use disorders include vomiting after drinking, blackouts and associated consequences, accidents, fights, injuries, unwanted sexual activity, emergency department evaluations, punishment from parents, and school or sport suspensions. Problems associated with mild to moderate marijuana use disorders include worsening academic performance, anxiety, depression, punishment from parents, trouble with police or school officials, feelings of paranoia, or occasionally hallucinations. An interview for problems using open-ended questions can quickly point to areas worthy of further exploration. Any problem reported by the patient should be followed up with open-ended questions such as *"Why did the police pull you over in the first place?"* or *"Tell me more about the time you "blacked out."* The clinician helps reflect back ambivalence and encourages a behavior change to avoid similar problems in the future with statements such as *"It seems as if you get really sick from drinking, and it can be embarrassing to throw up in front of your friends. How can you protect yourself better in the future?"* A key principle of motivational interventions is that the patient is in charge of making decisions while the clinician guides the process. We recommend encouraging the patient to make a concrete behavior change plan that may include a trial of complete abstinence, reducing quantity or frequency of use, and/or avoiding behaviors such as sexual intercourse after drinking.

Follow-up

Follow-up is an important component to brief motivational interventions. We recommend recording the details of the behavior change plan and asking the AYA to return after a few weeks to evaluate how well s/he was able to follow it. If the patient is not willing to return, following up the next time s/he returns to the office for any reason is recommended.

Severe SUD

Severe SUD, or addiction, is a chronic, relapsing neurological condition that results from a "re-wiring" of the brain's reward system in the nucleus accumbens resulting from exposure to psychoactive substances.[24] Patients with addiction lose control over their use of substances, and will often continue to use even after severe problems have developed and use no longer results in euphoria. Brain development that occurs during adolescence appears to make this age-group particularly vulnerable to developing addiction. AYAs with severe SUD may respond to brief motivational interventions (see section above). For this group, in addition to reducing use and high-risk behaviors, the target of the intervention should also include accepting a referral for more in-depth treatment. Several levels of care exist, including individual or group counseling with an allied counseling professional in a primary care setting, intensive inpatient stabilization programs, and long-term residential care, depending on the needs of the patient.

Referral to Treatment

Referral to treatment consists of two distinct clinical activities. The first is a brief motivational intervention or other brief counseling that recommends seeking treatment for a SUD (see above). The second component involves determining the appropriate treatment or level of care, identifying a referral source and facilitating referral completion. This second component may be particularly challenging as it requires alignment between patient, parent (if appropriate), insurance provider, community resources and availability; insurance and community resource availability is dependent on geographic location.

Table 68.3 describes available levels of care in detail. To help identify treatment options throughout the US, SAMHSA maintains a Substance Abuse Treatment Facility Locator on its Web site (see

resources below). This site also includes both a Buprenorphine Physician & Treatment Program Locator and an Opioid Treatment Program Directory. Table 68.4 describes quality elements for adolescent substance abuse programs. Table 68.5 describes treatment modalities that are the most commonly used in treatment for SUDs. Regardless of setting, most programs will include elements from these modalities.

Adolescents should receive treatment in programs designed specifically for their age-group and certainly should not be mixed with patients beyond young adulthood in age. In general, including parents in a discussion of the treatment plan is recommended whenever a referral is warranted. Few adolescents are able to successfully navigate identifying, entering, and continuing treatment without support from parents. Parent participation also improves outcomes. Engaging parents in counseling may be particularly attractive to adolescents who feel their parents are too punitive and may improve communication and family dynamics. The AAP has published guidelines on the optimal goals of SUD pediatric programs serving the pediatric population,[18] which are based on guidelines published by SAMHSA.[25] Some treatment facilities offer specialized programs for young adults. Patients aged 18 to 25 years may prefer these settings, which focus on the typical substances, use patterns, and problems for this age-group and facilitate peer support with those of similar age.

As with other disorders, patients with SUDs should be treated in the least restrictive environment possible. For most, outpatient programs are adequate, though enrollment may be challenging, as outpatient treatment, particularly intensive outpatient or partial hospitalization, requires daily transportation and may interfere with school, work, and/or parents' work schedules.

Some AYAs with severe SUDs benefit from residential treatment. In particular, adolescents who do not or cannot respond to house rules and parental limit setting, who are triggered to use substances by their home and/or school environments, and those with frequent contact with peers who use or sell substances may respond better to residential treatment. AYAs in unstable housing, at risk of homelessness or without available parents to partner in treatment, may also be better served in residential treatment.

An adolescent or young adult may be unwilling to engage in treatment for a SUD even when ongoing drug use poses a serious threat to safety—such as ongoing intravenous drug use. In all states, family members may seek an order for mandatory (involuntary) treatment through the court system. Voluntary treatment is always preferable to involuntary placement; counseling from a primary care clinician and close follow-up may be appropriate over a short period of time in an attempt to encourage an AYA in need of a higher level of care to accept a treatment referral.

Pharmacologic Treatment

Pharmacological treatment may be a useful adjuvant for patients with nicotine, alcohol, or opioid addiction, though all medications should be considered an adjuvant to psychosocial support and counseling aimed at helping patients identify and avoid triggers, learn new methods for coping with stress and other difficult emotions, improve communication skills, cope with cravings, and other long-term recovery skills. A full description of the pharmacology and use of these medications with adolescents is beyond the scope of this chapter; interested readers are referred to the Prescribers' Clinical Support System, a SAMHSA-funded organization that provides information and support particularly for the treatment of opioid dependence, for further details (see Ancillary Online Content).

Smoking Cessation

Nicotine replacement can be provided via patch, lozenge, chewing gum, or inhaler (see also Chapter 65). Patients under the age of 18 need a prescription for nicotine replacement. Recently,

TABLE 68.3

Substance Use Treatment

Outpatient

Individual Counseling	Adolescents with SUDs should receive specific treatment for their substance use; general supportive counseling may a useful adjuvant but should not be a substitute. Several therapeutic modalities (motivational interviewing, cognitive behavioral therapy, contingency management, etc.) have all shown promise in treating adolescents with SUDs.
Group Therapy	Group therapy is a mainstay of substance abuse treatment for adolescents with SUDs. It is a particularly attractive option because it is cost effective, and takes advantage of the developmental preference for congregating with peers. However, group therapy has not been extensively evaluated as a therapeutic modality for this age-group, and existing research has produced mixed results.
Family Therapy	Family-directed therapies are the best validated approach for treating adolescent substance abuse. A number of modalities have all been demonstrated effective. Family counseling typically targets domains that figure prominently in the etiology of SUDs in adolescents—family conflict, communication, parental monitoring, discipline, child abuse/neglect, and parental SUDs.
Intensive Outpatient Program	Intensive outpatient programs (IOP) serve as an intermediate level of care for patients who have needs that are too complex for outpatient treatment, but do not require inpatient services. These programs allow individuals to continue with their daily routine and practice newly acquired recovery skills both at home and at work. IOPs generally consist of a combination of supportive group therapy, educational groups, family therapy, individual therapy, relapse prevention and life skills, 12-step recovery, case management, and aftercare planning. The programs range from 2–9 h per day, 2–5 times a week, and last 1–3 mo. These programs are appealing because they provide a plethora of services in a relatively short period of time.
Partial Hospital Program	Partial hospitalization is a short-term, comprehensive outpatient program in affiliation with a hospital that is designed to provide support and treatment for patients with SUDs. The services offered at these programs are more concentrated and intensive than regular outpatient treatment as they are structured throughout the entire day and offer medical monitoring in addition to individual and group therapy. Participants typically attend sessions for 7 or 8 h a day at least 5 d a week for 1–3 wk. As with IOPs, patients return home in the evenings and have a chance to practice newly acquired recovery skills.

Inpatient/Residential

Detoxification	Detoxification refers to the medical management of symptoms of withdrawal. Medically supervised detoxification is indicated for any adolescent who is at risk of withdrawing from alcohol or benzodiazepines and may also be helpful for adolescents withdrawing from opioids, cocaine, or other substances. Detoxification may be an important first step but is not considered definitive treatment. Patients who are discharged from a detoxification program should then begin either an outpatient or residential substance abuse treatment program.
Acute Residential Treatment	Acute residential treatment (ART) is a short-term (days–weeks) residential placement designed to stabilize patients in crisis, often before entering a longer-term residential treatment program. ART programs typically target adolescents with co-occurring mental health disorders.
Residential Treatment	Residential treatment programs are highly structured live-in environments that provide therapy for those with severe substance abuse, mental illness, or behavioral problems that require 24-h care. The goal of residential treatment is to promote the achievement and subsequent maintenance of long-term abstinence as well as equip each patient with both the social and coping skills necessary for a successful transition back into society. Residential programs are classified by length of stay: less than 30 d is considered short term while long term is considered longer than 30 d. Residential programs generally consist of individual and group therapy sessions, plus medical, psychological, clinical, nutritional, and educational components. Residential facilities aim to simulate real living environments with added structure and routine in order to provide individuals with the framework necessary for their lives to continue drug and alcohol free upon completion of the program.[11]
Therapeutic Boarding School	Therapeutic boarding schools are educational institutions that provide constant supervision for their students by a professional staff. These schools offer a highly structured environment with set times for all activities, smaller more specialized classes, social and emotional support. In addition to the regular services offered at traditional boarding schools, therapeutic schools also provide individual and group therapy for adolescents with mental health or SUDs.

electronic or "e-cigarettes," which deliver nicotine via vaporization (and do not contain tobacco), have gained favor as a smoking cessation device, and have been gaining in market share among adolescents who smoke because of a perception that the product is safe because it does not involve smoke. This product remains controversial, especially for teens, because it contains highly addictive nicotine, and, unlike other nicotine replacement products, it is often the first nicotine exposure for adolescents. Bupropion, an atypical selective serotonin reuptake inhibitor, is also an effective medication to support smoking cessation. Varenicline is a Food and Drug Administration (FDA)-approved medication for smoking cessation in adults, though it is rarely used in adolescents because of the risk of associated mental health symptoms.

Alcohol Cessation

Three medications have been FDA approved to support alcohol cessation in patients with alcohol use disorders, though two of them (disulfuram and acamprosate) are not approved for children and are rarely used in adolescents. Naltrexone, which blocks the opioid receptor and may reduce the pleasure associated with drinking, is FDA approved for patients ages 18 and older. It is available as either an oral tablet or a 30-day intramuscular injection and may support reduced drinking or abstinence in adolescents with severe alcohol use disorder.

Opioid Addiction

Three medications are available to support patients with opioid addiction. Methadone has been available since the 1970s and has

TABLE 68.4
Criteria for the Selection of a Substance Abuse Treatment Program

1. View drug and alcohol abuse as a primary disease rather than a symptom.
2. Include a comprehensive patient evaluation and a developmentally appropriate management and treatment referral plan for associated medical, emotional, and behavioral problems identified.
3. Maintain rapport with the patient's primary care provider to facilitate seamless after care and primary care follow-up.
4. Adhere to an abstinence philosophy. Drug use is a chronic disease, and a drug-free environment is essential. Tobacco use should be prohibited, and nicotine cessation treatment should be provided as part of the overall treatment plan. Continued tobacco, alcohol, or other drug use should be viewed as a need for more treatment rather than discharge or refusal to treat.
5. Maintain a low patient-to-staff ratio.
6. Employ treatment professionals who are knowledgeable in both addiction treatment and child and adolescent behavior and development.
7. Ensure that professionally led support groups and self-help groups are integral parts of the program.
8. Maintain separate treatment groups for individuals at varying developmental levels (adolescents versus young adults versus older adults).
9. Involve the entire family in the treatment, and relate to the patients and their families with compassion and concern. Strive to reunify the family whenever possible.
10. Ensure that follow-up and continuing care are integral parts of the program.
11. Offer patients an opportunity to continue academic and vocational education and assistance with restructuring family, school, and social life. Consider formal academic and cognitive skills assessment, because unidentified weaknesses may contribute to emotional factors contributing to the substance use.
12. Keep the family apprised of costs and financial arrangements for inpatient and outpatient care and facilitate communication with managed-care organizations.
13. Be located as close to home as possible to facilitate family involvement, even though separation of the adolescent from the family may be indicated initially.

TABLE 68.5
Treatment Modalities

Therapeutic Modality	Description
Motivational interviewing	Motivational interviewing (MI) is a counseling style frequently used in primary care to support behavior change. The main premise of MI is that motivation to make and sustain a behavior change is not an intrinsic character trait, but rather a constantly changing state that is influenced by others—both positively and negatively. In MI, the counselor facilitates the patient's exploration of the benefits of a current behavior compared to the potential benefits of behavior change and in so doing helps a patient bring out his or her own inner motivation to change.[33]
Cognitive behavioral therapy	Cognitive behavioral therapy (CBT) is a structured, goal-oriented counseling style designed to teach patients specific skills that will help them remain abstinent by training patients to identify thoughts and feelings that precede drug use in order to learn either to avoid the situation or to substitute behaviors other than drug use. CBT is most effective when a patient is willing to practice newly acquired skills. CBT can be used in individual, family, or group therapy settings. It may be used alone or in combination with MI.[34,35]
Dialectical behavior therapy	Dialectical behavior therapy (DBT) is very similar to CBT. In this modality, patients are taught to regulate both emotion and behavior by identifying triggers that precede changes in emotional states that lead to dysregulated behavior. DBT is particularly effective for patients with co-occurring mental health disorders.[36]
Contingency Management	Contingency management is a treatment model that relies on reinforcement of desirable behaviors. It is often combined with drug testing (negative drug tests result in rewards or positive drug tests result in loss of privileges), though contingency management can be used with other target behaviors, such as participating in treatment, as well. Rewards may be gift certificates, small amounts of money, or in some cases approbation from a parent or counselor. Contingency management has been found to be effective in treating adolescents with substance use disorders and are a mainstay of drug courts, though few models using this modality have been developed for use in SUD treatment programs.[37–39]

a long track record of safety and efficacy for treating opioid addiction. Methadone is an opioid agonist with a long half-life that can help opioid-addicted patients achieve a constant, low level of opioid stimulation, and thus avoid the "highs" and "lows" associated with opioid use. Because it is a full opioid agonist, it has significant potential for abuse and diversion and is only available through highly monitored, specialty methadone programs, most of which do not accept patients under the age of 18. Buprenorphine is a partial mu-opioid agonist that is as effective as methadone in reducing relapse rates in opioid-addicted individuals. Compared to methadone, buprenorphine has a lower abuse and diversion potential. The Drug Abuse Treatment Act 2000 (DATA 2000) is a federal law that allows physicians with 8 hours of specialized training to apply for a waiver to prescribe buprenorphine as a treatment for opioid dependence from their offices. DATA 2000 has been successful at expanding treatment for opioid dependence, though to date, few pediatricians or clinicians who provide primary care for adolescents have been trained, leaving a treatment gap for this age-group. Naltrexone, an opioid antagonist with no significant potential for abuse or diversion, is also FDA approved as a treatment for opioid dependence and may be dispensed orally or as an intramuscular injection. Information about medication-assisted treatment for opioid use disorders and listings for buprenorphine waiver courses are available through the Providers Clinical Support System (see Ancillary Online Content).

BEYOND SCREENING: EVALUATING AYAs WITH BEHAVIORAL OR MENTAL HEALTH SYMPTOMS

SUDs may present with nonspecific signs and symptoms, such as change in school performance, loss of interest in hobbies or extracurricular activities, inability to keep a job, excessive moodiness, irritability, or other mental health symptoms. When any of these changes are reported by a patient or parent, the clinician should be particularly alert to the possibility of a SUD. In addition, any concerns about alcohol or drug use expressed by parents, school officials, coaches, or other adults should be taken seriously, even if a patient denies substance use. For young adults, a substance use evaluation may be mandated by the police or university. In these cases, the patient's report, including a thorough history that reviews the outside presenting concerns, collateral history from a parent if available, physical exam, and, in some cases, drug test results should all be triangulated to formulate a differential diagnosis. Even if drug use is "ruled out," new-onset behavioral or emotional symptoms should be fully evaluated as they may signal onset of a serious mental health disorder.

Physical Examination

A physical examination should be performed as part of a complete assessment of new-onset behavioral or mental health problems. Signs of chronic drug use are rare in teens, but should be noted if present. A list of physical findings associated with acute intoxication, withdrawal, and chronic drug use is presented in **Table 68.6**.

Drug Testing

Drug testing is a complicated procedure that when done correctly can be a useful part of an assessment for an SUD. Clinicians and parents should recognize that a single negative drug test result may support a history of no recent drug use, but does not rule out an SUD. Conversely, a single positive drug test result does not confirm a diagnosis of SUD. As with any other laboratory test, drug tests should be used in conjunction with and not instead of history and physical examination findings. In general, we do not recommend routine drug screening of AYAs without very specific indications. If a clinician recommends a drug screen as part of an evaluation, the adolescent or young adult should be informed that testing is to occur.

AAP policy guidelines state that physicians should obtain assent from competent adolescents before ordering a drug test; parental consent alone is not sufficient.[26] Ordering a drug test without explaining the procedure may decrease trust, impair communication, and make therapeutic alliance between the patient and clinician difficult. If a teenager refuses a drug test that is clearly indicated, the health care provider should counsel parents to use appropriate limit setting and consequences as they would with other behaviors. The same strategy can be used with young adults that continue to live with or be supported by parents. For example, a parent might suspend car privileges for a younger teen, or take a young adult off the car insurance policy, until s/he is reassured that a child is not using drugs. Ultimately, if a child refuses an indicated drug test, we recommend referral to a mental health or addiction specialist for further evaluation. Refusal should never prematurely terminate an evaluation for mental health or behavioral problems.

The authors recommend that the clinician, adolescent, and parent(s) discuss who will receive results and agree to a plan before a drug test is ordered. If the teen is not willing to share results with parents, the clinician should consider whether a test will be worthwhile, as a teen may have little incentive to make a behavioral change, engage in treatment, or accept a referral for further evaluation if parents do not receive results.

Source of Drug Testing Sample

Drugs and their metabolites can be detected in several biological matrices, including hair, saliva, breath, blood, and urine.[27] Urine drug testing has been well studied and is best standardized. Urine drug concentrations are relatively high and drugs and their metabolites are excreted in the urine for a period of time after acute

TABLE 68.6

Physical Signs of Drug Intoxication, Recovery from Intoxication, and Chronic Use[a]

Drug	Acute Intoxication	Recovery from Intoxication/Withdrawal	Chronic Drug Use
Alcohol	Fruity smelling breath, disinhibited or silly, clumsiness, vomiting	Headache, nausea, vomiting, dry mouth	Enlarged liver, increased liver enzymes, hypertension
Marijuana	Erythematous conjunctivae, tachycardia, dry mouth, increased talking, euphoria	Anxiety, nervousness	Chronic cough, wheezing Loss of interest in activities/apathy
Cocaine	Hyperalert state, increased talking, hyperthermia, nausea, dry mouth, dilated pupils, sweating, cardiac arrhythmias	Depression, anhedonia, insomnia, lethargy, mental slowing	Erosion of dental enamel, gingival ulceration, chronic rhinitis, perforated nasal septum, midline granuloma, cardiac arrhythmias, hypertension, paranoia, psychosis
Amphetamines	Similar acute intoxication effects as cocaine	Choreoathetoid movement disorders, skin picking, and ulcerations	Deficits in executive function, delusions, hallucinations, long term personality changes
Opioids	Constricted pupils, drowsiness ("nodding"), slowed respirations, bradycardia, slurred speech, slowed comprehension, constipation	Flu-like symptoms, muscle and joint aches, dilated pupils, coryza, lacrimation, sweating, abdominal cramps, nausea, vomiting, diarrhea, hot and cold flashes, piloerection, yawning, tremors, anxiety, irritability	Abscesses, cellulitis, phlebitis, and scarring (from injection use), chronic constipation, malnutrition
Benzodiazepines	Drowsiness, slowed respirations, slurred speech, slowed comprehension	Seizures (may be life threatening), anxiety, restlessness	Sleep difficulties, anxiety, personality changes
Hallucinogens	Toxic psychosis, paranoia, anxiety, tachycardia, hypertension, dry mouth, nausea, vomiting	Flashbacks, which may occur even after the effects of the drug have worn off, unpredictable or self-injurious behavior	Psychosis, depression, personality changes
Inhalants	Euphoria, slurred speech, ataxia, diplopia, lacrimation, rhinorrhea, salivation, irritation of the mucus membranes, nausea, vomiting, arrhythmias	Headaches, sleepiness, depression	Irritation of mucus membranes, changes in neurological examination
Ecstasy	Euphoria, decreased interpersonal boundaries, tachycardia, hypertension, hyperthermia, sweating, muscle spasms, bruxism, blurred vision, chills, nystagmus	Depression, anxiety, paranoia, dehydration	Cognitive deficits

[a]See also Chapter 67.

intoxication, making urine the most common biological matrix used for drug testing in the primary care setting.

There are two principle types of urine drug tests: enzyme-based immunoassay "screens" and more definitive mass spectrometry-based tests. Immunoassays are inexpensive, can test for a number of substances at the same time, and can be performed at home or in an office. However, they are relatively nonspecific and susceptible to false positives from cross-reacting substances. A recent review also found immunoassay screens to be less sensitive than mass spectrometry–based tests, even within the specified range of detection.[28] Mass spectrometry laboratory tests are relatively expensive and require more time for results. They can definitively identify a number of drugs or their metabolites and, as such, are the "criterion standard" for drug testing. Whenever an immunoassay test results in an unexpected or contested result, a mass spectrometry test should be used for confirmation. Mass spectrometry is also the procedure of choice for substances not detected on immunoassay screens. With newer, automated procedures, the expense of mass spectrometry testing has decreased and in some cases it may be practical to use this procedure as "first line," omitting an immunoassay screen entirely.

Substances detected on multi-panels vary; clinicians should be familiar with the panels offered by the laboratories they use. Immunoassay screens detect drug classes such as "opiates" or "benzodiazepines," but may not detect every drug in the class. For example, benzodiazepine panels detect oxazepam, a metabolite common to many, but not all, benzodiazpines. Clonazepam, a common substance of abuse, is not detected by a routine benzodiazepine screen. **Table 68.7** includes detailed information on immunoassay and mass spectrometry detection of different substances.

Clinicians should be cognizant of the multitude of methods for "defeating" urine drug tests in order to avoid incorrect results. Directly observed urine specimen collection provides the most reliable samples, though the invasiveness of the procedure and the potential impact of collecting a directly observed specimen on the relationship between the adolescent and his parents or clinicians must be considered. Regardless of the method of collection, urine tests should be checked for temperature, random creatinine level, and pH to minimize tampering. Some laboratories offer an "adulterant panel" to detect additives that may interfere with assays and may further reduce adulteration. We recommend considering any

sample with a random creatinine <20 mg/dL too dilute for proper interpretation.[29] Dilute samples may be spurious, or the result of an attempt to drive the concentration of a drug or metabolite below the detection threshold for the test. When this occurs, we recommend repeating the test using a first morning specimen.

Drug test results have both laboratory and clinical interpretations. The laboratory result will be negative whenever the drugs in the test panel are not detected in the sample provided. This can occur under three circumstances (**Table 68.8**): (1) a true negative (i.e., no recent substance use); (2) a "laboratory" false negative (i.e., dilute or adulterated sample); or (3) a "clinical" false negative (i.e., use of a substance longer ago than the window of detection, use of a substance not detected on the test panel, or a substituted sample). An immunoassay test will be positive whenever a molecule in the urine specimen reacts with the test panel, and this also must be interpreted with caution (**Table 68.9**). An immunoassay test may be positive if a chemical other than an illicit drug cross-reacts with the drug test panel. In this case, confirmatory mass spectrometry testing will be negative. Both immunoassay and mass spectrometry tests will be positive if an adolescent has consumed a detectable substance as a prescription or over-the-counter medication or in food. A careful patient history, including review of all prescription medications, recently used over-the-counter medications, and unusual food consumption may provide an explanation for the positive drug test result if the history is consistent with the result observed. Drug testing cannot distinguish between proper use and misuse of prescription medications.

Cannabis is lipid soluble and, with chronic use, significant stores can accumulate in fat tissue. Daily users of cannabis can have detectable urine cannabinoid levels for 10 days after discontinuing use, and chronic daily users can have detectable urine cannabinoid levels 30 days after discontinuing use.[30] The concentration of cannabinoid in the urine varies with urine concentration. Once use is discontinued, however, the ratio of urinary cannabinoids to urinary creatinine falls quickly over the first few days and then small amounts can be detected for long periods of time. A quickly decreasing ratio supports a history of discontinued use even in a patient with positive urine test results. Other substances with long half-lives, including long-acting benzodiazepines and opioids, can also remain positive for days to weeks after discontinuation (see Chapter 67 for details). As with cannabis, a declining metabolite:creatinine ratio supports a history of no recent use.

All patients with positive, dilute, adulterated, or substituted urine specimens should have the opportunity to discuss results privately before they are shared with parents. A private interview can help determine whether an explanation other than illicit drug use might account for the laboratory findings. Some teens will acknowledge drug use when a drug test result is positive, and this may provide an opportunity to have an honest conversation. If the adolescent is willing to abstain from drug use, repeat testing may be useful for monitoring and to help rebuild trust between parent and child. Some teens will deny drug use and insist that the laboratory is in error or offer another inconsistent explanation. In these cases, we recommend repeat drug testing. If subsequent drug tests are negative, either the original test was an error or the adolescent subsequently stopped using substances. If sequential tests are positive, they are unlikely to be the result of a laboratory "fluke," and referral for further assessment by an addiction or mental health specialist is warranted.

Parental involvement is an important part of intervention for many teens with SUDs and disclosing a positive drug test result to parents may be therapeutically useful. It is, however, important to respect the teen's burgeoning autonomy and, when possible, to protect the therapeutic alliance between the teen and the clinician. If a teen reports drug use that matches drug test results, discuss how the treatment plan will be altered and make this the focus of the discussion with parents. For example, let parents know if a teen has agreed to meet with a counselor to discuss drug use. If

TABLE 68.7
Detection of Drugs in Urine

Drug	Major Metabolites Detected in Urine	Window of Detection by Enzyme-Linked Immunosorbent Assay in Urine Following a Single Use
Methamphetamine	Amphetamine	1–4 d
Cocaine	Benzoylecgonine	2–4 d
	Ecognine methyl ester	2–4 d
Morphine	Morphine	2–3 d
Heroin	6-acetylmorphine	Up to 24 h
Phencyclidine	Phencyclidine	Up to 7 d
Benzodiazepines		
Diazepam	Nordiazepam, oxazepam, temazepam	Up to 10 d
Clonazepam	7-aminoclonazepam	Up to 5 d
Lorazepam	Lorazepam glucuronide	Up to 2 d
Oxazepam	Oxazepam glucuronide	Up to 2 d

TABLE 68.8

Interpretation of Negative Urine Drug Test Results

Screen Result	Laboratory Interpretation	Possible Clinical Interpretations	Next Step
Negative	Substance in question not detected in the urine. Substance may be either present at a concentration below the sensitivity level set for the test or not present	• Patient has not used the substance in question within the window of detection (24–48 h for most substances) • Patient has diluted, substituted, or adulterated the urine sample causing a false-negative result • Dilute samples should be repeated; multiple dilute samples should be considered positive	• Adulterated or substituted samples should be considered clinically positive

TABLE 68.9

Interpretation of Positive Urine Drug Test Results

Screen Result	Laboratory Interpretation	Possible Clinical Interpretations	Next Step
Positive	Substance in the urine has reacted with the substrate in the test panel	• True positive—patient has absorbed substance in question • False positive—chemical from an over-the-counter medication, prescribed medication, or food has cross-reacted with substrate in the test panel	• Order GC/MS to confirm result • If GC/MS is positive, discuss with the patient to determine if licit use of prescription or over-the-counter medications, or food consumption would explain a positive test result

GC/MS, gas chromatography/mass spectrometry.

the adolescent's history is not consistent with laboratory results, share the results with parents, and include the adolescent's report, an explanation that the two are not consistent, and treatment recommendations.

Negative results of drug tests done with proper collection and validation techniques provide good support for a history of no drug use, at least within the window of detection of the substances detected. Clinicians and parents must recognize, however, that even carefully done urine tests have limitations and cannot completely rule out drug use. Continued monitoring by parents, repeat drug testing, or referral to a mental health or addiction specialist may be indicated if signs and symptoms consistent with drug use, even in the context of a negative drug test result, are present.

Co-occurring Disorders

Co-occurring mental health disorders are common in AYAs with SUDs and a full psychosocial evaluation is recommended. In some cases it may be difficult to determine whether the symptoms are solely the result of drug use and the question of a co-occurring disorder cannot be fully resolved until the patient has had a period of complete abstinence. Severe symptoms, symptoms that antedate drug use, or positive family history of a similar disorder all suggest a co-occurring disorder, and concurrent treatment should be considered. In contrast, symptoms that began after the onset of drug use may resolve completely with abstinence, and patients may be observed and reassessed as necessary if symptoms are mild.

THE ROLE OF PARENTS

Parents play a vital role in the prevention and treatment of AYA substance use. Clinicians should encourage the parents of preteens to discuss drugs and alcohol, and to set clear family rules of no use. We recommend that clinicians encourage parents to set a good example by consuming alcohol only in moderation, never driving after drinking, and avoiding drug use.

Some AYAs with SUDs will not engage in treatment. In these cases, family or parent support counseling may be useful, even if the patient refuses to participate. Parents should be advised to set firm but logical limits and avoid enabling substance use. Limit setting refers to consequences designed by the parents, such as suspending privileges to spend time alone with friends, attend parties, or drive. For young adults, parents can insist on abstinence as a condition of supporting dormitory living expenses. We recommend consequences that are logically tied to substance use rather than merely punitive. For example, a parent may take away a cell phone or text service if an adolescent is using the phone to obtain drugs. Some parents may feel conflicted about enforcing rules and consequences. The clinician can support them by reminding them that it is the "job" of all parents to help correct their children when they engage in dangerous, unhealthy, or illegal behavior.

Enabling refers to any activity that intentionally or unintentionally assists the adolescent or young adult in obtaining or using drugs. Parents may unintentionally enable a child's drug use by providing money, cell phones, e-mail accounts, or a car that a child uses to obtain drugs. A review of sources of money, communication, and transportation may help parents identify enabling behaviors and eliminate them. If parents are unable to enforce their home rules with their minor children they may seek assistance from the court system, which can mandate services, including drug testing and counseling. It is important for parents to emphasize that consequences are intended to support the parents' rules, including "no drug use" and are not intended to make their children unhappy.

Ensuring that patients and parents feel welcome to return whenever they are ready may go a long way to ultimately assisting teens and families get the help they need. A supportive word may stay with the teen and encourage him or her to return for assistance in finding appropriate treatment even after a period of time.

REFERENCES

1. Johnston LD, O'Malley PM, Bachman JG, et al. *Monitoring the future national survey results on drug use, 1975–2012. Vol I: secondary school students.* Ann Arbor: Institute for Social Research: The University of Michigan, 2013.
2. Hingson RW, Heeren T, Winter MR. Age at drinking onset and alcohol dependence: age at onset, duration, and severity. *Arch Pediatr Adolesc Med* 2006;160(7):739–746. Available at http://www.ncbi.nlm.nih.gov/entrez/query.fcgi?cmd=Retrieve&db=PubMed&dopt=Citation&list_uids=16818840.

XIV

3. U.S. Preventive Services Task Force. *Screening and behavioral counseling interventions in primary care to reduce alcohol misuse: recommendation statement.* AHRQ publication No. 12-05171-EF-3, 2013. Available at http://www.uspreventiveservicestaskforce.org/uspstf12/alcmisuse/alcmisuserfinalrs.htm

4. Gogtay N, Giedd JN, Lusk L, et al. Dynamic mapping of human cortical development during childhood through early adulthood. *Proc Natl Acad Sci U S A* 2004;101(21):8174–8179. Available at http://www.pubmedcentral.nih.gov/articlerender.fcgi?artid=419576&tool=pmcentrez&rendertype=abstract. Accessed February 5, 2014.

5. NIAAA. *NIAAA alcohol screening and brief intervention for youth: a practitioners guide.* NIH Publication No. 11-7805, 2011. Available at http://pubs.niaaa.nih.gov/publications/Practitioner/YouthGuide/YouthGuide.pdf.

6. Committee on Substance Abuse. Alcohol use by youth and adolescents: a pediatric concern. *Pediatrics* 2010;125(5):1078–1087. doi:10.1542/peds.2010-0438.

7. Kelly SM, Gryczynski J, Mitchell SG, et al. Validity of brief screening instrument for adolescent tobacco, alcohol, and drug use. *Pediatrics* 2014;133(5). doi:10.1542/peds.2013-2346–. Available at http://pediatrics.aappublications.org/content/early/2014/04/16/peds.2013-2346.abstract?cited-by=yes&legid=pediatrics;peds.2013-2346v1#cited-by. Accessed May 9, 2014.

8. Levy S, Weiss R, Sherritt L, et al. An electronic screen for triaging adolescent substance use by risk levels. *JAMA Pediatr* 2014;168(9):822–828. Available at http://www.ncbi.nlm.nih.gov/pubmed/25070067.

9. American Psychiatric Association. *Diagnostic and statistical manual of mental disorders.* 5th ed. Arlington, VA: American Psychiatric Association, 2013.

10. Substance Abuse and Mental Health Services Administration (SAMHSA). *The TEDS report: substance abuse treatment admissions referred by the Criminal Justice System.* Rockville, MD: SAMHSA, 2009. Available at http://www.samhsa.gov/data/2k9/211/211CJadmits2k9.pdf.

11. Substance Abuse and Mental Health Services Administration. *Results from the 2012 National Survey on drug use and health: summary of national findings.* Rockville, MD: Substance Abuse and Mental Health Services Administration, 2013.

12. Wilson CR, Sherritt L, Gates E, et al. Are clinical impressions of adolescent substance use accurate? *Pediatrics* 2004;114(5):e536–e540. doi:114/5/e536 [pii] 10.1542/peds.2004-0098.

13. Skinner HA. The drug abuse screening test. *Addict Behav* 1982;7(4):363–371. Available at http://www.sciencedirect.com/science/article/pii/0306460382900053. Accessed February 28, 2015.

14. Van Cleave J, Gortmaker SL, Perrin JM. Dynamics of obesity and chronic health conditions among children and youth. *JAMA* 2010;303(7):623–630. doi:303/7/623 [pii] 10.1001/jama.2010.104.

15. Weitzman ER. Poor mental health, depression, and associations with alcohol consumption, harm, and abuse in a national sample of young adults in college. *J Nerv Ment Dis* 2004;192(4):269–277. doi:00005053-200404000-00003 [pii].

16. D'Amico EJ, Miles JNV, Stern SA, et al. Brief motivational interviewing for teens at risk of substance use consequences: a randomized pilot study in a primary care clinic. *J Subst Abuse Treat* 2008;35(1):53–61. Available at http://www.sciencedirect.com/science/article/pii/S0740547207002437.

17. Harris SK, Csemy L, Sherritt L, et al. Computer-facilitated substance use screening and brief advice for teens in primary care: an international trial. *Pediatrics* 2012;129(6):1072–1082. doi:peds.2011-1624 [pii] 10.1542/peds.2011-1624.

18. Committee on Substance Abuse. Substance use screening, brief intervention, and referral to treatment for pediatricians. *Pediatrics* 2011;128(5):e1330–e1340. doi:10.1542/peds.2011-1754.

19. Vasilaki EI, Hosier SG, Cox WM. The efficacy of motivational interviewing as a brief intervention for excessive drinking: a meta-analytic review. *Alcohol Alcohol* 2006;41(3):328–335. Available at http://www.ncbi.nlm.nih.gov/pubmed/16547122. Accessed February 7, 2014.

20. Pbert L, Flint AJ, Fletcher KE, et al. Effect of a pediatric practice-based smoking prevention and cessation intervention for adolescents: a randomized, controlled trial. *Pediatrics* 2008;121(4):e738–e747. doi:121/4/e738 [pii] 10.1542/peds.2007-1029.

21. Bernstein E, Edwards E, Dorfman D, et al. Screening and brief intervention to reduce marijuana use among youth and young adults in a pediatric emergency department. *Acad Emerg Med* 2009;16(11):1174–1185. doi:ACEM490 [pii] 10.1111/j.1553-2712.2009.00490.x.

22. Tait RJ, Hulse GK, Robertson SI, et al. Emergency department-based intervention with adolescent substance users: 12-month outcomes. *Drug Alcohol Depend* 2005;79(3):359–363. Available at http://www.sciencedirect.com/science/article/pii/S0376871605000943.

23. Monti PM, Barnett NP, Colby SM, et al. Motivational interviewing versus feedback only in emergency care for young adult problem drinking. *Addiction* 2007;102(8):1234–1243. Available at 10.1111/j.1360-0443.2007.01878.x.

24. Ries RK, David FA, Miller SC, et al., eds. *Principles of addiction medicine.* 4th ed. Philadelphia, PA: Lippincott Williams & Wilkins, 2009.

25. Center for Substance Abuse Treatment. *Treatment of adolescents with substance abuse disorders.* Rockville, MD: DHHS, 1999. Available at http://adaiclearinghouse.org/downloads/TIP-32-Treatment-of-Adolescents-with-Substance-Use-Disorders-62.pdf.

26. American Academy of Pediatrics Committee on Substance Abuse. Testing for drugs of abuse in children and adolescents. *Pediatrics.* In press.

27. Dolan K, Rouen D, Kimber J. An overview of the use of urine, hair, sweat and saliva to detect drug use. *Drug Alcohol Rev* 2004;23(2):213–217. Available at http://www.ncbi.nlm.nih.gov/pubmed/15370028. Accessed February 26, 2014.

28. Mikel C, Pesce AJ, Rosenthal M, et al. Therapeutic monitoring of benzodiazepines in the management of pain: current limitations of point of care immunoassays suggest testing by mass spectrometry to assure accuracy and improve patient safety. *Clin Chim Acta* 2012;413(15/16):1199–1202. Available at http://www.ncbi.nlm.nih.gov/pubmed/22484396. Accessed February 18, 2014.

29. Substance Abuse and Mental Health Services Administration (SAMHSA). *The U.S. mandatory guidelines for federal workplace drug testing programs current status and future considerations.* 2008. Available at http://www.gpo.gov/fdsys/pkg/FR-2008-11-25/pdf/E8-26726.pdf.

30. Mayo Medical Laboratories. *Drugs of abuse: approximate detection times table. 2011.* Available at http://www.mayomedicallaboratories.com/articles/drug-book/viewall.html. Accessed February 18, 2014.

31. Martino S, Grilo CM, Fehon DC. Development of the drug abuse screening test for adolescents (DAST-A). *Addict Behav* 2000;25(1):57–70. doi:S0306-4603(99)00030-1 [pii].

32. McCabe SE, Boyd CJ, Cranford JA, et al. A modified version of the drug abuse screening test among college students. *J Subst Abuse Treat* 2006;31:297–303.

33. Jensen CD, Cushing CC, Aylward BS, et al. Effectiveness of motivational interviewing interventions for adolescent substance use behavior change: A meta-analytic review. *J Consult Clin Psychol* 2011;79(4):433–440.

34. Waldron HB, Kaminer Y. On the learning curve: the emerging evidence supporting cognitive–behavioral therapies for adolescent substance abuse. *Addiction* 2004;99(s2):93–105.

35. Kaminer Y JB, R Goldberger. Cognitive-behavioral coping skills and psychoeducation therapies for adolescent substance abuse. *J Nerv Ment Dis* 2002;190(11):737–734.

36. Dimeff LA, Linehan MM. Dialectical behavior therapy for substance abusers. *Addict Sci Clin Pract* 2008;4(2):39–47. Retrieved from http://www.pubmedcentral.nih.gov/articlerender.fcgi?artid=2797106&tool=pmcentrez&rendertype=abstract

37. Lussier JP, Heil SH, Mongeon JA, et al. A meta-analysis of voucher-based reinforcement therapy for substance use disorders. *Addiction* 2006;101(2):192–203.

38. Stanger C. A randomized trial of contingency management for adolescent marijuana abuse and dependence. *Drug Alcohol Depend* 2009;105(3):240–247.

39. Stanger C, Budney A. Contingency management approaches for adolescent substance use disorders. *Child Adolesc Psychiatr Clin N Am* 2010;19(3):547–562.

🛜 **ADDITIONAL RESOURCES AND WEBSITES ONLINE**

PART XV

Mental Health

69

Depression and Anxiety Disorders

Daphne J. Korczak
Suneeta Monga

KEY WORDS

- Adjustment disorder
- Anxiety
- Depression
- Generalized anxiety disorder
- Psychopharmacology
- Psychotherapy
- Social anxiety disorder

Depression and anxiety disorders are highly prevalent among adolescents and young adults (AYAs): 75% of all lifetime cases will have started by age 24 years.[1] Social withdrawal, substance use, poor academic performance, decreased concentration, fatigue, and other somatic complaints may all indicate a new onset of a mental health issue. AYAs, collectively referred to as *youth* in this chapter, may also have limited awareness of the severity or functional impact of their symptoms, because of symptom chronicity or reluctance to acknowledge a mental health problem. Thus, clinicians working with youth must have a high index of suspicion for mental health disorders among this population. This chapter reviews the most frequently encountered mood and anxiety disorders of adolescence and young adulthood, and discusses the key causes, assessments, and diagnoses of, and treatments for, these conditions.

DEPRESSION IN YOUTH

Epidemiology

- According to the WHO, depression is a leading cause of disability globally.
- Clinically significant depressive illness occurs in about 5% to 8% of adolescents in the US, Canada, and Europe.
- Depressive symptoms are widely reported in community studies of youth. In one community survey of 9,863 adolescents in the US,[2] 18% of participants in early–middle adolescence reported depressive symptoms.
- About 25% to 50% of depressed youth have comorbid anxiety disorders; about 10% to 15% of anxious youth have depression.
- Gender: By mid-adolescence, the female predominance noted in adult samples is established: twice as many girls as boys are affected.
- Age of Onset: Although the mean age of onset of a first depressive episode is mid-20s, this age is decreasing with each generation; the prevalence of the pre-adult age of onset of major depressive disorder (MDD) is increasing. Many children experience subsyndromal and syndromal symptoms for years before coming to medical attention. Early identification of depression is important for healthy psychosocial and cognitive development and improved illness outcomes among youth.

- Onset of depression in adolescence is more likely to remain undetected for a longer period of time than onset in young adult or adulthood.
- Clinicians treating youth with depression play a critical role in altering lifelong developmental trajectories.

Course of Illness

Onset of depression in adolescence is associated with a more severe course of illness than onset in young adulthood or adulthood.[3,4] Affected adolescents are at greater risk of more depressive episodes, more severe episodes, increased suicidality, increased likelihood of dropping out of high school, poorer academic, occupational, and social outcomes, and greater psychiatric comorbidity than those who first experience depression as young adults or adults.

- About 60% to 70% of those who have a depressive episode in adolescence will have a recurrence within 5 years.
- Increased risk of recurrence is associated with greater episode severity, chronicity of symptoms, incomplete recovery, presence of dysthymia, comorbid anxiety, persistence of stressful life events, and parental history of depression.
- Early in the course of depression, a psychosocial stressor is frequently present and identified as a precipitant for the depressive episode. In contrast, depressive episodes later in adulthood may occur without any discernible precipitating stressful event.

Risk Factors

A number of biological, psychosocial, and social factors have been associated with increased risk of depression among youth (Table 69.1).

Biological

Children of parents with a history of depression are at increased risk of developing depression.

- Twin-study estimates of the heritability of MDD range from 0.36 to 0.70.[5,6]
- Family studies[7,8] estimate a 10% to 25% risk of MDD in first-degree relatives of MDD probands, two- to three times higher than that in controls.
- Youth with depression are more likely than adults to have a family history of depression in a first-degree relative.
- Offspring of parents with early-onset depression have about a four to five times higher risk of developing MDD (25% to 40% risk of MDD) than controls.
- An adopted person's risk of developing depression is increased if his or her biological parent had depression.

TABLE 69.1
Risk Factors for Depression among Youth

Biological Factors
- Female sex
- Older age
- Parent/family history of depression
- Comorbid chronic illness (e.g., diabetes, anxiety disorder, ADHD)
- Past history of depression
- Comorbid learning disorders
- Genetics (presence of specific serotonin-transporter gene variants)
- Certain medications (e.g., prednisone, isotretinoin [Accutane])
- Substance use

Psychosocial Risk Factors
- Family or peer conflict (e.g., bullying)
- Childhood neglect or abuse (physical, emotional, sexual)
- Poverty
- Recent loss, e.g., death of a loved one, break up of romantic relationship
- Academic difficulties or failure of the child
- Discrimination and social exclusion
- Poor (e.g., conflictual) home–school relationships
- Poor-quality (e.g., high conflict, low community support) neighborhoods

Psychological

Psychological factors that may contribute to the development of depression include:

- a tendency to respond to stress with unpleasant emotions, although many people with depression do not have strong emotional responses before the onset of depression
- a tendency to interpret emotionally neutral events as negative.

The experience of depressive illness during adolescence and young adulthood disrupts normative developmental growth of personality characteristics.

Social

A number of social factors also are risk factors for development of depression among youth:

- Bullying
- Poverty
- Poor physical health
- Perceived discrimination within the household (i.e., the perception of having less access to material and emotional supports than other children in the home)
- Increased daily-life stresses (e.g., excessive work or chores, academic difficulties)
- Early-life stress, such as childhood abuse and neglect. Evidence indicates that early-life stress can induce persistent changes in the responsiveness of the hypothalamic–pituitary–adrenal (HPA) axis to stress later in life that is associated with depression (see below).

Causality

The origin of depression is multifactorial: neurobiological, pathophysiological, psychological, and social factors contribute to the genesis of MDD.

- **Neurobiological.** Abnormalities of several brain structures are found in people with MDD, including the hippocampus, the hypothalamus, the amygdala, and the nucleus accumbens. Both structural and functional abnormalities have been described. Several neurotransmitter systems (serotonin, norepinephrine, dopamine) have also been implicated in the dysfunction reported in individuals with MDD, forming the basis for the use of the medication in treatment, as described below.

- **Pathophysiological.** Possible underlying pathological processes causing depression include dysfunction of the HPA axis, increased proinflammatory cytokines, and oxidative stress.

- **Psychological.** Numerous psychological theories about the basis of depression have been proposed. Both cognitive and interpersonal theories have led to specific treatment modalities for depressed youth (see treatment for depression). Other psychodynamic formulations of depression consider early developmental theories as a basis for understanding distress.[9] It is important that clinicians using psychotherapeutic treatment modalities are well versed in the psychological theories pertaining to the basis of depression and the treatment modality that they intend to employ.

ASSESSMENT

In contrast to the transitory aspects of a normal depressed mood in youth, depressive illness is characterized by the persistence of depressed mood and associated features. Pessimism, reduced ability to experience pleasure, and decreased energy and motivation are also frequently present. Experiences of helplessness, hopelessness, or worthlessness may occur. Together with associated depressive symptoms, the condition interferes with the ability to function at school, at home, and with friends.

Important Elements in the Assessment of Depression
Interviews and Collateral Information

Individual clinical interview of the youth and interviews with the parents or guardians (whenever possible) to obtain collateral information are essential in order to assess symptoms and their functional impact. This should include depressive symptoms, assessment of suicidality and self-harm behaviors, elucidation of precipitating stressors (e.g., breakup of a romantic relationship, bullying, new disclosure of homosexuality), and presence of additional symptoms (psychotic, anxious) or behaviors (substance use) required to ascertain an accurate diagnostic impression.

Youth must be made aware of the limits of confidentiality in this interview when disclosures may have a potential impact on the safety of the patient or others. Youth may downplay or misunderstand the basis of these symptoms and attribute them to problems with nerves, imbalance, or being physically unfit. Sleep disturbance and loss of energy are the most uniformly reported of depressive symptoms. Sadness may be denied at first, but later elicited through clinical interview or inferred from facial expression.

Assessment of Illness Characteristics

The severity of the current depressive episode (mild, moderate, or severe), the presence of associated illness specifiers (e.g., presence of psychotic features), and the nature of the overarching mood disorder (bipolar or unipolar) must be determined.

Consideration of Cultural Background

Cultural background may affect the type and intensity of affective expression.[10] Symptoms of depression share many similarities across cultures, but culture may affect the symptoms emphasized and the idioms used to describe distress.[10] For example, poor eye contact may be a symptom of emotional distress in cultures that stress individual autonomy, but may be a sign of respect in cultures that stress deference. In addition, patients may report symptoms of considerable suffering, but their restrained expression of distress may strain the credibility of the report. Conversely, they may describe symptoms in a highly expressive manner that seems exaggerated. In some cultures, somatic symptoms may constitute the presenting complaint.

Screening Tools for Depression

A number of self-report and clinician-administered instruments have been evaluated and validated for use in the screening and monitoring of depressive symptoms among youth. Self-report measures, in particular, have wide appeal because of their ease of administration, patient acceptability, and ability to translate symptom dimensions into quantifiable scores for evaluation. Although these instruments may be helpful supplementary tools for screening and monitoring depressive symptoms, they are not diagnostic instruments and cannot substitute for clinical assessment of depression. Although some measures have been validated in non–English-speaking youth, clinicians must be aware of individual cultural differences, intellectual or cognitive impairments, and comorbidity of depression with psychiatric and other chronic illnesses that may be pertinent and limit the generalizability of the measure's utility for their patient.

Commonly used depression-specific measures, with demonstrated reliability and validity in the populations outlined below, include (but are not limited to) the following:

Beck Depression Inventory-II

Beck Depression Inventory-II (BDI -II) is a 21-item self-report instrument that takes 10 to 15 minutes to complete by individuals 13 years of age and older. Each question is scored from 0 to 3. Higher scores indicate more severe depressive symptoms.

Children's Depression Inventory

Children's Depression Inventory (CDI-2) is a 28-item scale derived from the BDI used to assess depressive symptoms in children and adolescents. Questions from the BDI were modified to make them more appropriate for younger ages. The CDI-2 is a self-report measure that takes 15 to 20 minutes to complete by patients 7 to 17 years of age. Each item is scored from 0 to 3. In addition, two-scale (emotional problems and functional problems) and four-subscale scores can be computed. Higher scores indicate more severe depressive symptoms.

Children's Depression Rating Scale—Revised

This rating scale is a 17-item interviewer-administered instrument used to determine the presence and severity of depressive symptoms in children and adolescents. Each of the items is scored on a seven-point rating scale.

Patient Health Questionnaire

This questionnaire consists of nine self-report items that takes the adolescent or young adult about 5 to 10 minutes to complete. Originally developed for adults over 18 years of age, psychometric validity data also support its use among adolescent patients in primary care and pediatric hospital settings.

DEPRESSIVE DISORDERS AND THE DIAGNOSTIC AND STATISTICAL MANUAL OF MENTAL DISORDERS, FIFTH EDITION (DSM-5)

Major Depressive Episode[11]

- Five (or more) of the following nine symptoms must be present during the same two-week period.
- Symptoms must either be newly present or have clearly worsened when compared with those present before the person's current episode.
- Symptoms must persist for most of the day, nearly every day, for at least two consecutive weeks.
- At least one of the symptoms must be either (1) depressed mood or (2) loss of interest or pleasure.

1. Depressed mood, as indicated by either subjective or objective report, most of the day, nearly every day. For adolescents, the mood may be irritable.
2. Markedly diminished interest or pleasure in all, or almost all, activities most of the day, nearly every day

3. Significant weight loss when not dieting, weight gain, or change in appetite
4. Insomnia or hypersomnia nearly every day
5. Psychomotor agitation or retardation nearly every day, observable by others, not merely subjective feelings of restlessness or of being slowed down
6. Fatigue or loss of energy nearly every day
7. Feelings of worthlessness or excessive or inappropriate guilt (which may be delusional) nearly every day (not merely self-reproach or guilt about being sick)
8. Diminished ability to think or concentrate, or indecisiveness, nearly every day
9. Recurrent thoughts of death (not just fear of dying), recurrent suicidal ideation without a specific plan, suicide attempt, or a specific plan for committing suicide
   Note: symptoms must cause clinically significant distress or impairment in social, occupational, or other important areas of functioning. The episode cannot be attributable to the physiological effects of a substance or to another medical condition. All of these criteria must be met to represent a major depressive episode.

Adjustment Disorder

See Chapter 34.

Persistent Depression (Dysthymia)[11]

- Depressed mood that occurs for most of the day, for more days than not, for at least 2 years (or one year for adolescents). Youth whose depressed mood resolves consistently during the summer months, for example, do not have a persistent depressive disorder.
- At least two of six associated depressive neurovegetative or cognitive symptoms must be present.
- At times, the patient may have also experienced a major depressive episode.
- People with this disorder often describe years of feeling sad. Some youth may be unable to remember a time when they did not feel this way or attribute the experience to part of their personality.
- Youth with persistent depressive symptoms are at high risk of developing comorbid psychiatric illness, including substance use disorders and personality disorders. As a result, they may require treatment for these in addition to management of their depressive disorder.

Bipolar Depression[11]

Bipolar depression is differentiated from unipolar depressive illnesses by the presence of one or more periods of hypomania or mania during the course of illness. That is, bipolar depression refers to a Major Depressive Episode that occurs within the context of bipolar disorder.

- Youth with bipolar disorder, despite having suffered a hypomanic or manic episode in their lifetime, frequently experience much of the illness' morbidity as the result of either syndromal or subsyndromal depressive symptoms.
- A Major Depressive Episode in adolescence or young adulthood may be the index mood episode of bipolar disorder; the mean age of onset of the first mood episode is about 18 years of age.
- The presence of psychotic features, profound psychomotor retardation, or a family history of bipolar disorder should alert the clinician to the possibility of bipolar depression.
- Clinicians considering the diagnosis of bipolar depression should request psychiatric consultation to assess the potential of an underlying bipolar diathesis and obtain management suggestions because treatment algorithms are substantially different from those for unipolar depressive illness.

Youth with depressive disorders may also suffer from comorbid psychiatric illness (particularly, substance use, attention deficit hyperactivity disorder [ADHD], conduct and anxiety disorders). These disorders must also be identified to ensure safe and appropriate recommendations for treatment are made.

 TREATMENT

General Considerations

Ensure Safety

The single most important consideration in determining a treatment plan for depressed youth is to *assess for the risk for suicide* and ensure safety. Care providers must first decide whether the patient should be hospitalized or can be safely managed as an outpatient before proceeding with other treatment recommendations.

Provide Psychoeducation

Communication of the diagnosis of depression, eliciting patient and family conceptualizations of the illness, and the provision of psychoeducation about the symptoms, course, and treatments available for depression are key components to undertake before determining a treatment plan.

Identify and Address Stressors and Psychiatric Comorbidity

Additional components of a comprehensive treatment plan include discussing stressors that may be perpetuating depressive symptoms (e.g., ongoing family or peer conflict), and screening for and addressing comorbid psychiatric illness (e.g., substance use or anxiety disorders), as appropriate. It may be necessary to involve parents and/or guardians in order to address these factors.

Mild Depression

- For youth with mild depression, addressing perpetuating factors, providing active support, scheduling regular visits, and monitoring symptoms may help alleviate symptoms.
- Providing active, supportive strategies (e.g., encouraging involvement in enjoyable activities, ensuring sound sleep-hygiene routines, promoting routine physical activity, advocating for patients when they are having difficulties with academics or bullying at school) may relieve symptoms in as many as 20% of depressed youth.[12]
- Patients who do not respond to these strategies should begin a depression-specific treatment.

Moderate to Severe Depression

- Youth with moderate or severe depression should be referred to a specialist for assessment and management recommendations.
- Once assessed, primary care physicians may undertake management plans alone or in collaboration with a mental health specialist.
- Youth with moderate to severe symptoms are less likely to experience symptom remission without psychotherapy, medication, or combination treatment.

Psychotherapy

Cognitive Behavioral Therapy

Cognitive behavioral therapy (CBT) is a manualized treatment modality that can be delivered either individually or in groups, and administered in primary care settings. CBT is based on the cognitive theory of depression, which describes how people's perceptions of, or spontaneous thoughts about, situations influence their emotional, behavioral (and often physiological) reactions. Perceptions are often distorted when people are depressed, and a stream of seemingly spontaneous negative thoughts, called *automatic thoughts* may be experienced. Depressive automatic thoughts fall into one of three categories: negative thoughts about the self, the world or environment, and the future.

- CBT is an effective stand-alone treatment for depression in adolescents and a first-line treatment for depression of mild to moderate severity.[13]
- The combination of CBT and pharmacotherapy is reportedly more efficacious than either treatment modality alone for the treatment of adolescent depression.[14]
- The largest randomized placebo-controlled study to date, the Treatment for Adolescents with Depression Study,[14] compared placebo, CBT alone, fluoxetine alone, and combination fluoxetine plus CBT. Adolescent participants in the medication arms demonstrated significantly greater improvement in their depressive symptoms than those in either the CBT-alone or placebo arms. In this investigator-initiated study, patients with more severe and persistent depression benefited equally from medication alone or from combined medication and CBT. Another study,[12] however, found that the addition of CBT to antidepressant medication and routine specialist care did not further reduce depressive symptoms for more severely depressed adolescents.

CBT has been adapted for the treatment of depression by focusing on correcting cognitive distortions such as depressive negative self-cognitions (e.g., "I am worthless," "nobody likes me"), utilizing mood diaries to monitor symptoms, and expanding the behavioral component to include behavioral activation strategies (e.g., exercise, participation in group activities).

Interpersonal Therapy

Interpersonal therapy (IPT) is based on the interpersonal theory of depression, which suggests that people who are prone to depression are more likely to seek excessive reassurance in relationships. This support-seeking behavior tends to elicit support-giving behavior, which reinforces the depressive symptoms. The model further posits that this style of interpersonal communication may also occur more commonly in people with deficient social skills. People who excessively seek reassurance and may have poor social skills are theorized to have more interpersonal difficulties, including rejection, within their relationships, which further increases their depressive symptoms. As IPT was originally developed for the treatment of depression in adults, much of the evidence for its effectiveness comes from studies of adult populations, including young adults.

- IPT has since been adapted for administration in adolescents (interpersonal therapy for adolescents [IPT-A]).
- The central tenet of IPT is that depressive symptoms and interpersonal relationships are intertwined.
- Connections are made between the person's depressive symptoms and the practical life events that either precipitate or follow from the onset of the illness.
- Patients must be assessed as having one of four relational areas as a central theme to inform the therapy: role transitions (e.g., graduation, moving away to school), grief, role disputes (having conflictual relationships with important people in their lives), or interpersonal deficits (difficulty forming relationships with peers).
- Similar to CBT, IPT and IPT-A are structured, short-term, manualized therapies.
- In contrast to CBT for the treatment of adolescent depression, data supporting the efficacy of IPT-A is more limited.
- Comparison of the use of IPT-A to medication or in combination with medication to examine its comparative benefit has not been studied.

Nonspecific Psychotherapies

CBT and IPT (or IPT-A) are psychotherapies that may be indicated specifically for treatment of depressive symptoms among youth.

Youth with depression may also have *comorbid* psychiatric conditions or symptoms that are functionally impairing and highly problematic in their lives. The clinician may wish to consider using a psychotherapeutic modality that specifically targets these concerns, despite its lack of specificity for depressive symptoms, based on the difficulties that are the most distressing or impairing for the patient. For example, youth with highly conflictual family relationships may benefit from family therapy; those struggling with ongoing themes of past trauma may require a trauma-focused therapy. Motivational interviewing may address comorbid substance use; Dialectical Behavior Therapy may be required to address persistent thoughts and urges to engage in self-harm or suicidal behavior. Although these psychotherapies are not specific for the treatment of depression, the amelioration of the potentially perpetuating stressor or symptom may have nonspecific benefits in improving depressive symptoms.

Medication

Antidepressant medications are classified on the basis of their specific relation to brain neurotransmitters. Selective serotonin reuptake inhibitors (SSRIs) are a class of medications that include fluoxetine, sertraline, citalopram, escitalopram, fluvoxamine, and paroxetine (**Table 69.2**). SSRIs inhibit serotonin transporters, blocking reuptake and increasing the concentration of the serotonin neurotransmitter within the synapse. Within the broader class of SSRIs, specific medications may also influence other neurotransmitter systems (e.g., dopamine, norepinephrine), affecting the effectiveness and adverse effects of various SSRIs.

Laboratory Investigations

Laboratory investigations may be necessary to

- rule out alternate underlying causes of the presenting symptoms (e.g., hypothyroidism),
- assess comorbid medical conditions (e.g., hepatic impairment), or
- monitor therapeutic drug levels of medications used in combination with SSRIs (e.g., valproic acid).

However, laboratory investigations are not routinely required before initiating or maintaining SSRIs. Psychiatry consultation should be considered when the patient has a comorbid chronic medical illness or requires treatment with SSRIs in combination with other medications.

Evidence and Medication Use

In the US, the Food and Drug Administration (FDA) has approved fluoxetine and escitalopram for the treatment of depression for adolescents. Health Canada (HC) has not approved antidepressants (including SSRIs) for the treatment of depression for adolescents. It is important, therefore, that, when prescribing SSRIs for patients under the age of 18 years, physicians document relevant issues carefully.

TABLE 69.2
SSRI Medications: Half-Life and Dosing Schedules

Medication (Trade Name)	Mean Half-Life (h)	Dosing Schedule
Fluoxetine (Prozac)	96	Daily
Sertraline (Zoloft)	26	Daily
Fluvoxamine (Luvox)	15	Daily
Citalopram (Celexa)	35	Daily
Escitalopram (Cipralex)	30	Daily
Paroxetine (Paxil)	21	Daily

- Randomized double-blind placebo-controlled trials and systematic reviews suggest that SSRIs are effective for the treatment of adolescent depression; response rates range from 40% to 70%.[15,16]
- Response rates for patients receiving placebo are also considerable (30% to 60%). This indicates that the design of the study is important when evaluating the efficacy of antidepressant medications among youth.
- Clinical trials of fluoxetine have found the greatest difference between active drug and placebo.[15–17]
- Two randomized controlled trials (RCTs) showed the efficacy of escitalopram for the treatment of adolescent depression.[18,19]
- A single positive RCT for each of citalopram[20] and sertraline[21] reported greater benefits for these medications over placebo for the treatment of adolescent depression. A second RCT of citalopram demonstrated negative results in the treatment of adolescent depression.[22]
- Examination of paroxetine's efficacy in the treatment of child and adolescent depression has yielded negative results in three RCTs.[23–25]
- Among patients older than 18 years, several additional medications, including serotonin and norepinephrine reuptake inhibitors (e.g., venlafaxine), norepinephrine and dopamine reuptake inhibitors (e.g., buproprion), and others, have evidence for efficacy in the treatment of depression.[26]

Adverse Effects of Medications

- SSRIs are generally well tolerated. Common short-term side effects include gastrointestinal symptoms (e.g., stomach aches, nausea), sleep changes (either insomnia or somnolence, and sleep disturbances, including vivid dreams), restlessness, headaches, appetite changes, and sexual dysfunction.
- An increase in agitation or impulsivity (behavioral activation) may occur. If youth experience behavioral activation, then the clinician must ensure that early signs of hypomania are eliminated from the differential diagnosis.[27]
- SSRIs have rarely been associated with increased risk of bleeding and syndrome of inappropriate secretion of antidiuretic hormone.
- Serotonin syndrome may occur as a result of toxicity (e.g., overdose ingestion) and can include changes in mental status, myoclonus, ataxia, diaphoresis, fever, and autonomic dysregulation.
- Recently, both HC and the FDA have issued a health advisory or drug-safety communications about dose-dependent QT-interval prolongation and risk of arrhythmia with citalopram dosages of greater than 40 mg/day and escitalopram dosages greater than 20 mg/day.[28–30] They recommend that clinicians not exceed this dose. Further, patients with congenital long QT syndrome should not be treated with either citalopram or escitalopram. Patients with underlying heart disease or hepatic impairment (affecting citalopram metabolism), including a predisposition to cardiac arrhythmia because of electrolyte disturbances, should be treated with caution if receiving citalopram or escitalopram and monitored closely for cardiac adverse effects, including torsades de pointes.[28,31]

Suicide and SSRIs

When used appropriately, the potential benefits of SSRIs use outweigh the potential harms of untreated depression for youth with moderate to severe depression.

- Untreated moderate to severe depression is more likely to result in harm than appropriate SSRI use.
- Close initial monitoring, along with careful documentation of symptoms and adverse effects, is required.
- Suicidality lessens with effective treatment and improvement of depressive symptoms.[32]

Monitoring of Medications

For youth who begin a course of SSRI treatment, the goal should be to achieve the minimum effective dosage in 1 to 2 weeks of taking the starting dose. The FDA suggests clinical monitoring of patients at the following time points:

1. weekly (at least) for the first 4 weeks after initiation of SSRI medication
2. then, every 2 weeks for the next 2 weeks
3. then, at 12 weeks
4. then, as clinically indicated beyond the 12-week point.

The FDA notes that additional contact by telephone may be appropriate between face-to-face visits. Guidelines from the American Academy of Child and Adolescent Psychiatry[27] also encourage providers to follow the FDA monitoring schedule, although highlight the lack of evidence supporting an association between weekly face-to-face visits and suicide risk. Monitoring assessments should include evaluation of suicidal thoughts and behaviors, and the potential adverse medication effects described above. Overall adherence to medication should also be assessed over time; an abrupt discontinuation of SSRI medications (except fluoxetine) may lead to withdrawal symptoms and an abrupt worsening of depressive symptoms, including suicidality.

Maintenance of Medications

The goal of treatment is to achieve full remission of depression symptoms.

- Once an effective dosage is reached, symptoms should be re-assessed at four-week intervals to evaluate the effectiveness and tolerability of the current dosage and to determine the need to increase the dose.
- Once complete response is achieved, the medication should be continued for a minimum of 6 to 12 months to decrease the risk of depressive relapse.[27]
- Discontinuing an SSRI should consist of a slow taper of medication and occur during a relatively stress-free time (e.g., the summer months).
- For youth with a history of multiple depressive episodes, comorbid psychiatric illnesses, or complicated depressive episodes (e.g., with psychotic features), psychiatric consultation may be warranted before discontinuing medication.
- The presence of psychiatric comorbidity, including substance use disorders, may warrant further psychiatric assessment before embarking on a treatment plan.
- The relationship between ongoing substance use and depressive or anxious symptoms is frequently bidirectional. A substance use disorder should not necessarily exclude patients from receiving appropriate treatment for comorbid depression or anxiety disorders.

🔘 ANXIETY DISORDERS IN YOUTH

Anxiety disorders are delineated from normative anxiety and diagnosed when the anxiety is *excessive, persistent*, and *interferes* with day-to-day functioning. Typically, youth with anxiety disorders are unable to control or stop the worries and the worries prevent participation in activities such as school, work, and extracurricular or other social activities.

- Given that anxiety is normative along a developmental perspective, clinicians must evaluate the degree of anxiety in the context of normative development.
- Anxiety disorders are persistent, unlike transient anxiety, which is often stress-induced, therefore many anxiety disorders have time-based criteria (e.g., more than 6 months).
- Anxiety disorders are diagnosed based upon the main worry expressed by the individual.

Epidemiology

Anxiety disorders are the most common psychiatric disorders in youth, although they are not easily recognized and are often missed or undiagnosed especially in younger age groups.

- Prevalence rates for anxiety disorders are typically in the range of 10% to 20% for all youth.[33-35]
- Comorbidity among the anxiety disorders is the norm.[35] Many youth have symptoms for more than one anxiety disorder, although they may not meet full diagnostic criteria for each of the anxiety disorders.
- Comorbidity between anxiety disorders and other mental health conditions such as ADHD, depression, and substance abuse is common.[35]
- In general, most studies suggest that anxiety disorders are more common in females than in males (ratio about 2:1).[34]
- Many anxiety disorders typically develop in early childhood (median age is 6 years) although they may not be recognized or diagnosed until later. Many individuals however, may develop anxiety disorders in adolescence or young adulthood.

Course of Illness

- Anxiety disorders are chronic disorders although symptoms may wax and wane overtime.
- Evidence suggests that adolescents meeting criteria for an anxiety disorder have a moderate to high risk to meet criteria for an anxiety disorder in young adulthood.[34,36]
- Additionally, anxiety disorders may progress into mood (depression and bipolar disorder) or substance use disorders.

Risk and Prognostic Factors

Common risk factors for all anxiety disorders can be classified into three broad categories:

Temperamental Factors

Temperament describes the way in which a child approaches and reacts to the world, and interacts and behaves with others. Inborn traits such as a child's innate activity level, adaptability, response to new situations, sensitivity to surroundings, distractibility, and persistence are used to categorize children into various temperamental categories. *Behavioral inhibition* characterized by shyness, timidity, withdrawal, and fear of the unfamiliar appears to be relatively stable over the course of childhood and into adulthood and appears to be a risk factor for selective mutism (SM), social anxiety disorder (SAD), and generalized anxiety disorder (GAD).[33]

Environmental Factors

Nonspecific environmental factors include life stress, such as parental divorce, immigration, moves to a new school or neighborhood, loss (e.g., the death of a relative or pet), or an illness of a person or relative have been associated with the development of anxiety disorders. Childhood maltreatment and adversity may be risk factors for SAD. Interpersonal stressors, negative experiences with illicit or prescription drugs, and smoking are risk factors for panic attacks.

Parental factors such as overprotection and intrusiveness have been associated with separation anxiety disorder and GAD. Parental modeling of social hesitation or other symptoms of social anxiety are considered risk factors for the development of SAD.[33]

Genetic Factors

Evidence suggests that anxiety disorders are heritable disorders with involvement of multiple genes.

- Relatives of probands with anxiety disorders have strong family histories of both anxiety and mood disorders.
- Offspring of parents with anxiety, depressive and bipolar disorders have increased risk for the development of anxiety disorders.

- Studies suggest that anxious youth are more likely than non-anxious youth to have a parent with an anxiety disorder.
- Behavioral inhibition appears to have a strong genetic influence and is strongly associated with a variety of anxiety disorders, most commonly SAD and SM.[33]

Causality

- In general, the neurobiology and causes of anxiety disorders are less well understood than depressive disorders.
- Current neural system models emphasize the amygdala and related structures.
- Agents such as sodium lactate, caffeine, isoproterenol, yohimbine, carbon dioxide, and cholecystokinin more frequently provoke panic attacks in people with panic disorder than in healthy controls.
- Cigarette smoking and the use of various illicit and prescription drugs may precipitate panic attacks.

⬤ ASSESSMENT

Anxiety disorders are often missed and/or not recognized by clinicians and parents. Even youth may not recognize that their level of anxiety and/or worry is excessive. For the diagnosis of an anxiety disorder, the anxiety must interfere with the individual's day-to-day functioning and/or cause significant distress to the individual. Anxiety disorder assessments must therefore assess for the main type of worry experienced; assess the level of anxiety or worry and determine whether it is developmentally excessive; and most importantly, assess for the level of interference and/or distress caused by the anxiety symptoms.

Important Elements in the Assessment of Anxiety Disorders
Discussion of Confidentiality

As with depression, confidentiality is an essential component in the assessment of young people with an anxiety disorder (see above).

Interviews and Collateral Information

Similar to the assessment of mood disorders, individual clinical interviews of the youth and interviews with the parents or guardians (whenever possible) to obtain collateral information are helpful in order to assess for anxiety symptoms and functional impairment. It is important to ask the youth questions to obtain an understanding of the impact of, or the interference from, the anxiety symptoms. Questions such as "How does your anxiety cause problems for you?", "Does your anxiety prevent you from doing things you want to do?", "Do you avoid doing things with peers or in front of peers because of your anxiety?", and "How problematic is your anxiety for you?" are helpful questions.

Assessment of Illness Characteristics

The assessment of an anxiety disorder should include determination of the presence of:

- *medical conditions or factors* that could contribute to the anxiety symptoms (e.g., thyroid disease, excessive caffeine intake). Presence of such factors needs to be managed first and then anxiety symptoms reassessed before making an anxiety diagnosis.
- *external stressors* such as psychosocial stressors (e.g., family conflict); school stressors (e.g., learning or language deficits); social stressors (e.g., bullying or teasing); other medical stressors (e.g., hearing or visual difficulties) that may contribute to increased stress or transient anxiety. It is essential to determine whether the anxiety presents first or whether it is secondary to a stressor. For example, adolescents with undiagnosed learning issues may experience excessive anxiety and worry about their marks and academic performance, which, given their learning issues, would be normative or expected.

In this situation, when the anxiety is secondary to the learning issues, anxiety management would not be helpful until the primary cause is addressed. Further, if the anxiety is secondary to other stressors such as family conflict or bullying, these stressors must be addressed first, before anxiety management strategies can be effectively implemented.
- *physical symptoms* associated with anxiety (e.g., stomachaches, headaches, shortness of breath, dizziness or lightheadedness, nausea and/or vomiting, diarrhea, tingling, numbness, tightness in chest, back or neck, etc.).
- *specific worries and thoughts* to help identify the type of anxiety disorder.
- the *level of interference* and the persistence of the anxiety, in the context of developmentally normative worries.

Consideration of Cultural Background

Clinicians should consider cultural issues when diagnosing anxiety disorders. For example, clinicians should be mindful of the value some cultures place on interdependence among family members; the different cultural views on the role of adolescents; the potentially normative role of parental co-sleeping in some cultures; or expectations that adolescents be quiet and less interactive with their elders or other adults in other cultures.

Assessment of Comorbidity

There is high comorbidity among young people with anxiety disorders with about half (40% to 60%) of anxious youth meeting criteria for more than one anxiety disorder.[34,35]

- Comorbidity with other mental health disorders is high and therefore assessment warrants assessment for comorbid externalizing disorders (e.g., ADHD, oppositional defiant disorder [ODD]); mood disorders; and substance abuse disorders, all of which have implications for treatment.

Screening Tools for Anxiety Disorders

Self-report instruments may be quite helpful in assessing distress and the level of interference experienced by youth with anxiety disorders. These screening tools are generally well received by youth and are easy to administer; however, they are not diagnostic in and of themselves. Commonly used anxiety-specific measures, with demonstrated reliability and validity in the populations outlined below, include (but are not limited to) the following:

Beck Anxiety Inventory

The Beck Anxiety Inventory (BAI) is a 21-item self-report developed for adults that targets the severity of anxiety symptoms experienced during the previous week. Higher total scores indicate more severe anxiety symptoms. The BAI has good internal consistency and good 1-week test–retest reliability.[37] It is most useful in young adults.

Multidimensional Anxiety Screen for Children

The Multidimensional Anxiety Screen for Children (MASC) is a 39-item self-report targeted for adolescents that uses a 3-point rating scale. The MASC has four major factors: (1) physical symptoms (tense or restlessness and somatic or autonomic), (2) social anxiety (humiliation or rejection and public performance fears), (3) harm avoidance (perfectionism and anxious coping), and (4) separation anxiety. Stable across sex and age, the MASC shows excellent internal reliability and satisfactory to excellent test–retest reliability.[38]

Screen for Child Anxiety-Related Emotional Disorders/Parent Version and Child Version

This is a 41-item self-report instrument for parents and youth (targets children and adolescent 8 to 18 years old). Using a three-point scale, the Screen for Child Anxiety-Related Emotional Disorders (SCARED) consists of five factors that screen for panic disorder, GAD, separation anxiety disorder, SAD, and school refusal. The parent and child SCARED demonstrate good internal consistency, good test–retest reliability, and discriminates among the various anxiety disorders and between anxiety disorders and mood disorders.[39,40]

 ## ANXIETY DISORDERS AND THE DSM-5

Anxiety disorders are classified by the main fear or worry expressed (Table 69.3).

Major Changes to the Classification of Anxiety Disorders in the DSM-5

The DSM-5 has made several important changes in the classification of anxiety disorders.[11]

Obsessive-Compulsive Disorder

Obsessive-compulsive disorder (OCD) is now classified within a separate category of *obsessive-compulsive and related disorders*, which includes body dysmorphic disorder, hoarding disorder, trichotillomania (hair-pulling disorder), and excoriation (skin-picking) disorder, reflecting the increasing evidence for the relationship and high comorbidity seen among these disorders. OCD is characterized by the presence of obsessions (recurrent and persistent thoughts, urges, or images that are experienced as intrusive and unwanted or 'ego-dystonic') and/or compulsions (repetitive behaviors or mental acts in response to an obsession or in accordance with rules that must be applied rigidly). Typically, both obsessions and compulsions are present although cases with only obsessions or only compulsions can be seen.

Posttraumatic Stress Disorder

Posttraumatic stress disorder has also been placed within its own diagnostic category called *trauma- and stressor-related disorders* since exposure to a traumatic or stressful event is listed explicitly as a diagnostic criterion.

Selective Mutism

SM has now been recognized to be an anxiety disorder and has been added to the category of *anxiety disorders* (see below).

Generalized Anxiety Disorder

GAD is characterized by excessive anxiety and worry (apprehensive expectation) about numerous things for more than 6 months. Youth

with GAD can be conceptualized as *"worriers"* as they worry about 'anything and everything.' The intensity, duration, and frequency of the anxiety/worry are out of proportion to that expected. Controlling the worry is difficult and these worry thoughts interfere with psychosocial functioning. In addition to excessive worry, additional symptoms of restlessness, easy fatigue, difficulty concentrating, irritability, muscle tension, and/or sleep disturbance are required for the diagnosis of GAD. Adult GAD requires the presence of three or more of these additional symptoms, whereas child and adolescent GAD requires the presence of only one of these additional symptoms.

- Typical worries of GAD include worries about marks or grades, performance, catastrophic events (e.g., earthquakes, storms, world events), the future, the past, or things said or done. Generally, adolescents worry more about their competence (e.g., marks), quality of their performance, and punctuality, whereas adults worry more about finances, job performance, and the like. Worries tend to shift over the course of time.
- Normative worries of youth must be distinguished from GAD by the level of intensity and frequency (e.g., those without GAD can put the worry aside if need be, or are otherwise able to manage day-to-day functions despite their worries). The greater the number of worries, the more likely the diagnosis of GAD.
- Compared with normative anxiety, the majority of youth with GAD describe themselves as being anxious all the time.
- GAD is a chronic disorder; although symptoms may wax and wane over time, full remission is rare.
- Youth with GAD tend to be perfectionistic, overly conforming and often need to redo things because of dissatisfaction with their performance. They also often require excessive reassurance from parents and other adults.

Specific Phobias

Specific phobias are characterized by a fear of a specific object, which is often referred to as the phobic stimulus. Several subcategories of specific phobias exist including animal, natural environment, blood-injection-injury, and situation phobias. Other phobias such as fear of vomiting or costumed characters are often subsumed under the subcategory of 'other phobias.' Phobias typically develop in childhood with waxing and waning severity of symptoms; persistence of symptoms into young adulthood suggests low probability of remittance. Specific phobias are rarely seen in the medical clinical settings in the absence of other psychopathology; however, clinicians should screen for their presence when completing a thorough anxiety assessment and developing a management plan.

Social Anxiety Disorder

SAD is characterized by excessive or intense fear or anxiety about social situations. The specific worry is about *being embarrassed or humiliated* in front of others.

- In adolescents, the fear or worry must occur during interactions with same-aged peers rather than with adults only.
- For a diagnosis of SAD, the social situation must always cause fear or anxiety, although the degree and level of worry or fear may vary from situation to situation. Anticipatory anxiety may begin weeks before the actual event. Youth with SAD will avoid the social situation they fear or endure it with intense fear or anxiety.
- Difficulties such as eating in front of others, having their picture taken, performing in front of others, completing oral presentations, or public speaking may be noted.
- Over time, individuals with SAD may become more socially withdrawn and isolated as they lose contact with peers and have difficulties forming new relationships. Development of depression and substance abuse disorders may be sequelae of untreated SAD.
- Clinician judgment is important to determine whether the anxiety, especially in adolescents, is out of proportion to the

TABLE 69.3

Overview of the Different Anxiety Disorders

Anxiety Disorder	Main Worry Thought
GAD	Excessive worry about a number of things for 6 months or longer. Often referred to as "worrywarts." Additional symptoms must be present.
Panic disorder	Recurrent, unexpected attacks of anxiety—often "out of the blue."
SAD/social phobia	Worry about being laughed at or embarrassed or doing something humiliating in front of others.
SM	Excessive anxiety or inhibition about speaking to the point of mutism. Conceptualized as a variant of social anxiety.
Specific phobias	Consuming fear of a specific object. A variety of subcategories exist.
Separation anxiety disorder	Worry that something 'bad' will happen to them or their parent or primary caregiver when not together.

situation, given the normative preoccupation of adolescents with their peer groups and their often overestimation of the negative consequences of social situations.

- The onset of SAD typically occurs between 8 and 15 years of age. Although the disorder tends to emerge out of a history of shyness or social inhibition, it may follow a stressful or humiliating experience.

Selective Mutism

SM currently viewed as a variant of SAD is often seen in conjunction with symptoms or a diagnosis of SAD. Due to debilitating levels of anxiety, children with SM are unable to speak in social situations despite the absence of major language or learning issues. Therefore, despite speaking easily and comfortably in their own homes with immediate family members, children with SM do not initiate speech or reciprocally respond when spoken to by peers or adults; often not even being able to speak to less familiar relatives.

- The lack of speech with teachers and peers results in impairments in academic achievement and social relationships.
- Typical age of onset of SM is prior to age 5; however, given its association with SAD, it is important for clinicians working with older youth to inquire about the possibility of a previous diagnosis or symptoms of SM when assessing for SAD.
- Long-term consequences of SM are unknown. The assumption is that children outgrow the disorder over time; however, the symptoms or full diagnosis of social anxiety may persist.

Panic Disorder With and Without Agoraphobia

- *Panic disorder* is defined as the recurrence of panic attacks with at least 1 month or more of persistent concern or worry about having additional panic attacks or a significant maladaptive change in behavior related to the attacks.
- A *panic attack* is the occurrence of at least 4 of a total of 13 physical and cognitive symptoms developing abruptly and reaching a peak within a few minutes. Panic attacks can occur in the context of any anxiety disorder or other mental disorder and even some medical disorders. ***Expected panic attacks*** have an obvious cue or trigger, whereas ***unexpected panic attacks*** have no obvious cue or trigger and seem to occur for no reason or *"out of the blue."*
- The median age of onset of panic disorder is 20 to 24 years. Onset after age 45 years is unusual.
- A chronic course with waxing and waning of symptoms is typical. Comorbidity with other anxiety and mood disorders is common. Panic attacks and panic disorder are associated with higher rates of suicide attempts and suicidal ideations in the previous 12 months, even when other suicide risk factors are taken into account. Therefore, it is *critical to ask about suicidal ideations* in individuals presenting with panic disorder.
- **Agoraphobia** is characterized by marked fear or anxiety triggered by the risk of exposure to at least two of five situations, including using public transportation; being in open spaces; being in enclosed spaces; standing in line; being in a crowd; or being outside of the home.
- Individuals with agoraphobia usually avoid such situations although varying amounts of anxiety may be seen with different situations and proximity to the situation.
- Individuals with severe agoraphobia may become homebound.

Separation Anxiety Disorder

Separation anxiety disorder is an anxiety disorder of childhood in which the child's primary fear or worry is that *"something will happen to themselves or their parents/primary caregivers"* while not together.

- Although the full diagnostic criteria is uncommon in older adolescents and young adults, features of the disorder may be present in this age group at times of stress such as when young adults leave the parental home, enter into a romantic relationship, or become a parent themselves.
- Additionally, some evidence suggests that children with separation anxiety disorder may develop panic disorder as adolescents or young adults, therefore highlighting the importance of asking about the presence of previous separation anxiety disorder and/or symptoms when completing a full anxiety assessment of youth, especially those presenting with panic symptoms.

TREATMENT

General Considerations
Ensure Safety

Ensuring safety is important in the management of anxiety disorders, especially given the high comorbidity between anxiety disorders and mood disorders and/or substance abuse disorders.

Psychoeducation

Psychoeducation about anxiety and anxiety disorders is the first step in the management of anxiety disorders. It is important for youth and their families to understand what an anxiety disorder is and the impact it has on day-to-day functioning prior to the development of any management plan. Parental modeling of anxiety and/or facilitation of avoidance of situations causing anxiety must be curtailed. Youth and their families need to understand the importance of facing fears and learning coping strategies to do so in order to manage and treat the anxiety disorder.

Identify and Address Stressors and Psychiatric Comorbidity

Identification and treatment of other psychiatric comorbidities may take priority over the treatment of the anxiety disorder. For example, adolescents with untreated ADHD may benefit from management of the attentional difficulties before engaging in therapy for anxiety, similarly the young adult with comorbid depression may require a safety assessment and management of the depressive symptoms before starting therapy for the anxiety symptoms. Youth and families must be informed about substances that can exacerbate anxiety and they must learn to avoid use of these substances.

Mild Anxiety Disorders

Youths with mild anxiety disorders may be functioning quite well. They may benefit from psychoeducation and psychotherapy such as CBT. CBT has the strongest evidence base for the treatment of youth anxiety disorders.[11,35,41,42]

Moderate to Severe Anxiety Disorders

Youth with moderate to severe anxiety disorders may benefit from a referral to a specialist for assessment and management recommendations. In addition to psychotherapy, youth with moderate to severe anxiety disorders may benefit from the addition of medications such as the SSRIs.

Psychotherapy
CBT

CBT focuses on identifying, challenging, and revising anxious thoughts into more adaptive ones. CBT is a focused, time-limited therapy that can be conducted in individual or group formats. Therapy is focused on the 'here and now,' clearly focusing on the specific problems being worked on. Each hour-long session (usually in a series of 8 to 15 sessions) is structured so that skills are built incrementally on skills developed in previous sessions.

Therapy begins with psychoeducation, followed by support for recognizing and understanding feeling states and cues or triggers for anxiety. Relaxation strategies such as muscle-tension relaxation, diaphragmatic breathing, and imagery are taught to target autonomic arousal and physiological reactivity. Often an anxiety hierarchy or ladder of fears from least to most feared is created to allow for graduated, controlled exposure to these feared situations and stimuli, thereby helping to decrease and eliminate avoidant behaviors. Thought records are often used to help youth identify their automatic thoughts in various situations and learn to challenge these thoughts. Manualized treatments are available and used for youth. Strong evidence supports the use of CBT for youth.[34,40–42]

Exposure Therapy

Exposure therapy, also known as exposure-response-prevention (ERP) therapy, can be used as a stand-alone treatment, although it is often incorporated into a more general CBT approach. Exposure therapy involves learning to become less sensitive to a feared situation or phobic stimulus by gradually exposing the affected person to the stimulus over time.

Acceptance and Mindfulness-Based Therapies

Acceptance and commitment therapy gives the affected person the skills to accept unwanted thoughts, feelings, and sensations; place them in a different context; develop greater clarity about personal values; and commit to needed behavior change. In contrast to changing thoughts, mindfulness-based therapies encourage living in the moment and experiencing things without judgment, thereby seeking to change the relationship between the anxious person and his or her thoughts.

Other Psychotherapies

Increasingly, other therapies, including yoga and various forms of mindfulness and relaxation therapies, are being developed and used to treat anxiety disorders although there is limited evidence for their use. Various nonspecific psychotherapies may treat anxiety disorders in youth, such as family-based therapy for families who have high-tension or high-conflict relationships; behavioral and parent-management therapies to treat comorbid ODD or ADHD; and trauma-focused CBT for trauma-based anxiety. Supportive and psychodynamic psychotherapies may be beneficial for some cases of anxiety.

Medication
SSRIs

The mainstay of medication management for anxiety disorders is the use of the SSRIs, which can effectively alleviate anxiety in youth. The Child/Adolescent Anxiety Multimodal Study,[43] a large multisite, RCT, demonstrates that the most effective treatment for moderate to severe anxiety is the combination of medication (SSRIs) and CBT.

The guidelines for the use and monitoring of the SSRIs for anxiety disorders are similar to those for depressive disorders (see above). The side effects profile and dosing for anxiety are also similar to those for depressive disorders, although slow titration is critical in the treatment of anxiety disorders as lower doses are often quite effective in the management of youth anxiety disorders. The goal of treatment is to achieve remission of anxiety symptoms. Once an effective dose of the medication is reached, symptoms should be reassessed at four-week intervals to evaluate the effectiveness and tolerability of the current dosage, and to determine whether increased doses are necessary. Once complete response is achieved, medication should be continued for a minimum of 6 to 12 months to decrease the risk of relapse. Discontinuing an SSRI should consist of a slow tapering of medication and, as with depression, should occur during a relatively stress-free time (e.g., the summer months).

Benzodiazepines

Benzodiazepines have been used as an acute, short-term treatment for a variety of anxiety disorders primarily in adults. Although benzodiazepines can be helpful in the short-term management of severe cases of anxiety disorders (e.g., in the time frame before an

SSRI becomes effective or in the initial stages of CBT), they have concerning side effects, including addiction and misuse. Some individuals experience withdrawal symptoms, especially if the benzodiazepines are not tapered slowly. In addition, discontinuation of the benzodiazepines may cause return of the anxiety symptoms. Side effects include sedation and cognitive impairment; as well, behavioral disinhibition and, rarely, agitation. As a result, benzodiazepines should only be used for short-term, acute management of anxiety disorders, and only with an awareness and understanding of the potential adverse effects of these medications.

CONCLUSION

Anxiety and depression are serious, common mental health disorders of adolescence and young adulthood. It is critical that clinicians working with these individuals screen for these conditions. Comorbidity between anxiety and mood disorders is common; clinicians should assess youth for the presence of both conditions. Treatment approaches should include ensuring safety, providing psychoeducation about the disorder, and considering psychotherapy and pharmacotherapy management that is appropriate for the individual patient and family.

REFERENCES

1. Kessler RC, Berglund P, Demler O, et al. Lifetime prevalence and age-of-onset distributions of DSM-IV disorders in the National Comorbidity Survey Replication. *Arch Gen Psychiatry* 2005;62(6):593–602. doi:10.1001/archpsyc.62.6.593.
2. Saluja G, Iachan R, Scheidt PC, et al. Prevalence and risk factors for depressive symptoms among young adolescents. *Arch Pediatr Adolesc Med* 2004;158:760–765. doi:10.1001/archpedi.158.8.760.
3. Korczak DJ, Goldstein BI. Childhood onset major depressive disorder: course of illness and psychiatric comorbidity in a community sample. *J Pediatr* 2009;155(1):118–123.
4. Zisook S, Lesser I, Stewart JW, et al. Effect of age at onset on the course of major depressive disorder. *Am J Psychiatry* 2007;164:1539–1546.
5. Orstavik RE, Kendler KS, Czajkowski N, et al. Genetic and environmental contributions to depressive personality disorder in a population-based sample of Norwegian twins. *J Affect Disord* 2007;99:181–189. doi:10.1016/j.jad.2006.09.011.
6. Wray NR, Gottesman II. Using summary data from the danish national registers to estimate heritabilities for schizophrenia, bipolar disorder, and major depressive disorder. *Front Genet* 2012;3:118. doi:10.3389/fgene.2012.00118.
7. Lieb R, Isensee B, Hofler M, et al. Parental major depression and the risk of depression and other mental disorders in offspring: a prospective-longitudinal community study. *Arch Gen Psychiatry* 2002;59:365–374.
8. Weissman MM, Wickramaratne P, Merikangas KR, et al. Onset of major depression in early adulthood. Increased familial loading and specificity. *Arch Gen Psychiatry* 1984;41:1136–1143.
9. Busch FN, Rudden M, Shapiro T. *Psychodynamic treatment of depression.* Washington, DC: American Psychiatric Publishing, 2005.
10. Korczak DJ, Beiser M. In: Barozzino T, Hui C, eds. Depression. In: *Caring for kids new to Canada.* Ottawa, ON: Canadian Paediatric Society, 2013.
11. American Psychiatric Association. *Diagnostic and statistical manual of mental disorders.* 5th ed. Arlington, VA: American Psychiatric Publishing, 2013.
12. Goodyer IM, Dubicka B, Wilkinson P, et al. A randomised controlled trial of cognitive behaviour therapy in adolescents with major depression treated by selective serotonin reuptake inhibitors. The ADAPT trial. *Health Technol Assess* 2008;12(14):iii–iv, 1-60.
13. Korczak DJ. Use of selective serotonin reuptake inhibitor medications for the treatment of child and adolescent mental illness: Position Statement of the Canadian Paediatric Society. *Paediatr Child Health* 2013;18(9):487–491.
14. Emslie G, Kratochvil C, Vitiello B, et al. Treatment for Adolescents with Depression Study (TADS): safety results. *J Am Acad Child Adolesc Psychiatry* 2006;45:1440–1455. doi:10.1097/01.chi.0000240840.63737.1d.
15. Bridge JA, Iyengar S, Salary CB, et al. Clinical response and risk for reported suicidal ideation and suicide attempts in pediatric antidepressant treatment: a meta-analysis of randomized controlled trials. *JAMA* 2007;297:1683–1696. doi:10.1001/jama.297.15.1683.
16. Cheung AH, Emslie GJ, Mayes TL. Review of the efficacy and safety of antidepressants in youth depression. *J Child Psychol Psychiatry* 2005;46:735–754. doi:10.1111/j.1469-7610.2005.01467.x.
17. March J, Silva S, Petrycki S, et al. Fluoxetine, cognitive-behavioral therapy, and their combination for adolescents with depression: Treatment for Adolescents With Depression Study (TADS) randomized controlled trial. *JAMA* 2004;292:807–820. doi:10.1001/jama.292.7.807.
18. Emslie GJ, Ventura D, Korotzer A, et al. Escitalopram in the treatment of adolescent depression: a randomized placebo-controlled multisite trial. *J Am Acad Child Adolesc Psychiatry* 2009;48:721–729. doi:10.1097/CHI.0b013e3181a2b304.
19. Wagner KD, Jonas J, Findling RL, et al. A double-blind, randomized, placebo-controlled trial of escitalopram in the treatment of pediatric depression. *J Am Acad Child Adolesc Psychiatry* 2006;45:280–288. doi:10.1097/01.chi.0000192250.38400.9e.
20. Wagner KD, Robb AS, Findling RL, et al. A randomized, placebo-controlled trial of citalopram for the treatment of major depression in children and adolescents. *Am J Psychiatry* 2004;161:1079–1083.

21. Wagner KD, Ambrosini P, Rynn M, et al. Efficacy of sertraline in the treatment of children and adolescents with major depressive disorder: two randomized controlled trials. *JAMA* 2003;290:1033–1041. doi:10.1001/jama.290.8.1033.

22. von Knorring AL, Olsson GI, Thomsen PH, et al. A randomized, double-blind, placebo-controlled study of citalopram in adolescents with major depressive disorder. *J Clin Psychopharmacol* 2006;26:311–315. doi:10.1097/01.jcp.0000219051.40632.d5.

23. Berard R, Fong R, Carpenter DJ, et al. An international, multicenter, placebo-controlled trial of paroxetine in adolescents with major depressive disorder. *J Child Adolesc Psychopharmacol* 2006;16:59–75. doi:10.1089/cap.2006.16.59.

24. Emslie GJ, Wagner KD, Kutcher S, et al. Paroxetine treatment in children and adolescents with major depressive disorder: a randomized, multicenter, double-blind, placebo-controlled trial. *J Am Acad Child Adolesc Psychiatry* 2006;45:709–719. doi:10.1097/01.chi.0000214189.73240.63.

25. Keller MB, Ryan ND, Strober M, et al. Efficacy of paroxetine in the treatment of adolescent major depression: a randomized, controlled trial. *J Am Acad Child Adolesc Psychiatry* 2001;40:762–772. doi:10.1097/00004583-200107000-00010.

26. Lam RW, Kennedy SH, Grigoriadis S, et al. Canadian Network for Mood and Anxiety Treatments (CANMAT) clinical guidelines for the management of major depressive disorder in adults. III. Pharmacotherapy. *J Affect Disord* 2009;117 (suppl 1):S26–S43. doi:10.1016/j.jad.2009.06.041.

27. Birmaher B, Brent D; AACAP Work Group on Quality Issues, et al. Practice parameter for the assessment and treatment of children and adolescents with depressive disorders. *J Am Acad Child Adolesc Psychiatry* 2007;46:1503–1526. doi:10.1097/chi.0b013e318145ae1c.

28. *Association of CELEXA (citalopram hydrobromide) with Dose-Dependent QT Prolongation.* 2012. Available at http://www.healthycanadians.gc.ca/recall-alert-rappel-avis/hc-sc/2012/14672a-eng.php

29. Food and Drug Administration. *FDA drug safety communication: revised recommendations for Celexa (citalopram hydrobromide) related to a potential risk of abnormal heart rhythms with high doses.* 2011. Available at http://www.fda.gov/drugs/drugsafety/ucm297391.htm

30. Canada H. *Antidepressant Cipralex (escitalopram): updated information regarding dose-related heart risk.* 2012. Available at http://www.healthycanadians.gc.ca/recall-alert-rappel-avis/hc-sc/2012/13674a-eng.php

31. Food and Drug Administration. 2005. Available at http://www.fda.gov/drug/antidepressants/antidepressants_MG

32. Sakolsky D, Birmaher B. Developmentally informed pharmacotherapy for child and adolescent depressive disorders. *Child Adolesc Psychiatr Clin N Am* 2012;21:313–325, viii.

33. Connolly SD, Bernstein GA; Work Group on Quality Issues, et al. Practice parameters for the assessment and treatment of children and adolescents with anxiety disorders. *J Am Acad Child Adolesc Psychiatry* 2007;46(2):267–283.

34. Rapee RM, Schniering CA, Hudson JL, et al. Anxiety disorders during childhood and adolescence: origins and treatment. *Annu Rev Clin Psychol* 2009;5:311–341.

35. Connolly SD, Suarez L, Sylvester C, et al. Assessment and treatment of anxiety disorders in children and adolescents. *Curr Psychiatry Rep* 2007;13:99–110.

36. Bittner A, Egger HL, Erkanli A, et al. What do childhood anxiety disorders predict? *J Child Psychol Psychiatry* 2007;48:1174–1183.

37. Beck A.T, Steer RA, et al., *Manual for the Beck Anxiety Inventory.* San Antonio, TX: Psychological Corportation. 1990.

38. March JS, Parker JD, Sullivan K, et al. The Multidimensional Anxiety Scale for Childre (MASC): factor structure, reliability and validity. *J Am Acad Adolesc Psychiatry* 1997;36:554–565.

39. Birmaher B, Brent DA, Chiappetta, et al. Psychometric properties of the Screen for Child Anxiety Related Emotional Disorders (SCARED): scale construction and psychometric characteristics. *J Am Acad Child Adolesc Psychiatry* 1999;36:545–553.

40. Monga S, Birmaher B, Chiappetta L, et al. Screen for Child Anxiety-Related Emotional Disorders (SCARED): convergent and divergent validity. *Depress Anxiety* 2000;12:85–91.

41. Rapee RM, Lyneham HJ, Hudson JL, et al. Effect of comorbidity on treatment of anxious children and adolescents: results from a large combined sample. *J Am Acad Child Adolesc Psychiatry* 2013;52(1):47–56.

42. Compto SN, March JS, Brent D, et al. Cognitive-behavioral psychotherapy for anxiety and depressive disorders in children and adolescents: an evidence-based medicine review. *J Am Acad Child Adolesc Psychiatry* 2013;43(8):930–959.

43. Compton SN, Walkup JT, Albano AM, et al. Child/Adolescent Anxiety Multimodal Study (CAMS): rationale, design, and methods. *Child Adolesc Psychiatry Ment Health* 2010;4:1, 1–15.

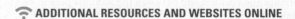 **ADDITIONAL RESOURCES AND WEBSITES ONLINE**

CHAPTER 70

Suicide and Suicidal Behavior in Adolescents and Young Adults

David A Brent
Candice Biernesser

KEY WORDS

- Assessment
- Psychotherapy
- Risk factors
- Suicide
- Suicide attempt
- Vulnerable populations

Suicide is the third leading cause of death in both adolescents and young adults (AYAs) aged 18 to 25 years.[1] In this chapter, we first offer standard definitions for different types of self-destructive behavior, describe some of the most commonly used models of suicidal risk, provide a framework for the assessment of key domains of suicidal risk and determination of imminent suicidal risk, identify some special populations of AYAs who are vulnerable to suicidal behavior, and provide guidelines for clinical management.

DEFINITIONS

The following set of definitions follow the widely accepted Columbia Classification Algorithm for Suicide Assessment[2]:

A. A *suicide attempt* is a self-inflicted injury with stated or inferred intent to die.
B. *Suicide* is a suicide attempt that results in a fatal outcome.
C. *Suicidal ideation* is present when the patient has thoughts of his or her own death without actually engaging in suicidal behavior. Ideation can range from "passive ideation," in which the patient thinks about his or her death, without any plan, to "active" suicidal ideation with an explicit plan and intent to act on suicidal thoughts. Intermediate to ideation and attempt are "aborted" and "interrupted" attempts.
D. *"Aborted attempts"* occur when a person begins to make a suicide attempt but stops him or herself before experiencing injury.
E. *"Interrupted attempts"* occur when the person is engaging in preparatory behavior of a suicide attempt, and another party intervenes prior to the occurrence of injury.
F. *Nonsuicidal self-injury* (NSSI) refers to purposeful, often repetitive or stereotyped self-injury with a motivation other than death, such as relief from emotional pain, self-punishment, or to gain attention.[3]

EPIDEMIOLOGY

Suicidal Ideation and Behavior

The incidence of suicidal ideation and suicidal behavior increases markedly after puberty and peaks in incidence during adolescence. The lifetime prevalence of suicide attempts in one recent survey of adolescents was 4.1%, with 4.0% having experienced suicidal ideation with a plan, and 12.1% having experienced any suicidal ideation.[4] The Youth Risk Behavior Survey[5] found somewhat higher 1-year incidences with 17.0% seriously considering suicide, 13.6% having a suicidal plan, and 8.0% having attempted suicide. The 1-year incidence of the spectrum of suicidal ideation and behavior is higher in females compared to males, Hispanics as opposed to other racial and/or ethnic groups, and younger versus older adolescents.[5] In the 2014 National College Health Association National College Health Assessment,[6] 8.1% of students seriously considered suicide (one-fourth under the influence of alcohol) and 1.3% made a suicide attempt.

Suicide

Suicide, that is, a suicide attempt that results in death, is much rarer than nonfatal suicide attempts.

- Age: Among US youth aged 10 to 14, 15 to 19, and 20 to 24 years, the suicide rates per 100,000 in 2009 were 1.3, 7.8, and 12.5, respectively.
- Gender: Suicide in males is twice as high as the rate in females in those 10 to 14 years old, 4 times as high in 15- to 19-year-olds, and five times higher in 20- to 24-year-olds.[7]
- Ethnicity: The suicide rate among Native Americans/Native Alaskans is 2.5 times higher than the rest of the population, and peaks in young adulthood, whereas suicide in most other ethnic groups tends to increase with age.[7]
- Method: The most common method for suicide in the US among 10- to 14-year-olds is hanging, but older AYAs most commonly use firearms to kill themselves.

MODELS OF SUICIDAL RISK

Diathesis Stress Models

This model hypothesizes that suicide and suicidal behavior are a result of a vulnerability to suicidal behavior, based on a tendency to act impulsively in the face of intolerable emotional distress. This vulnerability combined with stressors such as low mood, hopelessness, or loss lead to suicidal behaviors.[8] A variation of this model is the potential imbalance between distress (e.g., such as increased depression) and decreased restraint (e.g., loaded gun or intoxicated state).[9]

Interpersonal Theory of Suicide

This theory posits that suicide behaviors are a result of the convergence of perceived burdens, thwarted belongingness, and acquired capability for suicide.[10] According to this theory, NSSI leads to desensitization to physical pain and injury, which then results in an increased willingness to consider and to engage in suicidal behavior.

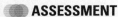

ASSESSMENT

Assessment of Suicidal Behavior Risk Factors

The most significant risk factors for suicidal behavior include past and current suicidal ideation and behavior, psychopathology, medical comorbidity, psychological traits, family and environmental factors, and availability of lethal agents.

Past Suicidal Ideation and Behavior

Past suicidal ideation and behavior are both risk factors for future suicide and suicide attempts.

- In adolescents, around 29% of those with suicidal ideation will make a suicide attempt within one year, whereas 56% of those with suicidal ideation with a plan will make an attempt during this time frame.[4]
- Among those with suicidal ideation, predictors of eventual suicide and suicide attempts are the most severe lifetime occurrence of suicidal ideation, as well as the frequency, intensity, and duration of current ideation.
- In those who have actually attempted suicide, the strongest predictors of suicide reattempt are regret about having survived and evidence of high suicidal intent, the latter of which refers to behavior indicative of a wish to die.[11] For example, evidence of high suicidal intent includes prior planning, arranging the attempt so as not to be discovered, and expressing or thinking that the goal of the attempt was death. Conversely, AYAs with strong reasons for living are less likely to engage in suicidal behavior, even in the face of strong suicidal risk.[12]

Motivation

AYAs often engage in suicidal behaviors for reasons other than to die, such as to escape psychological pain or painful circumstances, to get attention, to express hostility, or to try to get someone to change their mind about a relationship breakup or a punishment.[9] Precipitants for the suicidal behavior or ideation are important to ascertain, because part of the assessment for safety is determining if the precipitant is likely to recur. Table 70.1 provides common precipitants to suicidal behavior in children, younger adolescents, and older AYAs.

NSSI is usually motivated by a desire to relieve negative affect or a sense of numbness, but can also be a means to escape a stressful social or academic situation, or to engage in self-punishment.[3] Although the characteristics of those with NSSI are different than those who engage in suicide attempts, both behaviors share difficulties in emotion regulation and high levels of negative affect. Consequently, NSSI is a strong eventual predictor for a suicide attempt, perhaps even stronger than a previous suicide attempt.[13]

Psychopathology

Almost any psychiatric disorder can increase the risk for suicidal ideation and behavior.[5,11] Of all the disorders, depression is the most strongly associated with suicidal ideation. Suicidal behavior seems to occur as a result of a confluence of ideation related to depression or hopelessness; increased distress related to conditions such as panic disorder or posttraumatic stress disorder; and greater disinhibition that can occur with insomnia, alcohol and drug abuse, or behavioral disorders.[4,11] In AYAs, depression and especially bipolar disorder pose the highest risk for completed and attempted suicide. In later adolescence and young adulthood, eating disorders, psychotic disorders, alcohol and substance abuse, and impulsive aggressive personality traits increase the risk for completed and attempted suicide, especially when comorbid with mood disorders.[11]

Medical Comorbidity

The following medical conditions have been associated with an increased risk for suicidality.[11,14–16]:

- Symptoms of insomnia
- Symptoms of pain
- Medical conditions that affect the central nervous system, such as epilepsy and migraine
- Conditions that have an inflammatory component, such as asthma, inflammatory bowel disease, or obesity
- Traumatic brain injury, particularly in military populations

Psychological Characteristics

The following psychological conditions have been associated with an increased risk for suicidality:

- Hopelessness or pessimism about the future predicts treatment nonadherence, dropout, higher suicidal intent, and repetition of suicidal behavior.[11]
- Impulsive aggression or a tendency to engage in hostility or actual aggression in response to frustration or provocation is a strong predictor of suicidal behavior, is a precursor for mood disorder, and may explain some aspects of the familial transmission of suicidal behavior.
- Neurocognitive tests show that suicide attempters are more impulsive, less effective at generating alternatives solutions when faced with problems, and less able to engage in delayed gratification.[11]

Association with Health Risk Behaviors

Suicidal behavior is associated with a range of other health risk behaviors (e.g., having unprotected sex, weapon carrying), in part due to the common denominators of poor impulse control, difficulties with delayed gratification, and impaired ability to consider the longer-term consequences of behavior.[11]

Family and Environmental Risk Factors

- Parental history of suicidal behavior. Adoption, twin, and family studies show that a parental history of suicidal behavior increases the risk for suicidal behavior in offspring and that this relationship cannot be accounted for by the familial transmission of depression or by imitation.[11]
- Parental history of mental illness. Parental depression, alcohol and substance abuse, and antisocial disorder also contribute to risk for adolescent suicidal behavior.[17]
- Family climate. Family climate, discord, and abuse and neglect contribute to risk for suicidal behavior.
- Peer victimization. Bullying is a strong predictor of suicidal behavior.[18]
- Exposure to suicide. Exposure through media publicity or knowing someone who has attempted suicide has a modest but real increase on the risk for suicidal behavior and suicide.[19] The effect is less pronounced if the exposure is to completed rather than attempted suicide and if the exposee was a close friend of the suicide victim.[11]
- Protective factors include a positive relationship with at least one parent, adequate parental monitoring and supervision, a prosocial peer group, and strong connection to school.[11]

Availability of Lethal Agents

Particularly in AYAs, suicidal behavior tends to be more impulsive than suicide in older adults, and therefore the availability of

TABLE 70.1
Precipitants for Suicidal Behavior

Most Common Precipitants for Suicidal Behavior by Age-Group	
Older AYAs	Conflicts with peers and/or romantic partners
Younger adolescents	Conflicts with parents
Very young children	Child abuse

potentially lethal agents of suicide contribute to increased suicidal risk.[11] Case-control studies consistently show that having a gun in the home, particularly one that is loaded and unsecured, increases the risk for suicide in young people. Conversely, restricting access to guns has been shown to be associated with a lowered suicide rate. In Southeast Asia, availability of pesticides has an analogous effect on suicide risk.

Assessment of Imminent Risk

The task of the clinician assessing the suicidal AYAs is to determine whether there is imminent risk for suicidal behavior. Many of the factors noted above contribute to increased suicidal risk over a lifetime (e.g., family history of suicide) but do not necessarily increase a person's risk for suicide in the immediate present. Imminent suicidal risk is determined by factors that dramatically increase distress (depression, panic disorder, pain, acute loss), decrease restraint (intoxication, availability of a loaded gun), or both (insomnia, bipolar mixed state, psychosis).

Special Populations at Increased Risk for Suicide

Table 70.2 outlines the special populations at increased risk for suicide.

TABLE 70.2		
Special Populations at Increased Risk: Relationships with Suicidal Behavior		
LGBTQ	Effect	Sexual minority youth have consistently been found to have increased rates of substance abuse, depression, and suicidal behavior.
	Why?	The relationship between sexual minority status and suicidal behavior has been found to be mediated by parental rejection and peer victimization and may be in part explained by higher rates of early abuse among sexual minority youth.[20,21]
Incarceration	Effect	Suicidal behavior is increased in juvenile justice and prisons.
	Why?	Incarceration is highly stressful and is associated with past suicidal behavior and nonsuicidal self-harm, previous history of childhood trauma, and history of violence.[22,23]
Military	Effect	The suicide rate has increased dramatically in the American military, particularly among non-officers.
	Why?	Factors that contribute to suicidal risk in this population include posttraumatic stress disorder, sleep disturbance, marital and family stress, and traumatic brain injury.[16,24]
Indigenous peoples	Effect	Suicide and suicidal behavior are dramatically higher in indigenous than in European peoples across Westernized countries.
	Why?	Common contributing factors are erosion of tradition cultural values and social structures, economic deprivation, discrimination, and high unemployment, and high rates of alcohol and substance abuse.[25]

General Assessment

The clinical interview is the main tool available to clinicians when assessing an adolescent or young adult with suicidal ideation, although self-report questionnaires can be a helpful adjunct since some patients will disclose ideation on a questionnaire but not in an interview. The simplest self-report is the four-item Adolescent Suicide Questionnaire[26] that inquires about ideation and attempt. There is also a suicide ideation item on the nine-item Patient Health Questionnaire-9[27] that assesses for depression. The Columbia Suicide Severity Rating Scale[28] has both a self-report and interview form and assesses for recent ideation and behavior.

There is now evidence showing that asking about suicide does *not* put an adolescent or young adult at increased risk for suicide. Initially, the adolescent or young adult should be interviewed alone. Whenever possible, collateral history (e.g., family member or significant other) should supplement the interview. When conducting the interview, the clinician should keep in mind the general risk and protective factors associated with suicide. The initial encounter with a suicidal dolescent or young adult is critical and should include the following:

- Current suicidality
  - Recent attempt (especially if has regret about surviving)
  - Current ideation, frequency, intrusiveness, duration
  - Presence of plan and/or intent to carry it out
  - Reasons why the patient has **not** acted on suicidal thoughts
  - Past suicidal behavior and ideation, including worst
- Factors that increase distress, and suicidal risk
  - Depression
  - Hopelessness
  - NSSI (especially if frequent and with use of multiple methods)
  - Anxiety
  - Eating disorder
  - Chronic medical condition
- Factors that reduce inhibition
  - Sleep difficulties
  - Alcohol/substance abuse
  - Impulsivity and poor emotion regulation
  - Availability and storage of lethal agents (firearms, sharps, medication)
  - Exposure to friend who has attempted or completed suicide
- Factors that protect against suicide risk
  - Connection with parent, friends, school
  - Reasons for staying alive
  - Cultural or religious beliefs
- Contextual factors that increase suicide risk
  - Peer victimization
  - Lesbian, gay, bisexual, transgender, queer, questioning, intersex (LGBTQI), sexual orientation/identity
  - Parent child discord
  - Recent loss or humiliation
  - Parental depression or substance abuse
  - Interparental discord
  - Abuse, neglect, or exposure to domestic violence
- Availability of lethal means (e.g., access to a gun).

MANAGEMENT

Empirically Supported Treatment

Although depression is a significant risk factor for suicide, the treatment of depression, whether with antidepressants, psychotherapy, or both appears to be necessary, but not sufficient to prevent or relieve suicidal ideation and behavior.[29]

XV

Antidepressants

Antidepressants result in a slight, but statistically significant increase in suicidal events (suicide attempts or increase in suicidal ideation), compared to placebo in AYAs, but not in older adults; however, 11 times more depressed youth will respond to an antidepressant than will develop a suicidal event.[30] Pharmacoepidemiological studies find that there is an association between greater use of antidepressants and reduced rates of suicide in youth.[12]

Psychotherapy

In adults, the most widely studied intervention is dialectic behavior therapy (DBT), which focuses on learning emotion regulation (common in chronically suicidal individuals) and interpersonal effectiveness skills to cope with difficulties in distress tolerance. DBT has been shown to be more efficacious than expert treatment of borderline personality disorders and treatment as usual. However, when compared to similarly intense psychodynamic intervention, DBT showed similar efficacy.[29]

Another intervention that has been shown in one study to reduce recurrence of suicide attempts is a version of cognitive behavior therapy (CBT) that focuses on hopelessness and the cognitive distortions leading to suicidal ideation and behavior. In this treatment, which targeted a very ill, inner city, often homeless, and substance-abusing population, approximately nine sessions of CBT plus treatment as usual resulted in nearly half the rate of attempts compared to treatment as usual alone.[29]

In adolescents, there have been no large-scale positive intervention studies.[29] However, interventions that target family attachment, mentalization (conceptualization of actions in terms of thoughts and feelings), substance abuse, and family interaction have been shown to reduce ideation, self-harm, or actual suicide attempts. Interventions that have focused primarily on individual skills, or that have exclusively targeted safety, adherence, and follow-up have not been successful in reducing self-harm recidivism.[29]

Clinical Approach[9]

Determination of Level of Care

The first task of the clinician facing a suicidal adolescent or young adult is to determine what intensity and restrictiveness (e.g., inpatient versus outpatient care) of treatment best fits the degree of the patient's suicidal risk. The higher the clinician's assessment of imminent suicidal risk, the greater should be the intensity and restrictiveness of care. A safety plan, which is a set of strategies that the patient can implement to cope with suicidal urges, should be developed collaboratively with the patient and a trusted individual (e.g., parent for adolescents and a stable romantic partner for young adult) and can help the clinician determine the level of care required.[31] Specifically, the clinician should assess the extent to which the patient is able to engage collaboratively in the development of the plan and the likelihood that the patient will actually implement the plan. This will help determine if the patient can safely be treated as an outpatient.

Development of Safety Plan

The safety plan is developed on the basis of the clinician's knowledge of the precipitants, motivation, and emotional, behavioral, cognitive, and contextual triggers that led up to the suicide attempt and is implemented in a stepwise fashion:

- Recognize signs of distress.
- Take steps to reduce stress before it results in a suicidal crisis.
- If, suicidal, review reasons for staying alive.
- Engage in personal strategies that will distract from, or mitigate suicidal urges, for example, listening to music, going for a walk, looking at a picture of a favorite place, or deep breathing.
- Reaching out to pre-identified trusted individuals for support
- Professional contact with therapist, emergency department, crisis line, ambulance, or police

Chain Analysis and Development of a Treatment Plan

A chain analysis is a detailed review of the events, thoughts, feelings, behaviors, and contextual factors that led up to a suicidal crisis.[9,31] From the chain analysis, one can then identify different inflexion points that potentially could result in de-escalation of the suicidal crisis. By reviewing these possible strategies with the patient and a trusted support figure (e.g., parent for an adolescent or adult sibling, close friend, or romantic partner for young adult), the clinician can develop a hierarchy of interventions based on ease of implementation, likelihood that the patient/family perceives that the intervention will be practiced and used, and the likelihood that the intervention will contribute to reduction of suicidal risk. Those interventions that the patient is likely to use and that the therapist and patient think can reduce imminent suicidal risk should be deployed first.

Case Example

Courtney is a 15-year-old sophomore in high school who has been victimized by peers at school. Her parents and teachers have not been sympathetic, but think she ought to get more assertive and stand up for her rights. Your assessment finds that Courtney is shy, with social anxiety and depression. The main precipitant for her suicidal urges is being bullied at school, and then being told that she is not assertive enough by her parents and teachers. When assessing Courtney's reasons for living, she gives as reasons that she would like to be the head of a software company someday and also that she would not want to abandon her puppy. In meeting with Courtney and her parents, the clinician explains that the most effective approach to peer victimization is for the school to take steps to make it clear to the victimizers and their families that the school has a zero tolerance for bullying. In addition, the clinician, therapist, and parent come up with ways of responding to the victimization through self-talk and not showing a strong emotional reaction to the teasing. Furthermore, when the patient experiences suicidal urges, she is to carry a picture of her pet puppy, and also to carry a business card that shows her as the CEO of her own software company, whose motto is "Ingenious Solutions to Outrageous Problems." She identified a school nurse to whom she could go to if stressed at school, and, if previous strategies were not successful, could reach out to the clinician and emergency facilities for professional contact. The parents received education about the nature of peer victimization as well as the current limitations of their daughter given her social anxiety and helped them to project a more supportive response to their daughter's experience of victimization. The clinician coached parents and patient on how to get the school to take action against the victimizers.

The treatment plan included parental education about peer victimization and social phobia, ways to be supportive of their daughter, treatment that targeted the patient's social phobia, and intervention into the school situation to reduce or ideally eliminate the bullying. Specifically, the patient was taught techniques of distraction, distress tolerance, and emotion regulation to cope with peer teasing and her own social anxiety, as well as graduated exposure to building her confidence and competence in social situations.

Organization of Mental Health Services

There is evidence that the greater the extent that certain service elements and quality indicators for mental health care delivery were implemented in a given region, the greater the reduction in the suicide rate.[32] In regions in the United Kingdom, programs that implemented quality improvement in services, namely providing rapid access to emergency evaluation of suicidal individuals, assertive follow-up of those who were nonadherent, case management for the transition from inpatient to outpatient care, and integrated mental health and substance abuse treatment, showed significant declines in suicide.

Suicidal ideation and behavior are common and often emergent problems in adolescence and young adulthood and are significant risk factors for completed suicide, which is a major source of mortality in AYAs. Assessment of current and past suicidality, including frequency and intensity of ideation, suicidal intent, and the motivation and precipitant for suicidality, can help to shape safety and treatment plans. In addition, other relevant targets for treatment will likely include psychopathology, certain psychological traits, family and environmental stressors, and method restriction (removing or securing potentially lethal methods of suicide [e.g., firearms]). Efficacious treatments incorporate safety planning into their interventions, and have a focus on family, sobriety, and/or emotion regulation. More responsive, coordinated, and assertive follow-up care may also be effective in reducing the risk for suicide.

REFERENCES

1. Center for Disease Control Website. *10 leading causes of death, United States* Available at http://webappa.cdc.gov/cgi-bin/broker.exe. Accessed January 14, 2014.
2. Posner K, Oquendo MA, Gould M, et al. Columbia Classification Algorithm of Suicide Assessment (C-CASA): classification of suicidal events in the FDA's pediatric suicidal risk analysis of antidepressants. *Am J Psychiatry* 2007;164(7):1035–1043.
3. Nock MK. Why do people hurt themselves? New insights into the nature and functions of self-injury. *Curr Dir Psychol Sci* 2009;18(2):78–83.
4. Nock MK, Green JG, Hwang I, et al. Prevalence, correlates, and treatment of lifetime suicidal behavior among adolescents: results from the National Comorbidity Survey Replication Adolescent Supplement. *JAMA Psychiatry* 2013;70(3):300–310.
5. Kann L, Knichen S, Shanklin, S, et al. Youth risk behavior surveillance—United States, 2013. *MMWR Surveill Summ* 2013;63(4):11–13.
6. American College Health Association. *American College Health Association-National College Health Assessment II: Reference Group Executive Summary, Spring 2014.* Hanover, MD: American College Health Association, 2014. Available at http://www.acha-ncha.org/reports_ACHA-NCHAII.html
7. Crosby AE, Ortega L, Stevens MR, et al. Suicides—United States, 2005–2009. *MMWR Surveill Summ* 2013;62 (suppl 3):179–183.
8. Mann JJ, Waternaux C, Haas GL, et al. Toward a clinical model of suicidal behavior in psychiatric patients. *Am J Psychiatry* 1999;156(2):181–189.
9. Brent DA, Poling KD, Goldstein TR. Treating depressed and suicidal adolescents: a clinician's guide. New York, NY: Guilford Press, 2011.
10. Van Orden KA, Witte TK, Cukrowicz KC, et al. The interpersonal theory of suicide. *Psychol Rev* 2010;117(2):575–600.
11. Bridge JA, Goldstein TR, Brent DA. Adolescent suicide and suicidal behavior. *J Child Psychol Psychiatry* 2006;47(3/4):372–394.
12. Pinto A, Whisman MA, Conwell Y. Reasons for living in a clinical sample of adolescents. *J Adolesc* 1998;21(4):397–405.
13. Wilkinson PO. Nonsuicidal self-injury: a clear marker for suicide risk. *J Am Acad Child Adolesc Psychiatry* 2011;50(8):741–743.
14. Goldstein TR, Bridge JA, Brent DA. Sleep disturbance preceding completed suicide in adolescents. *J Consult Clin Psychol* 2008;76(1):84–91.
15. Scott KM, Hwang I, Chiu WT, et al. Chronic physical conditions and their association with first onset of suicidal behavior in the World Mental Health surveys. *Psychosom Med* 2010;72(7):712–719.
16. Bryan CJ, Clemans TA. Repetitive traumatic brain injury, psychological symptoms, and suicide risk in a clinical sample of deployed military personnel. *JAMA Psychiatry* 2013;70(7):686–691.
17. Gureje O, Oladeji B, Hwang I, et al. Parental psychopathology and the risk of suicidal behavior in their offspring: results from the World Mental Health surveys. *Mol Psychiatry* 2011;16(12):1221–1233.
18. Brunstein Klomek A, Sourander A, Gould M. The association of suicide and bullying in childhood to young adulthood: a review of cross-sectional and longitudinal research findings. *Can J Psychiatry* 2010;55(5):282–288.
19. Haw C, Hawton K, Niedzwiedz C, et al. Suicide clusters: a review of risk factors and mechanisms. *Suicide Life Threat Behav* 2013;43(1):97–108.
20. Marshal MP, Dietz LJ, Friedman MS, et al. Suicidality and depression disparities between sexual minority and heterosexual youth: a meta-analytic review. *J Adolesc Health* 2011;49(2):115–123.
21. Burton CM, Marshal MP, Chisolm DJ, et al. Sexual minority-related victimization as a mediator of mental health disparities in sexual minority youth: a longitudinal analysis. *J Youth Adolesc* 2013;42(3):394–402.
22. Humber N, Webb R, Piper M, et al. A national case-control study of risk factors for suicide among prisoners in England and Wales [corrected]. *Soc Psychiatry Psychiatr Epidemiol* 2013;48(7):1177–1185.
23. McReynolds LS, Wasserman GA. Self-injury in incarcerated juvenile females: contributions of mental health and traumatic experiences. *J Trauma Stress* 2011;24(6):752–755.
24. Nock MK, Deming CA, Fullerton CS, et al. Suicide among soldiers: a review of psychosocial risk and protective factors. *Psychiatry* 2013;76(2):97–125.
25. Clifford AC, Doran CM, Tsey K. A systematic review of suicide prevention interventions targeting indigenous peoples in Australia, United States, Canada and New Zealand. *BMC Public Health* 2013;13:463.
26. Horowitz LM, Bridge JA, Teach SJ, et al. Ask Suicide-Screening Questions (ASQ): a brief instrument for the Pediatric Emergency Department. *Arch Pediatr Adolesc Med* 2012;166(12):1170–1176.
27. Kroenke K, Spitzer RL. The PHQ-9: a new depression and diagnostic severity measure. *Psychiatric Annals* 2002;32:509–521.
28. Posner K, Brown GK, Stanley B, et al. The Columbia-Suicide Severity Rating Scale: initial validity and internal consistency findings from three multisite studies with adolescents and adults. *Am J Psychiatry* 2011;168(12):1266–1277.
29. Brent DA, McMakin DL, Kennard BD, et al. Protecting adolescents from self-harm: a critical review of intervention studies. *J Am Acad Child Adolesc Psychiatry* 2013;52(12):1260–1271.
30. Bridge JA, Iyengar S, Salary CB, et al. Clinical response and risk for reported suicidal ideation and suicide attempts in pediatric antidepressant treatment: a meta-analysis of randomized controlled trials. *JAMA* 2007;297(15):1683–1696.
31. Stanley B, Brown G, Brent DA, et al. Cognitive-behavioral therapy for suicide prevention (CBT-SP): treatment model, feasibility, and acceptability. *J Am Acad Child Adolesc Psychiatry* 2009;48(10):1005–1013.
32. While D, Bickley H, Roscoe A, et al. Implementation of mental health service recommendations in England and Wales and suicide rates, 1997–2006: a cross-sectional and before-and-after observational study. *Lancet* 2012;379(9820):1005–1012.

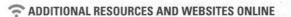 **ADDITIONAL RESOURCES AND WEBSITES ONLINE**

CHAPTER 71

Attention Deficit Hyperactivity Disorder and School Problems

Earl J. Soileau, Jr.

Attention deficit hyperactivity disorder (ADHD) has now been defined as a neurodevelopmental disorder that causes hyperactivity, impulsive behavior, and attention problems. The recent change in labeling underscores that while the disorder begins in childhood it can persist through adulthood for some people. As many as 10% of school children are affected with this disorder; however, the prevalence and incidence of those who have been diagnosed as adolescents and young adults (AYAs) are not clear. In AYAs with ADHD, the ratio of males to females is between 2 and 3 to 1. The evidence suggests that there is a lowered percentage of AYAs who meet diagnostic criteria.[1] Regardless, data are clear that many negative outcomes exist for those left untreated in the AYA years.[2] Treatment can provide enormous benefit and it is important for providers to have a clear understanding of the risks and benefits of treatment, as well as practical strategies to approach both the evaluation and management of this common disorder. In addition, clinicians should be aware that although school difficulties during adolescence and young adulthood may be the result of ADHD, one should also consider the possibility of learning disabilities, school phobias, avoidance, and other academic performance problems.

ATTENTION DEFICIT HYPERACTIVITY DISORDER

ADHD is characterized by the presence of the three major symptoms that include the following:

- Difficulty maintaining focus and paying attention
- Struggles with controlling impulsive behavior
- Troubles with hyperactivity

Often this cluster is evident in early childhood and persists throughout the child's life course. These major symptoms make it difficult for an adolescent or young adult to get along with others, make and maintain relationships, remember what they have learned, complete school work in a timely fashion, meet school and work deadlines, communicate with teachers and parents, organize their lives, resolve disagreements, and follow rules. Many individuals with ADHD have difficulty with the developmental tasks of adolescence and young adulthood such as developing independence, identity formation, and making career decisions. As would be expected, these failures often result in low self-esteem and depressive symptoms.[2,3] If motor overactivity or hyperactivity is present initially, this high activity level tends to subside in early adolescence. In contrast, impulse control and inattentive symptoms during childhood

persist in 60% to 80% of adolescents and upward of 50% continue to meet diagnostic criteria for ADHD into adulthood.[4,5] For many adults, mental overactivity or restlessness is a common manifestation. When motor overactivity is present in early adolescence, many will become normally active or underactive in adulthood.[6–8] Impulse control tends to improve during the middle adolescent years and resolves in many. Difficulty in the cognitive domains, for example, working memory, memory organization, perseverance in tasks, and distractibility, appears to continue in most, but not all. Young adults tend to continue to have difficulty in the cognitive domains, but may not be as symptomatic if they are occupied in jobs they find interesting and enjoyable. Among college students, these cognitive challenge requirements increase rather than decrease and most young adults become more symptomatic throughout the college years.

Etiology

At present, the etiology of ADHD is not clear, although studies suggest that ADHD results from a combination of genetic and environmental factors. Twin studies suggest a high heritability in ADHD with estimates near 80%.[9,10] Molecular genetic studies reveal that there are likely multiple gene systems that affect core symptoms.[11] Clearly, the environment plays a role and is superimposed on the genetic backdrop. For instance, there is evidence to suggest a potential link between cigarette smoking and alcohol use during pregnancy and ADHD. There is also evidence to suggest that individuals who have suffered a brain injury show some similar behaviors to those with ADHD.

Advances in brain imaging technology have shown structural and functional brain differences between individuals with and without ADHD.[12,13] Longitudinal brain imaging studies have shown that ADHD is characterized by a delay in structural brain maturation; although the brain matures in a normal pattern, it is delayed about 3 years.[12,13] This delay is associated with regions of the brain involved in thinking, attention, and planning.[13] Further studies using brain imaging and cognitive evaluation may help clarify how this disorder develops.

Diagnosis and Assessment

The diagnosis of ADHD is based on a clear picture of the adolescent or young adult's current function and history of difficulties. The provider should consider gathering information from three sources, that is, home, school, and the adolescent or young adult.[14,15] The parent, significant other, or close friend represents one source of information from the home and social sphere. To assess behavior in the school or work setting, information is gathered from teachers, employers, coaches, or coworkers. Clinicians should conduct a separate interview with adolescent or young adult as it allows the young person to self-report problems and concerns that they have been experiencing and it allows the clinician to identify signs or symptoms consistent with ADHD or suggestive of other serious comorbid disorders.

It is important for the provider to carefully evaluate descriptions of the problem(s) and to characterize the symptoms. The provider should determine if the symptoms occur frequently, interfere with functioning, and appear to be acute or chronic. Often it is helpful to seek out specific examples of such difficulties, for example, inability to complete homework or difficulty organizing simple tasks, to mention a few.

The evaluation should include a review of the medical and mental health history, psychosocial, and family histories.

Complete Medical History

A complete medical history, including prenatal exposures to tobacco, drugs, alcohol, perinatal complications or infections, developmental delay, central nervous system infection, head trauma, recurrent otitis media, and current or past medication use, should be determined. The history should include an exploration of hearing or visual impairments, sleep disturbances, thyroid abnormalities, and neurologic or cognitive impairments. This will help to distinguish ADHD from other medical conditions.

In addition, a review of current or past substance use should be determined.

It is particularly important to obtain a dietary history (i.e., appetite, picky eating), history of sleep patterns, and family cardiac history and cardiac review of systems before initiation of pharmacotherapy to avoid attributing preexisting problems to medications.

Family history of similar behaviors is important because ADHD is highly heritable. In addition, family history of other mental disorders can be helpful in determining the nature of comorbid disorders.

Questionnaires

Typically, representatives from all three domains are not present at the clinical encounter when assessing the adolescent or young adult, which requires the provider to rely on the use of some type of written report from the teacher or employer. Reliable standardized measures are available that enhance an accurate diagnosis (Table 71.1). Parents, teachers, and employers report their observations using various formats, and responses can be used to elucidate discussion as well as provide required documentation. In addition, there are self-report versions for AYAs to complete to ensure accurate and confirming information for each core domain. For young adults, documentation may be required by universities and athletic associations such as the National College Athletic Association, so that they can provide supportive classroom modifications and allow for the use of medication. It is important for the clinician to

remember that questionnaires and checklists are used as collateral information, but by themselves do not make a diagnosis.

The accepted standard for diagnosis remains the clinical interview. The interview delineates a persistent pattern of ADHD symptoms for more than 6 months and should use information from two or more informants who have exposure to the patient in at least two of the three domains.[14,15] Older AYAs may present for evaluation alone. For older youth, it may be difficult to obtain written reports or completed questionnaires from a teacher, employer, or parent, but it is an important component to confirm the diagnosis. Objective observers such as teachers, parents, or employers will see the older adolescent in limited situations such as in the classroom or home, and their input must be interpreted within this context. In these extreme cases where adult informants in key domains are not available, the use of peer observation may be helpful.

Differential Diagnosis

A number of disorders and factors may produce symptoms similar to those of ADHD; however, these are usually suggested by a thorough history and physical examination.

Medical

Medical conditions that may have similar clinical features or presentation to ADHD include hearing or visual impairment, lead poisoning, thyroid abnormalities, traumatic brain injury, sleep disorders (e.g., obstructive sleep apnea, restless-leg/periodic limb movement disorder), and medication effects (e.g., albuterol). Unlike the persistent symptoms of ADHD, the symptoms of an alternative condition may fluctuate with the disease course or exposure to medication. Neurologic or developmental conditions must also be considered, particularly learning disabilities and cognitive impairments, which can impair academic functioning and interfere with attending and task completion in school.

Mental Health

Mental illnesses such as depression (impairments in the ability to concentrate and in motivation), anxiety disorder (poor attention), bipolar disorder (impulsive or overactive behaviors and distractibility), oppositional defiant disorder (ODD), conduct disorder, obsessive compulsive disorder, posttraumatic stress disorder, and adjustment disorder may mimic or co-occur with ADHD. Problems with substance abuse, particularly cannabis and alcohol, can also mimic ADHD symptoms. Given that ADHD is characterized by an early onset of symptoms, it is important to assess the circumstances that prompt the adolescent or young adult and/or their families to seek assessment, particularly if there is not a history of ADHD symptomatology in the past.

TABLE 71.1

Paper -and -Pencil Instruments for ADHD Screening

ADHD Evaluation Instrument	Target Age	Cost	Source
Brown ADD Scales for Adolescents	Validated for Adolescents	Yes	http://www.pearsonclinical.com/education/products/100000456/brown-attention-deficit-disorder-scales-brownaddscales.html?Pid=015-8029-240
Vanderbilt ADHD Teacher Rating Scale	Validated for 6–12 y	No	http://peds.mc.vanderbilt.edu/VCHWEB_1/rating~1.html
Conners Wells Adolescent Self-Report Sclales	Validated for Adolescents	Yes	Amazon.com, ADD Wearhouse.com
World Health Organization ADHD Self-Report Scale (ASRS)	Validated for 18–44 y	No	http://www.hcp.med.harvard.edu/ncs/asrs.php
Wender Utah Rating Scale for ADHD in Adults	Validated for over 18 y	No	http://cairncenter.com/forms/Wender%20Utah%20Rating%20scale%20for%20ADHD.pdf

Psychosocial and Environmental Factors

Stressful home environment or an unsuitable educational environment can cause symptoms that may mimic ADHD or co-occur with it. In contrast to ADHD alone, these behaviors often occur only in one setting as opposed to being present in a number of different settings.

Physical Examination

The physical examination of most AYAs with ADHD will be normal. However, the examination is necessary to exclude other conditions in the differential diagnosis of ADHD. Important aspects of the examination include:

- Measurement of height and weight. Height and weight should be plotted on a growth chart for each individual. This will offer important information about the adolescent's growth, which may be affected by ADHD. It is not clear that medication has a major impact on growth.
- Measure vital signs (heart rate and blood pressure). This is important information as stimulant medications are likely to result in modest increases in heart rate and blood pressure.
- Assessment of dysmorphic features
- A complete neurologic examination, including assessment of neurocutaneous abnormalities as well as vision and hearing

Laboratory Studies

Laboratory evaluation may be helpful in the evaluation of other conditions that may be suggested by the history and physical examination. Likewise, electroencephalography and brain imaging may be indicated if there are symptoms or findings suggestive of another diagnosis. Professional practice guidelines do not recommend any specific laboratory studies or imaging before initiating ADHD medications in the absence of other symptoms.

Barriers to Evaluation

There are many barriers to the diagnosis and treatment of ADHD, including time required, use of multiple professionals and visits, as well as psychological testing. The key is to provide an efficient and comprehensive evaluation to ensure that the adolescent or young adult and family are not left untreated due to lengthy wait times for other professionals to conduct psychological or neuropsychology testing. Psychological, neuropsychological, and/or academic testing is not required to make a diagnosis of ADHD; however, these evaluations may be helpful in making a diagnosis and/or delineating comorbidities. In an effort to be efficient, the provider is encouraged to first screen for common comorbidities, and after a diagnosis is made and treatment initiated, subsequent referral for further diagnostic testing may be necessary. Since the adolescent or young adult may present due to a crisis situation in school such as failing multiple classes or behavioral problems that are precipitating suspension or expulsion, it is important for the clinician to evaluate all information presented including family history, the increased challenges in the to adolescent or young adult's life, reasons why this concern has not been diagnosed in the past, as well as comorbid conditions, that is, depression, anxiety, substance use, learning disabilities, or bipolar disorder.

CURRENT DIAGNOSTIC CRITERIA

The diagnostic criteria for ADHD have been modified in the Diagnostic Statistical Manual for Mental Disorders, Fifth Edition (DSM-5). In the DSM-5, ADHD is now included in the section on Neurodevelopmental Disorders, as this better reflects the way ADHD is currently conceptualized. The clinician should be aware that the inattentive or hyperactive/impulsive symptoms must be present prior to age 12 and adolescents who are >17 years can meet diagnostic criteria with 5 instead of 6 symptoms from the inattentive and hyperactivity/impulsivity categories, which must be present for >6 months.

The requirement that there be clear evidence that symptoms interfere with two domains, for example, social, academic, or occupational remains unchanged, but treatment should not be withheld because dysfunction does not exist in two life areas. In cases where interference of two domains is not present, diagnostically this can be accurately labeled as "Other Specified ADHD" or "Unspecified ADHD" depending on whether the dysfunction does not exist in the other domain, or if it is not uncovered as part of the assessment, respectively.

The ADHD diagnosis must be specified as mixed, primarily inattentive or primarily hyperactive, and impulsive. The severity rating of mild, moderate, or severe is optional. For those AYAs who have previously met diagnostic criteria, but some of these symptoms are no longer present, a notation of partial remission should be used.

Objective Testing

Recently, the Neuropsychiatric EEG-Based Assessment Aid (NEBA) System was approved by the US Food and Drug Administration (FDA) and takes about 15 to 20 minutes. This testing calculates ratios of theta to beta brain waves given off each second where the ratios are significantly higher in ADHD individuals. There is no widespread clinical experience with this diagnostic tool, but data suggest that combination of NEBA and the clinical evaluation together is superior to the clinical evaluation alone.[16] The FDA approval specifies that it is not to be used as a stand-alone diagnostic tool but as part of a clinical evaluation.[16]

Comorbidities

It is well established that ADHD frequently co-occurs with other psychiatric disorders. As many as 60% of AYAs with ADHD experience one or more of these comorbidities. Learning disorders are common as well as depressive, anxiety, and substance use disorders. Bipolar affective spectrum disorders are less common, but cause much more difficulty in many spheres of life and have many overlapping ADHD symptoms. ODD symptoms are common in younger adolescents with ADHD. ODD symptoms somewhat abate with pharmacotherapy, but those with ODD and emerging conduct disorders may be a subset of ADHD youth who have much more difficulty with accepting authority and following rules. Those youth with these comorbid disorders usually have increased family conflict, substance misuse, school failure, and truancy. Therefore, clinicians should be prepared to see a wide range of psychiatric symptoms when managing patients with ADHD.

If comorbidities are not apparent at diagnosis or a poor response to treatment is noted, the provider should examine for the presence of a comorbid condition that may be exacerbating ADHD symptoms or whether these symptoms are masking a different disorder. At times, there will be symptoms of anxiety or depression that appear to be related to the struggle with functional impairments of ADHD and may resolve when ADHD is effectively treated. If these other symptoms do not remit, consider the possibility of an independent psychiatric, neurodevelopmental, or other behavioral disorder.

MANAGEMENT

Management of ADHD can be broadly separated into two components: environmental and pharmacologic. Frequently, patients and their families have tried to adapt their environment before seeking outside help. Adapting or modifying the school and home environments may better allow for the completion of work and retention of material. Both are a powerful adjunct to medication use. Modification of the adolescent's or young adult's environment in combination with psychotherapy can provide improvements in concentration, organization, as well as coping. Medication use typically provides improved cognitive functioning in key areas: input information, increased task efficiency and completion, as well as retention.[13] Finally, for those patients with comorbid conditions including mood and anxiety symptoms, psychotherapy as well as psychotropic medication may be necessary to improve overall functioning.

Educational Modifications

Typically, it is necessary to provide modifications for most students with ADHD. In school settings this can be accomplished with minimal disruption to the student, but requires extra effort and support from school personnel. Common modifications include allowing extended time for completion of tests and projects, preferential seating so that the field of view between student and teacher is minimized, individual instruction, and provision of lecture notes. Because independent note taking can be very difficult for AYAs with ADHD, it is common for teachers to copy and provide their notes that have been used on overheads, whiteboards, or electronic screens, so that copying by the student is not required. Alternatively, other students who are proficient in taking notes could be asked to share their notes with the student with ADHD. Recording lectures may also be helpful. Finally, a quiet testing environment may also be required for some patients with ADHD to accurately assess their knowledge as they may be easily distracted by ambient classroom noise and activity.

Behavioral and Psychological Interventions

Helping the adolescent or young adult to cope with symptoms of anxiety, depression, and obsessive worrying through behavioral therapies may also improve academic performance as well as reduce the burden of ADHD symptoms. Behavioral and psychotherapeutic interventions, that is, counseling, behavioral modification, and psychotherapy are most helpful if they are targeted to the needs of the individual with ADHD.

While behavior modification may be challenging in adolescents, there is increasing evidence that cognitive behavioral therapy (CBT) improves functioning among AYAs with ADHD.[17,18] CBT is goal-directed and focuses on changing specific thoughts and patterns of behavior to obtain competency in particular situations. Successful behavioral interventions that have yielded significant improvement in ADHD outcomes when used as an adjunct to medication incorporate components that include psychoeducation, organizing/planning, coping with distractibility, and adaptive thinking elements. Two additional optional, but helpful, components include targeting strategies to reduce procrastination and relationship skill enhancement.[19]

Navigating Legal Rights

There are legal provisions available that ensure ADHD students' academic achievement is similar to students without these difficulties. In the United States, Title II of the Americans with Disabilities Act 504 modifications, **Individuals with Disabilities Education Act**, and the potential for an individualized education plan are all available to these students and their parents, if requested. However, the implementation and execution of these laws and policies may vary from school district to school district. At the college level, typically an Office for Students with Disabilities exists and can be helpful. Parents must advocate for their adolescent or young adult in order to ensure that all legal rights are afforded to their son or daughter. Young adults may also enlist other significant adults to navigate their legal rights within the school environment.

PHARMACOLOGIC TREATMENT OF ADHD

Dosing

Stimulant medications appear to improve cognitive functioning and functioning may be dose related. Unfortunately, most studies do not report dose range efficacy and instead report the use of arbitrary maximums. Thus, few data exist to guide dosing in clinical practice. The general principal is to advance the dose gradually until optimal benefit has been obtained with a minimum of side effects. If increasing the dose is not helpful or decreases function, an alternative medication may be needed. Moreover, when the number of days that the dose is taken consecutively is increased (e.g., 7 versus 5 days), side effects tend to be lessened.

Stimulants

Psychostimulants are usually first-line therapy for AYAs with ADHD. Stimulants used for the pharmacologic management of ADHD are of two main categories: dextroamphetamines and methylphenidates (**Table 71.2**). These medications have been available for over 50 years, with an excellent safety profile. Long-term side effects have not been reported with psychostimulant use and short-term side effects are usually brief and limited. One category of stimulant medication has not been shown to be clearly superior to the other, but an individual patient's response may differ. The reason for variations in medication response is unclear; however, studies have suggested that the differential response may be related to factors such as blood threshold levels or rate of rise of the stimulant in the bloodstream.

The goal of medication management should be to maximize performance during academic and/or occupational hours, 7 days a week, 365 days a year by reducing the sequelae of untreated or undertreated ADHD. The dose of medication should be titrated to optimize symptom control and minimize side effects. In younger adolescents, higher doses may be necessary because younger patients may metabolize these compounds more quickly than young adult patients. As the adolescent ages, the dosage may need to be decreased as medications are likely to be cleared more slowly with increasing age. Stimulant medications are generally safe at or near the recommended doses.[20] It would be helpful to prepare the prospective college student to be transitioned to care in the university setting by providing a summary of diagnosis and how it was arrived at as well as a medication treatment summary. In addition, universities and/or student health centers often have written policies that give clear guidelines for either obtaining medication prescriptions or educational accommodations.

Long-acting Stimulant Medication

Long-acting stimulant medications are generally preferred for the AYA population because less frequent dosing minimizes the risk of missed doses and should therefore improve symptom control. With sustained drug levels, patients may also experience fewer problems with side effects, cognition, and behavior. A long-acting stimulant should be initiated at a low dose to allow for medication adaptation and assess for side effects.

Long-acting preparations include lisdexamphetamine (Vyvanse) and the methylphenidates: osmotic controlled-release oral delivery system (OROS), methylphenidate (Concerta), transdermal methylphenidate (Daytrana Patch), and long-acting liquid methylphenidate (Quillivant XR). The usual duration of action for these formulations is about 12 hours, but the duration will vary among patients. For the transdermal release system, the duration of action is also dependent upon removal of the patch, with medication usually lasting for 1 to 3 hours after removal.

Lisdexamphetamine: Lisdexamphetamine should generally be initiated at a dose of 20 mg and titrated in 10 mg or 20 mg increments. Being a prodrug (e.g., medication administered in an inactive form that is converted through a normal metabolic process), it is not necessary to take it in the capsule to maintain the timed release nature of it. The capsule can be opened and the powder can be evened out between the two sides to make half capsules, which can be poured into an ounce of juice or milk. It may be difficult to have payors cover more than one capsule per day so a titration strategy like this can be used. The patient can take one 20 mg capsule daily, after 3 to 4 days increase to 30 mg (e.g., 1½ capsules), and 3 to 4 days later, increase to 40 mg. Further increase is based on reaching either optimal benefit or intolerable side effects.

TABLE 71.2

Stimulant Medications

Generic Class/ Brand Name	Dose Form	Typical Starting Dose	FDA Max/ Day	Off-Label Max/ Day	Comments
Amphetamine preparations					
Short-acting					Short-acting stimulants often used as initial treatment in small children (<16 kg), but have disadvantage of b.i.d.–t.i.d. dosing to control symptoms throughout day
Adderall[a]	5, 7.5, 10, 12.5, 15, 20, 30 mg tab	3–5 y: 2.5 mg q.d.; ≥6 y: 5 mg q.d.–b.i.d.	40 mg	>50 kg: 60 mg	
Dexedrine[a]	5 mg cap	3–5 y: 2.5 mg q.d.			
DextroStat[a]	5, 10 mg cap	≥6 y: 5 mg q.d.–b.i.d.			
Long-acting					Longer-acting stimulants offer greater convenience, confidentiality, and compliance with single daily dosing but may have greater problematic effects on evening appetite and sleep. Adderall XR cap may be opened and sprinkled on soft foods
Dexedrine Spansule	5, 10, 15 mg cap	≥6 y: 5–10 mg q.d.–b.i.d.	40 mg	>50 kg: 60 mg	
Adderall XR	5, 10, 15, 20, 25, 30 mg cap	≥6 y: 10 mg q.d.	30 mg	>50 kg: 60 mg	
Lisdexamfetamine	30, 50, 70 mg cap	30 mg q.d.	70 mg	Not yet known	
Methylphenidate preparations					
Short-acting	2.5, 5, 10 mg cap	2.5 mg b.i.d.	20 mg	50 mg	Short-acting stimulants often used as initial treatment in small children (<16 kg) but have the disadvantage of b.i.d.–t.i.d. dosing to control symptoms throughout day
Focalin	5, 10, 20 mg tab	5 mg b.i.d.	60 mg	>50 kg: 100 mg	
Methylin[a]	5, 10, 20 mg	5 mg b.i.d.	60 mg	>50 kg: 100 mg	
Ritalin[a]					
Intermediate-acting					Longer-acting stimulants offer greater convenience, confidentiality, and compliance with single daily dosing but may have greater problematic effects on evening appetite and sleep. Metadate CD and Ritalin LA caps may be opened and sprinkled on soft food
Metadate ER	10, 20 mg cap	10 mg q.a.m.	60 mg	>50 kg: 100 mg	
Methylin ER	10, 20 mg cap	10 mg q.a.m.	60 mg	>50 kg: 100 mg	
Ritalin SR[a]	20 mg	10 mg q.a.m.	60 mg	>50 kg: 100 mg	
Metadate CD	10, 20, 30, 40, 50, 60 mg	20 mg q.a.m.	60 mg	>50 kg: 100 mg	
Ritalin LA	10, 20, 30, 40 mg	20 mg q.a.m.	60 mg	>50 kg: 100 mg	
Long-acting					
Concerta	18, 27, 36, 54 mg cap	18 mg q.a.m.	72 mg	108 mg	Swallow whole with liquids. Nonabsorbable tablet shell may be seen in stool
Daytrana patch	10, 15, 20, 30 mg patches	Begin with 10 mg patch q.d., then titrate up by patch strength	30 mg	Not yet known	
Focalin XR	5, 10, 15, 20 mg cap	5 mg q.a.m.	30 mg	50 mg	
Selective norepinephrine reuptake inhibitor					
Atomoxetine Strattera	10, 18, 25, 40, 60, 80, 100 mg cap	Children and adolescents <70 kg: 0.5 mg/kg/d for 4 d; then 1 mg/kg/d for 4 d; then 1.2 mg/kg/d	Lesser of 1.4 mg/kg or 100 mg	Lesser of 1.8 mg/kg or 100 mg	Not a schedule II medication. Consider if active substance abuse or severe side effects of stimulants (mood lability, tics); give q.a.m. or divided doses b.i.d. (effects on late evening behavior); do not open capsule; monitor closely for suicidal thinking and behavior, clinical worsening, or unusual changes in behavior

[a]Generic formulation available.
FDA, US Food and Drug Administration; ADHD, attention deficit hyperactivity disorder.
From Pliszka S. Practice parameter for the assessment and treatment of children and adolescents with attention-deficit/hyperactivity disorder. *J Am Acad Child Adolesc Psychiatry* 2007;46(7):894-921.

OROS Methylphenidate: The starting dose of OROS methylphenidate is usually 18 mg with dose adjustment increases of 18 mg increments until an optimal response is observed. Dose changes should generally occur at intervals of 3 to 4 days.

Transdermal Methylphenidate: The transdermal patch has been FDA-approved for a wear time of up to 9 hours. It has a uniform delivery and the dose is titrated by changing the dosage form of the patch and can be further adjusted by varying the amount of contact that the patch has with the patient's skin. Any portion of the patch that is not in direct skin contact will not deliver medication. If the patient feels the dose is too high, he or she can pull the ends of the patch away from the skin to reduce the dosage. Thus, titration is slightly more variable. Occasionally, the patch and/or the medication may cause minor skin irritation.

Liquid Methylphenidate: Quillivant is a liquid preparation consisting of 20% immediate-release medication with 80% contained within polymeric diffusion particles. This medication is most helpful for those patients who may have difficulty swallowing pills as well as those who need a more exact method of titration.

Another group of long-acting stimulants, lasting 8 to 9 hours, include the mixed amphetamine salts extended-release capsules (Adderall XR), methylphenidate-beaded extended-release capsules (Metadate CD, Ritalin LA), and dexmethylphenidate extended-release capsules containing d-methylphenidate alone (Focalin XR). If taken in the morning, most of these medications will lose effectiveness by the evening hours. In this case, the use of a short-acting preparation may be needed in the afternoon to reduce ADHD symptoms while the adolescent or young adult attends to homework, employment, or other activities. While all these types of capsuled medications may be taken without the capsule, these compounds must not be chewed.

For many patients, missing 2 or more days of any stimulant causes a loss of tolerance to the medication; therefore, in such cases the medication should be reinitiated at a lowered dose and then increased to the full dose 2 days later.

Finally, for some AYAs, the full weekday dose may provide too great a response for less intense focus and persistence needs on weekend days and/or holidays. For these days, prescribing a partial dose is often preferred as the weekend/holiday challenge is less and side effects are minimized when returning to full dose after the weekend or holiday.

Short-acting Stimulant Medication

The short-acting medications include amphetamines such as mixed amphetamine salts (Adderall, Procentra liquid), dextroamphetamine (Dexedrine, Dextrostat), and methylphenidate (Ritalin, Methylin liquid). These medications typically have a duration of action of 3 to 5 hours with Adderall lasting closer to 5 hours and methylphenidate lasting 3 to 4 hours. Many college students may require medication lasting up to 16 hours/day. In these situations, short-acting medications may be taken at 3:00 or 4:00 p.m. and again at 6:00 or 7:00 p.m. They can also be useful on weekends when AYAs often sleep late and do not want to take long-acting medications upon arising in the late morning or early afternoon.

Other medications are used less commonly now and may be difficult to find in pharmacies, including Ritalin SR and Dexedrine Spansules. Ritalin SR is a wax matrix preparation that increases slowly in the bloodstream. Dexedrine spansules (capsules with medicines coated with materials having slow dissolving rates) contain a single enantiomer of amphetamine, the most active part of the mixed amphetamine salts. Some individuals seem to respond better to this than to mixed amphetamine salts. Both of these medications peak around noontime if taken in the morning, but neither is very effective alone due to very slow onset and not reaching therapeutic threshold in most. They are primarily used in combination with short-acting forms when newer long-acting stimulants are not available.[21]

Nonstimulant Medication

There are two types of nonstimulants that are indicated for ADHD: The first is the selective norepinephrine inhibitor, atomoxetine (Strattera), and the second are the α-2 agonists.

Atomoxetine

When compared to the stimulants, atomoxetine is less effective for the treatment of ADHD, but also has less impact on sleep and appetite than the stimulants. It has been studied and may have some dual effectiveness in populations with comorbid ADHD and anxiety. In general, atomoxetine should be considered a second-line medication, but may be first-line for AYAs with substance abuse or anxiety. It can be very useful for the patient who experiences intolerable side effects with stimulant medications. Atomoxetine may also be used off-label in combination with a stimulant medication to allow for a lower stimulant dose and improved efficacy.[22] For average-sized AYAs, atomoxetine is initiated at 25 mg/day and titrated to 40 or 50 mg/day with a maximum recommended dose of 100 mg, if needed. The clinician should allow intervals of at least a week before increasing the dose. As such, the clinician should be aware that the amount of time required to determine effectiveness is greater than for stimulant medication. Reported side effects are usually minimal, but sleepiness may occur if the dose is increased too quickly. Constipation and emotional lability are occasionally reported. It is prudent to monitor for suicidal ideation when prescribing atomoxetine as it has an FDA black box warning. Clinical trials have shown a 0.4% incidence rate of suicidal ideation in subjects taking atomoxetine compared to "no attempts" in those taking placebo.[23,24]

α-2-Adrenoceptor Agonists

The second type of nonstimulant medications is the α-2-adrenoceptor agonists, which includes clonidine and guanfacine. Immediate-release forms of these medications are not indicated for ADHD. The long-acting preparations (Intuniv, Kapvay) target symptoms of overactivity and impulsiveness and usually do not cause daytime sleepiness. For extended-release guanfacine, the duration of action is about 24 hours, and for clonidine extended release it is about 12 hours.[24] Both of these formulations exert a positive but small positive effect on working memory[25] and are not usually effective alone for ADHD symptoms, and the improvements in cognitive functioning are much less robust than the stimulant medications. Extended-release guanfacine and clonidine can be given as adjunctive therapy with a stimulant to boost the ability to maintain impulse control and decrease overactivity.[26,27] They are also approved for adjunctive therapy to assist with emotional regulation and aggression. While these medications are approved for ages 6 to 17 years and provide good response in most in 6- to 12-year-olds, one clinical trial suggested less efficacy in 13- to 17-year-olds.[28]

To initiate extended-release guanfacine, the clinician should begin with 1 mg each day and increase by 1 mg tablet every 4 to 7 days until optimal benefit or 4 mg is reached. In the event that the adolescent or young adult experiences sleepiness, the clinician should decrease the dose and maintain the lower dose for several days. If the patient does not report becoming drowsy after 45 minutes, the clinician may increase by 1 mg to facilitate the onset of sleep.

For extended-release clonidine, the initiation is similar but with twice-daily dosing. Extended-release clonidine is generally started at 0.1 mg twice a day and can be increased to 0.2 mg twice a day after 4 to 7 days. It can be given once a day or a smaller dose can be given in the morning (e.g., 0.1 mg in the morning and 0.3 mg in the evening) if sleepiness becomes problematic.

Other Medications

Although not approved by the FDA for this purpose, there are other medications that have been used in the treatment of ADHD. Bupropion, an antidepressant, has been used to treat ADHD symptoms, particularly in individuals with active substance abuse.[29] The slow-release preparations are much more helpful for these patients. Typical dosing is 150 mg SR/XL each morning for the first week and, if improvement is minimal, advance to 300 mg each morning with a maximum dose of 450 mg/day. Doses above 300 mg should be divided (e.g., 300 mg in the morning and 150 mg in the afternoon or evening). Because it may lower the seizure threshold, bupropion is contraindicated in AYAs with seizure disorder.

Side Effects
Cardiovascular

The use of stimulant medications is associated with modest increases in heart rate and systolic and diastolic blood pressure. Despite concerns, there does not appear to be an increased risk of sudden cardiac death among youth without structural heart disease who take psychostimulants. A large cohort study found that the incidence of serious cardiovascular events (including sudden death) among children, adolescents, and young adults taking stimulants for ADHD was similar to those of nonusers.[30] In reviewing the evidence from this and other studies, an FDA panel recommended that stimulant medications and atomoxetine should generally not be used in patients for whom an increase in blood pressure or heart rate would be problematic. Further, the FDA recommends that individuals with structural heart problems should not take stimulants (http://www.fda.gov/Drugs/DrugSafety/ucm279858.htm). An initial American Heart Association (AHA) recommendation in support of routine electrocardiogram (ECG) screening prior to the initiation of stimulant medication was challenged by the American Academy of Pediatrics who noted that such screening was not predictive of sudden cardiac death in AYAs.[31] Subsequently, the AHA and AAP issued a joint statement that ECG screening of youth without structural heart disease is not needed unless there is a family history or symptoms suggesting high risk of sudden cardiac death (http://newsroom.heart.org/news/american-academy-of-pediatrics-218228). Therefore, clinicians are advised to assess for cardiac conditions and symptoms in AYA patients before starting stimulant medication and to monitor for increases in heart rate and blood pressure after initiation of therapy.[32]

Tics

There is general consensus that stimulants do not cause tic exacerbation in most patients beyond the initial medication adjustment period.[32,33] When tics are present, medications should be initiated at low doses and advanced slowly. Once an effective dose has been achieved, the medication should be taken consistently, because tics can be exacerbated by starting and stopping medications abruptly. The more common contributor to the expression of tics is stress. Tics that are exacerbated by stress may actually diminish when the adolescent or young adult is functioning better in school, at work, or in relationships.

Epilepsy

Well-controlled seizure disorders do not preclude the use of stimulant medication where the benefit outweighs the risk.[34] However, stimulant medication in AYAs with uncontrolled seizures is not advised.

Priapism

Recently, the FDA posted a warning about the risk of long-lasting erections in males taking methylphenidate preparations. However, insufficient evidence exists to provide a "black box" warning. Prolonged, but not painful, erections are common in this age group with emerging pubertal changes. It is recommended by the FDA that clinicians provide education to all males with ADHD on the signs of priapism and when to seek emergent treatment.

Other Issues

The clinician should consider whether the stimulant dose is too high if an AYA voices concerns about lack of productivity at school. Stimulant doses that are too high may result in "over-focus,"

causing the adolescent or young adult to "think more and do less" leading to diminished productivity. Reducing the dose slightly may alleviate this problem.

Nonadherence to daily medication use is common, especially among young adults who are independent from their parent. AYAs who skip medication for 2 or more consecutive days and then reinitiate the stimulant may reexperience side effects of abdominal pain, diminished appetite, or stilted or subdued personality. The importance of medication adherence and strategies to improve adherence should be reviewed with AYAs taking stimulants. Some AYAs will object to taking medication on weekends. In these instances, a reduced dosage for weekends might be recommended to maintain their adaptation to using stimulant medication.

Diminished appetite is a common complaint,[32] especially among male adolescents who want to gain weight and develop a more muscular physique. While diminished appetite in the middle of the day is unlikely to go away, general suppression of appetite seems to dissipate with time; however, this may take 3 or more weeks to subside. While the midday meal may remain poorly eaten, these AYAs can increase their caloric intake before taking medication in the morning and/or in the late afternoon or early evening when medication effects are waning. The clinician should closely monitor for changes in growth in height and weight.[32]

Stimulant medications used to treat ADHD may disrupt sleep.[32] After initiation of stimulants, some AYAs will report sleeping better; however, a larger proportion report difficulty with sleep onset. The clinician should review sleep hygiene with the adolescent or young adult, including avoiding screen time for about an hour before attempting to sleep, engaging in calming presleep activities, and eliminating phone use including texting. If problems persist, some patients may benefit from the use of melatonin, which has been found to be helpful in various dosages up to 15 mg per evening at bedtime. The initial dose recommended is 1 to 2 mg with increases every other night of 1 mg until optimal sleep onset occurs. Melatonin side effects include morning sleepiness and vivid dreaming. If sleep-onset problems persist, clonidine may be used off-label to facilitate sleep initiation. Trazodone is another medication that facilitates sleep initiation and maintenance.[35,36] Mirtazepine is another medication that can be used for sleep for young adults, but can cause drowsiness in the morning and has the potential for increasing appetite leading to weight gain.[37]

Withdrawal/Misuse/Diversion

Addiction to ADHD medication rarely occurs. There is no defined withdrawal syndrome or cravings that occur after stopping these medications. Although depressed mood, hypersomnia, and increased appetite may occur, these symptoms are rarely significant enough to drive ongoing use of ADHD medications.[38] It is more common for AYAs to overuse ADHD medications during times of increased work requirements such mid-term or final exams because of the improvements they have experienced in their performance. Diversion of ADHD medications among AYAs is common and patients may provide medication to their peers in an effort to be helpful.

Use of stimulant medication without a prescription appears to be increasing among college students with lifetime prevalence ranging as high as 20%.[39–41] Stimulant use among young adults in college is commonplace and is used as a study aid and to increase concentration, especially during periods of high academic demand.[40] While students may purchase these medications on the black market, most commonly they are received from friends and peers who have been legitimately prescribed these medications.[42] Careful counseling and monitoring for misuse and diversion is warranted, especially among young adults.[41]

ACADEMIC PERFORMANCE PROBLEMS

It is not uncommon for AYA patients to seek care because of academic performance problems. While some patients have a long history of academic difficulties, other patients are just beginning to experience difficulties due to the increasing complexity of the school level and volume of information that must be mastered. As students increase in grade level, there is an increasing need to organize material, read and retain more, and acquire effective study skills. As the student increases in grade levels there is a greater demand to abstract and synthesize information and to apply this information to new learning situations. In addition, AYAs are faced with other opportunities such as romantic relationships, experimentation with alcohol or other substances, as well as typical extracurricular activities. Sometimes involvement in these "distracters" are the problem, but often the difficulty with school success makes other pursuits much more inviting, such as gang involvement and substance use. Motivational interviewing can be used to help them to come to conclusions about their motivation to continue in their education and see it to completion. Adults such as parents, guardians, or others interested in their success can be enlisted to help them remain motivated.

At preventive care and urgent visits, it is important for the provider to inquire with the adolescent or young adult about how school is progressing, achievement, and plans for the future. Drops in grades, behavior problems, emotional issues, and underperforming are all indicators of school failure. It is helpful to ask such questions as: "what do you need to be doing now that will help you get into college or a school to be a mechanic or a computer programmer?," "What can you do to help your grades move up enough to get into the school you would like to attend?" or "What do you have to do to get that kind of job you want when you are finished with high school?" Most often having a team consisting of patient, parents, and school representative such as teacher or coach is very helpful.

Causes of Poor Academic Performance

Medical

Physical difficulties with hearing or vision can cause academic problems as well as congenital conditions such as Fragile X, Turner syndrome, Klinefelter syndrome, and tuberous sclerosis. Many AYAs born with these conditions have intellectual limitations that become increasingly problematic as the student progresses in school. Those AYAs with chronic illnesses such as asthma, gastrointestinal disorders, heart disease, and/or diabetes mellitus may also experience academic difficulties secondary to their disease. Typically, this is largely due to absenteeism due to illnesses. Chronic sleep deprivation can also cause poor academic performance. Finally, many mental disorders such as mood disorders can also directly affect academic performance.

Learning Disorders

A learning disability is defined as a disorder with one or more of the basic psychological processes involved in the understanding of, or in the use of, language. Typically, these disorders interfere with an individual's ability to store, process, or produce information. For example, these conditions may manifest as an inability to read, write, spell, compute mathematical problems, or comprehend the spoken language. It does not include visual, hearing or motor disabilities, cognitive delays, emotional problems, cultural, economic or environmental problems.

It is important to note that a learning disability is defined through the educational system and is usually based on failing to meet academic expectations consistent with one's intellectual ability. That is, an adolescent with average intellectual abilities should be performing within a similar academic range. While there are several models used to determine the presence of a learning disability, it is usually defined as a discrepancy of two standard deviations, that is, 30 points between the full scale intelligence quotient (FSIQ) score and the standardized achievement score, for example, 115 FSIQ score and standardized score of 80 in reading comprehension. Unfortunately, many students who may

benefit from educational accommodations will not be afforded services due to this lack of significant discrepancy between actual and expected achievement.

Reading disorders are quite common and usually involve decoding words as well as understanding what the student has read. Dyslexia is a term that has been used interchangeably with a reading disability and typically refers to a decoding problem. A less common problem is the adolescent who can read the words, but does not understand what he or she has read.

Writing disorders entail difficulty with composing, punctuating, spelling, and organizing thoughts and concepts into a cohesive written story or paragraph. It often coexists with reading disorders; therefore, if a student has one disorder, the other also should be considered. As a student progresses in school, especially in high school or college, symptoms may become more problematic due to increased reading requirements. Writing disorders do not include the production of illegible handwriting, which is labeled as dysgraphia.

Math disorders refer to difficulties with simple calculations and may be severe enough that the young person is unable to do calculations. Applying math to common life situations may be very difficult. Word problems may be excruciatingly difficult for these students as well as problems with spatial orientation. In addition to educational testing to identify the presence of one or more learning disabilities, neuropsychological testing may be helpful to provide a better understanding of specific problems as well as assist in remediation or modification efforts.

While intellectual and academic testing is necessary and required for the identification of a specific learning disability, these tests alone may be insufficient to construct an effective education intervention. Wechsler Intelligence Scale for Children V is appropriate to test cognitive abilities in those up to 16 years of age and the Wechsler Adult Intelligence Scale, 4th edition is appropriate for those 16 years and older. Achievement tests are helpful in determining at what level of achievement a student is currently. Woodcock–Johnson III Test of Achievement, Wechsler Individual Achievement Test III, and Kaufman Test of Educational Achievement, 3rd edition are commonly used instruments.

To receive school-based assistance and interventions, at least within the United States, these disorders are determined by local school districts. Providers may be asked to provide information about the student's health, especially as it relates to comorbid conditions such as ADHD or depressive/anxiety disorders.

Behavioral

While family dysfunction, alcohol use or abuse, and parent–adolescent discord have traditionally been implicated in problems with academics, technological advances have yielded new challenges such as dysfunctional electronic dependence. Social interaction problems, bullying, and harassment also affect academic performance. Finally, cultural and economic differences also isolate and marginalize adolescents in middle and high school and cause additional challenges in maintaining academic success.

Common behavioral health concerns for the AYAs include depression, anxiety, and family conflict. While there are several screening measures that can be used to assess the presence of emotional and behavioral health difficulties, the following are recommended:

- Patient Health Questionnaire (PHQ)-9 as well as the PHQ-9 modified for adolescents (http://www.ncfhp.org/Data/Sites/1/phq-a.pdf) to assess symptoms of depression
- Screen for Child Anxiety Related Disorders to assess for anxiety (http://www.psychiatry.pitt.edu/sites/default/files/Documents/assessments/SCARED%20Child.pdf)
- To assess the presence of family problems, the Conflict Behavior Questionnaire can be useful (http://www.first5scc.org/sites/default/files/Conflict%20Behavior%20Questionnaire-TEEN-English%20v1.pdf)

In addition, the Beck Depression and Anxiety Inventories and the Mood Disorders Questionnaire (http://www.dbsalliance.org/pdfs/MDQ.pdf) can help the clinician assess the presence of depression, anxiety, or a mood disorder in AYAs.

School Avoidance

School avoidance is often used interchangeably with school refusal. Some have separated them into avoidance, being related to anxiety, and refusal, being the willful act of not going to school, such as truancy. The parents are usually aware that the adolescent is missing school with school avoidance, and they are usually not aware that their teen is not going to school with refusal/truancy.

School avoidance is defined as a persistent anxiety or fear of going to school, which can also be marked by calling from school to be picked up. For adolescents there are many stressors that can lead to the condition and include fear of undressing in gym class, being confronted by teachers or other students, poor grades, bullying, sexual orientation, or fear of poor academic performance. It is also possible that an anxiety disorder may be the underlying cause of failing to attend school. Typically, adolescents with significant social anxiety disorder (see Chapter 69) can experience difficulty attending school regularly, which is not unexpected. Regardless of diagnosis, cognitive behavioral treatment has shown efficacy as a first-line treatment strategy, but may not be available or affordable. Medications, in particular, the selective serotonin reuptake inhibitors, are very effective in reducing the anxiety symptoms and minimizing associated symptoms of depression. A school reentry treatment plan is essential and can be as simple as allowing the student to go to school for 2 hours a day at the onset. If the activity that provokes the most fear is approaching the school in the morning then it is advised to initiate school for the last 2 hours of the day. The gradual titration of attendance from 1 or 2 hours to 2 or 3, then 4, then 5, then the whole day can help to reintroduce the student to the full school environment.

Truancy

School truancy and dropping out of school are major problems for adolescents. In this case, the student is making a conscious decision not to go to school and is usually secretive about it, at least with parents. Failure to perform well in school is a major factor in truancy and dropout behavior. Getting a good school history from adolescents is helpful in recognizing someone who is not yet committed to dropping out. Often the adolescent does not see any chance of changing things or becoming successful in school. Many other options for passing time, such as substance use, sexual activity, criminal behavior, gangs, and violence, may appear more inviting. When the adolescent is experiencing difficulties in school and these have been long-standing, he or she may choose to leave school without graduating.

It is important for the provider to appreciate their local as well as regional dropout rates among adolescents attending high school. Within the United States, the average dropout rate can be as high as 50% of students leaving high school prematurely, especially in urban and economically disadvantaged areas. For students who drop out of school and do not obtain their high school diplomas, economic outcomes are much less favorable even if they do not become involved in gangs or engage in high-risk, self-destructive behaviors such as illicit drug use. Students who do not graduate have lower employability and less financial stability throughout their lifetime. It is also important for the clinician to inquire about family life among these students because the adolescent may leave school to help support the family or due to family conflict where the adolescent is told to leave the household. Finally, unintended pregnancy may also be cause for terminating school prior to graduation.

Intervention should occur as early as possible when school failure or a trajectory predicting school failure is recognized. ADHD or learning disabilities may cause chronic academic frustration and school failure in some AYAs. Support from the family and school is paramount to help young people achieve academic success and remain in school. Many school districts now have good alternatives for these students. Some academic instructions include special tracks that direct students into vocational training (i.e., mechanics, carpentry, cooking, and cosmetology), job training, and special skills training in areas that align with the young person's interests and abilities and ultimately improve their employability. Psychologists, whether private or through the school system, can develop an educational plan with realistic goals that are acceptable to the adolescent and the family.

The teen should be encouraged to continue in school, but the provider needs to understand that alternatives do exist, should the patient leave school. For example, is the student willing to complete a graduate equivalency program or complete an alternative high school program that does online educational classes? While all geographic locations may not provide multiple alternative high school programs, home study or Internet-based study programs can be very viable alternatives. All adolescents who are truant or experience school difficulties do not fit into the same pattern or present with the same life circumstances. Regardless, some adolescents can be very successful in adulthood even among those who leave school. If the adolescent can be lured into staying engaged and leaves high school with some type of diploma, he or she will have a much better chance of moving into a successful adulthood.

REFERENCES

1. Willcutt E. The prevalence of DSM-IV attention-deficit/hyperactivity disorder: a meta-analytic review. *Neurotherapeutics* 2012;9:490–499.
2. Klein R, Mannuzza S, Olazagasti M, et al. Clinical and functional outcome of childhood ADHD 33 years later. *Arch Gen Psychiatry* 2012;69:1295–1303.
3. Biederman J, Petty C, Evans M, et al. How persistent is ADHD? A controlled 10-year follow-up study of boys with ADHD. *Psychiatry Res* 2010;177:299–304.
4. Bernardi S, Faraone SV, Cortese S, et al. The lifetime impact of attention-deficit hyperactivity disorder: results from the national epidemiologic survey on alcohol and related conditions. *Psychol Med* 2012;42:875–887.
5. Wolraich ML, Wibbelsman CJ, Brown TE, et al. Attention-deficit/hyperactivity disorder among adolescents: a review of the diagnosis, treatment, and clinical implications. *Pediatrics* 2005;115:1734–1746.
6. Spencer T, Biederman J, Mick E. Attention-deficit/hyperactivity disorder: diagnosis, lifespan, comorbidities, and neurobiology. *Ambul Pediatr* 2007;7 (suppl):631–642.
7. Biederman J, Mick E, Faraone S. Age-dependent decline of symptoms of attention deficit hyperactivity disorder: impact of remission definition and symptom type. *Am J Psychiatry* 2000;157:816–818.
8. Hart EL, Lahey BB, Loeber R, et al. Developmental change in attention-deficit hyperactivity disorder in boys: a four-year longitudinal study. *J Abnormal Child Psychol* 1995;23:729–749.
9. Faraone S, Perlis R, Doyle A, et al. Molecular genetics of attention deficit/hyperactivity disorder. *Biol Psychiatr* 2005;57:1313–1323.
10. Franke B, Neale B, Faraone S, et al. Genome-wide association studies in ADHD. *Hum Genet* 2009;126:13–50.
11. Faraone S, Mick E. Molecular genetics of attention deficit hyperactivity disorder. *Psychiatr Clin North Am* 2010;33:159–180.
12. Rubia K, Alegria AA, Brinson H. Brain abnormalities in attention-deficit hyperactivity disorder: a review. *Rev Neurol* 2014;58 (suppl 1):S3–S18.
13. Friedman LA, Rapoport JL. Brain development in ADHD. *Curr Opin Neurobiol* 2014;30:106–111.
14. Pliszka S; The AACAP Work Group on Quality Issues. Practice parameter for the assessment and treatment of children and adolescents with attention-deficit/hyperactivity disorder. *J Am Acad Child Adolesc Psychiatr* 2007;46:894–921.
15. Subcommittee on attention-deficit/hyperactivity disorder, Stering Committee on Quliaty Improvement and Management. ADHD: clinical practice guideline for the diagnosis, evaluation, and treatment of attention-deficit/hyperactivity disorder in children and adolescents. *Pediatrics* 2011;128:1007–1022.
16. *De novo classification request for neuropsychiatric EEG-based assessment aid for ADHD* (**NEBA**) *system*. Available at http://www.accessdata.fda.gov/cdrh_docs/reviews/K112711.pdf. Accessed November 17, 2014.
17. Emilsson B, Gudjonsson G, Sigurdsson J, et al. Cognitive behaviour therapy in medication-treated adults with ADHD and persistent symptoms: a randomized controlled trial. *BMC Psychiatry* 2011;11:116.
18. Antshel K, Faraone S, Gordon M. Cognitive behavioral treatment outcomes in adolescent ADHD. *Focus* 2012;10:334–344.
19. Sprich S, Knouse L, Cooper-Vince C, et al. Description and demonstration of CBT for ADHD in adults. *Cogn Behav Pract* 2012;17(1).
20. Zosel A, Bartelson B, Bailey E, et al. Characterization of adolescent prescription drug abuse and misuse using the researched abuse diversion and addiction-related surveillance (RADARS®) System. *J Am Acad Child Adolesc Psychiatry* 2013;52:196–204.

21. Patrick KS, Straughn AB, Perkins JS, et al. Evolution of stimulants to treat ADHD: transdermal methylphenidate. *Hum Psychopharmacol* 2009;24(1):1–17.
22. Treuer T, Gau S, Mendez L, et al. A systematic review of combination therapy with stimulants and atomoxetine for attention-deficit/hyperactivity disorder, including patient characteristics, treatment strategies, effectiveness, and tolerability. *J Child Adolesc Psychopharmacol* 2013;23:179–193.
23. FDA Bulletin. *Public health advisory: suicidal thinking in children and adolescents being treated with Strattera (Atomoxetine)*. Available at www.fda.gov/Drugs/DrugSafety/PostmarketDrugSafetyInformationforPatientsandProviders/ucm051733.htm. Accessed September 29, 2005.
24. Sallee F, Kollins S, Wigal T. Efficacy of guanfacine extended release in the treatment of combined and inattentive only subtypes of attention-deficit/hyperactivity disorder. *J Child Adolesc Psychopharmacol* 2012;22:206–214.
25. Bidwell LC, Dew RE, Kollins SH. Alpha-2 adrenergic receptors and attention—deficit/hyperactivity disorder. *Curr Psychiatry Rep* 2010;12(5):366–373.
26. Spencer T, Greenbaum M, Ginsberg L, et al. Safety and effectiveness of coadministration of guanfacine extended release and psychostimulants in children and adolescents with attention-deficit/hyperactivity disorder. *J Child Adolesc Psychopharmacol* 2009;19:501–510.
27. Kollins S, Jain R, Brams M, et al. Clonidine extended-release tablets as add-on therapy to psychostimulants in children and adolescents with ADHD. *Pediatrics* 2011;127:e1406–e1413.
28. Biederman J, Melmed RD, Patel A. A randomized, double-blind, placebo-controlled study of guanfacine extended release in children and adolescents with attention-deficit/hyperactivity disorder. *Pediatrics* 2008;121(1),e73–e84.
29. Wilens T, Prince J, Waxmonsky J, et al. An open trial of sustained release bupropion for attention-deficit/hyperactivity disorder in adults with ADHD plus substance use disorders. *J ADHD Relat Disord* 2010;1:25–35.
30. Cooper WO, Habel LA, Sox CM, et al. ADHD drugs and serious cardiovascular events in children and young adults. *N Engl J Med* 2011;365:1896–1904.
31. Perrin JM, Friedman RA, Knilans TK; the Black Box Working Group, the Section on Cardiology and Cardiac Surgery. Cardiovascular monitoring and stimulant drugs for attention-deficit/hyperactivity disorder. *Pediatrics* 2008;122(2):451–454.
32. Cortese S, Holtmann M, Banaschewski T, et al. Practitioner review: current best evidence practice in the management of adverse events during treatment with ADHD medications in children and adolescents. *J Child Psychol Psychiatr* 2013;54:227–246.
33. Lyon GJ, Samar SM, Conelea C, et al. Testing tic suppression: comparing the effects of dexmethylphenidate to no medication in children and adolescents with attention-deficit/hyperactivity disorder and tourette's disorder. *J Child Adolesc Psychopharmacol* 2010;20:283–289.
34. Socanski D, Aurlien D, Herigstad A, et al. Epilepsy in a large cohort of children diagnosed with attention deficit/hyperactivity disorders (ADHD). *Seizure* 2013;22:651–655.
35. Efron D, Lycett K, Sciberras E. Use of sleep medication in children with ADHD. *Sleep Med* 2014;15:472–475.
36. Owen JA, Rosen CL, Mindell JA, et al. Use of pharmacotherapy for insomnia in child psychiatry practice: a national survey. *Sleep Med* 2010;11:692–700.
37. Adler LA, Reingold LS, Morrill MS, et al. Combination pharmacotherapy for adult ADHD. *Curr Psychiatry Rep* 2006;8:409–415.
38. Phillips KA, Epstein DH, Preston KL. Psychostimulant addiction treatment. *Neuropharmacology* 2014;87:150–160.
39. Brandt SA, Taverna EC, Hallock RM. A survey of nonmedical use of tranquilizers, stimulants, and pain relievers among college students: patterns of use among users and factors related to abstinence in non-users. *Drug Alcohol Depend* 2014;143:272–276.
40. Moore DR, Burgard DA, Larson RG, et al. Psychostimulant use among college students during periods of high and low stress: an interdisciplinary approach utilizing both self-report and unobtrusive chemical sample data. *Addict Behav* 2014;39:987–993.
41. Garnier LM, Arria AM, Caldeira KM, et al. Sharing and selling of prescription medications in a college student sample. *J Clin Psychiatry* 2010;71:262–269.
42. Vrecko C. Everyday drug diversions: a qualitative study of the illicit exchange and non-medical use of prescription stimulants on a university campus. *Soc Sci Med* 2015;131:297–304. doi:10.1016/j.socscimed.2014.10.016.

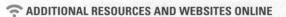

ADDITIONAL RESOURCES AND WEBSITES ONLINE

XV

72

Violence

Todd I. Herrenkoh
Paul Boxer
Anne McGlynn-Wright

Youth violence is a subcategory of interpersonal violence that involves the use of physical force or threats of force by a young person in which there is intent to cause another harm. Crimes typically associated with this definition include aggravated and simple assault, robbery with or without a weapon, and rape or sexual assault. In some reports, bullying and physical fighting are also included as examples of youth violence (http://www.cdc.gov/Violenceprevention/youthviolence/index.html). Those who commit violent acts, whether or not they are officially charged with a crime, are called *perpetrators* or *offenders*, terms used interchangeably throughout this chapter when summarizing research on the etiology and prevention of violence. While the mention of "youth" violence implies a focus on young people who are under the age of 18, research on the topic often applies to young adults aged 19 to 25 years (http://www.cdc.gov/violenceprevention/youthviolence/definitions.html). Thus, our reference to youth should be taken to include both adolescents and young adults (AYAs).

The World Health Organization[1] characterizes interpersonal violence as a "universal challenge" that affects every country and every community across the globe. Despite its pervasiveness, rates of the more serious forms of violent crime in the US, including crimes committed by juveniles and young adults, have actually declined in number over the past 30 years,[2] reasons for which are debated. Researcher suggests that the decline is due to targeted efforts at prevention. Others attribute the decline to better policing and an increasing intolerance of violence in the hardest hit communities (http://www.nij.gov/topics/law-enforcement/strategies/hot-spot-policing/Pages/welcome.aspx).

Still, others suggest that violent crime is less prevalent now than before only because population demographics have shifted and there are fewer young people now to commit violence. Regardless of the cause of the decline—and it is unlikely there is just one—the current trend is encouraging. Nonetheless, it is necessary to keep a focus on how to lessen violence so that this trend continues.

In this chapter, we briefly summarize the epidemiology of youth violence, and then provide information on its consequences, and the risk and protective factors for violence most documented in the research literature. We also provide information on assessment strategies for violent youth and give some information on promising prevention approaches at the community, school, and family levels.

 ## EPIDEMIOLOGY

Physical Assault and Other Violent Crime

Within the US, violent crime has become a topic of major concern for policy makers and program developers, partly because of the high-profile school shootings that have occurred in recent years and the outcry by the general public that has followed each event.[3] Statistics compiled by the Centers for Disease Control and Prevention (CDC)[4] indicate that young people under the age of 18 (i.e., those legally classified as juveniles) accounted for just under 14% of all violent crime arrests in 2010. Most arrests involve legal adults. However, among young people ages 15 to 24, homicide remains a leading cause of death. And, sadly, the majority of these deaths (82.8%) are linked to the use of firearms.

When less serious forms of violence are taken into account, rates of violence are even higher. According to the CDC, in 2009, nearly a third of all students in 9th to 12th grades had been in a physical fight and over 17.5% had carried a weapon in the past 30 days.[5] Among males, the prevalence of weapon carrying in 2013 was over 25%.

Statistics compiled from victimization records provide even more evidence of the widespread nature and harm caused by lethal and nonlethal forms of violence. In 2011, over 700,000 young people were treated by emergency room departments for injuries related to violence.[4] All the more alarming, these numbers capture only a fraction of the violent incidents that occur each year because many incidents go undocumented. A recent report suggests that in 2012 just under 60% of all violence-related injuries for all age groups were reported to police.[6]

Gender Differences

Many years of research have shown that physical violence is more common among males[7] and that males perpetrate more serious forms of violence than do similarly aged females.[8] Statistics compiled by the CDC show that 86% of youth homicide victims (age 10 to 24) in 2010 were male. Interestingly, a report by Chesney-Lind and Belknap[7] found that the gender gap in violent crime arrests may be narrowing, possibly due to changes in policing strategies that bring more young women into contact with authorities.

Racial and Ethnic Differences

In the US, the risk of perpetrating and being victimized by violence varies by age, race/ethnicity, and socioeconomic factors.[8] Victimization statistics show that Black youth are generally more involved in violence (as perpetrators *and* victims) than are youth of other racial groups.[8] At their peak rates of homicide victimization, Black men are nine times more likely than White men to become victims of homicide.[9] Nonlethal forms of violence that result in harm to victims, such as rape, robbery, and aggravated assault, are also higher among Blacks.[10] In 2012, more Blacks were victimized by violence than were Whites or Hispanics. Statistics show that Native Americans are also increasingly vulnerable.[11]

Some view these racial differences as an artifact of how violent crimes are documented and tallied. Others believe that they represent the lived realities of young people of color, such that they encounter violence more often. In fact, there is actually some consistency in trends shown in reports compiled from self-reports and official record data (e.g., police arrests and court processing documents), showing that young adult Black males are indeed the most likely to be impacted by violence.[4,12]

Leading hypotheses about these racial differences center on the socioeconomic disadvantages and poor living conditions of many Black families. Some scholars attribute disparate living conditions to discriminatory policies and practices that have reduced opportunities for upward social and economic mobility for certain youth.[13] It is most definitely the case that neighborhoods with highest crime rates are often those that have the fewest resources for young residents and their families.[13] High residential turnover and anonymity among residents in these neighborhoods can lead to a breakdown in the social fabric of the community that binds individuals together around a common set of values and norms against violence. As violence persists within the most disadvantaged neighborhoods, residents can be made to feel incapable of addressing the problem in any fundamental way, layering the appearance of resignation on top of the social disengagement many already experience. As problematic, violence can actually serve a useful purpose for some young people of color by allowing them a social standing among their peers.[13]

Consequences of Violence

That violence can bring about serious consequences for victims is well established and undisputed.[3] However, it is perhaps not as well known that those who perpetrate violence are also more likely to be victimized and harmed by violence themselves. A recent study by Chassin and colleagues[14] tracked a sample of youth offenders over a 7-year period into early adulthood and then analyzed why some offenders suffered an early death. They found that homicides and suicides were among the top causes of death for those who perpetrated crimes and then died in their 20s.

● RISK AND PROTECTIVE FACTORS ASSOCIATED WITH VIOLENCE

The etiology of violent offending of young people points to a range of risk and protective factors.[15] Risk factors are those that predict an increase in the likelihood of violence occurring, whereas protective factors are predictors of less violence. The risk factors most predictive of violence are similar across demographic groups and span a range of social environmental contexts or domains: family, school, neighborhood, peer, individual.[16]

Risk Factors

Risk factors for violence have been documented in a number of studies, including the Cambridge Study in Delinquent Development,[17] the Pittsburgh Youth Study,[18] the Rochester Youth Development Study,[19] and the Seattle Social Development Project,[16,20] to name a few. Findings of these studies show that there is considerable overlap in risk factors for violence and other youth problems, such as drug and alcohol abuse, teen pregnancy, and mental health disorders. Thus, many of these problems are rooted in similar causes and possibly preventable using similar strategies.[21] Table 63.2 (see Chapter 63) outlines some of the more well-established risk factors for youth problems, including violence.

Studies show that the likelihood of violence and other related problems is substantially higher for young people exposed to several risk factors in combination.[22] Therefore, prevention programs that target multiple risk factors are thought to have a higher likelihood of success than those more that are more narrowly focused on single risk factors in isolation from others.[20]

Firearms, Gang Involvement, and the Perpetuation of Violence

There are certain risk factors for violence worth emphasizing because they are discussed often in media reports and the popular literature. These include firearm availability, gang involvement, and child abuse or child maltreatment.

Firearms

In the aftermath of several tragic school shootings and mass killings involving guns, there has been a renewed interest in firearm control and gun safety.[23] One such event was a school shooting in 2012 perpetrated by a 20-year-old man in Newtown, Connecticut, which led to the deaths of many young children and the adults who tried to protect them. Following the event, there was a plea from gun control advocates to tighten restrictions on gun access. They warned of future tragedies and called upon elected officials to do more to keep children safe. At the same time, some in positions of influence cautioned against moving too quickly with any one corrective measure. And, others voiced strong opposition to any measure that would limit the rights of US citizens to own guns. Violence prevention researchers offered their own perspectives on what is needed to keep incidents like that in Newtown from happening again. For example, Kellermann and Rivara[23] called for an increasing investment of federal research funds in studies on firearm use, noting that there has been a deliberate attempt on the part of some in the government to block research for gun research because they feared political reprisal. Whether or not those who control research funds eventually choose to take a bold position on the issue, findings of the few studies that exist on the issue are rather convincing in showing that guns in the wrong hands can lead to terrible tragedy.[4]

Gang Involvement

Street gangs have been around for decades, and there is growing awareness that gang activity is more prevalent and entrenched now than previously thought.[24,25] It is estimated that about 25% of all middle and high school students in the US are aware of the presence of gangs in their schools,[24] and the most recent estimates by the National Gang Center[25] report that about 31% of all US cities, towns, suburbs, and rural communities encountered problems with gangs—all together, about 3,300 jurisdictions. This figure comprises approximately 782,500 gang members in 29,900 gangs, with most gang activity concentrated in urban areas. Slightly more than half of all gangs and three-quarters of all gang members are located in large cities, and the majority of gang-related homicides (87%) occur in these areas. Youth who participate in gangs are at a much higher risk for perpetrating and being victimized by violence.[26]

Although gang involvement poses a major risk for the youth involved, reasons why a young person joins a gang remain speculative. However, it is known that some of the same risk factors that predict youth violence also predict gang involvement,[27] suggesting the two are interrelated. Thus, it may be that gang-involved youth are more likely to perpetrate violence because they are reinforced for behavior that is already present.[28]

Child Maltreatment

Research provides compelling evidence that maltreated children are at a significantly higher risk to experience violence—as perpetrators and victims—than are other children.[3] Indeed, exposure to violence in the home, including interparental violence, conditions children to use violence in other contexts.[29] Children exposed to violence come to view it as a means to control the behaviors of

XV

others. It is also frequently the case that children in violent and unsafe homes are not afforded the opportunity to develop skills to handle conflict prosocially, or in other words, to learn nonviolent strategies to handle conflict that result in a resolution. Related findings have been produced by Widom[30] and others, who talk about a "cycle of violence" that continues across generations. This cycle occurs when violence is modeled by adults and then taken up by their children. Children, in turn, repeat the same pattern as adults. It is unfortunately the case that millions of children are abused each year in the US and elsewhere in the world.[31] And, even more children witness domestic violence in their homes, placing them at risk for repeating the behavior and also being revictimized.[29]

Protective Factors

Youth are more likely to engage in violence as their exposure to risk factors increases.[20] At the same time, a young person may encounter social and environmental influences that reduce his or her risk for violence. Protective factors include certain qualities and characteristics, such as a young person's social and interpersonal awareness and problem-solving abilities. Social supports in the environment, on the other hand, are generally protective. It is well established that adolescents benefit when adults and peers are warm and nurturing, and when they lend support in times of need (see Chapter 4). Having access to certain types of activities and groups, such as sports and extracurricular programming, can be very beneficial for young people of all ages, not just because of the learning they provide, but also the relationships they help form. Doing well in school (being committed to school) also is beneficial for obvious reasons.[20] For prevention, then, the goal is not just to reduce risk factors but also promote protective factors that improve youth development and early adult outcomes.[32]

⬤ ASSESSMENT OF RISK

Assessing risk and protective factors, and intervening to prevent and reduce violence, can take the form of large-scale, population- or group-level strategies, as well as individual- or family-level assessments. Other reports and research summaries attend very directly to group- and community-level risk assessments and procedures.[33] In this section, we focus on individual-level assessments and approaches because these may be of particular interest to individual practitioners.

Given the multidetermined nature of youth violence and tendency for individual, social, and environmental factors to converge and jointly influence behavior when conducting a risk assessment of youth, it is important that practitioners inquire about the following:

- *Risk domains*: Information about the risk domains previously mentioned (e.g., family, peers, school, community).[34]
- *Behavior*: Information on the behavior itself to determine when and where a young person encounters violence; when it was first observed; and for how long it has been an issue of concern (duration).
- *Family*: Information on factors such as whether there is a history of parental mental illness or substance use, whether parents are in conflict, whether there is abuse of any form in the home, and whether other siblings also exhibit conduct or other problems are also informative.
- *Environment*: Information on the surrounding environment most probably related to the presenting behaviors, such as negative peer or neighborhood influences and social or structural dynamics of the school to learn about factors that might reinforce and motivate the behavior in particular settings.[34]

All of these different aspects of the risk environment are important for intervention planning, particularly as one considers how or where to refer a young person for ongoing services or how to develop and implement an evidence-based prevention or intervention plan.

Mental Health Evaluation

Comprehensive psychological or psychiatric evaluations also may be needed if it is determined that an adolescent or young adult has a chronic, severe, and/or worsening conduct problem.[35,36]

Conduct Problem Assessment

As noted in a review of literature by McMahon and Frick,[36] the term "conduct problem" is used to describe a number of different behaviors that range in seriousness from those of a generally benign and harmless quality, such as yelling or teasing others, to those with which this chapter is more directly concerned, such as physical aggression and stealing. Many conduct disorders are also oppositional and defiant, although symptoms are not necessarily the same across all individuals with these comorbid problems. In fact, the way in which these behavioral dimensions converge varies to a point that researchers and practitioners now refer to different symptom clusters when diagnosing an adolescent, or when describing a particular group of young people for whom an evidence-based program would be recommended. The implication for assessment, according McMahon and Frick,[36] is a need to attend to the "number, types, and severity" of the problems of concern, as well as the level of impairment each has caused the individual and those around him/her. There are two discrete, but complimentary, approaches to conducting comprehensive assessments of conduct problems in youth: (a) a general risk assessment method and (b) a targeted risk assessment method.

- *General Risk Assessment*: In a general risk assessment, practitioners attend to risk factors by interviewing youth and other informants and by reviewing archival materials, such as psychiatric reports or, for older youth, juvenile justice records. Borum and Verhaagen (2006) refer to a number of structured risk assessment instruments that can be used for the purposes of assessing youth directly. One such tool is the Structured Assessment of Violence Risk in Youth (SAVRY),[37] which offers a manualized, checklist-type assessment of 24 different risk indicators over three domains—historical, social-contextual, and individual-clinical for youth between 12 and 18 years old. Practitioners are asked to incorporate multiple sources of information (e.g., personal interviews, reviews of records, consultation with information) to generate ratings of risk status on each item; once completed, the assessed information can help guide professional judgment in very specific ways.

  A variety of other similar instruments exist, some of which permit inferences from clinical "cut scores" for early adolescents (e.g., the Early Assessment Risk List)[38] and others that utilize an unscored but structured format similar to the SAVRY (e.g., Historical Clinical Risk Management-20).[39] A general risk assessment approach is typically used in cases where a youth's behavior has risen to a level of concern but not yet to a level where immediate intervention to address safety concerns is required.

- *Targeted Risk Assessment*: In a targeted risk assessment, there are usually discernible, sometimes immediate threats of violence made by an adolescent that require immediate action on the part of a trained clinician or other adults tasked with this responsibility in school or community context. In such cases, the first step is to gauge the level of risk involved and the likelihood a youth will carry through on a threat he or she has made. Reddy et al.[40] provide a model for this type of risk assessment that focuses on 10 areas of inquiry: (1) motivation for the referral behavior; (2) method of communicating threats; (3) "unusual interest" in targeted violence; (4) evidence for "attack-related behaviors and planning"; (5) mental status; (6) level of "cognitive sophistication" as applied to planning and executing a targeted violent act; (7) recent losses, including losses of status; (8) coordination of violent communications and related behaviors; (9) concern from collateral contacts about individual's propensity for violence; and (10) contextual and situational factors that increase or decrease the individual's propensity for violence. As with a general risk assessment approach, practitioners who conduct targeted risk assessments can use a variety of information sources to help formulate their plans (interviews, informant reports, etc.). However, in the case of targeted assessments, all information-gathering is predicated on concerns of immediate threat, often when plans to carry out the threat have also been voiced.

It is important to note that assessing an individual's risk or propensity for violence can be a daunting task that carries with it significant responsibilities, both legal and ethical, for practitioners. Those charged with assessing conduct-disordered and violent adolescents can find themselves in situations that require them not only to assess and stabilize the individual involved but also notify law enforcement or targeted third parties when there are credible threats of violence. Practitioners who inquire in the context of a comprehensive assessment about a young person's experience of domestic violence and child abuse might similarly need to file reports with authorities so that the safety of everyone involved can be assured. Thus, practitioners must be highly trained and versed on the protocols for accurately identifying and efficiently acting on threats of violence at the point they become known.

Prevention and Intervention

Reducing or eliminating risk factors and strengthening protective factors is a recommended, evidence-based strategy for reducing violence and other problems in youth.[22] In designing preventive interventions, even knowledge of predictors that are not malleable (e.g., gender, race, and ethnicity) can be useful because it helps to establish for whom prevention services are most needed. An understanding of the risk and protective factors most consistently related to youth violence is fundamental to the design and delivery of any program that focuses on prevention.

Violence prevention strategies, implemented at a group or population level typically, are organized around a public health model, which incorporates many of the risk and protective factors in the community, family, school, peer, and individual domains.[22] Public health prevention has traditionally been discussed using the terms primary, secondary, and tertiary prevention to designate where in the developmental progression of a problem and to which population a prevention program is most intended. Public health programs in prevention now fall under the headings of universal, selected, and indicated models, which categorize programs more so by risk level and population needs. *Universal* prevention programs focus on young people in the general population—those not yet manifesting signs of a problem of concern—with the intent of inoculating everyone against the influences most likely to cause violence. *Selected* programs focus on those at higher risk of a problem, but who have not yet begun to manifest signs of problem itself. And, *indicated* programs focus on those at highest risk for a problem like violence, including those who have already begun committing violence acts, although perhaps of a less serious nature. In that individuals in this category have not yet engaged in the most serious forms of violence, they are still considered candidates for prevention.[15]

Prevention programs are commonly implemented at the community, school, and family levels, less so at the individual youth level because it is recognized that individual predispositions and tendencies toward the use of violence are typically only acted upon when the social environment is conducive to that behavior, as is the case in dysfunctional (e.g., abusive and highly aversive)

families, or in schools or community settings in which norms support violence and control strategies are ineffectual. In addition, studies of clinical interventions targeting individual AYAs, such as psychotherapy for adolescents whose primary diagnosis is conduct disorder, have proven mostly ineffective if not combined with other interventions that focus also on the social environment.[41] In a review of research on psychosocial interventions for aggressive and violent youth, Connor[41] reported that of the more than 230 psychotherapies-available adolescents, a relatively small number had been evaluated, and of those that had, few produced consistent results for conduct problems. Far more evidence was available at the time of that review, and still to this day, point to the far greater benefits of other intervention modalities and approaches, and to multicomponent strategies that attend to several individual, social, and environment risk factors in combination.[3,41] Indeed, when cognitive-behavioral and social skills training programs (individual-level interventions) are embedded in programs that also attend to environmental influences related to families and peers, results are far more promising.[41] Moreover, it is now well recognized that the best chance of changing a young person's behavioral trajectory of aggression is to address the problem early: before age 8, according to some sources.[41] Research on programs like multisystemic therapy (MST), a rigorously evaluated, evidence-based program, shows, however, that well-designed interventions directed to older, high-risk and violence-prone youth in the middle and high school grades can in some cases change behavior for the better, even diverting delinquent youth from the criminal justice system.[42]

What about the Individual Practitioner in Practice?

For the individual practitioner, the goal following assessment is to:

1. become well acquainted with what the research shows about evidence-based prevention programs and
2. assist as much as possible in helping broker connections between families and service systems so that children, youth, and young adults have access to the best available options for intervention.

There are a number of ways that individual providers can access the latest information on evidence-based programs in violence prevention. One approach is to download materials from credible sources online, such as the CDC. The CDC's Division of Violence Prevention (http://www.cdc.gov/ViolencePrevention/index.html) provides excellent research summaries on a number of related topics, including child maltreatment, sexual assault, and elder abuse. Other online sources are also helpful for up-to-date information on best practices in youth violence prevention, such as the Blueprints for Health Youth Development website (http://www.blueprintsprograms.com/) and the MINCAVA electronic clearinghouse at the University of Minnesota (http://www.mincava.umn.edu/).

As for brokering connections between families and service systems, well-informed individual practitioners should focus on opening access to programs known to work (i.e., prevent violence) and to also discourage the use of programs and practices that have limited scientific support. As noted in a well-written review by Oesterle and colleagues,[43] for youth in the transition to young adulthood, relatively few rigorously evaluated prevention programs currently exist, making program selection for this particular age group possibly more challenging than for other ages. However, sourcebooks like that of the Institute of Medicine and National Research Council[44] on the well-being of young adults provides general guidance on developmental programs and approaches that are relevant to young people at risk for violence.

Evidence-Based Programs

A fuller discussion and review of evidence-based programs in youth violence prevention, including MST, can be found in online sources, which summarizes the goals and components of each program in some detail, their impacts on behavior, and also their benefits and financial costs. In the paragraphs below, we briefly review evidence on community-, school-, and family-based prevention models to provide some information for the individual practitioner.

Community-based prevention programs include a variety of approaches to reduce risk factors and enhance protective factors for young people. Programs can include community mobilizing and community policing, youth mentoring, and employment.[45] While promising in several ways, community-level prevention programs have proved difficult to evaluate because of the complex service delivery systems that surround youth programming in these contexts.[15,45] As a result, the field has amassed relatively little data to help guide program and policy makers to evidence-based models. There is, however, emerging evidence that certain approaches to crime reduction and prevention, like community mobilizing and neighborhood policing, can impact violence (http://www.ojjdp.gov/mpg).

Gang Involvement–Based Programs

Prevention and intervention programs focused on gang involvement are often organized at the community level, yet the dynamics of gangs are such that very specialized intervention approaches can be required.[46] Evidence-based practices shown to benefit violent and gang-involved youth tend to focus on reducing the violent behavior more so than extracting the youth from gangs, although models like the Office of Juvenile Justice and Delinquency Prevention's Comprehensive Gang Model provide some very specific guidance on strategies to engage gang-involved youth using outreach and other forms of social engagement to link young people to needed services and to expand their opportunities for education and employment. Unfortunately, when youth are involved in gangs, the very behaviors that are likely to harm others (and the youth involved) are precisely those that are encouraged and reinforced by gang culture.[47] Consequently, the effects of interventions that do not target gang involvement for violent adolescents are very likely to fall short of their intended goals related to reducing violence and improving public safety.[48]

School-Based Prevention Programs

According to a review of programs by Jenson and colleagues,[45] *school-based* violence prevention programs include classroom-based cooperative learning, small-group instruction, proactive classroom management, interactive teaching, and peer learning to create conditions that are conducive to positive behaviors and academic achievement among students. Social and emotional learning programs are also grouped under this general header. Meta-analytic reviews of school-based violence prevention programs have generally shown that effects on violence, aggregated across studies, point to relatively robust effects of these particular programs.[49] As noted by Wilson and Lipsey,[49] school prevention programs implemented with fidelity to the original design of a program model typically do better at preventing violence than do those implemented with less fidelity, likely because there is a reduction in the quality of implementation that occurs when programs stray from their original design.[49] Program duration also matters, according to meta-analytic reviews. That is, programs that continue over long periods of time generally produce more positive results with respect to a reduction in violence than do those of a shorter duration, all other factors being equal.

Family-Based Prevention Approaches

Family-based violence prevention approaches can include early childhood education, and parent training strategies, or programs to help build supports around families to lessen the burden of one or various stressors. Parent training programs are perhaps the most common in this domain. These programs focus on helping parents develop the knowledge and skills to think constructively about their children's behaviors, providing appropriate discipline, monitoring young people's whereabouts, and openly communicating with their children to avoid hostile conflicts that can escalate to violence. As noted by Jenson et al. (2011), findings from systematic and meta-analytic reviews of these approaches are also generally favorable, assuming they are implemented well.[49]

CONCLUSION

There is a considerable amount of information on the scope, causes, and consequences of youth violence, and also, strategies to assess and prevent violence in young people. Understanding risk and protective factors related to violence provides a starting point for developing preventive interventions to reduce risks and enhance protection for youth at risk, as well as those in the general population, so that the cycle of violence that can occur within families can be broken and lives saved as a result. Universal programs are necessary to attend to risks that all young people of a particular region or neighborhood experience, lessening the risk for violence by shifting broad social environmental factors away from violence and toward more prosocial ways of relating. Additionally, the use of evidence-based practices and programs in youth violence prevention is critical to address the problem and to reduce costs associated with ineffective or poorly implemented and low-quality programs.[50] For practitioners, having knowledge of which programs and approaches work best to prevent violence in real-world settings is an important goal.[48]

REFERENCES

1. World Health Organization. *World report on violence and health*, 2002. Geneva: World Health Organization, 2002.
2. Office of Juvenile Justice and Delinquency Prevention. *Juvenile arrests 2010*. Washington, DC: United States Department of Justice, Office of Justice Programs, 2013.
3. Herrenkohl TI, Aisenberg E, Williams JH, et al. *Violence in context: current evidence on risk, protection, and prevention*. New York, NY: Oxford University Press, 2011.
4. Centers for Disease Control and Prevention. *Youth violence facts at a glance*, 2012. National Center for Injury Prevention and Control, Division of Violence Prevention, Centers for Disease Control and Prevention.
5. Centers for Disease Control and Prevention. *Youth violence facts at a glance*, 2010. National Center for Injury Prevention and Control, Division of Violence Prevention, Centers for Disease Control and Prevention.
6. Truman JL, Rand MR. *Criminal victimization, 2009*. United States Department of Justice, 2010.
7. Chesney-Lind M, Belknap J. *Trends in delinquent girls' aggression and violent behavior: a review of the evidence*. In: Putallaz M, Bierman P, eds. *Aggression, antisocial behavior and violence among girls: a developmental perspective*. New York, NY: Guilford Press, 2004:203–220.
8. Puzzanchera C, Chamberlin G, Kang W. *Easy access to the FBI's Supplementary Homicide Reports: 1980–2011*. 2013.
9. Smith EL, Cooper A. *Homicide in the U.S. known to law enforcement, 2011*. 2013.
10. Harrell E. *Black victims of violent crime*, in *Bureau of Justice Statistics Special Report 2007*. Washington, DC: U.S. Department of Justice, Office of Justice Programs, 2007.
11. Truman JL, Langton L, Planty M. *Criminal victimization, 2012*. United States Department of Justice, 2013.
12. Williams JH, Bright CL, Petersen G. Racial and ethnic differences in risk and protective factors associated with youth violence. In: Herrenkohl TI, et al., eds. *Violence in context: current evidence on risk, protection, and prevention*. New York, NY: Oxford University Press, 2011.
13. Peterson RD, Krivo LJ. Macrostructural analyses of race, ethnicity, and violent crime: recent lessons and new directions for research. *Annu Rev Sociol* 2005;31:331–356.
14. Chassin L, Piquero AR, Losoya SH, et al. Joint consideration of distal and proximal predictors of premature mortality among serious juvenile offenders. *J Adolesc Health* 2013;52:689–696.
15. Fagan AF, Catalano RF. What works in youth violence prevention: a review of the literature. *Res Social Work Pract* 2013;23:141–156.
16. Herrenkohl TI, Maguin E, Hill KG, et al. Developmental risk factors for youth violence. *J Adolesc Health* 2000;26(3):176–186.
17. Farrington DP. Early predictors of adolescent aggression and adult violence. *Violence Vict* 1989;4(2):79–100.
18. Pardini DA, Loeber R, Farrington DP, et al. Identifying direct protective factors for nonviolence. *Am J Prev Med* 2012;43(2, suppl 1):S28–S40.
19. Browning K, Thornberry TP, Porter PK. *Highlights of findings from the Rochester Youth Development Study*. OJJDP Fact Sheet 1999, United States Department of Justice, Office of Justice Programs.
20. Hawkins JD, Herrenkohl TI, Farrington DP, et al. *Predictors of youth violence*. Juvenile Justice Bulletin, Office of Juvenile Justice and Delinquency Prevention, 2000.
21. Catalano RF, Haggerty KP, Hawkins JD, et al. Prevention of substance use and substance use disorders: the role of risk and protective factors. In: Kaminer Y,

Winters KC, eds. *Clinical manual of adolescent substance abuse treatment.* Washington, DC: American Psychiatric Publishing, 2011:25–63.

22. Institute of Medicine. *Reducing risks for mental disorders: frontiers for prevention intervention research.* Washington, DC: National Academy Press, 1994.

23. Kellermann AL, Rivara FP. Silencing the science on gun research. *J Am Med Assoc* 2013;309(6):549–550.

24. Dinkes R, Kemp J, Baum K, et al. *Indicators of school crime and safety: 2009 (NCES 2010-012).* Washington, DC: National Center for Education Statistics, Institute of Education Sciences, US Department of Education, 2009.

25. Egley A Jr, Howell JC. *Highlights of the 2011 National Youth Gang Survey.* Washington, DC: US Department of Justice, Office of Justice Programs, Office of Juvenile Justice and Delinquency Prevention, 2013.

26. Barnes JC, Beaver KM, Miller M. Estimating the effect of gang membership on nonviolent delinquency: A counterfactual analysis. *Aggress Behav* 2010;36:437–451.

27. Boxer P, Veysey B, Ostermann M, et al. Measuring gang involvement in a justice-referred sample of youth in treatment. *Youth Violence Juv Justice,* 2014. doi:1541204013519828.

28. Curry GD, Decker SH Egley A Jr. Gang involvement and delinquency in a middle school population. *Justice Quarterly* 2002;19:275–292.

29. Herrenkohl TI, Sousa C, Tajima EA, et al. Intersection of child abuse and children's exposure to domestic violence. *Trauma Violence Abuse* 2008;9(2):84–99.

30. Widom CS. The cycle of violence. *Science* 1989;244(4901):160–166.

31. World Health Organization. *Preventing child maltreatment: A guide to taking action and generating evidence.* Geneva: World Health Organization, 2006.

32. Herrenkohl TI, Chung IJ, Catalano RF. Review of research on predictors of youth violence and school-based and community-based prevention approaches. In: Allen-Meares P, Fraser MW, eds. *Intervention with children and adolescents: an interdisciplinary perspective.* Boston, MA: Allyn & Bacon,2004:449–476.

33. Hawkins JD, Catalano RF, Associates. *Communities that care: action for drug abuse prevention.* San Francisco, CA: Jossey-Bass, 1992.

34. Connor DF. *Clinical assessment, case formulation, and treatment planning.* In: *Aggression and Antisocial Behavior in Children and Adolescents.* New York, NY: The Guilford Press,2002:302–326.

35. Hoge RD. *Assessment in juvenile justice systems.* In: Hoge RD, Guerra NG, Boxer P, eds. *Treating the juvenile offender.* New York, NY: The Guilford Press, 2008.

36. McMahon RJ, Frick PJ. *Evidence-based assessment of conduct problems in children and adolescents.* J Clin Child Adolesc Psychol 2005;34:477–505.

37. Borum R. *Manual for the Structured Assessment of Violence Risk in Youth (SAVRY).* Odessa, FL: Psychological Assessment Resources, 2006.

38. Augimeri LK, Koegl CJ, Webster CD, et al. *Early assessment risk list for boys.* Toronto, ON: Child Development Institute, 2001.

39. Douglas KS, Hart SD, Webster CD, et al. *HCR-20V3: Assessing risk of violence—User guide.* Burnaby, Canada: Mental Health, Law, and Policy Institute, Simon Fraser University, 2013.

40. Reddy M, Borum R, Vossekuil B, et al. Evaluating risk for targeted violence in schools: comparing risk assessment, threat assessment, and other approaches. *Psychol Schools* 2001;38:157–172.

41. Connor DF. Psychosocial *interventions.* In: *Aggression and antisocial behavior in children and adolescents.* New York, NY: The Guilford Press, 2002:327–357.

42. Weiss B, Susan H, Vicki H, et al. An independent randomized clinical trial of multisystemic therapy with non-court-referred adolescents with serious conduct problems. *J Consult Clin Psychol* 2013;81(6):1027–1039.

43. Oesterle S. Background paper: pathways to young adulthood and preventive interventions targeting young adults. In: Institute of Medicine and National Research Council, ed. *Improving the health, safety, and well-being of young adults: workshop summary.* Washington, DC: The National Academies Press, 2013:147–176.

44. Institute of Medicine and National Research Council. *Investing in the health and well-being of young adults.* Washington, DC: National Academy Press, 2014.

45. Jenson JM, Powell A, Forrest-Bank S. Effective violence prevention approaches in school, family, and community settings. In: Herrenkohl TI, et al., eds. *Violence in context: current evidence on risk, protection, and prevention.* Oxford University Press, Series on Interpersonal Violence. New York, NY: Oxford University Press, 2011:130–170.

46. Arciaga M. *Overview of the OJJDP comprehensive gang model.* Tallahassee, FL: National Gang Center, 2010.

47. Boxer P. Negative peer involvement in multisystemic therapy for the treatment of youth problem behavior: exploring outcome and process variables in "real-world" practice. *J Clin Child Adolesc Psychol* 2011;40:848–854.

48. Pyrooz DC, Decker SH. Motives and methods for leaving the gang: Understanding the process of gang desistance. *J Criminal Justice* 2011;39: 417–425.

49. Wilson SJ, Lipsey MW. School-based interventions for aggressive and disruptive behavior update of a meta-analysis. *Am J Prev Med* 2007;33(2, suppl): S130–S143.

50. Lipsey MW. The primary factors that characterize effective interventions with juvenile offenders: a meta-analytic overview. *Vict Offenders* 2010;4(2):124–147.

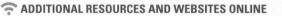 **ADDITIONAL RESOURCES AND WEBSITES ONLINE**

CHAPTER 73

Sexual Assault and Victimization

Vaughn I. Rickert
Dillon J. Etter
Mariam R. Chacko

SEXUAL ASSAULT

Sexual assault and victimization (SAV) among adolescents and young adults (AYAs) is of particular concern because of its high occurrence in this population, its infrequent disclosure, and the significant health consequences associated with this type of violence.[1] Slightly more than 25% of girls and about 6% of boys will experience some form of SAV before they turn 18.[2] Rates of SAV are four times higher among females aged 16 to 24 years compared to women in all other age-groups.[1] SAV estimates for gay, lesbian, or bisexual individuals suggest that these subgroups may also be at increased risk.[3] Sexual violence on college campuses is another area of concern, especially due to a recent increase in media exposure.

A history of SAV not only makes it more difficult for individuals to develop healthy intimate relationships as adults, but it also significantly increases the risk of negative health outcomes, including human immunodeficiency virus (HIV), depression, suicidal ideation, and substance abuse.[4] Health care providers play a key role in the early identification of victims of SAV and the prevention of subsequent negative health outcomes. SAV disclosure requires prompt medical and psychological intervention. When forensic evidence is required, providers who are willing to devote the time and support needed should examine the sexual assault victim. Thus, the clinician must be familiar with the proper protocol for intervention, including clinical, legal, and psychosocial techniques.

A victim of SAV is the object of a hostile, dehumanizing attack that can have long-lasting effects on concepts of self-worth and identity.[5] During adolescence, an individual is learning to manage feelings of sexual arousal, developing new forms of intimacy and autonomy, experiencing intimate interpersonal relationships, and building skills to control the consequences of sexual behavior. SAV or attempted SAV as a first or early sexual experience may cause confusion between intercourse and violence, jeopardizing the young person's sexual health. For young adults, SAV may initiate mental health problems, cause problems in future relationship decision making, increase psychological burden relative to self-attribution of the assault, and result in secondary victimization from family and friends.

Provider-initiated screening to detect sexual victimization represents an important public health strategy to overcome the difficulty that some AYAs face when disclosing these violent events.[6] Despite recommendations to screen AYA females and endorsement of screening acceptability by these young women, routine screening for SAV does not occur, especially among sexual minorities.[7]

The terms used to describe the range of victimizations included in sexual assault are sometimes used interchangeably, frequently unclear, and require definition. These labels have legal ramifications and reporting requirements that impact prevalence and incidence rates. Below is a summary of common terminology associated with SAV:

- "Sexual assault" can be defined as any act, either physical or verbal, of a sexual nature committed against another person that is accompanied by actual or threatened physical force.
- "Rape" is a legal term with a definition that varies widely. Generally, this term implies unlawful nonconsensual sexual activity carried out forcibly or under threat of injury against the will of the victim. Nonconsensual sex is divided into two categories—*stranger rape* is perpetrated by a stranger and *acquaintance rape* is perpetrated by someone known to the individual. *Date rape*, occurring between two people in a romantic relationship or potential sexual relationship, is a subset of acquaintance rape.
- "Sexual abuse" typically refers to the sexual victimization of a minor and is primarily a legal term. In certain contexts, the term can include consensual sex between minors or a minor and an adult (*statutory rape*).
- "Sex trafficking," as it pertains to children and adolescents, includes trafficking a minor for the purpose of sexual exploitation, exploiting a minor through prostitution, and exploiting a minor though survival sex.[8]
- "Prostitution" typically refers to sex in exchange for money.
- "Survival sex" is the exchange of sex for food, money, shelter, drugs, or other wants and needs.

Epidemiology

Trends of completed or attempted rape among all women from 1995 to 2010 have declined 58%.[9] The reporting of rape and sexual assault has also declined considerably in recent years from 56% in 2003 to 28% in 2012.[10] According to 2009 National Crime Victimization Survey (NCVS) data,[9] of the 106,100 rape and sexual assault cases where a female was the victim, only 31% of perpetrators were identified as strangers. Among the 19,820 male rape and sexual assault victims, a stranger perpetrated 52% of the attacks. Thus, for these data, which include all ages, female victims are five times more likely to know the perpetrator than male victims.

Data from the US Department of Justice[1] suggest a significant period of vulnerability for females between the ages of 12 and 24 years, with the largest number occurring between the ages of 16 and 24. Risk factors include female gender (age 16 to 24 years); history of abuse (sexual or other); for females, younger age at menarche, greater number of dating and/or sexual partners, and a sexually active peer group; for males, homelessness and disability (physical, cognitive, psychiatric); alcohol use by perpetrator or victim, especially in a dating situation; and dating relationships that include verbal or physical abuse.

Incidence

1. Gender: Across all age-groups, females experience significantly higher rates of SAV than males. Of AYAs aged 12 to 25, compared to males, females face 17 times the risk of SAV[11] (Fig. 73.1).
2. Age: For White and Black AYAs, females aged 18 to 25 experience the highest rates of SAV, followed closely by females aged 12 to 17. For Hispanic AYAs, females aged 12 to 17 experience the highest rates of SAV.[11]
3. Race: Black females experience the highest rates of SAV. Among AYAs aged 12 to 25, Black females are 62% and 200% more likely to experience SAV than White and Hispanic females, respectively.[11]
4. Eight percent of youth (11.8% of females and 4.5% of males) report that they have been forced to have sexual intercourse.[12]
5. Adults are responsible for relatively few victimizations (15% of general sexual victimizations and 29% of sexual assault) confirming that a vast majority of victimizations are perpetrated by peer acquaintances.[13]
6. Two-thirds of sexual assault victimizations reported to the police involve juvenile victims.
7. Adolescents ≤18 years who experience sexual victimization are twice as likely to experience a future assault during their college years.
8. Approximately 60% of sexual assaults occur at home or at the home of an acquaintance.

Sequelae

Most of the sexual violence that clinicians will encounter when treating AYA women has been perpetrated by an acquaintance, date, or a significant other. As a result, spontaneous disclosure by the victim is not likely—either because AYAs do not perceive it as sexual assault, they are embarrassed, or they believe it is their own fault.

AYAs who have been victimized experience significantly higher levels of depression and anxiety. Male and female high school–aged victims report decreased life satisfaction coupled with suicidal ideation and attempts. Moreover, the individual's sexual health is greatly impacted by victimization. Typically, sexually victimized youth engage in higher-risk sexual behaviors, have poorer attitudes and beliefs regarding sex, and demonstrate a greater prevalence of consequences from sexual activity, that is, unintended pregnancies and sexually transmitted infections (STIs). Common SAV responses include phobias, self-blame, loss of appetite, sleep disturbances, somatic responses, and drug and alcohol use. Sequelae, particular to date rape, may include self-blame, decreased self-esteem, and a difficult time maintaining relationships. Somatic responses can manifest as chronic pelvic pain or recurrent abdominal pain. In the most general case, the first 2 months postvictimization is a time of particular vulnerability for severe depression. Signs of stress disorder (PTSD) are not uncommon within the first year. Victimized AYAs can be two or even three times as likely to begin using illicit drugs, smoke, or regularly consume alcohol compared to their nonvictimized peers.[14]

SEXUAL ABUSE

Incidence

Sexual abuse accounted for almost 10% of all substantiated claims of child victimization, totaling 65,984 cases—29 of which resulted in death.[15] However, data from the National Incidence Survey 4 (NIS-4) suggest striking declines in both the rate and numbers of sexually abused children.[16] Indicators that should alert the provider to suspect abuse include the following:

1. STIs in a prepubertal adolescent or any adolescent with no history of sexual intercourse
2. Recurrent somatic complaints, particularly involving the gastrointestinal, genitourinary, or pelvic areas
3. Behavioral indicators, including significant changes in mood, onset of withdrawal from usual family, school, and social

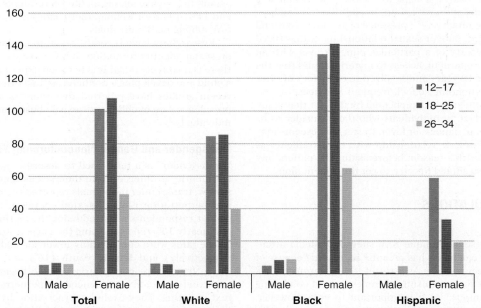

FIGURE 73.1 Sexual assault rates (per 100,000) by gender, race, and age-group, in the US, 2013. (From the Centers for Disease Control and Prevention. *Web-based Injury Statistics Query and Reporting System (WISQARS)* [Online], 2013.)

activities; patterns of disordered eating; running away from home; suicidal and self-injurious gestures; rapid escalation of alcohol and/or drug abuse; onset of promiscuous sexual activity; early adolescent pregnancy; and onset of sexual activity before age 13 years

Sequelae

The occurrence of sexual abuse during childhood has been linked to a variety of psychological and emotional problems during adolescence, with some continuing into adulthood. The relationship between severity of abuse, frequency of abuse, and subsequent mental health disorders remains elusive. Sequelae include depression, suicidal ideation and attempts, substance abuse, PTSD, eating disorders, and precocious sexual behaviors (e.g., earlier age at first coitus and greater number of lifetime partners). In addition, childhood sexual abuse for females has been linked to acquaintance and date rape in adolescence or young adulthood.

 SEX TRAFFICKING

Sex trafficking of AYAs for prostitution and other forms of sexual exploitation is an often-overlooked form of SAV. Sex trafficking of minors occurs daily and can lead to serious long-term consequences for victims as well as their families, communities, and society.[8] Sex trafficking can include commercial sex work (prostitution, exotic dancing, and pornography) as well as personal service (domestic or sexual servitude). This criminal endeavor is fast growing and is fueled by a growing demand by customers who pay for illicit sex.[17] Young women and adolescents are a particularly vulnerable group for international and domestic sex trafficking.[17–19] Experts estimate that there are currently at least 100,000 victims of sexual exploitation under the age of 18 in the US[20] and as many as 325,000 victims in the US, Canada, and Mexico.[21] Many victims report being sexually assaulted while they were trafficked.[22]

Victims of sex trafficking can be male, female, or transgender and can come from a variety of backgrounds and experiences. It is important to note that victims of sex trafficking can be much younger than victims of other forms of SAV, as the average age of entry into prostitution in the US is 12 to 14 years old.[22] Human trafficking victims are at increased risk for developing health problems due to substandard living conditions as well as physical, sexual, and emotional trauma. Warning signs for possible sex trafficking include those for victims of sexual assault in addition to homelessness and/or chronic running away[17]; presence of an older boyfriend or age disparity in an intimate or sexual relationship; tattoos (used to mark victim as property of a particular pimp); travel with an older male who is not a guardian; access to material things that the youth cannot afford; < 18 years and involved in or history of prior prostitution; and not attending school, frequent absences, or academic failures. Sex trafficking is complicated by the fact that many adolescents are trafficked by individuals who they consider to be their boyfriend/girlfriend, fiancée, or lover. In fact, adolescents may continue to have an intimate relationship with their trafficker as they are trafficked.[8] For this reason, before asking the patient any sensitive questions, you should first try to get the patient alone.

 SPECIAL POPULATIONS

College Students

College students represent a unique SAV subgroup. Media attention of SAV on college campuses has recently increased because of several high-profile occurrences. As a result, the government has focused considerable effort on raising awareness of and combating sexual violence on campus.[23,24] It is important to note, however, that hearing boards at colleges and universities operate under different procedural rules and evidence standards than the criminal justice system. The purpose of the judicial process at colleges and universities is to determine whether violations of student conduct occurred rather than determining criminal charges. These judicial processes to investigate occurrences of SAV vary considerably across campuses[25] and have recently been scrutinized for a lack of consequences for perpetrators of SAV.[26]

Incidence rates of SAV among college students differ from those of the general population and are likely underestimates.[27] Recent data suggests that, among college students in the US, 3.3% of males and 8.9% of females reported being sexually touched without their consent during the past 12 months.[28] About 1% of males and 4% of females reported a sexual penetration attempt without their consent, with 0.7% of males and 2.5% of females reporting actual penetration without their consent. Among college students who reported drinking alcohol, 1.2% of males and 2.6% of females reported someone having sex with them without their consent while drinking alcohol. In the context of dating, about 1% of males and 2% of females reported being in a sexually abusive intimate relationship within the past 12 months. Academic impact is evident, with 9.5% and 1% of college students reporting that relationship difficulties and sexual assault, respectively, impact their grades.

Males

Male adolescents who have been sexually abused are often overlooked and underserved. However, male sexual abuse is not uncommon and is significantly underreported. Since most perpetrators of sexual violence against adolescent males are male themselves, these victims may remain silent due to the homosexual nature of the assault. In addition, practitioners may fail to recognize and pursue this possibility because of their lack of awareness of this problem.

Lesbian, Gay, and Bisexual Youth

There is a significantly higher rate of childhood sexual abuse among individuals who identify as lesbian, gay, and bisexual (LGB).[4] Over the lifetime, gay and bisexual men were five times more likely to be sexually assaulted than heterosexual men, and lesbian and bisexual women were twice as likely to be assaulted than heterosexual women.[29] Another study reported a similar disparity in rates of SAV between heterosexual and LGB individuals. The median estimate of lifetime SAV was 30% for gay and bisexual men and 43% for lesbian and bisexual women. Given that estimates of lifetime sexual assault prevalence among all the US residents are 2% to 3% for men and 11% to 17% for women, these data suggest an increased risk for SAV among LGB individuals.

Researchers have recently begun to explore the impact of SAV on sexual identity formation. While most data clearly suggest that there is no direct *causal* link between experiencing sexual abuse as a child and developing a nonheterosexual orientation in adulthood, recent studies have reported that there is a 25% to 50% higher prevalence rate of childhood sexual abuse among nonheterosexual individuals.[4]

Transgender and Gender Nonconforming Youth

"Transgender" is a term used to describe individuals whose gender identity is different from their sex assigned at birth. In a large survey, transgender individuals reported the highest victimization and perpetration rates of sexual coercion.[30] Over 60% of transgender respondents reported being the victim of sexual coercion, and nearly 18% reported being the perpetrator of sexual coercion. These rates were considerably lower for male youth (9% and 4%, respectively) and female youth (16% and 1%, respectively).[30] These figures are particularly notable because they are limited to sexual coercion experienced or perpetrated within the context of dating. They exclude perpetration by strangers and other nonpartners, rates of which would likely increase the already-disproportionate prevalence of sexual coercion experienced by transgender AYAs.

"Gender nonconformity" is a less specific term that encompasses all individuals who do not conform to the expression typical of their biological sex. It is important to note that while gender nonconformity and sexual orientation are correlated, one does not necessarily predict the other.[31] Childhood gender nonconformity has been associated with increased prevalence of childhood sexual abuse.[32] In addition to SAV, children who are gender nonconforming in behavior or appearance may also be experiencing bullying, physical or emotional abuse at home, depressive symptoms, and other responses to victimization. Therefore, these children should be screened not only for SAV, but also for bullying, other types of abuse victimization, and mental health symptomatology.[32]

AYAs with Disabilities

AYAs with disabilities are at significantly higher risk for SAV than those without disabilities, and those with severe disabilities are at highest risk.[33,34] This increased risk has been attributed to a number of factors that increase the vulnerability of AYAs with disabilities. These factors could include decreased decision-making capacity, communication deficits, limited social environment, disempowerment of the disability community, poor or nonexistent sex education, misunderstanding of rights, and an increased volume of "touch" contact with others (especially if dependent on others for personal hygiene and basic care). Individuals with severe communication impairments might also experience extreme challenges when attempting to communicate their abuse to professionals. It is important to note that perpetrators of SAV against AYAs with disabilities are often family members, acquaintances, services providers, personal care staff, psychiatrics, or residential care staff. Therefore, speaking privately with AYAs who have disabilities might increase the likelihood of SAV disclosure.

Homeless/Street Youth

Rates of sexual assault for homeless youth in the US are greater than that of youth in the general population.[35] Due to their estrangement from family and friends, homeless and street youth are particularly vulnerable to victimization and violence, especially sex trafficking.[36] This population is more likely to be offered money, drugs, shelter, or food for sex,[37] increasing their risk for exploitation through survival sex. Although rates of survival sex in this population vary across studies, higher rates of engagement in survival sex are consistently reported by homeless gay, lesbian, and bisexual youth compared to heterosexual youth.[35,38] Decisions made by homeless and street youth about whether or not to seek care and report occurrences of SAV are often compounded by low perceived problem severity and barriers to engagement with health and support services.

SCREENING AND REPORTING

Screening

Disclosure of SAV is rarely spontaneous and is often deeply impacted by the adolescents' or young adults' beliefs surrounding their own victimization. Such sensitive information is more often revealed weeks or months after the assault than within a timeline in which emergency room care could be beneficial.[39] This lapse leaves primary care providers with an obligation to inquire about past and present sexual victimization in as sensitive a manner as possible.

Screening Measures

There are currently several useful screening measures that can be easily employed by a clinician and take <15 minutes.

1. Home, Education, Activities, Drugs, Depression, Suicidal ideation, Sex, Safety (HEEADSSS) inventory: As listed in Chapter 3, the HEEADSSS inventory is a helpful device to collect important psychosocial information.
2. Conflict in Adolescent Relationship Inventory[40] (for AYAs under the age of 19)
3. Sexual Experience Survey[41]
4. Date and Family Violence and Abuse Scale[42]
5. Revised Conflict Tactics Scales, Short Forms[43]

In addition, information pamphlets designed to help patients self-screen for dating violence or to increase awareness of sexual health issues can also be helpful. Some clinicians also find *anticipatory guidance,* a conversation centering on sexual health risk factors and warning signs for violence in partners, helpful in serving AYAs' needs.

Within the patient/clinician conversation, AYAs should be provided *accurate information* about the help they can receive from their social network, protective agencies, rape crisis centers, and hotlines. It is recommended that the screening take place in *a private, quiet space* where only the provider and the adolescent or young adult are present. An example of an icebreaker that prepares the patient for some of the questions they will be asked is,

> Because I want to help my patients, I ask everyone about topics that may be very sensitive or may make you uncomfortable. Sadly, some young adults come to my office having been hurt by people around them. It is important that I know those things to be able to help them out.

The concept of *limited confidentiality* should be introduced to the patient in a manner that conveys the legal obligations of the clinician, should any disclosure occur (see Chapter 4). Some providers choose to use a direct but nonthreatening statement similar to,

> Generally, what you say in here stays in here, but there are some exceptions. If I feel that you may hurt yourself or someone else, or that you have been abused by someone, I will need to talk to others to help make sure you get all the care you need.

Consistently asking AYAs about sexual history, even if negative answers were received in prior instances, can allow for this part of the examination to become more routine.

1. Sexual history: A sexual history includes sexual partners and experiences, any unwanted touch, or any previous victimization regardless of the patient's gender. It is also important to inquire whether the patient has obtained money, food, shelter, drugs, or clothing in exchange for sexual favors.
2. Examination: If the patient discloses that injuries were sustained, a thorough examination, consented to by the patient and described in detail in the section "Physical Examination," will be required. This consent must not be general. That is, the AYAs will need to know and consent to the specific purpose and procedures involved in the examination, including the various steps of evidence collection for a rape kit.

It should be noted that for AYAs who have experienced a recent victimization or are seeking treatment because of assault, it may be important to have *a family member or friend* present for the examination. Additionally, the provider can help the victim regain a sense of control over his or her body by encouraging him or her to make as many decisions during his or her examination as possible. It is crucial that the victim be informed that he or she is in control of what will be done and that, at any point, he or she can refuse treatment or stop the examination. For further clinical interventions in sexual violence, refer to the section "General Forensic Background."

Reporting

The following professional guidelines have been endorsed regarding the screening and reporting of sexual victimization.[44]

1. Sexual activity and sexual abuse are not synonymous. It should not be assumed that adolescents under the age of 18 who are sexually active are, by definition, being abused.
2. It is critical that all AYAs who are sexually active receive appropriate confidential health care and counseling.
3. Open and confidential communication between the health professional and the under-18 adolescent patient, together with careful clinical assessment, can identify most sexual abuse cases.
4. Physicians and other health professionals must know the laws in their geographic areas and report cases of sexual abuse to the proper authority after discussion with the adolescent and parent as appropriate.
5. Federal and state laws should support physicians and other health care professionals and their role in providing confidential health care to their patients <18 years.
6. In the US, federal and state laws should affirm the authority of physicians and other health care professionals to exercise appropriate clinical judgment in reporting cases of sexual abuse.

LEGAL ISSUES RELATED TO REPORTING OF SAV

In the US, every state mandates reporting of a reasonable suspicion of child abuse, including sexual abuse, to a designated authority. Mandated reporters of child abuse include virtually all medical and health professionals involved in the care of adolescents under the age of 18 years. The abuse does not need to be proven before being reported, and failure to report can result in civil liability or criminal penalties.

Many states have attempted to increase the reporting of sexually active minors under child abuse reporting laws, either through legislative and policy changes or enforcement of existing laws. These efforts have focused particular attention on younger adolescents who are sexually active. An area of potential confusion and controversy is the reporting of "statutory rape." Although this term does not appear in most states' laws, it is generally used to refer to sexual intercourse that is illegal even if it is consensual, and can refer either to sexual contact between two minors or between a minor and an adult. There are a variety of considerations that can have a bearing on when sexual activity, especially in a young adolescent, must be reported. These include use of coercion or pressure, force or threat of force, or a wide age difference between partners even if the adolescent and parent(s) consider the current relationship consensual and nonabusive. Owing to the variations in reporting laws among states, it is essential that health care providers consult their local legal and medical authorities regarding laws for their state and be aware of their institution's policies as they relate to the screening and reporting of SAV.

EVALUATION OF SEXUAL ABUSE AND ASSAULT: MEDICAL AND FORENSIC ASPECTS

Medical Evaluation

Facilitating an Appropriate Medical Examination

Clinicians and nurses have an obligation to care for those victims of alleged SAV. This involves being able to provide a legal defense in all cases, including those in which a rape kit may or may not have been completed. Medical professionals who conduct a forensic examination must have advanced training and clinical experience and are advised to use a team approach to providing victim-centered care.[45] Clinicians who have not received specialized training should refer these cases to programs and services that can appropriately conduct the examination of the AYA victim.

Individual jurisdictions determine the maximum time interval (36 hours to 1 week) in which evidence may be collected. Changing clothes, showering, and brushing teeth can change the yield of the forensic examination. If the adolescent or young adult declines a forensic examination, a speculum examination should not be undertaken to obtain STI tests until after 96 hours; a speculum examination conducted prior to forensic work will call into question the accuracy of evidence that may later be collected.

Anogenital Trauma—Gender-Specific Considerations
Females
* Complete hymenal clefts are not commonly associated with tampon use but may occur during painful insertion.[46] Thus, providers should interpret such data to the court in the context of a specific case with adequate and detailed history.[47]
* Estrogen affects the adolescent hymen by making it elastic and thereby permitting penile penetration without tearing. Therefore, while posterior hymenal notches or clefts strongly suggest trauma to the area, absence of hymenal notches or clefts should not exclude the possibility of vaginal penetration. Thus, even when penile–vaginal penetration is certain, definitive findings may not be present.[48]

Males
* Evidence of trauma is reported to occur in 20% to 37% of adolescent male sexual abuse/assault survivors.
* Most injuries from sexual abuse and assault involve the rectum, that is, tears and/or bruising and the penis with significantly fewer injuries occurring in the perineum, scrotum, or testes.[49]
* Rectal lacerations from sexual abuse or assault tend to be located at the 1, 5, 7, and 11 o'clock positions.[50]

Facilitating Appropriate Forensic Procedures

The *rape kit* enables collection of evidence such as semen, clothing, and debris for forensic examination. The earlier an examination is performed, the more likely the evidence of trauma will be noted. Thus, these cases should be given priority. Some jurisdictions, particularly those in rural and remote areas, are beginning to use technology for interactive video consultation to support examiners conducting examinations.[51]

The availability of deoxyribonucleic acid (DNA) amplification technology using polymerase chain reaction (PCR) is now used to identify assailants more accurately and allows for collecting evidence beyond the 72-hour period up to 4 days after the assault and possibly longer.[52,53] Since consensus on time limitations for forensic evidence is lacking, it is best to consult individual jurisdictions to determine the maximum time interval in which evidence may be collected.

Photography

The Department of Justice recommends photographs to supplement forensic documentation as they document significant genital injuries and fresh trauma (bloody tears and complete hymenal clefts). Findings such as erythema, swelling, or small labial tears are too subtle and may not be visualized by photographs. If photographs are taken, written consent must be obtained, the procedure explained, and photographs taken in a sensitive manner. A protocol for a secure and legal filing system should be in place.

Conducting the Medical History
* A brief description of the incident including body parts touched, orifices penetrated, the geographic location of the assault, identity of the assailant or alleged perpetrator (if known), whether a condom was used, whether any bleeding was noted from contact sites at the time of the abuse or assault, and method by which the assailant left the scene.
* Whether a weapon was used and any injuries sustained at the time of attack.
* Whether any illicit drugs or alcohol were used voluntarily or involuntarily (the latter may have been used to render the victim helpless and develop memory loss).
* Date of last menses and use of sanitary pads and/or tampons.

- Date and time of last voluntary coitus, other recent sexual experiences.
- History of previous STIs.
- History of prior pregnancy.
- Use of contraception.
- Any significant actions after alleged assault, such as showering or douching, rinsing of mouth, and brushing of teeth.

Physical Examination

- Prior to examining the patient, the provider should provide a step-by-step explanation of what he or she will be doing and why. Reassure the patient that she or he will be in control and that they can request someone to accompany during the physical examination.
- If a rape kit is to be completed, written consent needs to be obtained for the forensic examination, treatment, collection of evidence, and release of medical records.
- Collection of legally mandated tests for the rape kit has to be synchronized with the general physical examination, pelvic or genital examination, and hospital laboratory tests.
- Maintain personal contact with the patient, including verbal and eye contact throughout the examination. Proceed slowly with verbal directions to allow the patient to relax.

General Physical Findings

- General appearance, orientation, emotional state, and behavior should be recorded.
- Condition of patient's clothing should be observed and documented.
- All areas of the body should be explored for signs of trauma, especially at the neck, breasts, upper arms, where bruises resulting from forced restraint are apt to appear.
- Examine the throat.
- Check for abdominal crepitus; this may signify vaginal or rectal laceration with intra-abdominal bleeding.
- Conduct a genital examination for evidence of trauma.

Genital, Pelvic, and Rectal Examination

- Position: An examination on adolescent or young adult female is performed in the lithotomy position. Young and petite adolescent females and males can be examined in the knee-chest position for easier visualization of the anogenital area. The anal area in the larger and older male adolescent should be visualized with the adolescent lying in the lateral position and with one or both knees flexed.
- External genitalia: Note and record signs of blood secretions and sites of bruising, hematoma, ecchymoses, abrasions, lacerations and redness, and swelling in the external genitalia, including the hymen. Application of toluidine blue in the female will highlight local injuries of the fossa navicularis, posterior fourchette, and hymenal membrane, but this technique is not accepted by all the US jurisdictions. Colposcopic examination can enhance the ability to visualize milder genital trauma.
- Hymen: The hymen can be observed by using a cotton applicator swab moistened with water. Gently stretch the hymen all around to clearly define any partial or complete fresh hymenal tears and the amount of hymenal tissue present, especially at the 6 o'clock position of the posterior rim where acute hymenal tears are more likely to be found.[52] Of note, the absence of tears does not rule out previous penetration; therefore, the term "intact" hymen should be avoided.
- Anus: When anal penetration is reported in females or males, the perianal and anal area need to be inspected carefully for swelling with bluish discoloration consistent with bruising (not hemorrhoids), sphincter tears, fissures, scars, and distortion of the anus. Recurrent anal penetration should be suspected when there is anal laxity with dilatation. This observation is made when stool is absent in the vault. However, currently there is no consensus on the significance of anal laxity. An anoscopy or a proctoscopy is recommended when internal trauma and pathology (warts) are suspected. Internal trauma should be suspected when rectal bleeding, fever, or signs of an acute abdomen are present.
- Internal examination: An internal pelvic and rectal examination must be performed if there is pain, bleeding, a history of vaginal or rectal penetration, or signs of injury. A primary responsibility of the physician is to avoid further trauma to the patient in performing this part of the examination. General anesthesia may be indicated. In the young peripubertal adolescent, a small-sized metal speculum is preferred for easier insertion and visualization. Injuries such as ecchymoses and tears to the vagina and cervix must be noted.

Treatment for all significant trauma, including soft tissue injury as well as injury to the genital area, should precede collection of medicolegal information.

Collection of Specimens—Rape Kit

- The "chain of evidence" must be maintained when collecting forensic specimens by strictly following jurisdictional policies, rape kit protocols, and instructions, or evidence will likely be compromised.
- Legally mandated tests for evidence collection include specimen collection from various parts of the body for DNA testing. To reduce contamination of DNA, specimens should be collected using nonpowdered gloves.
- After evidence for the kit is collected, the sealed box is handed over to a police officer according to legal procedure.

Hospital Laboratory Tests

- STI tests: Trichomoniasis, bacterial vaginosis, chlamydia, and gonorrhea are the most common infections identified in a survivor of sexual assault. Nucleic acid amplification tests for chlamydia and gonorrhea infection should be obtained from the endocervix, rectum, and pharynx.[53]
- If genital ulcers or vesicles suspicious for herpes genitalis are present, a viral culture from the lesions should be sent for herpes simplex virus testing.
- Wet mount of vaginal secretions should be prepared and examined for evidence of trichomonas, bacterial vaginosis, and candidiasis. Alternatively, a point-of-care test for trichomonas can be obtained. The forensic examiner does not do the wet mount to detect sperm. If sperm are identified, the laboratory technician validates these findings with the examiner and/or a senior pathologist.
- Urine pregnancy test should be conducted on all peripubertal and postmenarcheal females.
- A serum sample should be obtained for (1) syphilis serology as a baseline test and repeated within 6 to 8 weeks; (2) HIV antibody/antigen (depending on the test available) at baseline and repeated at 4 to 6 weeks, 3 months, and 6 months; and (3) hepatitis B surface antigen and antibody.
- Routine toxicology screen is not recommended. However, the circumstances where urine or blood testing would be indicated include medical condition (including lack of recollection of events) suggesting alcohol or drug ingestion and reports from accompanying peers or adults that the victim may have been drugged.

Interpretation of Findings

A classification system has been developed by Adams[54] to assist clinicians in the interpretation of physical and laboratory findings and to provide an opinion as to the likelihood of sexual abuse or assault in adolescents (Table 73.1).

TABLE 73.1

Findings Diagnostic of Trauma and/or Sexual Contact[a]

1. Moderate specificity for abuse
   a. Acute lacerations or extensive bruising of labia, perihymenal tissues, penis, scrotum, or perineum (may be from unwitnessed accidental trauma)
   b. Scar of posterior fourchette (discrete, pale, off the midline). Scars are very difficult to assess unless acute injury at same location was documented.
   c. Fresh laceration of the posterior fourchette, not involving the hymen (must be differentiated from dehisced labial adhesion or failure of midline fusion, or may be caused by accidental injury)
   d. Perianal scar. Discrete, pale, off the midline (rare, difficult to assess unless acute injury at the same location was previously documented; may be due to other medical conditions such as Crohn disease, or previous medical procedures)
2. High specificity for abuse (diagnostic of blunt force penetrating trauma)
   a. Laceration (tear, partial or complete) of the hymen, acute
   b. Ecchymosis (bruising) on the hymen
   c. Perianal lacerations extending deep to the external anal sphincter (not to be confused with partial failure of midline fusion)
   d. Hymenal transection (healed). An area where the hymen has been torn through, to or nearly to the base, so there appears to be virtually no hymenal tissue remaining at that location, confirmed using additional examination techniques such as a swab, prone knee-chest position, Foley catheter, water to float the edge of the hymen. This finding has also been referred to as a *complete cleft* in sexually active adolescents and young women.
3. Presence of infection confirms mucosal contact with infected genital secretions; contacts most likely to have been sexual in nature
   a. Positive confirmed culture for gonorrhea, from genital area, anus, and throat, in a child outside the neonatal period
   b. Confirmed diagnosis of syphilis, if perinatal transmission is ruled out
   c. *Trichomonas vaginalis* infection in a child older than 1 year, with organisms identified (by an experienced technician or clinician) in vaginal secretions by wet mount examination or by culture
   d. Positive culture from genital or anal tissues for chlamydia. If child is older than 3 years at time of diagnosis, and specimen was tested using cell culture or comparable method approved by the CDC. Positive serology for HIV, if neonatal transmission and transmission from blood products have been ruled out.
4. Diagnostic of sexual contact
   a. Pregnancy
   b. Sperm identified in specimens taken directly from a child's body

[a]Findings which in the absence of a clear, timely, plausible history of accidental injury or nonsexual transmission should be reported to child protective services. HIV, human immunodeficiency virus.
Adapted from Adam J. Medical evaluation of suspected sexual abuse. *J Pediatr Adolesc Gynecol* 2004;17:191 (with permission).

Management

Clinicians must be sensitive to the likelihood of gastrointestinal side effects that can occur from multiple oral medications prescribed following a sexual assault evaluation. In this event, treatment should begin with emergency contraception and intramuscular medication for gonorrhea. Medications for other common STIs can begin after the emergency contraception regimen is completed.

- Patient instructions for managing any injuries including those to the genital area should be provided.
- Tetanus toxoid 0.5 mL intramuscularly (plus tetanus immune globulin if dirty wound) is indicated for severe or penetrating trauma.
- STI prophylaxis: Since compliance with follow-up visits is poor, prophylactic treatment for gonorrhea, chlamydia, and trichomonas infections should be provided. Recommended

regimens include Ceftriaxone 250 mg IM in a single dose *plus* metronidazole 2 g orally in a single dose *plus* azithromycin 1 g orally in a single dose *or* doxycycline 100 mg orally twice a day for 7 days.

- Prevention of pregnancy: Emergency contraception must be offered in all postmenarcheal females and may be provided without a speculum examination.[55] If the adolescent or young adult has not been using prescription methods of contraception, emergency contraception within 5 days of an incident should be discussed. A single-dose 30 mg tablet of ulipristal acetate (Ella) is approved by the Food and Drug Administration (FDA) for emergency contraception within 5 days of an incident. The levonorgestrel (progestin-only) pill (1.5 mg) is approved by the FDA for emergency contraception within 3 days of an incident: Plan B One Step (1.5-mg single-dose levonorgestrel) and other generic formulations which are available over the counter are preferred for teenagers as opposed to the two-tablet progestin-only regimen (0.75 mg each tablet). The latter is a prescription medication for minors, and therefore when this regimen is prescribed, it is recommended that the adolescent or young adult receives their first dose in the emergency room and the second dose 12 hours later. However, some hospitals and physicians do not offer or prescribe emergency contraception on religious and ethical grounds. In such circumstances, the provider should refer the young woman to a hospital or physician that does dispense or prescribe emergency contraception.
- Hepatitis B infection: The Centers for Disease Control and Prevention (CDC) recommends postexposure hepatitis B vaccine without hepatitis B immune globulin (HBIG) at the initial examination if the vaccine has not been received previously. Empiric treatment for hepatitis B with HBIG following sexual assault is controversial. Its efficacy in AYAs who are already immunized against hepatitis B infection is unknown.
- HIV postexposure prophylaxis (PEP): It is difficult to discuss PEP issues in the acutely traumatized survivor, and while HIV seroconversion has occurred in persons whose only risk factor is sexual assault/abuse, the frequency is low. The medical decision to recommend PEP is based on (1) the likelihood that the assailant has HIV; (2) any exposure characteristics that might increase risk for HIV transmission; (3) the time lapsed after the event; and (4) the potential benefits and risks associated with PEP. Determination of HIV status of the assailant at the time of the examination is determined on a case-by-case basis. The CDC recommends the following approach to the risk assessment: (1) whether the assailant is a male who has sex with males, uses injection drugs, or crack cocaine; (2) the local epidemiology of HIV/AIDS; and (3) exposure characteristics of the assault.
  - Exposure characteristics of the assault when HIV status of the assailant is unknown involves whether (a) vaginal or anal penetration occurred; (b) ejaculation occurred on mucous membranes; (c) multiple assailants were involved; (d) mucosal lesions were present on the assailant or the victim; or (e) any other characteristics of the assault, victim, or the assailant might increase risk for HIV transmission. Consult a specialist in HIV treatment in your local area if PEP is considered.
  - PEP is best started within 4 hours of the assault and should not be started after 72 hours postsexual assault. See Chapter 31 for more information.
  - If the victim is eligible for PEP, discuss antiretroviral prophylaxis, including toxicity and unknown efficacy.
  - Compliance with PEP is reported to be low (15% to 25%). Therefore, a family's ability to fill the prescription, obtain and afford medication refills, and keep follow-up appointments must be an integral part of starting PEP. Family support and a by a social worker should be a standard of care.

- If the victim accepts PEP, the best approach for an AYA would be to provide enough medication to him or her to last until the follow-up appointment in 3 to 7 days to assess tolerance of medication. Baseline complete blood count and serum chemistry should be obtained.
- Sleep aids: If needed, prescribed with a limited quantity.
- Medical follow-up: An appointment with a provider with expertise in sexual assault medical follow-up should be scheduled as indicated or within 14 to 21 days after the assault. A follow-up examination has been reported to change the interpretation of trauma likelihood in 15% of AYAs who have been sexually assaulted or victimized, and 5% were diagnosed with a new STI.[56] A third visit may be scheduled at 8 to 12 weeks to repeat initial serologic studies, including tests for syphilis, hepatitis B, or HIV infection. The young person should also be followed up and evaluated for psychological symptoms (i.e., PTSD, depression, and/or anxiety). Health care providers should determine the appropriate supports and treatment required.
- Written materials: Written materials regarding victims' rights, the rape experience, reporting rape, feelings about rape, and special reactions (the teenage victim, male victim, and the disabled victim) should be given before leaving the hospital. Providers can obtain this information from Web sites and their local District Attorney's Office. In addition, many urban centers have resources and organizations dedicated to providing support for sexual assault victims, but tend to be adult focused.

The Legal Investigative Process and Outcomes

The effort to prosecute sexual assault perpetrators has its own requirements. A single, dedicated individual who can ensure an unbroken chain of evidence during the forensic examination and is able to follow through with detailed, immediate documentation is essential for providing factual testimony in court.[45] In some areas, sexual assault nurse examiner (SANE) programs provide prompt access to emergency medical care by providing a dedicated examination room, a specially trained forensic examiner who is competent in collection of evidence for the investigation, expert witnesses, and a collaborative team approach. In large metropolitan areas, a community-based victim advocate can assist and counsel the victim and family.[57] In small towns and rural areas, such assistance is rarely available and is provided by the local law enforcement officer. Together, these factors can lead to successful prosecution.

⬤ ACKNOWLEDGMENT

The authors wish to acknowledge Owen Ryan, MPH, for his contributions to a previous version of this chapter.

REFERENCES

1. Bureau of Justice Statistics. *Criminal victimization in the United States, 2008 statistical tables*. Available at http://www.bjs.gov/content/pub/pdf/cvus0801.pdf. Accessed February 27, 2014.
2. Finkelhor D, Shattuck A, Turner HA, et al. The lifetime prevalence of child sexual abuse and sexual assault assessed in late adolescence. *J Adolesc Health* 2014;55(3):329–333. doi:10.1016/j.jadohealth.2013.12.026.
3. Rothman EF, Exner D, Baughman AL. The prevalence of sexual assault against people who identify as gay, lesbian, or bisexual in the United States: a systematic review. *Trauma Violence Abuse* 2011;12:55–66.
4. Walker MD, Hernandez AM, Davey M. Childhood sexual abuse and adult sexual identity formation: intersection of gender, race, and sexual orientation. *Am J Fam Ther* 2012;40:385–398.
5. Turner HA, Finkelhor D, Ormrod R. The effects of adolescent victimization on self-concept and depressive symptoms. *Child Maltreat* 2010;15:76–90.
6. Irwin Jr CE, Rickert VI. Coercive sexual experiences during adolescence and young adulthood: a public health problem. *J Adolesc Health* 2005;36:359–361.
7. Rickert VI, Davidson LL, Breitbart V, et al. A randomized trial of screening for relationship violence in young women. *J Adolesc Health* 2009;45:163–170.
8. Clayton EW, Krugman RD, Simon P. *Confronting commercial sexual exploitation and sex trafficking of minors in the United States*. Washington, DC: National Academies Press, 2014.
9. Truman J, Rand M. *Criminal victimization, 2009*. Available at http://www.bjs.gov/content/pub/pdf/cv09.pdf. Accessed March 7, 2014.
10. Langton L, Planty M, Truman J. *Criminal victimization, 2012*. Available at http://www.bjs.gov/index.cfm?ty=pbdetail&iid=4781. Accessed March 7, 2014.
11. Centers for Disease Control and Prevention. *Web-based Injury Statistics Query and Reporting System (WISQARS)* [Online], 2013.
12. Eaton DK, Kann L, Kinchen S. Youth risk behavior surveillance-United States, 2011. *MMWR* 2012;61:1–162.
13. Finkelhor D, Ormrod R, Turner H. The victimization of children and youth: a comprehensive, national survey. *Child Maltreat* 2005;10:5–25.
14. Diaz A, Simantov E, Rickert VI. Effect of abuse on health: results of a national survey. *Arch Ped Adolesc Med* 2002;156:811–817.
15. US Department of Health and Human Services. Administration for Children and Families. Administration on Children Youth and Families. Children's Bureau. *Child Maltreatment 2009*. Available at http://archive.acf.hhs.gov/programs/cb/pubs/cm09/cm09.pdf. Accessed March 7, 2014.
16. Sedlak AJ, Mettenburg J, Petta I, et al. *Fourth national incidence study of child abuse and neglect (NIS-4): report to Congress*. Washington, DC: US Department of Health and Human Services, 2010.
17. McClain NM, Garrity SE. Sex trafficking and the exploitation of adolescents. *J Obstet Gynecol Neonat Nurs* 2011;40:243–252.
18. Banks D, Kyckelhahn T. *Characteristics of suspected human trafficking incidents, 2008–2010*. Bureau of Justice Statistics, US Department of Justice, April 2011.
19. Logan TK, Walker R, Hunt G. Understanding human trafficking in the United States. *Trauma Violence Abuse* 2009;10:3–30.
20. Smith L. *Keynote address*, delivered at Catholic Charities Anti-Human Trafficking Training. San Antonio, TX: 2008.
21. Hughes D. *Enslaved in the USA*. National Review, 2007;30.
22. Williamson E, Dutch NM, Clawson HJ. *Medical treatment of victims of sexual assault and domestic violence and its applicability to victims of human trafficking*. Washington, DC: U.S. Department of Health and Human Services, 2010.
23. Calmes J. Obama seeks to raise awareness of rape on campus. *The New York Times*, January 23, 2014:A18.
24. Lombardi K. *Flurry of new legislation targets sexual assault on campus*. Center for Public Integrity, 2014. Available at http://www.publicintegrity.org/2014/07/30/15185/flurry-new-legislation-targets-sexual-assault-campus. Accessed April 11, 2015.
25. Amar AF, Strout TD, Simpson S, et al. Administrators' perceptions of college campus protocols, response, and student prevention efforts for sexual assault. *Violence Victims* 2014;29(4):579–593.
26. Lombardi K. *A lack of consequences for sexual assault*. Center for Public Integrity, 2014. Available at http://www.publicintegrity.org/2010/02/24/4360/lack-consequences-sexual-assault. Accessed April 11, 2015.
27. Yung CR. Concealing campus sexual assault: an empirical examination. *Psychol Public Policy Law* 2015;21(1):1.
28. American College Health Association. *American College Health Association-National College Health Assessment II: Reference Group Executive Summary Spring 2014*. Hanover, MD: American College Health Association, 2014.
29. Balsam KF, Rothblum ED, Beauchaine TP. Victimization over the life span: a comparison of lesbian, gay, bisexual, and heterosexual siblings. *J Consult Clin Psychol* 2005;73:477.
30. Dank M, Lachman P, Zweig JM, et al. Dating violence experiences of lesbian, gay, bisexual, and transgender youth. *J Youth Adolesc* 2013;1–12.
31. Rieger G, Savin-Williams RC. Gender nonconformity, sexual orientation, and psychological well-being. *Arch Sex Behav* 2012;41:611–621.
32. Roberts AL, Rosario M, Corliss HL, et al. Childhood gender nonconformity: a risk indicator for childhood abuse and posttraumatic stress in youth. *Pediatrics* 2012;129:410–417.
33. Mahoney A, Poling A. Sexual abuse prevention for people with severe developmental disabilities. *J Dev Phys Disabil* 2011;23(4):369–376.
34. Harrell E. *Crime against persons with disabilities, 2009–2012—Statistical tables*. Bureau of Justice Statistics, US Department of Justice, February 2014.
35. Heerde JA, Scholes-Balog KE, Hemphill SA. Associations between youth homelessness, sexual offenses, sexual victimization, and sexual risk behaviors: a systematic literature review. *Arch Sex Behav* 2015;44(1):181–212.
36. Shared Hope International. *The national report on domestic minor sex trafficking: America's prostituted children*. Vancouver, WA: Shared Hope International, 2009.
37. Edwards JM, Iritani BJ, Hallfors DD. Prevalence and correlates of exchanging sex for drugs or money among adolescents in the United States. *Sex Transm Infect* 2006;82:354–358.
38. Hein LC. Survival strategies of male homeless adolescents. *J Am Psychiatr Nurses Assoc* 2011;17(4):274–282.
39. Rickert VI, Wiemann CM, Vaughan RD. Disclosure of date/acquaintance rape: who reports and when. *J Pediatr Adolesc Gynecol* 2005;18:17–24.
40. Wolfe DA, Scott K, Reitzel-Jaffe D, et al. Development and validation of the conflict in adolescent dating relationships inventory. *Psychol Assessm* 2001;13:277.
41. Koss MP, Oros CJ. Sexual experiences survey: a research instrument investigating sexual aggression and victimization. *J Consult Clin Psychol* 1982;50:455.
42. Symons PY, Groër MW, Kepler-Youngblood P, et al. Prevalence and predictors of adolescent dating violence. *J Child Adolesc Psychiatr Nurs* 1994;7:14–23.
43. Straus MA, Douglas EM. A short form of the Revised Conflict Tactics Scales, and typologies for severity and mutuality. *Violence Vict* 2004;19:507–520.
44. American Academy of Family Physicians, American Academy of Pediatrics, and American College of Obstetricians and Gynecologists. Society for Adolescent Medicine. Protecting adolescents: ensuring access to care and reporting sexual activity and abuse. *J Adolesc Health* 2004;35:420–423.
45. U.S. Department of Justice Office on Violence Against Women. *National Training Standards for sexual assault medical forensic examiners, June 2006*. Available at https://www.ncjrs.gov/pdffiles1/ovw/213827.pdf. Accessed April 2, 2014.
46. Emans SJ, Woods ER, Allred EN, et al. Hymenal findings in adolescent women: impact of tampon use and consensual sexual activity. *Pediatrics* 1994;125:153–160.
47. Goodyear-Smith FA, Laidlaw TM. Can tampon use cause hymen changes in girls who have not had sexual intercourse? A review of the literature. *Forensic Sci Int* 1998;94:147–153.

XV

48. Kellogg ND, Menard SW, Santos A. Genital anatomy in pregnant adolescents: "normal" does not mean "nothing happened." *Pediatrics* 2004;113:e67–e69.
49. Doan LA, Levy RC. Male sexual assault. *J Emergency Med* 1983;1:45–49.
50. Kadish HA, Schunk JE, Britton H. Pediatric male rectal and genital trauma: accidental and nonaccidental injuries. *Pediatr Emerg Care* 1998;14:95–98.
51. US Department of Justice Office on Violence Against Women. *A national protocol on the sexual assault medical forensic examinations, adults/adolescents, 2013.* Available at https://www.ncjrs.gov/pdffiles1/ovw/241903.pdf. Accessed April 2, 2014.
52. Slaughter L, Brown CRV, Crowley S, et al. Patterns of genital injury in female sexual assault victims. *Am J Obstet Gynecol* 1997;176:609–616.
53. Fiore AE, Uyeki TM, Broder K, et al. Sexually transmitted diseases treatment guidelines, 2010. *MMWR* 59(RR-12):1–110.
54. Adams JA, Strickland J. Medical evaluation of suspected child sexual abuse. *J Pediatr Adolesc Gynecol* 2004;17:191–197.
55. Upadhya KK, Breuner CC, Trent ME, et al. Emergency contraception. *Pediatrics* 2012;130:1174–1182.
56. Gavril AR, Kellogg ND, Nair P. Value of follow-up examinations of children and adolescents evaluated for sexual abuse and assault. *Pediatrics* 2012;129:282–289.
57. Littel K. *Sexual assault nurse examiner (SANE) programs: improving the community response to sexual assault victims.* Washington DC: US Department of Justice, Office of Justice Programs, Office for Victims of Crime, 2001.

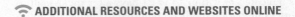 **ADDITIONAL RESOURCES AND WEBSITES ONLINE**

PART XVI

Special Populations

Introduction: Overview for Special Populations

Vaughn I. Rickert

The chapters in this section represent special populations of adolescents and young adults (AYAs). The health needs for AYAs from special populations can be challenging. These special populations include AYAs from the military or from families who are involved in the military; foster care or the juvenile justice system; homeless youth; immigrant youth and American Indian (AI) and Alaskan Native (AN) AYAs. These AYAs need assistance in overcoming barriers resulting from socioeconomic, cultural, political status, and psychosocial circumstances. Information provided in preceding chapters serves as a foundation for the care of AYAs, whereas the following chapters are designed to give providers a more nuanced understanding of the daily challenges these unique populations may experience.

Some of the special populations represented in the following chapters are relatively small in number, but collectively, these groups represent a sizeable population. For example, recent estimates suggest the following:

- Over 1 million international students are attending US academic or vocational institutions at the undergraduate and graduate levels.
- Over 1 million people 25 years and younger comprise the US military workforce, and another 600,000 family members between the ages of 13 and 25 years are living with a parent who is currently serving or has retired from military service.
- Approximately 5.2 million people partially identify as AI/AN, and 3 million identify only as AI/AN. Most AI/AN do not live on tribal reservations and have a younger median age than general population, that is, 22 versus 38 years.

Thus, these subgroups represent a wide range of differences in culture, geography, beliefs, politics, and physical characteristics, which will challenge those who care for these AYAs. Another group included in this section that has unique needs and systems of care is the large number of AYAs in college. As many as 24 million individuals in the United States are estimated to be enrolled in colleges and universities and that over half of these students will be between the ages of 14 and 24 years by 2020.

The contexts and situations of these young people are remarkable and impact their daily lives as well as their health. Annually, about 6 million youth are referred to social services for maltreatment in the United States, which results in 750,000 substantiated cases. Among youth 12 years or older, one-third of cases result in foster care placement. As might be expected, many of these youth are of color and are disproportionately represented in the foster care. On any given day, 150,000 youth are living in foster care environments, and approximately 20,000 young adults emancipate from this system annually. A related occurrence during this developmental period is the emergence of youth involved in the juvenile or criminal justice system. Data suggest that almost 1.5 million juveniles aged 18 and younger are arrested annually, with nearly 1.4 million delinquency cases being processed in juvenile courts. Slightly less than one-quarter are placed in detention facilitates, and less than 10% are sentenced to a term in juvenile prison. Of concern, more than 200,000 arrested juveniles faced prosecution in the adult criminal justice system. Homelessness and running away are yet additional outcomes of child maltreatment, involvement in the juvenile system, and growing up in families mired in chaos and dysfunction. The estimated size of the US homeless youth population ranges from 500,000 to 1.6 million depending on the definition employed. Many youth 18 years and older become homeless due to ageing out of much-needed youth services such as foster care or because of moving out of the juvenile justice system where their living situation was stable. Those who are disproportionately represented among the homeless population include former system youth; young adults recently released from prison or jail; veterans; lesbian, gay, and bisexual youth; transgender youth; immigrant and undocumented youth; and low-income ethnic minority youth.

One of the overarching themes that the provider will glean from these chapters on special AYA populations is the frequency of mental health concerns and problems that are likely to arise. For example, many of the wounds that returning combat veterans experience are invisible and often go unrecognized and untreated. As a result, suicide rates have dramatically increased among soldiers returning from deployment.

Another frequently unrecognized group in terms of mental health is the AI/AN population. Perhaps surprising to some, AI/AN adolescents have the highest rate of major depressive disorder when compared to other race/ethnicities. In fact, AI/AN males aged 15 to 24 had the highest suicide rate compared to same-age males of all other ethnic groups.

Sexual trauma among female veterans is also of concern as 15% of this population has screened positively for sexual trauma. Similarly, about one in five young women experiences sexual assault during her college years, many in her first year of college. Juvenile-justice involved youth and homeless youth also suffer disproportionately from negative health outcomes, including mental health and substance use disorders.

As providers will quickly recognize, the chief complaint expressed during a medical visit should be used as a mechanism to address a multitude of other issues, including housing, education/vocation, mental health, and social services. This strategy will enable providers to better confront the unique barriers to care, which may include linguistics, other systems of care, as well as cultural and legal concerns. It is important for providers to appreciate that most AYAs whose daily context is outside of the normal AYA experience are forgiving of "mistakes" as long as the provider conveys a genuine sense of caring and respect. Providers who are cognizant of community resources for these youth can be useful allies and advocates for these special populations. Health care providers' knowledge of the unique health needs of these populations will enable the provider to help the adolescent or young adult and their families navigating the system and the broad array of programs that can help meet their needs. Finally, providers are in an excellent position to promote the strengths and resiliencies and provide physical and mental resources that will support productive and meaningful lives of the youth who represent these special populations.

College Health

Sarah A. Van Orman
James R. Jacobs

More than 21 million students were enrolled in 2010 in the 4,495 colleges and universities in the US, with an anticipated 24 million by 2020. Over half (57%) of these students are in the 14- to 24-year-old age-group. College students comprise almost half the young adult population aged 18 to 24.[1] This young adult population comprises a unique population with specific health-related assets and vulnerabilities. While students are generally healthy, mental health conditions, substance use and misuse, injuries, and an increasing number of students with chronic illnesses represent significant health issues. The college campus is a unique health environment that creates risks and opportunities including efficient and effective delivery of health care services as well as opportunities for prevention through health promotion and public health initiatives. Colleges and universities, collectively referred to as institutions of higher education (IHEs), are important settings for the provision of health care as well as preventing or reducing health risks and enhancing well-being among a large portion of the young adult population. Understanding the campus environment and resources is critical when providing care for a college student. As care for college students is often shared between an on-campus student health service (SHS) and a hometown community provider, strong communication and collaboration are required to ensure the best possible care.

On-campus SHSs have as their mission the health and well-being of college students to support student academic success and retention, reduce institutional risk, and create healthier adults in the future. The last available survey data on health services on college campuses in 1988 estimated that there were approximately 1,600 colleges or universities that provide some level of health services, but the current actual number is unknown and likely much larger.[2] What specific services are offered varies widely in the US, ranging from part-time nurses providing triage and referral to comprehensive ambulatory health care centers providing medical and mental health care, public health, education and prevention services, and occasionally disability and recreational services.[3] Today's exemplary SHSs provide direct medical and mental health services, undertake population-based initiatives through health promotion and education, and are the public health leaders for their institutions, guiding campus health policy. Their overarching role is to create a healthy and safe campus environment, one that

helps make possible the learning, research, and teaching to which the institution is dedicated and which promotes student success. SHSs seek to reduce risk and reinforce behaviors that create health for the individual and for the community. The best practices in college health continually assess the student population on the particular campus to track their health status and identify service needs. This may involve assessing health status and promoting health in students who may never visit the SHS, through population-based primary prevention programs such as mandatory pre-matriculation alcohol education and campus vaccination outreach programs. SHS professionals frequently advise and help shape campus health policies, such as tobacco-free college campuses, and conduct surveillance of and lead responses to public health concerns.

Issues of college health are important to health care professionals serving adolescents and young adults (AYAs) for many reasons, including the following:

- Health care providers often perform precollege examinations or provide care during college years.
- Health care providers may communicate and collaborate with SHS providers and other student affairs professionals regarding the health care needs of a college student.
- SHS providers may be a source of ongoing referrals to other health care professionals of patients needing hospitalization or secondary and tertiary care consultations.
- Collaboration among SHS health care providers, other healthcare providers, insurance providers, local public health officials, and student affairs professionals can benefit all parties and especially students.
- Significant opportunities exist within SHSs for both teaching and research as well as employment and career opportunities.

DATA SOURCES ON COLLEGE STUDENTS AND COLLEGE HEALTH

American College Health Association Benchmark Survey

In 2006 and then again in the spring of 2010, the American College Health Association (ACHA) conducted a survey of campuses nationally regarding the utilization, staffing, and services available at SHSs, the ACHA-SHS Survey. SHSs nationally were invited to participate. While the number of campuses responding was small (N = 172) and overly representative of medium and large campuses, it does provide the only available limited data regarding the scope and nature of on-campus health services.

Morbidity Data

Comprehensive data on college students are limited in many areas; although age-group is easily identified in most data sets, current college enrollment is not always collected as part of standard demographic data.

ACHA-National College Health Assessment

One source of data regarding the health of the college student population is the ACHA-National College Health Assessment Survey (ACHA-NCHA). This survey began in the spring of 2000. Since its inception, over 1 million students have completed the ACHA-NCHA and the ACHA-NCHA II (starting in 2008). While the students sampled on any given campus are selected in a randomized manner, the participating IHE do not represent a random sample and the response rate is fairly low. The ACHA-NCHA data throughout the rest of this chapter are from the ACHA-NCHA's Undergraduate Students Reference Group Data Report Spring 2013. All NCHA surveys are available at http://www.achancha.org/.

NCHA 2013 Undergraduate Data Set

- Survey includes 153 IHEs (127, 4-year and 26, 2-year institutions) that chose randomly selected students (N = 94,911).
- Size of institution: 40 had more than 20,000 students; 42 had between 10,000 and 19,999; 39 had between 5,000 and 9,999; 16 had between 2,500 and 4,999; and 16 had less than 2,500.
- Gender: The sample of students was 65% female.
- Ethnicity: The ethnicity of the students was 67% White, 7% African American, 15% Hispanic, 12% Asian, 2% Native American/Alaskan Native/Native Hawaiian, 4% biracial, and 3% other.

Other Surveys of College Student Drug Use and Mental Health

- Monitoring the Future Study (since 1975) (http://monitoringthefuture.org/)
- Core Alcohol and Drug Survey (since 1989) (http://core.siu.edu/)
- The College Alcohol Study (1993, 1997, 1999, and 2001) (http://archive.sph.harvard.edu/cas/)
- The Cooperative Institutional Research Program (CIRP) Freshman Survey (http://www.heri.ucla.edu/cirpoverview.php)
- Mental health data are available through the Healthy Minds Study (since 2007) (http://healthymindsnetwork.org/)

KEY ASPECTS OF SHSs

Care at SHSs is informed by key aspects of the college student population.

- College student populations are generally young and healthy; 91% of students surveyed reported their health as good, very good, or excellent.[4]
- College students are very mobile and often have several residences throughout the year, including in their hometown, on campus, and perhaps in a foreign country or near a summer job or internship.
- The primary disease burden affecting students while in college is from mental health conditions and preventable accidents and injuries often associated with alcohol use.
- Short-term goals are student academic and personal success. The longer-term goal is the primary prevention of the diseases of later adulthood, including obesity and tobacco-related illnesses.[5]
- More young adults are entering college with chronic diseases. While some have medical conditions such as asthma, diabetes, and physical disabilities, the greatest increase has been in students with mental health disorders, learning disabilities, and pervasive developmental disabilities. Students with these chronic diseases need comprehensive services and case management to meet the goals not only of good health and

functioning, but also optimal long-term academic, vocational, and personal success.

- Many college students engage in behaviors that place them at increased health risk, including excessive alcohol use, prescription drug abuse, failure to engage in recommended physical activity, poor nutrition, failure to protect themselves against sexually transmitted infections (STIs), and high-risk recreational and vocational activities such as international travel.
- Relationship difficulties and interpersonal violence are frequently reported.[4]
- Mental health conditions and psychosocial stressors are frequent impediments to academic success. Of the top ten self-reported impediments to academic success only two are physical, while issues such as anxiety, sleep difficulties, and stress carry the greatest impact on student learning[4] (Fig. 74.1).

ENROLLMENT

In the academic year 2010, there were 21 million college students in the US. This is projected to rise to 21.9 million in 2015 and 23.5 million in 2020.[1] Enrollment has increased 32% between 2001 and 2011 (15.9 to 21 million). Although an increasing proportion of young adults below age 24 are enrolling, the greatest increase has been in students above age 25. College populations have become more diverse, including enrolling more first-generation students as well as both students of color and international students. Data and extensive tables regarding higher education enrollment are available from the National Center for Education Statistics at http://nces.ed.gov/programs/digest as well as the almanac issues of the Chronicle of Higher Education.

Trends

- Gender: Female enrollment has risen from 29% in 1947, to 37.6% in 1961, 41.8% in 1971, 51.7% in 1981, 54.7% in 1991, 56.3% in 2001, and 56.8% in 2012. Between 2001 and 2011, female enrollment rose 33% and male enrollment by 30%. Currently, approximately 43% of college students are male and 57% female.
- Age: Between 2001 and 2011, the number of 18- to 24-year-olds in the US rose from 28 million to 31.1 million (11%) while the percentage of this population enrolled in college increased from 36% to 42%. However, during this time period, the percentage increase has been even higher for students aged 25 and older (41% for those 25 and older and 35% for those under 25).

Within the last 12 mo, have any of the following affected your academic performance?	
Stress	30.7%
Sleep difficulties	21.4%
Anxiety	20.8%
Cold/flu/sore throat	16.7%
Work	15.5%
Depression	13.2%
Internet use/computer games	13.0%
Concern for a troubled friend or family members	11.2%
Relationship difficulties	10.4%
Participation in extra-curricular activities	9.8%

FIGURE 74.1 Top 10 impediments to academic performance reported on the National College Health Assessment. *American College Health Association-National College Health Assessment II: Reference Group Data Report, Spring 2013 Undergraduate Reference Group. Hanover, MD: American College Health Association, 2013.*

XVI

- Enrollment status: Between 2001 and 2011, undergraduate enrollment and postbaccalaureate enrollment both rose 32% (from 13.7 million to 18.1 million for undergraduate and from 2.2 million to 2.9 million for postbaccalaureate).
- Ethnicity: Between 1976 and 2011, the following changes have occurred among American college students:
  - Hispanic: Increased from 4% to 14%
  - Asian/Pacific Islanders: Increased from 2% to 6%
  - Black: Increased from 10% to 15%
  - Native American/Alaska Native: Increased from 0.7% to 0.9%
  - White: Decreased from 84% to 61%
- International students: The US enrolled the highest number of international students in its history to colleges and universities during the 2012 to 2013 school year (N = 819,644). This number has increased for 7 consecutive years and has increased by 40% in past 10 years.[6]

HEALTH CARE SERVICES

Medical Care

Most SHSs, 93% on the ACHA-SHS Survey, provide some level of care for students with acute and chronic medical problems. Fewer than 6% of campuses on the ACHA-SHS Survey, however, reported having an overnight infirmary or 24-hour care as they can no longer justify the cost, risk, and resources associated with these services.[7]

- Acute medical conditions such as minor infections (Epstein–Barr virus infections, genitourinary tract infections, upper respiratory tract infections, and acute gastroenteritis), musculoskeletal injuries, minor trauma, and skin problems are the most frequent conditions seen.
- Reproductive issues are common, including the screening, diagnosis, and treatment of STIs, contraceptive management, routine gynecology, men's health care, and unintended pregnancies.
- Most SHSs have active immunization programs, and many offer pretravel counseling and vaccinations.
- While only approximately 4% of college students surveyed report a chronic medical illness, many college undergraduate and older graduate students receive care at the SHS for these chronic medical conditions, including asthma, diabetes, seizure disorders, thyroid disorders, hypertension, eating disorders, and malignancies.[4] Given the 10% or more estimate of chronic illnesses in this age-group, it is likely that college students are underreporting their chronic diseases and may also be underutilizing health care services for this purpose.
- Integration of routine screening, brief intervention, and referral to treatment for depression, alcohol misuse, and tobacco use during all encounters, including acute care visits for minor conditions, has been a growing trend. These strategies should now be considered a standard of care for the college student population.[8]

Mental Health Care

Mental health symptoms, particularly depression and anxiety, are a frequently reported impediment to academic success, much more so than physical illnesses.[9] Common diagnoses in this population include stress-related symptoms, anxiety, depression, eating disorders, suicidality, chronic fatigue, substance abuse, and other disorders affecting academic performance such as attention deficit disorder. Approximately, 20.1% of NCHA respondents reported being diagnosed or treated for a mental health condition by a professional in the preceding 12 months.[4]

Other reported symptoms on the NCHA include the following:

- 84.3% reported feeling overwhelmed with all they had to do.
- 46.5% reported feeling hopeless.
- 51.3% reported overwhelming anxiety.
- 31.8% reported feeling so depressed it was difficult to function.
- 8% reported seriously considering suicide.
- 1.6% reported attempted suicide.

Given the significant impact of mental health on student well-being and academic success, almost all IHEs offer some level of mental health services. Services may be available through a stand-alone counseling service integrated into a larger umbrella unit which provides medical and mental health care or both. As mental health disorders have increased in both severity and prevalence and campus threats of violence have become more common, college mental health, historically based in a developmental model which focused on academic support and developmental concerns, has undergone a significant transition. Common now is the availability of psychiatric consultation and the creation of campus teams ("threat" assessment or behavioral intervention) with procedures to share information and develop interventions such as mandated mental health assessment for when students display behaviors of concern and are felt to pose a risk to self or others.[10]

In data from the National Longitudinal Study of Adolescent Health, young adults enrolled in school are more likely than their peers to receive mental health counseling, while health insurance status was not found to have a similar effect.[11] While the easy access provided by on-campus mental health services may play an important role in not on removing barriers to receiving care, significant treatment gaps remain. Evidence suggests that less than 25% of students with mental health diagnoses are currently receiving treatment.[12] More concerning are estimates that only one-third of students with depression and approximately half of students who report suicidal ideation are in treatment.[13] College students are less likely than their non-college-attending peers to receive alcohol and other drug treatment.[12] Adequacy of treatment may also be limited, with estimates that less than one-quarter of students in treatment are adequately treated.[13] Men, students of color (Black, Hispanic, and Asian), and international students are significantly less likely to report receiving mental health treatment than their female, White, and domestic student peers, respectively.[11,13,14]

These unmet mental health needs are a frequently cited concern of SHS providers and IHE staff. Most on-campus mental health services operate from a short-term model, referring students with complex or long-term needs to community providers. Lack of insurance coverage and a shortage of community providers are frequent barriers to students receiving care. To better meet the needs of students on campus, many SHSs are embracing novel approaches, including more closely integrating medical and mental health services.[15] Behavioral health programs offer brief, solution-focused mental health counseling integrated into primary care to address high-risk behaviors such as alcohol or tobacco use, treat stress and sleep disturbances, or as a bridge to more comprehensive mental health care. Delivered within the medical setting, these services are often acceptable to underserved students, male students, international students, and students of color.[16] SHSs are also enhancing support for students with chronic mental health conditions through the use of interdisciplinary teams for management of students with eating disorders and offering programs such as dialectical behavioral therapy.

Health Promotion, Wellness, Prevention

The campus environment presents a unique opportunity to use prevention strategies for optimal individual health and student academic success. Often referred to by the term "health promotion," most campuses have specific programs which advance student well-being through individual education and wellness programming as well as using environmental strategies such as broad health campaigns and changes to campus health policy. These health promotion and wellness functions are typically part of the SHS—70% on campuses on the ACHA-SHS Survey—or also may be a part of a closely aligned unit such as Division of Student Affairs or Student

Life.[7] These programs also conduct population-level assessments to determine areas of greatest need to focus their activities.

Healthy Campus 2020 provides a framework for improving the overall health status of a campus population and is utilized by many IHEs in evaluating campus health. Healthy Campus 2020 was developed by ACHA as a "sister" document to Healthy People 2020. Strategies suggested in Healthy Campus 2020 extend beyond traditional interventions of education, diagnosis, treatment, and health care within clinical setting and encourage collaborations between academic, student affairs, and administrative colleagues. Healthy Campus 2020 provides specific national health objectives for students and faculty/staff and utilizes an ecologic approach. This approach combines population-level and individual-level determinants of health and interventions as well as community-focused issues. Topic areas with Healthy Campus 2020 include impediments to academic success, health communications, injury and violence prevention, mental health, nutrition and weight, physical activity and fitness, STIs, family planning, immunizations, infectious disease, and substance abuse. IHEs can utilize Healthy Campus 2020 to set campus-specific goals and utilize measurable objectives to benchmark their performance nationally and internally[17] (Fig. 74.2).

Public Health and Communicable Disease Control

The close living and working conditions of a college campus create a high-risk environment for communicable disease outbreaks. The academic calendar brings large populations to campus from throughout the nation and world in short periods of time. Well-described outbreaks have included the following:

- Meningococcal disease—First year students residing on campus are at increased risk. Recent outbreaks have been associated with the Group B serotype. The Advisory Committee on Immunization Practices recommends that AYA aged 16–23 years may be vaccinated, preferably at 16 through 18 years old, with a serogroup B meningococcal vaccine to provide short-term protection against most strains of serogroup B meningococcal disease.
- Norovirus: This can be particularly difficult to contain and has led to outbreaks in the hundreds and in some cases over 1,000 cases in a short period of time on multiple campuses.
- Vaccine preventable disease outbreaks including mumps, measles, and varicella have been well described. Mumps outbreaks have been common on campuses over the past 10 years, with most cases in fully vaccinated individuals.

Reduce the Proportion of Students Who Report That Their Academic Performance Was Adversely Affected by Stress in the Past 12 mo	
Baseline	27.4% of students reported that stress adversely affected their academic performance in the past 12 mo in spring 2010
Target	24.7%
Target-setting method	10% improvement
Data source	American College Health Association-National College Health Assessment II (ACHA-NCHA II), Question 45D5
More information	Adverse academic performance is defined as receiving a lower grade on an examination or an important project; receiving a lower grade in a course; receiving an incomplete or dropping a course; or experiencing a significant disruption in thesis, dissertation, research, or practicum work

From American College Health Association. *American College Health Association-National College Health Assessment II: Reference Group Data Report Spring 2010.* Linthicum, MD: American College Health Association, 2010. Available at http://www.acha-ncha.org/reports_ACHA-NCHAII.html. Accessed June 2012.

FIGURE 74.2 Sample objective from Healthy Campus 2020 American College Health Association. (2012, June). *Healthy Campus 2020.* Available at http://www.acha.org/HealthyCampus/contact.cfm#usage. Accessed May 4, 2014.

- Pertussis: A potentially significant issue in young adults
- Bacterial conjunctivitis
- *Methicillin resistant Staphylococcus aureus:* Outbreaks have been particularly associated with athletic teams and recreational sports facilities.
- *Mycoplasma pneumoniae:* Recent outbreaks have been described on several campuses.
- Influenza and other upper respiratory viruses: These cause significant morbidity among college students, including increasing health care utilization and impacting academic performance.[19] The 2009 H1N1 influenza pandemic uniquely impacted campuses. Preferentially impacting young adult populations, SHSs across the nation experienced a profound health care surge that strained campus resources but also led to the creation of a stronger public health infrastructure on many campuses.[20]

Detection and control of communicable diseases, therefore, is one of the most critical roles played by SHSs and a public health framework in which the SHS is a kind of local public health agency is utilized on many campuses. Roles of the SHS in communicable disease control include primary prevention through immunization and health education campaigns, active surveillance for diseases, and detection of individual cases or suspect cases. For example, many SHSs are part of the Centers for Disease Control and Prevention sentinel influenza surveillance network. During an active outbreak or when managing individual cases of communicable diseases, the SHS may assist or have primary responsibility along with local public health authorities for case management and contact tracing. SHSs advise or coordinate public information campaigns for the campus community. Public health approaches are also now being utilized to address a variety of other chronic diseases and health risks among student populations, including high-risk alcohol use, mental health, interpersonal violence, and obesity.

BEHAVIORAL AND OTHER RISK FACTORS

Similar to other AYA populations, college students have a range of risk factors that must be considered when delivering health care. Screening and appropriate intervention can reduce short- and long-term health risks. Overall in the US, the highest risk factors are in emerging young adults 18 to 25 years old (www.usc.edu/thenewadolescents).

Alcohol

Alcohol remains one of the most serious public health problems facing college students in the US. College students are more likely than their noncollege peers to engage in heavy episodic drinking, also known as binge drinking, defined as 4 or more drinks in a row for women and 5 or more drinks in a row for men. While college students are not more likely to experience alcohol dependence than their noncollege peers, their alcohol use places them at risk for unintentional injury, victimization, and other health and personal consequences such as academic and legal difficulties.[21,22]

Surveys of college students consistently demonstrate high levels of alcohol use among undergraduates and its attendant consequences.

- Over 60% of students report any use within the past 30 days.[4]
- Approximately 40% report binge drinking within the past 2 weeks.[4]
- Of students who reported alcohol consumption, over 50% reported one or more consequences from their consumption within the past 12 months. Most commonly reported were doing something they later regretted, forgetting where they were or what they did, or having unprotected sex.[4]
- Serious consequences of alcohol use are consistently reported by a portion of college students: 22% driving after drinking, 16% a physical injury, 4% got in trouble with the police, 2.5%

considered suicide, and 2% having sex without giving their consent.[4] Alcohol-related unintentional injury deaths among college students increased from 1,440 in 1998 to 1,825 in 2005, primarily traffic related.[21]

- Rates of alcohol use vary widely among college students and among individual IHEs. Male students drink more heavily and frequently than female students, while White students drink more heavily than students from other racial and ethnic backgrounds.

Tobacco

While roughly one-third of college students report lifetime cigarette use and 15% report use within the last 30 days, daily use is infrequent (<5% of students).[4] Over half of college smokers report a pattern of "social" smoking associated only with socializing and alcohol use. While these smokers typically have low frequency of use and low levels of nicotine dependence, they also report less intention to quit and fewer quit attempts. While most of these "social smokers" become nonsmokers within 3 to 4 years, approximately 20% will progress to daily smoking. Understanding which students may be at risk and preventing this transition have important health implications as these students may not perceive themselves as smokers and therefore may not respond to traditional prevention messages and interventions.[23] Use of electronic nicotine delivery systems (ENDS) or e-cigarettes is growing, especially among young adults who perceive their health risks to be low. Young adult ENDS users may have never smoked combustible cigarettes, but view ENDS as safer and more attractive. The short- and long-term health risks of ENDS use are unknown.[24]

Other Drugs

Other drug use is also present and in some areas increasing, such as amphetamine use. Important drugs of abuse include marijuana and prescription stimulants and opioids. When compared with their same age-group 1 to 4 years postcollege, drug usage among college students in 2013 was similar, with 39% of college students reporting any drug use in the past 12 months. Amphetamine use continues to remain higher in college students. This is a major change from 2008 when amphetamine use was significantly higher in noncollege students.[25]

- Marijuana: Marijuana use is increasing, a trend which can be predicted to continue with legalization of marijuana use for individuals over age 18 in many states. Currently, 36% of students report annual and, of potential growing concern, 5.4% report being daily users.[25] IHEs are grappling with issues of medical marijuana use and legalization and are struggling to develop new campus policies to address medical marijuana use, use of marijuana within residence halls, and other emerging issues.
- Nonmedical use of prescription drugs: These drugs are the next most common drug abuse problem after alcohol, tobacco, and marijuana. Use by male students is typically higher than by female students. Within the past 12 months, the following drugs were used by students who were not prescribed these medications[4]:
  - 8.5% report use of stimulants (Adderall, Ritalin): As the number of students arriving on campus with a stimulant prescription has risen, diversion of stimulants has emerged as a troubling problem. Nonmedical use of prescription stimulants occurs in two distinct patterns, as a study aid and combined with alcohol to reduce its sedating effects in social settings.
  - 8% report use of prescription opioids (e.g., Vicodin, Oxy-Contin, codeine).
  - 4% report use of sedatives (e.g., Xanax, valium).
  - 3% report use of antidepressants.

Novel substances and patterns of substance use arise commonly and can spread quickly through individual campuses, as well as locally, regionally, and nationally. A popular recent example is consumption of alcohol beverages mixed with caffeine and other stimulants to overcome the sedative properties of alcohol. Other examples include novel ways to absorb alcohol such as through enemas or the conjunctiva, MDMA (3,4-methylenedioxymethamphetamine) previously known as Ecstasy, but more recently available in a purer form known as Molly, and various hallucinogens. Health care providers caring for college students need to be aware of trends and practices in their local area.

Sexual Assault, Dating Violence, and Stalking

Interpersonal violence including sexual assault, dating violence, and stalking remains part of a common and devastating reality on college campuses. Stalking is reported by 6% of college students.[4] It is estimated that one in five women will be sexually assaulted during college, most commonly during their first year.[26] New research suggests that these crimes are frequently perpetrated by serial offenders.[27] Alcohol can facilitate these crimes by reducing the capacity of a victim to respond as well as reducing the awareness of bystanders. It has been estimated that less than 10% of assaults are reported and in fewer cases are the perpetrators held responsible. Students who experience sexual assault are at risk for long-term physical and mental health problems. They may leave school and not complete their education. Sexual assault on college campuses has recently become the focus of national attention, and federal efforts are underway to make campuses safer through prevention, survivor response, and holding perpetrators responsible. IHEs are subject to multiple federal requirements, including the Clery Act and Title IX, to provide comprehensive prevention and response to these crimes. In January, 2014, President Barack Obama created a White House Task Force on Protecting Students from Sexual Assault, bringing national attention to the issue. Its report provides clearer guidance and expectations for IHEs (http://www.whitehouse.gov/sites/default/files/docs/report_0.pdf; https://www.notalone.gov/).

Relationship difficulties are also common among college students, with over 10% of students reporting an adverse academic impact in the past 12 months from a relationship difficulty. Abusive relationships are of particular concern: 10%, 2.5%, and 2% of college students report being in an emotionally, physically, or sexually abusive intimate relationship, respectively, within the past 12 months.[4]

Nutrition and Physical Activity

Poor nutrition, physical inactivity, overweight, obesity, and eating disorders are prevalent in college student populations. It is estimated that only 5% of college students consume the recommended 5 servings of fruits and vegetables daily and only 50% meet recommendations for physical activity.[4] The transition from adolescent to young adulthood is frequently associated with weight gain, and weight gain is common during the early and mid-20s. While the concept of the "freshman fifteen" is perhaps somewhat of a myth, studies suggest that students gain an average of 5 lb during the first 3 to 4 months in college and on average women have been estimated to gain 3.8 lb from freshman to senior year and men to gain 9.8 lb.[28] Dietary factors in the college setting can contribute to excess weight gain, including all you can eat on-campus dining facilities, greater intake of low-density nutrition ("junk") food, and frequent snacking (especially during late night hours to the extent many college students are felt to consume a fourth meal). Students may not have access to cooking facilities, lack basic cooking skills, and/or eat many meals out in fast-food restaurants. Physical activity levels decline at the transition to college and continue to decline throughout college. Alcohol intake can be an important contributor to overall calorie intake, and many students, especially young women, engage in patterns of restricting food intake to compensate for the calories they anticipate consuming when drinking alcohol. Addressing these patterns are important during the college years as research suggests that this is a critical time for the establishment of long-term health patterns and behaviors.[28]

Injury Prevention

As the leading cause of death among college students, unintentional injuries should remain a focus of prevention efforts. Alcohol related fatalities most often related, fatalities most often result from motor vehicle accidents, but falls, cold exposure, and drowning are also important mechanisms.[21] Only 30% of college students report mostly or always wearing a helmet when riding a bicycle.[4] In some urban campuses, bicycle injuries are a particular problem as riders are often inexperienced, riding without helmets, not observing traffic rules, and also texting at the same time.

Sexual and Reproductive Health

College students are at risk for STIs and unintended pregnancy. Nearly 70% of college students report having at least one sexual partner in the past 12 months, with a mean number of 2.3 partners. Only slightly more than 50% of students reported using a condom with last vaginal intercourse and only 30% with last anal intercourse. The most common forms of birth control reported by students are male condoms followed by birth control pills. Inadequate birth control, however, is common, with 30% of students reporting using withdrawal as a method the last time they had vaginal intercourse. Nearly 18% of sexually active college students or their female partners reported use of emergency contraception within the past 12 months. Long-acting reversible contraceptives (LARCs®) such as intrauterine devices (IUDs) and Implanon/Nexplanon are becoming increasingly popular and have the potential to provide more reliable contraception in this population. Approximately 6% of undergraduate women reported using an IUD in 2013, almost doubled from 2008.[4] In the past year, 2% of sexually active college students reported an unintended pregnancy.[4]

Sexual Minority Students

Heterosexism and homophobia result in health disparities for sexual minority college students. The experience of homophobia itself can impact self-image. Sexual minority youth much more commonly experience bullying and personal violence than their nonsexual minority peers. Parental rejection can have physical, emotional, and financial ramifications. As a result, sexual minority students have higher rates of depression, suicide attempts, substance abuse, and high-risk sexual behavior. Parental and community acceptance along with a safe school environment are important protective factors.

While reduction in overall societal stigma for some young people has resulted in young adults "coming out" at younger ages, often before starting college, many students feel comfortable disclosing their sexual orientation only after the age of 18. College is therefore an important time for many sexual minority students when they are first able to develop romantic relationships, be open in their community regarding their sexuality, and seek medical and mental health care confidentially. Sexual minority students are at risk for receiving inadequate health services unless health care providers and their staff provide an open and safe environment with providers knowledgeable and prepared to address their mental health and medical concerns.

Similarly, transgender students may first seek assistance with transitioning during college. Health care professionals caring for college students should be prepared to counsel and provide referrals to medical and mental health professionals knowledgeable and skilled in transgender care and the process of transition. Many SHSs have providers skilled in mental health assessment and the management of hormone therapy. Many young adults reject a binary notion of gender and may prefer the use of gender-neutral pronouns and language. Verbal questions and written questionnaires should be gender-neutral, and health care providers should address students based on their preference.

Sleep

Similar to other adult populations, college students frequently do not get adequate sleep. Only 10% reported getting enough sleep to feel rested in the morning on 6 or more days in the past week. Over 40% reported sleepiness was more than a little problem, a big problem, or a very big problem in the past 7 days.[4] Chronic sleep deprivation can lead to decreased cognitive performance, mood disturbance, and physical symptoms. It can be a risk factor for alcohol and marijuana use. While the most common sleep disorder in college students is inadequate sleep hygiene, delayed sleep phase disorder commonly has its onset in young adulthood and should be considered in a college student with sleep concerns.[29]

Many aspects of campus and college life contribute to altered sleep patterns and put college students at risk for poor sleep hygiene, including the cyclic nature of academic requirements leading to all-night study sessions, the adaptation to personal responsibility for sleep schedules when moving away from the family home, the highly stimulating social environment in an on-campus residence facility, a varied daily schedule, and frequent alcohol consumption.

Vocational Health Risks

College students in many fields may encounter health and safety risks that typically would fall under the category of occupational risks. Most common are students engaged in health care settings in a professional or preprofessional capacity. This includes medical, nursing, allied health professional, pharmacy, physical therapy, and athletic training students. It has been estimated that nearly one-quarter of health professions students experience a blood or body fluid exposure during their training and many of these events are unreported.[30] Other students at unique risk include veterinary students who experience frequent biologic exposures and physical injury, students engaged in laboratory research and study where biologic agents and/or chemical toxins are present, music students who are at risk for auditory damage and musculoskeletal injuries, architecture students with sharp injuries, and art students whose materials may contain toxins.

Because students are not employees, they are outside the protection provided through the Occupational Safety and Health Administration, even though they are often working within the same settings as employees. Similarly, they are often not covered by onsite employee health and occupational health services. Trainees may also be at higher risk due to a lower skill level when performing procedures, as well as possible fear of reporting accidents and injuries to their instructors. Younger workers typically experience more work-related injuries than their older counterparts in similar jobs. In addition to training and study-related risks, over half of college students are engaged in some level of part-time employment.[4] In one study of college students, 20% of working students had experienced an injury at work.[31]

Health care providers should consider incorporating an occupational risk assessment related to a student's course of study as well as any part-time or other employment and consider occupational and vocational hazards when evaluating injuries and illnesses. Health care students should receive the same preexposure immunizations, postexposure medical care, and training as other healthcare personnel. These include hepatitis B vaccination; screening for immunity to measles, mumps, rubella, and varicella; annual influenza vaccination; periodic tuberculosis screening; pertussis vaccination; and blood-borne pathogen and infection control training.

International Study

International study is increasingly part of today's college curriculum. Participation in study abroad programs has tripled over the past two decades. Nearly 10% of US undergraduates overall and nearly 15% of bachelor's students will study abroad during their degree program. The largest growth has been in programs outside of Europe including Asia, sub-Saharan Africa, Latin America, and the Caribbean. Almost 60% of students will stay for less than 8 weeks and 40% for approximately one semester, with a few students studying for an entire academic year.[6] The duration and nature of their travel means college students studying abroad are at risk not only for common travel-related illnesses, but also face unique risks. Students often reside in an apartment within the community or with a local family rather than a hotel and engage in different activities than a typical tourist. Young adults who stay abroad for extended periods are more likely to have new sexual partners, a significant risk factor for contracting a STI. Alcohol and drug use can endanger safety and place a student at legal risk. Occupational exposures such as needlesticks may occur in health professions students, a particular concern in countries with a high prevalence of human immunodeficiency virus (HIV) infection and limited access to postexposure prophylaxis. The greatest risk of serious illness and injury is from motor vehicle accidents and drowning. Another period of high risk is during academic breaks, especially spring break, when both international and domestic travel are combined with alcohol and drug use, high-risk sexual activity, and other behaviors that can lead to significant mortality and morbidity.

Students participating in study abroad experiences should, if possible, be evaluated by a medical provider with special skills in travel medicine and familiar with extended travel. They should receive information about health and safety in their travel destination, including food- and waterborne illnesses; STIs; insect-borne and other infectious diseases in the area; avoidance of unknown animals to reduce rabies risk; personal safety including crime prevention, food, and dietary customs (including availability of special diets); alcohol, tobacco, and other drug customs and laws; vehicular safety and injury/injury prevention; and availability of local medical and mental health care. In addition to standard travel prescriptions and immunizations, college students should receive birth control when appropriate and advance prescription of postexposure medications for HIV if working in a high-risk situation.

Otherwise stable mental health and medical conditions can worsen under the stress associated with life while abroad and access to local health care may be limited. Students with chronic illnesses, including mental health illnesses, should work with their health care provider to develop treatment plans including what to do during exacerbations during extended study abroad. Arrangements should be made for any prescription medications, medical supplies, and medical care. Most study abroad programs will have limited capability to assist students in managing chronic medical and mental health conditions and may not be able to accommodate all reported individual needs or circumstances.

Health care providers should be alert for the development of post-travel illnesses in college students by inquiring about foreign travel particularly during the evaluation of febrile, dermatologic, and gastrointestinal illnesses. Returning student travelers may not recognize the connection to current symptoms when several months have passed and may not provide a travel history unless questioned directly.

FUNDING AND SERVICE DELIVERY MODEL

Historically, SHS funding models relied on a combination of institutional or tuition support, designated SHSs fees paid directly to IHE from students, out-of-pocket service fees, and minimally on the billing of students' private health insurance. In the 2010 ACHA-SHS Survey, 57% of SHS respondents indicated that they received funding from a designated health fee (75% of public and 29% of private school respondents). While most respondents reported some revenue from billing, this was a relatively small part of total budget for most institutions: 50% of institutions reported receiving less than 10% of their budget from billed revenue, while only 16% received more than 50% from billed revenue.[7]

IHEs are now looking to reduce costs while freeing resources to make needed investments in new programs, technologies, and facilities. With transitions in both the US health care system from implementation of the Affordable Care Act (ACA) and in higher education from pressures to reduce costs of higher education, the service delivery and funding models for SHSs nationally are undergoing significant review. Outsourcing to noncampus service providers and growth of billing students' insurance carriers are potential changes in the financing and administration of SHSs. Given the rapid changes in the overall health care system that can be anticipated in the post-ACA period, much is still uncertain. ACA can provide students who are on a student health sponsored plan with access without copays or deductibles to covered clinical preventative services, including immunizations, contraception including LARC, and indicated screening tests such as screening for STIs. Insurance billing can provide incremental revenue to support some components of medical services and will be most viable if there is uniform comprehensive health insurance coverage for all students. At some IHEs, a portion of health services are now provided at or by a contracted noncampus health care provider. This can reduce the risk associated with and resources dedicated by campus administrators to manage their own SHS, potentially provide access to more comprehensive services, and provide needed investments in facilities and information technology. Contracted services have typically included only medical services, while both mental health services and health promotion/prevention services have remained with on-campus providers.

If strategies such as outsourcing and insurance billing are utilized and some traditional on-campus provided SHSs are integrated into other health care delivery systems, the unique needs of the college student population must be considered:

- Provisions must be made for uninsured and underinsured students to avoid disenfranchising them.
- Many students have primary insurance coverage through geographically limited health care networks and may not have access to services in all of the areas where they live, study, and work.
- Services provided at the SHS are easily accessible through their convenient location. Preservation of student confidentiality when receiving sensitive services is another advantage. If sensitive services are funded through health insurance or provided off campus, students may be reluctant to access them. Increased administrative barriers may deter young adults from receiving care.
- The type and geographic location of the IHE may play a critical role in this assessment. Those that do not have local health resources nearby and/or have a predominantly residential campus will likely need more services and more access to services.
- Communication and cooperation between medical and mental health providers can often best meet the needs of students with mental health illnesses. Models which integrate these services are emerging best practices. Outsourcing a portion of campus health services may fragment delivery of these services.
- At the core of the SHS model is population health. SHSs create a healthier student population through public health, prevention, and health promotion efforts that address risks such as communicable diseases, high-risk alcohol use, violence, obesity, nutrition, and mental health. Insurance billing does not provide a reliable funding mechanism for population health measures at the campus level. An additional funding stream for on-campus population-based measures and public health will be necessary.

Student Health Insurance

Prior to the passage of the ACA, estimates were that approximately 20% of college students were uninsured. While this is lower than the rate of the overall population of 19- to 29-year-olds, part-time students, students of color, and students from families with lower incomes were more likely than average to be uninsured. Uninsured young adults are more likely than insured young adults to delay seeking health care, skip recommended care, and are less like to receive recommended preventive services.[33,34] Under a key early provision of the ACA implemented in 2010, families were able to continue coverage of their dependent children until age 26. This provision had an immediate impact on health insurance coverage of young adults, with an estimated 6.6 million remaining covered during the first year of implementation who would previously not been covered.[33] The rate of uninsured young adults aged 18 to 25 dropped from 28% to 24% after implementation of utilization of parents insurance in 2010. For the next year, there was no decrease and the rate in January 2012 was 24.5% uninsured.[34]

Following full implementation of the ACA in 2014, college student options for health insurance have further expanded. In addition to remaining covered through a family health insurance policy, students may also choose individual policies through the health care marketplace, select a student health insurance plan (SHIP), or may be eligible for state-based Medicaid. Unfortunately, the focus on insurance in exchanges for young adults has been on catastrophic policies, which may not provide adequate coverage for the range of issues facing this population such as chronic mental health conditions. While there remains great uncertainty, emerging health insurance issues for college students include the predicted growth in high deductible plans with impact on student access, increasing cost to families to insure young adults through family plans, leading to discontinuation of coverage, and geographic and other network limitations potentially limiting coverage in the area in which students attend school or are residing in a job, internship, or study abroad. Current penalties for failure to have health insurance minimally impact student populations, and it is possible that many young adults in college will choose not to have health insurance. Student health insurance benefit plans (SHIP) may continue to be offered on many campuses. A form of individual insurance policy, a SHIP typically offers a broad national network. SHIP coverage may be less expensive than individual plans purchased through the marketplace, but currently they are not eligible for subsidies or tax credits.

OTHER ON-CAMPUS STUDENT SERVICES

IHEs provide a range of services to support student growth and development and their physical, mental, and emotional well-being. These services, collectively known as student services or less commonly student affairs, vary based on the size, type, and location of an institution. SHSs are often considered one of these services, and although organization varies widely between campuses, many SHSs institutionally report to a Chief Student Affairs Officer. SHSs as part of or in partnership with a comprehensive student affairs unit are often extensively involved in student affairs programs such as residential life, recreational sports, and orientation. The best practice of college health seeks such educational opportunities and promotes learning not just during the medical or mental health visit but throughout the campus culture. Wellness responsibilities may rest with the SHS or be part of a separate unit. Some SHSs report to the University Medical Campus or both to Medical School and Student Affairs. There are some SHSs that are also academic departments as well as reporting within Student Affairs. The academic component has the potential for synergy with university academic goals and may allow for involvement in teaching and college health clinical research. Other on-campus student affairs professionals are also often extensively involved when developing plans for serving students with mental or physical disabilities on campus. Students experiencing difficulties such as a severe eating disorder, mental health crisis, or drug or alcohol abuse may first come to the attention of a student affairs professional outside the SHS who may refer and coordinate intervention.

Common student affairs departments that support student health and well-being include the following:

- Academic services, including academic advising, career development, and judicial affairs. Judicial affairs (sometimes called student conduct) enforces community standards and campus codes of conduct, and may include ethical programs/education, disciplinary procedures, and mediation for academic or behavioral concerns.
- Campus life services, including campus safety/police, the student union, student activities, leadership, community service, parent programs, and Greek life.
- Diversity and inclusion including multicultural affairs, Lesbian, Gay, Bisexual, Transgender, and Queer (LGBTQ) student services, international student services, spirituality, faith, or religious services and disability support services. Disability support services typically coordinate services related to compliance with the Americans with Disabilities Act (ADA).
- Health and wellness including SHSs, counseling services, sexual assault and violence prevention, alcohol and other drug abuse prevention, and wellness education.
- Residence life (housing) and food services.
- New student enrollment and enrollment services, including admissions, student orientation, and financial aid.
- Sports and recreation, including intercollegiate athletics (at small and/or Division III institutions) and recreation, wellness and fitness programs.

DISEASE-SPECIFIC CONSIDERATIONS

For many specific circumstances, shared responsibility between the hometown health care provider, the SHS, other campus resources, and other community health care resources will ultimately provide the best experience for the student-patient. Students with chronic (e.g., diabetes) and subacute (e.g., rehabilitation following orthopedic surgery) medical conditions will face challenges, including resource limitations or policies of the SHS, availability of and transportation to specialists, out-of-network restrictions of the family's health insurance, the stresses of campus life, and the trials of emergence as an independent young adult. The hometown health care provider is uniquely positioned to help the student and his or her family to negotiate many of these transitions, and the goal of this section is to provide insights about some of the specific challenges.

- **Allergy immunotherapy.** Many, but certainly not all, SHSs will administer allergy shots, but few will initiate therapy, and fewer still have an allergist on staff. Students initiate therapy with the home allergist (the first and second injections) and then transfer the regimen to the SHS for subsequent injections, under orders submitted by the home allergist, who will also continue to supply sera as needed. Students will often transfer sera back and forth between the SHS and the home allergist during summers and other extended breaks from campus.
- **Food allergies.** Campus dining services are increasingly sophisticated in their ability to accommodate food allergies and other dietary needs (e.g., Kosher or vegan). Requests from the family or the health care provider to release the student from a required on-campus meal plan are typically not accepted or necessary, but if negotiation on this (or housing assignments) is intended, they should commence months in advance of matriculation.
- **Attention deficit hyperactivity disorder (ADHD).** Due to concerns about abuse and nonprescribed use of stimulant

medications, SHSs have become increasingly restrictive in initiating stimulant prescriptions and in continuing existing prescriptions. SHS expectations for disease documentation might, at minimum, be a letter from a psychiatrist or neurologist certifying the diagnosis and treatment history or, at the more extensive end of the spectrum, documentation of a formal psychoeducational assessment using standard evaluation, including raw test results. A letter from the primary care provider describing empiric diagnosis and several years of successful treatment will not usually be accepted. Students using stimulants and other controlled medications should be encouraged to investigate whether the residence hall or other living situation includes a lockbox or similar fixture where the medication can be secured. Students who take stimulants should be counseled regarding the legal and ethical ramifications of selling or giving away their medications.

- **Chronic pain.** Chronic pain patients attending college who require opioid medications may encounter significant obstacles. Few, if any, SHSs will prescribe long-acting opioids, again owing in at least small part to overall campus concerns about misuse and diversion of such medications, but also because this is regarded in many communities as within the purview of pain medicine and other specialists.

- **Disabilities.** Students with physical and mental disabilities, including ADHD, requesting campus or academic accommodations under the ADA will typically be required to submit appropriate documentation, in accordance with federal requirements. In general, the SHS (and/or counseling center) will not get involved in certifying disabilities because there is an inherent conflict of interest. Students and families should make requests for accommodations early as documentation needs may be extensive and updated testing and evaluation is sometimes requested. Educational accommodations required under the ADA are generally handled through a dedicated disabilities service office on campus. Other needs, such as a personal care attendant, which fall outside of the ADA requirements may not be provided through the school. The SHS can be helpful in locating community resources for these types of needs.

- **Asthma.** Many young adults underestimate the severity of their asthma or overestimate their degree of symptom control and arrive at college ill prepared for the bronchospasm that may ensue from changes in housing, allergens, temperatures, and climate. They may discover that the inhaler they last used 2 years ago has expired. Even the patient with rare exercise-induced wheezing deserves cautionary education and a new rescue inhaler prior to heading off to college.

- **Diabetes.** The insulin-dependent diabetic in college will be challenged by myriad opportunities for food and drink, irregular sleep, academic and professional stressors, and possibly even stigma. Students should be prepared with action plans for anticipated periods when blood glucose control becomes difficult. As a very practical matter, the student needs to determine campus options for sharps containers and appropriate disposal and a source for medication and supplies.

- **Physical therapy.** Even small minimally resourced SHSs often offer in-house physical therapy. This can be a convenient option, for example, for students who undergo an anterior cruciate ligament repair or other surgical procedure at home but who need to continue rehabilitation while at school.

- **National Collegiate Athletic Association (NCAA) Athletes.** Athletic programs often have sports medicine resources that are for the exclusive use of athletes and which are administratively wholly separate from the SHS. The culture and logistics of the athletic program will typically include written or unwritten rules about where the student-athlete should go for medical care. For example, female athletes might be directed to use the SHS for gynecologic services but to utilize

the sports medicine department for all other medical needs. Relevant to this chapter is that for students participating in NCAA athletics there might be yet another set of health care providers among which the student must navigate.

- **Bipolar and thought disorders.** Most SHSs will provide primary care management for mood disorders such as anxiety and depression, including medication management, ideally in collaboration with the on-campus counseling center or a community therapist. Few, however, will manage multidrug regimens or have resources to manage bipolar illnesses and thought disorders. Furthermore, on-campus access to a psychiatrist may be extremely limited, even when the SHS shares a campus with a major academic medical center. Students and their families should begin looking for resources early. While long-term care may not be available through the SHS or on-campus counseling center, these offices are often a good source for referrals and are knowledgeable about local resources.

- **Eating disorders.** Students with eating disorders can be particularly challenged by a campus environment. Resources on campus or within the local community may be limited. While many students with eating disorders are anxious to start college and to remain enrolled, this can be detrimental to their recovery. Students with eating disorders who are significantly underweight are newly diagnosed, or those who exhibit high levels of eating disorder behaviors frequently require more intensive treatment and support than what is possible as an enrolled student, particularly on a residential campus. Significant recovery is extremely challenging to impossible in this setting. To optimize the student's prospects for collegiate success and safety, patients with eating disorders entering college or returning to college after treatment should have achieved a significant level of recovery and have demonstrated an extended period of stability.

- **Substance abuse recovery.** There are increasing numbers of adolescents who have already endured significant substance abuse problems and who have entered recovery prior to arrival at college. The risk of relapse upon entering the collegiate environment is significant. Some campuses are addressing this issue directly, facilitating access to Alcoholics Anonymous, Narcotics Anonymous, and similar programs. Some campuses have created specific programs, Collegiate Recovery Communities, which offer academic and social support and in some cases residential housing. Prospective students in recovery may consider preferentially applying to a college with such a program.

- **Infusion medications.** The current era of immune modulators available for rheumatoid arthritis, asthma, psoriasis, inflammatory bowel disease, and other conditions can provide remarkable clinical benefits, but there are challenges for the patient on campus, especially if the medication is administered intravenously or if the formal labeling recommends administration in a specialty setting. Even for more familiar medications such as antibiotics, the SHS might have a policy prohibiting intravenous injections or might not have the expertise to infuse through a peripherally inserted central catheter (PICC line) or through a subcutaneous port. Whether in regard to acute or long-term administration of intravenous medications, each of the topics listed previously, or any of many other examples, the home provider or family should consult with the SHS well in advance of matriculation to determine whether the capacity exists on campus for administration of specialty medications or to enlist the SHS in helping to develop an alternative strategy that will meet the patient's need.

- **Chronic medical conditions.** In addition to diabetes and other disease states listed above, there are numerous additional chronic medical conditions that the late adolescent might be coping with as they enter college, including seizure disorders, organ transplants, cancer, cystic fibrosis, and inflammatory bowel disease. Although the SHS will usually be well able to provide episodic ambulatory care for many of these students, specialty care rarely will be available in the SHS, typically necessitating a relationship with a local specialist. The SHS will know the local specialty resources and will gladly make recommendations, but it is also desirable for the home provider or specialist to make a provider-to-provider connection.

ONGOING ENGAGEMENT WITH THE COLLEGE STUDENT

It is anticipated that many hometown health care providers who care for AYAs will have an ongoing (if sporadic) relationship with their patients during their college years. The final section of this chapter is orientated toward these providers who both prepare their patients to come to campus as well as continue to provide and coordinate care with campus resources including SHS providers.

Pre-matriculation

In addition to performing precollege physical examinations and signing vaccination compliance forms, there are many ways for the health care provider to engage with the patient preparing to enter college.

- **Managing ongoing health care while at college**: Importantly, there is also opportunity—ideally starting at least 1 year prior to any actual pre-matriculation visit—to engage in conversation about how the patient plans to manage ongoing health conditions while in college. Are the student and his or her family including medical considerations as they develop a short list of favorite colleges? What medical and counseling services are available on campus? Are appropriate specialists available in the community? The patient should be advised to ask such questions during campus visits. SHSs are generally happy to receive questions along the lines of "My daughter is considering your university to start as a freshman in the fall. Can she get allergy shots in your clinic?" "What about injections of omalizumab?" Is there a psychologist with whom she can talk with every week about her eating disorder?" "Is there a psychologist near campus whom you can recommend for long-term counseling?"
- **Discussion of substance use and abuse and reproductive health:** There is of course opportunity, and possibly parental expectation, for the clinician to engage the patient in pre-matriculation conversation and counseling regarding use of alcohol and other drugs, sexual identity and safer sexual practices, and the importance of medication adherence (e.g., anticonvulsants, insulin, antidepressants). A useful pamphlet produced by the Society for Adolescent Health and Medicine has been developed to review these key issues (www.adolescenthealth.org or www.adolescenthealth.org/Clinical-Care-Resources/Healthy-Student-Brochure.aspx).
- **Accomodation issues:** Once the choice of school is finalized, health care providers may be asked to write letters requesting special accommodations. In some cases, the requests from a student or his or her parents are not related to a documented disability, "He or she needs to be assigned a dormitory near the business school." "He or she needs to be granted special permission to have a car on campus." In considering writing such letters, be prepared for most such recommendations to be denied, as the university usually has philosophical, legal, and pedagogical reasons for randomized roommate assignments and so forth. Requests for accommodations should be sent to the on-campus disability service center.
- **Common access to health care issues:** There is also a compelling need to begin mentoring the patient (and her parents) as

a soon-to-be independent consumer of health care. Key topics might include the following:
- Keeping a medication list
- Carrying an insurance card
- Turning 18 and the implications for confidentiality
- Scheduling appointments
- Filling a prescription
- Providing a health care provider your family and personal medical history

Encourage young adults during their last year of high school to take responsibility for scheduling their own medical appointments, picking up prescriptions, and adhering to medication schedules. It is easier to learn these skills while they are still residing at home. Finally, when sending a patient with a complex medical history off to college, providers should write a comprehensive medical summary letter or other instrument that the student can provide to the SHS and any other care providers they encounter.
- **Health insurance:** Discuss with parents and soon-to-be college students their plans for health insurance coverage. Students should be able to access nonemergency care in the area where they will be attending school, if needed. Health insurance that may provide excellent coverage in the home community may be problematic if it does not cover care in the area where the student will be attending school. An insurance plan with no local in-network primary or specialty care may result in health compromise and much distress when the student cannot afford to obtain services until he goes home for a school break.
- **Consent and confidentiality:** Finally, most students starting college will be over the age of 18, with implications for confidentiality. Most SHSs will not accept an authorization signed a priori providing parent's wholesale access to the student's future medical record at the SHS. A college student's rapid development and growth makes this inappropriate. A student who signs such a release in August may feel very differently a few months later. This might seem frustrating for parents, but parents should be encouraged to allow their student to handle communications with health care providers independently, asking for advice and assistance from parents when needed. That being said, most SHS providers are willing and desirous to communicate with parents after obtaining student consent.

Matriculated Students

The ongoing connection of the hometown provider with a matriculated college student will likely depend on the nature of the pre-matriculation relationship, availability of health care resources at or near the school, proximity of the school to the practice, the nature of the student's health care issues, and the level of parental involvement.

Typically, the student will use the campus and home health care locations (and possibly others) to best advantage, relying on the SHS for episodic care and some primary care during the academic terms and returning home for ongoing specialty or primary care during school breaks. As an upperclassman and graduate student, the student will likely become increasingly dependent on the SHS and other health care providers in the community close to campus, as internships and other curricular demands limit the time available for trips home. Flexibility to use one site or another will also be influenced by the funding structure of the SHS (e.g., health fee versus fee-for-service), the restrictions of the student's health insurance coverage, and the relative incentive to use on-campus resources incorporated into health insurance plans offered by the university.

Negotiating this can be confusing, especially for students early in their undergraduate career. Consider the example of the student who has an incidental visit to an emergency department proximate to his or her college and upon discharge receives the ubiquitous instruction to "follow up with your primary care provider." The student might well consider his or her provider at home 1,000 miles

XVI

away to be the "primary care provider" and is tentative about how to incorporate the SHS, especially at centers with admittedly limited resources.

This can be conceptualized as the student navigating a "virtual medical home," where the home is not defined by geography or mutual participation within an identified health system but rather that use of the right resource at the right time results in the best experience for the student-patient. Unfortunately, this virtual medical home does not come with a shared health record, a shared philosophy, or, as suggested in this chapter, a universally standardized menu of on-campus services. The efficacy of this medical home depends on effective, proactive professional communication and collaboration and on an appreciation for the resources and role provided by the various players.

In a common scenario, the SHS provider identifies a medical condition in early November to which the student's response is, "I talked with my folks and they want me to wait to follow up with my regular doctor at home during Thanksgiving break." The SHS has a responsibility to provide the student with copies of relevant imaging studies or laboratory reports to have available for the home health care provider and to encourage the student (or his or her parent) to immediately get that appointment scheduled, since, almost by definition, such visits will occur around holidays, when the home practice also has limited availability. Likewise, significant interventions made by the home provider should be communicated back to the SHS if there is an expectation that there will be continuity of care when the student returns to campus. Most SHSs with laboratory or x-ray capabilities will gladly accept "outside" orders from a home provider if, for example, the patient desires for the home provider to have ongoing responsibility for monitoring thyroid-stimulating hormone or HgbA1C levels. A corollary of this is that the SHS will gladly do suture removal, dressing changes, and other primary care follow-up for procedures performed by a home provider, but it always goes more smoothly when there is a copy of a clinic note or other notification.

The student and his or her family will often have a long-standing relationship with the home provider and will hold his or her in a place of respect. This may predestine the SHS to a lesser position. The typical scenario is that of a student with an upper respiratory tract infection who is seen in the SHS and does not receive the antibiotic prescription he or she was anticipating. Rather than following the treatment plan offered by the college health provider and follow-up if needed, the immediate response may be to contact the home provider to request a sight unseen, long distance antibiotic prescription, the assumption being that the SHS was wrong. Clearly there are many opportunities for the various teams of providers to support each other and thereby provide optimal care for the mutual patient and his or her family. Provider-to-provider communication can often prevent such situations. Please call the SHS—they want to collaborate in the care of the mutual patient.

Leave of Absence

As a final consideration, the home provider is an important voice in helping a student or his family to come to peace with a decision to take a medical (understood to be inclusive of mental health concerns) leave of absence. Whether because of acute decompensation of an eating disorder, motor vehicle trauma requiring 2 weeks of hospitalization and then acutely limited mobility, or newly diagnosed insulin-dependent diabetes, there are times when the stressors of catching up with and sustaining school work will exacerbate the clinical condition and detract from participation in the treatment regimen. All of these factors can hinder academic performance and further increase the student-patient's stressors. It is very difficult for a student to remain academically productive while simultaneously managing a severe or chronic medical condition that is newly diagnosed or has become unstable. There are times when the best course is to take a leave for the rest of the

semester. Although the student and her family will also be receiving advice and options from the school, the family may look to the trusted home provider for endorsement of these difficult decisions.

More and more, universities are offering leave-of-absence insurance to refund some portion of tuition when a student takes a medical leave, which is another consideration to suggest during pre-matriculation counseling with patients with potentially labile medical conditions. Further, in some cases, the best advice might extend past a recommendation to take leave for the remainder of the current semester to include a recommendation to consider transferring to a school closer to home, to a campus in a contained urban setting rather than a sprawling rural setting, to a school with more extensive on-campus access to mental health services, or to one with better access to a subspecialist.

College students represent a significant portion of young adults. During the college years, students lay the foundations of their adult health habits and behaviors. Successful management of medical and mental health conditions along with mitigation of behavioral risk factors have a direct impact on students' educational and personal success. Strong partnerships with collaboration and communication between on-campus SHSs, student life professionals, students and their families, and outside health care providers combine direct medical and mental health care with population-based interventions. This comprehensive approach can significantly impact the short- and long-term health of these young adults as they complete this transition to adulthood.

● ACKNOWLEDGMENT

The authors would like to acknowledge Lawrence S. Neinstein, Paula L. Swinford, and James A.H. Farrow for their contributions to previous versions of this chapter.

REFERENCES

1. Digest of Education Statistics. *Total fall enrollment in degree-granting institutions, by attendance status, sex, and age: selected years, 1970 through 2020.* Alexandria, VA Institute of Education Sciences. National Center for Education Statistics. Available at http://nces.ed.gov/programs/digest/d11/tables/dt11_200.asp. Prepared September 2011. Accessed December, 15, 2013.
2. Patrick K. Student health. Medical care within institutions of higher education. *JAMA* 1988;260(22):3301–3305.
3. Boynton R. *Historical development of college health services.* American College Health Association, Thirty-ninth Annual Meeting, 1961. Detroit, MI.
4. American College Health Association. *American College Health Association-National College Health Assessment II: Reference Group Data Report Undergraduate Students Spring 2013.* Hanover, MD: American College Health Association, 2013.
5. World Health Organization. *The global burden of disease: 2004 update.* Available at http://www.who.int/healthinfo/global_burden_disease/GBD_report_2004update_full.pdf. Published 2008. Accessed December 28, 2013.
6. Institute of International Education. *Open doors 2013 fast facts.* Available at http://www.iie.org/Research-and-Publications/Open-Doors/Data/Fast-Facts. Published 2013. Accessed January 15, 2014.
7. McBride D, Van Orman S, Wera C, et al. *American College Health Association benchmarking report: 2010 survey on the utilization of student health services.* Available at http://www.acha.org/Topics/docs/ACHA_Benchmarking_Report_2010_Utilization_Survey.pdf. Published 2010. Accessed December 29, 2013.
8. Seigers DK, Carey KB. Screening and brief interventions for alcohol use in college health centers: a review. *J Am Coll Health* 2011;59(3):151–158.
9. Hysenbegasi A, Hass SL, Rowland CR. The impact of depression on the academic productivity of university students. *J Ment Health Policy Econ* 2005;8(3):145–151.
10. Shuchman M. Falling through the cracks—Virginia Tech and the restructuring of college mental health services. *N Engl J Med* 2007;357(2):105–110.
11. Yu JW, Adams SH, Burns J, et al. Use of mental health counseling as adolescents become young adults. *J Adolesc Health* 2008;43(3):268–276.
12. Blanco C, Okuda M, Wright C, et al. Mental health of college students and their non-college-attending peers: results from the National Epidemiologic Study on alcohol and related conditions. *Arch Gen Psychiatry* 2008;65(12):1429–1437.
13. Eisenberg D, Chung H. Adequacy of depression treatment among college students in the United States. *Gen Hosp Psychiatry* 2012;34(3):213–220.
14. Eisenberg D, Hunt J, Speer N, et al. Mental health service utilization among college students in the United States. *J Nerv Ment Dis* 2011;199(5):301–308.
15. American College Health Association. *Considerations for integration of counseling and health services on college and university campuses.* Available at http://www.acha.org/Publications/docs/Considerations%20for%20Integration%20of%20Counseling%20White%20Paper_Mar2010.pdf. Published March 4, 2010. Accessed January 23, 2014.
16. Colllins C, Hewson D, Munger R, et al. *Wade evolving models of behavioral health integration in primary care.* Available at http://www.milbank.org/uploads/documents/10430EvolvingCare/EvolvingCare.pdf. Milbank Reports. Published 2010. Accessed December 15, 2013.

17. American College Health Association. *Healthy Campus 2020*. Available at http://www.acha.org/healthycampus/. Accessed February 1, 2014.
18. http://www.cdc.gov/mmwr/preview/mmwrhtml/mm6441a3.htm
19. Nichol KL, D'Heilly S, Ehlinger E. Colds and influenza-like illnesses in university students: impact on health, academic and work performance, and health care use. *Clin Infect Dis* 2005;40(9):1263–1270.
20. Center for Infectious Disease Research and Policy. *H1N1 and higher ed lessons learned pandemic influenza tools, tips, and takeaways from the big 10 +2 universities*. Available at http://www.cidrap.umn.edu/sites/default/files/public/downloads/big102webfinal.pdf. Published 2010. Accessed May 23, 2014.
21. Hingson RW, Zha W, Weitzman ER. Magnitude of and trends in alcohol-related mortality and morbidity among U.S. college students ages 18–24, 1998–2005. *J Stud Alcohol Drugs Suppl* 2009(16):12–20.
22. Slutske WS. Alcohol use disorders among US college students and their non-college-attending peers. *Arch Gen Psychiatry* 2005;62(3):321–327.
23. Moran S, Wechsler H, Rigotti NA. Social smoking among US college students. *Pediatrics* 2004;114(4):1028–1034.
24. Pearson JL, Richardson A, Niaura RS, et al. e-Cigarette awareness, use, and harm perceptions in US adults. *Am J Public Health* 2012;102(9):1758–1766.
25. Johnston LD, O'Malley PM, Bachman, et al. *Monitoring the future national survey results on drug use, 1975–2013. Vol II. college students and adults ages 19–55*. Ann Arbor: Institute for Social Research, The University of Michigan, 2014:424.
26. Christopher P, Krebs CP, Lindquist CH, et al. College women's experiences with physically forced, alcohol- or other drug-enabled, and drug-facilitated sexual assault before and since entering college. *J Am Coll Health* 2009;57(6):639–649.
27. Swartout KM, Koss MP, White JW, et al. Trajectory analysis of the campus serial rapist assumption. *JAMA Pediatr* 2015; doi.10.1001/jamapediatrics.2015.0707.
28. Nelson MC, Story M, Larson NI, et al. Emerging adulthood and college-aged youth: an overlooked age for weight-related behavior change. *Obesity (Silver Spring)* 2008;16(10):2205–2211.
29. Kloss JD, Nash CO, Horsey SE, et al. The delivery of behavioral sleep medicine to college students. *J Adolesc Health* 2011;48(6):553–561.
30. Kessler CS, McGuinn M, Spec A, et al. Underreporting of blood and body fluid exposures among health care students and trainees in the acute care setting: a 2007 survey. *Am J Infect Control* 2011;39(2):129–134.
31. Balanay JA, Adesina A, Kearney GD, et al. Assessment of occupational health and safety hazard exposures among working college students. *Am J Ind Med* 2014;57(1):114–124.
32. US Government Accountability Office. *Most college students are covered through employer-sponsored plans, and some colleges and states are taking steps to increase coverage*. GAO-08-389. Available at http://www.gao.gov/assets/280/274105.pdf. Published March 28, 2008. Accessed December 30, 2013.
33. Collins SR, Robertson R, Garber T, et al. Young, uninsured, and in debt: why young adults lack health insurance and how the Affordable Care Act is helping: findings from the Commonwealth Fund Health Insurance Tracking Survey of Young Adults, 2011. Issue Brief (Commonw Fund). 2012;14:1–24.
34. Gallup-Healthways Well-Being. *Fewer young adults in U.S. lack health insurance in 2012*. Available at http://www.gallup.com/poll/160376/fewer-young-adults-lack-health-insurance-2012.aspx. Published February 11, 2013. Accessed August 9, 2014.

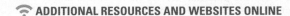 **ADDITIONAL RESOURCES AND WEBSITES ONLINE**

CHAPTER 75

Youth and Young Adults in the Military

Jeffrey W. Hutchinson
William P. Adelman

KEY WORDS

- Civilian
- Deployment
- Military
- Military anticipatory guidance
- Military eligibility
- Military service
- Predeployment
- Redeployment
- Reservist
- Resilience

The US military is an all-volunteer workforce that relies upon adolescents and young adults (AYAs) for its form and function. AYAs in the military include the nearly 800,000 people 25 years old and younger who actively serve in every branch and the 600,000 family members who are between the ages of 13 and 25 with a parent who is serving in, or has retired from, the military. These active duty personnel and family members are eligible for health care through the military health entitlement system TRICARE and may receive care at every military health facility. This chapter highlights the characteristics of, and requirements for, those who serve in the military, including the unique culture of military members and their families as they face deployment and relocation.

YOUNG ADULT SERVICE MEMBERS AND MILITARY CULTURE

Professional militaries have a service focus, an expert knowledge, a professional ethos, and a unique culture that exerts great influence upon individual military members and has unique health implications. Cultural sensitivity to the unique issues relevant to military service is a necessary and required skill for health care providers who deal with military populations. An appreciation and understanding of the unique experience of military members in the context of emerging issues of young adulthood allows the health care provider to provide optimal care.[1–3]

THE NEW RECRUIT

The US military is an all-volunteer force where applicants must meet mental, physical, and legal requirements to join the armed services.[1,4] Most young adults who join the military do not continue for a career. Instead, the military serves as a bridge between their adolescent experiences in their communities and secondary schools and their adult experiences in the labor market and higher education. As such, the military serves as a transition into adulthood for many Americans.[4]

Anticipatory Guidance for Military Service

Consistent with national recommendations, educational and vocational success is a desired outcome of reaching adulthood.[5] The provider can assist the potential service member and family with an assessment of military service suitability as a potential path to adult independence. Patient-centered anticipatory guidance regarding military service combines knowledge of AYA medicine with an understanding of military service.

Providing military guidance includes four steps: educate, articulate, navigate, and matriculate.[3] First, AYAs should educate themselves about the specific branch of the military, with information from multiple sources, such as the Internet, discussion with current or previous service members, and through a recruiter. If possible, the young person should speak to trusted friends or relatives with military experience. Second, the adolescent or young adult should articulate what the military offers, and what the military expects in return, and then be able to complete the sentence, "I plan to join the military because..." or "I decided against the military because..." Third, the interested adolescent or young adult should navigate the best individual path, considering whether to enlist directly out of high school or seek a commission after higher education, and if they prefer the Army or another service branch such as the Navy, Marines, or Air Force. Adolescents who enter the military for specific occupational training should take the Armed Services Vocational Aptitude Battery (ASVAB) before signing an enlistment contract. In this way, he or she would have a better understanding of his or her potential for acceptance into his or her preferred specialty or vocation. For example, an adolescent or young adult who wants to be in the medical field but scores poorly on the ASVAB would not qualify for training and assignment as a medic. Finally, the adolescent should matriculate only after discussion with family, as well as reviewing options with a service branch-specific recruiter who can facilitate the administrative and logistic elements of serving.

Common Disqualifying Conditions for the Military

The three primary reasons for disqualification in 2012 were

- excess weight (15.9%), which decreased from 21.6% the 4 years prior,
- poor visual acuity (12.5%), and
- the report of psychiatric conditions (12.3%), which increased almost 10% from 2007.[6]

Almost all of those who enlisted and were accepted into the military in 2012 had a high school diploma or greater. Those enlisting were required to take the standardized ASVAB to measure verbal, math, science, technical, and spatial abilities. Young adults entering the service as officer candidates through a service academy or Reserve Officer Training Corps (ROTC) scholarship qualify academically through their high school performance and do not take the ASVAB for placement.[7] Medical students who wish to join the military can qualify for the Health Professions Scholarship Program (HPSP), which requires a military commitment in exchange for medical school tuition. Commissioning after ROTC or service academy education requires successful completion of undergraduate studies and continued medical qualification. Medical students who are accepted into the HPSP are immediately commissioned into the reserves as officers during school if they meet the physical and legal requirements.

Physical standards are set by the Department of Defense, where applicants are screened with both standardized questions and a physical examination. Men must be between 60- and 80-inches tall and women 58- to 72-inches tall. Medical conditions such as asthma may be allowed in the service with a waiver. Individuals with other conditions may have a time requirement before eligibility. For instance, AYAs with attention deficit hyperactivity disorder (ADHD) treated with medication must maintain performance for 1 year without medication before acceptance into the service.[8] Before considering military service, AYAs should be aware of personal conditions that are disqualifying and the diagnoses that will not generally receive a waiver. **Table 75.1** highlights several conditions that are not favorable to military service and identifies common conditions that are associated with members leaving the service before completing their obligation. All applicants are screened with a background check to detect felonies and serious financial problems. Though a waiver may be possible for civic issues, most applicants with a criminal record are disqualified. In fact, applicants who give false information prior to entry may be dishonorably discharged after joining the service.

Recommendations for Providers Working with Recruits

Providers without military expertise may wish to further their own education before providing military guidance by using the resources in this chapter or discussing military service with others. Providers should also know individuals who are more qualified to clarify such issues. Important anticipatory guidance includes explaining weight standards, clarifying the significance of academics in military career opportunities, and encouraging the AYAs to research and speak openly about military service.

● ACTIVE DUTY/RESERVIST

General Information

Sovereign countries rely disproportionately upon their AYAs to make up their military population.[2,9] Demographic differences exist between active duty and selected reserve populations. With more than 2 million people on active duty and in the reserves, 43% and 33% respectively are ≤25 years. Enlisted members represent the backbone of the military, with a ratio of five enlisted personnel for every officer.[10,11] **Figures 75.1** and **75.2** depict the enlisted age distribution,

TABLE 75.1
Medical Conditions Not Typically Waivered

Psychological	**Systemic conditions**
• Bipolar disorder; panic disorders; sexual disorders; and severe personality disorders	• Diabetes mellitus type I or type II
	• History of cancer with treatment within 5 y (except basal cell carcinoma)
• Drug and/or alcohol abuse or diagnosed substance dependence	• Severe allergic reaction (anaphylaxis) to insects or food
• Eating disorders: anorexia nervosa and bulimia nervosa	• Single kidney
• Major depression, recurrent	
• Schizophrenia	

Musculoskeletal	**Neurologic**
• Loss of an arm, leg, or eye	• Headaches, recurrent, severe, which require prescription medication or interfere with daily activity
• Prosthetic replacement of joints	
• Severe orthopedic injuries that result in functional limitations secondary to residual muscle weakness, paralysis, or marked decreased range of motion	• Seizure disorder with seizure and/or medication within 5 y
	• Severe head injury within the past 5 y

Infectious diseases	**Gastrointestinal**
• AIDS, AIDS-related complex (ARC), HIV antibody, or history of any of the above	• Crohn's disease and ulcerative colitis (intestinal ulcers)
• Hepatitis, chronic: hepatitis B or hepatitis C carrier	• Intestinal bypass or stomach stapling surgery

highlighting the proportion of AYAs who are ≤25 years and are active military and selected reserves, respectively. The military is predominately male, with 85% men. Minorities comprise 30% and 24% who are active duty and in the selected reserves, respectively.

Physical injuries from both combat and training can affect the AYAs and their family. Overuse injuries as a consequence of training and recreational activities require prevention and treatment. Brain injuries, such as those caused by improvised explosive devices, are characteristic of the recent conflicts and can have long-lasting sequelae.

The invisible wounds of war are also critical to evaluate as suicide rates have increased among soldiers returning from deployment, and 15% of female veterans from Iraq and Afghanistan who have visited a Veterans Affairs (VA) facility have screened positively for sexual trauma.[12,13] Those returning from deployment may suffer from traumatic brain injury as well as psychiatric disorders,

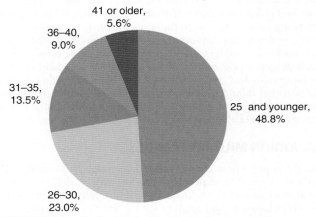

FIGURE 75.1 Age distribution of enlisted active duty personnel.

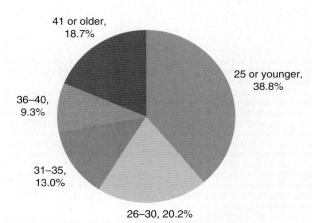

FIGURE 75.2 Age distribution of enlisted reserve personnel.

XVI

including posttraumatic stress disorder (PTSD) that may present without visible manifestations.

It is hard to obtain comparable data on health morbidity between young adults in the military compared to young adult civilians. There is the Department of Defense Survey of Health Related Behavior among Military Personnel. However, this is not consistent in questions asked or in the same time frame as some national surveys of nonmilitary young adults. However, **Table 75.2** is an attempt to provide some comparisons from the military surveys to the nonmilitary young adult survey. Of interest:

- Military young adults had similar smoking rates but far less illicit drug use.
- Heavy alcohol use was significantly higher in military young adults in all the years compared.
- Obesity was much lower in military young adults.

Some of this might be expected as exercise is far higher in the military than nonmilitary. In addition, illicit drug use/abuse would disqualify entry into the military and would also be potential grounds for expulsion.

Screening Considerations

Military culture values discipline, loyalty, and hard work, with high value placed on self-sacrifice, courage, and physical fitness.

TABLE 75.2
Comparison of Civilian and Military Risk-Taking Behavior

	2002		2008		2011	
	Civ (%)	Mil (%)	Civ (%)	Mil (%)	Civ (%)	Mil (%)
Cigarette smokers	40.8[a]	41.6[b]			31.9[a]	29.3[d]
Illicit drug use	19[b]	5.3[b]	20[c]	14[c]		
Heavy alcohol drinkers	15[a]	32.2[b]	16[c]	26[c]	12.9[a]	5.9[d]
						14.3[d]
Binge drinking past 30 d	41[a]	53.8[b]			39.5[a]	21.5[d]
						45.4[d]
Alcohol use (past month)	60.5[a]	66.6[b]			60.2[a]	41.1[d]
		83[b]				89.2[d]
Obese						0.4[d]
						7[d]
Overweight	24.1[a]	17.1[b]			28.7[a]	13[d]
						43[d]

[a]Park MJ, Scott JT, Adams SH, et al. Adolescent and young adult health in the US in the past decade: little improvement and young adults remain worse off than adolescents. *J Adolesc Health* 2014;55:3–16.
[b]Bray RM, Hourani LL, Rae CL, et al. *2002 Department of Defense Survey of health related behavior among military personnel.* Research Triangle Park, NC: Research Triangle Institute, 2003 (RTI/7841/006-FR). Available at http://oai.dtic.mil/oai/oai?verb=get Record&metadataPrefix=html&identifier=ADA431566. Accessed March 29, 2015.
[c]Bray RM, Pemberton MR, Hourani LL, et al. 2008 Department of Defense Survey of health related behaviors among active duty military personnel. Available at http://www.ncpgambling.org/files/public/Military/2008%20DoD%20Study%20risk%20taking%20section.pdf. Accessed March 29, 2014.
[d]Barlas FM, Higgins WB, Pflieger JC, et al. 2011 *health related behaviors survey of active duty military personnel.* Fairfax, VA: ICF International, 2013. Available at http://oai.dtic.mil/oai/oai?verb=getRecord&metadataPrefix=html&identifier=ADA582287. Accessed March 29, 2014.
Civ = civilian; Mil = Military

When these cultural influences combine with the perceived invulnerability and developing critical thinking typical of adolescence, medical conditions may be minimized or hidden from the provider. Young service members may underplay an injury or condition, especially if it is feared to negatively influence military advancement, fitness for duty, or unit reputation.[1,14] Therefore, providers must be diligent in seeking hidden agendas.

Physical Screening

The clinician should screen for signs of traumatic brain injury in war veterans and overuse injuries in all service members. Back and knee injuries are common. Burns, amputations, and hearing loss are other conditions seen in service members that require adjustment and may relate to psychosocial concerns and display physical manifestations of psychological conditions.[15]

Mental Health Screening Related to Combat

- *The Combat Experiences Scale* (CES) is a 7-item self-report scale (**Table 75.3**) from the Deployment Risk and Resilience Inventory (DRRI) which evaluates a soldier's experience in a combat situation, particularly when it involves direct conflict with the enemy or witnessing injury or death. Higher scores reflect greater combat exposure (i.e., ≤16: light; 17 to 32: moderate; ≥33: heavy) and can be helpful to identify the presence of PTSD.
- *The Posttraumatic Stress Disorder Checklist-Military Version* (PCL-M) is a 17-item instrument that allows military veterans to report their feelings that may be consistent with a diagnosis of PTSD. A score of ≥50 is considered positive for PTSD. Unlike the PCL-M, the CES inquires only about battlefield conditions. The PCL-M may offer a more rapid assessment to determine other needed services that may benefit the soldier.
- *The Personal Health Questionnaire* (PHQ-9) is a validated instrument that can be easily administered at each visit to screen for depression, with higher scores indicating greater severity.[12,16,17]

Psychosocial Screening

A modified HEEADSSS screening that addresses greater attention on alcohol use, resiliency, and sexual activity may be used for adolescent and young military members and veterans (**Table 75.4**).[18] Should the service member endorse concern about alcohol and/or drug use, the CRAFFT screening questionnaire should subsequently be used (see Chapter 64).[19] The provider should recall that a score ≥2 indicates a need for a more comprehensive assessment of substance abuse and misuse.

Recommendations

Providers must consider the physical and emotional traumas that may accompany military service through developing cultural sensitivity and an understanding of available resources. While there are significant causes of stress in the service such as family separation, injury, and training requirements, service members also benefit from resilience builders such as exercise, schedule predictability, esprit de corps (a common loyalty shared by members of a particular group), and group cohesion (e.g., Band of Brothers). Thus, the provider should evaluate service-related conditions at every encounter with a young adult who has served in the military, along with their coping abilities, and resilience.[1,14,18]

⬤ AYAs IN MILITARY FAMILIES

Military family life is characterized by service and sacrifice. Regardless of combat exposure, families with a military service member experience loss due to recurrent family separation, geographic relocation, and anxiety for the safety of the active duty member.

TABLE 75.3

Combat Experience Scale

Please circle the number that best describes your experience.

1. Did you ever go on combat patrols or have other dangerous duty?

1	2	3	4	5
No	1–3 ×	4–12 ×	13–50 ×	>50 ×

2. Were you ever under enemy fire?

1	2	3	4	5
Never	<1 mo	1–3 mo	4–6 mo	7 mo or more

3. Were you ever surrounded by the enemy?

1	2	3	4	5
No	1–2 ×	3–12 ×	13–25 ×	>25 ×

4. What percentage of soldiers in your unit were killed in action (KIA), wounded, or missing in action (MIA)?

1	2	3	4	5
None	1%–25%	26%–50%	51%–75%	>75%

5. How often did you fire rounds at the enemy?

1	2	3	4	5
Never	1–2 ×	3–12 ×	13–50 ×	>50 ×

6. How often did you see someone hit by incoming or outgoing rounds?

1	2	3	4	5
Never	1–2 ×	3–12 ×	13–50 ×	>50 ×

7. How often were you in danger of being injured or killed?

1	2	3	4	5
Never	1–2 ×	3–12 ×	13–50 ×	>50 ×

From Keane TM, Fairbank JA, Caddell JM, et al. Clinical evaluation of a measure to assess combat exposure. *J Consult Clin Psychol* 1989;1:53–55.

TABLE 75.4

Military HEEADSSS Additional Questions

Home: Where do you live? Do you feel like a valued member of your unit? Do you feel support by your leaders? Do you have someone you trust?

Employment: How long are you planning to serve in the military? What is your job in the Military?

Activity: What do you do on leave or free time? (video games, exercise, social media) Do you use supplements? Why?

Drugs: Do you drink alcohol more than you want to?

Safety/Suicide: Have you had any experiences that affect your life now? Do you have anyone you can talk to? Do you own a weapon? Have you ever thought about hurting yourself? Have you been deployed? How many times?

Demographics

There are more than 600,000 military family members aged 12 to 22 years with parents who are on active duty and another 300,000 with a parent in the reserves.[8] Children, until age 18, are eligible for care when their parent is on active duty or when a reservist is actively serving. A young adult who is a full-time student is eligible for health care until their twenty-third birthday. Under the Affordable Care Act, TRICARE for young adults, for a fee, is an option to extend health coverage up to age 26 years.

Screening

AYAs who have one or more members of their family in military services may present with physical or psychological complaints such as sleeping difficulties, substance use, anxiety, depression, social withdrawal, impotence, or headaches. Therefore, psychosocial screening must consider military service as a potential source of distress,[20-22] as well as other preventive health screening designed for this population.

Resiliency Factors

Resilience is defined as the successful adaptation following an adverse or traumatic event. Resilience for young adult family members grows with exposure to other cultures, military community, and navigating changing peer groups.[21,22] Both AYAs living in these families respond differently during different phases of deployment.

Predeployment is the time after a service member is selected to deploy; uncertainty and fear predominate negative feelings, especially among adolescents. The provider should encourage parents to discuss responsibilities and expectations during this time.

Deployment is the early period after the military member leaves home. It is a time characterized with feelings of loss and abandonment. Again, the provider must encourage families to continue traditions and develop new ones.

Sustainment is the time the family has established a routine after the service member has deployed. The AYAs living in the household may take on new roles. Families are challenged to establish support systems through extended family, friends, religious groups, and family support groups. Communication with the deployed service member via e-mail, phone, and letters will assist to maintain this relationship.

Postdeployment or redeployment is when the service member returns home. This is the period where reconnecting is important. The provider should stress to the families that it requires time to reacquaint themselves with one another and communication among and between members is key. Younger adolescents may be especially prone to feelings of guilt and be confused about their feelings. Parents can help by slowly making changes in routine and lowering holiday expectations. The returning parent must be helped back into the family circle.

Specific advice for parents of young and mid-age adolescents with a deployed parent includes the following:

1. Encourage conversations about deployment and war.
2. Help children keep in contact with the deployed parent.
3. Limit exposure or contact with media coverage of the conflict.
4. Maintain routines.
5. Do not expect teenagers to co-parent.
6. Continue the same discipline rules and consequences.
7. Encourage peer relationships and time with peers.
8. Be patient with expressions of anger, irritability, and withdrawal.
9. Encourage good nutrition, rest, and exercise.
10. Encourage journaling.
11. Use available resources.
12. Continue extracurricular and community activities.

REFERENCES

1. Hutchinson JW, Greene JP, Bryant CM, et al. Helping those who serve: care of the young adult veteran. *Adolesc Med State Art Rev* 2013;24(3):553–572.
2. Robinson CA, Hutchinson JW, Adelman WP. Military service: military culture and the adolescent. In: Elzouki AY, ed. *Textbook of clinical pediatrics.* 2nd ed. New York, NY: Springer, 2011:3897–3900.
3. Adelman WP. Basic training for the pediatrician: how to provide comprehensive anticipatory guidance regarding military service. *Pediatrics* 2008;121(4):e993–e997.
4. Institute of Medicine, National Research Council. *Investing in the health and well-being of young adults.* Washington, DC: The National Academies Press, 2014.
5. Hagan JF, Shaw JS, Duncan PM, eds. *Bright futures: guidelines for health care supervision of infants, children and adolescents.* 3rd ed. Elk Grove Village, IL: American Academy of Pediatrics, 2008. Available at www.brightfutures.org.
6. Accession Medical Standards Analysis & Research Activity (AMSARA). *Annual Report Published & Distributed 3th Quarter of Fiscal Year 2013.* 2013. Available at http://www.amsara.amedd.army.mil/Documents/AMSARA_AR/AMSARA%20AR%20 2013_final.pdf.
7. Naval Reserve Officers Training Corps—Military Service Requirements. Available at https://www.nrotc.navy.mil/requirements_new.aspx.
8. Office of the Deputy Under Secretary of Defense. 2012 Demographics profile of the Military Community. Available at http://www.militaryonesource.mil/12038/MOS/Reports/2012_Demographics_Report.pdf.
9. The Army Profession Pamphlet produced by the Center for the Army Profession and Ethic (CAPE). Available at http://cape.army.mil/repository/ProArms/Army%20 Profession%20Pamphlet.pdf.
10. Defense Manpower Data Center. *Active Duty Military Personnel Master File.* Arlington, VA: Defense Manpower Data Center, 2011.
11. Department of Defense, Office of the Assistant Secretary of Defense (Reserve Affairs). *Official guard and reserve manpower strengths and statistics.* Washington, DC: Department of Defense, 2011.
12. Briggs B. The enemy within: Soldier suicides outpaced combat deaths in 2012. January 4, 2013. Available at http://usnews.nbcnews.com/_news/2013/01/03/16309351-the-enemy-within-soldier-suicides-outpaced-combat-deaths-in-2012?lite.
13. Kimerling R, Street AE, Pavao J, et al. Military related sexual trauma among Veterans Health Administration patients returning from Afghanistan and Iraq. *Am J Public Health* 2010;100:1409–1412.
14. Greene-Shortridge TM, Britt TW, Castro CA. The stigma of mental health problems in the military. *Mil Med* 2007;172(2):157–161.
15. Baker DG, Heppner P, Afari N, et al. Trauma exposure, branch of service, and physical injury in relation to mental health among U.S. veterans returning from Iraq and Afghanistan. *Mil Med* 2009;174(8):773–778.
16. Pietrzak RH, Russo AR, Ling Q, et al. Suicidal ideation in treatment-seeking Veterans of Operations Enduring Freedom and Iraqi Freedom: the role of coping strategies, resilience, and social support. *J Psychiatr Res* 2011;45:720–726.
17. Pietrzak RH, Goldstein MB, Malley JC, et al. Risk and protective factors associated with suicidal ideation in Veterans of Operations Enduring Freedom and Iraqi Freedom. *J Affect Disord* 2010;123;102–107.
18. Hutchinson JW, Greene JP, Hansen SL. Evaluating active duty risk-taking: military home, education, activity, drugs, sex, suicide, and safety method. *Mil Med* 2008;173(12):1164–1167.
19. Knight JR, Sherritt L, Shrier LA, et al. Validity of the CRAFFT substance abuse screening test among adolescent clinic patients. *Arch Pediatr Adolesc Med* 2002;156:607–614.
20. Davis BE, Blaschke GS, Stafford EM. Military children, families, and communities: supporting those who serve. *Pediatrics* 2012;129:S3–S10.
21. Klein DA, Goldenring JM, Adelman WP. HEEADSSS 3.0: the psychosocial interview for adolescents updated for a new century fueled by media. *Contemp Pediatr* Jan 2014:1–16. http://contemporarypediatrics.modernmedicine.com/contemporary-pediatrics/news/probing-scars-how-ask-essential-questions?page=full
22. Aranda MC, Middleton LC, Flake E, et al. Psychosocial screening in children with wartime-deployed parents. *Mil Med* 2011;176(4):402–407.V

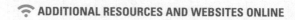 **ADDITIONAL RESOURCES AND WEBSITES ONLINE**

CHAPTER 76

The Health of Unaccompanied Homeless Minors and Young Adults

Colette L. Auerswald
Meera S. Beharry
Curren Warf

KEY WORDS

- Couch surfers
- Health status
- Homeless youth
- Literally homeless youth
- Runaways
- Street youth
- Systems youth
- Throwaways
- Trafficked youth

BACKGROUND

Homeless and runaway youth are a population of extraordinary vulnerability and potential who, like all youth, are faced with the challenges of accomplishing the developmental tasks of adolescence and young adulthood (see Chapter 2). However, many must accomplish these tasks hampered by dysfunctional familial environments, without the support of adult caretakers and without a stable roof over their heads.[1] This chapter focuses on the needs of homeless unaccompanied minors and of youth to age 26. Though the needs of minors and young adults on the street differ, a large percentage of homeless young adults were homeless as minors and continue to struggle with the similar challenges, while frequently having aged out of much-needed youth services such as foster care, juvenile justice, runaway services, and special education.

The Path to the Street

With varied paths to the streets and unique individual experiences, homeless youth are not a homogeneous population.[2] Generally, they have disproportionately experienced poverty; early childhood loss (such as parental death or incarceration); family chaos (including parental substance abuse and domestic violence); mental illness; emotional, physical, and/or sexual abuse and/or neglect; and resulting foster care placement.[1–6]

Population Size

The actual size of the homeless youth population in the US is unknown. Estimates have ranged from 500,000 to 1.6 million.[1,4,7] Obstacles to an accurate count include variability in definitions of homelessness; considerable methodological challenges; the hidden and intermittent nature of youth homelessness; youths' avoidance of services because of fear of authorities; and reluctance to identify as homeless due to stigma.[8–11]

Definitions and Terms

Youth homelessness is inconsistently defined in the medical literature and in federal legislation. The McKinney–Vento Homeless Education Assistance Act offers perhaps the most useful federal definition, defining homeless youth as those who lack "a fixed, regular, and adequate nighttime residence".[12]

The literature employs multiple, overlapping terms. *Runaways* are minors who have left home and lack adult supervision, commonly because of family conflict, abuse, and/or neglect. *Throwaways* are minors who have been ejected from their home by their families, frequently because of poverty, conflict, or familial substance abuse. *Couch surfers* migrate from one unstable housing situation to another, often falling through the cracks to find themselves without any shelter. *Literally homeless youth* live on streets or in parks with no access to housing. *Street youth* strongly identify with a local street-involved community of youth. *Systems youth* are youth who may become homeless after aging out of youth services, such as juvenile justice or foster care. We employ the term *homeless youth* for all these youth, recognizing that many youth would reject the label.[2]

Demographics

In most locations, the majority of homeless youth come from the local community or nearby. Some large metropolitan areas in North America such as New York, Denver, Los Angeles, San Francisco, Seattle, and Vancouver serve as gathering places for homeless youth from broader regions. However, even in these locations, a large percentage of homeless youth come from the local community. Minors and youth who are disproportionately represented among the homeless include former systems youth; young adults recently released from prison or jail; veterans; lesbian, gay, and bisexual youth; transgender youth; immigrant and undocumented youth; and low-income ethnic minority youth, particularly African American, Latino, and Native American youth.[4,13,14]

RISKY BEHAVIORS, MORBIDITY, AND MORTALITY

Risky Behaviors and Homeless Youth Health

Given their lack of familial support, society's failure to provide for them, and their underlying vulnerability, homeless youth have limited options to meet their basic needs for food, shelter, safety, emotional support and health care. Although adolescence is a developmental stage during which experimentation and exploration are normative (see Chapter 3), homeless youth often engage in behaviors considered particularly risky by providers in order to meet their basic needs and to bond with peers. Although this may be seen as dangerous within a medical paradigm, these behaviors may be quite rational from the standpoint of survival. To reduce their risk, youth require alternative means to meet their needs.

Violence and Abuse

Homeless youth are not only more likely than housed peers to have experienced trauma prior to being homeless, they are also at far greater risk than housed youth of experiencing additional episodes of violence, physical abuse, or sexual exploitation. In a multicity study of homeless youth, Bender and colleagues reported that 79% of youth recruited from homeless youth-serving agencies reported multiple types of childhood abuse and 29% reported street victimization.[15] Lesbian, gay, bisexual, and transgender (LGBT) youth report particularly high rates of victimization.[3,14,16] Youth may resist reporting or refuse services because of prior negative consequences resulting from reporting of past trauma (such as separation from family and removal from home), or because of economic dependence on a current abuser (such as a "pimp" or drug dealer). Providers should be guided by local laws and guidelines to ensure youth's safety (see Chapter 9). Furthermore, for minors who are being sexually exploited, guidelines regarding trafficked youth also apply.[17]

Substance Use and Abuse and Mental Health Concerns

Alcohol, tobacco, and other drug use and abuse are more prevalent among homeless youth than among housed youth. However, patterns of use vary greatly by geographic area. Injection drug use (IDU) is far more common among homeless youth and is a significant source of morbidity and mortality from overdose, addiction-related behaviors, drug effects, and blood-borne infections.[18] Venue-based samples of homeless youth in both San Francisco and Vancouver yielded a prevalence of IDU of 40%.[19,20] Community-based naloxone distribution has been found to be a life-saving measure.[21] Harm-reduction strategies that make clean syringes and drug-use paraphernalia available reduce the risk of negative consequences of IDU, including transmission of HIV/hepatitis C.[22] Methamphetamine use is also prevalent among homeless youth in many cities, with youth in a longitudinal study in Vancouver reported to have a incidence of methamphetamine initiation of 12.2 per 100 person-years.[23]

Homeless youth are more likely than their housed counterparts to suffer from psychiatric morbidity, including mood disorders (particularly depression and bipolar disorder), anxiety disorders (particularly generalized anxiety disorder), posttraumatic stress disorder, and suicidality.[3,15,16] The diagnosis of psychiatric disorders is often clouded by concurrent substance use, which may be an attempt at self-medication. Substance abuse treatment may be an important first step to treatment of underlying mental health disorders. Mental health services should not be deferred while youth continue to engage in drug or alcohol use.

Infectious Diseases, Including Sexually Transmitted Infections

Homeless youth are at greater risk for infectious diseases associated with marginalized status. The seroincidence rates of hepatitis C were 10.9 per 100 person-years among females and 5.1 per person-years among males in a study of illicit drug-using street-involved youth in Vancouver.[24] Street-based testing of homeless youth in San Francisco for gonorrhea and chlamydia yielded a 7.8% overall prevalence.[25] Homeless youth should routinely be screened for HIV, hepatitis C, chlamydia, gonorrhea, syphilis, and tuberculosis. A history of IDU, survival sex (sex in exchange for money, food, shelter, protection, or drugs), and/or of men having sex with men may further increase youth's risk and alter the indicated screening tests, as per current screening guidelines. Condoms, rapid testing, immediate linkage to care with no-cost antibiotics, and expedited partner therapy, as indicated, should be made available.[25,26]

Homeless youth are also susceptible to dermatologic infections associated with poor hygiene, IDU, or both, including cellulitis and abscesses. Methicillin-resistant *Staphylococcus aureus* should be strongly considered in this population.[27] Homeless youth are also more likely to be infected with parasitic infections, including lice and scabies.[28]

Reproductive Health

Homeless youth require no-cost, on-demand access to the full range of effective contraception methods, including postcoital contraception and therapeutic abortion. Homeless youth are far more likely than housed youth to experience an unintended pregnancy.[29] Women continuing pregnancy need prompt access to prenatal care, housing stabilization, counseling regarding the fetal risks of alcohol and other substance use, education about infant care and early childhood development, and family reconciliation when possible.[1] A pregnancy can expedite a departure from the street for youth, including the father.[29]

Other Medical Problems

Homeless youth have higher rates of common medical problems such as asthma, diabetes, and obesity. Additionally, their adverse childhood experiences put them at higher risk of lifelong poor health.[30]

Mortality

Mortality of homeless youth is significantly higher than among housed youth, largely due to preventable causes, particularly suicide, as well as drug overdose and accidental trauma.[31,32] Roy and colleagues in Montreal conducted two, 5-year prospective cohort studies with youth initially recruited from service agencies at ages 14 to 25.[31,32] They found a standardized mortality ratio (SMR) relative to the general population of Quebec of 15.3 in their first cohort tracked from 1995 to 2000 and a subsequent 79% mortality rate decrease to an SMR of 3.0 in their second cohort tracked from 2001 to 2006. They attributed the decrease to an improvement in local services to help the homeless and injection drug-using populations.

🔵 PRINCIPLES AND APPROACH TO CARE

Notwithstanding the trauma and lack of support they have faced, homeless and runaway youth often demonstrate great resilience and, at this critical developmental stage, commonly respond well to caring relationships with adults.

Guidelines for Providers

- Though it may seem minor in the eyes of clinicians, *the chief complaint* can serve as an opening to address issues of housing, education, mental health, and social services.[33]
- Recognize that *youth may avoid accessing care for multiple reasons*, including fear of being judged or treated disrespectfully, anxiety about the implications of a health problem, past negative experiences in the health care system, fear of being reported to child protective services (for minors), and concern regarding lack of coverage or inability to pay for care (for young adults).[34]
- *Foster trust and respect* through a nonjudgmental positive stance toward the homeless adolescent or young adult to maximize the potential for follow-up. Similarly, the clinician should recognize that although very high-risk behaviors, such as survival sex and IDU, are more common among homeless youth that assessment of an individual youth's risk should be based on a careful history and not on assumptions.[34]
- *Employ a harm-reduction approach* to encourage youth to reduce their risk behaviors to the degree they are able to minimize negative consequences.[35]
- *Help youth identify their own goals* and assist them in moving incrementally toward engagement, greater safety, and stability.

- *Utilize clinical encounters as opportunities to link youth to available resources* to address their needs, particularly housing, education, employment, and mental health services.

Guidelines for Clinics and Other Programs

- Concerns regarding *confidentiality, reporting, and consent* may be significant obstacles that both prevent youth from presenting for care and providers from making care available to homeless youth. In some US states, such as California, homelessness status alone is not, in and of itself, sufficient basis to report child abuse or neglect.[36] In most states, minors are entitled to confidentiality except when having an intent to die by suicide, kill another, or disclose physical, sexual, or severe emotional abuse by an adult.
- *Low barrier, no-cost health care* must be available to all homeless youth, including immigrant youth.
- Due to the lack of continuity in their care and the lack of stable and trustworthy adults in their lives to guide their access to medical care, homeless youth need *intensive case management.*
- Provide *drop-in and evening/weekend hours*, and praise youth for presenting for care without penalizing them for missing appointments.

Guidelines for Communities

To address the health of homeless youth, communities can address structural factors at the legislative, programmatic, and policy levels.[37,38]

- Provide housing on demand to youth as quickly as possible regardless of their engagement in services, as well as access on demand to developmentally appropriate substance use and mental health services.
- Ensure *youth's access to social services to which they are entitled*, such as housing, case management, education, vocational services, and primary health care.
- Promote *continuity of care* through collaboration among local and regional providers for homeless youth and access to a portable electronic records and documents system.[39]
- Oppose laws that criminalize homelessness (sit-lie or panhandling ordinances), minor offenses (such as marijuana possession), or informal care for the homeless by extended family or friends.
- Increase awareness of human trafficking, and encourage law enforcement to prosecute traffickers rather than youth.
- Eliminate rules that exclude youth and young adults from Section 8 housing or family shelters.
- Provide services tailored to the needs of specific high-risk populations, including lesbian, gay, bisexual, transgender, queer and questioning youth, and immigrant youth.
- Extend foster care services into young adulthood, including access to transitional housing, and extend such services to other transitional aged youth.[1]

REFERENCES

1. Institute of Medicine and National Research Council. *Investing in the health and well-being of young adults.* Washington, DC: The National Academies Press, 2014. Available at http://www.iom.edu/Reports/2014/Investing-in-the-Health-and-Well-Being-of-Young-Adults.aspx. Accessed April 13, 2015.
2. Hickler B, Auerswald CL. The worlds of homeless white and African American youth in San Francisco, California: a cultural epidemiological comparison. *Soc Sci Med* 2009;68:824–831.
3. Edidin JP, Ganim Z, Hunter SJ, et al. The mental and physical health of homeless youth: a literature review. *Child Psychiatry Hum Dev* 2012;43:354–375.
4. Toro PA, Dworsky A, Fowler PJ. *Homeless youth in the United States: recent research findings and intervention approaches.* Paper presented at: National Symposium on Homelessness Research; 2007. Available at http://www.huduser.org/portal/publications/homeless/p6.html. Accessed June 23, 2014.
5. Rew L, Whittaker TA, Taylor-Seehafer MA, et al. Sexual health risks and protective resources in gay, lesbian, bisexual, and heterosexual homeless youth. *J Spec Pediatr Nurs* 2005;10:11–19.
6. Cleverley K, Kidd SA. Resilience and suicidality among homeless youth. *J Adolesc* 2011;34:1049–1054.
7. National Alliance to End Homelessness. *An emerging framework for ending unaccompanied youth homelessness.* Washington, DC: National Alliance to End Homelessness, 2012.
8. Auerswald C, Lin J, Petry L, et al. *Hidden in plain sight: an assessment of youth inclusion in point-in-time counts of California's unsheltered homeless population.* Sacramento, CA: California Homeless Youth Project, 2013.
9. Milburn NG, Rosenthal D, Rotheram-Borus MJ, et al. Newly homeless youth typically return home. *J Adolesc Health* 2007;40:574–576.
10. Roman N. *Ending youth homelessness.* Washington, DC: National Alliance to End Homelessness, 2012.
11. United States Interagency Council on Homelessness. *Framework to end youth homelessness: a resource text for dialogue and action.* Washington, DC: United States Interagency Council on Homelessness, 2013.
12. The McKinney–Vento Homeless Assistance Act, §42 U.S.C. § 11301 (1987).
13. Fowler PJ, Toro PA, Miles BW. Pathways to and from homelessness and associated psychosocial outcomes among adolescents leaving the foster care system. *Am J Public Health* 2009;99:1453–1458.
14. Keuroghlian AS, Shtasel D, Bassuk EL. Out on the street: a public health and policy agenda for lesbian, gay, bisexual, and transgender youth who are homeless. *Am J Orthopsychiatry* 2014;84:66–72.
15. Bender K, Brown SM, Thompson SJ, et al. Multiple victimizations before and after leaving home associated with PTSD, depression, and substance use disorder among homeless youth. *Child Maltreat* 2015;20(2):115–124.
16. Cochran BN, Stewart AJ, Ginzler JA, et al. Challenges faced by homeless sexual minorities: comparison of gay, lesbian, bisexual, and transgender homeless adolescents with their heterosexual counterparts. *Am J Public Health* 2002;92:773–777.
17. National Research Council. *Confronting commercial sexual exploitation and sex trafficking of minors in the United States.* Washington, DC: The National Academies Press, 2013.
18. Evans JL, Tsui JI, Hahn JA, et al. Mortality among young injection drug users in San Francisco: a 10-year follow-up of the UFO study. *Am J Epidemiol* 2012;175:302–308.
19. Parriott AM, Auerswald CL. Incidence and predictors of onset of injection drug use in a San Francisco cohort of homeless youth. *Subst Use Misuse* 2009;44:1958–1970.
20. Kerr T, Marshall BD, Miller C, et al. Injection drug use among street-involved youth in a Canadian setting. *BMC Public Health* 2009;9:171. doi:10.1186/1471-2458-9-171.
21. Marshall BD, Milloy MJ, Wood E, et al. Reduction in overdose mortality after the opening of North America's first medically supervised safer injecting facility: a retrospective population-based study. *Lancet* 2011;377:1429–1437.
22. Vancouver Coastal Health. *Insite—supervised injection site.* Available at http://supervisedinjection.vch.ca/. Accessed April 13, 2015.
23. Uhlmann S, DeBeck K, Simo A, et al. Crystal methamphetamine initiation among street-involved youth. *Am J Drug Alcohol Abuse* 2014;40:31–36.
24. Puri N, DeBeck K, Feng C, et al. Gender influences on hepatitis C incidence among street youth in a Canadian setting. *J Adolesc Health* 2014;55:830–834.
25. Auerswald CL, Sugano E, Ellen J, et al. Street-based STD testing and treatment of youth are feasible, acceptable and effective. *J Adolesc Health* 2006;38:208–212.
26. Centers for Disease Control and Prevention. *Expedited partner therapy.* Available at http://www.cdc.gov/STD/ept/default.htm. Accessed April 13, 2015.
27. Pan ES, Diep BA, Charlebois ED, et al. Population dynamics of nasal strains of methicillin-resistant Staphylococcus aureus—and their relation to community-associated disease activity. *J Infect Dis* 2005;192:811–818.
28. Feldmann J, Middleman AB. Homeless adolescents: common clinical concerns. *Semin Pediatr Infect Dis* 2003;14:6–11.
29. Smid M, Bourgois P, Auerswald C. The challenge of pregnancy among homeless youth: reclaiming a lost opportunity. *J Health Care Poor Underserved* 2010;21:140–156.
30. Goodwin RD, Stein MB. Association between childhood trauma and physical disorders among adults in the United States. *Psychol Med* 2004;34:509–520.
31. Roy E, Haley N, Boudreau JF, et al. The challenge of understanding mortality changes among street youth. *J Urban Health* 2010;87:95–101.
32. Roy E, Haley N, Leclerc P, et al. Mortality in a cohort of street youth in Montreal. *JAMA* 2004;292:569–574.
33. Ensign J. Quality of health care: the views of homeless youth. *Health Serv Res* 2004;39:695–707.
34. American Academy of Pediatrics. *Reaching adolescents: strength-based communication strategies to build resilience and support healthy adolescent development.* Elk Grove Village, IL: American Academy of Pediatrics, 2014.
35. Ho J. *How using a harm reduction model for youth can help us accomplish the goal of ending youth homelessness.* Available at http://usich.gov/population/youth/harm_reduction_for_youth. Accessed June 20, 2014.
36. Child Abuse and Neglect Reporting Act: Homeless Children, AB652 (2013). Available at http://leginfo.legislature.ca.gov/faces/billNavClient.xhtml?bill_id=201320140AB652. Accessed April 13, 2015.
37. Marshall BD. The contextual determinants of sexually transmissible infections among street-involved youth in North America. *Cult Health Sex* 2008;10:787–799.
38. Viner RM, Ozer EM, Denny S, et al. Adolescence and the social determinants of health. *Lancet* 2012;379:1641–1652.
39. Dang MT, Whitney KD, Virata MC, et al. A web-based personal health information system for homeless youth and young adults. *Public Health Nurs* 2012;29:313–319.

XVI

📶 **ADDITIONAL RESOURCES AND WEBSITES ONLINE**

CHAPTER 77

Youth in Foster Care

Heather Taussig
Scott B. Harpin
William R. Betts
Lora Melnicoe
Gretchen J. Russo

KEY WORDS

- Child abuse and neglect
- Emancipation
- Foster care
- Medical home
- Mental health
- Transition care
- Trauma

Adolescents in foster care, the vast majority of whom have been abused and/or neglected, are at increased risk for physical and mental health problems throughout the developmental spectrum as evidenced by their involvement in multiple service systems, including juvenile justice, mental health, and special education. For young adults who have emancipated from foster care, the transition to independence may be especially challenging, as these young adults demonstrate high rates of substance use, early and multiple pregnancies, significant physical and mental health problems, criminal justice involvement, victimization, economic hardship, and homelessness. The consequences of maltreatment, early life instability, and trauma are far-reaching, leading to a cycle of both maltreatment and placement in foster care. Despite the many obstacles facing young people in foster care, there are opportunities to promote resilience through positive youth development.

EPIDEMIOLOGY

General Foster Care Statistics

- Each year, approximately 6 million youth are referred to social services for maltreatment, and three-quarters of a million have documented (e.g., substantiated report) evidence of abuse. This represents almost 1% of the population of youth aged 0 to 18.[1]
- Several hundreds of thousands of youth are in foster care each year; of those, 47% are in nonrelative foster homes, 28% are in kinship/relative care, 15% are in residential (congregate) care, and 10% are in other living arrangements.[1]
- Over a third of those in foster care are 12 years or older.[1]
- There is a fairly equal gender distribution among youth in foster care, but African American and multiracial youth are overrepresented relative to the population in the US.[1]
- Neglect is the most common type of maltreatment precipitating foster care placement, followed by physical abuse and sexual abuse. Many youth have experienced multiple forms of maltreatment, including emotional abuse.[2]

Health and Associated Problems

- Eye and dental problems are overrepresented among adolescents in foster care according to Medicaid claims.[3]

- The most frequent diagnoses for adolescents in foster care are attention deficit and conduct disorder. In addition, mood, anxiety, and adjustment disorders are two to three times higher than among nonfoster youth who receive Medicaid.[3]
- Outpatient and inpatient mental health service utilization is higher among adolescents in foster care, and they are more likely to be prescribed psychotropic drugs.[3]
- Approximately 20% to 40% of youth in foster care are in special education classes.[4]
- Despite high rates of service use, many youth in foster care do not receive needed physical health, mental health, or educational services.[5]

Emancipating Youth

- Approximately 23,000 adolescents "age out" of foster care each year.[1]
- These young adults are at high risk for unemployment, receipt of public assistance, incarceration, substance dependence, early childbearing, and significant mental health problems.[6]
- While some states allow young people to remain in foster care until age 21, many emancipating youth do not take advantage of this opportunity.
- Beginning in 2014, the Affordable Care Act (ACA) requires all states to provide Medicaid coverage for youth who emancipate from foster care at age 18 or older. This coverage lasts until the age of 26, but experts have concerns about these young adults navigating the enrollment procedures (http://www.pewtrusts.org/en/research-and-analysis/blogs/stateline/2014/04/30/states-enroll-former-foster-youth-in-medicaid).[7]
- Although many "independent living" programs exist to help with the transition to young adulthood for emancipating youth, none have demonstrated efficacy through rigorous research.[8]

ASSESSMENT AND TREATMENT

Current guidelines[9,10] suggest that the general physical examination and primary prevention efforts for adolescents entering foster care have the same components as a thorough well-adolescent examination.

Initial Assessment

An initial assessment should be conducted immediately after entry into foster care to screen for evidence of abuse or neglect, contagious diseases, chronic illnesses, substance use, and mental health issues, including suicidality, all of which may require immediate treatment. The health care provider should be especially cognizant of evidence of recent or past injuries, dental caries and pain, hygiene and nutritional problems, untreated congenital and chronic conditions, missing immunizations, and developmental delays.

Comprehensive Assessment

A comprehensive assessment is recommended within 30 days of placement, which must include obtaining a complete health history and evaluation of the youth's adjustment to care. Standardized screening tools for mental health and behavioral concerns, substance use, and psychological trauma should be administered. A confidential questionnaire which includes sexual history, risks for sexually transmitted infections (STIs), and need for contraception is essential.

Laboratory Studies

Laboratory studies should include urine screening for chlamydia and gonorrhea in all sexually active youth, and other STIs when indicated.

Other Screening

Obese youth should be screened appropriately for prediabetes and metabolic syndrome. If indicated by nutrition history, anemia and vitamin D screening should also be performed.

Periodic Care

Following the initial assessment, adolescents in care should be seen at least every 6 months for periodic preventive care visits to monitor and address any physical or mental health issues that arise while they are in placement.[9,10]

Mental Health and Substance Use

Screening for mental health and substance use problems should be conducted at every visit, as youth in foster care have often experienced early and chronic interpersonal trauma, which disrupts primary attachments and increases the risk for emotional dysregulation, social problems, poor self-concept, and cognitive difficulties, known as "complex trauma".[11] This complex trauma is not always recognized, and adolescents often receive other diagnoses, including attention deficit hyperactivity disorder, oppositional defiant disorder, depression/bipolar disorder, generalized anxiety disorder, and reactive attachment disorder. Treatment for these disorders can be unsuccessful because complex trauma-related clinical concerns and problems require longer-term interventions that are specialty focused for these diagnoses. As a result, long-term interventions may be at odds with the movement toward more time-limited clinical services due to limits of mental health care funding. Evidence has emerged suggesting the ineffectiveness of "generic" mental health services for youth involved or for those formerly involved with the child welfare system.[12] It is no longer sufficient to refer for generic mental health services and hope that the clinician will identify and implement services that effectively meet the adolescent's or young adult's needs.[13] Those youth and young adults with mental health needs should be referred to providers who have been trained in providing trauma-informed care.

● SPECIAL CONSIDERATIONS

There are many unique issues that make health assessments, interventions, and recommendations for adolescents in foster care and young adults with a history of foster care substantially more challenging. They include the following:

Barriers to Obtaining a Health History

When foster youth present for medical care, obtaining a health history can be challenging. Services are typically provided in the context of an open child welfare case in which permanency determinations are being made. This impacts youths' and families' willingness to disclose information and/or candidly report symptoms. Family members and current or previous foster parents

may be uncooperative or unable to provide health information, medications, or medical supplies and equipment. Sometimes the adolescent or young adult may be unwilling to share personal information, or may report incomplete or inaccurate information.

Inaccurate and Missing Records

Demographic and other identifying information (e.g., names) may be incorrect or may change due to adoption. Medical and school records are often incomplete or missing. In addition, it may be difficult to identify previous providers due to moves from one placement to another and inadequate documentation. Because of the fragmentation of health care that often happens in the child welfare system, many youth in foster care and young adults who grew up in foster care do not have access to their health records.

Consent and Confidentiality Issues

Foster youth can change placements and custody frequently, making it difficult for providers to know who has the legal authority to make decisions. Youth may seek confidential services that are contrary to their caseworker's or caregiver's approval. States differ on the age of consent for different services and who has decision-making power over different types of procedures and treatment, as well as who can receive the results of any testing.

System Issues

Because many youth are involved in multiple systems (child welfare, legal, educational, mental health, and/or juvenile justice), coordinating services and communication among multiple providers can be challenging. Providers and services may change abruptly due to placement changes or for legal reasons. The child welfare system often closes the cases of older chronic runaways, which may lead to their health information getting lost. Young adults may be unwilling to continue supportive services beyond the age of majority even when these services are available, in an attempt to distance themselves from the child welfare system.

Medication Management

Missing medications and the need for bridge prescriptions are common problems, as medications may not accompany youth from placement to placement.

Compliance with Procedures

Due to a history of trauma, adolescents in foster care and young adults who have emancipated may be especially sensitive to painful or invasive procedures such as blood draws, dental procedures, or pelvic examinations.

Challenges for Substitute Caregivers

Transportation to various and numerous appointments, child care for other children in their home, and service costs can be a challenge for families, as many foster parents care for multiple high-needs youth.

Cultural Issues

Lack of cultural awareness and sensitivity in service settings poses barriers, especially in regards to engaging youth and their families in services. Many youth in the child welfare system are placed far from their communities of origin. In addition, minor refugees in foster care who arrive without parents need translation services as well as community support.

● RECOMMENDATIONS

Care Delivery

A longer appointment time is needed for adolescents in foster care to allow discussion with the foster parent and/or caseworker, and additional paperwork is usually required for placement agencies. Between visits, extra time and effort are needed to gather and review health information from previous providers. Medical findings and treatment plans need to be communicated with the multiple individuals involved with foster youth, including the guardian ad litem (i.e., a guardian appointed by the court to represent the child's best interests), probation officer, and court and/or legal professionals.

Medical Home Model

Foster youth are a special-needs population, and a medical home model that provides coordinated, continuous, comprehensive, and culturally appropriate care is ideal. Health care professionals should be experienced in issues of child abuse and neglect, be familiar with child welfare processes, and understand the impact of trauma and foster care on adolescents. A case manager is invaluable to ensure that necessary health information is obtained and that recommended referrals and evaluations are scheduled and completed. If the foster home is not compliant with treatment recommendations, the child welfare caseworker needs to be notified so that they can intervene.

Health Care Coordination

Many adolescents in the child welfare system experience multiple placement moves. When these moves result in a change in health care providers, the adolescent's medical records often do not accompany them. Therefore, it is important to gather as comprehensive a medical, dental, and mental health history as possible on the initial visit and have resources available to track down prior records. For emancipating youth, anticipatory guidance should include a plan for obtaining primary care post-emancipation.

Establishing a Medical Record

Child welfare departments are charged with ensuring adequate health care for foster youth, and to accomplish this, they should either (1) have a designated medical team charged with acquiring health records and developing a health record or passport, which can accompany the youth as they move in and out of the child welfare system, or (2) ensure that the caseworker gathers and shares all relevant information, especially immunization records, that may require a search of previous schools and clinic sites. If a vaccination history cannot be obtained in 1 to 2 months post-initial placement, necessary immunization should take place. It is important that diagnostic and treatment information is well documented and available to the adolescent when they leave the child welfare system.

Monitoring Medication Use

When prescribing medication, providers must consider who can give medical consent for the medication, how the adolescents will access the medications, who will monitor the adolescents' compliance, and how the prescriptions will be refilled if the adolescent changes placement. When a decision is made to prescribe medication, especially psychotropic mediations, it is critical that the adolescent is informed about what they have been prescribed and why, the potential side effects or benefits, and the consequences of stopping the medication suddenly. For older adolescents, it is important to ensure they will have the ability to obtain medications once they leave the child welfare system.

Educating Foster Parents

Foster parent training through the child welfare system is not always consistent; therefore, health care providers should educate foster parents about typical adolescent reactions to trauma and foster care placement. Since many adolescents may not have previously had a regular source of medical care, health care providers should also be prepared to provide anticipatory guidance to both foster parents and adolescents on issues such as sleep, diet, sexual issues, and substance use. The discussion of normative adolescent development should include the teen's need for growth in autonomy as well as involvement in positive and healthy activities (e.g., sports, youth clubs).

Engaging Biologic Parents

As many adolescents will have ongoing contact with their biologic families, especially post-emancipation, it is important that health care providers include biologic families in treatment decisions, when appropriate and feasible. Youth may seek input from their biologic families when making medical decisions, especially regarding the use of psychotropic medications and reproductive decisions.

Relationship with the Child Welfare Agency

It is important to develop mechanisms of communication with the child welfare agency to enhance information sharing and treatment coordination. Caseworkers need to be aware of health issues that can impact placement stability, and ideally the medical team will be involved when making placement decisions and developing treatment plans.

Consent for Treatment

It is important for providers to educate themselves and abide by state statutes relating to who (i.e., biologic or foster parent, caseworker, adolescent, or emancipated youth) can consent for treatment of adolescents in foster care. Local clinics, agencies, and hospitals may differ in regards to consent practices, especially with regards to STIs, substance use, mental health, and access to testing results.

Confidentiality

While coordination of care for adolescents in the child welfare system is of critical importance, it is important that health care providers understand and respect the laws that govern the sharing of information. It is also important that they clearly explain to the youth information they can and cannot keep confidential so that provider trust can be established.

Post-Emancipation

When adolescents emancipate from foster care, results of medical evaluations, treatment plans, and ongoing recommendations should follow. Although young adults may be eager to leave the system, they risk focusing on basic needs other than health care, which can lead to negative physical and mental health outcomes. The transition from foster care should include the following:

- Access to health care coverage until age 26 through Medicaid or the ACA for eligible young adults
- Transfer of health care to an ongoing medical home
- Access to reproductive health services
- Resources for housing, education, and employment
- Mental health services
- Substance abuse treatment resources

Positive Youth Development Approach

There is often great focus on the multiple challenges or problem behaviors of youth in foster care, but all adolescents and young adults have strengths. Providers should take a positive youth development approach to health by identifying strengths in multiple domains (physical, intellectual, social, and emotional) and encouraging these young people to pursue their interests in these areas.[14] A book of community-based resources (e.g., mentoring programs, youth groups, Boys and Girls Clubs, YMCA programs, etc.) would support the practitioner in providing such referrals.

Empowering Youth

Foster youth and young adults who have emancipated from foster care report that a positive interaction with health care providers and having a voice in their treatment planning can empower them to take a more proactive role in their own care. Assisting youth to identify and achieve their goals can help them realize a healthy young adulthood.

REFERENCES

1. United States Department of Health and Human Services, Administration for Children and Families, Administration for Children, Youth, and Families. *AFCARS Data: Trends in Foster Care and Adoption (FY 2002-FY 2012)*. Available at http://www.acf.hhs.gov/sites/default/files/cb/trends_fostercare_adoption2012.pdf. Accessed February 2013.
2. United States Department of Health and Human Services, Administration for Children and Families, Administration on Children, Youth, and Families, Children's Bureau. *Child Maltreatment 2012*. 2012. Available at http://www.acf.hhs.gov/sites/default/files/cb/cm2012.pdf. Accessed February 15, 2014.
3. Center for Mental Health Services and Center for Substance Use Treatment. *Diagnoses and health care utilization of children who are in foster care and covered by medicaid*, HHS Publication No. (SAM) 13-4804. Rockville, MD: Center for Mental Health Services and Center for Substance Use Treatment, Substance Abuse and Mental Health Services Administration, 2013. Available at http://store.samhsa.gov/shin/content/SMA13-4804/SMA13-4804.pdf. Accessed February 14, 2014.
4. Scherr T. Educational experiences of children in foster care: meta-analyses of special education, retention and discipline rates. *School Psychol Int* 2007;28(4):419–436.
5. Burns BJ, Phillips SD, Wagner HR, et al. Mental health need and access to mental health services by youth involved with child welfare: a national survey. *J Am Acad Child Adolesc Psychiatry* 2004;43(8):960–970.
6. Courtney M, Dworsky A, Brown A, et al. *Midwest evaluation of the adult functioning of former foster youth: outcomes at age 26*. Chicago, IL: Chapin Hall at the University of Chicago, 2011.
7. English A, Scott J, Park MJ. *Fact sheet: impact of the ACA on vulnerable youth*. Chapel Hill, NC: Center for Adolescent Health & the Law; San Francisco, CA: National Adolescent and Young Adult Health Information Center, 2014.
8. Donkoh C, Underhill K, Montgomery P. Independent living programmes for improving outcomes for young people leaving the care system. *Child Youth Serv Rev* 2006;28(12):1435–1448.
9. American Academy of Pediatrics. *Fostering health: health care for children and adolescents in foster care*. 2nd ed. Elk Grove Village, IL: American Academy of Pediatrics, 2005.
10. Child Welfare League of America. *CWLA standards of excellence for health care services for children in out of home care*. Washington, DC: Child Welfare League of America, 2007.
11. Cook A, Spinazzola J, Ford J, et al. Complex trauma in children and adolescents. *Psychiatr Ann* 2005;35:390–398.
12. Bellamy JL, Gopalan G, Traube DE. A national study of the impact of outpatient mental health services for children in long-term foster care. *Clin Child Psychol Psychiatry* 2010;15(4):467–479.
13. McCrae JS, Barth RP, Guo S. Changes in maltreated children's emotional-behavioral problems following typically provided mental health services. *Am J Orthopsychiatry* 2010;80(3):350–361.
14. Centers for Disease Control and Prevention. *School connectedness: strategies for increasing protective factors among youth*. Atlanta, GA: U.S. Department of Health and Human Services, 2009.

 ADDITIONAL RESOURCES AND WEBSITES ONLINE

CHAPTER 78

Juvenile Detention and Incarcerated Youth and Young Adults

Matthew C. Aalsma
Cynthia L. Robbins
Katherine S. L. Lau
Katherine Schwartz

KEY WORDS

- Adult criminal justice system
- Detention
- Disproportionate minority contact
- Functional family therapy (FFT)
- Health care
- Health risk
- Incarceration
- Juvenile detention
- Juvenile justice
- Juvenile justice system
- Multisystemic therapy (MST)
- Multidimensional treatment foster care

When children reach adolescence and young adulthood, it becomes more likely that they will be involved in the justice system. In the US, youth offenders under the age of 18 are subject to the juvenile justice system, a process that is separate and distinct from that of adult criminals. For over 100 years, the juvenile justice system has been charged with protecting the community from delinquent youth through supervision and incarceration, but the system must also aid in the rehabilitation of these youth. Over time, society may vacillate toward either end of this continuum—law enforcement versus rehabilitation—but the political climate since the late nineties has increasingly favored limiting the incarceration of youth. Contributions to this societal shift may include recent research findings that highlight procedural injustice within the system, the unique characteristics and needs of youth offenders, and the health costs of incarceration to both individual youth and their communities. For example, much research has affirmed that youth of color are disproportionately involved in both the juvenile and adult criminal justice systems.[1] Through increased health screening efforts, it is evident that justice system–involved youth face both physical and mental health issues at higher rates than their nondelinquent peers.[2] As such, juvenile justice policy reform efforts continue.

Young adult offenders between the ages of 18 and 26 are not typically afforded the protections, however limited, associated with the juvenile justice system. In contrast, they are subject to the adult criminal justice system, where their experiences and needs are rarely separated from those of older adult offenders. Research on the health of young adult offenders as a distinct group is limited, though their physical and mental health issues may be similar to the needs of older adolescent offenders. Though the majority of youth offenders are no longer involved in the justice system after reaching adulthood, there is evidence that the criminal behavior of young adults is frequently a continuation of adolescent delinquency.[3] Researchers further suggest that young adult offenders are more similar to juvenile offenders than adults in both their physical and mental development as well as their criminal activity.[4] These findings are reflected in policy recommendations to extend the jurisdiction of the juvenile justice system to include young adults.[5]

EPIDEMIOLOGY OF JUSTICE SYSTEM INVOLVEMENT

Approximately 1.47 million juveniles <18 years were arrested in the US in 2011,[6] with nearly 1.4 million delinquency cases processed in juvenile courts in 2010.[7] Of these youth offenders, just under 300,000 (21%) were placed in detention (short-term, local secure placement prior to court) and over 98,000 (7%) were sentenced to a term in juvenile prison (longer-term incarceration at a state facility).[7] Further, it is estimated that more than 200,000 arrested juveniles faced prosecution in the adult criminal justice system.[8] In terms of young adults, more than 2.52 million individuals between the ages of 18 and 24 were arrested in 2013. This age range represents nearly a third of arrests, though they make up only 10% of the general population.[9]

Recidivism

The repetition of criminal behavior, recidivism, is a common outcome among detained adolescents; as many as 40% to 70% of adolescents recidivate within 1 year of release from detention.[10] Within the detained adolescent and young adult (AYA) populations, recidivism rates tend to be higher among males, minorities, youth younger at their first offense, those with prior criminal history, youth in unstable families, those with high rates of substance abuse, and those with a history of early childhood misbehavior or conduct problems.[11,12]

Disproportionate Minority Contact

Minority youth and adults are overrepresented in the justice system, which is defined as disproportionate minority contact. Over 60% of juvenile justice–involved youth are minority youth, though they make up only a third of the general population.[1] Not only are minority youth disproportionately represented within the juvenile justice system, they also tend to receive harsher sentences, including placement in adult prisons, and are more likely to be removed from their home environments than White youth.[13] Racial disparities are also prevalent throughout every stage of the adult criminal justice system.[14]

Mortality

Detained and incarcerated youth and young adults have increased rates of mortality in comparison to the general public. In a longitudinal study of detained youth, 15% of whom were tried in adult court, Teplin and colleagues found the mortality rate of detained youth to be four times that of the general population for males and eight times for females.[15] Most of these deaths result from gunshot wounds post-release.[9] Black, male, young adults are at greatest risk for violent death.[15] In a study of serious offenders with felony charges, 31% of whom were institutionalized, Chassin and colleagues found 3% of their sample died, which is similar to other studies of detained populations.[16]

Summary

It is likely that most providers will encounter patients involved in the justice system, especially providers who see minority youth and young adults. These individuals face much more troubled futures than the general population. Knowledge of high recidivism and mortality rates can have a direct effect on improving health by identifying factors that could lead to reinvolvement and screening for nonaccidental trauma risks, such as access to firearms. Advocacy is another way to intervene on behalf of young people; providers are in a unique role to advocate for youth as they are most knowledgeable about healthy adolescent development and conditions, such as substance abuse disorder, which are associated with continued delinquent behavior.

HEALTH ISSUES OF YOUNG PEOPLE IN THE JUSTICE SYSTEM

Youth and young adults involved in the justice system exhibit significant acute and chronic medical problems, whether precursors to, causes of, or direct and indirect effects of their system involvement. As examples, problems resulting from dog bites or drug use can be related to the reason for an individual's involvement in the system; other medical problems, such as poor dentition, may manifest frequently among AYA offenders because this population is largely medically underserved. Young people in custody are more likely than the general population to suffer diseases such as asthma, sexually transmitted infections (STIs), substance abuse, and other chronic conditions.[14]

Detention Conditions

The range of common health problems experienced by AYAs in the justice system presents unique challenges to health care providers, especially when their illnesses may arise as a direct result of confinement. Complaints related to stress and adaption to a new environment, such as somatic pain, are to be expected. Gastrointestinal complaints may result from a set menu of food that differs significantly from pre-detention diet (e.g., menus high in lactose). Communicable diseases are also a concern for youth in custody, since detained youth are often housed together in conditions that facilitate disease spread (e.g., crowded quarters, communal eating, and bathing) and because some diseases, such as tuberculosis, occur at high rates in correctional facilities.

The 2010 Juvenile Residential Facility Census collected information from 2,519 facilities in the US. The census is performed biennially. The 2010 census found crowding remains a common problem in facilities: 20% of facilities were either at or above capacity in 2010 and 3% of publically operated facilities were above bed capacity. Mechanical restraints and isolation (defined as locking a youth in a room for more than 4 hours) are used, respectively, in 41% and 47% of detention centers, and just over 20% of all facilities. Crowding and use of mechanical restraints and/or isolation can exacerbate health conditions. In addition, this census collected information on acute health events in custody. One-third of facilities utilized emergency room visits (most commonly for sports-related injuries and illness). While deaths were rare, 11 were reported in 2010 (five were suicides and four from illness or natural causes).[17]

Mental Health and Substance Use

Young people involved in the justice system suffer from mental health and substance use disorders at higher rates than the general population.[14,18] Among youth, studies have consistently found that, outside of externalizing problems (e.g., conduct disorder,

attention-deficit hyperactivity disorder), psychiatric disorders of the internalizing spectrum, such as major depression, anxiety, and posttraumatic stress disorder, are prevalent.[19] Unfortunately, most detention centers are not equipped to address the mental health needs of young people, and studies have found that even 5 years after release, at least 45% of male and 30% of female detainees experience one or more psychiatric disorders with associated impairment.[20] Substance use is also quite common among adolescents in the justice system, with approximately half of detained youth meeting the criteria for a substance use disorder and roughly 10% having a comorbid mental health and substance use disorder.[21]

Physical Health

Few national studies have described detainee health issues or how detention conditions specifically affect AYA in juvenile or adult facilities. The Survey of Youth in Residential Placement (SYRP)[22] and the National Commission on Correctional Health Care (NCCHC)[23] have both revealed higher rates of health problems among youth in detention when compared to the general population. The data regarding general health issues are reviewed in the following sections.

Preexisting Health Needs

The health needs of some youth in detention are related to neglected preexisting health conditions, which are common among this vulnerable population. For example, among a large sample of youth in an Alabama detention center, slightly more than 16% of youth had been hospitalized at some point before incarceration, and 10% presented with a significant medical problem that would require follow-up after release from detention. Again, physical health problems among detained youth are often a consequence of poor access to care before custody. No more than one-third of participating youth could identify a regular source of medical care, with only 20% of these youth identifying a private physician as their source of care.[24] A longitudinal study of almost 50,000 detained adolescents over more than a decade documented that almost half (46%) had an identifiable medical problem during their detention stay, more than 3,300 were admitted to the detention center infirmary, and 500 were transferred to a hospital for admission.[25]

Injuries

Physical injuries are common among juvenile justice system–involved youth. Some youth present with injuries upon detention center intake, which may be related to the crime committed or sustained during the process of being arrested. Unfortunately, injuries also commonly occur in custody. The SYRP directly and anonymously interviewed a large, nationally representative sample of youth in custody.[22,26] Safety concerns and injuries were frequently reported by youth, with 38% fearing attack by someone, most often other residents or a staff member (25% and 22%, respectively). Additionally, over three-quarters of youth in the SYRP reported that they would not know what to do in case of a fire.[26] Another longitudinal study conducted at a residential facility in North Carolina examined the rate of physical injuries, both intentional and unintentional, in juvenile detention. In this study, approximately half of youth presented a traumatic injury requiring medical care while detained. Sports and fights were the most common reasons for injury, but self-inflicted injuries and suicide attempts represented over 21% of injuries in this study.[27]

Sleep Disturbances

Youth in custody also experience sleep disturbances at higher rates than youth not in custody, exposing them to consequences of chronic sleep deprivation such as depression and school problems. Possibly an example of this fear, or representing another symptom of situational stress associated with being in custody, 34% of youth reported problems falling asleep in custody in the SYRP survey, compared to only 11% of the general population.[22]

XVI

Sexually Transmitted Infections

Youth and young adults involved in the justice system have high rates of STIs due to a combination of uncontrollable demographic factors such as age and race, and behaviors associated with STI acquisition that are more likely among young offenders. Regardless of involvement in the justice system, AYAs represent the age-group with the highest STI rates, with almost half of all new STI diagnoses occurring in this age-group.[28] Shared racial disparities between STI rates in the US (see Chapters 31, 57, 59, and 60) and the justice system population also impact these rates.

Correctional facilities, when considering the high rates of STI among the young Black individuals who are overrepresented in the system, should necessarily exhibit high rates of STIs. However, the actual rate of STI among this population is even higher than expected, making AYAs in the justice system among the highest risk groups in the US for STI. High rate of sexual abuse and sexual coercion in this population is one reason for this increased risk. Other behavioral factors likely account for the increased risk of STI among the juvenile justice population. In one of the only nationally representative studies of incarcerated youth and sexual activity, a survey comparison to Youth Risk Behavior Surveillance (YRBS) data found that youth offenders were more likely to be sexually active, used contraception at lower rates, and were more likely to report more than four lifetime partners when compared to their nondelinquent peers.[23] Prostitution and injection drug use, more common among the juvenile justice population, are other

behaviors that place juvenile justice–involved youth at higher risk for syphilis and human immunodeficiency virus (HIV). In fact, HIV risk behaviors, such as anal sex or having sex while drunk or high, have been reported to be high among juvenile justice–involved youth.[29] Unfortunately, data on HIV and syphilis rates are not available, likely due to the fact that many facilities do not screen for these infections. See Figures 78.1 and 78.2 for national rates of chlamydia and gonorrhea among youth entering the juvenile justice system.[30]

Other Reproductive Health Issues

In addition to the high rate of STIs among young offenders, detained youth have other serious reproductive health issues as well. Many of these adolescents are parents. SYRP found that one in five reported either having had or that they were expecting a child.[22] Unknown pregnancy and delayed prenatal care are potential health issues for many girls in custody. A 2004 census of 3,500 facilities in the US found that 25% of facilities housed pregnant teens, yet testing for pregnancy was reported in just under 18% of facilities.[31] Unintended pregnancy is a consequence of nonconsensual sex for some youth in the justice system, and other ramifications of sexual abuse, such as pelvic pain, are to be expected in this population. While consensual sexual activity is common among teens, sexual abuse is common among the juvenile justice population. Twelve percent of youth in the SYRP reported a history of sexual abuse, with more females than males reporting.[22]

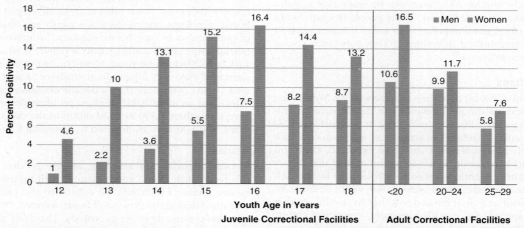

FIGURE 78.1 National chlamydia percent positivity of young people entering correctional facilities, by inmate age and sex. Source: 2008 Sexually Transmitted Diseases Surveillance: STDs in Persons Entering Correctional Facilities. 2008. Accessed October 13, 2015. Available at http://www.cdc.gov/std/stats08/corrections.htm.

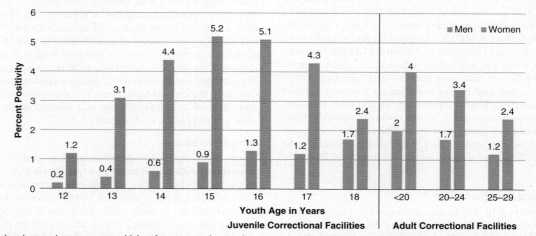

FIGURE 78.2 National gonorrhea percent positivity of young people entering correctional facilities, by inmate age and sex. Source: 2008 Sexually Transmitted Diseases Surveillance: STDs in Persons Entering Correctional Facilities. 2008. Accessed October 13, 2015. Available at http://www.cdc.gov/std/stats08/corrections.htm.

Dental

Dental problems have been well documented among juvenile justice system–involved youth. For example, 90% of youth had a dental need during their detention, including treatment for caries and fractured teeth. Forty-nine percent of youth had untreated dental decay[25] and only 14% had evidence of dental care (preventive sealants) in a study of 400 youth detained between 1999 and 2003.[32]

Summary

Young individuals involved in the justice system are likely to have serious health conditions, unfortunately some as consequences of their involvement. Familiarity with common conditions, such as reproductive health issues and substance abuse, is important to provide adequate care to AYAs in custody and after their release. Providers seeing these individuals should inquire about previous health care, including emergency room and dental visits, and be prepared to screen for substance abuse, STIs, and contraceptive needs. Recognition that many justice system–involved AYAs carry mental health diagnoses is especially important to connect them with care once released; few resources for treatment are available in secure facilities, and untreated mental health issues can lead to criminal recidivism (**Table 78.1**).

● ASSESSMENT AND TREATMENT ISSUES IN JUVENILE JUSTICE

Health care standards and recommendations for adolescents in custody exist. However, none are mandatory. Additionally, many of the physical and mental health standards are controlled and supervised by state and local government. This leads to wide system and geographic variability in services rendered. Variability in services received by youth and young adults in secure facilities is also exacerbated by cost and access to services, since federal Medicaid services cannot be billed while an individual is detained or incarcerated. Specific federal Medicaid law prohibits payment "with respect to care or services for any individual who is an inmate of a public institution" (except as a patient in a medical institution; 42 C.F.R 441.33 (a)(1), 435.1008(a)(1)).

Detention Care Guidelines, Mental Health Issues

Many juvenile justice facilities with limited resources are unable to meet the established standards for psychiatric care and provide minimal services.[33,34] In regards to mental health services, over one-third of facilities use correctional staff to administer mental health assessments and services, despite having little to no background or training.[33] In a survey of the mental health policies of juvenile detention facilities, Pajer and colleagues[35] reported that mental health treatment options primarily consisted of medication administration and management. Almost 70% of facilities provided counseling services. However, the services were commonly provided by staff members, rather than licensed mental health care professionals.[35]

Mental Health Assessment and Treatment Post-Detention Release

Multisystemic Therapy (MST), Functional Family Therapy (FFT), and Multidimensional Treatment Foster Care are three mental health interventions with strong empirical support for treating young offenders. These interventions have produced many positive outcomes, including better self-esteem, reduced psychiatric symptoms, reduced substance use, improved family functioning, decreased association with deviant peers, reduced number of rearrests and severity of charges, and delayed time of rearrest. Although evidence-based interventions exist for juvenile justice–involved youth, it is estimated that only 5% of adolescent offenders receive evidence-based interventions on an annual basis.[36]

Detention Care Guidelines, Physical Health Issues

The US NCCHC was founded by the American Medical Association to address the lack of national standards for health care in all jails and prisons and is supported by major health, law, and correctional organizations, including the American Academy of Pediatrics, American Bar Association, American Dental Association, and American Psychological Association. The most recent NCCHC Standards address nine general areas ranging from health services to medical-legal issues related to secure facilities. This document calls for a comprehensive health assessment (medical, mental health, dental history; tuberculosis screening; and physical examination) within 7 days of arrival, a mental health screening within 2 weeks, and an oral health screening within 7 days. It also provides standards for addressing new health concerns in custody and discharge planning, which can be ordered at http://www.ncchc.org/standards-for-correctional-health-services. The NCCHC offers voluntary accreditation, yet very few juvenile facilities are accredited. Many facilities fall short of these standards: A study comparing the NCHHC standards to Office of Juvenile Justice and Delinquency Prevention data of all US facilities reported poor adherence. For example, just under 40% of facilities were fully compliant with performing a health screening.[37] Other standards exist as well. The American Correctional Association is the largest correctional professional association and serves all disciplines within the correctional system. The American Correctional Association publishes 21 different manuals of standards, including one for juvenile facilities. These standards (available for purchase at http://www.aca.org/) cover physical and mental health care along with other aspects of the correctional system, such as food service and security. The Juvenile Detention Alternatives Initiative (JDAI), a project of the Annie E. Casey Foundation to reform juvenile justice, publishes standards based on "case law, statutes, professional standards, basic principles of humane treatment of youth, and JDAI's core values." These standards cover physical, mental, and dental health, and are available for purchase at

---

TABLE 78.1

Recommended Health Services for Youth Involved in Juvenile Justice

At intake
- Complete health history, including physical, dental, and mental health histories and visits to health care providers, including emergency services, in the past 3 y
- Review vaccination history
- Screen for reproductive health needs; include STI testing and discussion of contraception
- Screen for acute and chronic mental health problems, such as suicidality and substance abuse
- Perform physical examination, with attention to potential preexisting and/or unmet health needs, traumatic injuries, and signs of substance use withdrawal
- Assess for dental health needs, preferably via examination by a dentist

During detention/incarceration
- Manage treatment for acute and chronic health care needs
- Utilize support and resources from mental health care providers
- Emphasize discharge planning for appointments and continuation of medications

After release from detention
- Review health insurance status
- Review services received where the youth was detained
- Assess adaptation, distress, and new health problems present as a consequence of juvenile justice system involvement
- Screen for STIs
- Refer to affordable dentistry
- Inquire into mental health and substance abuse treatment needs; refer if indicated
- Give anticipatory guidance on mortality risks for juvenile justice–involved youth

XVI

http://www.aecf.org/KnowledgeCenter.aspx. Additional recommendations for health care in the juvenile justice system include policy statements from the American Academy of Pediatrics and Society for Adolescent Health and Medicine.[37]

Insurance Coverage during Detention and Post-Release

Insurance status may pose a significant obstacle to care once young individuals are released from secure facilities. Many young people in the justice system, and their families, are economically disadvantaged and living in poverty. As mentioned, Medicaid insurance may be terminated upon admission to detention facilities, jeopardizing inmate health care access once they are released. However, Medicaid rules do not state that individuals become ineligible or lose Medicaid once detained, just that Medicaid funds cannot pay for care while in custody. If suspended only, Medicaid can be quickly resumed once AYAs are released to cover health expenses, avoiding interruptions in care due to reenrollment and application times. Justice system programs serving AYAs may also have the ability to determine presumptive eligibility for Medicaid, allowing temporary Medicaid eligibility to cover health care pending final eligibility determinations. Finally, young offenders do not lose Medicaid eligibility upon involvement in the justice system and can be screened for eligibility and enrolled when entering the system, creating an opportunity to improve their health care access during detention.[38] This strategy may be especially important to consider with implementation of the Patient Protection and Affordable Care Act of 2010 (ACA). ACA implementation may help improve access to care for young people in the justice system by increasing insurance coverage in this population not only in states with Medicaid expansion, but also in states without. The ACA requires Medicaid coverage for all children through age 18 at a higher poverty level than previously allowed (now: 133% Federal Poverty Level). Justice system facilities can also help youth and young adults ineligible for Medicaid gain access to other health plans, many with subsidies to improve affordability of care.[39]

Young people receive no standard medical care while in custody, and services received vary greatly by geographic area, making it essential that providers know what care is available in their local jurisdiction. When centers are compliant with national standards, young people may receive very good care. However, most secure holding facilities are not in compliance, especially regarding mental health services standards. Medical coverage while AYAs are detained is often financed through the local court, as Medicaid cannot be billed for detention services in most cases. Unfortunately, as a result, health insurance coverage is sometimes canceled, creating significant barriers to these young people receiving care once they are released from detention into the community. Because most justice–involved AYAs are eligible for Medicaid or ACA subsidies, it is important to enroll or reenroll this population to connect them with regular and effective health care once released (Table 78.2).

TABLE 78.2
Clinical Summary

- Many juvenile justice–involved youth have poor or no access to health care prior to detention. Comprehensive screening for preexisting and chronic conditions should be performed with a full review of systems to identify unmet health needs.
- STIs are common. Teens should be offered confidential and complete screening, testing, and treatment. Vaccination against STIs (human papillomavirus and hepatitis A and B) is an intervention with great benefits to this population.
- Teen parents are often present in this population. Prenatal care, education on pregnancy prevention, parenting, and sexuality are necessary and valuable resources to employ.
- Dental problems are among the most commonly identified issues for this population and should be addressed while youth are in custody, as they are often an effect of poor pre-detention access to care.
- The majority of detained youth have a mental health and/or a substance abuse disorder. Differential diagnosis is important, as are referral and coordination of behavioral health treatment.
- Free and paid policy statements and standards are available to guide care.
- Insurance status may be interrupted during detention; prompt reenrollment is important for care upon release.

REFERENCES

1. Desai RA, Falzer PR, Chapman J, et al. Mental illness, violence risk, and race in juvenile detention: implications for disproportionate minority contact. *Am J Orthopsychiatry* 2012;82:32–40.
2. Teplin LA, Abram KM, McClelland GM, et al. Psychiatric disorders in youth in juvenile detention. *Arch Gen Psychiatry* 2002;59(12):1133–1143.
3. Piquero AR, Hawkins JD, Kazemian L. Criminal career patterns. In: Loeber R, Farrington DP, eds. *From juvenile delinquency to adult crime: criminal careers, justice policy and prevention*. New York, NY: Oxford University Press, 2012.
4. Loeber R, Farrington DP, Stouthamer-Loeber M, et al. *Violence and serious theft: development and prediction from childhood to adulthood*. New York, NY: Routledge, 2008.
5. Skeem JL, Scott E, Mulvey EP. Justice policy reform for high-risk juveniles: using science to achieve large-scale crime reduction. *Annu Rev Clin Psychol* 2014;10:709–739.
6. Puzzanchera C; U.S. Department of Justice, Office if Juvenile Justice and Delinquency Prevention. Juvenile arrests 2011. *Juvenile Offenders and Victims: National Report Series*. 2013. Available at http://www.ojjdp.gov/pubs/244476.pdf. Accessed March 3, 2014.
7. U.S. Department of Justice, Office of Juvenile Justice and Delinquency Prevention. *OJJDP statistical briefing book*. 2013. Available at http://www.ojjdp.gov/ojstatbb/court/qa06201.asp?qaDate=2010. Accessed July 20, 2013.
8. Griffin P, Addie S, Adams B, et al.; U.S. Department of Justice, Office of Justice Programs, Office of Juvenile Justice and Delinquency Prevention. Trying juveniles as adults: An analysis of state transfer laws and reporting. *Juvenile Offenders and Victims: National Resport Series Bulletin*. September 2011. Available at www.ncjrs.gov/pdffiles1/ojjdp/232434.pdf. Accessed March 1, 2014.
9. U.S. Department of Justice, Federal Bureau of Investigation, Criminal Justice Information Services Division. *Crime in the United States, 2013*. Available at http://www.fbi.gov/about-us/cjis/ucr/crime-in-the-u.s/2013/crime-in-the-u.s.-2013/persons-arrested/persons-arrested. Accessed December 17, 2014.
10. Cottle CC, Lee RJ, Heilbrun K. The prediction of criminal recidivism in juveniles: a meta-analysis. *Crim Justice Behav* 2001;28(3):367–394.
11. DeLisi M, Piquero AR. New frontiers in criminal careers research, 2000–2011: a state-of-the-art review. *J Crim Justice* 2011;39:289–301.
12. Grunwald HE, Lockwood B, Harris PW, et al. Influences of neighborhood context, individual history and parenting behavior on recidivism among juvenile offenders. *J Youth Adolesc* 2010;39:1067–1079.
13. Rodriguez N, Smith H, Zatz MS. Youth is enmeshed in a highly dysfunctional family system: exploring the relationship among dysfunctional families, parental incarceration, and juvenile court decision making. *Criminology* 2009;47:177–208.
14. Binswanger IA, Redmond N, Steiner JF, et al. Health disparities and the criminal justice system: an agenda for further research and action. *J Urban Health* 2012;89(1):98–107.
15. Teplin LA. Early violent death among delinquent youth: a prospective longitudinal study. *Pediatrics* 2005;115(6):1586–1593.
16. Chassin L, Piquero AR, Losoya SH, et al. Joint consideration of distal and proximal predictors of premature mortality among serious juvenile offenders. *J Adolesc Health* 2013;52:689–696.
17. Hockenberry S, Sickmund M, Sladky A. *Juvenile residential facility census, 2010: select findings*, Juvenile Offenders and Victims: National Report Series. Washington, DC: U.S. Department of Justice, Office of Justice Programs, Office of Juvenile Justice and Delinquency Prevention, 2013.
18. Fazel S, Doll H, Långström N. Mental disorders among adolescents in juvenile detention and correctional facilities: a systematic review and metaregression analysis of 25 surveys. *J Am Acad Adolesc Psychiatry* 2008;47:1010–1019.
19. Karnick NS, Soller M, Redlich A, et al. Prevalence of and gender differences in psychiatric disorders among juvenile delinquents incarcerated for nine months. *Psychiatr Serv* 2009;60:838–841.
20. Teplin LA, Welty LJ, Abram KM, et al. Prevalence and persistence of psychiatric disorders in youth after detention: a prospective longitudinal study. *Arch Gen Psychiatry* 2012;69:1031–1043.
21. Abram KM, Teplin LA, McClelland GM, et al. Comorbid psychiatric disorders in youth in juvenile detention. *Arch Gen Psychiatry*. 2003;60(11):1097–1108.
22. Sedlak AJ, McPherson KS; U.S. Department of Justice, Office of Juvenile Justice and Delinquency Prevention. Conditions of confinement: Findings from the Survey of Youth in Residential Placement. *Juvenile Justice Bull* 2010. Available at https://www.ncjrs.gov/pdffiles1/ojjdp/227729.pdf. Accessed Februray 26, 2014.
23. Morris RE, Harrison EA, Knox GW, et al. Health risk behavioral survey from 39 juvenile correctional facilities in the United States. *J Adolesc Health* 1995;17:334–344.
24. Feinstein RA, Lampkin A, Lorish CD, et al. Medical status of adolescents at time of admission to a juvenile detention center. *J Adolesc Health* 1998;22:190–196.
25. Hein K, Cohen MI, Litt IF, et al. Juvenile detention: another boundary issue for physicians. *Pediatrics* 1980;66:239–245.
26. Sedlak AJ, Bruce C. U.S. Department of Justice, Office of Juvenile Justice and Delinquency Prevention. Youth's characteristics and backgrounds: Findings from the Survey of Youth in Residential Placement. *Juvenile Justice Bulletin*. 2010. Available at https://www.ncjrs.gov/pdffiles1/ojjdp/227730.pdf. Accessed February 26, 2014.

27. Woolf A, Funk SG. Epidemiology of trauma in a population of incarcerated youth. *Pediatrics* 1985;75:463–468.

28. Workowski KA, Berman S; Centers for Disease Control and Prevention. Sexually transmitted diseases treatment guidelines, 2010. *MMWR Recomm Rep* 2010;59 (RR-12):1–110.

29. Romero EG, Teplin LA, McClelland GM, et al. A longitudinal study of the prevalence, development, and persistence of HIV/sexually transmitted infection risk behaviors in delinquent youth: implications for health care in the community. *Pediatrics* 2007;119:1126–1141.

30. Centers for Disease Control and Prevention. *2008 sexually transmitted diseases surveillance, STDs in persons entering corrections facilities.* Available at http://www.cdc.gov/std/stats08/corrections.htm. Accessed December 17, 2014.

31. Gallagher CA, Dobrin A, Douds AS. A national overview of reproductive health care services for girls in juvenile justice residential facilities. *Womens Health Issues* 2007;17:217–226.

32. Bolin K, Jones D. Oral health needs of adolescents in a juvenile detention facility. *J Adolesc Health* 2006;38:755–757.

33. Desai RA, Goulet JL, Robbins J, et al. Mental health care in juvenile detention facilities: a review. *J Am Acad Psychiatry Law* 2006;34:204–214.

34. Mulvey EP, Schubert CA. *Transfer of juveniles to adult court: effects of a broad policy in one court.* Washington, DC: U.S. Department of Justice, Office of Justice Programs, Office of Juvenile Justice and Delinquency Prevention, 2012.

35. Pajer KA, Kelleher K, Gupta RA, et al. Psychiatric and medical health care policies in juvenile detention facilities. *J Am Acad Child Adolesc Psychiatry* 2007;46:1660–1667.

36. Henggeler SW, Schoenwald SK. Social policy report: evidence-based interventions for juvenile offenders and juvenile justice policies that support them. *Sharing Child Youth Dev Knowl* 2011;25(1):1–28.

37. Committee on Adolescence. Health care for youth in the juvenile justice system. *Pediatrics* 20   11;128:1219–1235.

38. National Commission on Correctional Health Care. *Standards for health services in juvenile detention and confinement facilities.* Chicago, IL: National Commission on Correctional Health Care, 2004.

39. English A, Scott J, Park MJ; Center for Adolescent Health & the Law, National Adolescent and Young Adult Health Information Center. *Implementing the Affordable Care Act: how much will it help vulnerable adolescents & young adults?* 2014. Available at http://nahic.ucsf.edu/wp-content/uploads/2014/01/VulnerablePopulations_IB_Final.pdf. Accessed March 1, 2014.

ADDITIONAL RESOURCES AND WEBSITES ONLINE

IMMIGRANT AND REFUGEE HEALTH

International migration has become increasingly fluid, diverse, and common. Immigrants and refugees have health burdens that are often uniquely global and confront barriers to care, including linguistic, cultural, and legal issues as well as those that accompany poverty. In spite of this, many providers do not feel adequately equipped to provide the needed cross-cultural care.[1,2]

Worldwide, the migrant population has increased dramatically to more than 3% of the world's population.[3] The US became home to over 1 million newly arrived immigrants in 2012, representing a marked increase in immigration over the last century (www.migrationinformation.org/datahub/charts/final.fb.shtml),[4] and the US leads in countries welcoming foreign-born individuals (http://esa.un.org/unmigration/documents/The_number_of_international_migrants.pdf).[3] It is estimated that over 41 million US residents are foreign-born, representing just over 13% of the entire US population and more than half have noncitizen status[5] (http://www.pewhispanic.org/2013/01/29/statistical-portrait-of-the-foreign-born-population-in-the-united-states-2011/). Fifty-eight percent of new legalized immigrants reside in five states: California (19.4%), New York (13.5%), Florida (10.4%), Texas (9.4%), and New Jersey (5.4%).

Of particular interest is the increasing number of foreign-born adolescents and young adults (AYAs) who reside in the US, which is estimated to be over 4 million (aged 15 to 24).[6] In addition, 76% of Unaccompanied Alien Children (UAC, US Customs term) are between the ages of 14 and 18.[7]

Cultural Competency

A provider should:

- Acquire knowledge and information about the particular group(s) one is working with and/or develop a relationship with the medical interpreter or community health worker and utilize their knowledge for cultural and linguistic interpretation.
- Use a medical interpreter for all encounters with limited English proficient (LEP) patients.

- Approach each encounter with humility and respect, recognizing that each medical provider also has a cultural perspective from which the world is seen and may affect the perception of other cultures.
- Develop a comfort with differences that exist between one's own personal culture and the cultural values and beliefs of others.
- Remember that most immigrant AYAs are forgiving of cultural "mistakes" as long as the provider conveys a genuine sense of caring and respect.

Interpretation

Poor communication can be potentially devastating for patients seeking health care and also decreases access to health care.[8,9] LEP patients are at increased risk for medical errors. The US federal law mandates "linguistic accessibility to health care" under Title VI of the Civil Rights Act. Health care providers who receive federal funding are required to provide language access to LEP individuals who cannot communicate with their provider, but as might be expected, interpreters are often underutilized.[10,11] Useful tips for the use of medical interpreters can be found in **Table 79.1**[12] (www.health.state.mn.us/divs/idepc/refugee/guide/11interpreters.html).

In the event that an interpreter is not available, the use of a telephone interpreter service may be an option. It is important to provide information to the telephone interpreter regarding the setting prior to initiating the interview.

Legal Status

The legal status of migrants often complicates or influences an immigrant's ability to obtain medical insurance and their comfort to

TABLE 79.1
Guidelines for Using Medical Interpreters
1. Use qualified interpreters trained in medical interpretation.
2. Do not depend on children or other relatives and friends to interpret.
3. Have a brief preinterview meeting with the interpreter.
4. Address yourself to the interviewee, not to the interpreter. Maintain eye contact with the interviewee.
5. Avoid jargon and technical terms.
6. Keep your utterances short, pausing to permit the interpretation.

From the Minnesota Department of Health Refugee Provider Guide.

seek medical care. It is useful to understand the different classifications of foreign-born individuals to better appreciate barriers and their medical needs.

1. *Refugees* are designated by the United Nations High Commissioner for Refugees because they are forced to leave their country of origin owing to a well-founded fear of being persecuted for reasons of race, religion, nationality, membership of a particular social group, or political opinion and are living outside the country of nationality.[13] These individuals are recognized as refugees prior to arrival and typically are from countries experiencing significant violence and conflict. Refugees may apply for legal permanent resident (LPR) status after living in the US for 1 year.
2. *LPRs* are individuals who come to the US and are legally accorded the privilege of residing permanently.
3. *Unauthorized immigrants* arrive but do not have LPR status and face potential deportation and separation of families.
4. *Asylees* meet the definition of refugees, but are already in the US and are seeking admission at a port of entry.

Legal status has implication for access to health insurance. Refugees are provided with increased services through the US State Department in partnership with local Volunteer Resettlement Agencies (VOLAG). In addition to initial reception and placement, they are provided with medical assistance in the first 8 months after arrival in the US. Application for change in legal status to LPR necessitates a specific medical examination as required by the US Citizen and Immigration Service (USCIS). Unauthorized immigrants do not have access to health insurance and often do not seek medical attention for fear of deportation. Unauthorized immigrants are not eligible for change in legal status to LPR under the US federal law. Young adult immigrants (aged 16 to 26) are more likely to be unauthorized as compared to immigrants as a whole. In fact, nearly half of young adult immigrants are unauthorized. They are unique as compared to other marginalized young adults in that they are categorically excluded from programs, benefits, and services offered to other young adult groups.[14]

Health Screenings
Overseas Medical Screening

Overseas medical screening is required for all immigrants and refugees before entering the US. The purpose of this examination is to identify individuals with any disease of public health concern that renders the individual inadmissible. The evaluation is performed by panel physicians designated by the local US Embassy overseas. Guidelines for panel physicians are determined by the Centers for Disease Control and Prevention (CDC) Immigrant and Refugee Health.[15]

Excludable conditions of public health significance are Class A conditions and include the following:

- Active tuberculosis (TB)
- Syphilis
- Chancroid
- Gonorrhea
- Granuloma inguinale
- Lymphogranuloma inguinale
- Hansen disease (leprosy)
- Mental health disorder with associated harmful behaviors
- Substance-related disorder with associated harmful behaviors

The US Medical Screening

This is recommended by the CDC for all refugees and immigrants within 30 to 60 days upon arrival and aims to identify public health disease, promote and improve the health of the refugee/immigrant, and prevent disease and familiarize refugees with the US healthcare system.[16]

The health burden of refugees has been well documented,[17,18] and evidence-based recommendations for screening for refugee and immigrant AYAs include the following:

- A complete history (including detailed travel history)
- Review of all predeparture overseas documents including chest x-ray or predeparture presumptive treatment for malaria, schistosomiasis, or strongyloides

Complete physical examination should include the following:

- Height/weight/body mass index/nutritional assessment
- Vision/hearing screen
- Oral heath screen
- Scars suggesting previous injury/torture
- Genitourinary examination for both males and females. The genital examination may be deferred until the relationship with provider is developed and cultural implications are considered.

Evaluation recommended for both refugee and immigrant AYAs includes the following:

- Tuberculosis screening—tuberculin skin test (TST) or an interferon gamma-release assay (IGRA), such as *Quanti*FERON or T-SPOT, which may be preferred for those who have received Bacillus de Calmette Guérin
- Complete blood count (CBC) with differential and platelet count (identify iron deficiency, thalassemias and hemoglobinopathies, cell enzyme defects, eosinophilia)
- Hepatitis B surface antigen
- Gonorrhea and chlamydia nucleic acid amplification tests (NAATs)
- Human immunodeficiency virus (HIV)

Evaluation for refugees and targeted immigrants on the basis of symptoms, physical findings, predeparture treatment or living condition, and country of emigration includes the following:

- Stools for complete ova and parasites
- Urinalysis—(schistosomiasis, renal disease)
- Lead (adolescents 16 years of age or younger)
- Vitamin D
- Syphilis
- Malaria
- Serology for varicella, hepatitis A and B, measles
- Strongyloides
- Schistosomiasis

Screening for Adjustment of Legal Status

Application for LPR requires a specific medical examination, by USCIS. Medical information for this adjudication of status (I 693 Form) may be supplied by the medical provider, but should only be signed by an authorized civil surgeon.

Specific Health Issues
Immunizations

- Guidelines are found on the CDC Web site and consistent with the Advisory Committee on Immunization Practices (http://www.cdc.gov/vaccines/schedules/downloads/child/catchup-schedule-pr.pdf) and (http://www.cdc.gov/vaccines/schedules/hcp/imz/adult.html).
- Overseas immunizations are considered valid if documented with date of vaccination and given at the appropriate age and interval.
- Vaccination series do not need to be restarted because of time delay between immunization.
- If no written documentation is available, the youth is to be considered unvaccinated unless serum immunity is verified and must be immunized according to the "catch-up" schedule.
- TST can be applied before or on the same day that live virus vaccine is given (measles, mumps, rubella, varicella,

intranasal flu). However, if live virus vaccine is given on the previous day or earlier, the TST should be delayed for at least 1 month. Live measles vaccine given prior to the application of a TST can reduce the reactivity of the skin test because of mild suppression of the immune system.

- Consider obtaining serum immunology for varicella, measles, hepatitis A and B to verify immunity prior to immunizing.
- Proof of immunizations or positive serology is required for adjustment of legal status (human papillomavirus recommended but not required).

Tuberculosis

TB rates have declined in the US general population, but the rates among immigrants and refugees continue to increase at a rate 10 times higher than the rate of TB in US-born individuals.[19,20]

- Review predeparture medical records for TB testing, including chest x-ray.
- Obtain information regarding any prior treatment for TB, symptoms suggestive of TB (fevers, night sweats, cough >3 weeks, weight loss), or TB exposure.
- Perform TST or IGRA if no reliable documentation of predeparture testing.

- TST >5 is positive in a refugee with HIV or other immunosuppression, or if in close contact with someone with active TB, or if there are changes on chest x-ray consistent with prior TB. Induration >10 mm is positive on all other refugees.[21]
- Obtain chest x-ray on all positive TST or IGRA.
- Encourage treatment for latent tuberculosis infection (LTBI).
- Prompt referral to department of public health or infectious disease specialist for individuals with active pulmonary or extrapulmonary disease.

Parasitic Infections

- All refugees and at-risk immigrants should be screened for parasitic treatment. Common parasites include *Giardia*, *Ascaris*, *Hookworm*, *Trichuris* (whipworm), *Entamoeba histolytica*, and *Schistosoma*.[22]
- Collect two stool specimens (for ova and parasites separated by 24 hours) and CBC for eosinophilia (total eosinophil count >400).
- Confirm predeparture presumptive treatment, which will guide initial screening and treatment (Fig. 79.1).[23,24]

Malaria

- Individuals from sub-Saharan Africans and other highly endemic regions should receive presumptive treatment on

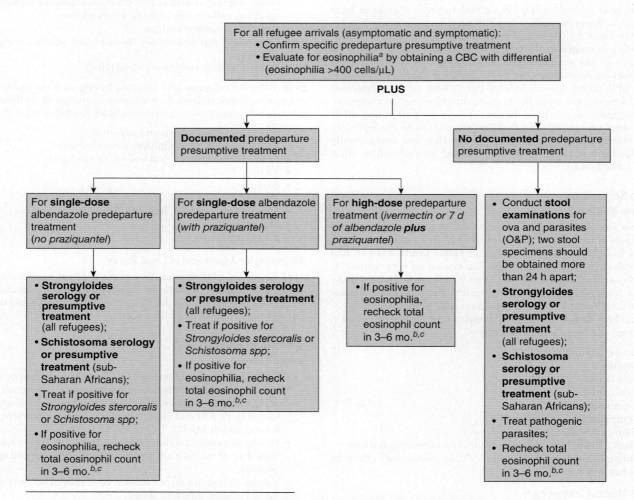

*a*Eosinophilia may or may not be present with parasitic infection; an absolute eosinophil count provides supplemental diagnostic information.
*b*Persistent eosinophilia or symptoms requires further diagnostic evaluation.
*c*If not positive for eosinophilia, further evaluation only if symptomatic.

FIGURE 79.1 Screening for parasitic infections and treatment. (From the Minnesota Refugee Health Provider Guide 2013—Parasitic Infections.)

arrival (if no documented predeparture treatment) or have laboratory screening.
- High index of suspicion for malaria in individuals from tropical or subtropical areas if they have fever of unknown origin or other symptoms suggestive of malaria.
- Laboratory evaluation includes malaria blood films (thick and thin smears) and rapid antigen testing. Polymerase chain reaction is more sensitive particularly in asymptomatic individuals and should be used if available.

Hepatitis B

- Screen all refugees and at-risk immigrants for hepatitis B virus (HBV), and immunize all AYAs without documentation of prior vaccination or immunity.

Lead

Lead exposure and toxicity are common in many countries of origin as well as continued exposures after arrival.[25]
- All young adolescent refugees (16 years of age or less) should be tested for lead upon arrival in the US.

Mental Health

Most refugee and immigrant AYAs display impressive resilience and a good ability to adjust and adapt in spite of significant adversity and trauma. However, as many as half of AYAs exhibit significant symptoms of posttraumatic stress disorder (PTSD), and up to 30% experience significant depression.[26–29] Predictors include the following:

- Experience prior to migration—trauma, separation from family members, death of loved ones, personal injury
- Experiences postmigration—adjustment to language and cultural differences, perceived discrimination, peer bullying, change in family hierarchy when adolescent becomes cultural broker for parents
- Lack of community social support, community violence, living arrangements

Common symptoms:

- Aggression and anger
- Depression
- Risky behaviors: illegal drug use, risky sexual behaviors
- Disturbing thoughts and images
- Concentration and school problems
- Somatic complaints

Intervention:

- Involvement in helping with important tasks for family/community
- Peer group activities
- Validation of experiences
- Culturally informed mental health services

NONIMMIGRANT FOREIGN-BORN AYAs

Nonimmigrant foreign-born individuals are granted temporary admission visas for a specific purpose such as academic and vocational study, temporary employment, business, and pleasure. Over a million students are actively attending academic or vocational institutions at the undergraduate as well as graduate levels. The most represented countries are China, South Korea, India, Saudi Arabia, and Canada[30] (http://www.ice.gov/doclib/sevis/pdf/quarterly_rpt.pdf).

Guidelines Include for Nonimmigrant Foreign-born AYAs

- All international students from high-incidence areas should be tested with TST or IGRA. High-incidence areas are considered 20 cases or more per 100,000 population and include most countries in Africa, Asia, Central America, Eastern Europe, and South America. The World Health Organization Global Health Observatory Data Repository is available for updates (http://apps.who.int/ghodata).
- American College Health Association (ACHA) guidelines for recommendations for institutional pre-matriculation immunizations may be found at the ACHA Web site (http://www.acha.org/Publications/Guidelines_WhitePapers.cfm#guidelines).
- All nonimmigrant visas require proof of medical health insurance.
- International nonimmigrant AYA students who seek adjustment of legal status to LPR must undergo a medical examination as required by the USCIS by a civil surgeon.
- Use of interpreters should be used with all LEP nonimmigrant AYAs, and guidelines for cultural competency (above) should be utilized.

SECOND-GENERATION IMMIGRANTS

Ambiguity surrounds the terminology regarding the generational description of immigrants and must be interpreted through context. First-generation immigrants can refer to foreign-born individuals who migrate to the US *or* to the first generation born in the US. Second-generation immigrants are those born of first-generation immigrants and thus the ambiguity persists. The term "1.5 generation" is commonly used to describe individuals arriving prior to adolescence.

It should be noted that the needs of immigrant foreign-born and US-born AYAs differ. The issues to consider include the following:

- Newly arrived immigrants to the US have increased acute illness such as infectious diseases, but in general have better health status when looking at chronic conditions and mortality. Mortality patterns for immigrants and for US-born adolescents vary considerably with immigrants experiencing lower mortality and is particularly true for young adults.[31] This health advantage seems to diminish with time and with generation. The reason for this discrepancy is unclear, but it is thought that it might, in part, be that healthier individuals migrate and that access to healthy lifestyle choices diminishes when in the US.
- Foreign-born immigrants and second-generation immigrants exhibit differences in health beliefs and behaviors.
  - Foreign-born young adults exhibit lower prevalence of smoking and tobacco use than US-born young adults, especially among Latino women.[32]
  - Pregnancy in 15- to 18-year-old foreign-born adolescents is more likely to be an intended pregnancy than for US-born Latino adolescents. There also appears to be an attitudinal difference between generations, with second and third generations more likely responding that teen pregnancy is a "bad thing for society" as compared to foreign-born.[33]
  - TB knowledge, attitudes, and beliefs vary between foreign-born and US-born LTBI patients. Foreign-born LTBI patients are less likely to acknowledge that they have LTBI and are more likely to feel protected from disease than US-born LTBI patients.[34] Since the majority of LTBI patients are foreign-born, the cultural differences need to be considered to improve outcomes.
  - US-born Latino youths go farther in school than do their foreign-born counterparts.[35]
  - Foreign-born Latinos (aged 16 to 25) are less likely to have been in a fight in the past year, know someone in a gang, carry a weapon during the last year, or be questioned by police.[35]
  - A more detailed review of social behaviors, values, and attitudes can be found elsewhere (http://www.pewhispanic.org/2009/12/11/between-two-worlds-how-young-latinos-come-of-age-in-america/).[35]

CONCLUSION

Global migration is more prevalent than ever. Providers who care for AYAs will need the tools to provide culturally appropriate medical care that addresses the specific needs of foreign-born young people.

REFERENCES

1. Weissman JS, Betancourt J, Campbell EG, et al. Resident physicians' preparedness to provide cross-cultural care. *JAMA* 2005;294(9):1058–1067.
2. Greer JA, Park ER, Green AR, et al. Primary care resident perceived preparedness to deliver cross-cultural care: an examination of training and specialty differences. *J Gen Intern Med* 2007;22:1107–1113.
3. Population Facts. *The number of international migrants worldwide reaches 232 million*. New York, NY: United Nations, Department of Economic and Social Affairs, Population Division, 2013:1–38. Available at http://esa.un.org/unmigration/documents/The_number_of_international_migrants.pdf.
4. Migration Policy Institute. Washington, DC. Available at www.migrationinformation.org/datahub/charts/final.fb.shtml. Accessed March 7, 2015.
5. Motel S, Patten E. *Statistical portrait of the foreign-born population in the United States, 2011*. Washington, DC: Pew Research Center, 2013. Available at http://www.pewhispanic.org/2013/01/29/statistical-portrait-of-the-foreign-born-population-in-the-united-states-2011/. Accessed March 8, 2015.
6. United Nations, Department of Economic and Social Affairs. *Trends in International Migrant Stock: Migrants by Age and Sex* (United Nations Database, POP/DB/MIG/Stock/Rev.2013). 2013
7. US Department of Health & Human Services; Office of Refugee Resettlement. About unaccompanied children's services. Available at http://www.acf.hhs.gov/programs/orr/programs/ucs/about#facts. Accessed March 8, 2015.
8. Flores G, Tomany-Korman SC. The language spoken at home and disparities in medical and dental health, access to care, and use of services in US children. *Pediatrics* 2008;121:1703–1714.
9. Cohen AL, Rivara F, Marcuse EK, et al. Are language barriers associated with serious medial events in hospitilized pediatric patients? *Pediatrics* 2005;116:575–579.
10. Grubbs V, Chen AH, Bindman AB, et al. Effect of awareness of language law on language access in the health care setting. *J Gen Intern Med* 2006;21:683–688.
11. Diamond LC, Schenker Y, Fernandez A, et al. Getting by: underuse of interpreters by resident physicians. *J Gen Intern Med* 2009;24:256–262.
12. Minnesota Department of Health; Refugee Health Provider Guide. Working with medical interpreters. Available at http://www.health.state.mn.us/divs/idepc/refugee/guide/11interpreters.pdf. Accessed February 16, 2014.
13. Office of the United Nations High Commissioner for Refugees. Available at http://www.unhcr.org/pages/49c3646c125.html. Accessed February 16, 2014.
14. Bonnie RJ, Stroud C, Breiner H, eds. *Investing in the health and well-being of young adults*. Washington, DC: Institute of Medicine and national Research Council of The National Academies Press, 2014:312–313.
15. Center for Disease Control and Prevention. Available at http://www.cdc.gov/immigrantrefugeehealth/exams/medical-examination. Accessed February 16, 2014.
16. Center for Disease Control and Prevention. Available at http://www.cdc.gov/immigrantrefugeehealth/guidelines/refugee-guidelines.html. Accessed February 16, 2014.
17. Museru OI, Vargas M, Kinyua M, et al. Hepatitis B virus infection among refugees resettled in the U.S.: high prevalence and challenges in access to health care. *J Immigr Minor Health* 2010;12:823–827.
18. Lifson AR, Thai D, O'Fallon A, et al. Prevalence of tuberculosis, hepatitis B virus, and intestinal parasitic infections among refugees to Minnesota. *Public Health Rep* 2002;117:69–77.
19. Barnett ED. Infectious disease screening for refugees resettled in the United States. *Clin Infect Dis* 2004;39(6):833–841.
20. Centers for Disease Control and Prevention. Trends in Tuberculosis—United States, 2007. *MMWR Morb Mortal Wkly Rep* 2008;57:281–285.
21. Center for Disease Control and Prevention. Available at http://www.cdc.gov/immigrantrefugeehealth/pdf/domestic-tuberculosis-refugee-health.pdf. Accessed February 16, 2014.
22. De Silva NR, Booker S, Hotez PJ, et al. Soil-transmitted helminth infections: updating the global picture. *Trends Parasitol* 2003;19:547–551.
23. Minnesota Department of Health Provider Guide. Available at http://www.health.state.mn.us/refugee/guide/. Accessed February 16, 2014.
24. Center for Disease Control and Prevention. Available at http://www.cdc.gov/immigrantrefugeehealth/guidelines/overseas/intestinal-parasites-overseas.html. Accessed February 16, 2014.
25. Eisenberg KW, van WijingaardenE, Geltman PL, et al. Blood lead levels of refugee children resettled in Massachusetts, 2000–2007. *Am J Public Health* 2011;101:48.
26. Fazel M, Reed RV, Panter-brick C, et al. Mental health of displaced and refugee children resettled in high-income countries: risk and protective factors. *Lancet* 2012;379(9812):266–282.
27. American Psychological Association. *Resilience & recovery after war: refugee children and families in the United States*. Washington, DC: American Psychological Association, 2010:1–96. Available at www.apa.org/pi/families/refugees.aspx.
28. Ellis BH, MacDonald HZ, Lincoln AK, et al. Mental health of Somali adolescent refugees: the role of trauma, stress, and perceived discrimination. *J Consult Clin Psychol* 2008;76(2):184–193.
29. Bronstein L, Montgomery P. Psychological distress in refugee children: a systematic review. *Clin Child Fam Psychol Rev* 2011;14:44–56.
30. Department of Homeland Security. Student and Exchange visitor information system: general summary quarterly review for the quarter ending March 31, 2012. Available at http://www.ice.gov/doclib/sevis/pdf/quarterly_rpt.pdf. Accessed February 22, 2014.
31. Singh GK, Siahpush M. All-cause and cause-specific mortality of immigrants and native-born in the United States. *Am J Public Health* 2001;91:392–399.
32. Lariscy JT, Hummer RA, Rath JM, et al. Race/Ethnicity, nativity, and tobacco use among US young adults: results from a nationally representative survey. *Nicotine Tob Res* 2013;15:1417–1426.
33. Guttmacher Institute. Teenagers' pregnancy intentions and decisions: a study of young women in California choosing to give birth. 1998. Available at http://www.guttmacher.org/pubs/or_teen_preg_survey.html. Accessed March 8, 2014.
34. Colson PW, Franks J, Sondengam R, et al. Tuberculosis knowledge, attitudes, and beliefs in foreign-born and US-born patients with latent tuberculosis infection. *J Immigr Minor Health* 2010;12:859–866.
35. Pew Research Center. *Between two worlds: how young Latinos come of age in America*. Washington, DC: Pew Research Center, 2013. Available at http://www.pewhispanic.org/2009/12/11/between-two-worlds-how-young-latinos-come-of-age-in-america/. Accessed March 8, 2014.

ADDITIONAL RESOURCES AND WEBSITES ONLINE

80

The Care of American Indian and Alaska Native Adolescents and Young Adults

Anthony H. Dekker
Roger Dale Walker
Dennis K. Norman
Raysenia L. James

KEY WORDS

- Aboriginal
- Alaska Native
- American Indian
- Indian Health Service
- Indigenous population
- Sun Dance
- Sweat lodge
- Traditional Indian Medicine

American Indian and Alaska Native (AI/AN) youth (aged 15 to 24) living in the US are at high risk for serious health, social, and educational disparities. Many AI/AN youth have demonstrated resilience and determination to succeed despite insurmountable odds.

DEMOGRAPHICS AND IDENTITY

Awareness of the unique cultural, historical, and political characteristics of the 566 nations that comprise the AI/AN communities will contribute to improved care of native youth. Of the 5.2 million people who identify themselves as AI/AN (including other ethnicities) in the 2010 US Census, about 3 million identified themselves as only AI/AN, with approximately 2 million reporting being members of federally recognized tribes.[1,2] Membership in a federally recognized tribe is a political identity defined by the citizenship of a sovereign nation. An excellent overview of these complicated regulations can be found at http://www.bia.gov/FAQs/. Federal, State, and Tribal legislation dictates several aspects of the care provided to these communities and populations. AI/AN population has experienced rapid growth, increasing by 39% since 2000.[2] Most (78%) AI/AN and their families live outside state or federal lands dedicated for reservation sites. There were over 200 Aboriginal languages before 1492, and more than 150 of these languages are still spoken today.

Although there are similarities with Indigenous Peoples of Canada (First Nations) and Aboriginal Communities of Mexico and Latin America, the term "AI/AN" is used to describe the indigenous people of the continental US. Many other nonfederally recognized groups exist (approximately 100), with many seeking federal recognition of their status including those tribes that are state, but not federally recognized.

HEALTH SERVICES

To effectively and competently provide behavioral and medical services for AI/AN adolescents and young adults (AYAs), it is critical to be cognizant of the diverse demographic and individual identity characteristics of the groups that make up North America's indigenous populations. AI/AN reside in all the US states and have a younger median age than general population, that is, 22 versus 38 years.[2] Slightly more than half reside in urban areas, with the remainder living in rural villages and small rural communities as well as on reservations.[3] Although many AI/AN youth are raised and practice traditional lifestyles, the actual rates of participation are unknown. The wide range of differences in culture, geography, spiritual beliefs, politics, and physical characteristics among AI/AN will challenge those who care for these AYAs.

HEALTH DELIVERY SYSTEM

The Indian Health Service (IHS), within the Department of Health and Human Services, annually provides inpatient and outpatient care to more than 2 million AI/ANs, through direct or contract services in 12 regional areas harboring approximately 772 facilities of hospitals, clinics, and satellite centers.[3] A relatively new but growing component administers social service and mental health programs. Because of varying and limited resources, service provision can range from exemplary to extremely lacking. Many facilities are not able to provide mental health services due to staff shortages of psychiatrists and other licensed behavioral health providers.[3,4]

The AI/AN health service delivery system is a complicated mixture of multiple service entities guided and impacted by jurisdictional boundaries that create significant problems in the delivery of needed medical and mental health services. The agencies directly responsible for service provision include the IHS, Bureau of Indian Affairs, as well as the Department of Veterans Affairs. Other federal programs that provide health services include the Department of Justice—Office for Victims of Crime and the Office of Juvenile Justice and Delinquency, Urban Indian Health Organization, state and local service agencies, as well as tribal health programs and traditional healing resources. Moreover, the system of behavioral health services in Indian country (land within an existing Indian reservation under the jurisdiction of the US government) is complex due to an inconsistent mixture of tribal, federal, state, local, and community-based services.[5] Often, there is little to no communication across these agencies, complicating an integrated health care network. The proliferation of services within the delivery structure outlined raises a large number of critical questions, the answers to which must guide greater efficacy in care for these youth.[6]

Treatment of youth varies widely across Indian country from having well-established medical centers to others having no trained service providers within a 200 mile range.[3] Lack of psychiatric services for families as well as youth for serious psychiatric disturbance is at a critical level. Eligibility criteria for individuals to obtain any type of health services from the IHS as well as gaining tribal benefits are even more confusing and vary with the provider agency in question. Indeed, this confusion prompted a study sponsored by the US Department of Education, Office of Indian Education, to determine workable definitions of "Indian."[7] Despite the "definition" of Indian study, bureaucratic ambiguity remains, employing tribally defined membership criteria (which differ across tribes), blood quantum (frequently one-fourth, genealogically derived), personal identification/community consensus, and various permutations.[8]

⬤ SPECIAL HEALTH ISSUES

While AI/AN AYAs experience similar health problems to their other ethnic peers, this is one of the highest at-risk subpopulations in the US because of the serious health disparities in a number of areas. In 2010, approximately 25% of AI/ANs lived on reservations or other US Census-defined tribal areas (http://www.census. gov/prod/cen2010/briefs/c2010br-10.pdf). Therefore, it is important for the provider to remember that the majority of AI/AN youth do not live on a federal reservation or on tribal lands, but will experience health conditions and problems at or above the rates reported by those AI/ANs living on tribal areas.

Physical Health
Obesity and Diabetes

The highest prevalence of obesity occurs in AI/AN children, with estimates at 31.2%, suggesting a realistic increase in the rates of obesity among the AYA AI/AN population.[9] In addition, the rates of type 2 diabetes among AI/AN youth are nine times the national average.[10–12] Among AI/AN, the prevalence and incidence of diabetes are much higher in older youth as compared to AI/AN children.[11,12] Specifically, among Navajo youth aged 15 to 19 years, 1 in 359 youth have diabetes and 1 in 2,542 develop diabetes annually. While the vast majority of diabetes among Navajo youth with diabetes is type 2, both AYAs with type 1 or type 2 diabetes are likely to experience poor glycemic control, a high prevalence of unhealthy behaviors, and evidence of severely depressed mood.[12]

Ear Infections and Hearing Loss

In general, AI/ANs have an extraordinarily high rate of middle-ear disease that progresses to chronic suppurative otitis media.[13] To date, there is no evidence of a genetic predisposition; however, it is likely that heredity plays an important role in the pathogenesis. Chronic ear infections can cause hearing loss, speech delay and, later, reading problems, and lower educational achievement. In 2005, AI/AN adults (6.4%) were nearly twice as likely as White adults (3.5%) and about four times as likely as Asian adults (1.8%) and Black adults (1.6%) to have trouble hearing or to be deaf.[14]

As many native youth have moved to metropolitan areas, higher rates of IgE-mediated allergy problems have been reported. This is likely multifactorial and due to genetic, environmental, and socioeconomic factors.

Sexual and Reproductive Health

Prior analyses of high school students suggest that AI/AN teens are more likely to engage in risky sexual behaviors, with reports of early sexual initiation and unintended pregnancy.[15]

- Among AI/AN aged 15 to 19 years, this group has the third highest birth, with rates of 31.1 per 1,000 after Black (39.0 per 1,000) and Hispanics (41.7 per 1,000).[16]
- Birth rates among AI/AN diminished by 11% compared to 2012 data, and the live birth rate for adolescents aged 10 to 14 and 15 to 19 years is 0.4 per and 31.1 per 1,000, respectively.[16]

Sexual health concerns among AI/AN youth compared to youth who reside in urban areas is striking.

- Young urban AI/AN females are having more unprotected first sex and more likely at first sex to have an older partners compared to non-Hispanic White youth.[17]
- A lower proportion of urban AI/AN teens are using contraception overall compared to non-Hispanic White teens.[17]
- Fewer urban AI/AN who have sex at younger ages are using condoms.[17]
- Urban AI/AN who had unprotected sex in the past year, had sex before age 15, and had more than two sex partners in the past 3 months are 77% more likely to have had an unintended

pregnancy than non-Hispanic Whites with the same sexual risk status.[17]

Sexually Transmitted Infections

- Chlamydia rates among AI/AN AYAs are almost 2.0 times higher than the average US rate, with age-specific rates among AI/AN men highest among the 20 to 24 cohort.[18]
- Gonorrhea rates are 4.2 times higher among AI/AN than for similar aged White youth, and in four IHS areas the gonorrhea rate is 1.3 to 6.0 times higher than the national average.[18]
- From 2009 to 2013, the rates of HIV infection for AI/AN have increased to 9.4 per 100,000 and 4.5 per 100,000, respectively.[18]
- Rates for AIDS have remained stable; although once diagnosed with AIDS, AI/AN have the lowest survival rates at 12, 24, and 36 months compared to all other ethnic groups.[19]

Access to reproductive health services for family planning and prevention of sexually transmitted infections (STIs) are highly variable, especially for those living in IHS areas. Among those living in urban areas, contextual factors including homelessness, isolation from cultural support systems, as well as distrust of medical and public health intuitions also inhibit access to needed sexual and reproductive health services.[15] Communities that have mobilized educational and traditional practices have been able to reduce unplanned pregnancies and STIs. For example, a longitudinal intervention conducted among young AI/AN adolescents found that an HIV prevention intervention increased HIV knowledge in the short term, but had no effect on sexual activity compared to those who did not receive intervention.[19] Despite this, there was a delay in onset of sexual activity among the youngest adolescents, with the greatest reduction of risk occurring in those receiving the curriculum early.

Substance Misuse and Abuse

Substance misuse and abuse is consistently cited as one of the most critical health concerns facing AI/AN communities.[20] Recent data suggest that:

- Among adults 18 years and older, AI/AN are 2.1 times more likely to suffer from any drug use disorder when compared to White youth and 3.8 times more likely to experience any drug dependence in the last 12 months.[21]
- The prevalence estimates of adults 18 years and older who met criteria for drug use disorder, drug abuse, or drug dependence in the last 12 months are 4.9, 2.3, and 2.6, respectively, all higher than other race/ethnicities.[21]
- Drinking alcohol before age 13 years is 1.6 times more likely when compared to White youth.[22]
- Binge drinking among AI/AN high school students is less likely when compared to their White peers 0.8 (0.7, 0.9), but 2.0 times more likely when compared to Black youth.[22]
- 40.1% report tobacco use, and 12.3% report illicit drug use.[23]
- The adjusted odds of ever having used marijuana, having tried marijuana for the first time before age 13 ears, and using marijuana on school grounds are 1.5 to 2.3 times higher among AI/AN than among White students.[22]
- The adjusted odds of ever having used cocaine, inhalants, heroin, methamphetamines, and ecstasy and having ever injected any illegal drug are between 1.4 and 2.1 times higher among AI/AN youth than among White youth and between 1.9 and 4.2 times higher than among Black youth.[22]

Recent research suggests that there are important differences in the normative environments for substance use between reservation-based American Indian youth and White youth who resided in the same area and attended the same schools.[24] Generally, the risk is higher for AI adolescents. These AI/AN students reported having more peer models for alcohol use compared to their White peers, and among the oldest AI/AN high school students, they perceive more adults are more accepting of alcohol use by male as compared to female adolescents. This perception of differential attitudes for use also occurs for marijuana use among older AI youth and across all grades for inhalants.

Little is known about factors that serve to protect AI/AN youth against developing a substance use problem.[20] For example, conflicting data have been reported about the effect of having a strong belief in the positive power of Indian cultural identity and participation. However, there is consistent evidence that bicultural competence, that is, the ability to alternate between one's ethnic and White identities in response to contextual cultural cues, decreases the risk for substance misuse.[20] In addition, data suggest that the time interval between the 8th and 10th grades is likely to be a critical period of risk for increased marijuana use and may be a key developmental period for monitoring and prevention efforts.[24]

Mental Health and Suicide

Research on mental health among AYA AI/AN is limited. This is due to the small sample size and heterogeneity of the population. Despite this, the existing literature suggests that AYA AI/AN suffer a disparate burden of mental health problems and high rates of suicide in AI/AN communities.[3]

- The most prevalent behavioral health concerns among AI/AN families include depression, substance use disorders, anxiety, and posttraumatic stress disorder.[25]
- AI/AN adolescents have the highest rates of major depressive disorder when compared to other race/ethnicities.[26]
- Forced assimilation across generations on tribal unity, family strength, and typical coping strategies has contributed to deterioration of mental health status in youth.[27]
- Suicidal ideation has been estimated to occur in almost 20% of AI/AN adolescents and is strongly associated with female gender, depressed mood, abuse, and substance use.[28] Among AI/AN young adults, suicidal ideation is 1.6 times more likely to be reported than by White young adults.[28]
- Compared with other racial groups, the rate of suicide among AI/AN males and females aged 15 to 24 in the US has increased.[29]
- AI/AN AYA males have the highest suicide rate compared to same-age males of all other ethnic groups.[29] Suicide was linked to ongoing behavioral health problems such as anxiety, substance abuse, trauma, and depression, as well as to underutilization of mental health services, high poverty, poor educational outcomes, substandard housing, and disease.[3,29]

Some key protective factors against suicide attempts as well as ongoing psychological distress among AI/AN youth include the following:

- Discussion of problems with family or friends[25,30]
- Connectedness to family[25,30]
- Emotional health[25,30]
- Spiritual orientation[25,30]

While a recent report found that over 80% of IHS and tribal facilities provide some type of mental health service, these services were inconsistent and limited across these facilities.[3] Moreover, inadequate staffing of providers because of geographic isolation can limit AI/AN access to behavioral health services. Improved public health funding from the IHS and tribal programs have had beneficial effects on improving mental health outcomes, especially when interventions are culturally sensitivity and span the transitional years into adulthood.[31–33]

Violence and Motor Vehicle Accidents

AI/AN and non-Hispanic Black youth fare worse in the rates of violent death and injury.[34] A recent congressional report found that several forms of violence challenge AI/AN youth, including simple assaults, violent threats, sexual assaults, gang violence, sex and drug trafficking, bullying, and homicide.[35]

- In 2009, the homicide rates were highest among non-Hispanic Blacks (19.9 deaths per 100,000), followed by AI/ANs (9.0 deaths per 100,000). This is most likely an underestimate because of the inadequate criminal investigation staff available to native communities.[35]
- Motor vehicle deaths are reported to be among the highest in AI/AN youth, with rates being 2 to 5 times higher in males and 2 to 4 times higher in females compared to the other races/ethnicities. Alcohol plays the predominant role in native motor vehicle deaths.[35]
- Gang activity has been reported in over 23% of AI/AN communities, compared to 20% of communities with similar demographics.[36]
- 15% of AI/AN youth are involved in gang activity, compared to 8% of Hispanic youth and 6% of Black youth.[36]

Often times the result of these occurrences requires federal interdiction because of long-standing Indian Citizen Act of 1924 requiring the Federal Government to play a central role in juvenile and criminal jurisdiction on the reservations and tribal lands. Thus, native AYAs are often forced into nonlocal judicial systems. Moreover, tribal law enforcement staff is often prohibited in the criminal processing of nonnative perpetrators. This system is expensive, complex, and is unable to address the needs in Indian country and further marginalizes the AI/AN young person.

SOCIAL DETERMINANTS OF HEALTH

A recent study was conducted by the Urban Indian Health Organization to assess the health status of AI/AN youth and families.[37] Although urban living may offer increasing numbers of opportunities, the departure of AI/AN AYAs from reservations has typically resulted in a loss of access to health care, historically provided by the IHS. Despite the increasing numbers of urban AI/AN, little is known about their health.

- Percentages of AI/AN with a 4-year college degree, both in urban service areas and nationwide, were less than half the percentages found for the corresponding general populations.[37]
- Similar disparities were observed in unemployment rates between urban AI/AN as well as AI/AN children were members of single-parent families.[37]
- In all Indian urban service areas, AI/AN rates of poverty, unemployment, and children living in single-parent families were highest. Thus, health disparities between groups reflect social inequalities, including inadequate education, disproportionate poverty, discrimination in the delivery of health services, and cultural differences.[37]

UNIQUE CONSIDERATIONS OF AI/AN YOUTH AND FAMILIES

Culture

Cultural strengths such as family and community, spirituality, connection to the past, traditional health practices, wisdom of elders, and group identity are key moderators of physical and mental health outcomes.[38] These strengths need to be considered and explored with the AYA AI/AN because they may provide the foundation for developing effective approaches and treatments.

Among AI/AN communities, there is a wide range of beliefs about illness, healing, and health.[38,39] Moreover, there are many different meanings and understandings about mental illness and why or how it develops within these communities. As a result, it is not uncommon for physical and psychological concerns to not be differentiated. And, the expression of these concerns by the AYA patient and families may not fit into standard diagnostic categories.[39]

If the adolescent or young adult or family requests that medical information be shared with a "traditional Indian" practitioner, an appropriate release of information is required. Providers should not view this traditional practitioner as competition or as an aversion to modern medicine. Collaboration is expected, and over 60% of AI/ANs use traditional services.[40] The spiritual, emotional, and mental impact on the patient is a critical part of the patient's and the family's healing.

Geographic Considerations

Providers in metropolitan areas need to conscientious about the AI/AN population because of recent migration patterns. Providers should obtain information from the AI/AN youth about their parents' migration to urban areas as the proportion of first-generation migrators suffer disproportionately from depression and substance abuse.[3]

Language

Many native youth are encouraged to speak their native language when they are among each other. Therefore, when the family is with the adolescent or young adult, the provider should not view this action as disrespectful. Native youth are often accompanied by grandparents and/or other relatives even when visiting the health provider, and these grandparents may use their primary language exclusively. However, some states have prohibited using the adolescent or young adult patient or other family members as translators. Many times the native family has given the responsibility of translation to the youth. This is especially true for translation to the grandparents who are non-English speakers. To disrespect this honor may cause a disruption in the provider–patient relationship.

Unfortunately, the US has a long history of eradication efforts of native language. Tribes have responded by encouraging language preservation. If an adolescent or young adult or family member requests or family member requests an interpreter, this request should be honored. Remember to address the adolescent or young adult patient, not the interpreter, for the medical evaluation and care provided.[41]

Eye Contact

As with most verbal communications between individuals, there also exists nonverbal components as well. The provider must be sensitive to the practices in some traditional native communities. For instance, members will not make eye-to-face contact with the speaker and instead look down or away to indicate and acknowledge respect to the speaker. This is particularly true of youth raised in more traditional AI/AN settings. Some youth have been taught that looking directly in someone's eyes while talking to them is disrespectful.[42] Thus, the provider needs to be aware of this communication style and not make assumptions or judgments about the patient's statements as not being truthful or embarrassed.

Consent and Confidentiality

Consent and confidentiality by the provider must take into consideration State and/or territorial laws of the practice location, as well as the tribal laws of the AI/AN AYAs' community, especially among those living on tribal lands. In addition, understanding the AYAs' perspective of their personal needs and their perceptions of their responsibilities to their family is critical. Often, laws designed to respect individual confidentiality are in direct conflict with cultural practices of communication within families. AYAs must provide informed consent for all invasive or intrusive procedures.

Time

In many native communities, time may not be concrete or fixed. This may challenge many providers who desire to keep schedules by the clock. Some providers may interpret lateness as disrespect or disinterest or make attributions to the patient and family as lazy, unmotivated, or irresponsible. Providers must remember that the AI/AN community ceremonies may not have concrete start and finish times. In addition, for those living on reservations, challenges in travel to and from the reservation to the clinic can be challenging, and hardships exist for many families. Many AI/AN families living on reservations do not have optimal travel options. Expectations relative to appointment times should be explained during the initial visit.[40]

Introductions

Each native community has their way of greeting in the healing setting. Members of some communities may not be comfortable with nonnative contact even in the medical setting. This may be based on the belief that they do not know who you are and/or do not want "negativity" to come to them. Native youth may not have the same feelings as their parents, but like most AYAs, first impressions are critically important. It is recommended that a at the start of any visit the provider introduce him or herself and ask, "How may I help you?" as opposed to a more direct and clinical approach. It is critical for the provider to actively listen to the patient's and family's response. As mentioned above, a key ingredient in a successful first visit is to be respectful and cognizant of the cultural issues in the community and family; this will improve the relationship between the provider and the patient and their community.[38]

Once the patient, family, and community achieve this trust, it is not uncommon for the provider to be embraced by the patient and/or family. A family member may deliver a breath in or near the provider's hands to deliver a "blessing" to bestow compassion, intelligence or good health.

History, Physical, and Screening

Native youth realize that health care providers utilize questions to better understand medically related issues. However, the provider must be aware that asking the details included in a typical social history may result in a perception of the provider being overly engaged in the patient's family and community. Creating a safe environment for the youth to be open is important, and similar to other AYAs, the provider should employ a style of open-ended questioning. Concentrate on the medical aspects of care, but if you need additional information, weave those themes into the issue of concern. The use of Traditional Indian Medicines and Ceremonies is a critical component of the care of native youth. The provider's nonverbal responses, that is, body language when these treatments and ceremonies are shared with the provider, will determine whether the youth and family will be open and forthcoming. Keep in mind there is federal legislation that protects the acquisition and utilization of Traditional Indian Medicine.

History taking should include the strengths and challenges faced by the youth as well as the patient's perceptions of the communication styles in the family and community. Social history of perceived threats and violence should be included as part of the history, and all patients should be appropriately screened for violence and violence exposure. With that screening, it is key that the provider be aware of tribal court processes and tribal child protective services because suspected maltreatment issues can become complicated. Federal and tribal laws are engaged if any crimes occur on tribal or federal lands. Anyone working close to native communities needs to be aware of the state, federal, and tribal regulations.

In most instances, the physical examination should be chaperoned, but conversation between the patient and family should confirm this practice for patients of both genders. In addition, all sexually experienced youth should be screened for STIs using nucleic acid amplification test as well as screening for syphilis.

For AI/AN youth, detecting suicidal ideations and intent is an important part of the history and physical. Some native communities have very high rates of suicide. The provider needs to be aware that suicide screening may be seen as intrusive in some communities. The word "suicide" is unspoken in some communities, and simply raising the topic may bring discomfort to the youth and their family. That said, the provider can ask very specific questions without using the word "suicide." "Are there times that you are worried about your safety? Do you feel you have a future that you can envision? Or "Are there times you feel your life is in danger" as examples.

Coming of Age and Other Ceremonies

Most native communities identify individual tribal members as healers and/or spiritual leaders. The provider must be sensitive to the native communities' ceremonial practices which cover the spectrum of life events and are officiated by the community's spiritual leader as a conduit from the Creator or Maker of All Things. For youth, this translates into important developmental events such as menarche as opposed to age-based occurrences, such as birthdays.[38] These coming of age experiences vary in each community and are typically requested by a tribal leader or family member. Often, these practices are conducted in the privacy of the AYAs' home or a designated place such as a sweat lodge. Other common ceremonies may include AYA who are suffering from an illness, may be pregnant or those in need of detoxification.[39] In fact, some medical disorders may be seen as caused by a loss of harmony or balance. Other AYAs and their families may believe that negative spirits or a loss of control will have an inevitable end point. Therefore, the provider must thoughtfully appreciate local customs and culture when providing care to native youth.

If an AYA is hospitalized, usually the ceremony will be conducted at the bedside. The provider needs to be aware that it is not uncommon for combustible materials to be part of a ceremony. The hospital administration typically has policies and procedures in place to maintain "smoke-free" facilities, and as a result, some negotiation about these ceremonies may be required. For example, local fire department notification is mandated as well as turning off of oxygen ports in the room are usual practices. Many facilities that provide care to native communities do recognize Traditional Indian Practitioners and provide access to patients and information similar to chaplains.[40]

⬤ UNIQUE MANAGEMENT CONSIDERATIONS

General

The medical provider needs to be aware of the special needs shared by AI/AN youth.[42] Understanding all local tribal beliefs, practices, and ceremonies are critical. In addition, potential conflicts relative to youth as well as the community's expectations of care will determine the success of how the AYAs utilize health care and their adherence to provider recommendations.

Traditional Indian Practices

Understanding cultural knowledge, traditional health practices and medicines, and collaborative practice with traditional healers will improve the acceptance of the provider's recommendations and the care delivered. Sweat lodge (also called purification ceremony or sweat, takes place in a typically dome-shaped hut made with natural materials and is used for purification, cleansing, and healing of the mind, body, emotions, and spirit), Sun Dance (a tribal ceremony that is considered to be a prayer for life or thanksgiving and may consist of a combination of various elements, including dance, song, traditional drum, sacred fire, praying with a pipe, fasting, and, in some cases, body piercing), prayer, ceremonial, and family rituals should be seen as contributing to the health of the youth and family. Therefore, it is critical when developing a care plan that the provider incorporates traditional knowledge of health,

spirituality, and related traditional practices in accordance with the AYA patient's cultural identity and level of acculturation.[42]

Provision and Access to Care

Shame is a powerful emotion, and the provider should not use or convey this feeling when the patient and/or families refuse services. Remember, missing appointments are a result of a variety of factors. Engaging the youth and family to maximize the benefit of the medical services is an ongoing process. Understanding the access to care and how to cancel appointments are important survival skills.[43]

Provision of Mental Health Care

Barriers to behavioral health services are multifaceted and are complicated by bureaucracy. While AI/AN adults and families report many problems, their use of services is similar to that of other race/ethnicities.[26] Regardless, treatment for serious mental and behavioral health difficulties including depression requires a care plan that accounts for environmental conditions as well as cultural background and should include the whole family or community.[26] The provider must also note that cultural identity, background, and preferences also impact on AI/AN's use of Western mental health care. Thus, AI/AN AYAs' and their families may first seek care from traditional or spiritual healers than from referred mental health providers.[26]

Taboos

Some native communities believe that medical equipment that has been used by other people (crutches, wheelchairs, etc.) may bring harm to the next youth who uses that equipment. Therefore, the provider should not be surprised when a patient or family member inquires about the name or person who previously used the equipment. Certain medications, especially psychiatric medications, may also be seen as taboo to some communities. Therefore, it is critical for the provider to work with the local Traditional Cultural Advocacy committee to obtain needed guidance in these areas.

When working within the native community, providers need to remember that in some communities pointing with fingers at individuals is disrespectful. Finally, in most native cultures, the elderly are highly respected and some feel to cross directly in front of an elder is disrespectful.[40]

Food Management

Many tribal leaders believe that the Western diet has brought great illness to native communities. Traditional AI/AN diets are landscape based, not pyramid based. There has been a resurgence of aboriginal diets, and the IHS has observed the positive effects in the reduction of diabetes. In some communities, it is disrespectful to refuse food when offered or to ask for food when it is not offered. Many native families and tribes offer food or beverage as a courtesy to their guests. Community gatherings are food based, and sharing promotes the cultural understanding of "give and take."

As mentioned previously, the provider must be aware that in many native communities, poverty is common. Many families rely on public assistance and commodity food and/or do not have fresh fruit and vegetables readily available. Many native communities are designated as food deserts (an area where it is difficult to buy affordable or good-quality fresh food). To advocate for improved nutrition, the provider may wish to consider attending local powwows or talking circles to see what AYA and their families traditionally eat and how it is prepared.[44]

Blood, Surgical Specimen, and Delivery By-Product Management

Many aboriginal communities believe that blood, surgical specimens, and other body parts that have been eliminated continue to have some effect on the health of an individual or community.

Providers should inquire whether AYA desires to keep any remaining body fluids or parts that have been removed. This is especially true of delivery by-products, umbilical cords, and placenta parts. It is recommended that all patients give permission to dispose of these body parts if they do not want to take ownership of the parts/fluids.[45]

Caring for Others

Most AI/AN communities are very family oriented, including extended family members. These extended family members may participate in the childrearing and care of the children and youth. Some families will expect the health professionals to respect the extended family member as a parent and therefore take on roles such as consent for services. This issue should be addressed during the first visits for care.

● SUMMARY AND CONCLUSION

Health care providers need to be aware of the increased morbidity and mortality rates of AI/AN AYAs and the disparities in risk-taking behavior. Attention to the cluster of mental health issues including suicide, violence, and alcohol use is vital. Providers should employ interventions specific to given conditions, but must also provide approaches that consider the social and historical context of the AYA AI/AN. The evaluation of AI/AN AYAs requires the provider to have an increased sensitivity to the individual, family, and community beliefs and practices. Collaboration with the local traditional practitioners and knowledge of family rituals will improve acceptance of the provider's recommendations. Awareness of the local tribal regulations and organizations will also optimize the integration of health services. There have been several national task forces that have specifically addressed the medical and mental health of AI/AN, including the President's Commission on Mental Health (PCMH) in 1978[9] and the report by the Office of the Inspector General.[2] These recommendations note that "at present services and service delivery systems to AI/AN people... are disjointed, disorganized, wasteful, fragmented, and counterproductive"[9] and call for an examination of ways in which to coordinate the delivery of health care more effectively.

While concern has been expressed over the lack of knowledge about the relative efficacy of nonindigenous forms of counseling and psychotherapy with AI/AN and families, it remains an important consideration in the treatment plan for youth with significant emotional health concerns. Thus, it is important for providers to integrate screening and treatment that are delivered in primary care as well as places not traditionally associated with mental health care, such as schools, in order to facilitate mental health services.[26] Ultimately, to provide the necessary care for these youth, an infrastructure must be developed to integrate physical with behavioral health care that is aligned with an AI/AN holistic approach that focused on wellness, reduces stigma and privacy concerns. Simultaneously, education and training of mental health providers in AI/AN cultural competence as well as evidence for treatment alternatives that are more consistent with a native wellness perspective are urgently needed.

Becoming part of the healing team for AI/AN youth should be seen as an honor and a privilege. Recognition of the individual, family, and community beliefs and practices are part of the caring process.

REFERENCES

1. United States Census Bureau Website. Available at http://www.census.gov/compendia/statab/. Accessed August 26, 2014.
2. U.S. Department of Health and Human Services, Office of Inspector General. *Access to mental health services at Indian Health Service and tribal facilities*, Publication No. OEI-09-08-00580. Rockville, MD: U.S. Department of Health and Human Services, 2011. Available at http://oig.hhs.gov/oei/reports/oei-09-08-00580.pdf. Accessed August 26, 2014.
3. Urban Indian Health Commission. *Invisible tribes: urban Indians and their health in a changing world*. Princeton, NJ: Robert Wood Johnson Foundation, 2007. Available at http://www.uihi.org/wp-content/uploads/2009/09/UIHC_Report_FINAL.pdf. Accessed August 28, 2014
4. Nelson SH, McCoy GF, Stetter M, et al. An overview of mental health services for American Indians and Alaska Natives in the 1990s. *Hosp Community Psychiatry* 1992;43:257–261.
5. Manson SM. Extending the boundaries, bridging the gaps: crafting mental health: culture, race, and ethnicity, a supplement to the surgeon general's report on mental health. *Cult Med Psychiatry* 2003;27:395–408.
6. U.S. Department of Health and Human Services. *Mental health: culture, race, and ethnicity—a supplement to mental health: a report of the surgeon general*. Rockville, MD: U.S. Department of Health and Human Services, Substance Abuse and Mental Health Services Administration, Center for Mental Health Services, 2001:77–97. Available at http://health-equity.pitt.edu/866/1/sma-01-3613.pdf. Accessed August 26, 2014.
7. U.S. Department of Education. Revised report on the definition of Indian. *A study of alternative definitions and measures relating to eligibility and service under Part A of the Indian Education Act*. Washington, DC: U.S. Department of Education, 1982. Available at http://www.eric.ed.gov/contentdelivery/servlet/ERICServlet?accno=ED226895. Accessed August 26, 2014.
8. Garroutte EM. The racial formation of American Indians: Negotiating legitimate identities within tribal and federal law. *Am Indian Quart* 2001;25:224–239.
9. Anderson SE, Whitaker RC. Prevalence of obesity among US preschool children in different racial and ethnic groups. *Arch Pediatr Adolesc Med* 2009;163:344–348.
10. Indiana Health Services website. Diabetes in American Indians and Alaska Natives. Facts at-a-glance. Available at http://www.ihs.gov/MedicalPrograms/Diabetes/ Home Docs/Resources/FactSheets/2012/Fact_sheet_AIAN_508c.pdf. Accessed October 25, 2015.
11. Dabelea D, Mayer-Davis EJ, Sayday S, et al. Prevalence of type 1 and type 2 diabetes among children and adolescents from 2001 to 2009. *JAMA* 2014;311:1778–1786.
12. Dabelea D, DeGroat J, Sorrelman C. Diabetes in Navajo youth: prevalence, incidence, and clinical characteristics: the SEARCH for Diabetes in youth study. *Diabetes Care* 2005;32 (Suppl 2):S141–S147.
13. Singleton RJ, Holman RC, Plant R, et al. Trends in otitis media and myringotomy with tube placement among American Indian/Alaska native children and the US general population of children. *Pediatr Infect Dis J* 2009;28:102–107.
14. Barnes PM, Adams PF, Powell-Griner E. Health characteristics of the American Indian and Alaska native adult population; United States, 1999–2003. Available at http://www.cdc.gov/nchs/data/ad/ad356.pdf. Accessed March 29, 2015.
15. Rutman S, Taualii M, Ned D, et al. Reproductive health and sexual violence among urban American Indian and Alaska Native young women: select findings from the National Survey of Family Growth (2002). *Matern Child Health J* 2012;16 (Suppl 2):347–352.
16. Martin JA, Hamilton BE, Osterman MJK, et al. Births: final data for 2013. *Natl Vital Stat Rep* 2015;64:1–65. Available at http://www.cdc.gov/nchs/data/nvsr/nvsr64/nvsr64_01.pdf.
17. Urban Indian Health Institute, Seattle Indian Health Board. *Reproductive health of Urban American Indian and Alaska native women: examining unintended pregnancy, contraception, sexual history and behavior, and non-voluntary sexual intercourse*. Seattle, WA: Urban Indian Health Institute, 2010. Available at http://www.uihi.org/wp-content/uploads/2010/09/nsfg-report_final_2010-09-22.pdf. Accessed March 30, 2015.
18. Centers for Disease Control and Prevention and Indian Health Service. *Indian Health Surveillance Report—Sexual Transmitted Diseases 2009*. Atlanta, GA: U.S. Department of Health and Human Services, 2012. Available at http://www.cdc.gov/std/stats/IHS/IHS-Surv-Report-2009.pdf.
19. Kaufman CE, Whitesell NR, Keane EM, et al. Effectiveness of circle of life, an HIV-preventive intervention for American Indian middle school youths: a group randomized trial in a Northern Plains tribe. *Am J Public Health* 2014;104:e106–e112.
20. Hawkins EH, Cummins LH, Marlatt GA. Preventing substance abuse in American Indian and Alaska native youth: promising strategies for healthier communities. *Psychol Bull* 2004;130:304–323.
21. Comptom WM, Thomas YF, Stinson FS, et al. Prevalence, correlates, disability, and comorbidity of DSM-IV drug abuse and dependence in the United States. *Arch Gen Psychiatry* 2007;64:566–576.
22. de Ravello L, Jones SE, Tulloch S, et al. Substance use and sexual risk behaviors among American Indian and Alaska native high school students. *J Sch Health* 2014;84:25–32.
23. U.S. Department of Health and Human Services, Substance Abuse and Mental Health Service Administration, Center for Behavioral Statistics and Quality. Results from the 2013 National Survey on drug use and health: summary of National Findings. Available at http://www.samhsa.gov/data/sites/default/files/NSDUHresultsPDF-WHTML2013/Web/NSDUHresults2013.pdf. Accessed March 29, 2015.
24. Swaim R, Stanley L, Beauvais F. The normative environment of substance use among American Indian students and white students. *Am J Orthopsychiatry* 2013;83:422–429.
25. American Psychiatric Association, Division of Diversity and Health Equity. Mental Health Disparities: American Indians and Alaska Natives. Available at http://www.psychiatry.org/american-indians-alaska-natives. Accessed March 29, 2015.
26. Urban Indian Health Institute, Seattle Indian Health Board. *Addressing depression among American Indians and Alaska Natives: a literature review*. Seattle, WA: Urban Indian Health Institute, 2012. Available at http://www.uihi.org/wp-content/uploads/2012/08/Depression-Environmental-Scan_All-Sections_2012-08-21_ES_FINAL.pdf. Accessed March 29, 2015.
27. Centers for Disease Control and Prevention, National Center for Injury Prevention and Control. Web based Injury Statistics Query and Reporting System (WISQARS). Available at http://www.cdc.gov/injury/wisqars/nonfatal.html. Accessed October 25, 2015.
28. Han B, McKeon R, Gfroerer J. Suicidal ideation among community-dwelling adults in the United States. *Am J Public Health* 2014;104:488–497.
29. Hummingbird LM. The public health crisis of Native American youth suicide. *NASN Sch Nurse* 2011;26:110–114.
30. Borowsky IS, Resnick MD, Ireland M, et al. Suicide attempts among American Indian and Alaska native youth: risk and protective factors. *Arch Pediatr Adolesc Med* 1999;153:573–580.
31. Gone JR, Alcántara C. Identifying effective mental health interventions for American Indians and Alaska Natives: a review of the literature. *Cultur Divers Ethnic Minor Psychol* 2007;13:356–363.

32. Indian Health Service Website. Behavioral health. Available at http://www.ihs.gov/newsroom/factsheets/behavioralhealth/. Accessed October 25, 2015.

33. Issacs MR, Huang LN, Hernandez M, et al. The road to evidence: the intersection of evidence-based practices and cultural competencies in children's mental health. Report to the National Alliance of Multi-ethic Behavioral Health Associations. Available at http://tapartnership.org/enterprise/docs/RESOURCE%20BANK/RB-CULTURALLY%20COMPETENT%20APPROACHES/General%20Resources/Intersection_of_EBP_and_CLC_Isaacs_et_al_2005.pdf. Accessed August 26, 2014.

34. Park MJ, Scott JT, Adams SH, et al. Adolescent and young adult health in the United States in the past decade: little improvement and young adults remain worse off than adolescents. *J Adolesc Health* 2014;55:3–16.

35. U.S. Department of Justice. *Attorney General's Advisory Committee on American Indian and Alaska Native children exposed to violence: ending violence so children can thrive.* Washington, DC: U.S. Department of Justice, 2014.

36. U.S. Department of Justice. *Youth gangs in Indian Country.* Washington, DC: Juvenile Justice Bulletin, 2004. Available at https://www.ncjrs.gov/pdffiles1/ojjdp/202714.pdf. Accessed March 29, 2015.

37. Castor ML, Smyser MS, Taualii MM, et al. A nationwide population-based study identifying health disparities between American Indians/Alaska Natives and the general populations living in select urban counties. *Am J Public Health* 2006;96:1478–1484.

38. Alvord LA, Van Pelt E. *The scalpel and the Silver Bear: The first Navajo woman surgeon combines Western medicine and traditional healing.* New York, NY: Bantam Books, 1999.

39. Berger LR, Rounds JE. Sweat lodges: a medical view. *Indian Health Serv Provid* 1998;23:6. Available at http://www.ihs.gov/provider/documents/1990_1999/PROV0698.pdf.

40. Rife JP, Dellapenna AJ. *Caring & curing: a history of the Indian Health Service.* Terra Alta, WV: Pioneer Press of West Virginia, 2009.

41. U.S. Department of Health and Human Services. Available at https://www.thinkculturalhealth.hhs.gov/pdfs/NationalCLASStandardsFactSheet.pdf. Accessed April 12, 2015.

42. Dixon M, Iron PE. *Strategies for cultural competency in Indian Health Care.* Washington, DC: American Public Health Association, 2006

43. McNeil J, Downer GA. Be safe: a cultural competency model for American Indians, Alaska Natives, and Native Hawaiians toward the treatment and prevention of HIV/AIDS. Available at http://aidsetc.org/resource/be-safe-cultural-competency-model-american-indians-alaska-natives-and-native-hawaiians. Accessed April 12, 2015.

44. Metropolitan Chicago Healthcare Council. Capes Memorandum No. 04-19 (November 18, 2004). Available at http://www.sswlhc.org/docs/MCHC-NativeAmericans.pdf. Accessed April 11, 2015.

45. Eastman CA (aka Ohiyesa). The soul of an Indian. In: Nerburn K, ed. *The soul of an Indian—and other writings from Ohiyesa.* Novato, CA: New World Library, 1993. Available at http://www.mountainman.com.au/eastman.html. Accessed April 12, 2015.

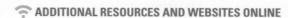

ADDITIONAL RESOURCES AND WEBSITES ONLINE

XVI

Index

665

Cetirizine, for urticaria, 222
Chamomile
    adverse effects of, 78
    clinical studies of, 78
    drug interactions, 78
    mechanism of action, 78
    uses of, 78
Chancroid, 508, 508f, 510t
Chantix. See Varenicline
Child abuse and neglect, 643
Child maltreatment, 605–606
Child welfare agency, foster care, 644
Childhood absence epilepsy, 233
Children's Depression Inventory (CDI-2), 580
Children's Depression Rating Scale–Revised, 580
Children's Health Insurance Program, 93
Childstats.gov, 17
Chiropractic
    complications of, 82
    health benefits of, 82
    theory of, 81
Chlamydia, 471, 475–484
    cases and incidence of, 476t
    epidemiology, 475–476
    etiology, 475
    gonorrhea and, 482
    homosexual youth, 338
    prevalence, 476–478
    screening of, 62, 472
    treatment, 482–484
Chlamydia pneumoniae, 269
Chlamydia trachomatis (C. trachomatis)
    and epididymitis, 457, 458
    and pelvic inflammatory disease, 486, 487, 488, 489
Chlamydial endocervicitis, in female, 481
Chlorazepate, pharmacological actions of various benzodiazepines, 559t
Chlordiazepoxide
    effect on contraceptives, 381
    pharmacological actions of various benzodiazepines, 559t
Chlorhexidine, 259t
    for folliculitis, 220
    for hidradenitis suppurativa, 225
Chlorpromazine, for acute episodic migraine, 240
Chlorthalidone, for hypertension, 165t
Cholesterol
    absorption inhibitor, hyperlipidemia, 138t, 140
    hyperlipidemia, pharmacologic treatment of, 135
    lipid physiology, 128–129
    women with PCOS, 422, 424
Cholestyramine (Questran), 139–140
Chronic abdominal pain, 322–326
    abdominal migraine, 326
    diagnosis, 325–326
    functional abdominal pain, 324t
    functional dyspepsia, 324t
    functional gastrointestinal disorders, 322–323
    irritable bowel syndrome, 324t
    organic causes, 323, 325
    treatment of, 326
Chronic daily headache, 316
    in AYA, 238
    treatment of, 241
Chronic diseases
    hypertension, 158
    mortality rates for, 26
    statistics and information on, 22
    young adults with, 623
Chronic fatigue syndrome (CFS), 315, 317–321
    definition of, 317, 318t
    epidemiology of, 317–318
    etiology of, 318–319
    evaluation of, 319

    management of, 319–320
    nonpharmacologic treatments of, 320
    pharmacologic treatment of, 320
    symptoms of, 318, 318t
Chronic health conditions
    adherence with treatment, 87
    in adolescent and young adults, 84–89
    adolescent development, interaction of, 85
    adolescent-friendly health care, 86–87, 86f, 87f
    AYA-friendly health care, 86
    definition of, 84
    health-related behaviors and states, social context of, 85–86
    prevalence of, 84–85
    sexual and reproductive health care, 87–88
    transition to adult health care, 88–89
    young adult friendly health care, 86–87, 87f
Chronic hip pain
    clinical manifestations of, 174
    differential diagnosis of, 174
    femoro-acetabular impingement, 174
    iliopsoas-related, 174
    labral tears, 174
Chronic illness, 87, 88
    and pubertal delay, 110, 111–112
    short stature, 103, 104
Chronic migraine headache, 238
Chronic sleep deprivation, 627
Chronic tension-type headaches, 238
Chronic Traumatic Encephalopathy (CTE), 207
Chylomicrons, 129
Cigarette smoking. See also Tobacco use
    Monitoring the Future (MTF) study of adolescents, 536
    risk assessment, 132–133
    in US adolescents, 11
Cimetidine, 467
    gynecomastia, 468t
    for warts, 220
Cipralex. See Escitalopram
Ciprofloxacin, 252
    chancroid, 510t
Citalopram (Celexa)
    and congenital long QT syndrome, 582
    for depression, 582, 582t
Civic engagement, social media and, 97–98
Civil Rights Act, Title VI, 652
Clarithromycin
    human immunodeficiency virus (HIV) infection, 291
    respiratory illness, 269, 270
Claviceps purpurea, 563
Clindamycin, 212, 213t
    bacterial vaginosis, 435
    breast, 463
    dental prophylaxis, 156t
    for folliculitis, 220
    for hidradenitis suppurativa, 225
Clinical Laboratory Improvement Amendments Program, 287
Clinics
    family-planning, 477
    guidelines for caring homeless youth, 641
    sexually transmitted infection, 477
    sleep disorder, 247
Clobazam (Onfi), 233
Clobetasol propionate, for psoriasis, 222
Clofibric acid, effect on contraceptives, 381
Clomiphene
    gynecomastia, 468
    to stimulate ovulation, 424
Clomipramine
    premenstrual disorders, 410
    for trichotillomania, 225

Clonazepam (Klonopin), 560
    effect on contraceptives, 380t
    pharmacological actions of, 559t
    seizure treatment, 233
Clonidine, 600. See also Extended-release clonidine
    for hypertension, 165t
    α-2-adrenoceptor agonists, 599
Clorazepate, seizure treatment, 233, 559
Clotrimazole
    for seborrheic dermatitis, 217
    for tinea pedis, 218
    for tinea versicolor, 218
    vaginitis, 435
    vulvovaginal candidiasis (VVC), 435
Cluster headaches, 237t, 238, 240
Co-occurring disorders, 575
Coagulopathies, 262t
Coarctation of aorta, 151t
Cocaethylene, 554
Cocaine, 519t, 522, 551–554
    acute overdose and treatment, 552, 554
    adverse effects of, 552
    athletes, 198
    and blood pressure, 162t
    chronic use of, 554
    epidemiology of, 551
    intoxication, effects of, 552, 573t
    medical use of, 551
    metabolism of, 551–552, 553t
    physiology of, 551–552, 553t
    preparation and dosage, 551
    prevalence of, 551
    residual cocaine, removal of, 552, 554
    teen pregnancy, 350
    tolerance of, 554
    withdrawal of, 554
Cognitive behavioral therapy (CBT), 320
    for anxiety disorder, 586–587
    for bulimia nervosa, 309
    for depression, 581
    for fibromyalgia, 314
    for marijuana use, 549
    for substance use disorder, 572t
    for suicidal ideation and behavior, 592
Cognitive development
    early adolescence, 39
    late adolescence, 40
    middle adolescence, 40
    younger adults, 41
Cognitive maturation, 85
Colchicine, for erythema nodosum, 224
Cold agglutinins, 269
College health program, 622–632
    behavioral and risk factors, 625–628
    consent and confidentiality, 631
    data sources on college students and, 622–623
    disease-specific considerations, 629–631
    enrollment, 623–624
    funding and service delivery model, 628–629
    health care services, 624–625
    on-campus student services, 629
    ongoing engagement with, 631–632
    SHS, key aspects of, 623
College students
    AYA pregnancy and birth rates, 346
    data sources on, 622–623
    inadequate sleep in, 627
    marijuana abuse, 547
    relationship difficulties among, 626
    at risk for STIs and unintended pregnancy, 627
    sexual assault and victimization, 612
    tobacco use among, 536–537
    young adults and, 529, 547
Columnar epithelium, 428

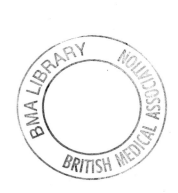